Study Guide
Christensen & Kockrow

Foundations and Adult Health Nursing

Sixth Edition

Patricia Ann Castaldi, RN, MSN, BSN
Director, Practical Nursing Program
Union County College
Plainfield, New Jersey

Kim D. Cooper, MSN
Nursing Department Program Chair
Ivy Tech Community College
Terre Haute, Indiana

Kelly Gosnell, RN, MSN
Associate Professor of Nursing
Ivy Tech Community College
Terre Haute, Indiana

Skills Performance Checklists

Barbara Lauritsen Christensen, RN, MS
Formerly, Nurse Educator
Mid-Plains Community College
North Platte, Nebraska

Elaine Oden Kockrow, RN, MS
Formerly, Nurse Educator
Mid-Plains Community College
North Platte, Nebraska

MOSBY
ELSEVIER

MOSBY
ELSEVIER

3251 Riverport Lane
St. Louis, Missouri 63043

STUDY GUIDE FOR FOUNDATIONS AND
ADULT HEALTH NURSING, SIXTH EDITION

ISBN: 978-0-323-05731-8

Notices

Knowledge and best practice in this field are constantly changing. As new research and experience broaden our understanding, changes in research methods, professional practices, or medical treatment may become necessary.

Practitioners and researchers must always rely on their own experience and knowledge in evaluating and using any information, methods, compounds, or experiments described herein. In using such information or methods they should be mindful of their own safety and the safety of others, including parties for whom they have a professional responsibility.

With respect to any drug or pharmaceutical products identified, readers are advised to check the most current information provided (i) on procedures featured or (ii) by the manufacturer of each product to be administered, to verify the recommended dose or formula, the method and duration of administration, and contraindications. It is the responsibility of practitioners, relying on their own experience and knowledge of their patients, to make diagnoses, to determine dosages and the best treatment for each individual patient, and to take all appropriate safety precautions.

To the fullest extent of the law, neither the Publisher nor the authors, contributors, or editors, assume any liability for any injury and/or damage to persons or property as a matter of products liability, negligence or otherwise, or from any use or operation of any methods, products, instructions, or ideas contained in the material herein.

Vice President and Publisher: Tom Wilhelm
Managing Editor: Jill Ferguson
Developmental Editor: Tiffany Trautwein
Associate Developmental Editor: Jennifer Hermes
Publishing Services Manager: Jeffrey Patterson
Senior Project Manager: Mary G. Stueck
Book Designer: Margaret Reid

Printed in the United States of America

Last digit is the print number: 9 8 7 6 5 4

To the Student

Understanding fundamental concepts and principles of nursing will prepare you for patient care experiences. By mastering the content of your *Foundations and Adult Health Nursing* textbook, you will have the necessary knowledge and skills for nursing practice. This Study Guide was created to help you achieve the objectives of each chapter in the textbook, establish a solid base of knowledge in the fundamentals of nursing, and evaluate your understanding of this critical information.

Each Study Guide chapter is organized into sections, each with its own topic and related objectives from the textbook. Different types of learning activities—definition of terms, short answer, multiple choice, fill-in-the blank, and true/false—assist you in meeting these content objectives. To maximize the benefits of this Study Guide and prepare for the learning activities:

1. Carefully read the chapter in the textbook and highlight, note, or outline important information.
2. Review the **Key Points,** access the **Additional Learning Resources,** and complete the **Review Questions for the NCLEX® Examination** at the end of each textbook chapter.
3. Complete the Study Guide exercises to the best of your ability.
4. Time and pace yourself during the completion of each exercise. You should spend approximately 1 minute for each multiple choice, true/false, and matching question, and approximately 2 minutes for completion activities or short answer questions.
5. After completing an exercise, refer to the textbook page references as needed. You can then repeat any exercises for additional practice and review. A complete Answer Key has been provided to your instructor.

ADDITIONAL LEARNING RESOURCES

Additional Learning Resources are available on the Companion CD in your textbook and on the Evolve website at http://evolve.elsevier.com/Christensen/foundationsadult.

Companion CD

- Body Spectrum Electronic Anatomy Coloring Book
- Fluids and Electrolytes Tutorial
- English/Spanish Audio Glossary
- Animations
- Video Clips
- Audio Clips

Evolve

- Review Questions for the NCLEX® Examination (for each chapter)
- Concept Map Creator
- Calculators
- Additional Animations
- Additional Video Clips

STUDY HINTS FOR ALL STUDENTS

- *Ask questions!* There are no bad questions. If you do not know something or are not sure, you need to find out. Other people may be wondering the same thing but may be too shy to ask. The answer could mean life or death to your patient, which certainly is more important than feeling embarrassed about asking a question.
- *Make use of chapter objectives.* At the beginning of each chapter in the textbook are objectives that you should have mastered when you finish studying that chapter. Write these objectives in your notebook, leaving a blank space after each. Fill in the answers as you find them while reading the

chapter. Review to make sure your answers are correct and complete, and use these answers when you study for tests. This should also be done for separate course objectives that your instructor has listed in your class syllabus.

- *Locate and understand key terms.* At the beginning of each chapter in the textbook are key terms that you will encounter as you read the chapter. Page numbers are provided for easy reference and review, and the key terms are in bold, blue font the first time they appear in the chapter. Phonetic pronunciations are provided for terms that might be difficult to pronounce.
- *Review Key Points.* Use the Key Points at the end of each chapter in the textbook to help you review for exams.
- *Get the most from your textbook.* When reading each chapter in the textbook, look at the subject headings to learn what each section is about. Read first for the general meaning, then reread parts you did not understand. It may help to read those parts aloud. Carefully read the information given in each table and study each figure and its caption.
- *Follow up on difficult concepts.* While studying, put difficult concepts into your own words to see if you understand them. Check this understanding with another student or the instructor. Write these in your notebook.
- *Take useful notes.* When taking lecture notes in class, leave a large margin on the left side of each notebook page and write only on right-hand pages, leaving all left-hand pages blank. Look over your lecture notes soon after each class, while your memory is fresh. Fill in missing words, complete sentences and ideas, and underline key phrases, definitions, and concepts. At the top of each page, write the topic of that page. In the left margin, write the key word for that part of your notes. On the opposite left-hand page, write a summary or outline that combines material from both the textbook and the lecture. These can be your study notes for review.
- *Join or form a study group.* Form a study group with some other students so you can help one another. Practice speaking and reading aloud, ask questions about material you are not sure about, and work together to find answers.
- *Improve your study skills.* Good study skills are essential for achieving your goals in nursing. Time management, efficient use of study time, and a consistent approach to studying are all beneficial. There are various study methods for reading a textbook and for taking class notes. Some methods that have proven helpful can be found in *Saunders Student Nurse Planner: A Guide to Success in Nursing School* by Susan C. deWit. This book contains helpful information on test-taking and preparing for clinical experiences. It includes an example of a "time map" for planning study time and a blank form that you can use to formulate a personal time map.

ADDITIONAL STUDY HINTS FOR STUDENTS WHO USE ENGLISH AS A SECOND LANGUAGE (ESL)

- *Find a first-language buddy.* ESL students should find a first-language buddy—another student who is a native speaker of English and is willing to answer questions about word meanings, pronunciations, and culture. Maybe your buddy would like to learn about your language and culture. This could help in his or her nursing experience as well.
- *Expand your vocabulary.* If you find a nontechnical word you do not know (e.g., *drowsy*), try to guess its meaning from the sentence (e.g., *With electrolyte imbalance, the patient may feel fatigued and drowsy*). If you are not sure of the meaning, or if it seems particularly important, look it up in the dictionary.
- *Keep a vocabulary notebook.* Keep a small alphabetized notebook or address book in which you can write down new nontechnical words you read or hear along with their meanings and pronunciations. Write each word under its initial letter so you can find it easily, as in a dictionary. For words you do not know or for words that have a different meaning in nursing, write down how they are used and sound. Look up their meanings in a dictionary or ask your instructor or first-language buddy. Then write the different meanings or usages that you have found in your book, including the nursing meaning. Continue to add new words as you discover them. For example:
  - *Primary*—Of most importance; main (e.g., *the primary problem or disease*); The first one; elementary (e.g., *primary school*)
  - *Secondary*—Of less importance; resulting from another problem or disease (e.g., *a secondary symptom*); The second one (e.g., *secondary school ["high school" in the United States]*)

Contents

Illustration Credits

Anthony, C.P. & Thibodeau, G.A. (1987). Textbook of anatomy and physiology. St. Louis: Mosby: Figures 45-1, 52-2, 54-2

Belcher, A.E. (1992). Cancer nursing. St. Louis: Mosby: Figure 57-1

Canobbio, M. (1990). Mosby's clinical nursing series: cardiovascular disorders. St. Louis: Mosby: Figure 48-1

Elkin, M. K., et al. (2004). Nursing interventions and clinical skills. (3rd ed.). St. Louis: Mosby: Figure 42-1

Herlihy, B. & Maebius, N.K. (2007). The human body in health and illness. (3rd ed.). Philadelphia: Saunders: Figure 41-1

Hockenberry, M.J. (2009). *Wong's essentials of pediatric nursing.* (8th ed.). St. Louis: Mosby: Figure 31-1

Lewis, S.M., et al. (2007). *Medical-surgical nursing: assessment and management of clinical problems.* (7th ed.). St. Louis: Mosby: Figure 22-1

Novak, J.C. & Broom, B.L. (1995). *Ingalls & Salerno's maternal and child health nursing.* (8th ed.). St. Louis: Mosby: Figure 26-1

Phipps, W., et al. (2007). Medical-surgical nursing: health and illness perspectives. (8th ed.). St. Louis: Mosby: Figures 44-2, 46-1

Potter, P.A. & Castaldo, P. (2003). *Study guide to accompany Potter: Basic nursing.* (5th ed.) St. Louis: Mosby: Figure 4-2

Potter, P.A. & Perry, A.G. (2009). *Fundamentals of nursing: concepts, process, and practice.* (7th ed.). St. Louis: Mosby: Figure 23-1

Thibodeau, G.A. & Patton, K.T. (1996). Anatomy and physiology. (3rd ed.). St. Louis: Mosby: Figure 51-1

Thibodeau, G.A. & Patton, K.T. (2003). Anatomy and physiology. (5th ed.). St. Louis: Mosby: Figures 43-2, 47-2, 53-1, 54-1

Thibodeau, G.A. & Patton, K.T. (2004). Structure and function of the body. (12th ed.). St. Louis: Mosby: Figures 44-1, 50-2, 52-1

Thibodeau, G.A. & Patton, K.T. (2005), The human body in health and disease. (4th ed.). St. Louis: Mosby: Figures 43-1, 47-1

Thompson, J.M., et al. (1997). *Mosby's clinical nursing.* (4th ed.). St. Louis: Mosby: Figure 31-2

Student Name______________________ **Date**______________

The Evolution of Nursing

chapter **1**

Answer Key: Textbook page references are provided as a guide for answering these questions. A complete answer key was provided for your instructor.

HISTORY OF NURSING

Objectives

- Describe the evolution of nursing and nursing education from early civilization to the 20th century.
- Identify the major leaders in the history of the development of nursing in America.

1. Nursing evolves along with changes in: ***(1)*** ______________________

2. In early civilization, care of the sick was primarily provided by: ***(2)*** ______________________

3. There is evidence that medical treatment existed in ancient Egypt; this treatment included: ***(2)***

4. Medicine progressed from the initial belief that illness was caused by: ***(2)***______________________

5. Discuss the monastic factors that influenced the practice of nursing. ***(2-3)***______________________

6. What factors influenced the evolution of nursing from occupation to profession? ***(4)*** ________________

7. Identify the six ways in which the "Nightingale nurses" improved patient care and advanced the practice of nursing. ***(4)***

8. Describe the effect that World War I and World War II had on nursing. ***(5-6)***________________

9. Identify the major events in America in the 19th century that led to the development of the current nursing education programs. ***(4)***

10. List the four major concepts that are the basis for nursing theories and models. ***(17-18)*** ________________

Multiple Choice

11. Hippocrates is credited with development of: ***(2)***
    1. a public system of health care.
    2. a public system of safety.
    3. a holistic approach to patient care.
    4. early guidelines for health care.

12. Phoebe, one of the first deaconesses, was known for providing: ***(2)***
    1. the first free hospital in Rome.
    2. care to the poor and sick in their homes.
    3. care for prisoners.
    4. care for those who were mentally ill.

13. Florence Nightingale applied the principles of nursing she learned in Germany to care of soldiers during the: ***(3)***
    1. Civil War.
    2. Spanish-American War.
    3. Great Plague.
    4. Crimean War.

14. Which of the following individuals is credited with the establishment and development of the Red Cross? *(5)*
    1. Dorothea Dix
    2. Florence Nightingale
    3. Clara Barton
    4. Lavinia Dock

15. Which of the following individuals crusaded for elevation of the standards of care for the mentally ill? *(5)*
    1. Dorothea Dix
    2. Mary Ann Ball
    3. Clara Barton
    4. Florence Nightingale

16. The American Society of Superintendents of Training Schools became a committee of the: *(5)*
    1. Association of Practical Nurse Schools.
    2. National Federation of Licensed Practical Nurses.
    3. National League for Nursing Education.
    4. American Nurses Association.

17. Orem's theory of nursing could be described as: *(17-18)*
    1. nursing care that becomes necessary when a patient is unable to fulfill biological, psychological, developmental, or social needs.
    2. a patient's environment is arranged to facilitate the body's reparative processes.
    3. caring is the central and unifying domain for nursing knowledge and practice.
    4. patients must adapt to circumstances based on physiologic, psychological, sociologic, and dependence-independence adaptive models.

NURSING ORGANIZATIONS

Objectives

- Identify the major organizations in nursing.
- Define the four purposes of NAPNES and NFLPN.

18. Identify the role of the NLN in nursing education. *(9)* ______________________________

____

____

19. List the purposes of NAPNES and NFLPN. *(9)* ______________________________

____

____

PRACTICAL NURSING

Objectives

- List the major developments of practical and vocational nursing.
- Define practical and vocational nursing.
- Describe the purpose, role, and responsibilities of the practical or vocational nurse.

20. Identify the major development or event that occurred in the given year and give a brief description of the change that it brought about in practical and vocational nursing. *(8)*

    a. 1892 ______________________________

    b. 1917 ______________________________

    c. 1941 ______________________________

    d. 1949 ______________________________

    e. 1957 ______________________________

    f. 1996 ______________________________

21. The definition that is adapted from NAPNES defines practical and vocational nursing as: *(9)*

    ____

    ____

22. Discuss the role and responsibilities of the practical or vocational nurse in today's health care system. *(18)*

    ____

    ____

23. Discuss the benefits of a professional appearance. *(6)* ______________________________

    ____

    ____

Multiple Choice

24. The duties and responsibilities of the LPN/LVN are determined by the: *(9)*
    1. National League of Nursing.
    2. American Nurses Association.
    3. Vocational Nursing Program.
    4. State Board of Nursing.

25. The content areas for the NCLEX-PN® are determined by the: *(9)*
    1. National League of Nursing.
    2. Council of State Boards of Nursing.
    3. American Nurses Association.
    4. Vocational Nursing Program.

26. Because of demographic changes in the population, increased need for nursing care is necessary in the care of: *(7)*
    1. newborns.
    2. adolescents.
    3. adults.
    4. the elderly.

27. Significant women's health care issues that have most recently guided nursing care include: *(7)*
    1. immunizations, such as the human papillomavirus (HPV) vaccine.
    2. the need for mammography.
    3. the importance of routine pap smears.
    4. the importance of prenatal care

28. Recognizing patients as individuals and making sure that they receive quality care is ensured by nurses providing care according to: *(7)*
    1. nurse practice acts.
    2. Patient's Bill of Rights.
    3. state boards of nursing guidelines.
    4. American Nurses Association recommendations.

29. Nurses are involved in disaster preparedness plans in which of the following ways? (Select all that apply) *(7)*
    1. Triaging of casualties
    2. Vaccination research
    3. Functioning as attendant nurses
    4. Crisis response team members

HEALTH CARE DELIVERY

Objectives

- Identify the components of the health care system.
- Identify the participants in the health care system.
- Describe the complex factors involved in the delivery of patient care.

30. Identify the participants in the health care delivery system and their roles and responsibilities. *(13)*

____

____

31. Identify three economic factors that influence contemporary health care delivery. *(13)* ______________

____

____

32. Provide a brief description of the following. *(14)*

    a. Malpractice insurance: ______________________________

    ____

    b. Cross-training: ______________________________

    ____

    c. Case management: ______________________________

    ____

33. What is the purpose of the Patient's Bill of Rights? *(15)* ______________________________

    ____

    ____

34. Briefly describe the concepts of health promotion and illness prevention. *(12)* ______________________________

    ____

    ____

Multiple Choice

35. Utilizing Maslow's Hierarchy of Needs, the nurse gives priority to which of the following problems of the patient? *(12)*
    1. Loneliness
    2. Inability to eat
    3. Anxiety
    4. Safety

36. Utilizing Maslow's hierarchy of needs, which of the following needs is basic and should be addressed first? *(12)*
    1. Safety and security
    2. Self-actualization
    3. Physiologic
    4. Love and belonging

37. Social factors that affect health and illness are: *(12)*
    1. smoking and stress.
    2. health care insurance and advanced technology.
    3. excessive body weight and alcoholism.
    4. lifestyle and personal financial hardship.

Student Name____________________ Date__________

chapter 2

Legal and Ethical Aspects of Nursing

Answer Key: Textbook page references are provided as a guide for answering these questions. A complete answer key was provided for your instructor.

LEGAL PROCESS

Objective

- Summarize the structure and function of the legal system.

1. The two basic categories of law are: ***(23)***______________________________

____

____

2. What is the difference between statutory and common law? ***(23)***______________________________

____

____

3. Identify the steps in the legal process for civil litigation. ***(23)*** ______________________________

____

____

4. Why would an appeal be filed in a lawsuit? ***(23)***______________________________

____

____

5. What does it mean to be *liable* for an action? ***(24)*** ______________________________

____

____

Multiple Choice

6. The function of criminal law is to: ***(23)***
   1. make the aggrieved person whole.
   2. restore the person to where he or she was.
   3. punish and prevent further crime.
   4. establish fault.

7. The function of civil law is to: ***(23)***
   1. establish fault.
   2. make the aggrieved person whole.
   3. punish and prevent further crime.
   4. prevent an appeal.

8. The individual who files the complaint in a civil litigation is referred to as the: ***(23)***
   1. defendant.
   2. respondent.
   3. plaintiff.
   4. prosecutor.

9. In a criminal case, the conduct or issue in question is considered to be a crime against: ***(23)***
   1. the court.
   2. the respondent.
   3. the plaintiff.
   4. society.

LEGAL RELATIONSHIPS

Objective

- Discuss the legal relationship existing between the nurse and the patient.

10. Discuss the concept of accountability and the legal relationship. ***(24)*** ________________

____

____

11. Discuss areas in which the nursing staff failed to follow standards of care in the case *Darling v. Charleston Community Memorial Hospital.* ***(24)***

____

____

Multiple Choice

12. It can be said that a nurse safeguards the nurse-patient relationship when he or she acts: *(24)*
    1. as a clinical nurse specialist with years of experience.
    2. as an experienced nurse in a specialty area.
    3. as other nurses with similar education and experience and in similar situations.
    4. in accordance with the law.

13. The nurse administers the wrong dose of a medication to a patient, and the patient experiences adverse effects as a result of this action. The nurse is considered: (Select all that apply) *(24)*
    1. liable.
    2. accountable.
    3. criminal.
    4. deliberate.

REGULATION OF PRACTICE

Objectives

- Explain the importance of maintaining standards of care.
- Give examples of ways the nursing profession is regulated.

14. What are the purposes of the standards of care? *(24)* ______________________________

____

____

15. Evidence that nursing standards are being or have been maintained includes: *(24)* ______________________________

____

____

16. How is nursing practice regulated by nurse practice acts and professional organizations? *(25)* ______________________________

____

____

17. Explain the interstate compact. *(25)* ______________________________

____

____

Multiple Choice

18. Select the action(s) that would be considered a breach in the standards of nursing care. (Select all that apply) ***(25)***
    1. Failure to take an accurate and thorough patient history
    2. Failure to notify physician of patient lab values in a timely fashion
    3. Failure to protect patient and prevent patient falls
    4. Failure to introduce self to patient and family members
    5. Failure to give appropriate discharge instructions to the patient

LEGAL ISSUES

Objectives

- Explain nursing malpractice.
- Give examples of ways the licensed practical or vocational nurse can avoid being involved in a lawsuit.
- Give examples of legal issues in health care.
- Discuss federal HIPAA (Health Insurance Portability and Accountability Act of 1996) regulations and the act's impact on the health care system.

19. Briefly define the following elements needed to establish malpractice. ***(26)***

    a. Duty: ____________________

    ____

    b. Breach of duty: ____________________

    ____

    c. Harm: ____________________

    ____

    d. Proximate cause: ____________________

    ____

20. Identify general ways that nurses can avoid involvement in lawsuits. ***(29)*** ____________________

    ____

    ____

21. Describe the nurse's role and responsibilities in relation to the following. ***(27)***

    a. Confidentiality: ____________________

    ____

b. Invasion of privacy: ____

____

c. Reporting of abuse: ____

____

d. Informed consent: ____

____

22. Discuss the nurse's primary duties in relation to HIPAA (Health Insurance Portability and Accountability Act of 1996). *(26)*

____

____

23. Discuss the nurse's responsibilities when obtaining an informed consent from a patient before a procedure. *(27)*

____

____

Multiple Choice

24. The nurse who uses unnecessary restraints on a patient may be charged with: *(24)*
    1. assault.
    2. battery.
    3. slander.
    4. defamation.

25. When providing first aid in an emergency situation outside a medical facility, it is important for the nurse to have knowledge of the: *(29)*
    1. Nurse Practice Act.
    2. Patient's Bill of Rights.
    3. Good Samaritan Act.
    4. Standards of care.

26. There are staffing issues throughout the medical center, and one of the nurses is "floated" to another unit where this nurse does not want to go. The nurse decides, after receiving the assignment, to leave the unit and go home. The nurse may be found liable specifically for: *(30)*
    1. fraud.
    2. malpractice.
    3. defamation.
    4. abandonment.

27. Select the nursing action that would be considered a breach of patient confidentiality. (Select all that apply) *(27)*
    1. The nurse answers questions asked by the bearer of the patient's health care power of attorney regarding the patient's condition.
    2. The nurse informs the patient's only living relative of the patient's scheduled procedure.
    3. The nurse, who is familiar with the patient's wife, answers her questions over the phone regarding the patient's lab results that have been pending.
    4. Upon being asked to do so by the patient, the nurse waits to explain a scheduled procedure until the patient's husband is present.

ETHICAL PRINCIPLES

Objectives

- Summarize how culture affects an individual's beliefs, morals, and values.
- Identify how values affect decision making.

28. The field of ethics involves the study of: *(31)* ____________________

____

____

29. Identify and briefly describe the five fundamental ethical principles. *(32)* ____________________

____

____

30. Discuss how values and beliefs are developed and how they affect behavior and decision making. *(31)*

____

____

31. Gaining insight into your own personal values is a process known as: *(31)* ____________________

32. List four ways the nurse can meet the needs of the patient while respecting the patient's cultural beliefs and practices. *(31)*

____

____

ETHICAL PRACTICE

Objectives

- Explain the meaning of a code of ethics.
- Differentiate between a legal duty and an ethical duty.
- Distinguish between ethical and unethical behavior.
- Explain the nurse's role in reporting unethical behavior.

33. A code of ethics serves to: *(32)* ______________________________

____

____

34. Indicate whether each of the following involves a legal or an ethical duty. *(31)*

    a. The nurse failed to perform in a reasonable and prudent manner. ______________________________

    ____

    ____

    b. The nurse failed to give the medication to the patient before he was discharged. ______________________________

    ____

    ____

    c. The nurse assigned to care for an AIDS patient requested to change patients with another nurse on the unit.

    ____

    ____

35. Describe the difference between ethical and unethical behavior. *(32)* ______________________________

____

____

36. List the priority nursing actions to be implemented in reporting unethical behavior. *(32)*______________________________

____

____

ETHICAL ISSUES

Objective

- Give examples of ethical issues common in health care.

37. Discuss the following ethical issues in health care. *(33)*

    a. Right to refuse treatment: ______________________________

    ____

    ____

    b. "Do not resuscitate" orders: ______________________________

    ____

    ____

    c. Refusal to treat: ______________________________

    ____

    ____

Student Name____ **Date**________________

Communication

chapter **3**

Answer Key: Textbook page references are provided as a guide for answering these questions. A complete answer key was provided for your instructor.

GOAL OF COMMUNICATION

Objective

- Recognize that communication is inherent in every nurse-patient interaction.

1. What is the goal of communication between the nurse and the patient? ***(40)***________________________

2. Describe the term "two-way communication," and identify when it would be used in a nurse-patient relationship. ***(37)***

Multiple Choice

3. When giving report during shift change, the night nurse should be aware that a patient may hear the information being exchanged. The patient hearing the information would be referred to as the: ***(36)***
   1. receiver.
   2. sender.
   3. unintended receiver.
   4. communicator.

4. In a nurse-patient relationship, when the nurse is communicating with the patient, the type of communication that is least effective is referred to as: ***(37)***
   1. two-way communication.
   2. one-way communication.
   3. nonverbal communication.
   4. open-ended communication.

TYPES OF COMMUNICATION

Objectives

- Discuss the concepts of verbal and nonverbal communication.
- Discuss the impact of nonverbal communication.
- Recognize assertive communication as the most appropriate communication style.

5. Identify the types of verbal and nonverbal communication. *(37-38)* ______________________________

____

____

6. Explain why consistency between verbal and nonverbal communication is important. *(37)*__________

____

____

7. Compare the characteristics of the following styles of communication. *(39)*

Assertive	Aggressive	Unassertive

Multiple Choice

8. An example of nonverbal communication is: *(37-38)*
   1. moaning.
   2. crying.
   3. grimacing.
   4. writing.

9. An example of verbal communication is: *(37-38)*
   1. writing.
   2. grimacing.
   3. smiling.
   4. frowning.

10. Nonverbal communication involves the use of cues. Which of the following is an example of a nonverbal cue? ***(38)***
    1. Symbols
    2. Written words
    3. Reading
    4. Physical appearance

11. In the English language, the denotative meaning of the term "hospital" refers to: ***(37)***
    1. a facility that generally provides long-term care to patients.
    2. a facility that provides health care treatment to a patient by trained staff.
    3. an organization that depends on volunteers to provide services.
    4. an organization that provides care in the patient's familiar surroundings, such as the patient's home.

12. Choose the term(s) that best describe(s) nonverbal cues. (Select all that apply) ***(38)***
    1. Jargon
    2. Tone of voice
    3. Touch
    4. Reading
    5. Rate of voice

THERAPEUTIC COMMUNICATION

Objectives

- Use various therapeutic communication techniques.
- Recognize trust as the foundation for all effective interaction.

13. Discuss tips for building rapport with the patient. ***(40)*** ____________________

    ____

    ____

14. Provide examples of the following therapeutic communication techniques. ***(43-44)***

    a. Closed questioning: ____________________

    ____

    b. Stating observations: ____________________

    ____

    c. Offering information: ____________________

    ____

    d. Use of humor: ____________________

    ____

e. Touch: ____

____

f. Silence: ____

____

15. When using the communication technique of ______________________, the nurse acknowledges listening to the patient by nodding or using eye contact. ***(43-44)***

Multiple Choice

16. The following is an example of which therapeutic technique? The patient states, "I am worried and don't know what to expect after my biopsy." The nurse replies, "Are you feeling anxious about the results of your biopsy?" ***(43-44)***
    1. Reflection
    2. Clarification
    3. Restatement
    4. Paraphrasing

17. An example of activity involving the personal zone is when the nurse: ***(46)***
    1. bathes the patient.
    2. sits in a chair and speaks with the patient.
    3. speaks to a small group of expectant parents.
    4. gives a lecture to a large auditorium filled with newly hired staff members.

18. The nurse is aware that providing an opportunity for receiving feedback from the patient is a way of maintaining therapeutic communication. This is an example of which of the following therapeutic communication techniques? ***(42)***
    1. Active listening
    2. Therapeutic silence
    3. Minimal exchange
    4. Conveying acceptance

19. The patient will be discharged from the hospital tomorrow. During the discharge teaching, the patient states, "I don't know how I will be able to care for myself after I leave the hospital." The nurse responds, "You don't know how you will take care of yourself when you leave the hospital?" This is an example of which technique? ***(43)***
    1. Restating
    2. Reflection
    3. Paraphrasing
    4. Summarizing

20. In completing the patient's history, the nurse asks the patient, "What type of surgeries have you had in the past?" This is an example of which of the following therapeutic communication techniques? ***(43-44)***
    1. Clarifying
    2. Paraphrasing
    3. Restating
    4. Open-ended questioning

FACTORS THAT AFFECT COMMUNICATION

Objectives

- Identify various factors that can affect communication.
- Discuss potential barriers to communication.

21. Identify the factors that may affect communication, and provide an example of each. ***(46)***____________

____

____

22. For each of the following blocks to communication, provide an example of a response that should be avoided by the nurse. ***(51)***

    a. Giving advice: ________________________________

    ____

    b. Defensiveness: ________________________________

    ____

    c. Value judgment:________________________________

    ____

Multiple Choice

23. When communicating with an older adult, the nurse is aware that it is important to: ***(48)***
    1. speak loudly.
    2. allow time for processing information.
    3. provide a dark, quiet environment.
    4. avoid hearing the patient's stories.

24. When communicating with a patient of an unfamiliar culture, the nurse knows that: (Select all that apply) ***(47-48)***
    1. formal names are preferred in most cultures.
    2. there may be differences in the interpretation of social versus clock time.
    3. the practice and meaning of touch varies among cultures.
    4. the meaning that eye contact conveys may differ among cultures.

COMMUNICATION IN SPECIAL SITUATIONS

Objectives

- Apply the nursing process to patients with impaired verbal communication.
- Apply therapeutic communication techniques to patients with special communication needs.

25. Identify at least five nursing interventions for a patient with impaired communication. *(52)*__________

____

____

26. A 58-year-old man was admitted to the medical-surgical unit with a diagnosis of left-sided CVA (stroke). During the admission process, the nurse observed that the patient's speech was unclear and his words were slurred. The nurse also observed that when the patient was asked a question that could be answered with a "yes" or "no" response, he could answer the question by moving his head to imply "yes" or "no." Apply the nursing process to the given situation. *(52)*

    a. Identify problems observed by the nurse during the admission process. __________

    ____

    b. Write a nursing diagnosis based on the identified problems.__________

    ____

    c. Write a realistic goal for the nursing diagnosis. __________

    ____

    d. Identify at least two nursing actions that can be implemented.__________

    ____

    e. Write a statement that reflects the evaluation of the outcome.__________

    ____

Multiple Choice

27. The patient tells the nurse, "I'm supposed to check my blood sugar at least three times each day, but I can't always find the test sticks and they're very expensive." The nurse uses which specific therapeutic technique of clarification when responding: *(43)*
    1. "When did you last check your blood sugar?"
    2. "I'll speak with the physician about your situation."
    3. "I see that you know how important it is to check your blood sugar."
    4. "Let me make sure I understand what your concern is with the blood sugar testing."

28. When communicating with a patient who has expressive aphasia, the nurse is aware that it is important to: *(52)*
    1. ask open-ended questions.
    2. ask questions that can be answered with a "yes" or "no."
    3. refer to the family members for information.
    4. allow a short time for the patient to respond.

Student Name____ **Date**__________________

chapter **4**

Vital Signs

Answer Key: Textbook page references are provided as a guide for answering these questions. A complete answer key was provided for your instructor.

PURPOSE AND GUIDELINES

Objectives

- Discuss the importance of accurately assessing vital signs.
- Discuss methods by which the nurse can ensure accurate measurement of vital signs.
- Identify the guidelines for vital signs measurement.
- Discuss frequency of vital signs measurement.
- State the normal limits of each vital sign.
- List the factors that affect vital signs readings.
- Identify the rationale for each step of the vital sign procedures.

1. Accurate assessment of vital signs provides the nurse with: ***(56)*** ______________________________

   ____

   ____

2. A myocardial contraction that occurs at a regular rhythm but at a rate greater than 100 beats per minute is known as ____________________________. ***(70)***

3. The second blood pressure reading that is a result of the decreased pressure in the arteries when the ventricles are resting is known as ____________________________. ***(78)***

4. For the following vital signs, identify factors that may influence them and how they are affected.

   a. Temperature: ***(62)*** ____

   ____

   b. Pulse: ***(70)*** ____

   ____

   c. Respirations: ***(76)*** _______________________________________

   ____

   d. Blood pressure: ***(79)*** _____________________________________

   ____

5. What are the general guidelines for taking vital signs? ***(59)*** ________________________________

____

____

Multiple Choice

6. The nurse is aware that in an acute care facility, the patient's vital signs are measured a minimum of: ***(59)***
   1. every 2 hours.
   2. every 4 hours.
   3. every 8 hours.
   4. every 12 hours.

7. The purpose of baseline vital signs includes: (Select all that apply) ***(59)***
   1. comparison with vital signs obtained later.
   2. an indication of the patient's normal range of vital signs.
   3. identification of a change in vital signs.
   4. an indication of the patient's past medical history.

TEMPERATURE

Objective

- Accurately assess oral, rectal, axillary, and tympanic temperatures.

8. The ________________________________ site is considered the *least* accurate site for temperature measurement. ***(69)***

9. Identify the sites for temperature measurement and the expected temperature reading for each. ***(69)***

____

____

10. Convert the following temperature readings. ***(61)***
    a. 37° C = ________° F
    b. 101.2° F = ________° C
    c. 39.2° C = ________° F
    d. 97.8° F = ________° C

11. Identify signs and symptoms associated with an elevated temperature. ***(62)***________________________

____

____

12. What should the nurse do if the patient's temperature is above normal? ***(62)*** ________________________

____

____

Multiple Choice

13. A patient's temperature is 93.2° F. This temperature is referred to as: ***(62)***
    1. fever.
    2. hyperthermia.
    3. hypothermia.
    4. pyrexia.

14. Normal body cells are at risk for damage when the temperature exceeds: ***(62)***
    1. 100.4° F (38° C).
    2. 104.0° F (40° C).
    3. 105.0° F (40.5° C).
    4. 110.0° F (43.3° C).

15. Normal body temperature can change throughout the day. It is important for the nurse to know that the lowest body temperature can occur between the hours of: ***(61)***
    1. 4 PM and 6 PM.
    2. 3 PM and 6 PM.
    3. 2 AM and 9 AM.
    4. 1 AM and 4 AM.

16. It is important for a nurse to know that normal body temperature can range from: ***(61)***
    1. 96° F to 98.2° F (35.6° C to 36.8° C).
    2. 98.2° F to 99° F (36.8° C to 37.2° C).
    3. 97° F to 99.6° F (36.1° C to 37.5° C).
    4. 96.2° F to 100.2° F (35.7° C to 37.9° C).

17. When obtaining a rectal temperature from an adult, the nurse inserts the electronic thermometer probe into the rectum approximately: ***(66)***
    1. ½ inch.
    2. 1½ inches.
    3. 2 inches.
    4. 3 inches.

PULSE

Objectives

- List the various sites for pulse measurement.
- Accurately assess an apical pulse, a radial pulse, and a pulse deficit.

18. Identify the anatomical site for apical pulse measurement. ***(75)*** ______________________

19. On the figure, identify the names and sites for assessment of peripheral pulses. *(74)*

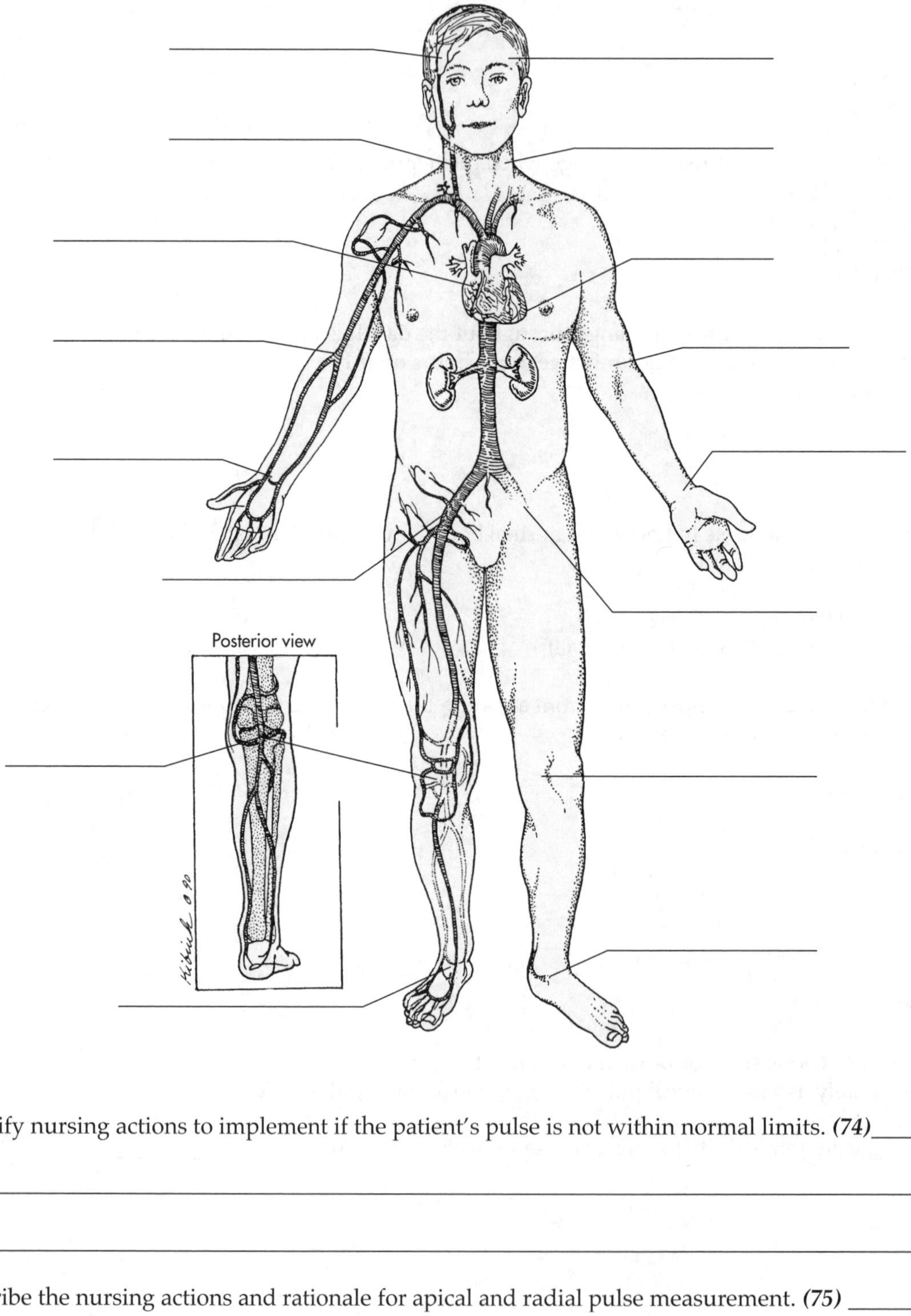

20. Identify nursing actions to implement if the patient's pulse is not within normal limits. *(74)*____________

____

____

21. Describe the nursing actions and rationale for apical and radial pulse measurement. *(75)* ____________

____

____

Multiple Choice

22. Pulse deficit is described as the difference between the radial and: *(73)*
    1. femoral pulse rates.
    2. brachial pulse rates.
    3. apical pulse rates.
    4. carotid pulse rates.

23. The patient's pulse is difficult to assess and disappears with slight pressure. The pulse strength is described as: *(71)*
    1. absent.
    2. weak.
    3. thready.
    4. abnormal.

24. The patient's pulse is easily palpable but disappears when moderate pressure is applied. The pulse strength is described as: *(71)*
    1. thready.
    2. weak.
    3. normal.
    4. abnormal.

25. When assessing the apical pulse, the nurse counts the pulse rate for: *(75)*
    1. 20 seconds and multiplies by 3.
    2. 60 seconds and does not multiply.
    3. 30 seconds and multiplies by 2.
    4. 15 seconds and multiplies by 4.

26. The nurse determines that further teaching is required when the student is observed: (Select all that apply) *(71)*
    1. palpating the carotid pulses bilaterally.
    2. assessing the apical pulse for a full minute.
    3. measuring the popliteal artery at the dorsum of the foot.
    4. using the pads of the index and middle fingers to obtain a radial pulse.

27. The average adult heart rate is: *(70)*
    1. 40 to 80 beats per minute.
    2. 60 to 100 beats per minute.
    3. 80 to 120 beats per minute.
    4. 100 to 140 beats per minute.

RESPIRATION

Objective

- Describe the procedure for determining the respiratory rate.

28. In determining the respiratory rate, the nurse counts for __________ seconds. *(78)*

29. A rapid respiratory rate is described as ______________________________. *(76)*

30. The respiratory rate may be increased by: *(76)*______________________________

____

____

31. Describe the nursing actions and the rationale for measurement of respirations. *(78)* ______________

____

____

32. What should the nurse do if the patient's respirations are rapid and labored? *(77)* ______________

____

____

Multiple Choice

33. Respiratory rate is controlled by the: *(76)*
    1. cerebellum.
    2. spinal cord.
    3. medulla oblongata.
    4. cerebrum.

34. The nurse is aware that a patient's respiratory rate may be increased by: *(76)*
    1. narcotics.
    2. acute pain.
    3. hypothermia.
    4. brainstem injury.

35. The best time for the nurse to count respirations is: *(77)*
    1. immediately after the patient wakes up.
    2. following any strenuous activity.
    3. before and after each meal, and before administering medications to the patient.
    4. immediately following measurement of the radial pulse while the fingers are still in place over the artery.

BLOOD PRESSURE

Objectives

- Accurately assess the blood pressure.
- Describe the benefits of and precautions to follow for self-measurement of blood pressure.

36. When obtaining the patient's blood pressure, the cuff is deflated at a rate of
    ______________________. *(83)*

37. The pulsating sounds that are heard when assessing the patient's blood pressure are known as
    __________________________ sounds. *(80)*

38. When should the blood pressure be assessed in the lower extremities? *(82, 84)* ____________________

____

____

39. Describe the nursing actions and the rationale for measurement of blood pressure. *(82-83)* ____________

____

____

40. What nursing actions should be implemented if the patient's blood pressure is below normal? *(79-80)*

____

____

41. Identify on the aneroid gauge where the Korotkoff sounds were heard for a blood pressure of 136/78 mm Hg. *(81)*

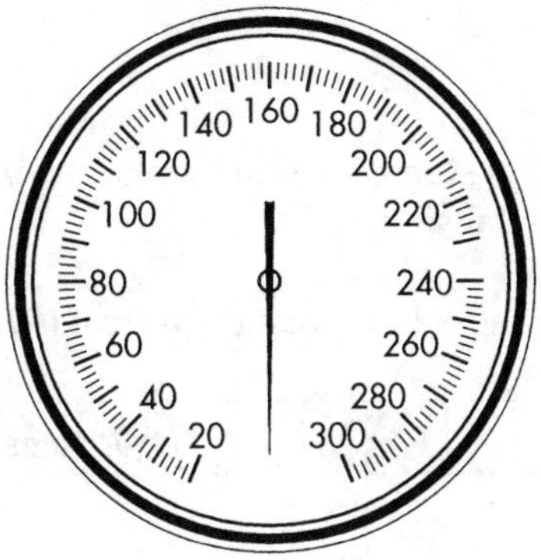

Multiple Choice

42. A high blood pressure reading may result if the blood pressure cuff is: *(82)*
    1. too large.
    2. too small.
    3. placed low on the arm.
    4. placed high on the arm.

HEIGHT AND WEIGHT

Objective

- Accurately assess the height and weight measurements.

43. To obtain an accurate weight measurement, the nurse should: *(87)* ____________________

____

____

44. Describe the nursing actions and rationale for measurement of height and weight. ***(87)*** ______________

____

____

45. It is important for the nurse to know how to convert a weight in pounds to the equivalent in kilograms. *(87)*
    a. A patient who weighs 44 lbs weighs ____________ kg.
    b. A patient who weighs 210 lbs weighs ____________ kg.

46. Fluid balance may be assessed by weighing the patient. If the patient weighs 1 kg less today than yesterday, how much fluid was lost? *(87)*

____

____

DOCUMENTATION AND REPORTING

Objectives

- Accurately record and report vital signs measurements.
- State the normal limits of each vital sign.

47. Identify the expected vital signs for the following age groups. ***(60)***

	Pulse	Respirations	Blood Pressure
a. Neonate			
b. Toddler			
c. Adolescent			
d. Adult			

48. In most health care facilities, vital signs are documented on a __________________. ***(61, 63)***

49. What vital signs measurements should be reported immediately? ***(59)*** ______________

____

____

Multiple Choice

50. The nurse receives the end-of-shift report from another staff member. Based on the following assessment information for the adult patients on the unit, it is a priority for the nurse to visit which patient first? ***(60)***
    1. BP–120/80, P–68, R–16
    2. BP–110/74, P–72, R–14
    3. BP–130/90, P–80, R–18
    4. BP–120/90, P–62, R–10

51. The nurse documents a pulse that feels full and springlike, even with pressure, as: ***(71)***
    1. 1+.
    2. 2+.
    3. 3+.
    4. 4+.

Student Name______________________________ **Date**______________

Physical Assessment

chapter
5

Answer Key: Textbook page references are provided as a guide for answering these questions. A complete answer key was provided for your instructor.

DISEASE AND DIAGNOSIS

Objectives

- Discuss the difference between a sign and a symptom.
- Compare and contrast the origins of disease.
- List the four major risk categories for development of disease.
- Discuss frequently noted signs and symptoms of disease conditions.
- List the cardinal signs of inflammation and infection.

1. Identify the difference between a sign and a symptom. ***(93-94)*** ______________________________

____

____

2. Identify whether each of the following is a sign or a symptom. ***(93-94)***

   a. Headache: ______________________________

   b. Nausea: ______________________________

   c. Anxiety: ______________________________

   d. Vomiting: ______________________________

   e. Drainage: ______________________________

3. Identify at least five possible etiologies of disease. ***(93)*** ______________________________

____

____

4. The four major risk categories for the development of disease are: ***(95)*** ______________________________

____

____

5. The cardinal signs of infection and inflammation are: ***(95)*** ______________________________

____

____

6. ______________________ is a sign comprising an abnormal "swishing" sound heard over an artery. ***(110)***

Multiple Choice

7. The nurse recognizes that an example of a hereditary disease is: ***(95)***
   1. mitral valve prolapse.
   2. tuberculosis.
   3. cystic fibrosis.
   4. congestive heart failure.

8. Congenital diseases: ***(94)***
   1. appear at birth.
   2. are transmitted from parent to child.
   3. have unknown etiology.
   4. are a result of infection.

9. Deficiency diseases are a result of: ***(94)***
   1. lack of nutrients.
   2. abnormal growth of tissue.
   3. exposure to microorganisms.
   4. harmful substances.

10. The risk factor that can lead to the development of coronary artery disease is: ***(95)***
    1. osteoporosis.
    2. cancer.
    3. trauma.
    4. diabetes.

11. A lifestyle risk that can lead to the development of lung disease is: ***(95)***
    1. air pollution.
    2. asbestos.
    3. smoking.
    4. malnutrition.

12. While obtaining the vital signs, the nurse observed that the patient was sweating profusely. The term used to describe this sign is: ***(96)***
    1. diaphoresis.
    2. cyanosis.
    3. ecchymosis.
    4. pruritus.

13. When assessing the patient's skin color, the nurse noted that the skin and the mucous membranes had a bluish discoloration. The term used to describe this sign is: ***(96)***
    1. jaundice.
    2. pallor.
    3. cyanosis.
    4. ecchymosis.

14. While transferring the patient from the stretcher to the bed, the nurse observed that the patient was experiencing difficulty breathing. The term used to describe this sign is: ***(96)***
    1. orthopnea.
    2. dyspnea.
    3. tachypnea.
    4. asthenia.

15. The patient's oral temperature is 101.2° F. The term used to describe this sign is: ***(96)***
    1. edema.
    2. fever.
    3. pruritus.
    4. jaundice.

16. The patient informed the nurse that she was not hungry and had been experiencing loss of appetite for several days. The term used to describe this symptom is: ***(96)***
    1. lethargy.
    2. dyspnea.
    3. anorexia.
    4. erythema.

17. When assessing the older adult, the nurse is aware that slumping, irritability, or sighing can indicate that the patient is exhibiting signs related to the symptom of: ***(106)***
    1. dyspnea.
    2. fatigue.
    3. orthopnea.
    4. erythema.

18. Choose the data that are considered objective data. (Select all that apply) ***(93)***
    1. Pulse
    2. Nausea
    3. Pain
    4. Fear
    5. Cyanosis

19. Choose the data that are considered subjective data. (Select all that apply) ***(93-94)***
    1. Blood pressure
    2. Edema
    3. Pain
    4. Erythema
    5. Pruritus

MEDICAL EXAMINATION

Objectives

- Describe the nursing responsibilities when assisting a physician with the physical examination.
- List equipment and supplies necessary for the physical examination and assessment.

20. When assisting the physician with the physical examination, the nurse is responsible for: *(97)* ____________

____

____

21. For the following parts of the examination, identify the position(s) of the patient. *(99)*

    a. Head and neck: ____________

    b. Thorax: ____________

    c. Abdomen: ____________

    d. Female genitalia: ____________

    e. Musculoskeletal system: ____________

22. Identify the equipment needed to assess or examine the following. *(98)*

    a. Vital signs: ____________

    b. Lung sounds: ____________

    c. Reflexes: ____________

23. Discuss the nursing responsibilities related to the psychological preparation of the patient for a physical examination. *(97)*

____

____

NURSING ASSESSMENT

Objectives

- Explain the necessary skills for the physical examination and nursing assessment.
- Discuss the nurse-patient interview.
- List the essentials to obtaining a patient's health history.
- Discuss the sequence of steps when performing a nursing assessment.
- Explain ways to develop cultural sensitivity.

24. Provide examples of questions that may be asked by the nurse to obtain information during a review of systems. *(103)*

    a. Respiratory: ____________

    ____

    b. Endocrine: ____________

    ____

c. Gastrointestinal: ______________________________

____

25. When preparing to check the patient's pupillary reflexes, the nurse must first ______________. ***(109)***

26. Identify the skills used in the physical examination and nursing assessment and the purpose of each one. ***(106-107)***

____

____

____

____

27. Identify two elements that can enhance the nurse-patient interview. ***(101)***______________

____

____

28. The objectives of obtaining the nursing health history are: ***(101-102)*** ______________

____

____

29. List the essential information obtained in a health history that will assist the nurse in developing the patient's plan of care. ***(102-106)***

____

____

30. Identify ways that the nurse may develop cultural sensitivity in relation to the physical examination. ***(104)***

____

____

31. What does each letter or word represent in the mnemonic device for assessing patients? ***(108)***

a. A: ______________________________

b. B: ______________________________

c. C: ______________________________

d. In: ______________________________

e. Out: ______________________________

f. P: ______________________________

g. S: ______________________________

32. Identify areas included in a cardiovascular assessment. ***(113-115)*** ______________________________

____

____

Multiple Choice

33. The nurse uses the OPQRST method for obtaining the most information about the patient's present health concerns. The P in the OPQRST method refers to the: ***(102)***
    1. quality of the concern.
    2. cause of the concern.
    3. severity of the concern.
    4. beginning of the concern.

34. The most frequently used skill in the physical nursing assessment is: ***(107-108)***
    1. inspection.
    2. palpation.
    3. percussion.
    4. auscultation.

ASSESSMENT FINDINGS

Objective

- Discuss normal assessment findings in the head-to-toe assessment.

35. Identify whether the following findings are expected or unexpected. ***(107-118)***

a. Decreased skin turgor: ______________________________

b. Fruity breath: ______________________________

c. Pupils round and reactive to light: ______________________________

d. Barrel chest: ______________________________

f. Two-second capillary refill: ______________________________

g. Adventitious breath sounds: ______________________________

h. No abdominal sounds: ______________________________

i. Bilateral, palpable pedal pulses: ______________________________

DOCUMENTATION

Objective

- Describe documentation of the physical examination and nursing assessment.

36. How are physical assessment results usually documented? *(117-118)* ______________________________

____

____

37. What is important for the nurse to do when documenting findings? *(117-118)* ____________________

____

____

Multiple Choice

38. The nurse documents that the patient has crackles. This is determined by the nurse as a result of auscultating: *(111-112)*
    1. short, discrete, bubbling sounds on inspiration.
    2. high-pitched musical sounds on inspiration.
    3. grating sounds on expiration.
    4. coarse gurgling on expiration.

Student Name____ **Date**__________________

Nursing Process and Critical Thinking

chapter **6**

Answer Key: Textbook page references are provided as a guide for answering these questions. A complete answer key was provided for your instructor.

PHASES OF THE NURSING PROCESS

Objectives

- Explain the use of each of the six phases of the nursing process.
- List the elements of each of the six phases of the nursing process.

1. The six phases of the nursing process are: ***(122)***____

____

____

2. "Readiness for enhanced nutrition" is an example of a ________________ nursing diagnosis. ***(126)***

Multiple Choice

3. The nursing process: ***(121)***
   1. provides the patient with quality care.
   2. focuses on a specific patient-related problem.
   3. provides a framework for the practice of nursing.
   4. ensures positive outcomes.

4. The patient's information and data are collected during the: ***(122)***
   1. assessment phase.
   2. planning phase.
   3. implementation phase.
   4. evaluation phase.

5. During which phase of the nursing process does the nurse identify the health problems? ***(123-124)***
   1. Assessment
   2. Diagnosis
   3. Planning
   4. Implementation

6. The nurse sets priorities for nursing intervention in the: *(128)*
   1. assessment phase.
   2. diagnosis phase.
   3. planning phase.
   4. implementation phase.

7. The nurse instructs the patient on the use of her inhaler. During which phase of the nursing process does this take place? *(131)*
   1. Diagnosis
   2. Planning
   3. Implementation
   4. Evaluation

ASSESSMENT

Objective

- Describe the establishing of the database.

8. What sources are used to obtain information for the patient database? *(122-123)* ____________________

____

____

9. Explain the difference between objective and subjective data. *(122)* ____________________

____

____

Multiple Choice

10. After collecting and validating the data, the nurse organizes and clusters the data. Data clustering refers to: *(123)*
    1. the evaluation of the patient data.
    2. focusing on the patient's problems.
    3. the grouping of related cues.
    4. the analysis of related outcomes.

11. It is best to perform a focused assessment when a patient is: (Select all that apply) *(122)*
    1. admitted to a long-term care facility.
    2. critically ill.
    3. disoriented.
    4. unable to respond to the nurse.

12. During a patient assessment, biographical data would include: *(123)*
    1. the patient's medications taken at home.
    2. the reason for the patient's admission to the facility.
    3. age, obtained weight, and place of employment.
    4. a history of any medical conditions.

DIAGNOSIS

Objectives

- Discuss the steps used to formulate a nursing diagnosis.
- Differentiate among types of health problems.

13. Identify the four components of a nursing diagnosis. ***(124-126)*** ________________

14. Write a possible nursing diagnosis based upon the following situations. ***(126)***

    a. A 52-year-old patient is admitted after episodes of severe vomiting. ________________

    b. A 75-year-old patient with right hemiparesis arrives seeking care following a cerebral vascular accident (stroke).

15. What are the four types of nursing diagnosis statements? ***(126)*** ________________

Multiple Choice

16. The nursing diagnosis is defined as: ***(124)***
    1. the identification of a disease or condition that involves problems with structures.
    2. problems that nurses cannot prescribe a treatment for.
    3. a clinical judgment about individual, group, or community responses to actual or potential health problems.
    4. problems that are identified as a result of the planning phase.

17. At the completion of the nursing assessment phase, the nursing diagnosis statement is formulated and a possible diagnosis statement may be written by the nurse. The possible or "risk diagnosis" statement is written when the: ***(126)***
    1. actual factors are present in a circumstance.
    2. factors are predicted to occur in a circumstance.
    3. medical aspects of a circumstance are unsafe.
    4. cues obtained from the patient indicate no problems exist.

18. Based on the definition of a collaborative problem, which of the following problems would be an example of one? ***(126)***
    1. Pain
    2. Anxiety
    3. Coping
    4. Edema

OUTCOMES IDENTIFICATION, PLANNING, AND IMPLEMENTATION

Objectives

- Describe the development of patient-centered outcomes.
- Discuss the creation of nursing orders.

19. Identify Maslow's hierarchy of needs beginning with the ones that are given highest priority in patient care situations. ***(128)***

    ____

    ____

20. Patient-centered outcomes should be statements that are: ***(127-128)*** ______________________________

    ____

    ____

21. Write possible patient-centered outcomes using the following terms. ***(127-128)***

    a. Describe: ______________________________

    ____

    b. Verbalize: ______________________________

    ____

    c. List: ______________________________

    ____

    d. Demonstrate: ______________________________

    ____

22. What is included in a nursing order? ***(129-130)*** ______________________________

    ____

    ____

23. Write an example of a nursing order. ***(129-130)*** ______________________________

____

____

24. Provide examples of possible nursing actions that may be implemented for a patient with a nursing diagnosis of "Risk for impaired skin integrity, due to loss of mobility on right side." ***(129-130)***

____

____

Multiple Choice

25. A nursing order is created to provide: ***(129-130)***
    1. specific written instructions for all caregivers.
    2. a general statement that conveys information.
    3. a statement providing general information for nursing interventions.
    4. information for the formulation of a care plan.

26. Which of the following are nursing interventions? (Select all that apply) ***(129)***
    1. Monitoring the patient for problems or complications
    2. Performing an activity for a patient
    3. Teaching the patient or family about health maintenance
    4. Advising a patient on the type of medication necessary for the patient's condition

EVALUATION

Objective

- Explain the evaluation of a nursing care plan.

27. Describe the steps in the evaluation of the nursing care plan. ***(131-132)*** ______________________________

____

____

28. What are the possible evaluation outcomes? ***(131-132)*** ______________________________

____

____

CARE PLANS AND CLINICAL PATHWAYS

Objectives

- Demonstrate the nursing process by writing a nursing care plan.
- Describe the use of clinical pathways in managed care.

29. Identify the purpose and advantages of clinical pathways. *(133)* ______________________________

____

____

30. Write a nursing care plan for the following patient situation. *(133)*

Ms. M., 48 years of age, is admitted to the medical-surgical unit after an abdominal hysterectomy. Her vital signs are stable. The IV in her left forearm is patent, without swelling or tenderness. The dressings are dry and intact. Ms. M. has a Foley catheter in place that is draining clear, yellow urine. Ms. M. was just transferred from the surgical recovery unit. Ms. M. is expressing severe pain.

____

____

____

____

____

____

GROUPS

Objective

- Explain the activities of NANDA, NIC, and NOC.

31. Describe the general activities of NANDA, NIC, and NOC. *(124-125)* ______________________________

____

____

32. Identify at least two benefits of using the standardized language of NANDA, NIC, and NOC. *(124-125)*

____

____

CRITICAL THINKING

Objective

- Discuss critical thinking.

33. Provide specific examples of how critical thinking is applied in clinical nursing situations. ***(134-135)***

____

____

34. Describe the term "evidence-based practice." ***(131)*** _______________________

____

____

Student Name______________________________ **Date**______________

chapter
7
Documentation

Answer Key: Textbook page references are provided as a guide for answering these questions. A complete answer key was provided for your instructor.

PURPOSES

Objectives

- List the five purposes for written patient records.
- Explain the relationship of the nursing care plan to care documentation and patient care reimbursement.

1. The person who is appointed to examine patients' charts and health records to assess quality of care is known as ____________________. ***(139-140)***

2. The ____________________ is a system used to consolidate patient orders and care needs in a centralized, concise way. ***(145)***

3. The five basic purposes of written patient records are: ***(138-139)*** ____________________

4. Explain how home health care documentation relates to reimbursement. ***(151)*** ____________________

Multiple Choice

5. A system that is used by Medicare for reimbursement of patient care services is: ***(139)***
   1. focused medical factor–related grouping.
   2. diagnosis-related group.
   3. quality assurance or improvement.
   4. problem-oriented diagnosis-related group.

6. The most accurate definition of *the patient's chart* is: ***(138)***
   1. a system used to consolidate patient orders and care needs in a centralized, concise way.
   2. a legal record used to meet the many demands of the health system.
   3. written information contained in the patient records.
   4. subjective and objective assessment, plan, evaluation; in this more compact form, the care given or action taken is included in the plan notations.

METHODS AND FORMS

Objectives

- Describe the differences between traditional and problem-oriented medical records.
- Describe the purpose of and the relationship between the Kardex and the nursing care plan.
- Describe the differences in documenting care using activities of daily living and physical assessment forms, and narrative, SOAPE, and focus formats.
- Discuss issues related to computerization in documentation.
- Discuss documentation and clinical pathways.

7. Explain the major differences between a traditional patient record and a problem-oriented (POMR) record. ***(142-143)***

____

____

8. a. What is the purpose of an incident report? ***(145)*** ______________________

____

____

   b. Is the incident report included in the patient's record? ***(148)*** ______________________

____

____

9. Describe the relationship between the Kardex and the patient chart. ***(145)***______________________

____

____

10. What are the advantages and disadvantages of computer documentation? ***(152-153)*** ______________________

____

____

11. Identify the primary benefit of documenting with clinical pathways. ***(149, 151)***______________________

____

____

Multiple Choice

12. Focus charting contains: ***(144)***
    1. nursing action and patient response.
    2. a description of the patient's present condition.
    3. objective and subjective assessment data.
    4. nursing diagnosis, action, and patient's response.

13. Charting by exception: ***(145)***
    1. provides comprehensive nurse's notes.
    2. provides a more organized flow in the nurse's notes.
    3. decreases the time needed to complete the nurse's notes.
    4. summarizes the information in the nurse's notes.

14. What type of charting format usually requires the most time to complete? ***(142)***
    1. SOAP
    2. Focus
    3. PIE
    4. Narrative

15. What type of charting format most reflects the nursing process? ***(144)***
    1. Narrative
    2. Traditional
    3. Focus
    4. PIE

16. What documentation is included in the "P" when using the PIE method of charting? ***(145)***
    1. Patient response
    2. Problem list
    3. Assessment
    4. Plan

17. The POMR is divided into which four major sections? ***(142)***
    1. History and physical examination, physician's orders, nurse's notes, and progress notes
    2. Database, problem list, plan, and progress notes
    3. Subjective data, objective data, diagnostic tests, and progress notes
    4. Physician's orders, nurse's notes, lab reports, and progress notes

18. The problem-oriented medical record: ***(142)***
    1. uses a patient problem list as index for chart documenting.
    2. uses a narrative format for documenting in the nurse's notes.
    3. uses care plans for documenting in the nurse's notes.
    4. emphasizes the use of specific forms for charting.

19. The charting format most commonly used for documentation of clinical pathways is: ***(149, 151)***
    1. focus charting.
    2. traditional charting.
    3. charting by exception.
    4. narrative charting.

GUIDELINES

Objectives

- Describe the basic guidelines for and mechanics of charting.
- State important legal aspects of chart ownership, access, confidentiality, and patient care documentation.

20. The essential elements of documentation are: ***(138)*** ______________________

____

____

21. What are the basic guidelines for charting? ***(140-141)***______________________

____

____

22. Confidentiality of the patient's medical record is guaranteed by: ***(152)***______________________

____

____

23. Identify the important legal aspects for the following. ***(152)***

    a. Record ownership:______________________

    ____

    b. Access:______________________

    ____

    c. Confidentiality: ______________________

    ____

24. Military time is used in most hospitals to document the time care is given. Convert the following civilian times to military time. ***(151)***

    a. 3:00 PM = ________
    b. 7:30 PM = ________
    c. 6:00 PM = ________
    d. Midnight = ________

Multiple Choice

25. When an error is made by the nurse in charting: ***(140)***
    1. it is reported to the charge nurse, and the nurse continues with the charting.
    2. Wite-out (correction fluid) is used to correct the error, and the nurse continues with the charting.
    3. the charting is started over on a new sheet.
    4. a line is drawn through the error and initialed, and then the nurse continues with the charting.

26. Confidentiality is most often maintained with use of computer charting through the: ***(155)***
    1. assignment of individual passwords.
    2. legal signature of the nurse.
    3. use of patient code names.
    4. use of assigned individual patient unit numbers.

27. The patient can gain access to his or her records or chart: ***(152)***
    1. in all states.
    2. immediately upon request of the information.
    3. through a formal written request.
    4. by following established procedures of the facility or institution.

28. Inadequate documentation that is commonly involved in cases of malpractice include: (Select all that apply) ***(140-141)***
    1. documenting incorrect data.
    2. charting nursing actions in advance.
    3. charting incorrect times at which events occurred.
    4. failing to record verbal orders or failing to have them signed.

HEALTH CARE SITES

Objectives

- Discuss long-term health care documentation.
- Discuss home health care documentation.

29. In relation to documentation, the Omnibus Budget Reconciliation Act (OBRA) of 1987 requires: ***(152)***

    ____

    ____

30. Briefly identify how long-term care and home health care documentation are different from acute care (hospital) documentation. ***(151-152)***

    ____

    ____

Student Name______________________________ Date______________

chapter 8

Cultural and Ethnic Considerations

Answer Key: Textbook page references are provided as a guide for answering these questions. A complete answer key was provided for your instructor.

CULTURE AND ETHNICITY

Objective

- Describe ways that culture affects the individual.

1. The term that describes learned beliefs, customs, and practices shared by a group and passed to another generation is ______________________. *(158)*

2. A group of people who share common social and cultural heritage based on traditions and national origin is referred to as ______________________. *(161)*

Multiple Choice

3. The nurse anticipates that the older adult patient will be: *(160)*
   1. more tolerant of other cultures.
   2. moving away from traditions and rituals.
   3. farther removed from their religious beliefs and practices.
   4. resistant to attempts to change trusted home remedies and practices.

4. A group that shares primary characteristics with another but has some different behaviors and ideas describes a(n): *(158)*
   1. ethnic group.
   2. dominant group.
   3. subculture.
   4. race.

CULTURALLY RELATED ASSESSMENTS

Objectives

- Explain how personal cultural beliefs and practices can affect nurse-patient and nurse-nurse relationships.
- Identify and discuss cultural variables that may influence health behaviors.

5. Describe how the following cultural variables influence health behaviors. ***(159-160)***

   a. Family structure and roles: ______________________________

   ____

   b. Religious beliefs: ______________________________

   ____

   c. Health-practice traditions: ______________________________

   ____

6. Compare and contrast two different cultural groups in relation to the following. ***(163-164)***

   a. Time orientation: ______________________________

   ____

   b. Dietary preferences: ______________________________

   ____

   c. Birth rites: ______________________________

   ____

Multiple Choice

7. Which of the following statements reveals the influence of culture on health beliefs? (Select all that apply) ***(170-171)***
   1. Western cultures have traditionally used the biomedical method of treating illness.
   2. All cultures value traditional medicine.
   3. The response to health and illness varies among different cultures.
   4. Based on cultural data, the nurse makes certain assumptions about the patient.

8. Which of the following religious groups believes that blood transfusions violate God's laws? ***(165-169)***
   1. Quakers
   2. Mennonites
   3. Jehovah's Witnesses
   4. Roman Catholics

9. The nurse caring for a diverse group of patients anticipates that special intervention at the time of death will be provided for the patient who is: ***(165-169)***
   1. Eastern Orthodox.
   2. Pentecostal.
   3. a Disciple of God.
   4. Seventh Day Adventist.

NURSING PROCESS

Objectives

- Identify the importance of transcultural nursing.
- Explain how the nurse can use cultural data to help develop therapeutic relationships with the patient.
- Discuss the use of the nursing process when caring for culturally diverse patients.

10. How does the nurse integrate transcultural nursing into practice? ***(159-160)***____________________

11. List considerations related to cultural differences that nurses need to be aware of when caring for an older adult. ***(160)***

12. Identify nursing interventions that may be used to communicate with a non–English-speaking patient. ***(162)***

13. In order to assist the patient to meet his or her needs, the nurse wants to complete an accurate assessment. How should the nurse ask the patient about the following? ***(162-163)***

    a. Language: ____________________

    b. Illness: ____________________

    c. Family structure: ____________________

    d. Dietary practices: ____________________

    e. Use of folk medicine: ____________________

14. Write a nursing diagnosis that can be modified to reflect the problems of a culturally diverse patient. ***(171-172)***

____

____

Multiple Choice

15. Transcultural nursing is: ***(159-160)***
    1. nursing care that is given to a group of patients who share specific beliefs.
    2. nursing care based on a specific group's behavior and needs.
    3. the implementation of culturally appropriate nursing care.
    4. the implementation of generalized standards of care to meet needs of all patients.

16. When communicating with a patient who has a limited grasp of English, the nurse should: ***(162-163)***
    1. speak loudly.
    2. keep questions brief and simple.
    3. use sign language and get an interpreter.
    4. provide detailed directions.

17. In assisting a female patient who is Muslim American, the nurse anticipates her cultural needs during a physical examination by: ***(168)***
    1. covering body parts as much as possible.
    2. examining her in the presence of her husband.
    3. maintaining close eye contact throughout the examination.
    4. requesting that a male physician perform the entire examination.

18. In reviewing the dietary needs of a group of patients, the nurse notices that there is a shared restriction for patients who are of the Pentecostal, Church of the Nazarene, and Mormon faiths. This dietary restriction includes: ***(168-169)***
    1. mixing of dairy and meat products.
    2. ingestion of pork and corn-based flour products.
    3. use of alcohol and tobacco.
    4. ingestion of caffeinated beverages.

19. When communicating with a patient, the nurse knows that eye contact may have to be avoided with which cultures? (Select all that apply) ***(175)***
    1. Italian American
    2. elderly Native American
    3. Hispanic
    4. Middle Eastern

Student Name______________________________ Date______________

Life Span Development

chapter **9**

Answer Key: Textbook page references are provided as a guide for answering these questions. A complete answer key was provided for your instructor.

FAMILY

Objectives

- Differentiate among the types of family patterns and their functions in society.
- Describe different types of stresses that commonly affect today's families.

1. Conception (fertilization) can be described as the union between ____________ and ____________. ***(181)***

2. Families are composed of two or more people who are united by __________________. ***(182-183)***

3. List the four family patterns and describe how each one functions. ***(183-184)*** ______________________

   ____

   ____

4. Identify factors that have contributed to the changes that families of today have undergone and are still undergoing. ***(183)***

   ____

   ____

5. Discuss the qualities of functional families. ***(184)*** ______________________________

   ____

   ____

6. Three common causes of family stress are: ***(186-187)*** ______________________________

   ____

   ____

Multiple Choice

7. The nuclear family is: ***(183)***
   1. biological parents, offspring, and grandparents.
   2. biological parents, offspring, grandparents, aunts, and uncles.
   3. biological parents and their offspring.
   4. traditional family and some additional family members.

8. A social contract family consists of: ***(184)***
   1. remarried adults and children.
   2. same-sex couple with foster or adoptive children.
   3. the family unit with adopted children.
   4. an unmarried couple living together and sharing roles and responsibilities.

9. The nurse is assessing how the patient's family functions. The nurse determines that the family is primarily autocratic based upon the observation of the: ***(184)***
   1. mother assuming primary dominance in decision making.
   2. parents implementing strict rules and expectations.
   3. uncle controlling the finances.
   4. children participating in negotiations.

10. The disengagement phase of parenthood can be best described as: ***(186)***
    1. beginning at the birth or adoption of the first child.
    2. extending from the wedding up until the birth of the first child.
    3. the period of family life when the grown children depart from the home.
    4. the last stage of the life cycle, which requires the individual to cope with a large range of changes.

GROWTH AND DEVELOPMENT

Objectives

- Describe the physical characteristics at each stage of the life cycle.
- List the psychosocial changes at the different stages of development.
- Discuss Erikson's stages of psychosocial development.
- Describe Piaget's four stages of cognitive development.

INFANCY, TODDLERHOOD, PRESCHOOL AGE, SCHOOL AGE

Objective

- Describe the cognitive changes occurring in the early childhood period.

11. ____________________ is a function or gradual process of change from simple to complex. ***(188-189)***

12. Children may be affected by stress. Identify at least five common signs of stress in children. ***(186)***

    ____

    ____

13. Identify the major physical and psychosocial changes that occur from infancy through school age. ***(189-198)***

	Physical Changes	Psychosocial Changes
a. Infant		
b. Toddler		
c. Preschooler		

Multiple Choice

14. Height increases approximately _____ a month for the first 6 months of life. ***(189)***
    1. ½ inch
    2. 1 inch
    3. 2 inches
    4. 3 inches

15. By the time an infant is 1 year of age, the child will have: ***(189)***
    1. doubled his or her birth weight.
    2. gained 1 lb per month.
    3. tripled his or her birth weight.
    4. gained 3 lbs per month.

16. Weight gain after 8 months is attributed to gains in: ***(189)***
    1. fat and muscle.
    2. fat and bone.
    3. fat and increased fluid volume.
    4. muscle and bone.

17. Obvious growth in the long bones and increase in height of approximately 2 inches per year for both boys and girls are physical characteristics of: ***(198)***
    1. preschoolers.
    2. toddlers.
    3. school-age children.
    4. adolescents.

18. By the age of 2½ years, the toddler has: ***(189)***
    1. complete primary dentition, 20 teeth.
    2. approximately 16 teeth.
    3. approximately 12 teeth.
    4. approximately 30 teeth.

19. The infant uses the senses to learn about self and environment in the: ***(190)***
    1. formal operational stage.
    2. preoperational stage.
    3. sensorimotor stage.
    4. concrete operational stage.

20. The toddler gradually begins to "de-center" (becomes less egocentric and understands other points of view) in the: ***(194)***
    1. formal operational stage.
    2. preoperational stage.
    3. sensorimotor stage.
    4. concrete operational stage.

21. The school-age child is able to think about abstractions and hypothetical concepts and is able to move in thought "from the real to the possible" in the: ***(200)***
    1. formal operational stage.
    2. preoperational stage.
    3. sensorimotor stage.
    4. concrete operational stage.

22. The preoperational thought stage of early childhood extends from: ***(194)***
    1. 1 to 3 years of age.
    2. 2 to 7 years of age.
    3. 5 to 9 years of age.
    4. 9 to 12 years of age.

23. The parent tries to hand the child over to a caregiver at the day care center, but the child reacts by crying and clinging. The nurse anticipates this behavior will begin in children at the age of: ***(190)***
    1. 3 months.
    2. 8 months.
    3. 1 year.
    4. 2 years.

24. The nurse is teaching the parents of an infant what the principles are for introduction of foods. The nurse provides accurate information when informing the parents that: (Select all that apply) ***(191)***
    1. citrus fruits may be given before the infant is 6 months of age.
    2. foods should be mixed together for improved taste.
    3. cereals should be started before vegetables and meats.
    4. it is best to introduce only one new food at a time, allowing several days between new foods.

ADOLESCENCE

Objective

- Discuss the developmental tasks of the adolescent period.

25. Identify at least five developmental tasks of the adolescent. ***(204)*** ______________________

____

____

Multiple Choice

26. The second major period of rapid physical growth is observed in the: ***(201)***
    1. school-age child.
    2. adolescent.
    3. young adult.
    4. middle adult.

27. The most critical indicator of severe depression is: ***(204)***
    1. a change in appetite.
    2. an inability to concentrate.
    3. a preoccupation with death.
    4. a verbalization of thoughts of harming oneself.

28. The nurse is working with a group of parents of high school students. During the discussion, the following statements are made by the parents. Based on an understanding of the needs of adolescents, which statement requires follow-up by the nurse? ***(202)***
    1. "We try to set reasonable limits on dating."
    2. "The car has to be back home by 9:00 PM on school nights."
    3. "We think that there should be as much experimentation and freedom as possible."
    4. "The number of after-school activities are tremendous, so we discuss how many things are realistic."

YOUNG AND MIDDLE ADULTHOOD

Objectives

- List the developmental tasks for early adulthood.
- Describe the developmental tasks for middle adulthood.

29. Provide examples of the developmental tasks for the early and the middle adult. ***(204, 206)*** ____________

____

____

30. A leading cause of death for the young adult is ____________________. ***(206)***

Multiple Choice

31. Generativity can best be defined as: ***(208)***
    1. the ability to relate one's deepest hopes and concerns to another person.
    2. the task of reorganization, reevaluation, and acceptance.
    3. accepting responsibility for and offering guidance to the next generation and adapting to physical and role changes.
    4. a time of satisfaction and pleasure.

32. Developmental tasks of early adulthood include: (Select all that apply) ***(204)***
    1. development of career and job satisfaction.
    2. acceptance of self and others.
    3. maximizing personal worth and identity.
    4. making decisions regarding careers, marriage, and children.

LATE ADULTHOOD

Objectives

- Define aging.
- Discuss theories of aging.
- Describe the normal age-related changes affecting the major body systems.
- Discuss the effect of the aging process on personality, intelligence, learning, and memory.

33. A form of discrimination and prejudice against older adults is referred to as ____________________. ***(209)***

34. Define the aging theory of biological programming: ***(210)***____________________________________

____

____

35. Describe the physical changes that occur in each of the following systems as a result of the aging process. ***(212-213)***

    a. Sensory:____

    ____

    b. Integumentary:____

    ____

c. Cardiovascular: ______________________________

____

d. Respiratory: ______________________________

____

e. Gastrointestinal: ______________________________

____

f. Genitourinary: ______________________________

____

g. Musculoskeletal: ______________________________

____

h. Neurologic: ______________________________

____

36. What influence does the aging process have on the following? ***(213-215)***

a. Personality: ______________________________

____

b. Intelligence and learning: ______________________________

____

c. Memory: ______________________________

____

Multiple Choice

37. Aging is best defined as a: ***(209-210)***
    1. period of decline in social activities.
    2. period in which senility increases.
    3. normal condition of human existence that can be affected by health habits and family.
    4. normal state in which changes in physiological conditions are universal and inevitable.

38. The nurse is assessing an older adult patient and recognizes that the following is an unexpected finding associated with the aging process: ***(212)***
    1. Presbyopia
    2. Opacity of the lens
    3. Decreased depth perception
    4. Slowed accommodation

Student Name______________________________ Date______________

Loss, Grief, Dying, and Death

chapter **10**

Answer Key: Textbook page references are provided as a guide for answering these questions. A complete answer key was provided for your instructor.

GRIEF AND LOSS

Objectives

- Explain how the concept of loss affects the grief reaction.
- Recognize the five aspects of human functioning and how each interacts with the others during the grieving and dying process.

1. The condition of being subject to death is known as ______________________. ***(219)***

2. Grief is a pattern of physical and emotional responses to bereavement, separation, or ______________________. ***(218)***

3. Briefly describe the concepts of loss and grief. ***(218)***______________________

4. Identify at least seven factors that influence the experience of loss. ***(220)***______________________

5. Discuss how physical and social aspects of human functioning influence the grieving process. ***(220-223)***

6. Describe grief therapy. When was it introduced? ***(219)*** ______________________

Multiple Choice

7. Maturational loss is best defined as: ***(219)***
   1. a loss occurring suddenly in response to a specific external event.
   2. any significant loss that requires adaptation through the grieving process.
   3. a loss resulting from normal life transitions.
   4. events such as the death of a loved one, divorce, the breakup of a relationship, or the loss of a job.

8. Situational loss can best be defined as: ***(219)***
   1. a loss occurring suddenly in response to a specific external event.
   2. any significant loss that requires adaptation through the grieving process.
   3. a loss resulting from normal life transitions.
   4. events such as the death of a loved one, divorce, the breakup of a relationship, or the loss of a job.

STAGES OF GRIEF AND DYING

Objectives

- Describe the stages of dying.
- Identify needs of the grieving patient and family.
- Discuss support for the grieving family.
- Discuss approaches to facilitate the grieving process.

9. Identify Kübler-Ross's stage of dying in each of the following examples of patient responses. ***(223)***

   a. "No, not me." ______________________________

   b. "I just want to live until my daughter gets married." ______________________________

   c. "It's not fair. I can't stand this!" ______________________________

10. Identify the nursing assessments and interventions for the patient and/or family experiencing death and grieving. ***(224-228)***

	Assessment	Interventions
a. Physical needs		
b. Emotional needs		
c. Spiritual needs		

11. A sign, symptom, or behavior associated with dysfunctional grieving (unresolved grief) is ________________________________. ***(222-224)***

12. It is important that the nurse have knowledge and an understanding of survivors' reactions to be able to identify and meet the needs of the grieving family. List and describe Martocchio's manifestations of grief or survivors' reactions. ***(244)***

____

____

Multiple Choice

13. Following the loss of a loved one, an individual may experience a sense of presence. These perceptions typically manifest by which of the following experiences? (Select all that apply) ***(221)***
    1. Dreams
    2. Hallucinations
    3. Perceptions of smell
    4. General feelings of the deceased's presence

NURSING PROCESS

Objectives

- Identify unique physical signs and symptoms of the near-death patient.
- Discuss nursing interventions for the dying patient.
- Describe techniques in assisting the dying patient to say good-bye.
- Identify how the changes in the health care system affect nursing interventions for the dying patient.
- Describe nursing responsibilities in the care of the body after death.

14. Write a nursing diagnosis, patient outcome, and nursing interventions based on the following situation. ***(224-225, 229)***

    The patient lost her husband in an automobile accident a year ago. She is still experiencing insomnia and feelings of worthlessness and anger, and she continues to avoid family and social functions.

____

____

____

____

15. Provide examples of how nurses cope with grief when they deal with their dying patients. ***(221-222)***

____

____

16. What are the priority needs of the dying patient? ***(240)*** ____________________

____

____

17. What are some techniques that nurses may use to assist patients to say good-bye? ***(237-238)*** ____________________

____

____

18. Number the following nursing actions in the order that they should be done for postmortem care, from first to last. ***(241-243)***
    - ______ Remove all tubing and other devices.
    - ______ Wash hands and don gloves.
    - ______ Place patient in supine position.
    - ______ Bathe patient as necessary.
    - ______ Close patient's eyes and mouth if needed.
    - ______ Allow family to view body and remain in the room.

Multiple Choice

19. Signs and symptoms that the nurse would expect to assess in the patient nearing death include: (Select all that apply) ***(239-240)***
    1. lowered blood pressure.
    2. rapid, bounding pulse.
    3. irregular respiratory pattern.
    4. constricted and fixed pupils.

SPECIAL SUPPORTIVE CARE

Objective

- List nursing interventions that may facilitate grieving in special circumstances.

20. Identify nursing interventions in the following special circumstances. ***(231-233)***

    a. Perinatal death: ____________________

    ____

    b. Pediatric death: ____________________

    ____

    c. Gerontologic death: ____________________

    ____

d. Suicide: ____

____

ISSUES RELATED TO DEATH AND DYING

Objectives

- Explain advance directives, which include the living will and the durable power of attorney.
- Explain concepts of euthanasia, do-not-resuscitate (DNR) orders, organ donations, fraudulent methods of treatment, and the Dying Person's Bill of Rights.

21. Provide examples of fraudulent methods of treatment that may be offered to the dying patient or family. ***(237)***

____

____

Multiple Choice

22. The terminally ill patient has been experiencing severe pain and has requested that the doctor assist her to end her suffering. The appropriate term used when referring to the action of ending this patient's life is: ***(233)***
    1. euthanasia.
    2. passive suicide.
    3. brain death.
    4. mercy killing.

23. The patient in Room 318 has a DNR order. The licensed vocational nurse knows that a DNR order means: ***(234)***
    1. withholding of nutrition.
    2. administering pain medication.
    3. not administering CPR if the patient stops breathing.
    4. discontinuing all intravenous lines (IVs).

24. The Uniform Anatomical Gift Act: ***(235-236)***
    1. stipulates that physicians who certify death shall not be involved in removal or transplant of organs.
    2. prohibits selling or purchasing organs.
    3. facilitates this area of medical and nursing research.
    4. stipulates that at the time of death a qualified health care provider must ask family members to donate organs.

25. The goal of the Dying Person's Bill of Rights is to: ***(236)***
    1. assist the nurses in providing appropriate care.
    2. list the treatment options of the patient.
    3. provide guidelines for the health care agencies.
    4. ensure death with dignity for the patient.

26. An advance directive: ***(235)***
    1. appoints a health care surrogate to make decisions in the event the patient or individual is incompetent.
    2. provides for decisions related to the patient's financial needs.
    3. describes the patient's wishes about his or her estate when death is near.
    4. describes the patient's wishes about his or her care when death is near.

27. The nurse is working in a pediatric outpatient clinic. There is an 8-year-old child whose grandfather has just died. The nurse anticipates, based on the developmental level, that the child will respond by saying the following: ***(223, 232)***
    1. "Grandpa will come back soon."
    2. "Grandpa was old and supposed to die."
    3. "I was bad at school and talked back to Mom. That's why Grandpa died."
    4. "It was better that Grandpa died quickly and didn't have to suffer a long time."

28. Durable power of attorney: ***(234)***
    1. appoints a health care surrogate to make decisions in the event the patient or individual is incompetent.
    2. provides for decisions related to the patient's financial needs.
    3. describes the patient's wishes about his or her estate when death is near.
    4. describes the patient's wishes about his or her care when death is near.

Student Name____ Date____________________

chapter **11**

Admission, Transfer, and Discharge

Answer Key: Textbook page references are provided as a guide for answering these questions. A complete answer key was provided for your instructor.

PATIENT RESPONSE TO HOSPITALIZATION

Objectives

- Describe common patient reactions to hospitalization.
- Identify nursing interventions for common patient reactions to hospitalization.

1. Provide examples of nursing interventions for the following reactions to hospitalization. ***(248-249)***

   a. Fear of the unknown: ____________________

   ____

   b. Loss of identity: ____________________

   ____

   c. Disorientation: ____________________

   ____

   d. Separation anxiety and/or loneliness: ____________________

   ____

Multiple Choice

2. The practical or vocational nurse is aware that separation anxiety can be expressed in older adults by: ***(249)***
   1. quietness.
   2. crying.
   3. calling for the nurse.
   4. fear.

3. The nurse is aware that separation anxiety can be expressed in children by: ***(248-249)***
   1. quietness.
   2. crying.
   3. calling for the nurse.
   4. fear.

4. Fear of the unknown can be related to Maslow's need for: ***(248)***
   1. self-esteem.
   2. self-actualization.
   3. safety.
   4. belonging.

5. Loss of identity can be related to Maslow's need for: ***(249)***
   1. self-esteem.
   2. self-actualization.
   3. safety.
   4. belonging.

ADMISSION

Objective

- Discuss the nurse's responsibilities in performing an admission.

6. Provide the rationale for each of the following nursing actions related to the admission of the patient to the care unit. ***(249-250)***

   a. Checking and verifying of ID band: ______________________________

   ____

   b. Assessing immediate needs: ______________________________

   ____

   c. Explaining hospital routines, such as visiting hours, mealtime, and morning wake-up: __________

   ____

7. List the information that should be included when orienting the patient to the room. ***(251)***__________

   ____

   ____

TRANSFER

Objective

- Describe how the nurse prepares a patient for transfer to another unit or facility.

8. When transferring a patient to another unit or facility, the nurse should ________________. ***(257)***

DISCHARGE

Objectives

- Discuss discharge planning.
- Explain how the nurse prepares a patient for discharge.
- Identify the nurse's role when a patient chooses to leave the hospital against medical advice.

9. Ideally, discharge planning begins ______________________________. *(259)*

10. Identify two examples of health care disciplines other than nursing that are involved in referrals, and explain their role in the discharge process. *(260-262)*

    ____

    ____

11. Provide the rationale for each of the following nursing actions in the discharge of a patient. *(262-263)*

    a. Makes certain there is a written discharge order: ______________________________

    ____

    b. Arranges for patient and family to visit the business office and check to see that a release has been given:

    ____

    c. Notifies the family or person who will be transporting the patient to home: ______________

    ____

    d. Gathers equipment, supplies, and prescriptions that the patient is to take home: ____________

    ____

    e. Assists the patient in dressing and packing items to go home: ____________________

    ____

Multiple Choice

12. When a patient wishes to leave the hospital against medical advice (AMA), the nurse's first responsibility is to: *(263)*
    1. notify the physician.
    2. document the incident thoroughly in the nurse's notes.
    3. detain the patient.
    4. request that the patient sign the special release form (AMA form).

13. After the patient has been discharged AMA, the nurse: *(263)*
    1. notifies the accounting department.
    2. notifies the supervisor.
    3. documents the incident thoroughly in the nurse's notes.
    4. reports the AMA to the risk manager.

NURSING PROCESS

Objectives

- Identify guidelines for admission, transfer, and discharge of a patient.
- Discuss the nursing process and how it pertains to admitting, discharging, and transferring the patient.

14. Discuss factors that the nurse should consider when admitting, transferring, or discharging an older adult patient. ***(249)***

____

____

15. Identify at least two guidelines that can be used when communicating with patients from various cultural backgrounds during the admission, transfer, or discharge process. ***(250)***

____

____

16. Provide an example of a general nursing diagnosis that may be appropriate for a patient during the admission, transfer, or discharge process. ***(256-257)***

____

____

17. The nurse is aware that admission to a health care facility evokes anxiety and fear in many patients; therefore, the nurse should convey _______________ towards the patient, as evidenced by the nurse recognizing, understanding, and to some extent sharing the emotions that the patient is experiencing. ***(249)***

Multiple Choice

18. Planning the discharge of a patient should begin: ***(259)***
    1. the day of discharge.
    2. the day before discharge.
    3. as soon as possible after admission.
    4. two to three days after admission.

19. During the admission of a patient to a health care facility, the responsibilities of the admitting clerk or secretary include: (Select all that apply) ***(249-250)***
    1. obtaining identifying information from the patient.
    2. giving the patient information on Health Information Portability and Accountability Act (HIPAA) guidelines.
    3. placing the correct ID band on the patient's wrist.
    4. obtaining the list of current medications from the patient.

20. An elderly Chinese-American male patient is admitted to Room 412, which is a semiprivate room, at 1:00 PM. The patient demonstrates signs of being very anxious, most likely in relation to: ***(250)***
    1. separation from his children.
    2. sharing the room with a roommate.
    3. being admitted to a room containing the number "4."
    4. being admitted during a busy part of the hospital day.

Student Name________________________ Date____________

chapter 12

Medical-Surgical Asepsis and Infection Prevention and Control

Answer Key: Textbook page references are provided as a guide for answering these questions. A complete answer key was provided for your instructor.

TERMS

Objective

- Define the key terms listed.

1. Define the following terms.

   a. Carrier: *(271)*________________________

   ____

   b. Endogenous: *(275)*________________________

   ____

   c. Exogenous: *(275)*________________________

   ____

   d. Fomite: *(272)*________________________

   ____

   e. Vector: *(272)*________________________

   ____

ASEPSIS

Objectives

- Explain the difference between medical and surgical asepsis.
- Identify principles of surgical asepsis.

2. Describe the difference between medical and surgical asepsis. ***(267)***____________________

3. Identify the seven major principles of sterile technique, and for each principle provide at least one example of how the nurse implements it. ***(292)***

INFECTION AND INFLAMMATION

Objectives

- Discuss the events in the inflammatory response.
- Describe the signs and symptoms of a localized infection and those of a systemic infection.

4. Describe an inflammatory response and the stages of the infectious process. ***(273-274)***________________

5. Identify the differences between localized and systemic responses to infection. ***(273)*** ________________

CHAIN OF INFECTION

Objectives

- Explain how each element of the chain of infection contributes to infection.
- List five major classifications of pathogens.
- Differentiate between *Staphylococcus aureus* and *Staphylococcus epidermidis* in terms of virulence.
- Discuss nursing interventions used to interrupt the sequence in the infection process.
- Discuss examples of how to prevent infection for each component in the chain of infection.

6. For the chain of infection, identify how each component contributes to infection and nursing interventions to prevent or control the spread of infection. ***(267-273)***

	Contribution to Infectious Process	Nursing Actions
a. Infectious agent		
b. Reservoir		
c. Exit route		
d. Method of transmission		
e. Entrance		
f. Host		

7. Identify the five major classifications of pathogens and one example of a microorganism for each. ***(268-271)***

____

____

8. How do *S. aureus* and *S. epidermidis* differ from each other in terms of virulence? ***(269-270)***____________

____

____

9. Identify the normal body defense mechanisms and factors that may alter each. ***(274)***

   a. Skin: ______________________________

   ____

   b. Respiratory tract: ______________________________

   ____

   c. Gastrointestinal tract: ______________________________

   ____

10. The nurse recognizes that the best way to interfere with the transmission of microorganisms is ______________________. ***(277-278)***

Multiple Choice

11. The patient has a large midline abdominal incision. With the specific purpose of reducing a possible reservoir of infection, the nurse: ***(271)***
    1. wears gloves and mask at all times.
    2. isolates the patient's personal articles.
    3. has the patient cover the mouth and nose when coughing.
    4. changes the dressing when it becomes soiled.

HEALTH CARE–ASSOCIATED INFECTION

Objective

- Explain conditions that promote the onset of health care–associated infections.

12. Describe a health care–associated infection, and identify conditions that may lead to its development. ***(274-275)***

    ____

    ____

INFECTION CONTROL

Objectives

- Demonstrate the appropriate procedure for 2-minute hand hygiene.
- Discuss the recommended guidelines of isolation precautions for the health care facility, referred to as standard precautions.
- Demonstrate technique for gowning and gloving.
- Demonstrate the procedure for double-bagging contaminated articles.
- Correctly don and remove sterile gloves using the open technique.
- Describe the accepted techniques of preparation for disinfection and sterilization.
- Discuss health promotion in patient teaching for infection control.

13. Identify at least five miscellaneous guidelines for standard precautions. ***(276-277)*** ________________

____

____

14. Discuss at least four areas for patient teaching to prevent the spread of infection in the home environment. ***(304)***

____

____

15. You discover that your nursing colleague has an allergy to latex. What should you suggest? ***(291)***

____

____

16. You are observing the nursing assistant performing routine hand hygiene. Identify whether the following actions are appropriate or require more instruction. ***(278-279)***

    a. Hands are kept higher than the elbows.________________

    b. Faucets are turned off with a dry paper towel.________________

    c. Care is taken to wash around jewelry. ________________

17. What is the proper method for disposal of sharps? ***(272)***________________

____

____

18. For the following patients on isolation precautions, identify the type of room that should be selected. ***(286)***

    a. A patient with an active infectious disease:________________

    b. A patient with an immunosuppressive problem:________________

19. Identify the basic principles of isolation. ***(290)***________________

____

____

20. Identify the proper steps for donning and removing sterile gloves. ***(298-301)***________________

____

____

21. Describe the procedure for gowning for contact isolation. ***(283-284)*** ______________________

____

____

22. Articles from the patient's isolation room require double-bagging. Identify if the following actions by the nurse are appropriate or inappropriate. ***(284-285)***

    a. Bag is removed completely from the patient's room.______________________

    b. Contaminated bag is dropped into a second bag without touching the edges of the second bag.

    ____

    c. Gown, gloves, and mask are removed before double-bagging.______________________

23. Describe the steps for opening a wrapped sterile package. ***(295-296)*** ______________________

____

____

24. Explain how sterile solutions should be poured onto a sterile field. ***(295, 297)*** ______________________

____

____

25. Provide an example of a patient who would require the following precautions. ***(286)***

    a. Airborne precautions: ______________________

    b. Droplet precautions: ______________________

    c. Contact precautions: ______________________

26. Identify the major differences between routine hand hygiene and surgical handwashing. ***(280)***

____

____

27. Identify at least two specific considerations for the older adult patient regarding the infectious process. ***(273)***

____

____

28. Specify two possible nursing diagnoses for a patient who is susceptible to or affected by an infectious process. *(305)*

____

____

Multiple Choice

29. The nurse is preparing a room for a patient with herpes simplex virus. In particular, this type of precaution means that the care should include: *(286)*
    1. a private room with negative air flow.
    2. hand hygiene after filtration masks are removed.
    3. use of gloves and gown upon entering the room.
    4. use of a surgical mask on the patient during transfers.

30. The nurse is preparing a teaching plan for patients about rubella. The nurse informs them that this virus may be transmitted by: *(286)*
    1. mosquitoes.
    2. droplet nuclei.
    3. blood products.
    4. improperly handled food.

31. The nurse is working on a unit with a number of patients who have infectious diseases. One of the most important methods for reducing the spread of microorganisms is: *(277)*
    1. sterilization of equipment.
    2. the use of gloves and gowns.
    3. maintenance of isolation precautions.
    4. hand hygiene before and after patient care.

32. The assignment today for the nurse includes a patient with tuberculosis. In caring for a patient on airborne precautions, the nurse should routinely use: *(287)*
    1. regular masks and eyewear.
    2. gowns and gloves.
    3. surgical handwashing and gloves.
    4. particulate respirator masks and gowns.

33. The nurse is observing the new staff member who is preparing to do a sterile dressing. The nurse determines that the staff member requires correction and additional instruction if observed: *(293, 295-297)*
    1. opening the closest flap of the sterile wrapped package first.
    2. placing the cap of the sterile solution inside up on a clean surface.
    3. opening sterile items and dropping them directly onto the sterile field.
    4. maintaining a 1-inch border around the sterile drape.

34. The nurse is aware that the body has normal defenses against infection. An acidic environment is one defense mechanism that is characteristic of which of the body systems? (Select all that apply) *(274)*
    1. Respiratory system
    2. Gastrointestinal system
    3. Reproductive system
    4. Urinary system

Student Name________________________________ Date______________

chapter 13

Surgical Wound Care

Answer Key: Textbook page references are provided as a guide for answering these questions. A complete answer key was provided for your instructor.

ASSESSMENT

Objectives

- Discuss the body's response during each stage of wound healing.
- Discuss common complications of wound healing.
- Differentiate between healing by primary and secondary intention.

1. Provide an example for each of the following wound classifications. *(311)*

    a. Clean: ______________________________

    b. Clean-contaminated: ______________________________

    c. Contaminated: ______________________________

2. Describe the following aspects of the stages of wound healing. *(311)*

	Time Frame	Cellular/Tissue Activity
a. Inflammatory phase		
b. Reconstruction phase		
c. Maturation phase		

3. Describe the following types of wound healing. ***(311-312)***

   a. Primary: ______________________________

   b. Secondary: ______________________________

   c. Tertiary: ______________________________

4. Identify factors that may impair wound healing. ***(313)*** ______________________________

5. Describe the complications that may occur with wound healing and the nursing assessment and intervention for each. ***(313)***

   ____

6. The trend for care of a postoperative sutured clean wound is to: ***(314)*** ______________________________

WOUND CARE, SUPPORT, AND COMFORT MEASURES

Objectives

- Explain the procedure for applying sterile dry dressing and wet-to-dry dressings.
- Identify the procedure for removing sutures and staples.
- Discuss care of the patient with a wound drainage system such as Hemovac or Davol suction or T-tube drainage.
- Identify the procedure for performing sterile wound irrigation.
- Describe the purposes of and precautions taken when applying bandages and binders.
- List nursing diagnoses associated with impaired skin integrity.

7. What is the purpose of each of the following types of dressings? ***(315-316)***

   a. Gauze: ______________________________

   b. Semiocclusive: ______________________________

   c. Occlusive: ______________________________

8. For the following dressings, identify the type of wound that it can be used on. ***(316-321)***

   a. Dry dressing: ______________________________

   b. Wet-to-dry: ______________________________

   c. Transparent: ______________________________

9. You are observing a new staff member perform a sterile dry dressing change. How would you correct the following actions, if you observe them? ***(317-318)***

   a. The tape is loosened in a direction away from the incision. ______________________________

   ____

   ____

   b. Clean gloves are used to remove the old dressing. ______________________________

   ____

   ____

   c. The area surrounding the incision is cleansed, and then the incision is cleansed using a back-and-forth stroking motion.

   ____

   ____

   d. Montgomery straps are used. ______________________________

   ____

   ____

10. The new staff member proceeds to do a wet-to-dry dressing change. How would you correct the following actions, if you observe them? ***(319-320)***

    a. The old dressing is moistened for easy removal. ______________________________

    ____

    ____

    b. The new dressing is left dripping wet. ______________________________

    ____

    ____

c. The deep wound is packed using forceps.____________________

d. A dry dressing is applied over the wet gauze. ____________________

11. The nurse is preparing to implement wound irrigations. ***(321-323)***

a. The purpose of wound irrigation is:____________________

b. The equipment needed for irrigation includes:____________________

c. The position of a syringe for irrigation is: ____________________

d. The direction of cleansing is: ____________________

e. A hand-held shower is positioned:____________________

12. The nurse is assessing the amount of drainage that the patient has from a surgical wound and finds that 650 mL has drained from 9:00 AM until now, 11:40 PM. What should the nurse do? ***(327)***

13. The patient has a T-tube in place following an abdominal cholecystectomy. The nurse anticipates that the expected output of bile will be ____________________. ***(329-330)***

14. Discuss the specific interventions for irrigating a deep wound. ***(322-323)*** ____________________

15. For staple or suture removal, indicate the correct options. *(324-325)*
    a. Sterile or clean procedure? _____
    b. All of the staples are removed at once? _____
    c. Steri-Strips are applied to the site? _____
    d. Intermittent sutures are snipped at skin level away from the knots? _____

16. Identify two nursing diagnoses and patient outcomes associated with wound healing. *(338-340)*________

17. What is the difference between a Penrose drain and a Hemovac or Jackson-Pratt drainage system? *(328-329)*

18. What nursing assessment and patient teaching are necessary for a patient with a wound drainage system? *(328-329)*

19. Identify at least three home care considerations for wound care. *(339)*________

20. The patient has a wound vacuum-assisted closure. Describe the correct options for the following aspects of this system. *(330-333)*
    a. Type of foam used: ________
    b. Periwound skin care:________
    c. Maintenance of occlusive seal:________
    d. Pressure range or average pressure: ________
    e. The alarm sounds when:________
    f. A leak is present if the nurse:________

21. Before a bandage or binder is applied, what should the nurse assess? *(334)* ________

22. Identify at least five guidelines for bandage and binder application. ***(337)***________________________

____

____

23. Identify the type of bandage turns that should be used for the following body areas. ***(336)***

    a. Finger or wrist:____

    b. Calf or thigh:____

    c. Joints:____

    d. Scalp:____

24. The patient is to have an abdominal binder applied. What is an important consideration for the nurse when implementing this application? ***(335)***

____

____

Multiple Choice

25. A binder is used for a patient to: ***(334)***
    1. reduce ventilatory capacity.
    2. assist in ambulation.
    3. increase circulatory stasis.
    4. provide support.

26. The nurse is preparing to remove the patient's staples. Upon assessment, the nurse determines that the staples should not be removed because: ***(325)***
    1. the wound edges are separated.
    2. there is no drainage from the incision.
    3. the patient is anxious about their removal.
    4. a negative cosmetic result could occur.

27. The nurse is preparing to change the patient's dry sterile dressing. Upon attempting the removal of the old dressing, it is found to be adhered to the site. The nurse should: ***(316)***
    1. notify the physician.
    2. leave the dressing in place.
    3. pull the dressing off quickly.
    4. moisten the dressing with saline.

28. The nurse notes that the patient's abdominal surgery dressing is saturated with red, watery drainage. The best description of this exudate is: ***(314)***
    1. serous.
    2. purulent.
    3. serosanguineous.
    4. sanguineous.

29. A postoperative patient after total abdominal hysterectomy develops a wound evisceration. The nurse's first response is: ***(324)***
    1. notify the physician.
    2. make the patient NPO (nothing-by-mouth status).
    3. place the patient in a low Fowler's position with the knees flexed.
    4. cover the wound with a dressing moistened with saline.

30. If, during the postoperative period, a patient develops internal abdominal bleeding that progresses to hypovolemic shock, the signs and symptoms the nurse would expect to see include: (Select all that apply) ***(324)***
    1. a drop in blood pressure.
    2. an increased pulse rate.
    3. an increase in urinary output.
    4. the abdomen becoming rigid and distended.

Student Name____ **Date**__________________

Safety

chapter **14**

Answer Key: Textbook page references are provided as a guide for answering these questions. A complete answer key was provided for your instructor.

TERMS

Objective

- Define the key terms as listed.

1. Define or describe the following.

   a. Disaster situation: ***(346)*** ____

   ____

   b. Hazard Communication Act: ***(357)*** __________________________________

   ____

   c. RACE: ***(359)*** ____

   ____

   d. Safety reminder device (SRD): ***(361)*** _______________________________

   ____

   e. Bioterrorism: ***(363)*** ____

   ____

ENVIRONMENT

Objective

- Discuss necessary modifications of the hospital environment for the left-handed patient.

2. The patient who has just been admitted to the unit is left-handed. What special instructions will you provide to the nursing assistant for modification of the patient's environment? ***(354)***

PROMOTION OF SAFETY

Objectives

- Relate the Occupational Safety Health Administration's (OSHA's) guidelines for violence protection programs to the workplace.
- Summarize safety precautions that can be implemented to prevent falls.

3. Identify at least five risk factors for work-related violence in the health care agency and three ways in which the nurse can be involved in violence prevention. ***(356)***

4. A patient in the long-term care facility has a history of falls in the home. Identify nursing interventions that may be implemented to prevent falls while the patient resides in the facility. ***(344-345)***

5. The patient is using an older thermometer at home that contains mercury. The thermometer is dropped and breaks, releasing mercury onto the floor. A priority nursing action with a mercury spill is to: ***(355)***

6. For the nursing diagnosis *risk for injury/falls,* identify a patient outcome and three nursing interventions. ***(365-366)***

Multiple Choice

7. An older adult patient in the extended care facility has been wandering around outside of the room during the late evening hours. The patient has a history of falls. The nurse intervenes by: ***(344-345)***
   1. obtaining an order for a bed and chair alarm.
   2. keeping the light on and the television playing all night.
   3. reassigning the patient to a room close to the nurse's station.
   4. having the family members come and check on the patient during the night.

SPECIFIC SAFETY CONCERNS

Objectives

- Relate specific safety considerations to the developmental age and the needs of individuals across the life span.
- Identify nursing interventions that are appropriate for individuals across the life span to ensure a safe environment.
- Identify safety concerns specific to the health care environment.

8. For the following age groups, identify a specific safety concern and a nursing intervention to prevent injury. *(345-346)*

	Safety Concern	Nursing Intervention
a. Infant		
b. Toddler		
c. Older adult		

9. Identify basic precautions that may be implemented by the nurse to promote overall safety in the health care environment. *(344)*

____

____

10. Describe how the nurse can promote safe ambulation for the patient in a health care facility. *(344-345)*

____

____

11. Identify three additional factors that influence the safety of the older adult in the home or health care environment. ***(346)***

____

____

12. What are some of the safety risks to the nurse working within the health care environment? ***(355-357)***

____

____

Multiple Choice

13. A male patient of average body build resides in the extended care facility and requires assistance to ambulate down the hall. The nurse has noticed that the patient has some weakness on the left side. The nurse assists this patient to ambulate by standing at his: ***(344-345)***
    1. left side and holding his arm.
    2. right side and holding his arm.
    3. left side and holding one arm around his waist.
    4. right side and holding one arm around his waist.

SAFETY REMINDER DEVICES

Objectives

- Describe safe and appropriate methods for the application of safety reminder devices.
- Discuss nursing interventions that are specific to the patient requiring a safety reminder device.
- Detail measures to create a restraint-free environment.

14. Identify the related principles for the application and the maintenance of safety reminder devices. ***(346-353)***

    a. Medical orders: ______________________________

    ____

    b. Patient assessment: ______________________________

    ____

    c. Maintenance of skin integrity and circulation: ____________________

    ____

    d. Documentation: ______________________________

    ____

15. Describe how the nurse may implement a restraint-free environment for a patient. *(347)*______________

____

____

Multiple Choice

16. The patient is newly admitted to the extended care facility and appears to be disoriented. There is a concern for the patient's immediate safety. The nurse is considering the use of a safety reminder device to prevent an injury. When using an SRD the nurse should: (Select all that apply) *(346-353)*
    1. obtain a physician's order.
    2. explain purpose of the SRD to the patient.
    3. explain the purpose of the SRD to the family.
    4. be sure that all of the nursing staff agree that the SRD is necessary.

FIRE SAFETY

Objective

- Cite the steps to be followed in the event of a fire.

17. In the event of a fire in a health care agency, the nurse's top priority is: ____________________ *(358)*

18. The nurse is planning to teach a community group about fire safety in the home. What information should be included in the presentation? *(360)*

____

____

19. There is a fire in the health care agency. Identify the nursing interventions for the following individuals. *(357-358)*

    a. A patient who is close to the area of the fire but is unable to ambulate: ____________________

    ____

    b. Visitors who have gone over to use the elevators: ______________________________

    ____

    c. A patient who has oxygen in use: ____

    ____

20. For the following fires, identify the extinguisher that should be used. ***(359)***

    a. Paper in a wastebasket: ____________________

    b. A liquid anesthetic: ____________________

    c. An electric intravenous (IV) infusion pump: ____________________

Multiple Choice

21. While walking through the hallway in the hospital, the nurse notices smoke coming from the wastebasket in the patient's room. Upon entering the room, the nurse finds that there is a fire that is starting to flare up. The nurse should first: ***(358)***
    1. extinguish the fire.
    2. remove the patient from the room.
    3. contain the fire by closing the door to the room.
    4. turn off all of the surrounding electrical equipment.

DISASTER PLANNING

Objective

- Discuss the role of the nurse in disaster planning.
- Discuss high-risk syndromes of bioterrorism.

22. Explain the difference in focus between an internal and an external disaster. ***(361)*** ____________________

____

____

23. What is the role of the nurse in disaster planning? ***(361-362)*** ____________________

____

____

24. Indications that alert the nurse to a possible bioterrorism-related outbreak include: ***(363)*** ____________________

____

____

25. A role of the nurse during a bioterrorist attack is to: ***(363-364)*** ____________________

____

____

26. Identify the signs and symptoms associated with acute radiation syndrome. ***(355)***

    a. Hematopoietic: ______

    b. Gastrointestinal: ______

    c. Cerebrovascular and/or central nervous system: ______

Multiple Choice

27. It is suspected that a patient has been exposed to cyanide gas. The nurse is alert to the presence of which one of the following indications? ***(364-365)***
    1. Erratic behavior
    2. Nausea and vomiting
    3. Respiratory distress
    4. Vesicle formation

ACCIDENTAL POISONING

Objective

- Describe nursing interventions in the event of accidental poisoning.

28. Identify the specific risks for and prevention of accidental poisoning for each group. ***(360-361)***

	Risks	Preventive Measures
a. Children		
b. Older adults		

29. A patient is suspected of having ingested a poisonous substance. The nurse should: ______________________________ ______________________________ ***(360-361)***

Multiple Choice

30. A mother calls the poison control center after a child has ingested a bottle of baby aspirin. The mother should be instructed to: ***(360-361)***
    1. identify the amount of substance ingested.
    2. give the age-appropriate amount of syrup of ipecac.
    3. position the child, lying down, with the head tilted back.
    4. drive the child herself to the nearest emergency department.

31. During a type IV hypersensitivity allergic reaction to latex, the signs and symptoms that nurse would expect the patient to exhibit include: (Select all that apply) ***(354)***
    1. hives.
    2. generalized edema.
    3. difficulty breathing.
    4. skin redness and itching.

Student Name____ **Date**____________________

Body Mechanics and Patient Mobility

chapter **15**

Answer Key: Textbook page references are provided as a guide for answering these questions. A complete answer key was provided for your instructor.

BODY MECHANICS

Objectives

- State the principles of body mechanics.
- Explain the rationale for using appropriate body mechanics.

1. Identify four principles of body mechanics for health care workers and the rationale for each one. *(370-371)*

____

____

2. The nurse is observing a colleague performing patient care. Identify whether the following techniques are appropriate or inappropriate body mechanics. *(370-372)*

    a. Facing away from the work: ______________________________

    b. Positioning the feet 6 to 8 inches apart: ________________________

    c. Keeping the knees straight: ______________________________

    d. Keeping the head down:________________________________

    e. Sliding heavy objects: ________________________________

    f. Relaxing the abdominal muscles: ___________________________

POSITIONING

Objective

- Demonstrate execution of Fowler's, supine (dorsal), Sims', side-lying, prone, dorsal recumbent, and lithotomy positions.

3. For the following patient positions, identify the position of the bed and the equipment needed and its placement for patient alignment. *(372-375)*

	Bed Position	Equipment and Placement for Patient Support
a. Fowler's		
b. Supine		
c. Sims'		
d. Side-lying		
e. Prone		
f. Dorsal recumbent		
g. Lithotomy		

4. What is the rationale for the use of the following devices? *(377)*

   a. Hand rolls: ____________________

   ____

   b. Foot boots: ____________________

   ____

   c. Side rails: ____________________

   ____

   d. Wedge pillows: ____________________

   ____

RANGE OF MOTION

Objective

- Explain range-of-motion (ROM) exercises.

5. Identify the purpose, as well as the principles related to performance, of range-of-motion exercises. *(378-379)*

   ____

   ____

6. Describe the range-of-motion exercises that are performed with the following body areas. *(380-381)*

   a. Knee: ____________________

   ____

   b. Hip: ____________________

   ____

   c. Wrist: ____________________

   ____

MOVING PATIENTS

Objective

- Relate appropriate body mechanics to the techniques for turning, moving, lifting, and carrying the patient.

7. Before turning or transferring patients, what patient assessment and preparations should be made? ***(387)***

____

____

8. For the following situations, identify the appropriate nursing intervention. ***(382-387)***

   a. A patient who is going to ambulate after not being out of bed for a while: _______________

   ____

   b. A patient who is in bed and has a serious head and neck condition needs to be turned: _______________

   ____

   c. A patient with left-sided weakness is to move from the bed to a chair: _______________

   ____

Multiple Choice

9. The nurse is working with a patient who is only able to minimally assist the nurse in moving from the bed to the chair. The nurse needs to help the patient up. The correct technique for lifting the patient to stand and pivot to the chair is to: ***(384-386)***
   1. keep the legs slightly bent.
   2. maintain a narrow base with the feet.
   3. keep the stomach muscles loose.
   4. support the patient away from the body.

10. The patient has had a surgical procedure and is getting up to ambulate for the first time. While ambulating down the hallway, the patient complains of severe dizziness. The nurse should first: ***(376)***
    1. call for help.
    2. lower the patient gently to the floor.
    3. lean the patient against the wall until the episode passes.
    4. support the patient and move quickly back to the room.

IMMOBILITY

Objectives

- Discuss the complications of immobility.
- State the nursing interventions to prevent complications of immobility.
- Identify complications caused by inactivity.

11. Identify the complications of immobility and nursing interventions that may be implemented to prevent their occurrence. *(376)*

____

____

12. For the following situations, identify the nursing intervention. *(376-377)*

    a. The patient develops a reddened area on the sacrum.____________________

    ____

    b. While transferring the patient from the bed to a chair, the patient starts to fall.____________

    ____

    c. The patient with right-sided weakness following a cerebrovascular accident (CVA or stroke) is unable to perform range of motion of the right extremities.

    ____

13. The patient has a cast on the lower left leg. Upon completion of a neurovascular assessment, the nurse believes that the patient may be experiencing compartment syndrome as a result of finding ____________________. *(377-378)*

14. Identify a nursing diagnosis for a patient who has had a CVA with resulting right-sided paresis. *(389-390)*

____

____

Multiple Choice

15. It is known that the patient will be immobilized for an extended period. The nurse recognizes that there is a need to prevent respiratory complications and intervenes by: *(376)*
    1. suctioning the airway every hour.
    2. changing the patient's position every 4 to 8 hours.
    3. using oxygen and nebulizer treatments regularly.
    4. encouraging deep breathing and coughing every hour.

16. Patients who are immobilized in health care facilities require that their psychosocial needs be met along with their physiological needs. The nurse recognizes these needs when telling the patient: *(376)*
    1. "Visiting hours will be limited so you can rest."
    2. "We will help you do everything so you don't have to worry."
    3. "Let's talk about what you used to do at home during the day."
    4. "A private room can be arranged for you."

17. The patient experienced a CVA (stroke) that left her with severe left-sided paralysis and very limited mobility. To prevent prolonged dorsiflexion, the nurse uses a: ***(377)***
    1. foot boot.
    2. bed board.
    3. trapeze bar.
    4. trochanter roll.

18. When assessing the neurovascular status of a patient, an expected finding is: ***(377-378)***
    1. capillary refill after 8 seconds.
    2. pulses strong and easily palpated.
    3. loss of sensation peripheral to an affected area.
    4. localized discomfort.

19. The ROM that can be safely performed on the neck includes: (Select all that apply) ***(379)***
    1. flexion.
    2. supination.
    3. lateral flexion.
    4. rotation.

20. A contracture is defined as: ***(376-377)***
    1. abnormal extension and fixation of a joint.
    2. abnormal flexion and fixation of a joint.
    3. abnormal hyperextension of a joint.
    4. abnormal lateral movements of a joint.

21. When moving or transferring older adults, it is important to avoid pulling them across bed linens because this puts them at risk for: ***(383)***
    1. dislocation of a joint.
    2. increased stress to the joints.
    3. abnormal hyperextension of a joint.
    4. shearing or tearing of the skin.

Student Name________________________ Date____________

chapter 16

Pain Management, Comfort, Rest, and Sleep

Answer Key: Textbook page references are provided as a guide for answering these questions. A complete answer key was provided for your instructor.

TERMS

Objective

- Define the key terms listed.

1. Define or describe the following.

   a. Endorphin: ***(396)*** ________________________________

   ____

   b. Gate control theory: ***(396)*** ________________________________

   ____

   c. Noxious: ***(395)*** ________________________________

   ____

   d. Patient-controlled analgesia (PCA): ***(402)*** ________________________________

   ____

   e. Transcutaneous electrical nerve stimulation (TENS): ***(398)*** ________________________________

   ____

COMFORT AND DISCOMFORT

Objective

- List 10 possible causes of discomfort.

2. Identify at least 10 different causes of discomfort that the nurse should be aware of for the patient in the health care or the home environment. *(394)*

DESCRIPTIONS AND THEORIES OF PAIN

Objectives

- Explain McCaffery's description of pain.
- Explain the implications of the gate control theory on the selection of nursing interventions for pain relief.
- Discuss the synergistic relationship of fatigue, sleep disturbance, and depression with perception of pain.

3. McCaffery's description of pain is: *(395)*

4. Using the gate control theory of pain, identify the most effective types of nursing interventions. *(396)*

5. Identify how the patient's perception of pain is influenced by factors such as fatigue, sleep disturbance, and depression. *(395)*

ASSESSMENT OF PAIN

Objectives

- Identify subjective and objective data in pain assessment.
- Discuss the concept of making pain assessment the fifth vital sign.
- Explain several scales used to identify intensity of pain.

6. What is the difference between acute and chronic pain? ***(396)*** ______

7. Identify at least five objective signs that the patient is experiencing pain. ***(408)*** ______

8. What different types of pain intensity scales are used to assess a pain for adults and children? ***(406-407)***

9. What subjective data may the nurse obtain from the patient regarding his or her pain experience? ***(405)***

10. What is the rationale for making pain assessment the fifth vital sign? ***(397)*** ______

11. Identify examples of cultural and ethnic considerations for pain assessment and management. ***(407)***

12. The patient has identified to the nurse that she is experiencing pain. What should the nurse do to fully assess the patient's pain? ***(405-408)***

PAIN THERAPY

Objectives

- Discuss pain mechanisms affected by each analgesic group.
- List six methods for pain control.

13. a. Management of pain is required by the ______________________ (organization). ***(397)***

    b. Identify three of the key concepts included in the standards that are applied to health care facilities. ***(397)***

    ____

    ____

14. Identify at least five guidelines for individualizing pain therapy. ***(408-409)*** ______________________

    ____

    ____

15. Provide two examples of noninvasive pain relief measures. ***(399)*** ______________________

    ____

    ____

16. For the following drug classifications, identify an example of a specific medication and how the drug affects the pain mechanism. ***(399-401)***

	Drug Example	Pain Relief Mechanism
a. Nonopioids		
b. Opioids		
c. Adjuvant medication		

Multiple Choice

17. The patient had a surgical procedure this morning and is requesting pain medication. The nurse assesses the patient's vital signs and decides to withhold the medication based on the finding of: ***(400)***
    1. pulse = 90/min.
    2. respirations = 8/min.
    3. blood pressure = 130/80 mm Hg.
    4. temperature = 99° F rectally.

18. The visiting nurse is working with a patient who has arthritis. The patient has no known allergies to any medications, so the nurse anticipates that the physician will prescribe: ***(399)***
    1. propoxyphene (Darvon).
    2. diphenhydramine (Benadryl).
    3. ibuprofen (Motrin).
    4. morphine (MS Contin).

NURSING INTERVENTION IN PAIN MANAGEMENT

Objectives

- Discuss the responsibilities of the nurse in pain control.
- Identify nursing interventions to control painful stimuli in the patient's environment.

19. What problem(s) can occur if the nurse does not respond to and treat the patient's pain? ***(395)***__________

____

____

20. What is the role of the nurse in the administration of epidural analgesia? ***(403)*** ____________________

____

____

21. Identify nursing interventions that may be implemented to reduce or eliminate the patient's pain. ***(408)***

____

____

22. Several patients on the medical unit are experiencing varying degrees of discomfort. What criteria are used to determine whether the patient is a candidate for PCA? ***(402-403)***

____

____

23. The nurse wishes to intervene and reduce the discomfort experienced by an older adult patient. What special considerations for pain control does the nurse have to make for a patient in this age group? ***(400)***

____

____

Multiple Choice

24. The patient is receiving epidural analgesia. The nurse is alert for a complication of this treatment and observes the patient for: ***(403)***
    1. diarrhea.
    2. hypertension.
    3. urinary retention.
    4. an increased respiratory rate.

SLEEP AND REST

Objectives

- Describe the differences and similarities between sleep and rest.
- Discuss the sleep cycle, differentiating between non–rapid eye movement (NREM) and rapid eye movement (REM) sleep.

25. Compare and contrast sleep and rest. ***(409)*** ______________________________

____

____

26. Identify and briefly describe the usual phases and stages of the sleep cycle. ***(411)*** ______________

____

____

NURSING ASSESSMENT

Objectives

- List six signs and symptoms of sleep deprivation.
- Identify two nursing diagnoses related to sleep problems.

27. The nurse suspects that a patient is experiencing sleep deprivation when observing the following signs and symptoms: ***(411-412)***

____

____

28. Identify at least two nursing diagnoses related to sleep problems. ***(413)***______________________

____

____

29. For each of the following factors, identify how sleep may be affected and why. ***(410)***

	Effect on Sleep	Reason
a. Physical illness		
b. Anxiety		
c. Drugs		
d. Environment		
e. Nutrition		
f. Exercise		

NURSING INTERVENTIONS

Objective

- Outline nursing interventions that promote rest and sleep.

30. The patient is experiencing difficulty sleeping while in the hospital. Identify nursing interventions that may be implemented to promote sleep. ***(412)***

___

___

Multiple Choice

31. The nurse enters the patient's room at 3:00 AM and finds that the patient is awake and sitting up in a chair. The patient tells the nurse that she is not able to sleep. The nurse should first: ***(412)***
    1. obtain an order for a hypnotic.
    2. instruct the patient to return to bed.
    3. provide a glass of warm milk with honey.
    4. ask about ways that have helped her to sleep before.

32. An older adult patient diagnosed with osteoarthritis suffers from chronic pain. Based on the patient's age, which pain medications will the physician most likely avoid? (Select all that apply) ***(401)***
    1. Meperidine
    2. Acetaminophen
    3. Morphine sulfate
    4. Nonsteroidal antiinflammatory drugs

Student Name____ **Date**__________________

Complementary and Alternative Therapies

chapter **17**

Answer Key: Textbook page references are provided as a guide for answering these questions. A complete answer key was provided for your instructor.

TERMS

Objective

- Define the key terms listed.

1. Define or describe the following.

   a. Imagery: ***(426)***____

   ____

   b. Meridians: ***(423)*** ______________________________________

   ____

   c. Qi: ***(423)***____

   ____

TYPES OF THERAPIES

Objectives

- Differentiate between complementary and alternative therapies and allopathic (conventional) medicine.
- Describe how herbs differ from pharmaceuticals.
- Explain the scope of practice of chiropractic therapy.
- Describe the principles behind acupuncture and acupressure.
- Explain the difference between acupuncture and acupressure.
- Explain how essential oils may be used to provide aromatherapy.
- Discuss the therapeutic results of yoga.
- Explain the theory of reflexology.
- Describe the possible benefits of magnetic therapy.
- Discuss animal-assisted therapy.
- Describe safe and unsafe herbal therapies.
- Describe the health benefits of t'ai chi.

2. It is estimated that __________% of the population in the United States uses one or more forms of complementary and alternative therapy. ***(416)***

3. What are some of the general benefits for the use of complementary and alternative therapies? ***(416-417)***

4. How do herbs differ from pharmaceutical agents? ***(418)***

5. What are some of the positive and negative aspects of herbal therapy? ***(418)***

6. Identify at least two commonly taken herbs and their uses. ***(419-420)***

7. The patient asks the nurse what the chiropractic doctor will do for him. Describe the role of the chiropractic physician as you would to the patient. ***(423)***

8. What is the difference between acupuncture and acupressure? What are the principles underlying these therapies? ***(423-424)***

9. Identify two essential oils used in aromatherapy and their uses. ***(422)***

10. The principle behind reflexology is: ***(424-425)***

11. The patient asks the nurse if "those magnets they sell in the store are really any good?" The nurse responds by telling the patient that magnetic therapy is thought to: ***(426)***

____

____

12. What are the benefits of the use of imagery? ***(426)*** ______________________

____

____

13. The patient is preparing to take a yoga class because she has heard that the positive effects include: ***(428)***

____

____

14. A positive outcome of animal-assisted therapy is: ***(427-428)*** ______________________

____

____

15. How can older adults benefit from t'ai chi? ***(428-429)*** ______________________

____

____

NURSING ASSESSMENT AND INTERVENTIONS

Objectives

- Explain why a thorough health history is important for a patient using complementary and alternative therapies.
- List three conditions when therapeutic massage may be contraindicated.

16. The nurse is obtaining a patient's health history. What should the nurse ask the patient about in regard to complementary and alternative therapies, and why is it important to ask? ***(417-418)***

____

____

17. The patient is asking about including complementary and/or alternative therapies in the treatment regimen. What information should the nurse include in teaching this patient? ***(421)***

18. The nurse is preparing the patient for a therapeutic massage. How should the environment be prepared? ***(424)***

19. What assessment findings by the nurse will contraindicate the use of a therapeutic massage? ***(424)***

20. When is reflexology used with caution or contraindicated for the patient? ***(424-425)***

21. Patients with the following health problems should be instructed to avoid the use of magnets: ***(426)***

22. The nurse is preparing to demonstrate relaxation techniques to the patient. What types of behaviors will the nurse be teaching? ***(426-427)***

23. What is the role of the nurse in the use of complementary and alternative therapies? ***(429-431)***

24. Identify two cultural considerations that arise in relation to complementary and alternative therapies. ***(431)***

Multiple Choice

25. The patient has a history of congestive heart failure and receives a prescription for digoxin. The nurse cautions the patient against the use of which of the following herbs? ***(419-420)***
    1. Evening primrose oil (*Oenothera biennis*)
    2. Goldenseal (*Hydrastis canadensis*)
    3. St. John's wort (*Hypericum perforatum*)
    4. Kava (*Kava-Kava*)

26. A pregnant patient in the maternal/child clinic asks the nurse if there are herbs that are safe to take during the pregnancy. The nurse responds accurately by telling the patient that the following herb has shown no definitive problems for pregnant women: ***(419-420)***
    1. Ginger (*Ginkgo biloba*)
    2. Asian ginseng (*Panax ginseng*)
    3. Echinacea (*Echinacea pallida*)
    4. Chamomile

27. The patient asks why her physician prefers to prescribe medications for her hypertension rather than treating her with only herbal preparations. The most likely reason the physician has made this decision is: ***(418-420)***
    1. physicians receive a bonus for the number of prescriptions written.
    2. patients tend to be more compliant when taking prescription medications.
    3. prescription medications are less expensive than herbal preparations.
    4. herbal preparations are not subject to the same testing and manufacturing regulations as pharmaceuticals.

Student Name________________________ Date____________

Hygiene and Care of the Patient's Environment

chapter 18

Answer Key: Textbook page references are provided as a guide for answering these questions. A complete answer key was provided for your instructor.

ENVIRONMENT

Objective

- Discuss the therapeutic hospital room environment.

1. What does the nurse need to do to prepare a therapeutic hospital room environment? ***(436-437)*** ________

2. What is the recommended room temperature for an adult patient? What should the nurse keep in mind regarding the room temperature for infants and older adults? ***(436)***

HYGIENIC CARE

Objectives

- Describe personal hygienic practices.
- Discuss variations of the bath procedure determined by the patient's condition and physician's orders.
- Perform the procedure for the bed bath.
- Perform the procedures for oral hygiene; shaving; hair care; nail care; and eye, ear, and nose care.
- Perform the procedure for perineal care for the male patient and the female patient.
- Perform the procedure for the back rub.

3. Describe the usual daily hygienic care schedule. ***(435)***________

4. What factors influence a patient's personal hygiene? ***(435)*** ______

______

______

5. For the following patients, identify how bathing may be affected or altered. ***(435, 438)***

   a. The patient is extremely fatigued. ______

   ______

   b. The patient is on complete bed rest. ______

   ______

   c. The patient has right-sided paralysis following a cerebrovascular accident (CVA, or stroke). ______

   ______

   d. There is inflammation of the perianal tissue. ______

   ______

   e. The patient is an East Indian Hindu. ______

   ______

   f. The patient is an older adult who is incontinent. ______

   ______

6. Supply examples of nursing actions to achieve the following while giving a bed bath. ***(440-448)***

   a. Provision of privacy and patient dignity: ______

   ______

   b. Promotion of warmth: ______

   ______

   c. Reduction in the spread of microorganisms: ______

   ______

7. In preparing to perform a back rub, the nurse will begin at the patient's ______. The types of strokes to use are ______. ***(447-448)***

8. Oral hygiene for the unconscious patient includes: ***(453-454)*** ______

______

______

9. When is shaving the patient with a straight (blade) razor contraindicated? ***(455)*** ______________________

____

____

10. What equipment is needed to provide hair care for the bed-bound patient? ***(455-456)*** ______________

____

____

11. Describe what information is included in a teaching plan on foot care for a patient newly diagnosed with diabetes mellitus. ***(470)***

____

____

12. The nurse is evaluating the eye care that has been delegated to and is being provided by a new staff member. Identify whether the following actions are appropriate or inappropriate. ***(460-461)***

    a. Removing dried secretions with a dampened cotton ball or gauze: ______________________

    ____

    b. Using soap and water on a washcloth: ______________________________

    ____

    c. Cleansing the eyes from the outer to the inner canthus: ______________________

    ____

    d. Washing plastic eyeglass lenses with a special cleaning solution: ________________

    ____

13. The nurse observes the patient performing the following ear care. Identify which behaviors are incorrect and indicate that teaching is necessary. ***(461)***

    a. Cleaning the internal auditory canal with a cotton-tipped swab: ________________

    b. Leaving the hearing aid turned off when not in use: ______________________

14. What aspects of hygienic care should not be delegated to assistive personnel? ***(439)*** ______________

____

____

15. Describe what should be included in teaching care of the nose. ***(461)*** ______________________

____

____

16. When providing perineal care, provide examples of nursing actions to achieve the following. ***(457-460)***

 a. Promotion of privacy and minimal embarrassment: ______________________

 ____

 b. Facilitating the performance of the procedure: ______________________

 ____

 c. Preventing the spread of microorganisms for the male and female patient: ______________________

 ____

17. What patient assessment is completed by the nurse just before performing perineal care? ***(458)*** ______________________

____

____

Multiple Choice

18. The patient in the hospital requires foot care. The nurse should include in the care provided: ***(457)***
 1. cutting away corns and calluses.
 2. filing toenails straight across.
 3. instructing the patient to wear loose shoes.
 4. using alcohol for dryness between the toes.

19. The nurse is caring for an older adult patient in the extended care facility. The patient wears dentures, and the nurse will delegate the denture care to the nursing assistant. The nurse instructs the assistant that the patient's dentures should be: ***(454)***
 1. cleaned in hot water.
 2. left in place during the night.
 3. brushed with a soft toothbrush.
 4. wrapped in a soft towel when not worn.

20. The nurse is working out the patient assignment with the nursing assistant. In delegating the morning care for the patient, the nurse expects the assistant to: ***(439)***
 1. cut the tangles from the patient's hair.
 2. use soap to wash the patient's eyes.
 3. wash the patient's legs with long strokes from the ankle to the knee.
 4. place the unconscious patient in high Fowler's position to provide oral hygiene.

SKIN ASSESSMENT AND SPECIAL CARE

Objectives

- Discuss the procedures for skin care.
- Identify nursing interventions for the prevention and treatment of pressure ulcers.

21. Identify the stages of pressure ulcers. ***(449-450)***____________________

____

____

22. Identify possible risk factors for development of pressure ulcers. ***(448-449)***____________________

____

____

23. How can the nurse prevent the development of pressure ulcers? ***(448-449)***____________________

____

____

24. Identify general guidelines for care of pressure ulcers. ***(450)***____________________

____

____

Multiple Choice

25. The nurse determines, after completing the assessment, that an expected outcome for a patient with impaired skin integrity will be that the skin: ***(469-470)***
    1. remains dry.
    2. has increased erythema.
    3. tingles in areas of pressure.
    4. demonstrates increased diaphoresis.

26. While completing the bath, the nurse notices a reddened area on the patient's sacrum. The nurse should first: ***(469-470)***
    1. cleanse the skin with alcohol.
    2. wash the area with hot water and soap.
    3. massage the area vigorously.
    4. assess for any other areas of erythema.

BED MAKING

Objectives

- Perform the procedure for making the unoccupied bed.
- Perform the procedure for making the occupied bed.

27. How can the nurse make the bed as clean and comfortable as possible for the patient? ***(462-465)***________

____

____

28. What are the principles of medical asepsis as they relate to bed making? ***(465)***________

____

____

NURSING INTERVENTION TO ASSIST WITH ELIMINATION

Objective

- Discuss assisting the patient in the use of the bedpan, the urinal, and the bedside commode.

29. What equipment is necessary to assist the patient who is not able to use the bathroom facilities? ***(465-467)***

____

____

30. How can the nurse assist the patient with elimination? ***(466)*** ________

____

____

31. Identify whether the following characteristics of urine and stool are expected or unexpected. ***(466)***

    a. Pink-tinged urine: ________

    b. Urine negative for protein and ketone bodies: ________

    c. Clay-colored stool: ________

    d. Frequency of stool three times per day: ________

32. List at least two nursing diagnoses related to hygienic care. ***(469)*** ________________________________

____

____

Multiple Choice

33. Risk factors for skin impairment include: (Select all that apply) ***(448-449)***
    1. adequate hydration.
    2. incontinence.
    3. immobility.
    4. advanced age.

Student Name________________________________ Date________________

Specimen Collection and Diagnostic Examination

chapter **19**

Answer Key: Textbook page references are provided as a guide for answering these questions. A complete answer key was provided for your instructor.

PURPOSE AND GUIDELINES FOR SPECIMEN COLLECTION

Objectives

- Explain the rationales for collection of each specimen listed.
- Discuss guidelines for specimen collection.

1. Identify the rationale for the collection of specimens identified in the chapter. ***(479-517)*** ______________

____

____

2. Identify the general guidelines for specimen collection and diagnostic examinations. ***(478, 494)***________

____

____

NURSING ASSESSMENT AND INTERVENTIONS

Objectives

- Identify the role of the nurse when performing a procedure for specimen collection.
- Discuss patient teaching for diagnostic testing.
- Describe appropriate labeling for a collected specimen.
- Discuss the nursing interventions necessary for proper preparation of a patient having a diagnostic examination.
- List the diagnostic tests for which the nurse should determine whether the patient is allergic to iodine.

3. What are the general responsibilities of the nurse in specimen collection? ***(493-494)*** ________________

____

____

4. Describe the nursing responsibilities in the general preparation of the patient before diagnostic testing. ***(477)***

____

____

5. In addition to the interventions associated with specimen collection or preparation for a diagnostic examination, the nurse should also assess the patient for the following: ***(478)***

____

____

6. Identify considerations for the older adult in regard to specimen collection and diagnostic testing. ***(476)***

____

____

7. a. What procedures require that the patient be assessed for an allergy to iodine? ***(478)*** ____________

____

____

   b. If the patient does develop an allergic reaction to the dye used in a diagnostic test, what signs and symptoms will be observed? ***(478)***

____

____

   c. What is the treatment for this allergic reaction? ***(478)*** ____________

____

____

8. The nurse is performing a gastric secretion analysis. For this procedure, identify the following: ***(501-502)***
   a. Specimen is obtained by ____________.
   b. The amount of specimen to obtain for analysis is ____________.
   c. To perform the analysis, the nurse applies ____________ to the slide.
   d. A positive monitor is indicated by ____________.
   e. A negative monitor is indicated by ____________.

9. Identify at least four diagnostic procedures that require the patient to remain on nothing-by-mouth status (NPO) beforehand. ***(479-493)***

____

____

10. Proper labeling of specimens requires the following: ***(499)*** ____________________

____

____

11. a. During a bronchoscopy, the most important observation is the patient's ____________________ ____________________. ***(481-482)***

    b. Following the bronchoscopy, the patient needs to be assessed for ____________________ ____________________. ***(481-482)***

12. For the following diagnostic tests, identify at least one preprocedural and one postprocedural nursing intervention that should be implemented. ***(479-493)***

	Preprocedure	**Postprocedure**
a. Arteriography		
b. Barium enema		
c. Bone scan		
d. Cardiac catheterization		
e. Colonoscopy		
f. Glucose tolerance		
g. Intravenous pyelogram		
h. Liver biopsy		
i. Lumbar puncture		
j. Magnetic resonance imaging		
k. Paracentesis		
l. Ultrasound		

13. Of the following specimen collections, which ones are usually possible to delegate to assistive personnel? ***(516)***
    a. Urine and stool _____
    b. Gastric secretion analysis _____
    c. Venipuncture _____
    d. Sputum specimen by suctioning _____
    e. Blood glucose _____
    f. Wound cultures _____

Multiple Choice

14. The nurse is using a commercially prepared tube for the collection of an aerobic wound specimen for culture. After collecting the specimen with the swab, the nurse should: ***(502, 505)***
    1. place the swab into the collection tube, close it tightly, and keep the specimen warm until it is sent to the laboratory.
    2. take the swab and mix it with the special color-changing reagent in the collection tube.
    3. place the swab into the collection tube and add the liquid culture medium.
    4. crush the ampule at the end of the tube and put the tip of the swab into the solution.

15. Following a lumbar puncture, the patient tells the nurse that he has a headache. The nurse: ***(488-489)***
    1. reduces the patient's fluid intake.
    2. places the patient in low Fowler's position.
    3. informs the patient's physician immediately.
    4. instructs the patient to lie flat for up to 12 hours.

16. The patient is to have a thoracentesis performed. The nurse assists the patient to which position for this test? ***(492)***
    1. Dorsal recumbent
    2. Supine with the arms held above the head
    3. Sitting up and leaning over a table
    4. Side-lying with the knees drawn up

17. The physician has ordered a magnetic resonance imaging (MRI) study for the patient. The patient is concerned about the procedure and requests information from the nurse. The nurse informs the patient to expect: ***(489)***
    1. having nothing to eat or drink for 4 hours before the test.
    2. hearing humming and loud thumping sounds.
    3. minor discomfort to the area being tested.
    4. frequent position changes.

GLUCOSE TESTING

Objectives

- List the proper steps for teaching blood glucose self-monitoring.
- List the nursing responsibilities for the glucose tolerance test.

18. What information is necessary to include in the teaching plan for a newly diagnosed diabetic patient who needs to monitor blood glucose levels? ***(498)***

____

____

19. a. The patient is scheduled to have a glucose tolerance test. How will you explain this procedure and how to prepare for it to the patient? ***(486)***

____

____

b. What are the nurse's responsibilities during the glucose tolerance test? ***(486)*** _______________

____

____

Multiple Choice

20. The nurse is teaching the patient how to collect a specimen for blood glucose monitoring. The patient demonstrates correct technique when: ***(498)***
    1. using the center of the finger for the puncture.
    2. holding the finger upright after puncture.
    3. vigorously squeezing the fingertip after puncture.
    4. touching only the blood to the pad on the test strip.

URINE AND STOOL SPECIMENS

Objectives

- Discuss the procedure for obtaining stool specimens.
- List the proper steps when obtaining urine specimens.

21. What are the purposes of obtaining stool specimens? ***(499-500)*** _______________

____

____

22. How does urine specimen collection differ depending on the test to be done? ***(494-496)*** _______________

____

____

23. a. During a 24-hour urine collection, one of the patient's samples is accidentally discarded. What should the nurse do? ***(496-497)***

____

____

b. A positive patient outcome for this procedure is: ***(496-497)*** ________________

____

____

Multiple Choice

24. Instruction to the patient for collection of a midstream sample includes: ***(495)***
    1. use of a clean specimen cup.
    2. collection of 200 mL of urine for testing.
    3. voiding some urine first and then collecting the sample.
    4. washing the perineal area with Betadine before collection.

25. When obtaining a urine specimen from a patient with an indwelling catheter, the nurse should: ***(496)***
    1. apply sterile gloves for the procedure.
    2. clamp the drainage tubing for 30 minutes before specimen collection begins.
    3. disconnect the catheter from the drainage tubing and collect the urine in a specimen cup.
    4. insert a small-gauge needle directly into the catheter tubing to draw up the urine.

26. The patient will be catheterized for residual urine. Which of the following demonstrates correct technique for this procedure? ***(494)***
    1. Catheterize the patient when the bladder is full.
    2. Obtain an order for an indwelling catheter.
    3. Catheterize the patient within 10 minutes of voiding.
    4. Use clean technique to obtain the sample.

ADDITIONAL SPECIMEN COLLECTION

Objectives

- State the correct procedure for collecting a sputum specimen.
- Identify procedure for performing a phlebotomy.
- Identify procedure for performing the electrocardiogram.

27. The nurse is to perform an electrocardiogram (ECG). Explain the purpose of the test and describe the usual position of the patient and placement of the electrodes. ***(516-517)***

____

____

28. For the collection of a sputum specimen: ***(503-505)***

    a. Identify the steps of the procedure and the rationale for each step. ______________________________

    ____

    ____

    b. Specify what type of collection device or equipment is needed. ______________________________

    ____

    ____

29. Before performing a venipuncture, the nurse selects and assesses the site to be used. What criteria does the nurse use to determine that the site is acceptable? ***(509-510)***

    ____

    ____

30. How does the nurse apply aseptic technique during a venipuncture? ***(511-512)***______________________

    ____

    ____

31. The best time to collect a throat specimen is the following: ***(506)***______________________________

    ____

    ____

32. The specific procedure for determination of bacteremia is the following: ***(506-508)*** __________________

    ____

    ____

Multiple Choice

33. A risk factor to be considered when performing a venipuncture on a patient is: ***(507)***
    1. blood glucose level.
    2. platelet count.
    3. diuretic use.
    4. sex.

34. A tourniquet is used when performing a venipuncture. The nurse is aware that the tourniquet should be: ***(511)***
    1. tied into a knot.
    2. left in place no more than 1 to 2 minutes.
    3. placed 6 to 8 inches above the selected site.
    4. tight enough to occlude the distal pulse.

DOCUMENTATION

Objective

- Document the patient's condition before, during, and after a laboratory or diagnostic test.

35. After a procedure is completed, what general evaluations of patient status should the nurse perform? ***(476-478, 519)***

____

____

36. Give an example of how the nurse should document that a specimen has been obtained or a procedure completed. ***(477)***

____

____

Multiple Choice

37. The patient is suspected to have a urinary tract infection (UTI). The physician has ordered a urine specimen for culture and sensitivity testing. The patient asks the nurse, "What is the purpose of this test?" The nurse's best response is: ***(494)***
    1. "This is just a routine test for any patient suspected of having a UTI."
    2. "Your physician must feel that this test is necessary in determining your diagnosis."
    3. "It is best if you speak with your physician if you have questions regarding this test."
    4. "This test will determine the bacteria causing your UTI and the best antibiotic for your physician to prescribe to treat the infection."

38. When performing a Hemoccult slide test to determine the presence of occult blood in a stool specimen, the nurse would be correct in using which of the following interventions? (Select all that apply) ***(499-501)***
    1. Using two separate areas of the stool when obtaining the specimen
    2. Obtaining the specimen from the toilet bowl
    3. Performing the test control on the slide immediately after performing the test on the specimen obtained
    4. Documenting a positive result if a blue color appears on or at the edge of the smear after the developer as been applied

Student Name________________________________ Date______________

Selected Nursing Skills

chapter **20**

Answer Key: Textbook page references are provided as a guide for answering these questions. A complete answer key was provided for your instructor.

IRRIGATIONS

Objectives

- Identify the procedure for irrigating the eye and the ear.
- Explain the procedure for external and internal vaginal irrigation (douche).
- Discuss the procedure for nasal irrigation.

1. For an eye and ear irrigation, identify the following: ***(525-528)***

	Eye Irrigation	Ear Irrigation
a. Position of patient		
b. Position of irrigating equipment		
c. Flow of solution		
d. Postprocedure care		

2. The nurse is preparing to perform a vaginal irrigation for a patient. ***(583-584)***
   a. Perineal care is required before the irrigation if the patient has: ______________________.
   b. The patient is positioned in bed on a: ______________________.
   c. The temperature of the irrigating solution is: ______________________.
   d. Which type of asepsis is used, medical or surgical? ______________________
   e. While inserting the irrigating nozzle, the nurse should: ______________________.

3. A nasal irrigation is being performed on a patient by a nursing colleague. Which steps are appropriate? ***(529-530)***
   a. Positioning the patient with the head back _____
   b. Informing the patient not to speak or swallow during the procedure _____
   c. Inserting the tip of the irrigating device ½ inch to 1 inch _____
   d. Having the patient blow the nose immediately after the irrigation _____

HOT AND COLD APPLICATIONS

Objective

- Discuss heat and cold therapy and procedures.

4. Provide examples of the types of heat and cold applications that may be used. ***(532-536)***______________________

____

____

5. When is the use of heat or cold therapy contraindicated for a patient? ***(533)*** ______________________

____

____

6. Identify at least four safety measures to be considered when applying heat or cold therapy. ***(533)***

____

____

7. Before a hot moist compress is applied to an open wound, the nurse may apply ______________________ around the wound to protect the skin. ***(533)***

8. What materials can the patient use in the home to make a quick ice pack? ***(534)***______________________

____

____

Multiple Choice

9. A cold application is ordered for the patient. The nurse is aware that a positive effect of this treatment is: ***(531)***
   1. vasodilation.
   2. local anesthesia.
   3. reduced blood viscosity.
   4. increased capillary permeability.

10. There are principles to consider when using heat and cold therapy for patients. The nurse recognizes that the: ***(532)***
    1. application usually lasts only 10 to 20 minutes.
    2. patient should be able to adjust the temperature settings.
    3. patient should be able to move the application around.
    4. application is positioned so that the patient cannot move away from the temperature source.

PARENTERAL THERAPY

Objectives

- Summarize the nurse's responsibilities for the patient receiving intravenous therapy and procedures.
- Explain the nurse's responsibility when administering blood therapy.
- Discuss the complications of intravenous therapy.
- Discuss the complications of blood therapy.

11. Identify three guidelines for monitoring and maintaining intravenous (IV) therapy. ***(536)*** ____________

____

____

12. Before a venipuncture, what does the nurse have to assess? ***(536, 541)*** ____________

____

____

13. What documentation is necessary following insertion of an IV device? ***(540)*** ____________

____

____

14. The patient has an IV infusion. What assessments at the insertion site would indicate that the infusion should be discontinued? ***(545-546)***

____

____

15. For the following situations, what should the nurse do? ***(538-554)***

    a. There is less than 100 mL left in the IV bag. ______________________________

    ____

    b. Blood components will be given by IV route to the patient.______________________________

    ____

    c. The nurse is unsuccessful in the venipuncture attempt. ______________________________

    ____

    d. The patient asks if the IV insertion will hurt. ______________________________

    ____

16. What are the priority nursing responsibilities for a blood transfusion? ***(546-547)***______________________________

    ____

    ____

17. a. The nurse determines that the patient is having a transfusion reaction. What signs and symptoms did the patient most likely exhibit to lead the nurse to this determination? ***(548)***

    ____

    ____

    b. What should the nurse do first for the patient with a reaction? ***(548)***______________________________

    ____

    ____

18. Most severe transfusion reactions occur as a result of ______________________________. ***(548)***

19. The nurse is going to change the dressing of the peripheral IV line. Select all of the following actions that represent correct technique for this procedure. ***(549-550)***
    a. Palpate the catheter site after the old dressing is removed. _____
    b. Leave the tape in place that secures the IV catheter to the skin. _____
    c. Discontinue the infusion if there is erythema or edema at the site. _____
    d. Cover the insertion site with tape. _____
    e. Place tape over the transparent dressing. _____
    f. Label the dressing with the date, the time, and the nurse's initials. _____

Multiple Choice

20. Just before IV line insertion, the nurse should: ***(538)***
    1. shave the hair from the selected site.
    2. select a proximal site on the upper extremity.
    3. apply a tourniquet 4 to 6 inches above the site to be used.
    4. vigorously massage the extremity to be used.

21. Upon assessment of the IV insertion site, the nurse suspects that the patient has phlebitis. This is based upon the observation of: ***(546)***
    1. edema at the site.
    2. erythema along the vein path.
    3. cool skin around the insertion site.
    4. an increase in systemic blood pressure and pulse.

22. A blood transfusion is prepared for the patient. In setting up the IV, the nurse is aware that an acceptable piggyback solution for the set is: ***(546-547)***
    1. normal saline.
    2. 5% dextrose in water.
    3. 10% dextrose in water.
    4. Ringer's solution.

OXYGENATION

Objectives

- Discuss nursing interventions and procedures for the patient receiving oxygen.
- Discuss care of (procedures for) a patient with a tracheostomy.
- Differentiate among oropharyngeal, nasopharyngeal, and nasotracheal suctioning.
- Develop nursing diagnoses for the patient on oxygen therapy.

23. Identify at least four safety precautions for oxygen use in the hospital and home environment. ***(555-560)***

____

____

24. The patient is to receive oxygen. What assessments should be made by the nurse? ***(556-557)*** __________

____

____

25. When performing tracheostomy care, the nurse is aware of the following. ***(562-564)***

    a. Cleansing solution to be used: ______________________________

    b. Rinsing solution to be used: ______________________________

    c. The part that is removed for cleaning: ______________________________

    d. Safety measures: ______________________________

26. What can the nurse do to reduce possible sensory deprivation for the patient with a tracheostomy? ***(564)***

____

____

27. What criteria are used for the reinflation of a tracheostomy cuff? ***(566)***_______________________

____

____

28. In preparing to suction a patient, the nurse implements the following. ***(567-569)***
    a. Position of patient, if patient is able:_______________________
    b. Appropriate vacuum pressure for adult patient: _______________________
    c. Check the patency of suction catheter tubing by:_______________________
    d. Lubricant used on tubing: _______________________
    e. Length of insertion for nasotracheal suctioning for adult patient:_______________________
    f. Suctioning performed for _____ seconds.

29. Identify at least two signs or symptoms of hypoxia. ***(556)***_______________________

____

____

30. The patient is to receive oxygen. ***(557-559)***
    a. The nurse is aware that the usual flow rate of oxygen via a nasal cannula is: _____________.
    b. Comfort measures that should be implemented for the patient receiving oxygen by nasal cannula include: _______________________.
    c. The usual flow rate for the patient who is to receive oxygen via a face mask is: _____________.

Multiple Choice

31. The patient requires suctioning of pulmonary secretions. An appropriate nursing diagnosis for this patient is: ***(565)***
    1. fluid volume excess.
    2. ineffective breathing pattern.
    3. diminished respiratory ability.
    4. ineffective airway clearance.

32. The nurse is working in the special care nursery and will be suctioning the airways of infants. For this age group, the pressure of the wall suction should be set at: ***(567)***
    1. 5 to 15 mm Hg.
    2. 20 to 40 mm Hg.
    3. 50 to 95 mm Hg.
    4. 100 to 120 mm Hg.

33. Preparation for tracheostomy care in the acute care environment includes: ***(562)***
    1. using clean technique and supplies for cleaning.
    2. placing the patient in supine position.
    3. removing and cleaning the outer cannula.
    4. preparing cotton swabs with hydrogen peroxide and saline.

URINARY ELIMINATION

Objective

- Discuss management of the patient with an indwelling catheter:
  - Male catheterization
  - Female catheterization
  - Discontinuing an indwelling catheter
  - Catheter irrigation
  - Urostomy care

34. Identify at least five nursing interventions for patients with urinary drainage systems. ***(570, 579)*** _______

____

____

35. For urinary catheterization of male and female patients, identify the following. ***(571-575)***

	Male	Female
a. Position of patient		
b. Method of cleansing before insertion		
c. Length of portion of catheter to be inserted		

36. The nurse is inserting a urinary catheter and encounters the following situations. What should be done? ***(571-575)***

    a. Resistance is met: ______________________________

    ____

    b. The male patient has an erection: ______________________________

    ____

    c. The catheter is inserted into the vagina: ______________________________

    ____

37. The catheter itself is checked before insertion by doing the following: ***(572)*** ______________________________

    ____

    ____

38. After catheter removal, the nurse assesses the patient for the following: ***(583)*** ______________________________

    ____

    ____

39. Describe catheter care for a male and female patient. ***(576-577)*** ______________________________

    ____

    ____

40. a. The patient who self-catheterizes at home uses ____________________ technique. ***(579-580)***

    b. The nurse teaches this patient the signs and symptoms of a urinary tract infection, which include: ***(579-580)***

    ____

    ____

41. What are the different methods of bladder irrigation? ***(577-579)*** ______________________________

    ____

    ____

42. The patient is receiving continuous bladder irrigation through a three-way indwelling urinary catheter. Prescribed: 350 mL of normal saline irrigating solution infused. There are 475 mL in the urinary drainage bag. What is the patient's urinary output? ***(577-579)***

    ____

    ____

43. The primary concern for a patient with a urostomy is: *(595)*______________________________________

____

____

44. Identify two nursing diagnoses for a patient with a urinary disorder. *(581)*________________________

____

____

Multiple Choice

45. The nurse has inserted the catheter into the patient, and while the balloon is being inflated the patient expresses discomfort. The nurse should: *(573)*
    1. remove the catheter and begin the procedure again.
    2. pull back on the catheter to determine tension.
    3. draw fluid back out from the balloon and move the catheter forward.
    4. continue to inflate the balloon since discomfort is expected.

46. The nurse is providing instruction to the nursing assistant on catheter care for the patient. An appropriate instruction is to: *(576-577)*
    1. maintain strong tension on the external catheter tubing.
    2. empty the drainage bag every 24 hours.
    3. keep the drainage bag on the bed or attached to the side rails.
    4. clean from the urinary meatus down the catheter.

47. When inserting a urinary catheter into a female patient, the nurse knows that it should be inserted: *(573)*
    1. 2 to 4 inches.
    2. 4 to 6 inches.
    3. 6 to 8 inches.
    4. 8 to 10 inches.

48. The charge nurse delegates the removal of an indwelling urinary catheter to a new staff member. The charge nurse goes in to observe the procedure and recognizes that correction is required if the new staff member is observed doing which of the following? *(582)*
    1. Explaining that there may be a burning sensation felt with the first voiding
    2. Obtaining a urine specimen from the port
    3. Cutting the catheter near the connection to the drainage bag
    4. Using clean gloves and performing perineal care

BOWEL ELIMINATION

Objectives

- Identify the procedures for promoting bowel elimination:
  - Administering an enema
  - Inserting a rectal tube
  - Performing ostomy and stoma care
  - Removing a fecal impaction
- Describe nursing care required to maintain structure and function of a bowel diversion.

49. How can the nurse promote normal bowel functioning for the patient in a hospital or extended care facility? *(589)*

____

____

50. The nurse is observing the patient at home performing colostomy care. What areas require further teaching? *(598)*
    a. The patient says he is not concerned about the swelling of the stoma. _____
    b. Alcohol and skin cream are used around the stoma. _____
    c. The patient is blotting the skin dry around the stoma. _____
    d. The skin barrier and pouch are being changed twice daily. _____
    e. The patient is leaving $\frac{1}{16}$-inch clearance between the stoma and the skin barrier. _____
    f. 750 mL of warm water is prepared for the irrigation. _____
    g. The irrigation cone is pushed forcefully into the stoma to create the fit. _____

51. For the administration of an enema, the nurse is aware of the following parameters. *(593-594)*
    a. Preferred position of patient: _______________
    b. Temperature of prepared solution: _______________
    c. Maximum volume of solution for an adult patient: _______________
    d. Patient instruction for relaxation of external sphincter: _______________
    e. Height of fluid container: _______________
    f. Length of insertion of tube for adult patient: _______________
    g. Patient complaints of cramping: _______________
    h. Documentation required: _______________

Multiple Choice

52. Before the digital removal of a fecal impaction, the nurse checks the medical record. Because of the possible effect of the digital manipulation, a patient with a history of which of the following will have to be observed especially closely during the procedure? *(595)*
    1. Cardiac disease
    2. Abdominal discomfort
    3. Urinary infection
    4. Diabetes mellitus

ENTERAL THERAPY

Objectives

- Explain nursing interventions for the patient with nasogastric intubation.
- Discuss gastric and intestinal suctioning care.
- Identify the procedure for nasogastric tube removal.

53. What is the purpose of nasogastric (NG) tube insertion? *(583)* ____________________

____

____

54. The nurse is preparing to perform a NG tube insertion and is aware of the following. *(585-587)*

    a. Measurement procedure for insertion: ____________________

    ____

    b. Position of patient for insertion: ____________________

    ____

    c. Instructions for patient during insertion: ____________________

    ____

    d. Most reliable determination of tube placement: ____________________

    ____

    e. Securing of NG tube: ____________________

    ____

55. The patient is not able to talk after the NG tube is inserted. The nurse suspects the following: *(587)*

____

____

56. You are evaluating the new staff member's performance of an NG tube irrigation. Which actions indicate that further instruction is needed? *(588)*
    a. The nurse draws up 100 mL of tap water for the irrigation. _____
    b. The solution is instilled slowly. _____
    c. The solution is withdrawn and measured. _____
    d. Solution is forced down afterward to clear the tubing. _____

57. The patient is to have gastric or intestinal suctioning applied. Identify the appropriate nursing interventions. *(589-590)*

    a. Pressure to set the wall suction at: ____________________

    ____

    b. Assessment of the patient: ____________________

    ____

c. Method to determine patency of the Salem sump: ______________________________

____

d. Abnormalities to report to the physician: ______________________________

____

58. While removing the NG tube, the patient begins to gag. The nurse should do the following: ***(590)*** ______

____

____

59. A priority nursing diagnosis for the patient with an NG tube is the following: ***(585)*** ______________

____

____

60. A priority action for the nurse to implement before performing any skill is to check the following: ***(524)***

____

____

61. Identify how the nurse achieves the following actions before, during, and after the performance of a procedure. ***(524-525)***

a. Identify the patient: ______________________________

____

b. Reduce the spread of microorganisms: ______________________________

____

c. Provide privacy: ______________________________

____

d. Ensure the patient's safety: ______________________________

____

62. Although policy and procedure can vary from agency to agency, what are some of the skills that may, in general, be delegated to assistive personnel? ***(532, 538, 565, 569, 589, 597)***

____

____

Multiple Choice

63. The physician has ordered the application of a warm compress to a patient's leg wound. The patient asks, "What is a compress?" The nurse's best response is: ***(532)***
    1. "We will be soaking your leg in a warm solution."
    2. "We will be wrapping your leg with a device similar to a heating pad."
    3. "We will be applying a hot water bottle to your leg and then wrap a towel around it to keep the heat application constant."
    4. "We will be applying a sterile, moist gauze dressing to the wound, then wrap it with a warm aquathermia pad in order to maintain the warmth of the compress."

64. Upon assessment of a patient's IV site, the nurse determines that the site has become infiltrated. The signs and symptoms that the nurse assessed include: (Select all that apply) ***(546)***
    1. warmth at the insertion site.
    2. swelling at and above the insertion site.
    3. redness at the insertion site.
    4. coolness upon palpation of and above the insertion site.

65. The maximum amount of fluid that should be administered to an adult during a tap water enema is: ***(593)***
    1. 150 to 250 mL.
    2. 250 to 500 mL.
    3. 500 to 700 mL.
    4. 750 to 1000 mL.

Student Name________________________________ Date______________

Basic Nutrition and Nutrition Therapy

chapter 21

Answer Key: Textbook page references are provided as a guide for answering these questions. A complete answer key was provided for your instructor.

TERMS

Objective

- Define the key terms listed.

1. Define the following terms.

   a. Anabolism: ***(612)*** ________________________________

   ____

   b. Basal metabolic rate (BMR): ***(631)*** ________________________________

   ____

   c. Catabolism: ***(612)*** ________________________________

   ____

   d. Essential nutrients: ***(608)*** ________________________________

   ____

   e. Nitrogen balance: ***(612)*** ________________________________

   ____

   f. Vegan: ***(612)*** ________________________________

   ____

ESSENTIAL NUTRIENTS

Objectives

- List the six classes of essential nutrients, and identify those that provide energy.
- List the functions and food sources of protein, carbohydrates, and fats.
- List food sources and possible health benefits of dietary fiber.

- Distinguish between saturated, unsaturated, and trans fats and cholesterol; identify current recommendations for dietary intake of fats and cholesterol.
- Discuss key vitamins and minerals, their role in health, and their food sources.

2. Identify the six classes of nutrients and their general function. ***(608)***____________________

3. What are the calories provided and the recommended percentage of intake for each of the following nutrients? ***(608)***

   a. Protein: ____________________

   b. Carbohydrates: ____________________

   c. Fats: ____________________

4. Identify the following for carbohydrates. ***(608-609)***

   a. Role in the body: ____________________

   b. Types: ____________________

5. Identify an example of a simple and a complex carbohydrate. ***(608)*** ____________________

6. What is the difference between these types of fiber? ***(609)***

   a. Insoluble fiber: ____________________

   b. Water-soluble fiber: ____________________

7. What do fats provide for the body? ***(610)*** ____________________

8. Identify examples of food sources for the following. ***(610)***

   a. Saturated fats: ____________________

   b. Unsaturated fats: ____________________

9. In considering food choices, the nurse recognizes that cholesterol is found mainly in ________________ ____. *(610-611)*

10. Lipoproteins have been talked about in the news. Which ones are important in cardiovascular disease? *(611)*

____

____

11. What is the role of protein in the body? *(611)* ____

____

____

12. Define and identify possible food sources for a complete protein. *(612)* ________________________

____

____

13. For the following types of protein-kilocalorie malnutrition states, describe the problem and the signs and symptoms exhibited by the patient. *(612-613)*

    a. Kwashiorkor: ____

    ____

    b. Marasmus: ____

    ____

14. What is the general function of vitamins? *(613)* ____

____

____

15. What are the two main types of vitamins? *(613)* ____

____

____

16. How do minerals differ from vitamins? *(613)* ____

____

____

17. For each of the following vitamins, identify a food source, its function in the body, and signs and symptoms of a deficiency and toxicity (if applicable). ***(614-615)***

    a. Vitamin C: ____________________

    b. Vitamin D: ____________________

    c. Vitamin K: ____________________

    d. Folic acid: ____________________

    e. Niacin: ____________________

18. The patient tells the nurse that he has heard about antioxidants but is not sure what they are. The nurse responds by telling the patient that antioxidants are: ***(613)***

    ____

19. For a patient older than 50 years of age, vitamin __________ is recommended. ***(615-616)***

20. For each of the following minerals, identify a food source, its function in the body, and signs and symptoms of a deficiency and toxicity (if applicable). ***(616-617)***

    a. Calcium: ____________________

    b. Potassium: ____________________

    c. Iron: ____________________

    d. Iodine: ____________________

    e. Zinc: ____________________

21. a. Identify factors that enhance the absorption of iron. ***(619)*** ______________________________

____

____

b. Patients with the greatest risk for iron deficiency anemia are: ***(619)*** ______________________________.

22. What is the function of water in the body and the recommended daily intake? ***(619)***______________________________

____

____

Multiple Choice

23. The vitamin to be used with caution for a patient who is taking anticoagulants is vitamin: ***(615)***
    1. A.
    2. D.
    3. K.
    4. B complex.

24. Patients who have an inadequate intake of vitamin C may develop: ***(615)***
    1. bleeding gums.
    2. liver damage.
    3. depression.
    4. convulsions.

25. The patient has been diagnosed with pernicious anemia. The nurse expects that the patient will receive: ***(616)***
    1. vitamin B_1.
    2. vitamin B_6.
    3. vitamin B_{12}.
    4. niacin.

26. The nurse is working with a patient who requires an increase in complete proteins in the diet. The nurse will recommend the intake of: (Select all that apply) ***(612)***
    1. chicken.
    2. eggs.
    3. peanuts.
    4. beans.

27. A patient in the clinic is asking the nurse about vitamin supplements. The nurse cautions the patient about potential toxicity and not to exceed the guidelines for: ***(613)***
    1. vitamin A.
    2. vitamin B.
    3. vitamin C.
    4. folic acid.

28. The patient tells the nurse that the ads on television are talking about zinc and its importance. The patient says that he doesn't know anything about zinc and would like to find out what foods have it. The nurse tells the patient that a good source of zinc is: ***(616)***
    1. fruit.
    2. liver.
    3. poultry.
    4. cheese.

DIET MODIFICATIONS

Objectives

- Identify standard hospital diets and modifications for texture, consistency, and meal frequency.
- List medical/surgical conditions that require a high-kilocalorie and high-protein diet, and suggest ways to increase kilocalories and protein in the diet.
- Define obesity. List components of an effective weight management program.
- Describe the diet in the management of type 1 and type 2 diabetes mellitus.
- Distinguish among anorexia nervosa, bulimia nervosa, and binge eating disorder.
- List conditions requiring a fat-modified diet, and identify foods and food preparation methods that should be limited.
- Identify medical/surgical conditions requiring modifications in sodium, potassium, protein, or fluid intake, and describe the dietary adjustments necessary in these conditions.

29. Identify what health problems the following diets are used for. ***(630-631)***

    a. Soft, and low residue: ______________________________

    b. High kilocalorie: ______________________________

30. What is the body mass index (BMI) used for? Calculate your own BMI. ***(632)*** ______________________________

    ____

    ____

31. Identify the risks associated with obesity. ***(631-632)*** ______________________________

    ____

    ____

32. What is the general dietary approach for the obese patient? ***(632, 634)*** ______________________________

    ____

    ____

33. Identify the similarities among the eating disorders. ***(635)*** ______________________________

    ____

    ____

34. What physiologic signs and symptoms should the nurse be alert for that may indicate an eating disorder? *(636)*

____

____

35. What are the general dietary guidelines for a patient with type 2 diabetes mellitus? *(637-638)* __________

____

____

36. The patient with diabetes mellitus is diaphoretic, weak, and breathing shallowly. What should the nurse do? *(639-640)*

____

____

37. What is the 15/15 rule for diabetic patients? *(639)* __________

____

____

38. Describe dumping syndrome and ways that the patient may avoid it. *(640)* __________

____

____

39. Fat-controlled diets are used for patients with __________. *(640)*

40. How is the patient able to modify the intake of the following fats? *(641)*

    a. Eggs: __________

    b. Meats: __________

41. A protein-restricted diet is used for patients with: __________ __________. *(643)*

42. A sodium-restricted diet is used for patients with: __________ __________. *(643)*

43. Identify the dietary modifications for patients with the following health problems. *(645)*

    a. Acquired immunodeficiency syndrome (AIDS): __________

    ____

b. Constipation: ____________________

____

c. Hiatal hernia: ____________________

____

44. Develop a plan for the distribution of fluids for a patient on a 24-hour 1000-mL fluid restriction. ***(644)***

____

____

Multiple Choice

45. A patient in the hospital who is placed on a clear liquid diet may have: ***(630)***
    1. fruit juice.
    2. gelatin.
    3. sherbet.
    4. strained soup.

46. The nurse recognizes that the diet for a patient diagnosed with diabetes mellitus will be: ***(637)***
    1. fat modified.
    2. sodium restricted.
    3. protein restricted.
    4. carbohydrate modified.

47. A patient who is lactose intolerant needs to avoid: ***(640)***
    1. meat.
    2. fish.
    3. cheese.
    4. vegetables.

ENTERAL THERAPY

Objective

- Define enteral nutrition and parenteral nutrition and list medical and surgical conditions in which nutrition support may be indicated.

48. What are the indications for the use of enteral feeding? ***(646)*** ____________________

____

____

49. What are the possible complications of enteral feeding? ***(647)*** ________________

50. What is parenteral nutrition, and when is it used? ***(652-653)*** ________________

51. Complications of parenteral nutrition include the following: ***(653)*** ________________

52. Identify the nursing assessments and interventions for enteral feeding and the following situations. ***(648-652)***

    a. Patient assessment before feeding: ________________

    b. Assessment of gastric aspirate: ________________

    c. Gastric residual above 150 mL: ________________

    d. Formula is cold: ________________

    e. Occlusion of the tubing is suspected: ________________

    f. After feeding is given: ________________

    g. Documentation: ________________

53. What is included in the care of a gastrostomy or jejunostomy site? ***(652)*** ________________

54. Positive outcomes for patients with enteral tube feedings are the following: ***(646)*** ____________________

____

____

Multiple Choice

55. Patients with nasogastric (NG) tubes may develop otitis media. In order to prevent this occurrence, the nurse will: ***(647)***
    1. increase fluid intake.
    2. remove and reinsert the tube every 24 hours.
    3. suction the nose and mouth.
    4. turn the patient side to side every 2 hours.

56. A patient on the unit has an NG tube in place with continuous feedings. When the nurse enters the room, the patient says that he is having stomach cramps. The nurse should first: ***(651)***
    1. cool the formula.
    2. remove the NG tube.
    3. use a different type of formula.
    4. decrease the administration rate.

NURSING ASSESSMENT AND INTERVENTIONS

Objectives

- Discuss the role of the nurse in promoting good nutrition.
- Explain how to use diet planning guides in the assessment and planning of a diet.
- Discuss changes in nutrient needs throughout the life cycle, and suggest ideas to ensure adequate nutrition during each stage of life.
- Identify the effects of common medications on nutritional status.

57. Identify the role of the nurse in promoting nutrition. ***(605)*** ____________________

____

____

58. In the MyPyramid guide, the emphasis is on ____________________. ***(605)***

59. Identify the number of daily servings recommended in the pyramid for a 2000-calorie diet: ***(605)***

    a. Vegetables: ____________________

    b. Meat, beans: ____________________

    c. Milk: ____________________

60. An active teenage girl asks the nurse how many calories she should have every day and what types of food she should eat. The nurse provides the following information. ***(605)***

 a. Calorie intake: ______

 b. Servings of bread: ______

 c. Servings of vegetables: ______

 d. Servings of fruit: ______

 e. Servings of milk: ______

 f. Servings of meat: ______

61. A patient is asking about a vegetarian diet. Explain the positive and negative aspects of this diet for the patient. ***(612)***

______

______

62. There is an increased need for nutrients during pregnancy because: ***(619, 621)*** ______

______

______

63. Increased intake of which vitamins is recommended for the pregnant patient? ***(620)*** ______

______

______

64. The nurse teaches the pregnant woman to avoid the following foods and lifestyle activities: ***(621-623)***

______

______

65. In teaching a new parent about nutritional guidelines for the infant, the nurse explains that the following foods should be avoided during the first year: ***(623)***

______

______

66. Identify ways to encourage good dietary habits in children. ***(626)*** ______

______

______

67. A common nutritional problem in adolescence is that a large part of the diet may be comprised of the following: ***(626)***

____

____

68. Nursing home residents may have nutritional problems as a result of the following: ***(627)*** ____________

____

____

69. You are evaluating the nursing assistant feeding a patient. Which of the following actions indicate a need for correction? ***(655-656)***
    a. Offering the patient the bedpan before the meal. _____
    b. Placing the patient in low Fowler's position. _____
    c. Using a straw for liquids. _____
    d. Directing food toward the patient's paralyzed side. _____
    e. Talking with the patient during the feeding. _____

70. Identify at least two foods or fluids that are allowed on each of the following diets. ***(630)***
    a. Clear liquid: ____
    b. Full liquid: ____
    c. Soft: ____

Multiple Choice

71. The mother asks the nurse about giving strained fruits to her infant. The nurse tells the mother that this food should be introduced at around: ***(623)***
    1. 2 months.
    2. 5 months.
    3. 8 months.
    4. 12 months.

72. The patient is taking a diuretic medication every day. The nurse observes the patient for signs of a decrease in: ***(618)***
    1. vitamin K.
    2. vitamin C.
    3. phosphorus.
    4. potassium.

Student Name________________________________ Date____________

Fluids and Electrolytes

chapter **22**

Answer Key: Textbook page references are provided as a guide for answering these questions. A complete answer key was provided for your instructor.

FLUID AND PARTICLE MOVEMENT

Objectives

- List, describe, and compare the body fluid compartments.
- Discuss active and passive transport processes, and give two examples of each.

1. a. Identify the body fluid compartments in the body. ***(661)*** ____________________

   ____

   ____

   b. Most of the body fluid in an adult is located in the ____________________compartment. ***(661)***

2. What is the relationship of body weight to fluid? ***(660)*** ____________________

   ____

   ____

3. For the following types of fluids, identify the how the fluid will move when administered to the patient intravenously. ***(664)***

   a. Hypertonic solution: ____________________

   b. Hypotonic solution:____________________

4. Provide examples for each of the following processes in the body. ***(664-665)***

   a. Diffusion:____________________

   ____

   b. Filtration:____________________

   ____

c. Osmosis: ____

____

d. Active transport: ____

____

5. The minimum hourly urinary output is ______, and the minimum daily output ______. ***(662)***

ELECTROLYTES

Objectives

- Discuss the role of specific electrolytes in maintaining homeostasis.
- Describe the cause and effect of deficits and excesses of sodium, potassium, chloride, calcium, magnesium, phosphorus, and bicarbonate.

6. a. The major extracellular electrolyte is ______________________________. ***(665)***

   b. The major intracellular electrolyte is ______________________________. ***(665)***

7. Identify the most common signs and symptoms of hyponatremia, and nursing interventions for the imbalance. ***(666)***

____

____

8. Identify the most common signs and symptoms of hypokalemia, and nursing interventions for the imbalance. ***(668)***

____

____

9. What are the most serious problems associated with hyperkalemia, and what are the nursing interventions for the imbalance? ***(669)***

____

____

10. The role of calcium in the body is the following: ***(669-670)*** ______________________________

____

____

11. a. Identify the most common signs and symptoms of hypocalcemia, and the nursing interventions for the imbalance. ***(670-671)***

____

____

b. In the illustrations, what assessments are being performed to determine the presence of this imbalance? ***(670-671)***

i. ____

ii. ____

i.

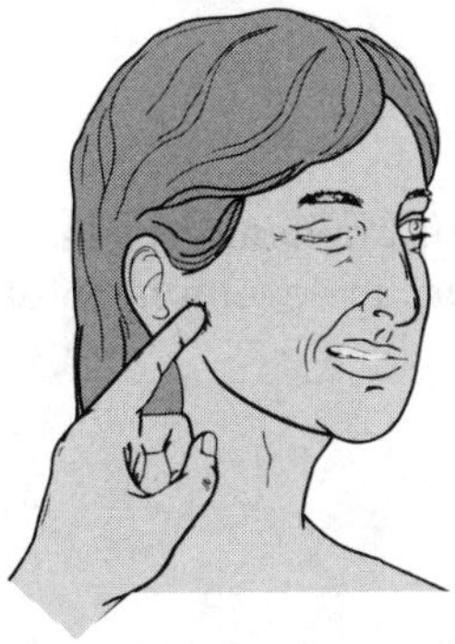

ii.

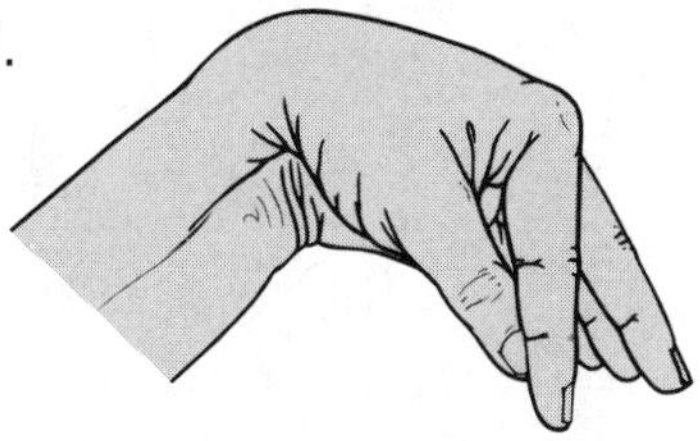

12. Identify possible causes of hypomagnesemia, its common signs and symptoms, and nursing interventions for the imbalance. ***(672)***

____

____

13. For the following laboratory results, identify the electrolyte imbalance.

a. Serum sodium 127 mEq/L: ***(665)*** ______________________

b. Serum potassium 5.6 mEq/L: ***(666)*** ______________________

c. Serum calcium 3.8 mEq/L: ***(669)*** ______________________

d. Serum magnesium 2.7 mEq/L: ***(672)*** ______________________

14. Select all of the following that can contribute to hypokalemia. ***(668)***
    a. Vomiting _____
    b. Diarrhea _____
    c. Diuretic use _____
    d. Metabolic acidosis _____
    e. Chemotherapy _____
    f. Deficiency of vitamin D _____
    g. Thyroid surgery _____

Multiple Choice

15. The patient is experiencing hyperkalemia. The nurse anticipates that the treatment will include: ***(669)***
    1. intravenous (IV) calcium.
    2. fluid restrictions.
    3. foods high in potassium.
    4. administration of diuretics.

16. Following an auto accident and a significant hemorrhage, the patient was given a large infusion of citrated blood. The patient is assessed for the development of: ***(671)***
    1. urinary retention.
    2. poor skin turgor.
    3. increased blood pressure.
    4. positive Chvostek's sign.

17. Good food sources for both calcium and potassium are: ***(667, 670)***
    1. meats.
    2. cranberries.
    3. whole grains.
    4. green, leafy vegetables.

ACID-BASE

Objectives

- Differentiate between the roles of the buffers, the lungs, and the kidneys in maintenance of acid-base balance.
- Compare and contrast the four major types of acid-base imbalances.

18. The normal pH range of the blood is ________________________. ***(673)***

19. a. In determining acid-base balance, the base substance that increases or decreases in the blood is ________________________. ***(673-674)***

    b. The acid substance is ________________________. ***(673-674)***

    c. The ratio of these two substances is ________________________. ***(673-674)***

20. What are the three body systems that regulate acid-base balance in the body? ***(673-674)*** ______________

____

____

21. a. If carbonic acid increases in the blood, the pH will ______________________. ***(674)***

    b. The respiratory system will respond by ____________________. ***(674)***

22. If the pH of the blood increases, the kidneys will respond by ____________________. ***(674)***

Multiple Choice

23. The patient has experienced a prolonged episode of diarrhea. The nurse is observing the patient for signs of: ***(676)***
    1. metabolic acidosis.
    2. metabolic alkalosis.
    3. respiratory acidosis.
    4. respiratory alkalosis.

24. The patient has had emphysema for a number of years. Which of the following arterial blood gas values indicates that the patient is in respiratory acidosis? ***(675)***
    1. pH 7.35, $Paco_2$ 40, HCO_3 22
    2. pH 7.40, $Paco_2$ 45, HCO_3 30
    3. pH 7.30, $Paco_2$ 50, HCO_3 24
    4. pH 7.48, $Paco_2$ 55, HCO_3 18

25. While in the delivery room with his wife, the father-to-be begins to develop an anxiety reaction and lightheadedness. Nursing intervention to prevent respiratory alkalosis is: ***(676)***
    1. lay him down.
    2. provide nasal oxygen.
    3. have him breathe into a paper bag.
    4. have him cough and deep-breathe.

26. A child has gotten into the medicine cabinet in the home and ingested the remaining contents of an aspirin bottle. The problem that may occur as a result of this ingestion is: ***(676)***
    1. metabolic acidosis.
    2. metabolic alkalosis.
    3. respiratory acidosis.
    4. respiratory alkalosis

27. The patient has had continuous gastric suction. The nurse suspects a specific acid-base imbalance that can occur with this treatment. This is confirmed by the following findings: ***(677)***
    1. pH elevated, $Paco_2$ normal, and HCO_3 elevated.
    2. pH elevated, $Paco_2$ elevated, and HCO_3 decreased.
    3. pH decreased, $Paco_2$ decreased, and HCO_3 decreased.
    4. pH decreased, $Paco_2$ normal, and HCO_3 decreased.

NURSING

Objectives

- Discuss the role of the nursing process for fluid, electrolyte, and acid-base balances.
- Discuss how the very young, the very old, and the obese patient are at risk for fluid volume deficit.

28. How does body fluid change as an individual ages and grows? ***(660-661)***

29. Identify at least two considerations for the older adult patient regarding fluid and electrolyte and acid-base balance. ***(661)***

30. The nurse is monitoring the patient's intake and output (I&O). What should be counted as part of the output? ***(662)***

31. What are the signs and symptoms of respiratory acidosis? ***(675)***

32. The nurse anticipates that the treatment for respiratory acidosis will include the following: ***(675)***

33. Identify possible causes of and interventions for metabolic acidosis and alkalosis. ***(676-677)***

34. Identify possible nursing diagnoses and outcomes for patients experiencing fluid, electrolyte, or acid-base imbalances. ***(677)***

35. What are the general nursing interventions that should be implemented for patients with fluid, electrolyte, or acid-base imbalances? ***(678)***

____

____

Multiple Choice

36. The best way for the nurse to determine the patient's fluid balance is to: ***(663)***
    1. assess vital signs.
    2. weigh the patient daily.
    3. monitor IV fluid intake.
    4. check diagnostic test results.

37. For the patient with intracellular dehydration, the nurse anticipates that the patient will receive a(n): ***(664)***
    1. hypotonic solution.
    2. hypertonic solution.
    3. isotonic solution.
    4. parenteral feeding.

38. A postoperative patient is receiving an isotonic IV solution. The patient asks the nurse why he is receiving this solution. The nurse's best response is: ***(664)***
    1. "This fluid will expand your body's fluid volume that has been lost from your surgery."
    2. "This is a solution that will pull fluid from your cells into your circulatory system."
    3. "This solution will pull fluid from your circulatory system into your cells, where it is needed."
    4. "Since the physician ordered this IV, it would be best if you discussed the reason with your physician."

39. The nurse is aware that electrolytes serve a variety of purposes, including: (Select all that apply) ***(665)***
    1. maintenance of normal body metabolism.
    2. regulation of water balance in the body.
    3. regulation of water and electrolyte contents within cells.
    4. formation of hydrochloric acid in gastric juice.

40. The patient has been placed on a low-sodium diet to assist in the treatment of hypertension. The nurse perceives that the patient has understood diet teaching when the patient states: ***(665)***
    1. "Cheese is a good between-meal snack for me."
    2. "It is okay for me to eat at my favorite seafood restaurant."
    3. "In order for me to eat enough vegetables, I can prepare canned peas and corn."
    4. "I love cooked frozen broccoli. I'm glad I will still be able to eat it."

41. The nurse realizes that the patient's bicarbonate level is significant in maintaining: ***(673)***
    1. electrolyte balance.
    2. fluid balance.
    3. acid-base balance.
    4. serum potassium levels.

Student Name______________________________ **Date**________________

chapter

23

Mathematics Review and Medication Administration

Answer Key: Textbook page references are provided as a guide for answering these questions. A complete answer key was provided for your instructor.

CALCULATION

Objectives

- Confidently use basic mathematical skills to solve dosage problems accurately.
- Set up and work problems using the following formula: (desired dose/available dose) = amount.
- Set up and work problems using the proportion method.
- Use "key" equivalents of metric and apothecary measurement systems in dosage problems.
- Convert measurement units within the metric system.
- Convert between measurement units of the metric system and the apothecary system.
- Determine the appropriateness of dosage orders for children by the use of Young's, Clark's, and Fried's rules and the body surface area.

1. For fractions, provide examples of the following. *(682-683)*

   a. Numerator: _________

   b. Denominator: _________

   c. Proper fraction: _________

   d. Improper fraction: _________

   e. Mixed fraction: _________

2. Change the following improper fractions to mixed numbers. *(682)*

   a. $8/5$ = _________

   b. $12/7$ = _________

   c. $7/6$ = _________

   d. $100/13$ = _________

   e. $30/4$ = _________

   f. $97/8$ = _________

3. Change the following mixed numbers to improper fractions. ***(682)***

   a. $7\frac{5}{8}$ = ________

   b. $8\frac{1}{5}$ = ________

   c. $15\frac{1}{4}$ = ________

   d. $9\frac{1}{3}$ = ________

   e. $6\frac{5}{7}$ = ________

   f. $25\frac{2}{3}$ = ________

4. Reduce the following fractions to their lowest terms. ***(682-683)***

   a. $\frac{4}{8}$ = ________

   b. $\frac{3}{9}$ = ________

   c. $\frac{21}{3}$ = ________

   d. $\frac{15}{30}$ = ________

   e. $\frac{25}{100}$ = ________

   f. $\frac{5000}{1000}$ = ________

   g. $\frac{8}{40}$ = ________

   h. $\frac{4}{16}$ = ________

   i. $\frac{18}{3}$ = ________

   j. $\frac{75}{50}$ = ________

5. Identify which is the largest fraction in the each group. ***(683)***

   a. $\frac{6}{14}$ $\frac{8}{14}$ $\frac{13}{14}$: ________

   b. $\frac{3}{4}$ $\frac{4}{5}$ $\frac{7}{8}$: ________

6. Add the following fractions, and reduce the sum to its lowest term. ***(683-684)***

   a. $\frac{1}{2} + \frac{5}{2} + \frac{3}{2}$ = ________

   b. $\frac{2}{5} + \frac{1}{3} + \frac{7}{10}$ = ________

   c. $\frac{1}{3} + \frac{1}{5}$ = ________

   d. $\frac{2}{12} + \frac{5}{12} + \frac{9}{12}$ = ________

   e. $2\frac{1}{3} + 5\frac{1}{4}$ = ________

7. Subtract the following fractions, and reduce the answer to its lowest term. ***(684)***

   a. $\frac{4}{5} - \frac{1}{5} =$ ________

   b. $\frac{1}{2} - \frac{1}{3} =$ ________

   c. $2\frac{3}{4} - 1\frac{1}{2} =$ ________

   d. $\frac{4}{5} - \frac{1}{7} =$ ________

   e. $\frac{3}{4} - \frac{1}{4} =$ ________

8. Multiply the following fractions, and reduce the product to its lowest term. ***(684)***

   a. $\frac{1}{3} \times \frac{3}{12} =$ ________

   b. $2\frac{7}{8} \times 3\frac{1}{3} =$ ________

   c. $\frac{1}{2} \times \frac{1}{5} =$ ________

   d. $\frac{2}{5} \times \frac{1}{7} =$ ________

   e. $41 \times \frac{3}{4} =$ ________

   f. $\frac{6}{5} \times 1\frac{2}{3} =$ ________

9. Divide the following fractions, and reduce the answer to its lowest term. ***(685)***

   a. $\frac{1}{2} \div \frac{1}{3} =$ ________

   b. $\frac{21}{4} \div \frac{1}{7} =$ ________

   c. $\frac{5}{8} \div \frac{3}{4} =$ ________

   d. $\frac{5}{3} \div \frac{5}{3} =$ ________

   e. $\frac{3}{10} \div \frac{5}{25} =$ ________

10. Add the following decimals. ***(685)***

    a. 5.4 + 6.9 = ________

    b. 4.25 + 3.217 = ________

    c. 22.1 + 0.75 = ________

    d. 4.297 + 1.919 = ________

    e. 2.2 + 1.68 = ________

    f. 57.629 + 14.22 = ________

11. Subtract the following decimals. ***(685)***

a. $0.089 - 0.0057 =$ ________

b. $2.69 - 1.678 =$ ________

c. $1.5 - 0.22 =$ ________

d. $15.6 - 1.2 =$ ________

e. $75.1 - 24.2 =$ ________

f. $26 - 6.225 =$ ________

12. Round the following decimals to hundredths and then to tenths. ***(686)***

a. $5.753 =$ ________ ________

b. $4.215 =$ ________ ________

c. $3.178 =$ ________ ________

d. $52.371 =$ ________ ________

e. $0.604 =$ ________ ________

f. $152.772 =$ ________ ________

13. Multiply the following decimals. ***(686)***

a. $4.2 \times 5.75 =$ ________

b. $64.75 \times 22.9 =$ ________

c. $33.1 \times 25.95 =$ ________

d. $2.197 \times 0.93 =$ ________

e. $22.5 \times 50 =$ ________

f. $154.5 \times 14.2 =$ ________

14. Divide the following decimals, and round to the nearest hundredth. ***(686)***

a. $5.6 \div 6.97 =$ ________

b. $2.9 \div 0.218 =$ ________

c. $45.62 \div 1.4 =$ ________

d. $0.02 \div 0.0007 =$ ________

e. $75 \div 2.2 =$ ________

f. $32.7 \div 15.952 =$ ________

15. Convert the following fractions into decimals. ***(686)***

a. $\frac{1}{4}$ = ________

b. $\frac{1}{2}$ = ________

c. $\frac{1}{5}$ = ________

d. $\frac{3}{4}$ = ________

e. $\frac{4}{8}$ = ________

f. $\frac{7}{12}$ = ________

16. Convert the following fractions into percents. ***(687)***

a. $\frac{75}{100}$ = ________

b. $\frac{1}{3}$ = ________

c. $\frac{42}{100}$ = ________

d. $\frac{5}{10}$ = ________

e. $\frac{20}{100}$ = ________

f. $\frac{33}{100}$ = ________

17. In the following ratios, solve for X. ***(687)***

a. $20 : 40 = X : 5$ X = ________

b. $\frac{1}{150} : 2 = \frac{1}{250} : X$ X = ________

c. $X : 9 = 4 : 12$ X = ________

d. $\frac{1}{2} : 2 = \frac{1}{3} : X$ X = ________

e. $X : 1 = 0.4 : 6$ X = ________

18. Complete the following equivalents. ***(689)***

a. 30 mL = ________ ounces

b. 1000 mL = ________ L

c. 1 L = ________ quarts

d. 500 mL = ________ pints

e. 60 mg = ________ g

f. 1 kg = ________ pounds

g. 400 mL = ________ L

h. 2 mcg = ________ mg

i. 4 mg = ________ g

j. 44 pounds = ________ kg

k. 5 mg = ________ mcg

19. What are the differences among Young's rule, Clark's rule, and Fried's rule? ***(690-691)*** ________________

____

____

20. Calculate the patient's total fluid intake for breakfast: 8 ounces of milk, 6 ounces of juice, and 10 ounces of coffee. ***(689)*** ________ mL

21. The prescription is for Tegretol 200 mg po tid. ***(687-690)***
Available—Tegretol 100-mg tablets
How many tablets should be given per dose? ________

22. The prescription is for Aldomet 250 mg po bid. ***(687-690)***
Available—Aldomet 125-mg tablets
How many tablets should be given per dose? ________

23. The prescription is for V-Cillin K suspension 500,000 units po. ***(687-690)***
Available—V-Cillin K suspension 200,000 units/5 mL
How much should be prepared? ________

24. The prescription is for morphine 4 mg IM prn for pain. ***(687-690)***
Available—morphine 10 mg/mL
The nurse prepares ________ mL.

25. The prescription is for heparin 5000 units subQ. ***(687-690)***
Available—heparin 10,000 units/mL.
How much should be given? ________

26. The prescription is for Solu-Medrol 50 mg IV. ***(687-690)***
Available—Solu-Medrol 125 mg/2 mL.
How much is prepared? ________

27. Using Young's rule, identify the dose for a child who is 3 years old when the adult dose is 75 mg. ***(690)***

____

28. Using Clark's rule, identify the dose for a child who weighs 30 pounds when the adult dose is 50 mg. ***(691)*** ________

29. Using Fried's rule, identify the dose for a child who is 10 months old when the adult dose is 100 mg. ***(691)***

____

30. Using the body surface area calculation, identify the dose for a child with a body surface area of 1.1 m^2 when the adult dose is 10 mg. ***(691)*** ________

Multiple Choice

31. A prescription for codeine gr ½ is written for the patient. The medication is supplied in mg. The nurse should administer: ***(687-690)***
    a. 3 g.
    b. 30 g.
    c. 3 mg.
    d. 30 mg.

DRUG ACTION

Objectives

- Explain each phase of drug action.
- Explain the importance of decreased hepatic and renal functioning.

32. Identify the two general types of drug actions. ***(692)*** ______________________

____

____

33. Describe possible responses that patients may have to medications. ***(692-693)*** ______________________

____

____

34. Provide two examples of how older adults may respond to medications, and nursing interventions to prevent the occurrence or reduce the severity of these responses. ***(694)***

____

____

DRUG DOSAGE

Objectives

- Discuss drug dosage.
- Discuss minimal dosage.
- Discuss maximal dosage.
- Discuss toxic dosage.
- Discuss lethal dosage.
- Discuss potentiation.
- Explain the importance of an antagonist counteracting an agonist.
- Describe five factors that affect drug action in patients.

35. What are the terms used to describe drug dosage? ***(692)*** ______________________________

____

____

36. What factors can influence a patient's response to a medication? ***(693-694)*** ______________________________

____

____

37. Provide an example of a drug interaction. ***(692)*** ______________________________

____

____

MEDICATION ORDERS

Objectives

- Describe factors to consider in choosing routes of administration of medication.
- Describe the importance of accurate transcription of medication orders.
- Give the order of priority in the following terms: *stat, ASAP, now,* and *prn.*
- Explain what is meant by a *controlled substance.*
- List three ways medication orders are given.
- Discuss the use of The Joint Commission's abbreviations to prevent medication errors.

38. What is the difference between the trade name and the generic name of a drug? ***(695)*** ______________________________

____

____

39. A medication order should include the following: ***(696)*** ______________________________

____

____

40. Put the following terms in order of priority. ***(696)***
    a. prn _____
    b. now _____
    c. stat _____
    d. ASAP _____

41. Provide an example of a controlled substance and the special nursing considerations for storage and administration. *(696)*

____

____

42. Identify the different types of medication orders. *(696, 698)* ____

____

____

43. Identify the meaning of the following abbreviations. *(699)*

a. bid: ____

b. tid: ____

c. qid: ____

d. pc: ____

44. Provide an example of a form of medication for each of the following routes. *(702, 707, 712)*

a. Enteral: ____

b. Percutaneous: ____

c. Parenteral: ____

NURSING

Objectives

- Discuss the nurse's role and responsibilities in medication administration.
- List the "six rights" of drug administration.
- Discuss "Safety Tips from Nurse-Experts."

45. What are the "six rights" of medication administration? *(698-700)* ____

____

____

46. For the following situations, identify what the nurse should do. *(702)*

a. The prescriber's handwriting on the medication order sheet is hard to read. ____

____

____

b. One nurse asks another to administer to her patient the medications she has prepared. ___________

c. The dosage of the medication prescribed appears high. ___________

47. What are some of the guidelines for documentation of medication administration? ***(700-701)***___________

48. To prevent errors in the administration of medications, the nurse should do the following: ***(701-702)***

49. Identify home health safety information that should be included in a teaching plan for medication administration. ***(702)***

50. The nurse is preparing to administer oral medications to the patient. How are the following prepared? ***(703-704)***

a. Pills from a multidose vial: ___________

b. Tablets in unit-dose packages: ___________

51. The nurse is preparing to administer a liquid medication to the patient. ***(704-705)***

a. What equipment is needed? ___________

b. How is the liquid poured? ___________

c. How is the dosage amount checked? ____

____

52. The site selected for a transdermal patch application should be ____________________. *(707)*

53. Medication is to be administered via a nasogastric tube. *(705-706)*

a. It is critical for the nurse to check ____.

b. Equipment needed includes____

____

c. Medication administration is followed by ______________________________.

54. An example of a sublingual medication is ______________________________. *(712)*

55. For a rectal suppository, the nurse places the patient in ____________________ position and prepares the suppository for insertion by ______________________________. *(706-707)*

56. The nurse is evaluating the patient's administration of eye drops that are prescribed as gtt ii daily OD. Identify which actions indicate a need for correction: *(709)*
a. The patient touches the tip of the bottle to the eyelid. _____
b. One drop is administered to the left eye. _____
c. The drop is placed in the conjunctival sac. _____

57. In preparing to give ear drops to an adult patient, the nurse will pull the earlobe ____________________ ______________________________. *(710)*

58. For the following, identify the type of syringe or needle required. *(715-716, 726)*

a. Administration of 0.25 mL of medication: ____

b. An IM injection of 1.5 mL of a nonviscous medication to an average-sized adult: ____________________

____

c. Identify the angles of insertion and the types of injections that are administered in the following illustration.

i. ______________________________

ii. ______________________________

iii. ______________________________

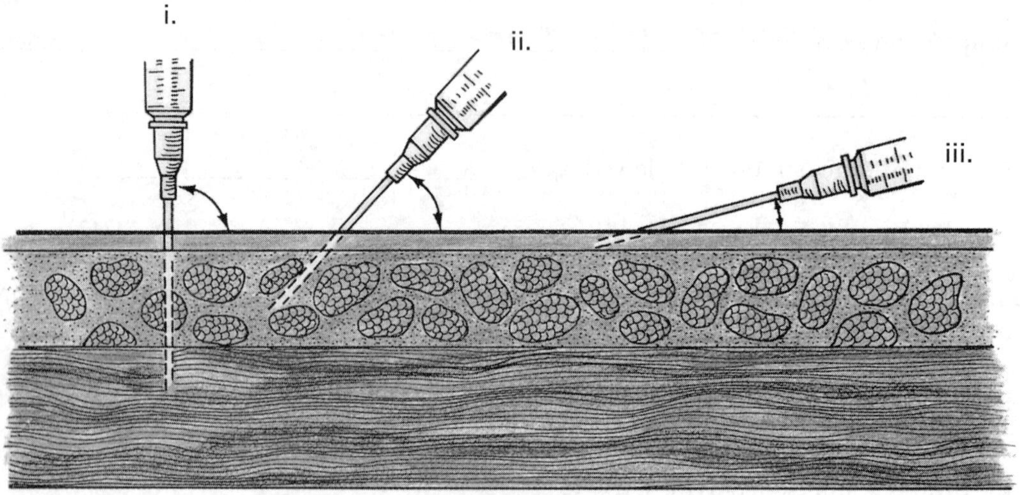

59. How can needlesticks be prevented? ***(718)*** ______________________________

____

____

60. What information should be included in a teaching plan for a patient who requires a metered-dose inhaler without a spacer? ***(713-714)***

____

____

61. What sites can be used for a subcutaneous injection? ***(724, 726)*** ______________________________

____

____

62. For a buccal medication, identify which action is correct: ***(714-715)***
   a. Placing the medication between the cheek and the gum _____
   b. Following the medication with a glass of water _____

63. Identify the common medications that are used in patient-controlled analgesia (PCA), and the nurse's responsibilities associated with this administration. ***(729-730)***

____

____

64. What is the procedure for mixing two medications in one syringe? ***(720)***______________________

____

____

65. A microdrip IV set delivers __________ drops/mL. ***(730-731)***

66. What are the responsibilities of the nurse in monitoring IV therapy? ***(731-732)***__________________

____

____

67. An IV is prescribed to infuse at 75 mL/hr. The drip factor is 10 gtt/mL. The rate of infusion should be ________________ gtt/min. ***(731)***

68. An IV is prescribed to infuse at 30 mL/hr with a microdrip set. The rate of infusion should be ________________ gtt/min. ***(731)***

69. An IV of 1000 mL is to infuse over 6 hours. The drip factor is 15 gtt/mL. The rate of infusion should be ________________ gtt/min. ***(731)***

70. For an IM injection, identify the following. ***(725)***

    a. Preparation of the site: ______________________________

    ____

    b. Action to take if blood is returned on aspiration: ______________________

    ____

71. What problem does polypharmacy pose for the older adult? ***(732)*** ______________________

____

____

Multiple Choice

72. An IV of 500 mL D_5W is to infuse over 4 hours. The administration set is 15 gtt/mL. How many gtt/min should the infusion run? ***(731)***
    1. 19 gtt/min
    2. 24 gtt/min
    3. 31 gtt/min
    4. 42 gtt/min

73. The nurse determines the location for an injection by identifying the greater trochanter of the femur, the anterosuperior iliac spine, and the iliac crest. The injection site being used by the nurse is the: ***(722)***
    1. rectus femoris.
    2. ventrogluteal.
    3. dorsogluteal.
    4. vastus lateralis.

74. Upon getting the assignment for the evening, the nurse notices that two patients on the unit have the same last name. The best way to prevent medication errors for these two patients is to first: ***(702)***
    1. ask the patients their names.
    2. check the patients' ID bands.
    3. ask another nurse about their identities.
    4. verify their names with the family members.

75. The nurse is working in the newborn nursery and will be giving vitamin K injections to the babies. The site preferred for these injections is the: ***(721)***
    1. deltoid.
    2. dorsogluteal.
    3. ventrogluteal.
    4. vastus lateralis.

76. When preparing a narcotic medication, the nurse drops the pill on the floor. The nurse should: ***(696)***
    1. discard the medication.
    2. notify the pharmacy.
    3. wipe off the medication and administer it.
    4. have another nurse witness the disposal of the pill.

77. The Z-track technique is used by the nurse when the patient is: ***(724)***
    1. extremely obese.
    2. less than 5 years old.
    3. receiving an irritating medication.
    4. having a large dosage of medication given.

78. A Mantoux skin test will be given to the patient. In selecting the site for this intradermal injection, the nurse assesses the: ***(724)***
    1. upper outer aspect of the arm.
    2. anterior aspect of the forearm.
    3. middle third of the anterior thigh.
    4. 2-inch diameter around the umbilicus.

79. How does the nurse determine what the drip factor is for an IV set? ***(731)***
    1. Ask the primary nurse.
    2. Calculate the IV rate.
    3. Look in a reference book.
    4. Check the IV tubing box.

80. The nurse is observing the patient self-administer medication with a metered-dose inhaler (MDI). What action by the patient requires correction and further instruction? ***(713-714)***
    1. Inhaling slowly
    2. Inhaling one puff with each inspiration
    3. Spraying the back of the throat
    4. Using an aerochamber spacer for a better fit

81. The nurse is aware that certain types of medications cannot be crushed for ease in administration. These medications include: (Select all that apply) ***(703-704)***
    1. timed-release capsules.
    2. tablets.
    3. sublingual tablets.
    4. enteric-coated tablets.

82. A patient being seen in an outpatient clinic asks the nurse why the hypnotic medication he was prescribed causes him to be awake most of the night. The nurse responds: "Sometimes medications have an unexpected response in an individual." What type of response to a medication is the nurse describing? ***(693)***
    1. Synergistic
    2. Antagonist
    3. Idiosyncratic
    4. Potentiative

83. Which route of drug administration will achieve the fastest onset of action? ***(712)***
    1. Intradermal
    2. Buccal
    3. Subcutaneous
    4. Enteral

Student Name________________________________ Date______________

chapter 24

Emergency First Aid Nursing

Answer Key: Textbook page references are provided as a guide for answering these questions. A complete answer key was provided for your instructor.

TERMS

Objective

- Define the key terms as listed.

1. Define the following terms.

   a. Cyanosis: ***(746)*** ________________________________

   b. Ecchymosis: ***(750)*** ________________________________

   c. Embolism: ***(748)*** ________________________________

   d. Epistaxis: ***(749)*** ________________________________

   e. Flail chest: ***(752)*** ________________________________

   f. Hematemesis: ***(750)*** ________________________________

   g. Pneumothorax: ***(751)*** ________________________________

   h. Stridor: ***(745)*** ________________________________

NURSING

Objectives

- List the priorities of assessment to be performed when arriving at a situation requiring first aid.
- Discuss moral, legal, and physical interventions of performing first aid.

2. How are the Good Samaritan laws related to emergency situations? *(738)*________________________

____

____

3. What is the nursing responsibility in assessment and treatment of a victim in an emergency? *(738-739)*

____

____

Multiple Choice

4. You arrive outside of the public library and find a person lying on the ground. The first action to take is to: *(738)*
   1. check if the victim is unconscious.
   2. check the carotid or brachial pulse.
   3. move the victim to a flat, hard surface.
   4. call to have someone activate the emergency medical system (call 911).

CARDIOPULMONARY RESUSCITATION (CPR)

Objectives

- List the reasons cardiopulmonary resuscitation (CPR) should be performed.
- Discuss the legal implications of CPR.
- List the steps in performing one-rescuer and two-rescuer CPR on the adult victim.
- List the steps in performing CPR on the infant and child.

5. When is CPR performed? *(739)*____

____

____

6. What are the "ABCs" for assessing the emergency patient? *(740)* ________________________

____

____

7. a. The nurse opens the patient's airway by doing the following: ***(740)***_______________

____

____

   b. If a neck injury is suspected, the nurse opens the airway by doing the following: ***(740)***_______________

____

____

8. What is the proper rate of mouth-to-mouth ventilation for an adult victim? ***(742)*** _______________

____

____

9. For CPR, provide the following information. ***(741-742)***

   a. Check the pulse at the: _______________.

   b. If no pulse is found:_______________.

   c. Placement of hands: _______________

   d. Depress the sternum for an adult:_______________.

   e. Ratio of compressions to breaths: _______________

10. Number the steps for one-rescuer adult CPR in the order that they should be performed. ***(742)***
   a. Check for obstruction if unable to ventilate. _____
   b. Determine breathlessness. _____
   c. Reevaluate the victim after four full cycles. _____
   d. Call for help. _____
   e. Position the victim and open the airway. _____
   f. Begin compressions. _____
   g. Determine unresponsiveness. _____
   h. Provide two slow breaths. _____
   i. Determine pulselessness. _____

11. Breaths are given at _________ seconds each to minimize the chance of _______________
_______________. ***(741)***

12. For pediatric CPR, if help cannot be obtained right away, the rescuer should first _______________
_______________. ***(743)***

13. For pediatric CPR, identify the following. ***(743-744)***

	Infant	Child
a. Where the pulse is checked		
b. Ratio of compressions to breaths		

Multiple Choice

14. For CPR to an adult victim, a single rescuer provides breaths at a rate of: ***(742)***
    1. 8 per minute.
    2. 12 per minute.
    3. 20 per minute.
    4. 24 per minute.

AIRWAY

Objectives

- Name the steps in performing the Heimlich maneuver on conscious and unconscious victims.
- Discuss management of airway obstruction in the child and the infant.

15. In a situation involving a possible airway obstruction, the victim is coughing. What should the nurse do? ***(744)***

____

____

16. a. Describe the procedure for the Heimlich maneuver for a conscious adult victim. ***(745)*** _______________

____

____

b. What is the difference in the procedure for an unconscious victim? ***(745)*** _______________

____

____

17. How is the airway clearance procedure for an infant different? ***(745-746)*** _______________

____

____

Multiple Choice

18. A sign or symptom of a foreign body airway obstruction that necessitates immediate attention is the: *(744-745)*
    1. ability of the victim to speak.
    2. ability of the victim to cough forcefully.
    3. presence of wheezing between coughs.
    4. presence of a high-pitched inspiratory noise.

19. When performing the Heimlich maneuver, the fist should be placed: *(745)*
    1. over the ribs.
    2. over the sternum.
    3. slightly above the navel.
    4. over the xiphoid process.

20. For an unconscious adult victim with a foreign body airway obstruction, a nurse should: *(745)*
    1. apply a series of three quick chest thrusts.
    2. repeat chest thrusts continuously 10 times.
    3. perform finger sweeps between abdominal thrusts.
    4. attempt to ventilate the victim after each abdominal thrust.

SHOCK

Objectives

- Discuss the signs and symptoms of shock.
- List nursing interventions to treat shock.

21. Identify the different types of shock. *(746)* ______________________________

____

____

22. What assessments lead the nurse to believe that a victim or patient is in shock? *(746-747)* ____________

____

____

23. Select all of the following interventions that are appropriate for a victim or patient who is in shock. *(747)*
    a. Establish airway. _____
    b. Control bleeding. _____
    c. Keep the head elevated. _____
    d. Cover the patient. _____
    e. Provide fluids. _____
    f. Administer over-the-counter analgesics. _____

INJURY

Objectives

- Discuss three methods of controlling hemorrhage.
- Define four types of wounds.
- Discuss treatment of wounds.
- Discuss methods of treating three common types of poisonings.
- List the characteristics of assessment of bone, joint, and muscle injuries.
- Discuss emergency care for suspected injuries.

24. If the victim has a suspected head, neck, or spinal injury, the nurse rescuer should: *(760)* ____________

____

____

25. What are the effects of blood loss on the body? *(747)* ____________

____

____

26. What are the nursing interventions for a victim or patient who is bleeding? *(748-750)* ____________

____

____

27. a. Epistaxis is fairly common. What are the nursing interventions for an individual experiencing this problem? *(749)*

____

____

b. Identify signs and symptoms that are specific to internal bleeding. *(749)* ____________

____

____

28. The individual has a closed wound. What are the appropriate nursing interventions? *(750)* ____________

____

____

29. For the treatment of the following types of open wounds, provide an example of a specific nursing intervention. ***(751)***

    a. Puncture wound: ______________________________

    b. Avulsion: ______________________________

30. The victim had an accident and now has a piece of wood protruding from the chest. The nurse should: ***(751-752)***

    ____

31. What interventions should be taken for an individual with a sucking wound to the chest? ***(751-752)***

    ____

32. What is the first action to take when there is a suspected poisoning? ***(753-754)*** ______________________________

33. For the a victim of a poisoning, identify the assessments that may be made for the following body systems. ***(753)***

    a. Respiratory: ______________________________

    b. Neurologic: ______________________________

    c. Gastrointestinal: ______________________________

34. The nurse is instructed to provide water to a poisoning victim to dilute the substance ingested. Identify how much water should be given to an adult and how much to a child. ***(753-754)***

    ____

35. The nurse is instructed to give syrup of ipecac to a poisoning victim. Identify the amounts of ipecac that should be given to an adult and to a child. *(753-754)*

____

____

36. Vomiting is not induced if an individual has ingested ____________________. *(753-754)*

37. An employee has been exposed to a chemical that may be absorbed through the skin. The nurse should assist by ______________________________. *(754)*

38. After assessing the ABCs in a victim with a bone injury, the nurse should ____________________ ______________________________. *(758)*

39. What are the interventions associated with the following acronym? *(759)*

R ____

I ____

C ____

E ____

40. Identify areas that should be included in a teaching plan for safety and response to emergency in the home environment. *(765)*

____

____

Multiple Choice

41. An appropriate action for a patient having a severe reaction to an insect bite is to first: *(754-755)*
    1. apply a constricting band proximal to the wound.
    2. wash the wound carefully with mild soap and water.
    3. keep the affected part elevated above the level of the heart.
    4. remove the stinger, if visible, with tweezers.

THERMAL INJURY

Objectives

- Define three types of burns.
- Discuss the nursing interventions in the first aid treatment of burns.
- Describe the nursing interventions of heat and cold emergencies.

42. a. What are the signs and symptoms of heat exhaustion? *(756)* ____________________

____

____

b. A priority nursing action for the victim of heat stroke is: *(756)* ____________________

____

____

43. a. What are the signs and symptoms of hypothermia? *(757)* ____________________

____

____

b. For the conscious victim with hypothermia, intervention includes: *(757)* ____________________

____

____

44. Describe the three different types of burns. *(759-760)* ____________________

____

____

45. What are the nursing interventions for a patient or victim with a moderate burn? *(760-761)* ____________________

____

____

Multiple Choice

46. An adult patient has severe burns to the anterior and posterior thorax and both upper extremities. Using the rule of nines, how much of the body surface is burned? *(759)*
    1. 18%
    2. 36%
    3. 54%
    4. 63%

TERRORISM AND BIOTERRORISM

Objectives

- Discuss features that should alert you to the possibility of a bioterrorism-related outbreak.
- Discuss high-risk syndromes of bioterrorism.

47. A group of signs and symptoms resulting from a common cause that presents a clinical picture of a disease is known as ____________________________. ***(762)***

Multiple Choice

48. The nurse working in a local health department knows that a bioterrorist attack that can occur via foodborne route is: ***(762)***
    1. anthrax.
    2. botulism.
    3. plague.
    4. smallpox.

Student Name______________________ Date__________

Health Promotion and Pregnancy

chapter 25

Answer Key: Textbook page references are provided as a guide for answering these questions. A complete answer key was provided for your instructor.

TERMS

Objective

- Define the key terms as listed.

1. Define the following terms.

   a. Amniocentesis: ***(783)*** ______________________________

   ____

   b. Gravida: ***(788)*** ______________________________

   ____

   c. Morula: ***(769)*** ______________________________

   ____

   d. Para: ***(788)*** ______________________________

   ____

   e. Teratogenic agent: ***(770)*** ______________________________

   ____

   f. Ectopic pregnancy: ***(769)*** ______________________________

   ____

PHYSIOLOGY

Objectives

- Explain the physiology of conception.
- Discuss the anatomical and physiologic alterations that occur during pregnancy.

2. Fertilization occurs in the ___________. The new cell is called the ______________. *(768-769)*

3. Enzymes are secreted by the _______________ to allow for implantation. Implantation occurs in the ______________________ of the uterus. *(769)*

4. The embryonic stage of development lasts for _______ weeks. After this initial stage, the embryo is called the ______________________. *(769-770)*

5. What is the role of the placenta? *(770)* ____

____

____

6. Identify the usual time that the following developments occur in the mother or the fetus. *(771-780)*

    a. Morning sickness: ____

    b. Genitalia are defined: ____

    c. Swallowing and sucking begin: ____

    d. Stretch marks, redness, and darkening of the skin occur: ______________________________

    e. Surfactant forms in the lungs: ____

7. What is the function of amniotic fluid? *(770, 781)* ____________________________________

____

____

8. What maternal antibodies are usually transferred to the fetus? *(779)* _________________________

____

____

9. What is the highest level of the uterus at full term? *(785)* ______________________________

____

____

10. The usual duration of an uncomplicated pregnancy is ___________. This time is divided into _________________. *(785)*

Multiple Choice

11. The woman asks the nurse when the baby's heartbeat can be heard. The nurse responds by saying, "The heartbeat can be heard by week _____." *(781)*
    1. 6
    2. 8
    3. 10
    4. 16

12. The very first fetal movements, characterized as "bubbling through a straw" in the stomach, may be experienced at: *(773)*
    1. 4 weeks.
    2. 6 weeks.
    3. 10 weeks.
    4. 18 weeks.

13. The woman has entered her sixteenth week of pregnancy and asks the nurse, "How is the baby growing?" The nurse provides accurate information by informing the mother that the baby will have: *(773)*
    1. development of head hair.
    2. attained a weight of about 27 ounces.
    3. settled into a favorite position.
    4. formed all organs and structures.

HEALTH ASSESSMENT

Objectives

- Differentiate among the presumptive, possible, and positive signs of pregnancy.
- Discuss the common discomforts of pregnancy.
- List the danger signs that might occur during pregnancy.
- Discuss cultural practices and beliefs that may affect ongoing health care during pregnancy.
- Identify the components of antepartal assessment.

14. The mother asks the nurse why she is having such terrible backaches. The nurse responds by telling the woman that: *(780)*

    ____

    ____

15. A basic prenatal examination usually includes: *(786)* ______________________________

    ____

    ____

16. What are the important aspects of genetic counseling? *(785-786)* ______________________

    ____

    ____

17. An obstetric nursing assessment should include information on the following about the patient: ***(786)***

____

____

18. In determination of pregnancy, identify if the following are presumptive, probable, or positive signs of pregnancy. ***(786-787)***

    a. Uterine enlargement: ______________________

    b. Quickening: ______________________

    c. Positive pregnancy test: ______________________

    d. Amenorrhea: ______________________

    e. Nausea and vomiting: ______________________

    f. Goodell's sign: ______________________

    g. Visualization: ______________________

    h. Breast changes: ______________________

    i. Hegar's sign: ______________________

19. The patient had her last menstrual period (LMP) on August 18. Using Naegele's rule, when is the estimated date of birth (EDB)? ***(787)***

____

____

20. What is the usual preparation for an ultrasound? ***(782)*** ______________________

____

____

21. What tests are used to determine the well-being of the fetus? ***(781)*** ______________________

____

____

22. Define the parity of the following woman using the GTPAL system: She has been pregnant four times, delivered three full-term infants, had no abortions or preterm deliveries, and has three living children. ***(788)***

____

____

23. Describe some of the common skin changes that occur during pregnancy. ***(783)***________________

____

____

24. Psychological aspects that should be considered during the pregnancy are: ***(795-796)***________________

____

____

Multiple Choice

25. The patient believes that she is pregnant. On examination, Chadwick's sign is found. This is: ***(786)***
    1. a sensation of fetal movement.
    2. softening of the cervix.
    3. darkened pigmentation of the cheeks.
    4. purplish discoloration of the vagina, vulva, and cervix.

26. An early amniocentesis is performed to determine: ***(783)***
    1. fetal distress.
    2. fetal lung maturity.
    3. presence of intrauterine infection.
    4. presence of biochemical abnormalities.

NURSING

Objectives

- Describe nutritional requirements during pregnancy.
- Identify nursing diagnoses relevant to care of the prenatal patient.

27. What interventions are appropriate for the following maternal discomforts? ***(771-780)***

    a. Morning sickness: ________________

    ____

    b. Headaches: ________________

    ____

    c. Leg cramps: ________________

    ____

    d. Indigestion: ________________

    ____

28. Identify five drugs that the mother should avoid during pregnancy. ***(771-780)*** ______________________

____

____

29. Identify the areas of counseling for self-care on the trimester checklist. ***(788)*** ______________________

____

____

30. What signs and symptoms should the nurse instruct the woman to report during the pregnancy? ***(790)***

____

____

31. In addition to selected medications, the nurse instructs the woman to avoid the following during the pregnancy. ***(771-780)***

____

____

32. For the following systems, identify common problems that may develop during pregnancy and interventions to relieve them. ***(793)***

    a. Gastrointestinal: ______________________

    ____

    b. Urinary: ______________________

    ____

33. a. Identify two common discomforts experienced during the third trimester, and the teaching for self-care for each one. ***(792)***

    ____

    ____

    b. Provide examples of complementary and alternative therapies that a woman may use to relieve discomfort. ***(792)***

    ____

    ____

34. The usual position of comfort for the woman to sleep or rest is ______________. ***(794)***

35. What counseling is appropriate regarding sexual activity for the pregnant woman? *(794-795)* ________

____

____

36. Identify an example of a cultural or ethnic consideration for pregnancy. *(798)* ________

____

____

37. Identify at least three general prenatal nursing interventions. *(800)* ________

____

____

38. Formulate a nursing diagnosis, patient outcome, and nursing interventions for a woman experiencing a nonrisk pregnancy. *(798-799)*

____

____

____

____

Multiple Choice

39. The nurse informs the patient to report which of the following during the pregnancy? *(790)*
    1. Reddened palms
    2. Urinary frequency
    3. Swelling of the face
    4. Dilated capillaries on the skin

40. The patient asks the nurse what can be done specifically about the ptyalism that the physician told her about. The nurse instructs the patient to: *(790)*
    1. eat small, frequent meals.
    2. suck on hard candy.
    3. sit up after eating.
    4. avoid eating spicy foods.

41. Which of the following should be included in a plan for prenatal exercise? *(795)*
    1. Exercise one time per week.
    2. Exercise for 30 minutes, then rest.
    3. Keep moving after exercising.
    4. Reduce exercise sharply 4 weeks before the due date.

42. The pregnant patient has been instructed to count fetal movements (kick count). The patient demonstrates understanding of the procedure if she states: (Select all that apply) ***(790)***
    1. "I should count all movements during a 24-hour period."
    2. "I should choose a time of the day when I can sit or lie down quietly to count the movements."
    3. "My baby should move at least 10 times in a 12-hour period."
    4. "I should feel the baby move at least 4 times after I have eaten a meal."

43. After teaching the patient how to perform Kegel exercises, the patient asks the nurse how often she should perform these exercises. The nurse's best response is: ***(794)***
    1. "The exercises are most beneficial if you perform them 10 times in a row, at least 3 times a day."
    2. "If you could perform the exercises 100 times in a row you will only have to do them once a day."
    3. "As many times as you think will help you."
    4. "Every patient is different, so we will need to discuss this with your doctor."

Student Name______________________________________ **Date**____________________

Labor and Delivery

chapter **26**

Answer Key: Textbook page references are provided as a guide for answering these questions. A complete answer key was provided for your instructor.

IMPENDING LABOR

Objectives

- Explain the five factors that affect the labor process.
- Discuss the signs and symptoms of impending labor.
- Distinguish between true and false labor.

1. Identify the signs of impending labor. ***(805-806)*** ____

2. Provide a few examples of true versus false labor. ***(806)*** ____

3. The woman is asking about delivering somewhere other than a hospital. The nurse provides the following information: ***(804)***

PROCESS OF LABOR AND DELIVERY

Objectives

- Discuss fetopelvic disproportion.
- Describe the "powers" involved in labor and delivery.
- Identify the mechanisms of labor.
- Identify the stages of labor.

4. The five P's of labor are: ***(807)*** ____

5. What influence does the passageway have on labor and delivery? ***(807-808)***________________________

6. What is meant by each of the following? ***(809-810)***

   a. Fetal attitude: ________________________

   b. Fetal lie: ________________________

   c. Fetal presentation: ________________________

   d. Fetal position: ________________________

7. How is the position of the fetus determined? ***(809)***________________________

8. a. Identify what the following abbreviations indicate. ***(810)***

   i. ROP: ________________________

   ii. LOA: ________________________

   iii. LSA: ________________________

   b. What position is illustrated? ________________________

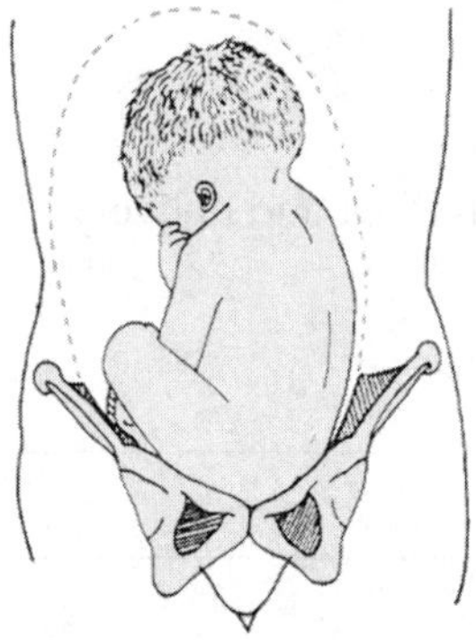

9. a. What is the normal fetal heart rate? _______________ *(822)*

   b. What do the following changes in fetal heart rate indicate?

      i. Late deceleration: ______________________________

      ii. Variable deceleration: ______________________________

10. What signs precede the delivery of the placenta, and what is done after the delivery of the placenta? ***(817, 819)***

    ____

    ____

11. What is the usual frequency and duration of uterine contractions, and what is their purpose? ***(818-819)***

    ____

    ____

12. What position(s) are most effective for the first and second stages of labor? ***(818-819)***______________

    ____

    ____

13. Put the following steps in the mechanism of labor in the order in which they occur for vertex positions. ***(816)***
    a. Extension _____
    b. Flexion _____
    c. Descent _____
    d. Internal rotation _____
    e. Expulsion _____
    f. Engagement _____
    g. External rotation and restitution _____

Multiple Choice

14. On examination, the patient is found to be 8 cm dilated with contractions every 3 minutes that last for 70 seconds. She also does not want to communicate with the nurse or her coach. This is point in labor is described as: ***(818)***
    1. early latent phase.
    2. mid to active phase.
    3. transitional phase.
    4. second stage.

15. A woman who is in the mid to active phase of labor will be expected to have: ***(818)***
    1. 2-cm cervical dilation.
    2. contractions every 4 minutes.
    3. a desire to ambulate.
    4. very mild, easily controlled pain.

16. The second stage of labor begins at the: *(818)*
    1. onset of contractions.
    2. rupture of the amniotic sac.
    3. dilation of the cervix to 10 cm.
    4. delivery of the placenta.

17. When coaching the patient through the early or latent phase of labor, the nurse uses the breathing technique of: *(819)*
    1. shallow panting.
    2. slow, deep chest or abdominal breathing.
    3. acceleration through contractions.
    4. holding the breath for 5 seconds and exhaling.

18. The nurse informs the mother that the membranes have ruptured if the results of the nitrazine test are: *(805)*
    1. yellow, pH 4.0.
    2. olive yellow, pH 5.5.
    3. olive green, pH 6.0.
    4. blue green, pH 6.5.

INTERVENTIONS—NURSING AND MEDICAL

Objectives

- Describe the assessment for labor and delivery.
- Explain breathing techniques beneficial for the patient in labor.
- Identify nursing diagnoses relevant to the woman in labor.
- Outline medical interventions related to labor and delivery.
- Discuss nursing interventions related to labor and delivery.

19. The admission assessment to the labor area includes: *(828)* ______________________________

____

____

20. How is fetal status monitored? *(819-826)* ______________________________

____

____

21. The nurse suspects fetal distress because of the presence of: *(826)*______________________________

____

____

22. The monitor indicates a late deceleration. The patient is positioned: ***(822)***

23. Identify the interventions for a prolapsed cord. ***(838)***

24. For regional anesthesia during labor, what are the possible effects on the fetus and the appropriate nursing interventions? ***(833)***

25. The patient requires an emergency cesarean section and will be given general anesthesia. The nurse is aware that the adverse effects of this type of anesthesia include: ***(833)***

26. The nurse's response to the husband or coach is very important. How can the nurse provide a positive experience for the mother's support person? ***(830)***

27. Nursing assessment of a patient's status throughout labor includes: ***(835)***

28. a. What is the goal of the breathing techniques that are used throughout labor? ***(837)***

    b. The patient should avoid the following type of breathing during pushing: ***(837)***

29. Medical intervention during labor includes induction. Why is this implemented, and what methods are used? *(836)*

30. Identify two nursing diagnoses for a woman in labor. *(835)*

31. a. Identify a nursing diagnosis for a woman who has had a cesarean delivery. *(838)*

    b. Identify a priority goal for a patient with this nursing diagnosis. *(838)*

32. What is the purpose of an episiotomy? *(819)*

33. For the fourth stage of labor, what are the nursing assessments, and how often are they done? *(819)*

34. Provide at least one example of a medication commonly used for pain relief during labor, possible side effects, and associated nursing interventions. *(820-822)*

35. The baby is assessed after birth and the following are noted: heart rate 124/minute; respiratory effort good, crying; some flexion of the extremities; grimacing; body pink, extremities bluish. Based on this information, what is the Apgar score? *(827)*

36. Care of the baby after birth includes: ***(826-827)*** ______________________________

____

____

37. Complications of a precipitous labor are: ***(834)*** ______________________________

____

____

Multiple Choice

38. The nurse recognizes that which of the following is an acceptable practice in labor and delivery? ***(828)***
    1. Maintenance of a full bladder
    2. Maintenance of supine position
    3. Ambulation before membrane rupture
    4. Administration of enemas to a patient with vaginal bleeding

39. The patient is receiving intravenous (IV) Pitocin for the stimulation of labor. The nurse notes that the fetal heart rate (FHR) is dropping below 100/min. The nurse should: ***(837)***
    1. stop the infusion.
    2. slow down the infusion.
    3. monitor the FHR for 5 to 10 full cycles of contractions.
    4. do nothing as this is an expected response.

40. Assessment of the amniotic fluid reveals yellow staining. The nurse is aware that this is associated with: ***(826)***
    1. intrauterine infection.
    2. fetal hemolytic disease.
    3. abruptio placentae.
    4. meconium passage with a breech birth.

41. A birth plan includes the discussion of possible options related to: (Select all that apply) ***(804)***
    1. labor.
    2. delivery.
    3. the postpartum period.
    4. when to plan on becoming pregnant.

42. The patient demonstrates understanding of prenatal class discussions regarding the term "lightening" when she states: ***(805)***
    1. "I should be alarmed if I feel like the baby has "dropped" into my pelvis a couple of weeks before my due date."
    2. "During the end of my first trimester I will feel movement of the fetus."
    3. "About 2 weeks before my delivery I can expect to feel the baby settle into my pelvis."
    4. "The presence of meconium is a dangerous sign."

43. The nurse is aware that the pregnant patient will often experience an irregular tightening of the uterus beginning in the first trimester and continuing throughout the pregnancy, known as: ***(806)***
    1. restitution.
    2. Braxton-Hicks contractions.
    3. effacement.
    4. engagement.

Student Name____________________ Date__________

chapter 27

Care of the Mother and Newborn

Answer Key: Textbook page references are provided as a guide for answering these questions. A complete answer key was provided for your instructor.

POSTPARTUM

Objectives

- Describe postpartum assessment of the mother.
- Identify the physiologic changes that occur in the postpartum period.
- Discuss the psychosocial adaptations that occur postpartum.
- Explain parent-child attachment (bonding).

1. Identify the height of the fundus through the process of involution. ***(842)***

    a. Immediately after delivery: ____________________

    b. 12 hours after delivery: ____________________

    c. 24 to 48 hours after delivery: ____________________

    d. 1 week after delivery: ____________________

    e. 6 weeks after delivery: ____________________

2. Identify the types of lochia and the characteristics from delivery through the first 14 days after delivery. ***(842-843)***

3. What type of nonlochia bleeding should be reported right away? ***(843)*** ____________________

4. What physiologic processes are involved in lactation? ***(844)*** ____________________

5. Identify the changes that occur in the following body systems after delivery. ***(844-846)***

   a. Cardiovascular: ______________________________

   ____

   b. Urinary: ______________________________

   ____

   c. Gastrointestinal: ______________________________

   ____

   d. Endocrine: ______________________________

   ____

   e. Integumentary: ______________________________

   ____

6. Identify postpartum danger signs. ***(847)***

   a. Maternal: ______________________________

   ____

   b. Parent-child: ______________________________

   ____

7. What are the basic nutritional needs of the postpartum patient? ***(851)*** ______________________________

   ____

   ____

8. For hygienic care: ***(851-852)***

   a. Following a vaginal delivery, women should avoid ______________________________.

   b. Following a cesarean delivery, women should avoid ______________________________.

9. A slight temperature within 24 hours of delivery is usually indicative of ______________________________. ***(853)***

10. After delivery, the mother's sleep and rest is usually disturbed by ______________________________. ***(854)***

11. Provide an example of a specific cultural practice that occurs during the postpartum period. ***(864)***

    ____

    ____

Multiple Choice

12. The mother has lost a large volume of blood and appears to be in hypovolemic shock following the delivery. The nurse implements an appropriate action by: ***(843)***
    1. raising the head of the bed to 80 degrees.
    2. discontinuing the oxytocic agent in the intravenous (IV) infusion.
    3. massaging the uterus firmly and continuously.
    4. providing oxygen by face mask at 8 to 10 L/min.

NEWBORN

Objectives

- Describe the assessment of the normal newborn.
- Identify the physical characteristics of the normal newborn.
- Identify normal reflexes observed in the newborn.
- Explain common variations that may be observed in the newborn.
- Describe the behavioral characteristics of the newborn.
- Discuss nutritional needs and feeding of the newborn.

13. For newborn assessment, specify the normal parameters of the following. ***(866-872)***

    a. Relationship of head to chest circumference: ____________________

    b. Temperature: ____________________

    c. Pulse: ____________________

    d. Respirations: ____________________

    e. Blood pressure: ____________________

14. Indicate for the following assessment findings whether they are expected (normal) or unexpected. ***(866-872)***

    a. Acrocyanosis within the first 7 days: ____________________

    b. Jaundice within the first 24 hours: ____________________

    c. Lanugo: ____________________

    d. Milia: ____________________

    e. Nevus flammeus: ____________________

    f. Palpable posterior fontanelle: ____________________

    g. Low-set ears: ____________________

    h. Epstein's pearls: ____________________

    i. Molding: ____________________

j. Two-vessel umbilical cord: ____________________

k. Syndactyly: ____________________

l. Gynecomastia: ____________________

m. Asymmetric popliteal folds: ____________________

15. a. Identify some of the important safety measures that should be implemented when working with a newborn. *(865)*

____

____

b. To prevent infant abduction, what measures are implemented? *(865)* ____________________

____

____

16. Match the terms in Column A with the appropriate definition or description in Column B. *(870-872)*

Column A	**Column B**
_____ Moro's reflex	a. Toes fan out with stroking of the foot.
_____ Tonic neck reflex	b. Trunk is flexed and pelvis swings to the side on which the spine is stimulated.
_____ Babinski's reflex	c. Change in equilibrium causes flexion and abduction of the extremities.
_____ Galant's reflex	d. Arm and leg extend on side of the body toward which the head is turned.

17. What are the daily nutritional and fluid needs of the infant? *(874)* ____________________

____

____

18. For feeding the newborn: *(874)*

a. What should be done if the baby is allergic to a milk-based formula? ____________________

____

____

b. What is the purpose of burping the baby? ____________________

____

____

19. How can the nurse reduce the heat loss in a newborn? *(875)* ______________________________

____

____

20. Urine and bowel elimination is expected in the newborn within _______ of the delivery. *(876)*

21. Identify the characteristics of the newborn's bowel elimination. *(876)*

    a. Meconium: ______________________________

    ____

    b. Transitional: ______________________________

    ____

    c. Breastfed: ______________________________

    ____

    d. Abnormal: ______________________________

    ____

22. Most newborns sleep ________ hours each day. *(877)*

23. What is the infant's form of communication? *(877)* ______________________________

____

____

Multiple Choice

24. The nurse identifies that the mother requires additional teaching if, for the care of the umbilicus, she: *(875)*
    1. gives a tub bath in the first 3 days after delivery.
    2. uses alcohol on the stump daily.
    3. folds the diaper down from the umbilicus.
    4. reports a foul odor or redness from the stump.

25. Care of the circumcision includes: *(875-876)*
    1. removing the yellow crusting right away.
    2. fan-folding the diaper.
    3. applying alcohol to the area.
    4. using petroleum gauze under the Plastibell.

26. An appropriate technique to teach the new mother about the baby's bath is: *(875)*
    1. vigorous removal of the vernix caseosa.
    2. use of plain water on the perineal area.
    3. washing the baby twice daily.
    4. having the bath water at 100° F.

NURSING

Objectives

- Discuss the nursing responsibilities during the postpartum period.
- Explain the importance of teaching personal and infant care.
- Discuss nursing interventions for the circumcised newborn.

27. The nurse assesses the episiotomy for the following: *(845)* ______________________________

____

____

28. Before checking the fundus, the nurse asks the patient to ____________________. *(857)*

29. Before ambulating a patient for the first time after delivery, the nurse should do the following: *(853)*

____

____

30. What types of medications are given to the mother and the newborn in the postpartum period? *(855-856)*

____

____

31. How can the nurse assess the amount of lochia? *(857)* ______________________________

____

____

32. Engorgement is treated as follows. *(857-858)*

    a. Breastfeeding mother: ______________________________

    ____

    b. Nonbreastfeeding mother: ______________________________

    ____

33. The patient asks the nurse if breastfeeding is really better for the baby. The nurse informs the patient that the benefits of breastfeeding are the following: *(859)*

____

____

34. What does the acronym BUBBLE-HE for postpartum assessment mean? *(858)*____________________

____

____

35. Describe assessment of the fundus during the recovery period for each of the following cases. ***(854-857)***

    a. Technique for cesarean delivery:________________________________

    ____

    b. Atony is noted:____

    ____

36. The emotional state of the mother changes in the postpartum period. What are the phases that many women go through? ***(860-861)***

____

____

37. What assessment findings would lead the nurse to believe that the patient is having postpartum emotional problems? ***(860)***

____

____

38. Identify two nursing diagnoses and outcomes for the postpartum patient. ***(862)*** ____________________

____

____

39. What behaviors, if observed by the nurse, indicate that the parents are bonding with the infant? ***(847)***

____

____

Multiple Choice

40. The nurse is discussing sexuality with the new mother. Appropriate information to provide is that: ***(848)***
    1. menses usually returns in 3 to 5 months.
    2. breastfeeding acts as an effective contraceptive.
    3. ongoing discomfort and bleeding are expected with sexual activity.
    4. resumption of sexual activity should wait until after the first postpartum office visit.

41. In teaching the patient about breastfeeding, the nurse informs the mother to: ***(850)***
    1. use only one breast during each feeding.
    2. have the baby nurse for 5 minutes.
    3. put as much of the areolar tissue into the baby's mouth as possible.
    4. pull the breast straight away from the baby's mouth to break the suction seal.

42. The nurse is teaching the patient about the signs and symptoms that should be reported to the health care provider. The patient is instructed to notify the physician if, after 5 days from the delivery date, the patient experiences: ***(849)***
    1. a temperature of 99° F.
    2. lochia that is light pink-brown in color.
    3. breast tenderness and redness.
    4. a fundus that feels like a softball.

43. The patient has opted to bottle feed her newborn. The nurse is confident that the patient has understood discharge teaching related to breast engorgement when the patient states: (Select all that apply) ***(857)***
    1. "I will most likely not experience breast engorgement if I wear a firm-fitting bra."
    2. "If I experience engorgement, I should use ice to try to get some relief."
    3. "Engorgement will most likely occur about 3 days from my delivery date."
    4. "Breast engorgement is not really very common for most women after delivering their baby."

44. The nurse is caring for an infant that was born at 30 weeks of gestation. The mother asks the nurse, "What is all that hair on my baby's body called?" The correct response is: ***(867)***
    1. vernix caseosa.
    2. lanugo.
    3. lochia.
    4. fontanelle.

45. A normal variation in the physical characteristics of a newborn that the parents should not be alarmed in seeing is: (Select all that apply) ***(866-872)***
    1. acrocyanosis in an infant that is 5 days old.
    2. the harlequin sign in a 2-day-old infant.
    3. jaundice during the first 24 hours after delivery.
    4. Epstein's pearls on the hard palate of a 2-week-old infant.

Student Name____ **Date**__________________

chapter 28

Care of the High-Risk Mother, Newborn, and Family with Special Needs

Answer Key: Textbook page references are provided as a guide for answering these questions. A complete answer key was provided for your instructor.

TERMS

Objective

- Define the key terms as listed.

1. Define the following terms.

   a. Cerclage: ***(890)*** ____

   b. Erythroblastosis fetalis: ***(918)*** ____

   c. Hydramnios: ***(894)*** ____

   d. Kernicterus: ***(918)*** ____

   e. Tocolytic therapy: ***(890)*** ____

   f. TORCH: ***(902)*** ____

HIGH-RISK PREGNANCY

Objectives

- List those conditions that increase maternal and fetal risk.
- Discuss bleeding disorders that can occur during pregnancy.
- Identify diagnostic tests used to determine high-risk situations.

- Describe the HELLP syndrome.
- Discuss pregnancy-induced hypertension.
- Identify preexisting maternal health conditions that influence pregnancy.
- List the infectious disease most likely to cause serious complications.
- Discuss the care of the pregnant adolescent.

2. Identify examples of high-risk factors in pregnancy for the following areas. ***(883)***

   a. Biophysical: ____________________

   ____

   b. Psychosocial: ____________________

   ____

   c. Sociodemographic: ____________________

   ____

   d. Environmental: ____________________

   ____

3. Identify factors that place the postpartum mother and infant at risk. ***(884)*** ____________________

   ____

   ____

4. For hyperemesis gravidarum, identify the signs and symptoms, medical treatment, and nursing interventions. ***(884)***

   a. Signs and symptoms: ____________________

   ____

   b. Medical treatment: ____________________

   ____

   c. Nursing interventions: ____________________

   ____

5. The mother has just had twins, a boy and a girl. This is the result of the fertilization of ____________________. The term for this is ____________________. ***(885-886)***

6. What are the maternal and the fetal risks in a multifetal pregnancy? ***(886)*** ____________________

   ____

   ____

7. Assessment of the presence of a hydatidiform mole is based on: ***(886-887)*** ________________________

____

____

8. Ninety-five percent of ectopic pregnancies occur in the ________________________. ***(887)***

9. For an ectopic pregnancy, identify the signs and symptoms, the medical treatment, and the nursing interventions. ***(888)***

   a. Signs and symptoms: ________________________

   ____

   ____

   b. Medical treatment: ________________________

   ____

   ____

   c. Nursing interventions: ________________________

   ____

   ____

10. A spontaneous abortion may be the result of: ***(888-889)*** ________________________

____

____

11. The nurse instructs the patient on the treatment for a threatened abortion, which includes: ***(889)*** ________

____

____

12. Treatment for an incompetent cervix usually includes: ***(890)*** ________________________

____

____

13. a. Diagnosis of placenta previa is made when the patient exhibits: ***(891)*** ________________________

   ____

   ____

b. The nurse instructs the patient to expect that treatment for placenta previa may include: ***(891)*** ______

______

______

14. a. Medical management of abruptio placentae includes: ***(892-893)*** ______

______

______

b. A priority nursing diagnosis and interventions for a patient with abruptio placentae are: ***(892-893)***

______

______

15. What are the classic signs and symptoms of pregnancy-induced hypertension (PIH)? ***(896)*** ______

______

______

16. Medical management and nursing interventions for PIH usually include: ***(897, 899-900)*** ______

______

______

17. a. The nurse is assessing the postpartum patient and suspects a hemorrhage as a result of observing: ***(894-895)***

______

______

b. Treatment for postpartum hemorrhage includes: ***(894-895)*** ______

______

______

18. a. What signs and symptoms may be exhibited by the patient who is experiencing disseminated intravascular coagulation (DIC)? ***(893-894)***

______

______

b. What diagnostic tests are usually performed to determine the presence of DIC? ***(893-894)*** __________

____

____

19. a. In HELLP syndrome, what happens to the platelet, aspartate transaminase (AST), and alanine transaminase (ALT) levels? ***(900-901)***

____

b. What is a priority of care for a patient with HELLP? ***(900-901)*** __________

____

20. What complications should the nurse be alert for when the mother is experiencing gestational diabetes? ***(905-906)***

____

____

21. The patient with gestational diabetes should anticipate that the following diagnostic tests may be performed: ***(906)***

____

____

22. Postpartum care of the adolescent mother focuses on: ***(910-911)*** __________

____

____

23. A 45-year-old woman is pregnant. She wants the nurse to tell her what complications of pregnancy are more common for women of her age and if the baby is at risk. The nurse recognizes that the risks for an older woman during pregnancy are: ***(912)***

____

____

Multiple Choice

24. The patient being seen in the obstetrician's office has a missed abortion. The nurse recognizes that this means the patient will have: ***(889)***
    1. malodorous bleeding, increased temperature, and cramping.
    2. expelled some, but not all, of the products of conception.
    3. fetal death and cessation of uterine growth.
    4. increased bleeding and a rupture of membranes.

25. The nurse notes that the most appropriate outcome for a woman experiencing hyperemesis gravidarum is: ***(885)***
    1. relief of painful uterine contractions.
    2. absence of fetal withdrawal symptoms.
    3. platelets and prothrombin time and partial thromboplastin time (PT/PTT) values within normal limits.
    4. adequate caloric intake for maternal and fetal health.

26. The difference in the diagnosis of placenta previa and abruptio placentae is that abruptio placentae is associated with: ***(891-892)***
    1. decreased vaginal bleeding.
    2. sudden uterine pain and rigidity.
    3. occurrence before 20 weeks gestation.
    4. decreased uterine size and poor contractions.

27. The nurse's assignment on the postpartum unit includes patients with the following assessment data. Which patient should the nurse see first? ***(896)***
    1. The patient has saturated one feminine pad within the last 2 hours.
    2. The patient has a blood glucose of 160 mg/dL.
    3. The patient had a spontaneous abortion and is experiencing moderate dark bleeding.
    4. The patient has had a continuous headache, upset stomach, and blurred vision.

28. The patient is assessed by the nurse to be hyperglycemic as a result of the patient's: ***(906)***
    1. pallor.
    2. hunger.
    3. depressed reflexes.
    4. diaphoretic state.

HIGH-RISK NEWBORN

Objectives

- Discuss the problems created by alcohol and drug abuse.
- Identify concerns related to preterm infants.
- Explain the hemolytic disease of the newborn.

29. How can human immunodeficiency virus and acquired immunodeficiency syndrome (HIV/AIDS) in the mother affect the fetus? ***(904)***

    ____

    ____

30. What are the characteristic physical manifestations of a preterm infant? ***(917)*** ____________

    ____

    ____

31. a. Signs and symptoms of newborn respiratory distress include: ***(917)*** ______________________

____

____

b. Treatment for respiratory distress includes: ***(917)***______________________

____

32. a. What is a problem seen in infants who are small for gestational age (SGA)? ***(918)***______________

____

b. What tool can be used to estimate gestational age? ***(918)*** ______________________

____

33. Hemolytic disease occurs when: ***(918)***______________________________

____

____

34. Diagnostic tests that are used to determine possible hemolytic disease are: ***(919)***______________

____

____

35. Fetal alcohol syndrome (FAS) may result in the newborn experiencing withdrawal symptoms. What will the nurse will observe for? ***(921)***

____

____

Multiple Choice

36. The nurse recognizes that the chance of a hemolytic disease in the newborn is very low if which of the following findings are present? ***(918)***
    1. Mother blood type O, infant blood type A
    2. Mother Rh negative, father Rh negative
    3. Mother Rh negative, infant Rh positive
    4. Mother blood type B, infant blood type A

NURSING

Objective

- Discuss nursing diagnoses related to high-risk conditions of the mother and newborn.

37. Identify the nursing assessment that should take place if the patient experiences bleeding during the pregnancy. ***(892)***

____

____

38. Identify possible nursing diagnoses for patients experiencing the following complications.

   a. Postpartum hemorrhage: ***(895)*** _______________

   ____

   b. Gestational diabetes: ***(906-907)*** _______________

   ____

39. What teaching should be done about the prevention of an infection during pregnancy? ***(902)*** _______________

____

____

40. a. What interventions are planned by the nurse for a pregnant patient with a preexisting cardiac condition? ***(907-908)***

   ____

   ____

   b. What is the primary difference in cardiopulmonary resuscitation (CPR) technique for the pregnant woman? ***(907-908)***

   ____

   ____

41. Identify a nursing diagnosis that may be formulated for an adolescent patient during her first experience in labor and delivery. ***(910)***

____

____

42. General nursing interventions for preterm infants include: ***(917-918)*** _______________

____

____

43. Identify a nursing diagnosis that may be formulated for a preterm infant. ***(917-918)*** _______________

____

____

44. Identify the nursing interventions for a patient with mastitis. ***(902)*** ______________________________

____

____

Multiple Choice

45. The nurse is alert to a significant sign of pregnancy-induced hypertension (PIH), which is: ***(896-897)***
    1. edema.
    2. bradycardia.
    3. weight loss.
    4. hypoglycemia.

46. The nurse anticipates that the medication to be given to the patient who is experiencing severe PIH will be: ***(897-899)***
    1. meperidine (Demerol).
    2. heparin (Lovenox).
    3. oxytocin (Pitocin).
    4. magnesium sulfate.

47. The nurse is working with an adolescent mother with her first child. A likely nursing diagnosis that is formulated for this patient is: ***(910)***
    1. knowledge deficit.
    2. fluid volume deficit.
    3. ineffective parenting.
    4. cardiac output, decreased.

48. The nurse is teaching the pregnant woman about prevention of infection. In discussing toxoplasmosis with the patient, the nurse specifically highlights: ***(903)***
    1. hand hygiene after using the bathroom.
    2. vaccination with an attenuated virus.
    3. reduction of sexual relations.
    4. avoidance of cat litter.

49. The nurse suspects that a postpartum patient, being seen for her 6-week postdelivery check-up, is experiencing postpartum depression (PPD) as evidenced by the patient's signs and symptoms of: (Select all that apply) ***(921-922)***
    1. showing little interest in her baby.
    2. talking extensively about her labor experience.
    3. discussing her level of fatigue due to getting limited sleep.
    4. stating that she is finding that she has limited maternal feeling towards her baby.

Student Name____________________________ Date____________

chapter **29**

Health Promotion for the Infant, Child, and Adolescent

Answer Key: Textbook page references are provided as a guide for answering these questions. A complete answer key was provided for your instructor.

TERMS

Objective

- Define the key terms as listed.

1. Define the following terms.

   a. Anticipatory guidance: ***(926)*** ____________________________

   b. Botulism: ***(935)*** ____________________________

   c. Nursing bottle caries: ***(936)***____________________________

HEALTH PROMOTION

Objectives

- Identify the 10 "Leading Health Indicators" cited in *Healthy People 2010.*
- List three benefits of regular physical activity in children.
- State American Academy of Pediatrics recommendations for immunization administration in healthy infants and children.
- State three strategies to promote dental health.
- Identify six health benefits associated with exercise, activity, and sports.

2. Identify the "Leading Health Indicators" from *Healthy People 2010.* ***(926)***____________________________

3. What are the target goals for the following health indicators? ***(927)***

   a. Physical activity: ______________________________

   b. Substance abuse: ______________________________

   c. Responsible sexual activity: ______________________________

   d. Immunizations: ______________________________

4. What are the benefits of physical activity? ***(927)*** ______________________________

5. How can the nurse promote physical activity for children? ***(927-928)*** ______________________________

6. a. What factors contribute to obesity in children and adolescents? ***(927)*** ______________________________

   b. What are the criteria to determine that a child is overweight or obese? ***(927)*** ______________________________

7. The single most preventable cause of death and disease in the United States is ______________________________. ***(929)***

8. Identify social problems associated with substance abuse. ***(929)*** ______________________________

9. What information should be taught about responsible sexual behavior? ***(930)*** ______________________

____

____

10. What is the newest guideline regarding immunization for children aged 2 to 23 months? ***(932)*** __________

____

____

11. Identify strategies to promote dental health for the following age groups. ***(935-936)***

    a. Infant: ______________________________________

    ____

    b. Preschooler: _________________________________

    ____

    c. Adolescent: __________________________________

    ____

12. Identify at least one nutritional consideration for the following age groups. ***(928)***

    a. Infant: ______________________________________

    b. Preschooler: _________________________________

    c. Adolescent: __________________________________

SAFETY MEASURES

Objectives

- State the causes and prevention of accidental poisonings.
- Describe four strategies to prevent aspiration of a foreign body.
- Discuss the proper use of infant safety seats in motor vehicles.
- List 10 safety precautions important in educating parents to prevent environmental injuries to children.

13. Identify measures to teach parents regarding vehicular safety for children. ***(930-931)*** ________________

____

____

14. What strategies may be implemented to prevent accidental poisoning? ***(936-938)*** ____________________

____

____

15. Identify at least five strategies that may be implemented to prevent burns. ***(938-939)*** ____________________

____

____

16. For the nursing diagnosis *risk for poisoning, related to lack of knowledge of safeguards,* identify at least three interventions or areas for teaching. ***(938)***

____

____

17. Identify strategies that may be implemented to prevent foreign body aspiration. ***(938)***____________________

____

____

Multiple Choice

18. Of the following, which age group is most at risk for foreign body aspiration? ***(938)***
    1. 1 to 5 months
    2. 6 to 12 months
    3. 1 to 2 years
    4. 2 to 4 years

19. The nurse is developing a nutrition plan with the parents of an overweight 12-year-old child. The parents demonstrate an understanding of the plan by stating: (Select all that apply) ***(928)***
    1. "Our child's calories from saturated fats should be no more than 7% daily."
    2. "We should not allow our child to drink milk that is less than 2% milk fat."
    3. "Our child should participate in some type of physical activity for at least 60 minutes a day."
    4. "We should be sure our child consumes foods from all the food groups except for grains."

20. Parents should be advised to monitor television shows that their children are viewing since _____ of these transmissions contain violence: ***(929-930)***
    1. 21%
    2. 41%
    3. 61%
    4. 81%

Student Name________________________ Date____________

Basic Pediatric Nursing Care

chapter **30**

Answer Key: Textbook page references are provided as a guide for answering these questions. A complete answer key was provided for your instructor.

TERMS

Objective

- Define the key terms as listed.

1. Define the following terms.

   a. Birth defect: ***(941)***________________________

   b. En face position: ***(943)***________________________

   c. Mortality: ***(952)***________________________

   d. Weaning: ***(955)***________________________

HISTORICAL EVENTS

Objectives

- Identify events that had a significant impact on the health care of children in the United States in the twentieth century.
- Discuss the works of Dr. Abraham Jacobi and Lillian Wald.
- Describe the purposes and outcomes of the White House Conferences on Children from 1901 to the 1980s.

2. Identify the activities associated with the following people or events and their impact upon the development of pediatric care. ***(941-942)***

   a. Dr. Abraham Jacobi: ____________________

   b. Lillian Wald: ____________________

   c. President Theodore Roosevelt (1909): ____________________

   d. President Franklin Roosevelt (1937): ____________________

   e. President Ronald Reagan (1987): ____________________

ROLE OF THE PEDIATRIC NURSE

Objectives

- Discuss the personal characteristics and professional skills of a pediatric nurse.
- Identify key elements of family-centered care.
- Describe areas in which growth and development principles are used by the pediatric nurse.

3. Identify the main purpose of pediatric nursing. ***(943)*** ____________________

4. What are the characteristics and role of a pediatric nurse? ***(943)*** ____________________

5. Identify the key elements in family-centered care. ***(944)*** ______________________________

____

____

6. How are the principles of growth and development used by the nurse? ***(946-947)***______________

____

____

7. Children with special needs are those children with: ***(944)*** ____________________________

____

____

ASSESSMENT

Objectives

- Discuss the physical assessment of a child using the head-to-toe method.
- Describe metabolism and its relationship to nutrition in the child.

8. Identify the guidelines for performing a physical assessment on a child. ***(948)***______________

____

____

9. a. The temperature of a 6-month-old is higher ______ or lower ______ (check one) than the temperature of an adolescent. ***(949-950)***

   b. The preferred method of temperature measurement for a child is ______________________
   ____________________________________. ***(949-950)***

10. How does the vision of a child change from infancy to preschool age? ***(952)***______________

____

____

11. The nurse is teaching the parents about the development of teeth. The nurse instructs the parents that there are __________(number) of primary teeth that are usually all in place by the age of _________ years. The permanent teeth usually appear by age _________. ***(952)***

12. The nurse is preparing to auscultate the child's lungs. Describe methods that can be used to have the child assist in this procedure. ***(953)***

____

____

13. What spinal abnormalities may be found on an assessment of a child or adolescent? ***(953-954)***______________________________

____

____

14. a. What is the usual specific gravity of the child's urine? ***(954)*** ______________________________

____

____

b. What is the usual urinary output for a 6-month-old? ***(954)*** ______________________________

____

____

15. Identify the average time frame for the following foods or nutritional activities to be introduced. ***(954-955)***

a. Whole milk: ______________________________

b. Solid foods (cereals): ______________________________

c. Fruits and vegetables: ______________________________

d. Table food:______________________________

e. Weaning: ______________________________

16. Energy requirements for an infant are highest during ______________________________. ***(955-956)***

Multiple Choice

17. When assessing the child, the nurse knows that the expected annual rate of growth for a 4-year-old is: ***(948)***
    1. 18 to 22 cm.
    2. 14 to 18 cm.
    3. 8 cm.
    4. 5 cm.

18. The temperature measurement site of choice for an infant is: ***(950)***
    1. oral.
    2. rectal.
    3. tympanic.
    4. axillary.

19. When measuring the vital signs of a 2-year-old, the nurse expects that they will be close to the average findings for that age, which are: ***(950)***
    1. P 110, R 25, BP 94/66.
    2. P 100, R 20, BP 110/80.
    3. P 90, R 22, BP 108/70.
    4. P 70, R 24, BP 120/76.

20. It is expected that the vocabulary for a preschooler will be characterized by: ***(956-957)***
    1. three or four familiar words.
    2. 25 to 50 words.
    3. more than 250 words.
    4. full, complete sentences.

21. When measuring the vital signs of a 12-year-old, the nurse expects that they will be close to the average findings for that age, which are: ***(950)***
    1. P 114, R 25, BP 94/66.
    2. P 100, R 20, BP 100/80.
    3. P 88, R 20, BP 110/70.
    4. P 70, R 24, BP 120/76.

22. The nurse is reviewing infant development and recognizes that an expected finding for this age group is: ***(952)***
    1. having a visual acuity of 20/100 at birth.
    2. enjoying "peek-a-boo" games.
    3. controlling bladder elimination by 10 months.
    4. tripling of birth weight by 6 months.

23. The nurse is preparing to administer medication to a 4-year-old child in the pediatric clinic. The best communication with this child is: ***(956-957)***
    1. "This may feel like a pinch."
    2. "Don't move when I give you this."
    3. "Do you want to take this medicine now?"
    4. "I will be coming back to give you a shot."

NURSING INTERVENTIONS

Objectives

- List general strategies to consider when talking with children.
- Outline several approaches for making the hospitalization of children a positive experience for them and their families.
- Discuss pain management in infants and children.
- Explain the needs of parents during their child's hospitalization.
- Discuss common pediatric procedures.
- Discuss administration of pediatric medications.
- Identify each category of age/behavior, accident/hazard, and prevention in the pediatric child.

24. Describe how the nurse would explain the sensations of blood pressure measurement to a child. ***(957-958)***

____

____

25. Identify strategies that should be used when communicating with children. ***(958)***_______________

____

____

26. What should the nurse do to reduce anxiety for the child and the parents when the child is admitted to the hospital? ***(958-959)***

____

____

27. Identify an example of an age-related concern or need of a hospitalized child, the child's possible response, and the positive parent or nurse responses. ***(961)***

    a. Concern or need: ____

    ____

    b. Child's response: ____

    ____

    c. Parent or nurse response: ____

    ____

28. Pain is often underestimated in children. What can the nurse do to better assess the child's pain? ***(960, 962)***

____

____

29. What methods in addition to pain medication can be used for relief or reduction of the child's pain? ***(960, 962)***

____

____

30. How can the nurse increase the trust and participation of the parents in the care of the hospitalized child? ***(963-964)***

____

____

31. a. The recommended approach for preparing children for procedures is to ____. ***(964-965)***

    b. When is it best to prepare younger children for a procedure? ***(964-965)*** ____

    ____

32. The nurse is evaluating the bath given to the infant by the adult caregiver. Identify what actions indicate a need for additional teaching. ***(965)***
    a. Using soap around the eyes _____
    b. Using a cotton-tipped swab to clean the ear canal _____
    c. Supporting the head while bathing the infant in a tub _____
    d. Washing the extremities after washing the face _____
    e. Washing the perineum in an anterior to posterior direction _____
    f. Retracting the foreskin of the male infant _____

33. How is gavage feeding for the infant provided? ***(966-967)*** ______________________________

____

____

34. What are the different types of safety reminder devices that are used for children? ***(967-968)*** __________

____

____

35. How can urine be collected from an infant? ***(968-969)*** ______________________________

____

____

36. Following a lumbar puncture, what should the nurse do for each of the following patients? ***(970)***

    a. Young child: ______________________________

    ____

    b. Adolescent: ______________________________

    ____

37. Delivery of oxygen to a small infant is best provided with: ***(970)***______________________________

____

____

38. What assessment findings by the nurse would indicate a need for the child's airway to be suctioned? ***(971)***

____

____

39. When suctioning a child, the nurse should: ***(971-972)***
    a. Set wall suction pressure at ____________________.
    b. Insert the tubing ____________________ (distance).
    c. Suction for ____________________ seconds.
    d. Suction no more frequently than every ____________________.

40. When monitoring intake and output for a child who is not toilet-trained, how is the urinary output measured? ***(972)***

____

____

41. What can the nurse offer that will increase the fluid intake and provide variety for the child? ***(972)***

____

____

42. The nurse is to administer an intramuscular (IM) injection to a 10-year-old patient. Identify the following parameters. ***(974-975)***

    a. Site(s) to use: ______________________________

    b. Needle selection: ______________________________

    c. Pain reduction: ______________________________

43. What intravenous (IV) site is used for children younger than 9 months of age? ***(975)*** ______________

____

____

44. For enema administration to each of the following patients, identify the type and amount of solution to use as well as the procedure for tube insertion. ***(977)***

	Type of Solution/Amount	Tube Insertion
a. 2 to 4 years old		
b. 11 years old		

45. Identify at least two strategies for administering oral medication to children. ***(973)***______________

____

____

46. Provide examples of behaviors, accidents or hazards, and preventive measures from at least two different age groups. ***(977-979)***

____

____

Multiple Choice

47. An older school-age child will be having surgery with anesthesia. The nurse intervenes to reduce anxiety by: ***(964)***
    1. showing the child the mask that will be used for the anesthesia.
    2. introducing the child to a peer and having them discuss the procedure.
    3. reassuring the child that only the procedure that is supposed to be done will be completed.
    4. explaining the special type of sleep that will occur with the anesthetic.

48. The nurse is discussing nutritional needs of the toddler with his mother. She asks the nurse how to get him to eat right. The nurse responds appropriately by telling the mother that: ***(966)***
    1. food should be left around the house where the child can pick it up when he feels like it.
    2. the child should be restrained in the high chair for meals.
    3. the child should sit at the table for scheduled meals.
    4. meals should be arranged about every 5 hours for the child.

49. A medication is to be administered to a child who has a body surface area (BSA) of 0.94 m^2. The recommended adult dose is 10 to 20 mg. What is the dosage range that is safe for this child? ***(972-973)***
    1. 5.5 to 11 mg
    2. 9.4 to 18.8 mg
    3. 10 to 20 mg
    4. 11 to 22 mg

50. The nurse is confident that health promotion teaching has been successful when the mother of a 3-month-old states: (Select all that apply) ***(946)***
    1. "My baby's birth weight should be doubled at the age of 6 months."
    2. "My baby's vision now is about 20/100."
    3. "My baby should enjoy parallel play by the age of 8 months."
    4. "My baby should enjoy toys that bang, shake, or can be pulled."

51. The nurse can calculate the normal systolic blood pressure of a 5 year old by adding: ***(951)***
    1. 90 to the age in years.
    2. 83 to double the age in years.
    3. 50 to the age in years.
    4. 20 to triple the age in years.

52. The nurse prepares to give an injection to an infant in the vastus lateralis muscle. The father of the infant asks why the nurse is giving the infant an injection in the leg. The nurse is correct in responding: (Select all that apply) ***(974-976)***
    1. "This is the easiest area to expose on the baby."
    2. "This site is a preferred site for infants because it is not close to vessels or nerves."
    3. "We have found in our clinic that this site is the least painful site for injections for infants."
    4. "This leg muscle is the most developed muscle in an infant, so it is a preferred site for injections."

Student Name____ Date__________________

Care of the Child with a Physical Disorder

chapter **31**

Answer Key: Textbook page references are provided as a guide for answering these questions. A complete answer key was provided for your instructor.

CARDIOVASCULAR—HEMATOLOGIC—IMMUNE SYSTEM

Objectives

- Describe the etiology / pathophysiology, types of defects, clinical manifestations, diagnostic tests, and medical management of congenital heart defects.
- Describe the etiology / pathophysiology, clinical manifestations, diagnostic tests, medical management, nursing interventions, and patient teaching for children with iron deficiency anemia, sickle cell anemia, and aplastic anemia.
- Discuss the etiology / pathophysiology, clinical manifestations, diagnostic tests, medical management, nursing interventions, patient teaching, and prognosis for children with the coagulation disorders of hemophilia and idiopathic thrombocytopenia purpura.
- Describe the etiology / pathophysiology, clinical manifestations, diagnostic tests, medical management, nursing interventions, patient teaching, and prognosis for children with leukemia.
- Demonstrate an understanding of the etiology, pathophysiology, clinical manifestations, diagnostic tests, medical management, nursing interventions, patient teaching, and prognosis for children with acquired immunodeficiency syndrome (AIDS).
- Discuss the etiology / pathophysiology, clinical manifestations, diagnostic tests, medical management, nursing interventions, patient teaching, and prognosis for children with juvenile rheumatoid arthritis.

1. Identify the four categories of congenital heart disease and an example of a disorder from each category. *(985-992)*

____

____

2. What are the general clinical manifestations of congenital heart disease? *(987)*______________________

____

____

3. Identify two nursing diagnoses for a child with congenital heart disease. *(987-989)* __________________

____

____

4. What are the four defects found in tetralogy of Fallot? ***(990)***

5. Identify the clinical signs and symptoms associated with tetralogy of Fallot and the medical management for the disorder. ***(991)***

6. The child has a coarctation of the aorta. The nurse expects that the blood pressure measurement will be: ***(992)***

7. For the following children, identify the signs and symptoms that may be manifested.

   a. Child with a hemoglobin (Hgb) value of 8 g/dL: ***(992)***

   b. Child with a Hgb value of 4.5 g/dL: ***(992)***

8. a. What is the etiology of iron deficiency anemia? ***(992)***

   b. What information should be provided to the parents of the child who is to receive a liquid iron supplement? ***(992)***

9. Identify an example of a type of sickle cell crisis and the treatment that should be implemented. ***(995)***

10. Children who have hemophilia and idiopathic thrombocytopenic purpura (ITP) have similar problems. What common information can be provided to the parents of these children? ***(995-997)***

____

____

11. Identify a nursing diagnosis for a child with leukemia and nursing interventions that may be implemented. ***(998)***

____

____

12. Provide the following information regarding HIV infections. ***(999-1001)***

    a. The majority of children are infected:_______________________

    b. The greatest physical threat is:_______________________

13. The mother of a child with HIV infection asks if the child should receive routine immunizations. The nurse responds by saying: ***(1000-1001)***

____

____

14. What are the priority nursing diagnoses and outcomes for a child with juvenile rheumatoid arthritis? ***(1003)***

____

____

Multiple Choice

15. A common sign or symptom of patent ductus arteriosus and septal defects is: ***(987, 989-999)***
    1. murmur.
    2. chest pain.
    3. hypotension.
    4. headache.

16. The nurse recognizes that the majority of congenital heart defects are treated with: ***(987-992)***
    1. diet.
    2. exercise.
    3. surgery.
    4. medication.

17. Screenings are being conducted on children for blood disorders. The nurse is aware that the most prevalent blood disorder is: ***(992)***
    1. hemophilia.
    2. sickle cell anemia.
    3. iron deficiency anemia.
    4. idiopathic thrombocytopenic purpura.

18. The nurse instructs the parents of a child with iron deficiency anemia that iron absorption may be enhanced by: ***(993)***
    1. giving the supplement with milk.
    2. giving the supplement with citrus juice or fruits.
    3. offering a chewable form once each day.
    4. waiting until the child has a full stomach to administer.

19. HIV testing for a child who is younger than 18 months of age is done with a: ***(1000)***
    1. Western blot test.
    2. reticulocyte test.
    3. polymerase chain reaction (PCR) test.
    4. enzyme-linked immunosorbent assay (ELISA).

RESPIRATORY

Objective

- Discuss the etiology/pathophysiology, clinical manifestations, diagnostic tests, medical management, nursing interventions, patient teaching, and prognosis for children with disorders of the respiratory system, including respiratory distress syndrome, bronchopulmonary dysplasia, pneumonia, sudden infant death syndrome, upper respiratory tract infections, tonsillitis, croup, bronchitis, respiratory syncytial virus, pulmonary tuberculosis, cystic fibrosis, and bronchial asthma.

20. When do the signs and symptoms of respiratory distress syndrome (RDS) become apparent? ____. ***(1003)***

21. Treatment for RDS includes: ***(1003-1004)*** ____

    ____

    ____

22. Identify the common nursing interventions that are implemented for children experiencing respiratory disorders. ***(1004-1005)***

    ____

    ____

23. The largest percentage of pneumonia in children is caused by ____. ***(1005)***

24. The priority nursing intervention for parents of children with sudden infant death syndrome (SIDS) is: ***(1007)***

____

____

25. The new parent asks the nurse what the "Back to Sleep" campaign is all about. The nurse explains this campaign: ***(1006)***

____

____

26. a. Acute pharyngitis is treated with _______________________. ***(1007)***

    b. Diagnosis is based on _______________________. ***(1007)***

    c. Nursing measures include _______________________. ***(1007)***

27. What is a classic sign of croup (laryngotracheobronchitis)? ***(1008-1009)*** _______________________

____

____

28. What discharge instructions should be provided to the parents of a child who has had a tonsillectomy? ***(1008)***

____

____

29. Describe the medical treatment for epiglottitis. ***(1009)*** _______________________

____

____

30. a. What is the pathophysiology involved in cystic fibrosis? ***(1011-1012)*** _______________________

    ____

    ____

    b. What is the medical management for this disorder? ***(1011-1012)*** _______________________

    ____

    ____

31. One of the most frequent causes of bronchial asthma is _______________________ _______________________. ***(1013)***

32. For bronchial asthma, identify the following. ***(1013-1014)***

    a. Signs and symptoms: ______________________________

    ____

    b. Diagnostic tests: ______________________________

    ____

    c. Medical treatment: ______________________________

    ____

    d. Nursing interventions: ______________________________

    ____

GASTROINTESTINAL

Objective

- Describe the etiology/pathophysiology, clinical manifestations, diagnostic tests, medical management, nursing interventions, patient teaching, and prognosis for children with disorders of the gastrointestinal system, including cleft lip and cleft palate, dehydration, diarrhea, gastroenteritis, constipation, gastroesophageal reflux, hypertrophic pyloric stenosis, intussusception, and Hirschsprung's disease.

33. a. The child is born with a cleft lip and palate. What are the primary problems for this child and the parents? ***(1016-1017)***

    ____

    ____

    b. What is included in the postoperative care of the child after a repair of a cleft lip and/or palate? ***(1016-1017)***

    ____

    ____

34. Identify the signs and symptoms of dehydration. ***(1018)*** ______________________________

    ____

    ____

35. Children with gastrointestinal disorders are susceptible to fluid and electrolyte imbalances. Identify the nursing assessments and interventions that should be implemented by the nurse for these children. ***(1019-1020)***

    ____

    ____

36. Identify a nursing diagnosis for a child with diarrhea and/or dehydration. ***(1019)*** ____________________

____

____

37. Identify how the diet may be modified for the following children who are experiencing constipation. ***(1020)***

    a. Newborn: ____

    ____

    b. Older infant: ____

    ____

38. The primary sign that is seen in children with hypertrophic pyloric stenosis is ____________________ ____. ***(1022)***

39. The hallmark sign of intussusception is ______________________________. ***(1023)***

40. Treatment for intussusception includes: ***(1023-1024)*** ______________________________________

____

____

41. A neonate is suspected of having Hirschsprung's disease (megacolon) when ____________________ ______________________________________. ***(1024)***

42. The usual surgical treatment for Hirschsprung's disease (megacolon) involves: ***(1024-1025)*** __________

____

____

43. What are general nursing measures that can be implemented for children experiencing gastrointestinal disorders? ***(1015-1025)***

____

____

44. The nurse is aware that cultural practices related to hernias may include: ***(1026)*** ____________________

____

____

Multiple Choice

45. For the child experiencing gastroenteritis with diarrhea, the nurse anticipates that treatment will include: ***(1019)***
    1. nothing-by-mouth status (NPO).
    2. oral rehydration.
    3. no solid foods for 48 hours.
    4. traditional BRAT diet.

46. There are several different types of hernias that children may experience. The type of hernia that usually has spontaneous closure by the time the child is 2 years old is: ***(1026)***
    1. hiatal.
    2. inguinal.
    3. umbilical.
    4. diaphragmatic.

47. The most severe type of hernia that is found within hours of delivery and requires immediate surgical repair is: ***(1026)***
    1. hiatal.
    2. inguinal.
    3. umbilical.
    4. diaphragmatic.

48. The nurse anticipates that a child who is receiving pharmacologic treatment for gastroesophageal reflux will receive: ***(1021)***
    1. Compazine (prochlorperazine).
    2. Mylanta (calcium chloride).
    3. Tagamet (cimetidine).
    4. Cerebyx (fosphenytoin).

GENITOURINARY

Objectives

- Discuss the parent teaching necessary to prevent urinary tract infection in infants and children.
- Discuss the etiology / pathophysiology, clinical manifestations, diagnostic tests, medical management, nursing interventions, and patient teaching for children with disorders of the genitourinary system, including nephrotic syndrome, acute glomerulonephritis, and Wilms' tumor.

49. What are the signs and symptoms manifested by the child who has nephritic syndrome (nephrosis)? ***(1027)***

    ____

    ____

50. a. Acute glomerulonephritis is most often the result of ______________________________
    ______________________________. ***(1028)***

    b. What diagnostic tests are performed to determine the presence of glomerulonephritis? ***(1028)*** ______

    ____

    ____

51. For acute glomerulonephritis, identify the following. ***(1028)***

    a. Signs and symptoms: ______________________________

    ____

    b. Treatment: ______________________________

    ____

52. Wilms' tumor (nephroblastoma) is usually found by the parents when ______________________________
______________________________. ***(1029)***

53. Treatment for Wilms' tumor includes: ***(1029)*** ______________________________

____

____

Multiple Choice

54. The nurse is aware of the disease process and treatment for nephrosis. It is anticipated that treatment for the child will include: ***(1027)***
    1. prevention of infection.
    2. increased sodium.
    3. decreased protein.
    4. diuretics.

55. The nurse expects that the treatment for a child with cryptorchidism will include: ***(1030)***
    1. circumcision.
    2. fixation of the testes.
    3. extension of the urethra.
    4. bladder neck reconstruction.

ENDOCRINE

Objective

- Discuss the etiology/pathophysiology, clinical manifestations, diagnostic tests, medical management, nursing interventions, and patient teaching for children with disorders of the endocrine system, including hypothyroidism, hyperthyroidism, and diabetes mellitus.

56. What are the signs and symptoms associated with acquired hypothyroidism? ***(1030)*** ______________________________

____

____

57. The dietary needs of the child with hyperthyroidism include: ***(1031)*** ______________________________

____

____

58. a. Most children with diabetes mellitus require ______________________________. ***(1032-1033)***

    b. A laboratory test that is used to diagnose diabetes mellitus is ______________________________. ***(1032-1033)***

59. What information is necessary to include in a teaching plan for a newly diagnosed diabetic child and the parents? ***(1033)***

____

____

Multiple Choice

60. The nurse recognizes that hyperthyroidism is most common in which one of the following age groups? ***(1031)***
    1. Neonates
    2. Toddlers
    3. Preschoolers
    4. Adolescents

MUSCULOSKELETAL

Objective

- Discuss the etiology / pathophysiology, clinical manifestations, diagnostic tests, medical management, nursing interventions, and patient teaching for children with disorders of the musculoskeletal system, including hip dysplasia, Legg-Calvé-Perthes disease, osteomyelitis, talipes, Duchenne's muscular dystrophy, and septic arthritis.

61. In the illustration, identify what the nurse is assessing the infant for. ***(1034-1035)*** ______________________________

____

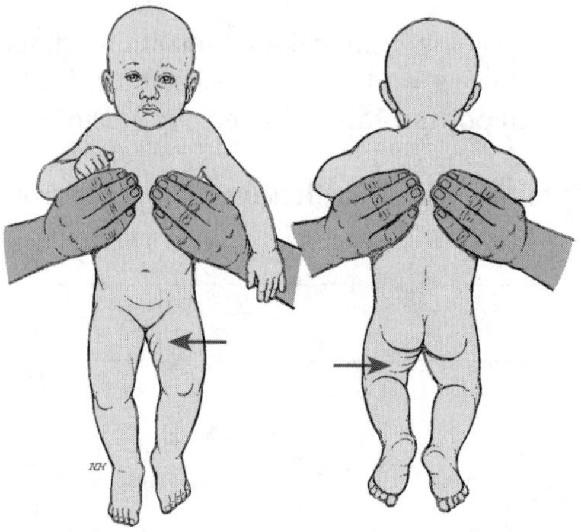

62. Identify the interventions that are important in the care of a cast or corrective device. ***(1036)*** ____________

____

____

63. A child with Legg-Calvé-Perthes disease usually exhibits the following: ***(1036)*** ____________

____

____

64. a. What condition is present in the individual in the following illustrations? ***(1038)*** ____________

____

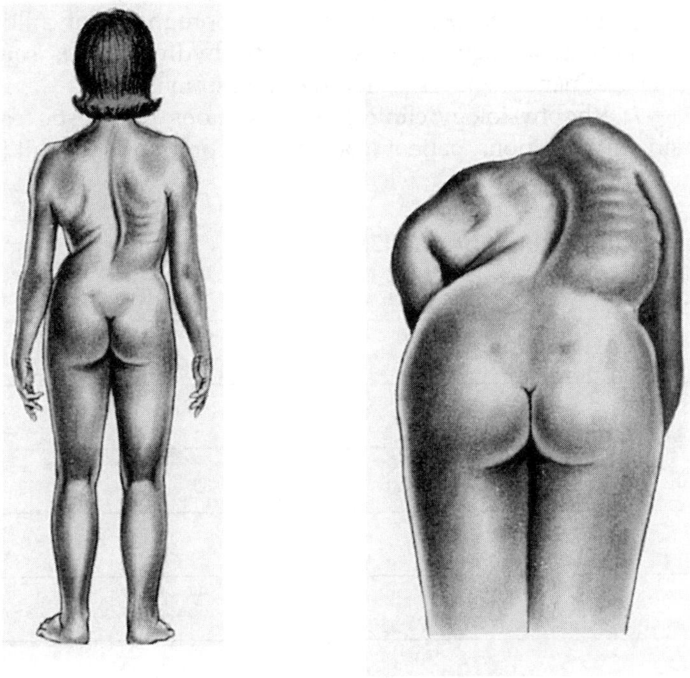

b. This condition is most often seen in what age group? ***(1038)*** ____________

c. Treatment usually includes: ***(1038)*** ____________

65. The goals of treatment for a child with Duchenne's muscular dystrophy are: ***(1039)*** ____________

____

____

Multiple Choice

66. For a child with talipes equinovarus, the nurse explains to the parents that treatment usually includes: ***(1038)***
    1. oxygen administration.
    2. medication therapy.
    3. skeletal traction.
    4. cast applications.

NEUROLOGIC

Objectives

- Discuss the etiology / pathophysiology, clinical manifestations, diagnostic tests, medical management, nursing interventions, patient teaching, and prognosis for children with disorders of the nervous system, including meningitis, encephalitis, hydrocephalus, cerebral palsy, seizures, spina bifida, neonatal abstinence syndrome, and neuroblastoma.
- Describe the etiology / pathophysiology, clinical manifestations, diagnostic tests, medical management, nursing interventions, patient teaching, and prognosis for children with lead poisoning.

67. For meningitis, identify the following. ***(1040-1042)***

    a. Most common cause: ______________________________

    ____

    b. Classic signs and symptoms: ______________________________

    ____

    c. Diagnostic test: ______________________________

    ____

    d. Medical treatment: ______________________________

    ____

    e. Preventive measure: ______________________________

    ____

68. What are the antenatal factors that may contribute to the development of cerebral palsy? ***(1044)*** ________

    ____

    ____

69. What are the nursing goals for a child with cerebral palsy? ***(1045-1046)*** ______________________

____

____

70. Identify whether the following interventions during a child's seizure are appropriate or require correction. ***(1046-1047)***
    a. Keeping the side rails padded _____
    b. Moving the child to the bed when the seizure begins _____
    c. Loosening restrictive clothing _____
    d. Turning the child's head to the side _____
    e. Pushing a tongue blade between the teeth _____
    f. Staying with the child throughout the seizure _____

71. Nursing care for a child with a myelomeningocele includes: ***(1047)*** ______________________

____

____

72. For lead poisoning, identify the following. ***(1049-1050)***

    a. Sources of lead: ______________________________________

    ____

    b. Prevention: ______________________________________

    ____

    c. Screening: ______________________________________

    ____

    d. Parent guidelines to reduce lead levels: ______________________

    ____

INTEGUMENTARY/COMMUNICABLE DISEASE

Objective

- Discuss the etiology / pathophysiology, clinical manifestations, diagnostic tests, medical management, nursing interventions, patient teaching, and prognosis for children with disorders of the integumentary system, including contact dermatitis, diaper dermatitis, eczema, seborrheic dermatitis, acne vulgaris, herpes simplex virus type I, tinea infections, candidiasis, and parasitic infections.

73. Identify some of the common areas for parent teaching for children with contact dermatitis, diaper rash, and eczema. ***(1050-1052)***

____

____

74. The skin disorder most commonly associated with adolescents is _______________ _______________. ***(1053)***

75. For an adolescent taking Accutane (isotretinoin), there will be specific monitoring for _______________ _______________ levels. ***(1055)***

76. Identify a nursing diagnosis appropriate for a child with an integumentary disorder. ***(1054)***_______________

____

____

77. Identify actions that may be implemented to prevent traumatic injuries. ***(1056)***_______________

____

____

78. For a bacterial infection of the skin, identify an example of a nursing intervention. ***(1057)***_______________

____

____

79. The nurse is presenting information on parasitic infections to parents at a parent-teacher association (PTA) meeting. What information should be included? ***(1058)***

____

____

80. Which childhood communicable diseases may have cardiac complications? ***(1059-1060)*** _______________

____

____

Multiple Choice

81. A possible etiology associated with atopic dermatitis (eczema) is: ***(1051-1052)***
    1. food allergy.
    2. bacterial infection.
    3. exposure to poison ivy.
    4. increased sebaceous gland activity.

82. The nurse determines that the child has varicella as a result of observing: ***(1059)***
    1. pinpoint red spots with white specks in the buccal cavity.
    2. a pinkish-red maculopapular rash that began on the face.
    3. a rose-pink macular rash on the trunk.
    4. vesicles on an erythematous base.

SENSORY

Objective

- Discuss the etiology/pathophysiology, clinical manifestations, diagnostic tests, medical management, nursing interventions, and patient teaching for children with disorders of the sensory system, including otitis media, refractive errors (myopia, hyperopia), strabismus, periorbital cellulitis, and allergic rhinitis.

83. For otitis media, identify the following. ***(1058, 1060-1062)***

    a. Reason for common occurrence in children: ____________________

    ____

    b. Signs and symptoms: ____________________

    ____

    c. Nursing interventions: ____________________

    ____

84. What behaviors usually indicate that a child may be having difficulty with vision? ***(1063)***____________

    ____

    ____

85. Children experiencing health deviations and their parents may be referred to community agencies, organizations, and support groups. Identify at least three examples of available community resources. ***(983-1066)***

    ____

    ____

86. A symptom of meningitis is ______________, which manifests as pain and stiffness in the neck. ***(1041)***

87. ____________________ is a condition caused by a decreased blood supply to the femoral head in children ages 3 to 12 years of age. ***(1036)***

Multiple Choice

88. The nurse is assessing a school-age child for signs of scoliosis. Clinical manifestations for this disease include: (Select all that apply) ***(1036-1037)***
    1. unequal hip and shoulder height.
    2. scapular and rib prominence.
    3. protrusion of the spine in the lumbar region.
    4. posterior rib hump that is visible when the child bends forward at the waist.

89. The parent of a child with strabismus demonstrates an understanding of the disorder by stating, "If we don't get treatment for this problem, my child may develop: ***(1063)***
    1. myopia."
    2. hyperopia."
    3. presbyopia."
    4. amblyopia."

90. The nurse notices that a patient is constantly scratching the skin as a result of atopic dermatitis. The nurse knows that the scratching may lead to: ***(1052)***
    1. subluxation.
    2. lichenification.
    3. pica.
    4. priapism.

Student Name______________________________ Date______________

chapter 32

Care of the Child with a Mental or Cognitive Disorder

Answer Key: Textbook page references are provided as a guide for answering these questions. A complete answer key was provided for your instructor.

TERMS

Objective

- Define the key terms as listed.

1. Define the following terms.

   a. Cognitive impairment: ***(1067)*** ______________________________

   b. Failure to thrive: ***(1073)*** ______________________________

   c. Intelligence quotient (IQ): ***(1067)*** ______________________________

   d. Somatization disorder: ***(1077)*** ______________________________

COGNITIVE DISORDERS

Objectives

- Identify six possible causes of cognitive impairment.
- Describe the clinical manifestations of Down syndrome.
- Discuss the appropriate nursing interventions required for caring for a patient with autism.

2. How are cognitive impairments classified? ***(1067)*** ______________________________

3. For cognitive impairments, identify the following. ***(1067-1068)***

   a. Possible etiology: ____________________

   ____

   b. Clinical manifestations: ____________________

   ____

   c. Diagnostic testing: ____________________

   ____

   d. Nursing interventions: ____________________

   ____

4. In 95% of the instances, Down syndrome is the result of ____________________. ***(1069)***

5. Identify the clinical manifestations of Down syndrome. ***(1069-1070)*** ____________________

   ____

   ____

6. Medical care for the child with Down syndrome involves: ***(1070)*** ____________________

   ____

   ____

7. a. Identify the clinical manifestations of autism. ***(1071)*** ____________________

   ____

   ____

   b. Select all of the appropriate interventions for a child with autism. ***(1071)***
      i. Encourage the parents to bring in favorite possessions. _____
      ii. Teach the parents about the cure for the disease. _____
      iii. Avoid establishing routines. _____
      iv. Provide brief, concrete communication with the child. _____
      v. Promote increased amounts and frequency of auditory and visual stimulation. _____

CHILD ABUSE

Objective

- State five physical and behavioral indicators that should arouse suspicion of child abuse.

8. Identify the different types of neglect. ***(1072)*** ______________________________

____

____

9. a. What situational factors may contribute to child abuse? ***(1072)*** ______________________________

____

____

b. What cultural practices may be misinterpreted as abuse? ***(1072)*** ______________________________

____

____

10. What is the role of the nurse regarding child abuse? ***(1072-1074)*** ______________________________

____

____

11. Identify at least one behavioral and one physical indicator for each of the following. ***(1073)***

a. Physical neglect: ______________________________

____

b. Physical abuse: ______________________________

____

c. Sexual abuse: ______________________________

____

d. Emotional neglect and abuse: ______________________________

____

LEARNING/BEHAVIORAL DISORDERS

Objectives

- Demonstrate an understanding of the medical management and the nursing interventions for the child with a learning disability.
- Describe four nursing interventions for the child with attention deficit hyperactivity disorder.

12. The nurse believes that the child is experiencing school avoidance. What physiologic and psychological assessment findings would lead to that belief? ***(1074)***

____

____

13. How can the nurse assist and support the parents if the child is experiencing school avoidance? ***(1074)***

____

____

14. For learning disabilities, identify the following. ***(1074-1075)***

    a. Possible etiology: ____

    ____

    b. Clinical signs and symptoms: ____

    ____

    c. Medical and nursing intervention: ____

    ____

15. Management of an attention deficit hyperactivity disorder (ADHD) includes: ***(1075-1076)*** ____________

____

____

16. Nursing interventions for a child with ADHD include: ***(1076)*** ____

____

____

MENTAL DISORDERS

Objectives

- Identify six clinical manifestations of depression in children.
- Discuss three nursing interventions for the child who is suicidal.

17. Describe depression and how it is diagnosed. ***(1076-1077)*** ____

____

____

18. In addition to medication, what treatment is provided for children who are depressed? ***(1077)***__________

19. Identify a nursing diagnosis for a child who is depressed. ***(1077)*** __________

20. The nursing interventions for a child who is threatening or has attempted suicide include the following: ***(1078-1079)***

21. The occurrence of recurrent abdominal pain (RAP) is mostly associated with: ***(1079)*** __________

Multiple Choice

22. The nurse anticipates that the child who is depressed will receive which one of the following medications? ***(1077)***
    1. Prozac (fluoxetine)
    2. Ritalin (methylphenidate)
    3. Benadryl (diphenhydramine)
    4. Dexedrine (dextroamphetamine)

23. The nurse is alert to careful screening for signs of suicidal thoughts or behaviors. The age group that is most prone to suicide is: ***(1077)***
    1. 5 to 7 years.
    2. 8 to 11 years.
    3. 12 to 14 years.
    4. 15 to 19 years.

24. The parents of a child with an IQ of 40 demonstrate an understanding of the child's capabilities by stating: (Select all that apply) ***(1067)***
    1. "Our child is considered to have severe cognitive impairment."
    2. "Our child can be taught activities of daily living tasks and perform them on his own."
    3. "Our child is considered to have moderate cognitive impairment."
    4. "Our child will most likely never be able to perform self-care tasks, like bathing, on his own."

25. The school nurse is aware that the incidence of depression among high school girls is approximately: ***(1076)***
    1. 15%.
    2. 25%.
    3. 35%.
    4. 45%.

Student Name____ Date____________________

Health Promotion and Care of the Older Adult

chapter **33**

Answer Key: Textbook page references are provided as a guide for answering these questions. A complete answer key was provided for your instructor.

OVERVIEW OF AGING

Objectives

- Discuss health and wellness in the aging population of the United States in relation to the aims of *Healthy People 2010*.
- Identify some of the common myths concerning the older adult.
- Describe biological and psychosocial theories of aging.

1. It is estimated that by the year 2030, ________% of the population will be older than 65 years of age. ***(1082)***

2. Identify health promotion measures for the older adult. ***(1083-1084)*** ____________________

3. There are many myths about older adults. Identify at least two of these myths. ***(1086)*** ____________________

4. The screenings that are recommended specifically for men older than age 50 are: ***(1084)*** ____________________

5. The first major legislation for financial support of older adults was the ____________________. This legislation established the programs for ____________________. ***(1087)***

6. The two most frequent indicators of elder abuse are ____________________ and ____________________. ***(1116-1117)***

7. The main goals of *Healthy People 2010* related to older adults are: ***(1085)*** ____________________

8. Erikson's developmental stage for an older adult is ____. *(1086)*

Multiple Choice

9. The theory of aging that presumes the personality of older adults remains the same and behavior becomes more predictable is: *(1086)*
   1. activity theory.
   2. exchange theory.
   3. continuity theory.
   4. programmed aging.

PHYSIOLOGIC CHANGES THAT OCCUR WITH AGING

Objectives

- Describe changes associated with aging for each of the body systems.
- Discuss methods of assessment used for each body system.
- Compare how older adults differ from younger individuals in their response to illness, medications, and hospitalization.
- Discuss changes that occur with aging in intelligence, learning, and memory.

10. Identify at least three changes in the integumentary system that occur with aging. *(1088)* ____________

11. Why is the older adult more susceptible to pressure ulcers? *(1089)* ____________

12. Identify at least three changes in the gastrointestinal system that occur with aging. *(1090)* ____________

13. Why is the older adult more susceptible to the following complications? *(1090-1091)*

    a. Dehydration: ____________

    b. Obesity: ____________

c. Weight loss: ____

____

14. The older adult may experience problems with oral hygiene, such as ____. ***(1091-1092)***

15. a. Identify at least three changes in the urinary system that occur with aging. ***(1094-1095)*** ______________

____

____

b. Provide an example of a medication that may be prescribed for urinary incontinence. ____ ***(1094-1095)***

16. Identify at least three changes in the cardiovascular system that occur with aging. ***(1096)*** ______________

____

____

17. a. Identify at least three changes in the respiratory system that occur with aging. ***(1098)*** ______________

____

____

b. A musculoskeletal change that occurs with aging and has an influence on respiratory function is ____. ***(1098)***

18. Identify at least three changes in the musculoskeletal system that occur with aging. ***(1100)*** ______________

____

____

19. Identify at least three changes in the endocrine system that occur with aging. ***(1103)*** ______________

____

____

20. The majority of older adults experience ______________ diabetes. ***(1103)***

21. Identify at least three changes in the reproductive system that occur with aging. ***(1104)*** ______________

____

____

22. Identify the changes that occur with the aging process in the following sensory areas. ***(1105)***

    a. Vision: ______________________________

    ____

    b. Hearing: ______________________________

    ____

    c. Taste and smell: ______________________________

    ____

23. An age-related change in the neurologic function of the older adult is ______________________________
______________________________. ***(1108)***

24. The goals for the patient with Alzheimer's disease are: ***(1109-1110)***______________________________

    ____

    ____

25. What is the difference between a transient ischemic attack (TIA) and a cerebrovascular accident (CVA)? ***(1111-1112)***

    ____

    ____

26. What changes occur in the pattern of rest and sleep for the older adult? ***(1108-1109)***______________________________

    ____

    ____

27. Metabolism of medications is decreased in the older adult as a result of: ***(1115-1116)***______________________________

    ____

    ____

Multiple Choice

28. A change that occurs in the integumentary system of the older adult is: ***(1088)***
    1. decreased capillary fragility.
    2. increased hair pigmentation.
    3. increased sweat gland function.
    4. decreased vascularity of the dermis.

29. The recommended caloric intake for an average older adult is: ***(1090)***
    1. 1000 to 1200 kcal/day.
    2. 1200 to 1500 kcal/day.
    3. 1800 to 2400 kcal/day.
    4. 3000 or more kcal/day.

30. Inadequate arterial circulation to the lower extremities of an older adult is usually evident with the presence of: ***(1096-1097)***
    1. edema.
    2. excessive warmth.
    3. bounding pulses.
    4. cramping of the calf muscles.

31. The effects of medications given to older adults may be altered as a result of: ***(1115-1116)***
    1. decreased adipose tissue.
    2. increased gastric secretions.
    3. increased total body water.
    4. increased sensitivity of brain receptors.

PSYCHOSOCIAL CHANGES THAT OCCUR WITH AGING

Objectives

- Describe ways finances and housing are major concerns for the older adult.
- Discuss common psychosocial events that occur to the older adult.
- Identify ways to preserve dignity and to increase self-esteem of the older adult.

32. Social reminiscence involves: ***(1111)*** ______________________________

    ____

    ____

33. Identify the concerns of the older adult related to the following. ***(1113-1114)***

    a. Finances: ______________________________

    ____

    b. Housing: ______________________________

    ____

34. Specify whether the following statements are true (T) or false (F). ***(1086)***
    a. Cognitive abilities decrease in old age. _____
    b. Medication dosages for older adults may have to be reduced. _____
    c. The majority of older adults reside in nursing homes. _____
    d. A primary factor in the decreased sexual activity of the older adult is the lack of a sexual partner. _____

35. Losses experienced by the older adult may include: ***(1087)***________________________________

____

____

36. A common response to loss in the older adult is ________________________. ***(1087)***

37. Evaluate whether the following communication is appropriate. ***(1120)***
    a. Calling the older woman "Grandma" _____
    b. Addressing the older adult by the first name _____

NURSING INTERVENTIONS

Objectives

- Identify nursing diagnoses appropriate to common health concerns of the older adult.
- Describe appropriate nursing interventions for common health concerns of the older adult.

38. For the following systems, describe the nursing assessment of the older adult. ***(1088-1109)***

    a. Integumentary:____

    ____

    b. Cardiovascular: ____

    ____

    c. Respiratory: ____

    ____

    d. Gastrointestinal:____

    ____

    e. Urinary:____

    ____

    f. Musculoskeletal: ____

    ____

    g. Neurologic:____

    ____

39. Identify nursing interventions that may be implemented for the older adult who is experiencing constipation. ***(1093-1094)***

____

____

40. What nursing interventions may be implemented for the patient with peripheral vascular disease? ***(1097)***

____

____

41. Identify a possible nursing diagnosis and interventions for an older adult experiencing respiratory changes. ***(1099)***

____

____

42. What interventions should be implemented by the nurse to reduce the chance of falls for the older adult in an acute or long-term care setting? ***(1114)***

____

____

43. How can the nurse promote an older adult's sexuality? ***(1105)***______________________

____

____

44. Measures that should be used by the nurse to promote the patient's vision and hearing are: ***(1107)***

____

____

45. Reality orientation includes: ***(1109)*** ______________________________

____

____

46. Identify the nursing interventions for the older adult who is taking the following medications. ***(1115-1116)***

    a. Antihypertensives: ______________________________

    ____

    b. Diuretics:______________________________________

    ____

c. Opioids and narcotics: ____

____

47. Upon visiting the patient at home following hospital discharge, the nurse determines that the individual is at risk for the effects of polypharmacy, as evidenced by finding ________________________________ ________________________. ***(1115-1116)***

Multiple Choice

48. For the patient who is experiencing nocturia, the nurse intervenes by: ***(1095)***
    1. restraining the patient.
    2. giving diuretics after 7:00 PM.
    3. providing fluids at bedtime.
    4. keeping the call bell within reach.

49. The older adult is experiencing pruritus. The nurse should: ***(1089)***
    1. apply water-based lotions.
    2. use an antibacterial soap.
    3. increase the frequency of bathing.
    4. administer regular alcohol rubs.

50. For the older adult patient with dysphagia, the nurse should: ***(1092)***
    1. add thickeners to liquids.
    2. feed the patient quickly to reduce fatigue.
    3. place the patient in low Fowler's position for meals.
    4. distract the patient by putting on music or the television.

51. The nurse anticipates that the patient who has osteoporosis will receive: ***(1102)***
    1. raloxifene (Evista).
    2. amantadine (Symmetrel).
    3. tacrine (Cognex).
    4. trihexyphenidyl (Artane).

52. The patient is taking a nonsteroidal antiinflammatory agent for arthritis. Appropriate teaching includes instructing the patient to: ***(1100)***
    1. take the medication with food.
    2. monitor blood glucose levels.
    3. observe for changes in hearing acuity.
    4. take the medication daily in the early morning.

53. The nurse is performing an admission assessment on a new resident in a long-term care facility. The nurse notes that the resident has kyphosis. This means that the resident an abnormal curvature in the: ***(1102)***
    1. cervical spine.
    2. thoracic spine.
    3. lumbar spine.
    4. entire spine.

54. The nurse has been performing patient and family teaching for a male patient who has suffered a stroke. The family demonstrates an understanding of their loved one's condition of difficulty in speaking by stating: ***(1112-1113)***
    1. "We hope the aphasia will improve as his condition improves."
    2. "Suffering from dysphasia is going to put him at risk for developing pneumonia."
    3. "Presybyopia is a difficult condition to deal with."
    4. "Having akinesia is going to make care at home very challenging."

55. During the integumentary assessment, the nurse notes that the patient suffers from pruritus. To help the patient with this condition, the nurse should encourage the patient to: (Select all that apply) ***(1089)***
    1. avoid antibacterial soap during bathing.
    2. apply water-based lotions after bathing.
    3. bathe or shower daily using only warm water.
    4. be sure to rinse all soap from skin.

Student Name______________________ **Date**______________

chapter

34

Basic Concepts of Mental Health

Answer Key: Textbook page references are provided as a guide for answering these questions. A complete answer key was provided for your instructor.

BASIC CONCEPTS

Objectives

- Describe the mental health continuum.
- Identify defining characteristics of persons who are mentally healthy and those who are mentally ill.
- Describe the parts of personality.
- Describe the factors that influence an individual's response to change.

1. What is the emphasis of mental health nursing? ***(1122)*** ______________________

2. In relation to treatment of mental illness, identify a major development or historical figure associated with the following time periods or events. ***(1123-1125)***

   a. Greco-Roman period: ______________________

   b. Dark Ages: ______________________

   c. Late 1700s to 1800s: ______________________

   d. 1940s: ______________________

   e. 1970s: ______________________

   f. Omnibus Budget Reconciliation Act (OBRA): ______________________

3. What is meant by a *mental health continuum*? ***(1125)*** ______________________

4. Identify some general characteristics that are associated with mental illness. ***(1125)*** ______________________

5. For the following theorists, identify the basic concepts of personality development. ***(1126)***

   a. Erikson: ____________________

   b. Freud: ____________________

6. Identify the following parts of the self. ***(1126)***

   a. The part that strives for perfection and morality: ____________________

   b. The part that demands constant gratification: ____________________

   c. The part that decides when and how to act: ____________________

ALTERATIONS IN MENTAL HEALTH

Objectives

- Identify factors that contribute to the development of emotional problems or mental illness.
- Identify barriers to health adaptation.
- Identify sources of stress.
- Identify stages of illness behavior.
- Identify major components of a nursing assessment that focuses on mental health status.
- Identify basic nursing interventions for those experiencing illness or crisis.

7. What are the types and the effects of stressors on a person? ***(1127)*** ____________________

8. Identify the typical responses to the following types of anxiety. ***(1127)***

   a. Mild anxiety: ____________________

   b. Moderate anxiety: ____________________

   c. Severe anxiety: ____________________

   d. Panic: ____________________

9. Describe how motivation, frustration, conflicts, and coping abilities affect an individual. ***(1128)*** ____________________

10. What are possible coping responses that may be used by individuals? ***(1128)*** ____________________

11. Common behaviors seen in illness are: ***(1130)*** ____________________

____

____

12. Identify examples of nursing diagnoses and patient outcomes that may be used in mental health nursing. ***(1130)***

____

____

13. a. What are the goals of crisis intervention? ***(1131)***____________________

____

____

b. Put the following steps of crisis intervention in order. ***(1131)***
   i. Implement the plan of interventions. _____
   ii. Begin anticipatory planning. _____
   iii. Assess the situation and the individual involved. _____
   iv. Obtain assistance from significant others. _____

14. What considerations should be made for the older adult in regard to mental health? ***(1130)*** ____________________

____

____

15. Assessment of the patient's emotional state includes: ***(1132)***____________________

____

____

Multiple Choice

16. The nurse is assessing an individual's use of defense mechanisms. One of the parents has had a bad day at work and comes home and shouts at the children. This is an example of: ***(1129)***
   1. projection.
   2. displacement.
   3. identification.
   4. reaction formation.

17. Regressive behavior is identified by the nurse when observing: ***(1129)***
   1. the victim of sexual abuse who laughs while telling about the incident.
   2. an adolescent who participates in a lot of competitive sports.
   3. an 80-year-old acts as if an incident of incontinence did not occur.
   4. an 8-year-old begins sucking his thumb and wetting the bed when hospitalized for the first time.

18. An adolescent female patient tells the nurse that she often feels very "uneasy" but can't identify any specific reasons for this feeling. This patient is experiencing: ***(1127)***
    1. stress.
    2. anxiety.
    3. crisis.
    4. mental illness.

19. A mentally healthy individual is capable of: (Select all that apply) ***(1122)***
    1. adapting successfully to change.
    2. setting realistic goals.
    3. problem solving.
    4. enjoying life's activities.

20. Deinstitutionalization occurred in the 1950s as a result of: ***(1124)***
    1. electroconvulsive therapy.
    2. the National Health Act.
    3. insulin shock therapy.
    4. the introduction of psychotherapeutic drugs.

Student Name________________________ Date____________

chapter

35

Care of the Patient with a Psychiatric Disorder

Answer Key: Textbook page references are provided as a guide for answering these questions. A complete answer key was provided for your instructor.

MENTAL DISORDERS

Objectives

- List the five axes of *DSM-IV-TR* used to examine and treat mental illnesses.
- Identify and describe the major mental disorders.
- List five warning signs of suicide.

1. What is the difference between neurosis and psychosis? ***(1135)*** ____________

____

____

2. What is the purpose of the *Diagnostic and Statistical Manual of Psychiatric Disorders, IV-TR*? ***(1135-1136)***

____

____

3. What is the difference between anorexia nervosa and bulimia nervosa? ***(1148)***____________

____

____

4. For organic mental disorders, what is the difference between delirium and dementia? ***(1136)*** ____________

____

____

5. For the following, identify the classification of major mental disorder. ***(1136-1139)***

   a. Dementia: ____________

   b. Bizarre behavior, delusions, hallucinations: ____________

   c. Mood swings with manic episodes: ____________

d. Irrational fear of a specific object or situation: ________________

e. Poor impulse control, manipulation of others: ________________

6. The inability for a person to experience happiness or joy is known as ________________ ________________. *(1141)*

7. The patient with schizophrenia suffers from ________________, which is characterized by the inability to interpret information being received. *(1140)*

8. ________________ often affects patients with schizophrenia, leaving them with a reduced content of speech. *(1140)*

9. The patient with schizophrenia shows little or no nonverbal expression of emotions. The nurse documents this as the patient displaying a ________________. *(1141)*

10. ________________ is exhibited by a person showing a lack of caring or a state of indifference to the world around him or her. *(1140)*

11. Identify the following types of delusions that are exhibited. *(1140)*

a. "The man on the radio is telling me to buy that car." ________________

b. "That other patient put the idea in my head." ________________

c. "They are listening to my conversations through the intercom." ________________

12. What are the subtypes of schizophrenia? *(1141)* ________________

____

____

13. Identify the warning signs of suicide. *(1142)* ________________

____

____

14. What are the signs and symptoms of a panic attack? *(1145)* ________________

____

____

15. Identify the different types of personality disorders. *(1147)* ________________

____

____

16. Behavior that indicates a persistent desire to be the opposite sex is termed ________________ ________________. *(1147)*

TREATMENT

Objectives

- Identify basic interventions for patients experiencing various mental health problems.
- Describe the general care and treatment methods for patients experiencing mental health problems.
- Name two alternative medicines used for mental disorders.

17. What are some of the commonalities in nursing interventions for patients with mental disorders? ***(1136-1139)***

____

____

18. Identify at least two considerations for older adult patients with mental disorders. ***(1140)***_______________

____

____

19. For a patient with a mood or anxiety disorder, the nurse can decrease stimuli by: ***(1138-1139)***_______________

____

____

20. What are specific treatments for patients who are depressed? ***(1143)***_______________

____

____

21. Identify precautions that should be taken for patients who are suicidal. ***(1142)***_______________

____

____

22. Identify whether the following statements are appropriate when preparing a patient for electroconvulsive therapy (ECT). ***(1143)***
    a. Pain will be experienced. _____
    b. Confusion will decrease after a few hours. _____
    c. Grand mal seizures are experienced. _____
    d. Temporary memory loss is experienced after treatment. _____
    e. Most patients are kept in the hospital for 2 to 3 days afterward. _____

23. What medications are typically used for depression? ***(1143)*** _______________

____

____

24. Identify possible patient outcomes for an individual who is experiencing depression. ***(1144-1145)***______

______

______

25. The patient in the clinic escaped the World Trade Center disaster on September 11, 2001. ***(1146)***

 a. The nurse is alert to the possible development of: ______.

 b. Signs and symptoms of this disorder are: ______

______

______

26. The patient has come to the physician's office with nausea, vomiting, and stomach pain. The patient tells the nurse that she just got a new job with a lot of responsibilities, many people to supervise, and two projects that are due within the month. The nurse suspects that this patient may be experiencing: ***(1148)***

______

______

27. The nurse who is working with patients with sexual disorders should first: ***(1147)*** ______

______

______

28. While completing an admission history, the patient asks the nurse not to tell anyone that he wants to end his life. The nurse should respond by: ***(1150)***

______

______

29. What are the different types of psychotherapy? ***(1149-1150)*** ______

______

______

30. a. For the following, identify examples of medications, side effects, and nursing actions. ***(1151-1152)***

 i. Antipsychotics: ______

______

 ii. Antidepressants: ______

______

b. The nurse anticipates that intervention for tardive dyskinesia will include: ***(1151-1152)*** ____________

____

31. Identify examples of alternative therapies and their uses. ***(1154)*** ____________________

____

____

32. A serious problem that can occur with selective serotonin reuptake inhibitors (SSRIs) is ____________ ____________________. ***(1153)***

Multiple Choice

33. Communication with a patient who is in the manic phase of a bipolar affective disorder should: ***(1138)***
    1. reinforce assertive behaviors.
    2. provide focus and consistency.
    3. offer verbal reminders of the day and date.
    4. encourage lengthy expression of thoughts and feelings.

34. The nurse anticipates that the patient with an obsessive-compulsive disorder will receive: ***(1151-1152)***
    1. Lithobid (lithium carbonate).
    2. Haldol (haloperidol).
    3. Thorazine (chlorpromazine).
    4. Anafranil (clomipramine).

35. The nurse is aware that a patient who is receiving lithium therapy needs to have an adequate intake of: ***(1151-1152)***
    1. calcium.
    2. sodium.
    3. magnesium.
    4. potassium.

36. A patient tells you that he is hearing voices right now that are telling him not to eat. The nurse's best response is: ***(1137)***
    1. "What did the voices tell you not to eat?"
    2. "Did the voices say that you couldn't even eat snacks?"
    3. "I don't think that the voices would tell you not to eat anything."
    4. "I don't hear any voices. Tell me what you are experiencing now."

37. The nurse is given the assignment for the day. Based on the report provided, the nurse prioritizes and decides to see which one of the following patients first? ***(1142)***
    1. The patient had ECT therapy 30 minutes ago.
    2. The patient has refused to take the prescribed medication.
    3. The patient has said, "I am going to end this suffering."
    4. The patient identified that "voices" told him not to eat the food today.

38. The patient experiencing drug-induced psychosis complains to the nurse while on the behavioral health unit that he has been smelling natural gas in the air for the past 2 days. This patient is experiencing: ***(1140)***
    1. delusions.
    2. depression.
    3. mania.
    4. hallucinations.

39. Signs and symptoms of schizophrenia typically include: (Select all that apply) ***(1140)***
    1. phobias.
    2. delusions.
    3. mania.
    4. paranoia.

40. Which patient statement would indicate a compulsion? ***(1146)***
    1. "I can't stop thinking about my hand towels in the bathroom being out of place on the towel rack."
    2. "I had to drive back home 8 times this morning to be sure I locked my front door."
    3. "Those voices in my head are driving me crazy. Can you make them stop?"
    4. "It terrifies me to think about going fishing this weekend because I know there may be spiders in the boat."

41. Mrs. B. suffers from bipolar disorder and is displaying an outgoing personality, productivity in her work, and great optimism. What phase of bipolar disorder is she experiencing? ***(1143)***
    1. Manic
    2. Depressive
    3. Cyclothymic
    4. Hypomanic

42. A wife complains that her husband must be neurotic. What signs and symptoms would you expect the husband to display? (Select all that apply) ***(1135)***
    1. Nervousness
    2. Low self-esteem
    3. Psychosis
    4. Phobias

Student Name____ Date______________

chapter 36

Care of the Patient with an Addictive Personality

Answer Key: Textbook page references are provided as a guide for answering these questions. A complete answer key was provided for your instructor.

ADDICTION

Objectives

- Name two traits attributed to an addictive personality.
- Describe the three stages of dependence.
- Describe one legal effort that has decreased the incidence of substance abuse.

1. What are the four elements of addiction? ***(1158)*** ____________________

____

____

2. a. An amazing statistic is that ________% of children who begin drinking at or before the age of 14 develop alcoholism. ***(1158)***

   b. ________% of all motor vehicle accident deaths and fatal injuries are associated with alcohol. ***(1159)***

3. In relation to drugs, how has federal law influenced the health care provider? ***(1159)*** ____________________

____

____

4. Provide examples of behaviors seen in the early, middle, and late stages of dependence. ***(1159)*** ________

____

____

5. Provide examples of the subjective and objective data that typically emerge in the course of completing a nursing assessment that may be indicative of substance abuse. ***(1162)***

____

____

6. What diagnostic tests may be used to determine the possibility of substance abuse? ***(1162)*** ____________

____

____

7. Give examples of possible nursing diagnoses and outcomes for addicted patients who have physical and emotional needs. ***(1163)***

____

____

8. What support groups are available for individuals who are seeking to stop their addictive behavior? ***(1164-1165)***

____

____

9. The goal of treatment centers is ____________. ***(1165)***

ALCOHOLISM

Objectives

- Describe three disorders associated with alcoholism.
- Explain the two phases of recovery: detoxification and rehabilitation.

10. a. What are some of the possible contributing factors to alcoholism? ***(1160)*** ____________

____

____

b. A questionnaire that is helpful in determining alcohol abuse is: ____________
____________. ***(1161)***

11. Alcohol is classified as a ____________. ***(1160)***

12. One of the reasons that binge drinking by college students is such a hazard is because rapid, large-quantity consumption of alcohol can lead to ____________
____________. ***(1161)***

13. Identify the electrolyte and nutritional imbalances that may occur with alcoholism and the reason they occur. ***(1160-1161)***

____

____

14. What complications or problems are associated with fetal alcohol syndrome? ***(1161)*** ______

15. For the following disorders associated with alcoholism, identify the signs and symptoms and when they usually begin to be seen. ***(1161)***

    a. Alcohol withdrawal syndrome: ______

    b. Delirium tremens: ______

    c. Korsakoff's psychosis and Wernicke's encephalopathy: ______

16. Identify the effects that alcohol has on the following body systems. ***(1162)***

    a. Gastrointestinal: ______

    b. Hepatic: ______

    c. Cardiovascular: ______

    d. Respiratory: ______

    e. Musculoskeletal: ______

17. For the phases of recovery, identify the nursing interventions that should be implemented. ***(1163)***

    a. Acute or detoxification: ______

    b. Rehabilitation: ______

Multiple Choice

18. A patient has a blood alcohol level of 475 mg/dL (0.475%). The nurse expects that this patient will exhibit: ***(1161)***
    1. stupor or coma.
    2. stumbling and blurred vision.
    3. clumsiness and emotional changes.
    4. mild sedation with pleasant, relaxed attitude.

DRUG ABUSE

Objective

- Identify six types of drugs of abuse.

19. Substance abuse affects what part of the brain? ***(1160-1161)*** ______________________

    This may alter the person's ______________________.

20. Identify the signs and symptoms of central nervous system (CNS) depressants. ***(1167)***______________________

    ____

    ____

21. Identify at least six commonly abused drugs. ***(1166)***______________________

    ____

    ____

22. What drugs have been associated with "date rape"? ***(1167)*** ______________________

    ____

    ____

23. The most widely abused opioid is______________________. ***(1167)***

24. For opioids, identify the signs and symptoms of an overdose and withdrawal. ***(1167)*** ______________________

    ____

    ____

25. a. What is the use of methadone? ***(1167)*** ______________________

    ____

    ____

    b. What drug is being used to obtain better effects than methadone? ***(1167)***______________________

26. Identify the different types of stimulants. ***(1167-1168)*** ____________________

____

____

27. What are the signs and symptoms of stimulant use? ***(1168)*** ____________________

____

____

28. Medications that are used to decrease the craving for cocaine are: ***(1168)*** ____________________

____

____

29. The nurse is assessing a patient who is suspected of chronic cocaine abuse. The nurse will expect to find: ***(1168)***

____

____

30. What are the complications of amphetamine use? ***(1168)*** ____________________

____

____

31. A patient has been abusing a hallucinogen. What serious problems may this patient develop? ***(1168-1169)***

____

____

32. a. What signs and symptoms may be seen with the use of ecstasy (methylenedioxymethamphetamin, or MDMA)? ***(1169)***

____

____

b. What makes this drug so dangerous for abuse? ***(1169)*** ____________________

____

____

33. a. Cannabis is also known as____________________. ***(1170)***

b. Identify possible effects of its use: ***(1170)*** ______________________________

____

____

34. Identify examples of gateway drugs. ***(1158-1170)*** ______________________________

____

____

35. What are some of the common effects of inhalant use? ***(1170-1171)*** ______________________________

____

____

Multiple Choice

36. A co-worker states that he has had too much caffeine and wants to eliminate it from his diet. He should be advised to drink: ***(1168)***
    1. coffee.
    2. cola drinks.
    3. orange juice.
    4. hot chocolate.

37. The patient is quitting smoking cigarettes. The withdrawal from nicotine may result in the patient having: ***(1168)***
    1. lethargy.
    2. improved concentration.
    3. decreased heart rate.
    4. decreased appetite.

38. The nurse is working with patients who have abused the following substances. The nurse is *not* anticipating to see withdrawal signs and symptoms with the patient who uses: ***(1168-1169)***
    1. cannabis.
    2. CNS stimulants.
    3. CNS depressants.
    4. hallucinogens.

39. A college student who has used marijuana since early high school is diagnosed with amotivational cannabis syndrome. Characteristics of this disorder include: (Select all that apply) ***(1170)***
    1. unusual irritability.
    2. frequent mood swings.
    3. depression.
    4. psychosis.

40. Upon admission to a rehabilitation unit, a patient states that he has noticed that he must smoke more marijuana to "get high" than he used to. This patient is exhibiting: ***(1170)***
    1. bruxism.
    2. tolerance.
    3. addiction.
    4. withdrawal.

41. Addiction can occur with which of the following substances? (Select all that apply) ***(1158-1159)***
    1. Alcohol
    2. Tobacco
    3. Caffeine
    4. Antidepressants

42. Methylenedioxymethamphetamine (MDMA) is an example of which classification of drugs? ***(1169)***
    1. Opioids
    2. Amphetamines
    3. Depressants
    4. Hallucinogens

IMPAIRED NURSE

Objective

- Describe steps taken to help the chemically impaired nurse.

43. The chemically impaired nurse may exhibit the same signs and symptoms of abuse as any other individual who is addicted. What are the specific role-related signs or behaviors that may be seen by co-workers? ***(1173)***

    ____

    ____

44. Identify the assistance that is available for the chemically impaired nurse. ***(1173)*** ____________

    ____

    ____

45. What is the Healthcare Integrity and Protection Data Bank (HIPDB)? ***(1173)***____________

    ____

    ____

Student Name______________________________ Date______________

chapter 37 Home Health Nursing

Answer Key: Textbook page references are provided as a guide for answering these questions. A complete answer key was provided for your instructor.

TERMS

Objective

- Define the key terms as listed.

1. Define the following terms.

 a. Medicare: ***(1187)***______________________________

 ____

 b. Medicaid: ***(1187)***______________________________

 ____

OVERVIEW AND TRENDS

Objectives

- List at least three types of home health agencies.
- Discuss new developments that are occurring in home health care, including remote electronic monitoring.

2. Identify the historical developments in home health care associated with the following dates. ***(1178-1179)***

 a. 1600s: ______________________________

 ____

 b. 1796: ______________________________

 ____

 c. 1893: ______________________________

 ____

d. 1909: ______________________________

____

e. 1935: ______________________________

____

f. 1965: ______________________________

____

g. 1983: ______________________________

____

3. What special considerations are made by the nurse in regard to the older adult and home care? ***(1179)***

____

____

4. For the following types of home health agencies, provide an example and state who the agency is governed by. ***(1181)***

a. Voluntary: ______________________________

____

b. Official: ______________________________

____

c. Proprietary: ______________________________

____

5. What are some of the regulations that must be followed by home health agencies? ***(1179-1180)*** ________

____

____

6. Identify at least two of the changes that are occurring in home health care. ***(1180, 1182)*** ________

____

____

7. What factors have increased the need for home health care? ***(1180, 1182)*** ________

____

____

8. Discuss telemonitoring in home health care. ***(1180)*** ____________________

____

____

SERVICES

Objectives

- Describe how home health care differs from community and public health care services.
- List at least four services that may be provided by home health care.
- Describe two major ways home care differs from hospital care.
- Define skilled nursing services.
- Describe the role of the LPN/LVN in the delivery of skilled nursing care.
- Relate the nursing process to home health care practice.
- Relate seven steps to breaking through cultural barriers to communication.

9. Identify the types of services that are provided by home health agencies. ***(1182)*** ____________________

____

____

10. What is meant by *skilled nursing care*? ***(1182)*** ____________________

____

____

11. The service goals of home health nursing are: ***(1182)*** ____________________

____

____

12. The role of the LPN/LVN in home health care is: ***(1183)*** ____________________

____

____

13. Where do home health care referrals usually come from? ***(1185)*** ____________________

____

____

14. What are the steps in the home health care process once the patient is referred? ***(1185)*** ____________________

____

____

15. Identify what is included in the admission of a patient to the home health care agency. ***(1185-1186)***______

____

____

16. What type of documentation is used in home health care, and what methods may be used to complete it? ***(1186)***

____

____

17. The major principles of total quality management or quality improvement are: ***(1187)*** ______________

____

____

18. Identify at least two steps that may be taken to break through the cultural barriers to communication. ***(1189)***

____

____

19. What activities may be delegated to a home health aide? ***(1185)***______________________________

____

____

Multiple Choice

20. The home health nurse will refer the patient who requires promotion of independence with the use of a self-help device to the: ***(1184)***
    1. social worker.
    2. physical therapist.
    3. home health aide.
    4. occupational therapist.

21. The home health nurse should provide safety information to the patient and family members for home oxygen use. The information should include: (Select all that apply) ***(1183)***
    1. the use of petrolatum-based lubricant on the lips is allowed.
    2. "No Smoking" signs should be posted on the front and back doors.
    3. frequent oral hygiene is necessary owing to the drying of mucous membranes.
    4. only wool blankets should be used by the patient.

REIMBURSEMENT

Objectives

- Summarize governmental financing for home health nursing.
- List two sources of reimbursement for home care services.

22. Identify the effect that federal financing has had on home health care since 1997. ***(1179)***_______________

____

____

23. Medicare and Medicaid require that the plan of treatment is: ***(1187)***____________________

____

____

24. What are the Medicare requirements for the following services? ***(1184-1185)***

    a. Physical therapy: ____

    ____

    b. Speech therapy: ____

    ____

    c. Home health aide: _______________________________________

    ____

Student Name________________________________ Date______________

Long-Term Care

chapter **38**

Answer Key: Textbook page references are provided as a guide for answering these questions. A complete answer key was provided for your instructor.

REGULATIONS AND REIMBURSEMENT

Objectives

- Discuss federal and state regulations related to long-term care.
- Identify the sources of reimbursement for long-term care services.

1. What did the Omnibus Budget Reconciliation Act of 1987 (OBRA) do for long-term care? ***(1201)*** ________

____

____

2. What did OBRA do for the LPN/LVN in long-term care? ***(1201)*** ________________

____

____

3. Identify the legal and ethical issues related to long-term care. ***(1201)*** ________________

____

____

4. What sources of reimbursement are available for long-term care facilities? ***(1201)*** ________________

____

____

5. Describe what is provided under the Program of All-Inclusive Care for the Elderly (PACE). ***(1196)***

____

____

PATIENTS AND SERVICES

Objectives

- Describe settings of long-term care services.
- Identify patients of long-term care services.
- Define chronic and acute health services.
- Describe goals of long-term care health services.
- Describe long-term care nursing services.
- Describe services available from each type of agency: home health agency, hospice agency, adult day care, assisted living facility, continuing care community, long-term care facility.

6. What are some of the cultural and ethnic considerations for long-term care? ***(1194)***__________________

____

____

7. Identify the different settings for long-term care, and provide an example of each type. ***(1194-1199)***

____

____

8. For the patient who has a terminal disease, the appropriate referral is to a: ***(1196)*** __________________

____

____

9. The patient requires stimulation and supervision while her daughter is at work. What type of setting is recommended? ***(1196-1197)***

____

____

10. Assisted living offers what types of services for its residents? ***(1197)***__________________________

____

____

11. How does a continuing care retirement community differ from an assisted living community? ***(1198)***

____

____

12. Identify the advantages or benefits associated with subacute care. ***(1198)*** ______________________

____

____

13. What is the profile of the patient who requires long-term care in an institutional setting? ***(1199)***

14. Explain how the administration of medications can differ in long-term care facilities. ***(1200)***

15. What is the purpose of a resident assessment instrument (RAI), and what is involved in the assessment? ***(1202)***

16. How does documentation in a long-term care facility differ from that in a hospital setting? ***(1202)***

17. Identify a nursing diagnosis for a resident in a long-term care facility who has safety needs. ***(1203)***

18. Identify the usual time frame for the following nursing activities in a long-term care facility. ***(1199-1200)***
    a. Making rounds to monitor residents:
    b. Reviewing the plan of care:
    c. Charting for a resident who has no change in status:

19. What are two ethical issues that may arise in relation to long-term care? ***(1201)***

Multiple Choice

20. The nurse is assisting in training a new certified nurse assistant (CNA) at a long-term care facility. The nurse would be correct in describing activities of daily living (ADLs) as: (Select all that apply) ***(1195)***
    1. bathing.
    2. brushing teeth.
    3. exercise.
    4. ambulating.

21. Mr. M. is requiring extensive wound care and intravenous antibiotics due to an infection in his surgical wound. A _________ will best meet his needs. ***(1198)***
    1. long-term care facility
    2. subacute unit
    3. residential care facility
    4. hospice unit

22. _________ defines requirements for the quality of care given to residents and covers many aspects of institutional life, including nutrition, staffing, and qualifications required of personnel. ***(1201)***
    1. Medicare
    2. HCFA
    3. OBRA
    4. Medicaid

23. The adult children of an elderly couple are concerned about their parents and feel that the parents, at times, need assistance with bathing, dressing, and taking their medication. Both of the parents are alert and oriented at all times. They are mobile, but suffer from arthritis. The setting that the parents would most benefit from would be: ***(1197)***
    1. a skilled nursing facility.
    2. a subacute unit.
    3. an adult day care facility.
    4. an assisted living community.

24. The interdisciplinary team at a long-term care facility is meeting to discuss the care plan of one of the residents, Mrs. H. Who should attend this meeting? (Select all that apply) ***(1199-1200)***
    1. Mrs. H.
    2. The activities director
    3. The director of nursing
    4. The nursing unit manager

Student Name______________________ Date______________

Rehabilitation Nursing

chapter **39**

Answer Key: Textbook page references are provided as a guide for answering these questions. A complete answer key was provided for your instructor.

TERMS

Objective

- Define the key terms as listed.

1. Define the following terms.

   a. Interdisciplinary rehabilitation team: ***(1209)*** ______________________

   b. Multidisciplinary rehabilitation team: ***(1209)*** ______________________

   c. Transdisciplinary rehabilitation team: ***(1210)*** ______________________

REHABILITATION NURSING

Objectives

- Define the philosophy of rehabilitation nursing.
- Describe the interdisciplinary rehabilitation team concept and the function of each team member.
- Discuss specialized practice characteristics of the rehabilitation nurse.

2. State the philosophy of rehabilitation nursing. ***(1206)*** ______________________

3. What are the different needs for rehabilitation? ***(1206-1207)*** ______________________

4. Identify at least two focus areas related to chronic illness and disability from *Healthy People 2010*. ***(1207)***

____

____

5. Identify a general goal of rehabilitation. ***(1209)*** ______________________

____

____

6. a. Who are the members of the rehabilitation team, and what are their roles? ***(1210)*** ________

   ____

   ____

   b. Describe the role of the rehabilitation nurse. ***(1210)*** ______________________

   ____

   ____

7. The comprehensive rehabilitation plan has the following characteristics. ***(1211)***

   a. The plan is started: ______________________________.

   b. The plan is reevaluated: ______________________________.

   c. The plan is developed based upon: ______________________________.

Multiple Choice

8. Two patients are admitted to a rehabilitation hospital. Both have the same medical condition, but one patient is not able to manage, physically or emotionally, the adaptation that is required. This patient is best described as having a: ***(1207)***
   1. disability.
   2. handicap.
   3. chronic illness.
   4. functional limitation.

DISABLING DISORDERS

Objectives

- Discuss two major disabling conditions.
- Provide nursing diagnoses, goals, interventions, and evaluation and outcome criteria for two major disabling conditions.

9. a. Discuss characteristics of chronicity. ***(1207)***

   b. What are two of the major disabling conditions? ***(1207)***

10. Define the following terms. ***(1214)***

    a. Quadriplegia:

    b. Paraplegia:

    c. Paresis:

11. For the following problems associated with spinal cord injuries, describe what happens, the signs and symptoms that are seen, and the nursing interventions. ***(1217)***

    a. Postural hypotension:

    b. Heterotopic ossification:

12. What are the two types of head injuries? ***(1217)***

13. Identify the characteristic rehabilitation needs of patients who have suffered traumatic brain injuries. ***(1218-1219)***

14. In the rehabilitative assessment of a patient following a traumatic brain injury (TBI), the nurse may expect to find: ***(1218)***

____

____

15. For patients with a spinal cord injury or a traumatic brain injury, identify possible nursing diagnoses and outcomes. ***(1216-1219)***

____

____

Multiple Choice

16. The patient experienced a spinal cord injury at the T6–T9 level. The nurse anticipates that the patient should be able to: ***(1216)***
    1. assist with activities of daily living (ADLs).
    2. ambulate independently.
    3. drive with hand controls.
    4. control bowel and bladder function.

17. The construction worker sustained an injury to C7 after a fall at a work site. The nurse anticipates that this patient will be: ***(1216)***
    1. nonambulatory.
    2. ADL-independent.
    3. independent in bladder care.
    4. returning to prior job responsibilities.

18. The emergency squad brought in the patient following an accident at home. One of the squad members tells the nurse that the patient, according to the spouse, was unconscious for 1½ hours. This head injury is described as: ***(1218)***
    1. mild.
    2. moderate.
    3. severe.
    4. catastrophic.

19. The patient has a spinal cord injury above the level of T5. While assisting with hygienic care, the nurse notices that the patient is diaphoretic and shivering, and he states that he has a headache. Upon assessment, it is found that his blood pressure is elevated. The nurse's next action should be to: ***(1217)***
    1. position the patient flat.
    2. provide analgesic medication.
    3. check for bladder distention.
    4. cover the patient with blankets.

20. The nurse anticipates that treatment for the patient with a spinal cord injury and deep-vein thrombosis will include: (Select all that apply) ***(1217)***
    1. fluid restriction.
    2. assessment for postural hypotension.
    3. application of heat.
    4. prescription of anticoagulants.

ISSUES IN REHABILITATION

Objectives

- Discuss the importance of returning home and preparing for community reentry.
- Recognize the importance and significance of family-centered care in rehabilitation.
- Recognize the uniqueness of pediatric and gerontologic rehabilitation nursing.

21. Differentiate between polytrauma and posttraumatic stress disorder (PTSD). ***(1213-1214)*** __________

22. Identify the cornerstones of rehabilitation. ***(1209)*** __________

23. Identify the key elements of family-centered care. ***(1212)*** __________

24. How are pediatric and gerontologic rehabilitation different from adult rehabilitation? ***(1212-1213)*** __________

Student Name________________________ Date____________

Hospice Care

chapter **40**

Answer Key: Textbook page references are provided as a guide for answering these questions. A complete answer key was provided for your instructor.

PHILOSOPHY AND ORGANIZATION

Objectives

- Discuss the philosophy of hospice care.
- Differentiate between palliative care and curative care.
- Name the members of the interdisciplinary team and explain their roles.
- Discuss the role of hospice in families' bereavement period.

1. What was the origin of the concept of hospice care? ***(1222)*** ____________________

____

____

2. The focus and the goals of hospice care are: ***(1224)*** ____________________

____

____

3. Identify the professionals in the core interdisciplinary hospice team and their roles. ***(1225)*** ____________________

____

____

4. What is the purpose of the bereavement team? ***(1226)*** ____________________

____

____

HOSPICE PATIENTS AND COMMON SYMPTOMS

Objectives

- Discuss four criteria for admission to hospice care.
- List three common symptoms related to a terminal illness.

- Discuss the usefulness of pain assessments and when assessments should be completed.
- Develop a care plan with patient goals related to these symptoms.

5. The usual criteria for admission of a patient to hospice are: ***(1224)*** ______

______

______

6. What is included in a pain assessment? ***(1228)*** ______

______

______

7. In addition to assessment, what are the other nursing responsibilities for management of a hospice patient's pain? ***(1227-1229)***

______

______

8. For pain relief or reduction, identify the types of medications that may be used for the following. ***(1227)***

   a. Mild to moderate pain: ______

   b. Severe pain: ______

   c. Long-lasting results: ______

9. In addition to pharmacologic therapy, the nurse recognizes that the following measures may also be implemented to relieve or reduce pain. ***(1229)***

______

______

10. For the other common symptoms of a terminal illness, identify the nursing interventions. ***(1229-1232)***

   a. Nausea and vomiting: ______

   ______

   b. Constipation: ______

   ______

   c. Anorexia and malnutrition: ______

   ______

   d. Dyspnea or air hunger: ______

   ______

e. Weight loss, dehydration, and weakness: ____________________

____

11. An appropriate response for the hospice nurse in determining the patient's spiritual needs is to: ***(1222)***

____

____

12. Identify signs and symptoms of approaching death and the appropriate nursing interventions. ***(1233)***

____

____

ISSUES

Objective

- Discuss two ethical issues in hospice care.

13. Identify ethical and legal issues that are associated with hospice care. ***(1234)*** ____________________

____

____

Multiple Choice

14. The patient asks the nurse what the criteria are for admission to a hospice. The nurse responds correctly when informing the patient that: ***(1224)***
    1. a nurse can certify the patient's condition.
    2. the patient must have a prognosis of fewer than 2 to 3 months to live.
    3. the patient and family must understand and be willing to participate in the planning of care.
    4. the patient will agree that life support measures will be performed routinely if needed.

15. The family of a dying patient is feeling physically and emotionally exhausted while taking shifts to care for their loved one 24 hours a day. This family could best benefit from the hospice service of: ***(1226)***
    1. respite care.
    2. palliative care consultation.
    3. bereavement counseling.
    4. the hospice ethics committee.

16. The physician orders additional medications as adjuvant therapy to the oral narcotics the terminally ill patient is taking for pain control. Examples of adjuvant medications include: (Select all that apply) ***(1228)***
    1. anticholinergics.
    2. anticonvulsants.
    3. pain medication patches.
    4. nonsteroidal antiinflammatory medications.

17. The wife of a terminally ill patient asks the hospice nurse why she gives different amounts of pain medication to her husband rather than the same dose each time. The nurse's best response is: (Select all that apply) ***(1229)***
    1. "Determining the right dose of medication is difficult. We must try different amounts to determine a safe dose."
    2. "It is difficult to determine how much pain medication is a safe dose for someone who is dying. I want to be sure we get the right dose."
    3. "Finding the correct dose for pain medication is by trial and error. Every patient is different with how he or she responds to the medication."
    4. "I am titrating his medication amount so that we can best manage his pain while keeping him alert enough to interact with you and your family."

Student Name________________________________ Date________________

chapter

41

Introduction to Anatomy and Physiology

Answer Key: Textbook page references are provided as a guide for answering these questions. A complete answer key was provided for your instructor.

ANATOMY AND PHYSIOLOGY

Objective

- Define the difference between *anatomy* and *physiology*.

Multiple Choice

1. The nursing instructor is planning a short in-service for nursing students. After completion of the program, the nursing instructor administers a short quiz to assess the participants' understanding of the information provided. Which of the following responses indicates the need for further education? ***(1237)***
    1. "There is little difference between anatomy and physiology."
    2. "*Anatomy* refers to the structures of the body."
    3. "The study of anatomy includes study of the organs of the body."
    4. "Physiology focuses on the functions of the body structures."

Objectives

- Define the term *anatomical position.*
- List and define the principal directional terms and sections (planes) used in describing the body and the relationship of body parts to one another.

2. The patient is in the anatomical position. Next to each body part, label the relationships of that part to the right hand and to the head. Also list the plane where the body part is located. ***(1237-1239)***

Body Part	Relationship to Right Hand	Relationship to Head	Plane of Body Part
a. Left hand			
b. Right foot			
c. Left shoulder			
d. Right knee			
e. Left elbow			

(Continued next page)

Body Part	Relationship to Right Hand	Relationship to Head	Plane of Body Part
f. Chin			
g. Right pelvic area			
h. Left posterior buttock			
i. Right heel			
j. Left thigh			

ANATOMICAL TERMS

Objective

- Use each word in a given list of anatomical terms in a sentence.

3. Insert the correct choice from the following word bank into the blank in each sentence: *above, anterior, caudal, cranial, distal, inferior, lateral, medial, proximal,* and *superficial.* ***(1237-1238)***

   a. When facing forward, the patient is considered to be in a ____________________ position.

   b. The nurse knows the brain to be in the ____________________ portion of the body.

   c. The patient indicates the presence of pain toward the lower portion of the back. The nurse is aware that the distal region of the spine is ____________________.

   d. The nurse is reviewing the medical record in which the physician has documented that the patient's pain is superior to the shoulders. This means the pain is ____________________ the level of the shoulders.

   e. After being in an automobile accident, the patient has many abrasions near the surface of the skin. These are considered to be ____________________ lacerations.

   f. The knees are below the hips and are considered to be ____________________ to them.

   g. The nurse is preparing to document the patient's reports of pain in the center of the chest. Pain in this location can be termed ____________________.

   h. The patient asks for assistance to turn on to the right side. The nurse recognizes this to be a ____________________ lying position.

   i. The elbow is ____________________ to the forearm.

   j. The nurse is performing an assessment on the feet of a client who has reported to the clinic with an injury to the right heel. The nurse notes swelling in the toes. The toes are ____________________ to the heels.

BODY SYSTEMS

Objectives

- List and discuss the levels of organization of the body, in order of complexity.
- Differentiate among tissues, organs, and systems.

4. Describe the relationship among tissues, organs, and systems. Begin with most basic level of organization, and advance to more complex organizations. ***(1240-1241)***

____

____

CELL ART

Objective

- Identify and define three major components of the cell.

5. Label the parts of the cell. ***(1241)***

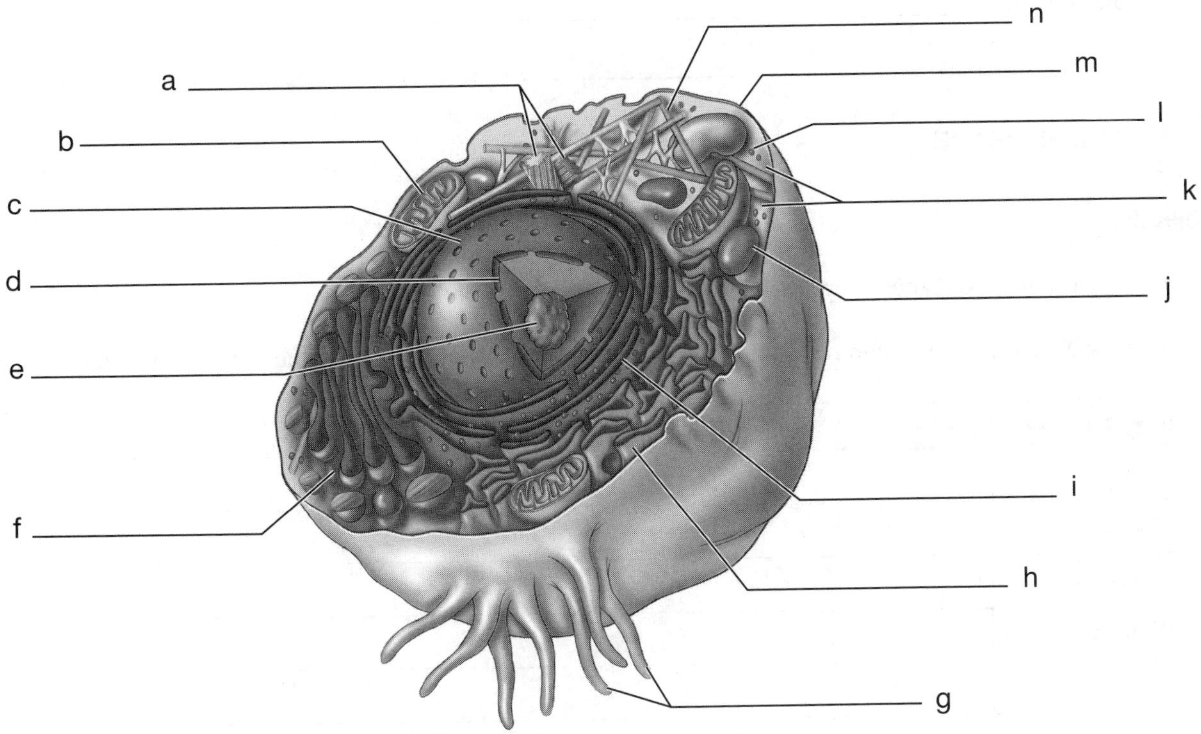

STAGES OF MITOSIS

Objective

- Discuss the stages of mitosis and explain the importance of cellular reproduction.

6. Next to each stage of mitosis, explain what happens to the chromosomes; also explain the significance of this type of reproduction. ***(1243-1244)***

   a. Prophase: ______________________________

   ____

   b. Metaphase: ______________________________

   ____

   c. Anaphase: ______________________________

   ____

   d. Telophase: ______________________________

   ____

   e. Significance: ______________________________

   ____

TYPES OF MEMBRANES

Objective

- Discuss the two types of epithelial membranes.

7. Identify each type of membrane that is present on the body surface listed in the left column. ***(1248)***

Body Surface	Type of Membrane
a. Nose	
b. Lungs	
c. Intestines	
d. Bladder	
e. Mouth	
f. Vagina	
g. Heart	
h. Knee	
i. Elbow	

MAJOR SYSTEMS—PATIENT OBSERVATION

Objective

- List the 11 major organ systems of the body and briefly describe the major functions of each major organ system.

8. When entering a patient's room for the first time, list the major systems that one would need to observe, one body part of that system, and why it would be important to make that observation. ***(1248-1249)***

Major System	One Body Part of that System	Importance of Observation
a.		
b.		
c.		
d.		
e.		
f.		
g.		
h.		
i.		
j.		
k.		

TYPES OF MUSCLES

Objective

- Describe the four types of body tissues.

9. Identify the types of muscles, and provide an example of the location of each type. ***(1247)***

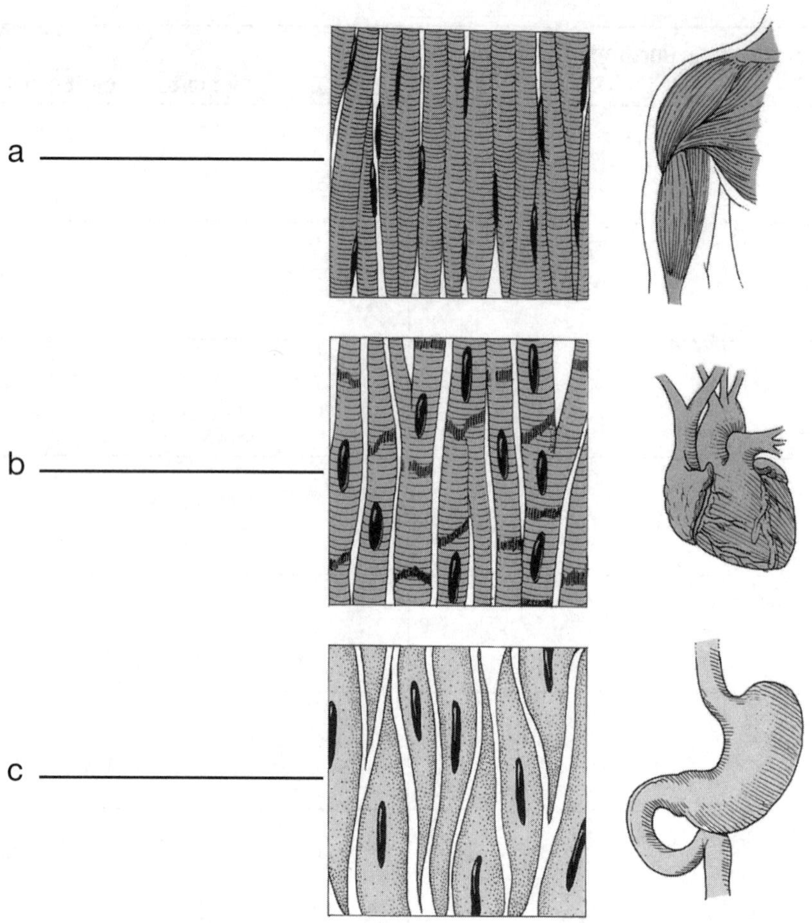

MOVEMENT

Objective

- Differentiate between active and passive transport processes that act to move substances through cell membranes, and give two examples of each.

10. List three types of active and three types of passive transport processes, and give two examples of each. ***(1244-1245)***

Active Transport	Example	Example
a.		
b.		
c.		
Passive Transport	**Example**	**Example**
d.		
e.		
f.		

FACING THE PATIENT

Objective

- List the nine abdominopelvic regions and the four abdominopelvic quadrants.

11. Standing at the foot of the supine patient's bed, establish the locations of the patient's major organs. Below, next to each of the nine abdominopelvic regions and the abdominopelvic quadrants, identify a major organ system and one part of that system. ***(1239)***

Region	Major Organ System	Part of that System
a. Right hypochondriac		
b. Epigastric		
c. Left hypochondriac		
d. Right lumbar		
e. Umbilical		
f. Left lumbar		
g. Right iliac (inguinal)		
h. Hypogastric		
i. Left iliac (inguinal)		

(Continued next page)

Quadrant	Major Organ System	Part of That System
j. Right upper		
k. Left upper		
l. Right lower		
m. Left lower		

12. Arrange the phases of mitosis in order of occurrence. ***(1244)***
    _____ Prophase
    _____ Telophase
    _____ Metaphase
    _____ Anaphase

MULTIPLE CHOICE

13. The production of enzymes and other proteins is the responsibility of the: ***(1241-1242)***
    1. mitochondria.
    2. ribosomes.
    3. nucleus.
    4. lysosomes.

14. Osmosis refers to: ***(1245)***
    1. the movement of water and particles through a membrane due to the force of either pressure or gravity.
    2. the passage of water across a selectively permeable membrane.
    3. a process in which solid particles in a fluid move from an area of higher concentration to an area of lower concentration.
    4. the passage of plasma across a selectively permeable membrane.

15. Examples of active transport processes include which of the following? (Select all that apply) ***(1244-1245)***
    1. Calcium pump
    2. Sodium pump
    3. Phagocytosis
    4. Pinocytosis

16. The nurse is reviewing a list of the functions of epithelial tissue. Which of the following should be included on this list? (Select all that apply) ***(1247)***
    1. Hormone production
    2. Protection
    3. Absorption
    4. Removal of wastes

Student Name________________________________ Date____________

chapter 42

Care of the Surgical Patient

Answer Key: Textbook page references are provided as a guide for answering these questions. A complete answer key was provided for your instructor.

PURPOSES OF SURGERY

Objective

- Identify the purposes of surgery.

1. Determine whether each statement below is true or false. ***(1254)***

   ______ a. The restoration of function to a lacerated arm is considered constructive surgery.

   ______ b. Removal of the appendix is an ablative type of surgery.

   ______ c. A breast biopsy is a palliative surgery.

   ______ d. A diagnostic surgery allows the physician to confirm a diagnosis.

   ______ e. A colostomy usually will not produce a cure.

   ______ f. Total hip replacement is a type of transplant surgery.

   ______ g. Closure of an atrial septal defect in the heart is constructive surgery.

   ______ h. Internal fixation of a right fibula is reconstructive surgery.

   ______ i. Removal of a mole that has an abnormal appearance is reconstructive surgery.

   ______ j. An ablative surgery is a removal of a diseased body part.

SURGERY URGENCY

Objective

- Distinguish between elective, urgent, and emergency surgery.

2. Explain the urgency of the following types of surgeries. List a surgical procedure for each. ***(1254)***

   a. Elective: ____

   ____

b. Emergency: ______________________________

____

c. Urgent: ______________________________

____

PERIOPERATIVE NURSING

Objective

- Explain the concept of perioperative nursing.

3. The surgical suite offers a variety of roles to the nurse. Obtain an index card. Divide the card into three separate areas. Designate areas for preoperative, intraoperative, and postoperative phases of the surgical experience. List three to five responsibilities of the nurse during each of the phases. ***(1254, 1255, 1260, 1261, 1264, 1269, 1277, 1281)***

TOLERANCE FACTORS

Objective

- Discuss the factors that influence an individual's ability to tolerate surgery.

Activity 1

4. Each of the following factors will affect how a patient will tolerate surgery. Explain what difference each one can make in a patient's reaction to surgery. ***(1255-1256)***

   a. Serious illness: ______________________________

   ____

b. Nutrition: ____

____

c. Socioeconomic and cultural needs: ____

____

d. Education and experience: ____

____

Objective

- Discuss considerations for the older adult surgical patient.

Activity 2

5. Discuss five unique challenges an older adult may experience when undergoing surgery. ***(1256, 1262)***

a. ____

____

b. ____

____

c. ____

____

d. ____

____

e. ____

____

PREOPERATIVE INFORMATION

Objective

- Describe the preoperative checklist.

6. Read each of the statements and indicate if it is true or false. ***(1277)***

_____ a. The preoperative checklist is completed by staff in the holding area of the surgical department.

______ b. The primary purpose of the preoperative checklist is to ensure that preoperative medications are administered on time.

______ c. The preoperative checklist must be completed by a licensed nurse.

______ d. The preoperative checklist provides a means of documenting the disposition of the patient's jewelry.

______ e. The Joint Commission requires surgical facilities to use a standardized preoperative checklist.

TURNING, COUGHING, DEEP-BREATHING, AND LEG EXERCISES

Objective

- Explain the procedure for turning, coughing, deep-breathing, and leg exercises for postoperative patients.

7. Develop an index card that will prompt you during your patient teaching for turning, coughing, deep-breathing, and leg exercises. Include major steps and enough information to remind you about what to teach your patient. ***(1266-1269)***

INFORMED CONSENT

Objective

- Explain the importance of informed consent for surgery.

8. Name the formal requirement that a patient provide informed consent before having a specific test or surgery. ***(1260-1261)***

____

____

9. What is established by the patient's signing the consent form? *(1260)*____________________

10. What four elements are required to be included in the information provided to the patient before a procedure? *(1260)*

11. To what does the witness attest by signing the consent? *(1260)* ____________________

12. Under what circumstances should informed consent not be obtained? *(1260)*____________________

13. What is done in the event of an emergency when the patient is unable to give informed consent? *(1261)*

14. What should be done if the patient does not understand the procedure or reports discrepancies from what he or she was told by the physician? *(1261)*

ANESTHESIA DURING THE SURGICAL EXPERIENCE

Objectives

- Differentiate among general, regional, and local anesthesia.
- Explain conscious sedation.

Multiple Choice

15. The patient is in the induction stage of anesthesia. Which of the following activities will most likely be taking place? *(1274)*
    1. Positioning the patient to perform the surgical procedure
    2. Decreasing the dosage(s) of anesthetic agent(s)
    3. Skin preparation
    4. Endotracheal intubation

16. During the preoperative teaching session, a patient voices concerns about waking up during surgery. What response by the nurse is indicated? *(1274)*
    1. "The anesthesia given during surgery will not wear off and allow you to wake up."
    2. "The anesthesiologist is able to monitor for this and will provide medications as needed."
    3. "Waking up is a risk you will face during the surgical procedure."
    4. "Emergence from anesthesia is a rare complication of surgery."

17. The patient is scheduled to undergo a urologic procedure in the surgical suite. The patient will be conscious during the procedure. Which of the following types of anesthesia will most likely be used? *(1275-1276)*
    1. Nerve block
    2. Epidural anesthesia
    3. Spinal anesthesia
    4. Local anesthesia

18. The patient is scheduled to undergo the removal of a benign cyst from his hand in the physician's office. The nurse is aware that the physician will most likely use which of the following types of anesthesia? *(1275-1276)*
    1. Regional anesthesia
    2. Local anesthesia
    3. Conscious sedation
    4. Intrathecal anesthesia

19. The nurse is preparing to assist the physician who is performing a procedure using conscious sedation. Which activity will be included in the nurse's responsibilities during the procedure? *(1276)*
    1. Monitoring of intake and output.
    2. Administration of the medication under the direction of the physician.
    3. Placement of the electrodes on the patient's chest to monitor cardiac activities.
    4. Assessment of vital signs.

20. The nurse is preparing an in-service for nursing staff on the unit. When discussing conscious sedation, which of the following statements should be included in the presentation? *(1276)*
    1. The recovery from the procedure is often risky.
    2. The patient undergoing conscious sedation is only intubated for a short time.
    3. There must be close access to resuscitation equipment.
    4. Conscious sedation is most appropriate for procedures such as biopsies or cosmetic procedures.

21. Skills of the nurse assisting with a conscious sedation procedure include: (Select all that apply) *(1276)*
    1. knowledge of normal and abnormal vital signs.
    2. ability to administer the medications to achieve conscious sedation under the direction of the physician.
    3. ability to initiate resuscitative actions.
    4. knowledge of pharmacologic principles related to anesthetic agents.

NURSE'S RESPONSIBILITIES

Objective

- Describe the roles of the circulating nurse and the scrub nurse during surgery.

22. Next to each task, indicate with a "C" if it is the circulating nurse's duty, an "S" if it is the scrub nurse's duty, or "CS" if it is both nurses' responsibility. ***(1280)***

Duty	Nurse
a. Performs surgical hand scrub	
b. Performs and confirms patient assessment	
c. Counts sponges, needles, and instruments	
d. Gowns and gloves surgeon	
e. Provides supplies as needed	
f. Assists by tying gowns	
g. Checks medical record for completeness	
h. Documents operative records and nursing notes	
i. Checks instruments for proper functioning	
j. Assists with surgical draping of patient	
k. Identifies and handles surgical specimens	
l. Observes progress of surgical procedure	
m. Observes sterile field closely for any breaks in aseptic techniques and reports accordingly	
n. Sends for patient at proper time	
o. Transfers patient to gurney for transport to recovery	
p. Maintains neat and orderly sterile field	
q. Prepares operating room with necessary equipment and supplies and ensures that equipment is functional	

ORAL AIRWAY

Objective

- Describe the roles of the circulating nurse and the scrub nurse in maintaining the airway during surgery.

23. Label the parts of the airway when the oral airway has been inserted. ***(1275)***

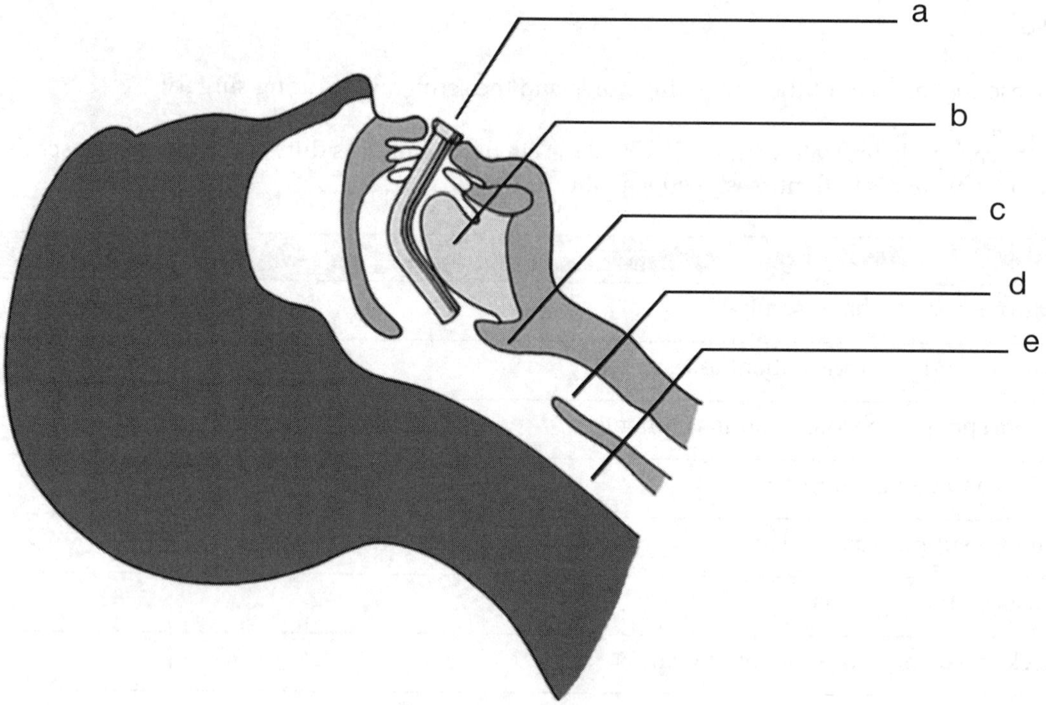

POSTOPERATIVE CARE

Objective

- Discuss the initial nursing assessment and management immediately after transfer from the postanesthesia care unit (PACU).

24. The patient has just returned from gastric surgery. Next to each assessment, list what normal findings the nurse would expect and how frequently he or she would do data collection. ***(1280-1287)***

Assessment	Normal Findings	Frequency
a. Vital signs		
b. Incision		
c. Ventilation		
d. Pain		

e. Urinary function		
f. Venous status		
g. Activity		
h. Gastrointestinal function		
i. Fluids and electrolytes		

RATIONALE FOR NURSING INTERVENTIONS

Objective

- Identify the rationale for nursing interventions designed to prevent postoperative complications.

25. The patient has just returned from surgery. List the rationale for each nursing intervention to prevent postoperative complications for this patient. ***(1280-1287)***

Nursing Intervention	Rationale
a. Vital signs	
b. Incision	
c. Ventilation	
d. Pain	
e. Urinary function	
f. Venous status	
g. Activity	
h. Gastrointestinal function	
i. Fluids and electrolytes	

NURSING PROCESS

Objectives

- Discuss the nursing process as it pertains to the surgical patient.
- List the assessment data for the surgical patient.

26. For each phase of the nursing process, indicate how it relates specifically to the surgical patient. ***(1287-1291)***

    a. Assessment: ______________________________

    b. Nursing diagnoses: ______________________________

    c. Planning: ______________________________

    d. Implementation: ______________________________

    e. Evaluation: ______________________________

PREPARATION FOR DISCHARGE

Objective

- Identify the information needed by the postoperative patient in preparation for discharge.

27. Develop an index card that contains the major information included in discharge planning for a surgical patient. ***(1291)***

MULTIPLE CHOICE

28. When developing the plan of care for an Arab American undergoing surgery, what cultural consideration may be of concern? ***(1257)***
    a. The culture's stoicism with regard to pain
    b. The often submissive role of woman
    c. The need for a written consent for surgery
    d. The high level of modesty

29. Preoperative teaching is ideally provided: ***(1255, 1260)***
    a. 1 to 2 days before surgery.
    b. the morning of surgery.
    c. at least 2 weeks preoperatively.
    d. any time, since there is no best time to teach preoperative care.

30. In which of the following conditions is use of GoLYTELY contraindicated? (Select all that apply) ***(1261)***
    a. Patients having a history of nausea and vomiting after surgery
    b. Patients experiencing gastric retention
    c. Patients having a history of bowel perforation
    d. Patients having had a hysterectomy

31. Before surgery of the bowel, neomycin, sulfonamides, or erythromycin may be given to: ***(1261)***
    a. reduce the risk of bowel perforation.
    b. reduce the risk of urinary tract infections.
    c. detoxify and sterilize the gastrointestinal tract.
    d. reduce the risk of pneumonia.

32. The nurse is providing care for a patient in the PACU who had an unexpected surgical procedure performed. As the nurse reviews the medical history, he notes the patient has a long-standing history of taking prescriptions for hypertension. Based upon this information, for what side effects that might be tied to the used of antihypertensive medications should the nurse monitor the patient? (Select all that apply) ***(1274)***
    a. Tachycardia
    b. Hypotension
    c. Bradycardia
    d. Hypothermia
    e. Diaphoresis

33. The patient preparing for surgery questions why he will be unable to continue to take ibuprofen in the days leading up to surgery. What information should be included in the nurse's response to the patient? (Select all that apply) ***(1274)***
    a. "Ibuprofen is associated with increased bleeding and will have to be avoided before surgery."
    b. "The medication may result in impaired healing during the postoperative period."
    c. "The medication can be associated with impaired functioning of the platelets."
    d. "The use of this medication is associated with an increase in postoperative infections."

34. Surgery is scheduled for an 81-year-old patient. A mastectomy is planned. Which of the following nursing diagnoses will of the highest priority during the immediate postoperative period? ***(1280-1281)***
    a. Knowledge deficit
    b. Potential for ineffective airway clearance
    c. Alteration in comfort
    d. Anxiety

CRITICAL THINKING ACTIVITIES

Activity 1

35. A 35-year-old woman reports to the physician's office with complaints of itching; hives on her arms, neck, and chest; and sore throat. She further reports that these symptoms occur when she is at work. Further assessment reveals she works in a local nursing home in the housekeeping department. Her health history is uneventful. She is diagnosed with a latex allergy.

    Discuss latex allergies. Include types, influencing factors, and methods of prevention. ***(1259, 1262-1263)***

    ____

    ____

    ____

    ____

Activity 2

36. The nurse is assigned to care for a 78-year-old patient of Southeast-Asian ethnicity who is scheduled to undergo bowel surgery in the morning. He speaks little English. What interventions should be incorporated into the plan of care when performing preoperative teaching? ***(1260)***

    ____

    ____

    ____

    ____

Activity 3

37. A 54-year-old woman of American-Indian descent is recovering from an appendectomy. Discuss actions that should be included in the postoperative assessment unique to this patient. ***(1284)***

    ____

    ____

    ____

    ____

Student Name________________________________ Date______________

Care of the Patient with an Integumentary Disorder

chapter **43**

Answer Key: Textbook page references are provided as a guide for answering these questions. A complete answer key was provided for your instructor.

PROTECTION

Objective

- Discuss the primary functions of the integumentary system.

1. List the five functions of the skin. ***(1295-1296)***

   a. ______________________________

   b. ______________________________

   c. ______________________________

   d. ______________________________

   e. ______________________________

STRUCTURES OF THE SKIN

Objective

- Describe the differences between the epidermis and the dermis.

2. Label the structures of the skin. *(1296)*

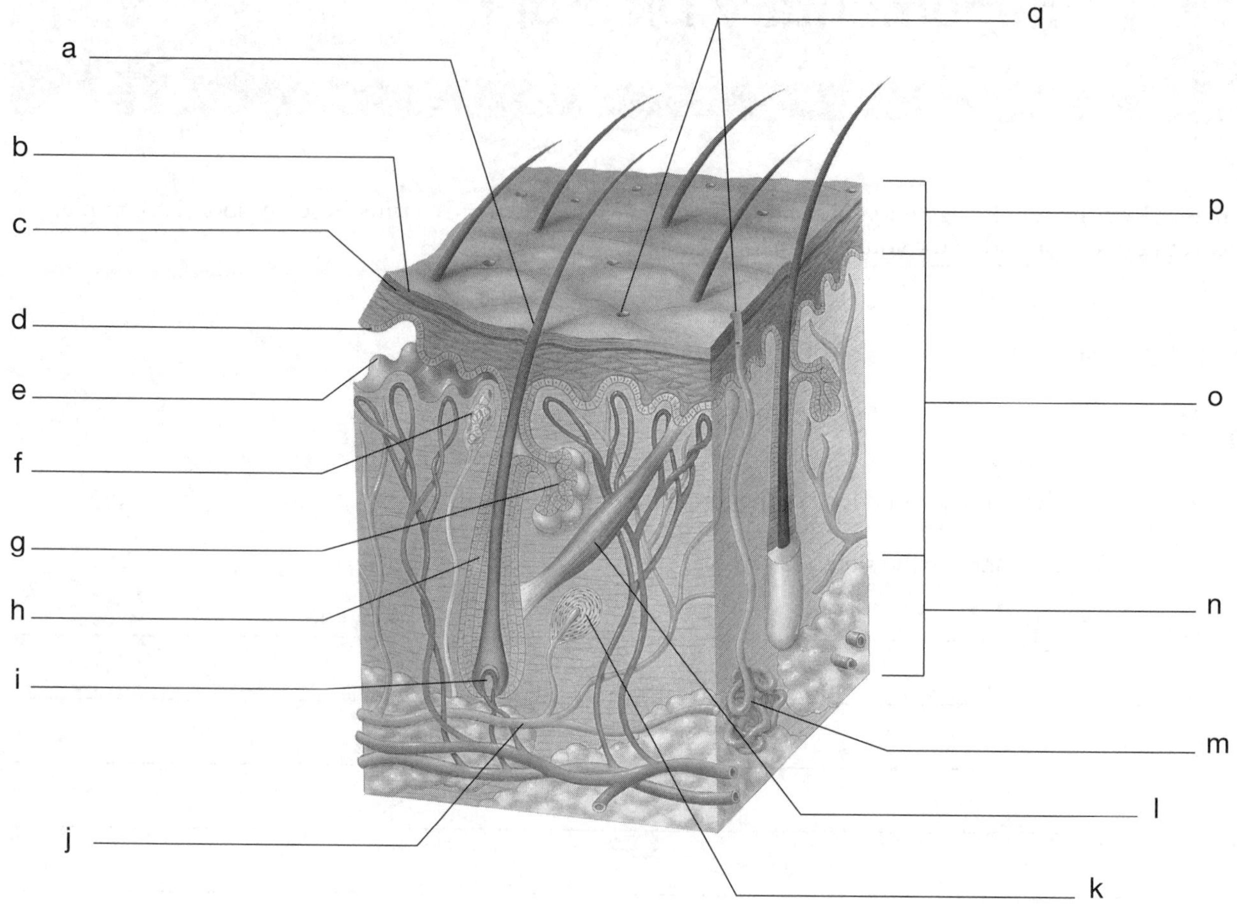

LAYERS OF SKIN

Objective

- Describe the differences between the epidermis and the dermis.

3. For each layer of the skin, identify the components and their function. *(1296-1297)*

Layer	Components	Function
a. Epidermis		
i. Stratum germinativum		
ii. Stratum corneum		

b. Melanocyte		
c. Dermis		
d. Superficial fascia		

MAJOR GLANDS IN THE SKIN

Objective

- Discuss the functions of the three major glands located in the skin.

4. Lubrication of the skin and the hair is a primary function on which skin appendage? ***(1297)***__________

____

____

5. The sudoriferous (sweat) glands are responsible for secreting sweat. What are the components of this discharge? ***(1297)***

____

____

6. The glands responsible for the secretion of cerumen are known as ____________________. ***(1297)***

ASSESSING SKIN DISORDERS

Objectives

- Discuss general assessment of the skin.
- Discuss how to use the nursing process in caring for patients with skin disorders.
- Identify general nursing interventions for the patient with a skin disorder.

7. Pallor in the dark-skinned individual should be assessed in what locations? ***(1303)*** __________

____

____

8. Assessment of a rash in the darker-skinned patient should be assessed using what technique? ***(1303)***

____

____

9. When performing an assessment of an integumentary complaint, what should be included? (Hint—use "PQRST") *(1303)*

____

____

10. When performing an assessment of a mole, what characteristics should be included? (Hint—use "ABCDE") *(1304)*

____

____

11. List the physiologic factors that influence skin color. *(1304)* ______________________

____

____

VIRAL DISORDERS OF THE SKIN

Objective

- Discuss the viral disorders of the skin.

12. Compare and contrast herpes simplex and herpes zoster. Include cause, clinical manifestations, medical management, nursing care, and prognosis. *(1304-1309)*

____

____

BACTERIAL, FUNGAL, AND INFLAMMATORY DISORDERS OF THE SKIN

Objective

- Discuss the bacterial, fungal, and inflammatory disorders of the skin.

13. List three bacterial disorders of the skin. Identify their clinical manifestations and treatments. *(1310-1312)*

Disorder	Clinical Manifestations	Treatment
a.		
b.		
c.		

14. Develop an index card comparing and contrasting the following fungal inflammatory disorders of the skin: tinea capitis, tinea corporis, tinea cruris, and tinea pedis. ***(1314-1315)***

PARASITES

Objectives

- Identify the parasitic disorders of the skin.
- Identify general nursing interventions for the patient with a skin disorder.

15. List two parasitic disorders of the skin. Identify their clinical manifestations and treatments. ***(1323-1326)***

Disorder	Clinical Manifestations	Treatment
a.		
b.		

TUMORS

Objective

- Describe the common tumors of the skin.

16. List the four common benign tumors of the skin, and identify their underlying causes and clinical manifestations. ***(1326-1329)***

Common Tumors	Underlying Cause	Clinical Manifestations
a.		
b.		
c.		
d.		

DISORDERS OF THE APPENDAGES

Objectives

- Identify the disorders associated with the appendages of the skin.
- Identify general nursing interventions for the patient with a skin disorder.

Multiple Choice

17. The nurse is caring for a patient who has complaints of excessive hair growth. Which of the following terms is used to describe this condition? ***(1330)***
    1. Alopecia
    2. Hirsutism
    3. Hypotrichosis
    4. Paronychia

18. The physician has diagnosed a patient with paronychia. When planning care, the nurse recognizes that it will likely be managed with: (Select all that apply) ***(1330)***
    1. chemical depilation.
    2. wet dressings.
    3. surgical debridement.
    4. antibiotic therapy.
    5. antiviral therapy.

19. The LPN/LVN is assisting the registered nurse to prepare the plan of care for the patient with alopecia. Which of the following nursing diagnoses will be most appropriate to include? ***(1330)***
    1. Alteration in comfort
    2. Pain
    3. Potential for infection
    4. Impaired body image

20. A patient arrives to be seen at the physician's office with complaints of hypotrichosis. The nurse recognizes that potential causes for the disorder include: ***(1330)***
    1. excessive dietary fat intake.
    2. iron deficiency anemia.
    3. malnutrition.
    4. diabetes mellitus.

EXPLANATION OF BURN INJURY

Objective

- State the pathophysiology involved in a burn injury.

21. The patient has a severe burn over 20% of her body. She has asked the nurse what will be happening to the area that has been burned. In the space below, provide the nurse's explanation to her, in order of occurrence, of the pathophysiologic process that ensues after a burn. ***(1330-1331)***

    ____

    ____

STAGES OF BURNS

Objectives

- Discuss the stages of burn care with appropriate nursing interventions.
- Discuss how to use the nursing process in caring for the patient with a skin disorder.
- Identify general nursing interventions for the patient with a skin disorder.

22. List the major nursing interventions for each stage of burn care. ***(1333-1339)***

Phase	Major Nursing Interventions
a. Emergent phase	
b. Acute phase	
c. Rehabilitation phase	

RULE OF NINES

Objective

- Identify the methods used to classify the extent of a burn injury.

23. Label the body with the rule of nines. ***(1332)***

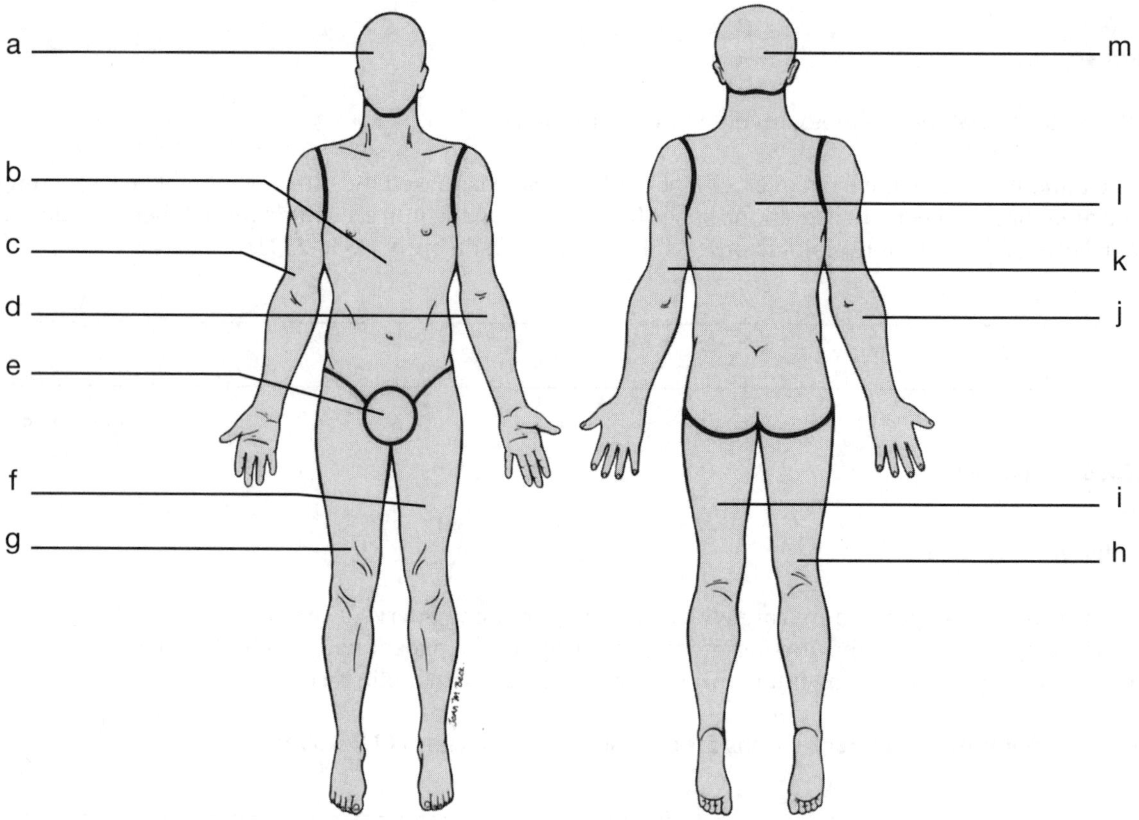

24. Calculate the percentage of burns for each of the situations listed below. ***(1332-1333)***
    a. Nine-year-old child old was burned while playing with fireworks. She has burns on both of her arms (anterior and posterior) and her anterior chest. __________%
    b. A 70-year-old man was burned when he backed up into an open-flame heater. He has burns on the posterior of his body from his ankles to his head. He also has burns on the anterior portion of his legs. __________%
    c. The patient, who has diabetes mellitus, stepped into a hot shower and has burns on his back and buttocks. __________%

MULTIPLE CHOICE

25. A patient is admitted with complaints of pain and tenderness in his lower right leg. The nurse's assessment reveals that the extremity is warm, swollen, and has a slightly pitted appearance. Based on the nurse's knowledge, what medical diagnosis can be anticipated? ***(1310-1311)***
    1. Cellulitis
    2. Impetigo
    3. Herpes zoster
    4. Folliculitis

26. When assisting a mother to plan meals for a child recently diagnosed with eczema, the nurse should advise her that common allergies for a patient with this diagnosis may include: ***(1318)***
    1. chocolate, strawberries, and cured sandwich meats.
    2. eggs, rye-containing products, and preservatives.
    3. orange juice, wheat, and eggs.
    4. rye, wheat, and bananas.

27. A 16-year-old questions why the physician has prescribed Accutane for her acne. The nurse advises her that the medication will: ***(1319)***
    1. reduce the scarring associated with acne.
    2. reduce the formation of blackheads.
    3. counteract the overactive hormones of adolescence associated with acne.
    4. reduce the production of sebum.

28. Which of the following factors is associated with aging of the integumentary system? (Select all that apply) ***(1339)***
    1. Localized clusters of melanocytes surrounded by areas of decreased pigmentation
    2. Loss of pigmentation
    3. Reduced thickness of the skin
    4. Reduced incidence of seborrheic dermatitis of the scalp

CRITICAL THINKING ACTIVITIES

29. A 17-year-old patient reports concerns about her ongoing skin breakouts. The assessment reveals papulopustular skin eruptions on her face and neck. There is also evidence of scarring from previous breakouts. ***(1319-1320)***

    a. The nurse would anticipate a diagnosis of what integumentary disorder? ____________________

    ____

    b. Identify three nursing diagnoses that would apply to this patient. ____________________

    ____

    ____

    ____

c. Identify treatment options for this patient. ______________________________

____

____

____

____

d. Identify five teaching topics for this patient. ______________________________

____

____

____

____

Student Name________________________________ Date________________

Care of the Patient with a Musculoskeletal Disorder

chapter **44**

Answer Key: Textbook page references are provided as a guide for answering these questions. A complete answer key was provided for your instructor.

FUNCTIONS OF THE MUSCULOSKELETAL SYSTEM

Objective

- List the five basic functions of the skeletal system.

1. List five functions of the skeletal system. ***(1345-1346)***

   a. ______________________________

   b. ______________________________

   c. ______________________________

   d. ______________________________

   e. ______________________________

BONES: LOCATION AND SKELETAL DIVISION

Objectives

- Describe the location of major bones of the skeleton.
- List the two divisions of the skeleton.

2. List the bones that are present within each body part, and identify the division in which each of the bones is located. ***(1346)***

Body Part	Bones	Skeletal Division
a. Skull		
b. Chest		

(Continued next page)

Body Part	Bones	Skeletal Division
c. Abdomen		
d. Arms		
e. Legs		
f. Hands		
g. Feet		

LOCATION OF MUSCLES

Objective

- Describe the location of the major muscles of the body.

3. Next to the body part, list the major muscles present in that part. ***(1348)***

Body Part	Muscles
a. Skull	
b. Chest	
c. Abdomen	
d. Arms	
e. Legs	

MOVABLE JOINTS

Objective

- List the types of body movements.

4. Label the structures of a freely movable (diarthrotic) joint. ***(1346)***

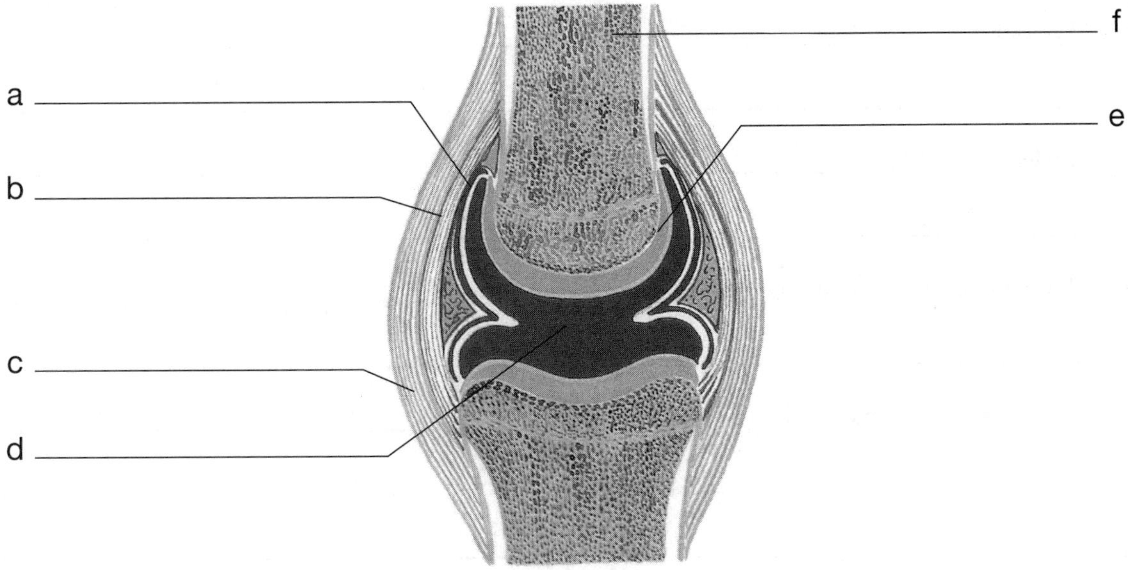

FUNCTIONS

Objective

- Describe three vital functions that muscles perform when they contract.

5. List three functions that muscles perform when they contract. ***(1346-1349)***

   a. ______________________________

   b. ______________________________

   c. ______________________________

DIAGNOSTIC PROCEDURES

Objective

- List diagnostic procedures pertinent to musculoskeletal function.

6. Explain the following types of diagnostic studies. ***(1349-1353)***

    a. Laminography: ______________________________

    b. Scanography: ______________________________

    c. Myelogram: ______________________________

    d. Nuclear scanning: ______________________________

    e. Magnetic resonance imaging (MRI): ______________________________

    f. Computed axial tomography (CT or CAT scan): ______________________________

    g. Bone scan: ______________________________

    h. Arthroscopy: ______________________________

    i. Endoscopic spinal microsurgery: ______________________________

    j. Aspiration: ______________________________

    k. Arthrocentesis: ______________________________

    l. Electromyogram (EMG): ______________________________

ARTHRITIS

Objective

- Compare the medical regimens for patients suffering from gouty arthritis, rheumatoid arthritis, and osteoarthritis.

7. List the four goals of medical regimens for patients suffering from gouty arthritis, rheumatoid arthritis, and osteoarthritis. *(1355)*

    a. ______________________________

    b. ______________________________

    c. ______________________________

    d. ______________________________

NURSING INTERVENTIONS

Objectives

- Discuss the nursing interventions appropriate for rheumatoid arthritis.
- Describe the nursing interventions appropriate for degenerative joint disease (osteoarthritis).

8. Next to each nursing diagnosis, list the nursing interventions that would be appropriate for rheumatoid arthritis and osteoarthritis. *(1359)*

Nursing Diagnosis	Nursing Interventions
a. Pain related to joint inflammation	
b. Pain related to disease process	
c. Self-esteem, chronic low, related to negative self-evaluation about self or capabilities	
d. Self-esteem, chronic low, related to body image change	
e. Knowledge deficit related to lack of information concerning medication and home care management	

LIFESTYLE

Objective

- List at least four healthy lifestyle measures a person can practice to reduce the risk of developing osteoporosis.

9. Discuss osteoporosis. Include a definition of the disorder, risk factors, and actions a patient can take to reduce the risk of developing osteoporosis. ***(1364-1365)***

   a. Definition: ______________________________

   ____

   b. Risk factors: ______________________________

   ____

   c. Methods of prevention: ______________________________

   ____

SURGERY

Objective

- Describe the surgical intervention for arthritis of the hip and knee.

10. The patient has had arthritis of the hip and knee for many years. The medical regimen has failed to relieve the patient's significant pain, resulting in loss of movement. List five reasons why surgical intervention would benefit the patient. ***(1369)***

   a. ______________________________

   b. ______________________________

   c. ______________________________

   d. ______________________________

   e. ______________________________

TOTAL HIP OR KNEE REPLACEMENT

Objective

- Describe the nursing interventions for the patient undergoing a total hip or knee replacement.

11. The patient has decided to take the doctor's advice and have a total knee replacement. Underneath each of the interventions, list the specific nursing actions needed to provide care for the patient after surgery. ***(1370)***

    a. Positioning:

       i. ______________________________

       ii. ______________________________

    b. Wound care:

       i. ______________________________

       ii. ______________________________

       iii. ______________________________

    c. Activity:

       i. ______________________________

       ii. ______________________________

       iii. ______________________________

       iv. ______________________________

       v. ______________________________

       vi. ______________________________

    d. Pain control:

       i. ______________________________

       ii. ______________________________

    e. Discharge teaching:

       i. ______________________________

       ii. ______________________________

FRACTURES

Objective

- Discuss nursing interventions appropriate for a patient with a fractured hip after ORIF and bipolar hip prosthesis (hemiarthroplasty).

12. Label each type of fracture. *(1373)*

a ______________________________

b ______________________________

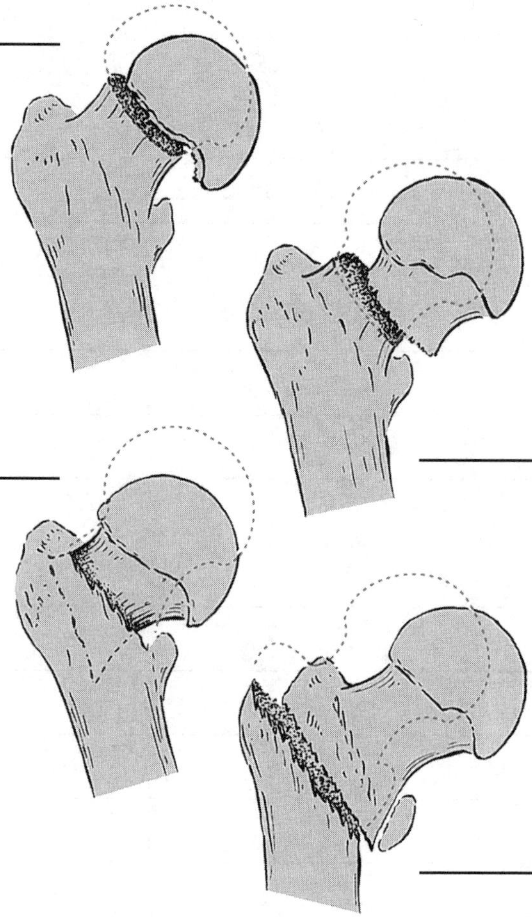

______________________________ d

______________________________ c

FRACTURE HEALING

Objective

- Discuss the physiology of fracture healing (hematoma, granulation tissue, and callus formation).

13. Next to each step of fracture healing, explain the physiology of fracture healing. *(1380)*

   a. Hematoma: ______________________________

   ____

   b. Granulation tissue: ______________________________

   ____

   c. Callus formation: ______________________________

   ____

FRACTURE COMPLICATIONS

Objectives

- Describe the signs and symptoms of compartment syndrome.
- List nursing interventions appropriate for a fat embolism.

14. List seven potential complications of a fracture. Include the signs and symptoms of each. ***(1384)***

    a. ____________________

    b. ____________________

    c. ____________________

    d. ____________________

    e. ____________________

    f. ____________________

    g. ____________________

TRACTION

Objective

- List at least two types of skin and skeletal traction.

15. Discuss the rationale for the use of traction. Discuss the differences between skin and skeletal traction. ***(1392)***

16. List two types each of skin and skeletal traction in the spaces provided. ***(1392)***

Skin Traction	Skeletal Traction
a.	
b.	

DATA COLLECTION

Objective

- Compare methods for assessing circulation, nerve damage, and infection in a patient who has a traumatic insult to the musculoskeletal system.

17. The patient has just returned from an application of a long leg cast to her right leg. She fell while hanging wallpaper in her kitchen and broke her right tibia just below her knee. Explain the correct method of determining adequate circulation, possible nerve damage, and infection in her right leg. ***(1389-1390)***

____

____

BONE CANCER

Objective

- List four nursing interventions appropriate for bone cancer.

18. The patient has just returned from surgery to remove a large tumor of the left arm. Make an index card of nursing interventions to prompt the nurse during care of this patient. ***(1403)***

PHANTOM PAIN

Objective

- Describe the phenomenon of phantom pain.

19. The patient had his left lower leg surgically amputated 2 days ago. Since that time, he has been complaining of pain in the missing limb. Discuss why the phantom pain phenomenon takes place. ***(1404-1405)***

____

____

MEDICAL TERMINOLOGY VERSUS PATIENT TERMINOLOGY

Objective

- Describe the following conditions: lordosis, scoliosis, and kyphosis.

20. Define the following terms using medical terminology. In the last column, indicate how the nurse would explain the meaning of that term to a patient. ***(1406)***

Term	Medical Terminology	Patient's Terminology
a. Lordosis		
b. Scoliosis		
c. Kyphosis		

MULTIPLE CHOICE

21. A patient is prescribed colchicine to treat gout. What potential side effects associated with the medication should the nurse be assessing for? ***(1363)***
    1. Diarrhea, nausea, and vomiting
    2. Elevated blood pressure and pulse
    3. Hypotension and elevated temperature
    4. Rash

22. When assisting in planning meals for a 59-year-old woman concerned about her risk of osteoporosis, which of the following foods can the nurse recommend as good sources of calcium? (Select all that apply) ***(1366-1367)***
    1. Milk
    2. Leafy green vegetables
    3. Potatoes
    4. Sardines

23. While the nurse is performing discharge teaching to the parents of a 6-year-old child with a greenstick fracture of the left arm, the parents request clarification about this type of fracture. The nurse explains that the: ***(1380)***
    1. bone is splintered into three or more fragments at the site of the break.
    2. fracture extends completely through the bone.
    3. break coils around the bone.
    4. fracture line extends only partially through the bone.

24. A 32-year-old woman diagnosed with fibromyalgia syndrome questions the nurse about what causes the condition. The nurse explains that: ***(1367-1368)***
    1. there is an unfortunate correlation between the condition and anxiety disorders.
    2. it is associated with a diet lacking protein and calcium.
    3. the exact cause is still unknown.
    4. she will need to discuss these questions with her physician.

25. The nurse is providing care for a patient who has just had a hip replacement. Which comments from the patient indicate the need for further education? (Select all that apply) ***(1371-1372)***
    1. "To ensure my hip replacement is successful, I will need to be on bed rest for the first 72 hours."
    2. "I will need to obtain a seat riser for my toilet at home."
    3. "I must limit time spent sitting with crossed legs to no more than 1 hour per day."
    4. "My limitations in positioning my hip in a flexed position will remain in place for 2 to 3 months."

CRITICAL THINKING ACTIVITIES

Activity 1

26. A patient reports that after exercising for the first time in months, he has begun to experience pain and stiffness in his thigh muscles. Does the nurse anticipate his diagnosis will be a strain or a sprain? Why? What should his plan of care include? ***(1396-1397)***

    ____

    ____

    ____

    ____

Activity 2

27. A patient has been diagnosed with carpal tunnel syndrome. Discuss the teaching plans for this patient. Include the cause, risk factors, signs and symptoms, and treatment options. ***(1400)***

____

____

____

____

Activity 3

28. A patient diagnosed with rheumatoid arthritis reports she is confused. After further questioning, she states she has heard of two types of arthritis. She asks about the differences between rheumatoid arthritis and osteoarthritis. Compare and contrast rheumatoid arthritis and osteoarthritis. Include cause, clinical manifestations, treatment options, and prognosis. ***(1354-1363)***

____

____

____

____

Student Name______________________________ Date______________

Care of the Patient with a Gastrointestinal Disorder

chapter **45**

Answer Key: Textbook page references are provided as a guide for answering these questions. A complete answer key was provided for your instructor.

DIGESTIVE ORGANS

Objectives

- List in sequence each of the component parts or segments of the alimentary canal and identify the accessory organs of digestion.
- Discuss the function of each digestive and accessory organ.

1. Label the digestive organs. *(1412)*

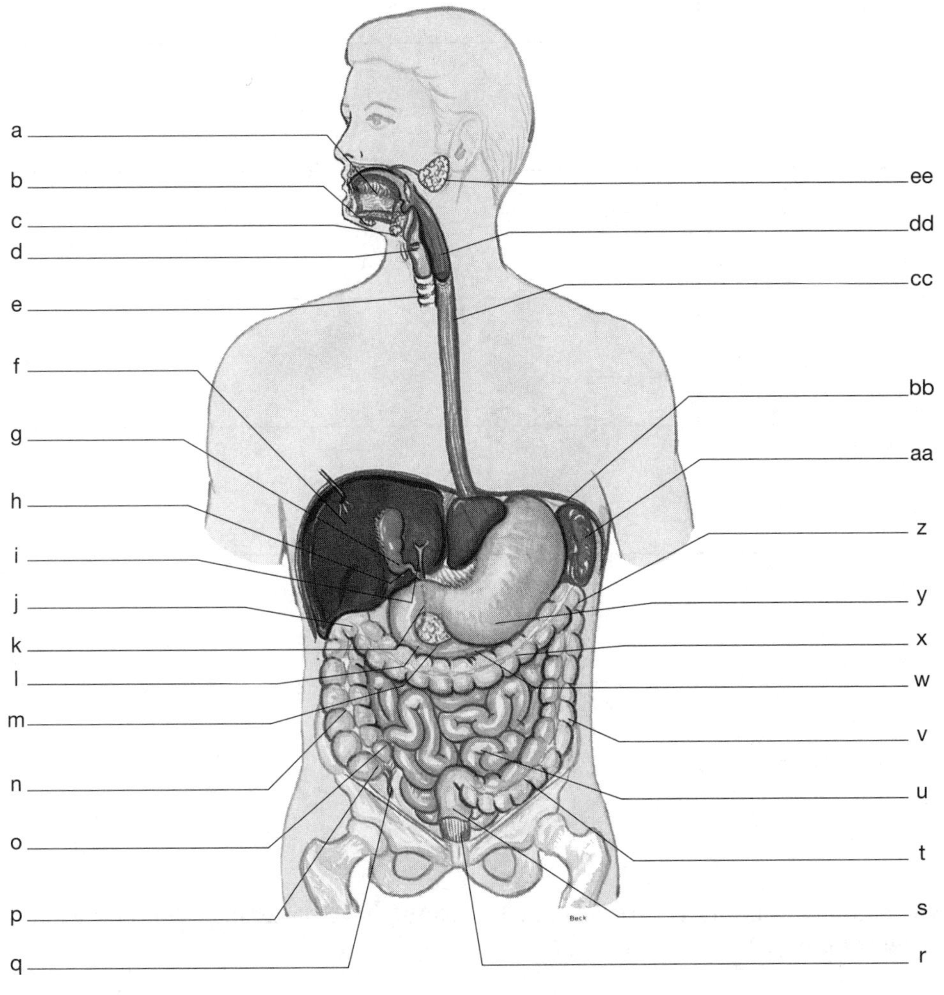

FOOD'S JOURNEY

2. A patient has just eaten a piece of cherry pie. List each component part or segment of the alimentary canal and its function as the bite of pie passes through the digestive tract. Be sure to include the accessory organs. ***(1412-1415)***

Component Part	Function
a.	
b.	
c.	
d.	
e.	
f.	
g.	
h.	
i.	

DIAGNOSTIC PROCEDURES

Objective

- Discuss the laboratory and diagnostic examinations and give the nursing interventions for patients with disorders of the gastrointestinal tract.

3. Choose six diagnostic procedures and list nursing interventions that a nurse would use when taking care of patients with disorders of the gastrointestinal tract. ***(1416-1419)***

Diagnostic Procedure	Nursing Interventions
a.	
b.	
c.	
d.	
e.	
f.	

DISORDERS OF THE MOUTH

Objective

- Explain the etiology and pathophysiology, clinical manifestations, assessments, diagnostic tests, medical-surgical management, and nursing interventions for the patient with disorders of the mouth, esophagus, stomach, and intestines.

4. Identify three potential causes of dental decay. ***(1419)*** ______________________________

____

____

5. List or formulate two nursing diagnoses for a patient with severe dental caries. ***(1420)*** ______________

____

____

6. Candidiasis can also be referred to by what other terms? ***(1420)*** ______

7. Identify patients who may be more susceptible to candidiasis. ***(1420)*** ______

8. The majority of malignancies of the oral cavity are of what type? ***(1420)*** ______

9. Why is the rate of metastasis elevated in cancer of the tongue? ***(1420)*** ______

10. What factors are associated with the increase in mouth and throat cancers? ***(1420)*** ______

11. What is the survival rate for oral cancer? ***(1421)*** ______

NURSING PROCESS FOR ESOPHAGEAL DISORDERS

Objective

- Explain the etiology and pathophysiology, clinical manifestations, assessments, diagnostic tests, medical-surgical management, and nursing interventions for the patient with disorders of the mouth, esophagus, stomach, and intestines.

12. For each phase of the nursing process, indicate specifically how that phase relates to patients with esophageal disorders. ***(1423)***

    a. Assessment: ______

b. Nursing diagnoses and planning: ______________________

____

c. Implementation: ______________________

____

d. Evaluation: ______________________

____

GASTRIC SURGERY

Objective

- Identify nursing interventions for preoperative and postoperative care of the patient who requires gastric surgery.

13. For each subject, list the nursing interventions appropriate for a patient who is having gastric surgery. ***(1426)***

a. Preoperative

i. Preparation: ______________________

____

ii. Knowledge: ______________________

____

b. Postoperative

i. Knowledge: ______________________

____

ii. Pain: ______________________

____

iii. Noncompliance: ______________________

____

iv. Nutrition: ______________________

____

INTESTINAL DISORDERS

Objective

- Compare and contrast the inflammatory bowel diseases of ulcerative colitis and Crohn's disease, including etiology and pathophysiology, clinical manifestations, medical management, and nursing interventions.

14. List the common causes, clinical manifestations, diagnostic tests, medical management, and nursing interventions for patients who have ulcerative colitis and Crohn's disease. Then list specific information that distinguishes each disorder from the other. ***(1441-1442)***

Common Information	
a. Etiology	
b. Clinical manifestations	
c. Diagnostic tests	
d. Medical management	
e. Nursing interventions	
Ulcerative Colitis	**Crohn's Disease**
f.	

FECAL DIVERSION

Objective

- Identify five nursing interventions for the patient with a stoma for fecal diversion.

15. List five nursing interventions for the patient who has a stoma for fecal diversion. ***(1450-1451)***

   a. ______________________________

   ____

   b. ______________________________

   ____

c. ______________________________

____

d. ______________________________

____

e. ______________________________

____

ACUTE ABDOMINAL INFLAMMATIONS

Objective

- Discuss the etiology and pathophysiology, clinical manifestations, assessment, diagnostic tests, medical management, and nursing interventions for the patient with acute abdominal inflammations (appendicitis, diverticulitis, and peritonitis).

16. Identify the anatomical structure that becomes inflamed during appendicitis. ***(1448)*** ______________

____

____

17. List the most common causes of appendicitis. ***(1448)*** ______________

____

____

18. List diagnostic tests that may be used to confirm appendicitis. ***(1448)*** ______________

____

____

19. Peritonitis is a complication associated with appendicitis. Discuss events that may cause this complication to occur. What should the nurse review to ensure prompt diagnosis of the condition? ***(1449)***

____

____

20. The nurse is providing information to a patient diagnosed with diverticulitis. When discussing dietary recommendations, what facts should be included? ***(1450)***

____

____

HERNIAS

Objective

- Discuss the etiology and pathophysiology, clinical manifestations, assessment, diagnostic tests, medical management, and nursing interventions for the patient with external hernias and hiatal hernia.

Activity 1

21. Hernias can be attributed to what causes? ***(1452)*** ______________________________

____

____

22. Define the following hernia-related terms. ***(1452)***

    a. Reducible: ______________________________

    ____

    b. Irreducible: ______________________________

    ____

    c. Strangulation: ______________________________

    ____

23. What data should be collected when assessing an abdominal hernia? ***(1452)***______________

____

____

24. If complications arise involving the strangulation of an abdominal hernia, what signs and symptoms might be observable? ***(1452)***

____

____

25. What tests can be used to diagnose hernias? ***(1453)*** ______________________________

____

____

Activity 2

26. Under each type of hernia, list the cause and surgical and nursing interventions for that type of condition. ***(1452-1453)***

	Abdominal	Hiatal
a. Cause		
b. Surgical interventions		
c. Nursing interventions		

INTESTINAL OBSTRUCTIONS

Objective

- Differentiate between mechanical and nonmechanical intestinal obstruction, including causes, medical management, and nursing interventions.

27. The nurse is providing care to a patient suspected of having an intestinal obstruction. Answer the following questions pertaining to this patient. ***(1453-1456)***

    a. When performing an assessment on the patient, what objective data should be included?

    ____

    ____

    b. What diagnostic tests may be performed to confirm the presence of an intestinal obstruction?

    ____

    ____

    c. What are the goals of treatment for an intestinal obstruction? ______________

    ____

    ____

d. Compare and contrast a mechanical and a nonmechanical intestinal obstruction.________________

____

____

CANCER

Objective

- Describe the etiology and pathophysiology, clinical manifestations, assessment, diagnostic tests, medical management, surgical procedures, and nursing interventions for the patient with colorectal cancer.

28. The nurse is taking care of a patient who has had a bowel resection as a result of cancer of the colon. Develop an index card that will prompt the nurse with information regarding clinical manifestations, surgical procedures, and nursing interventions for the patient. ***(1456-1459)***

FECAL INCONTINENCE

Objective

- Explain the etiologies, medical management, and nursing interventions for the patient with fecal incontinence.

Multiple Choice

29. The nurse caring for a patient with fecal incontinence recognizes that common causes of the disorder include which of the following? (Select all that apply) ***(1462)***
    1. Aging
    2. Anal intercourse
    3. Trauma
    4. Childbirth

30. The nurse is caring for a patient with a motor paralysis. When planning care for the patient, the nurse understands which of the following facts about the patient's defecation status? ***(1462)***
    1. Motor paralysis will automatically result in an inability to control defecation.
    2. Bowel training is possible in patients with a motor paralysis.
    3. Reflex defecation cannot be stimulated in the patient with motor paralysis.
    4. Continued ability to control defecation is possible in patients with upper motor neuron dysfunction but not patients with lower motor neuron dysfunction.

31. The most effective bowel training programs will include: ***(1462)***
    1. biofeedback.
    2. surgery.
    3. enema use to prevent constipation.
    4. the daily administration of glycerin suppositories.

32. The patient practicing a bowel training program will benefit from a diet rich in ____________. ***(1462)***
    1. Protein
    2. Calcium
    3. Fiber
    4. Iron

MULTIPLE CHOICE

33. A patient being treated with Zantac for a peptic ulcer asks how the medication will help her condition. The nurse explains that the medication will: ***(1429)***
    1. reduce the acidity of the stomach contents.
    2. inhibit the secretion of gastrin.
    3. decrease acid secretions by blocking the histamine H_2 receptors.
    4. reduce gastric motility.

34. A patient being treated for pernicious anemia after her total gastrectomy asks why she has developed this disorder. This disorder has resulted because: ***(1432)***
    1. the lack of intrinsic factor normally produced by the stomach has resulted in a failure of absorption of vitamin B_{12}.
    2. vitamin B_{12} is no longer produced in her body because of the gastric surgery.
    3. the lack of vitamin B_{12} is causing the intrinsic factor to be malabsorbed.
    4. the diarrhea associated with the gastric surgery has resulted in dehydration and a loss of vitamin B_{12}.

35. The risk of cancer of the stomach is associated with which of the following? (Select all that apply) ***(1436)***
    1. Hyperkalemia
    2. Hypochlorhydria
    3. Chronic atrophic gastritis
    4. Diet high in smoked and preserved foods

36. When caring for a patient diagnosed with Crohn's disease, the nurse may anticipate which of the following signs and symptoms to be present? (Select all that apply) ***(1446)***
    1. Nausea, vomiting, and diarrhea
    2. Diarrhea, fatigue, and abdominal pain
    3. Weight gain, lactose intolerance, and vomiting
    4. Weight loss, fever, and anemia

37. The nurse is providing care to a patient suspected of having an acute appendicitis. Which interventions may be included in care? (Select all that apply) ***(1449)***
    1. Apply heating pad to the abdomen.
    2. Maintain bed rest.
    3. Administer mild antacids to promote comfort.
    4. Monitor temperature.

CRITICAL THINKING ACTIVITIES

Activity 1

38. A 49-year-old obese male truck driver reports to the clinic complaining of rectal itching. After the medical examination, a diagnosis of hemorrhoids is made. ***(1460)***

    a. What caused this condition? ______________________________

    ____

    ____

    b. What nonsurgical approaches can the nurse teach the patient to help manage the condition?

    ____

    ____

Activity 2

39. An 18-year-old male reports to the emergency room complaining of lower abdominal pain and tenderness and an elevated temperature. ***(1448)***

    a. Concerned, the patient asks what other tests may be done to assess for an appendicitis. How would the nurse respond?

    ____

    ____

    b. The patient requests a narcotic to relieve his pain. Discuss an appropriate response to this request.

    ____

    ____

Student Name______________________________ Date_______________

chapter **46**

Care of the Patient with a Gallbladder, Liver, Biliary Tract, or Exocrine Pancreatic Disorder

Answer Key: Textbook page references are provided as a guide for answering these questions. A complete answer key was provided for your instructor.

NURSING INTERVENTIONS

Objective

- Discuss nursing interventions for the diagnostic examinations of patients with disorders of the gallbladder, liver, biliary tract, and exocrine pancreas.

1. Next to each of the diagnostic examinations, indicate appropriate nursing interventions for that examination. *(1467-1472)*

Diagnostic Examination	Nursing Interventions
a. Cholecystography	
b. Computed tomography of abdomen	
c. Endoscopic retrograde cholangiopancreatography	
d. Gallbladder scanning	
e. Hepatitis virus studies	
f. Liver biopsy	

(Continued next page)

Diagnostic Examination	Nursing Interventions
g. Liver enzyme analysis	
h. Radioisotope liver scanning	
i. Serum ammonia determination	
j. Serum amylase determination	
k. Serum bilirubin determination	
l. Serum lipase determination	
m. Serum protein determination	
n. T-tube cholangiography	
o. Ultrasonography (echogram)	
p. Ultrasonography of pancreas	
q. Urine amylase determination	

SIGNS AND SYMPTOMS

Objective

- Define *jaundice* and describe signs and symptoms that may occur with jaundice.

2. Explain to a patient with hepatitis what jaundice is, and list the objective data that one might observe. ***(1473)***

____

____

VIRAL HEPATITIS

Objectives

- State the six types of viral hepatitis, including their modes of transmission.
- List the subjective and objective data for the patient with viral hepatitis.

Activity 1

3. List the types of hepatitis, and state how they are transmitted. ***(1479)***

Type of Viral Hepatitis	Mode of Transmission
a.	
b.	
c.	
d.	
e.	
f.	

Activity 2

4. Identify three causes of hepatitis. ***(1479)*** ______________________________

____

____

5. Discuss the basic shared pathophysiology of the six forms of hepatitis. ***(1479)*** ____________________

____

____

6. When considering a diagnosis of hepatitis, what diagnostic tests can be anticipated? ***(1479)*** __________

____

____

7. Discuss the reasons a patient suffering from hepatitis may experience pruritus. ***(1479)***______________

____

____

8. Identify the subjective signs and symptoms of hepatitis. ***(1479)***________________________

____

____

9. Identify the objective signs and symptoms of hepatitis. ***(1479)***________________________

____

____

10. What dietary support and interventions may be needed by the patient with hepatitis? ***(1481)***_________

____

____

11. What populations are considered to be at risk for contracting hepatitis B? ***(1479)***________________

____

____

12. Discuss the immunization process for hepatitis B. ***(1481)*** ________________________

____

____

CIRRHOSIS

Objectives

- Explain the etiology, pathophysiology, clinical manifestations, complications, medical management, and nursing interventions for the patient with cirrhosis of the liver, carcinoma of the liver, hepatitis, liver abscesses, cholecystitis, cholelithiasis, pancreatitis, and cancer of the pancreas.
- Discuss specific complications and teaching content for the patient with cirrhosis of the liver.

Activity 1

13. Discuss each topic as it pertains to a patient diagnosed with cirrhosis of the liver. ***(1472)***

   a. Cause and pathophysiology: ______________________________

   ____

   b. Clinical manifestations: ______________________________

   ____

   c. Medical management: ______________________________

   ____

   d. Nursing management: ______________________________

   ____

   e. Patient teaching: ______________________________

   ____

Activity 2

14. What serum diagnostic examinations may be ordered to diagnose cirrhosis? ***(1472)*** ______________

____

____

15. What visual examinations may be used to diagnose cirrhosis? ***(1472)*** ______________________

____

____

16. List and discuss complications that may accompany cirrhosis. ***(1472)***____________________

17. List two nursing diagnoses for the patient with cirrhosis. ***(1472)*** ____________________

18. Discuss the prognosis for the patient with cirrhosis. ***(1472)***____________________

19. Discuss the cultural and ethnic implications associated with cirrhosis. ***(1472)***____________________

LIVER, PANCREAS, AND GALLBLADDER

Objective

- Explain the etiology, pathophysiology, clinical manifestations, medical management, and nursing interventions for the patient with cirrhosis of the liver, carcinoma of the liver, hepatitis, liver abscesses, cholecystitis, cholelithiasis, pancreatitis, and cancer of the pancreas.

20. Describe the common causes and pathophysiology, clinical manifestations, medical management, and nursing interventions for (1) carcinoma of the liver and pancreas, (2) acute and chronic pancreatic disease, and (3) gallbladder disease. Then, under each disorder, list the specific information that differentiates that disorder from the others, and identify the prognosis. ***(1467-1494)***

	Common Information
a. Causes and pathophysiology	
b. Clinical manifestations	
c. Medical management	
d. Nursing interventions	

	Carcinoma of the Liver and Pancreas	Acute and Chronic Pancreatic Disease	Gallbladder Disease
e. Specific information			
f. Prognosis			

COMMON SITES FOR GALLSTONES

Objective

- Discuss two methods of surgical treatment for cholecystitis and cholelithiasis.

21. Label the common sites for gallstones. ***(1484)***

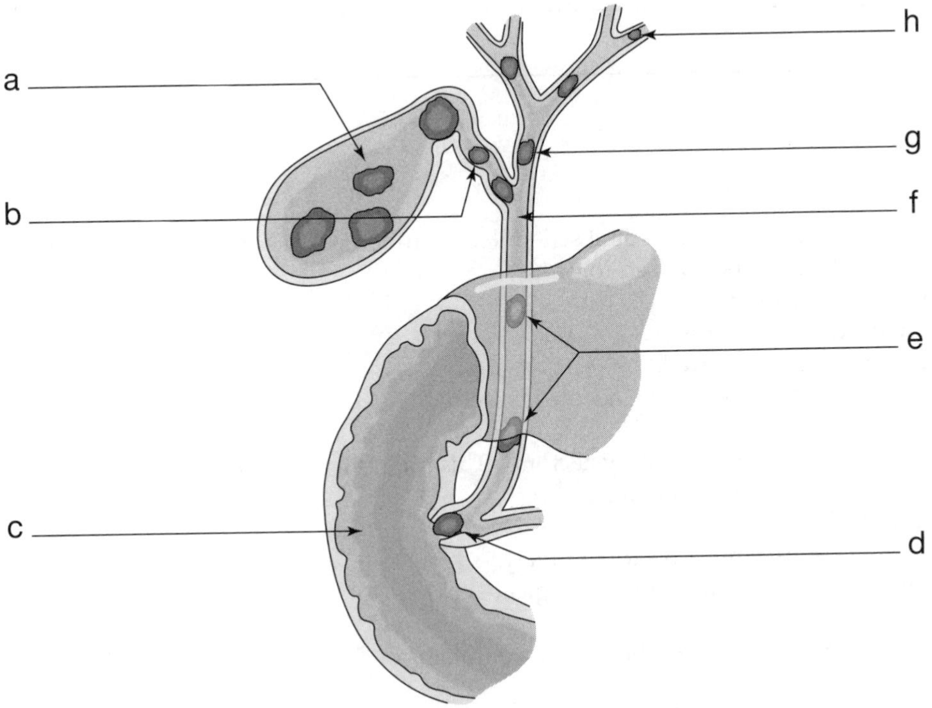

LIVER TRANSPLANTATION

Objective

- Discuss the indicators for liver transplantation and the immunosuppressant drugs to reduce rejection.

22. List indications for liver transplantation. ***(1481)*** ______________________________

____

____

23. Rejection of liver transplants has decreased in recent years. What factors are associated with this decrease? ***(1481)***

____

____

24. Discuss the use of cyclosporine in the management of patients who have undergone a liver transplant. ***(1482)***

____

____

MULTIPLE CHOICE

25. The nurse is providing teaching to a patient scheduled to undergo a needle liver biopsy. During the examination, the patient should be advised to: ***(1469)***
    1. inhale as the needle is inserted.
    2. cough as the needle is withdrawn.
    3. inhale after the needle is inserted.
    4. exhale before and not breathe as the needle is inserted.

26. A T-tube may be inserted during a cholecystectomy. This tube is inserted to: ***(1489)***
    1. keep the duct open and allow drainage.
    2. reduce inflammation.
    3. reduce the patient's discomfort postoperatively.
    4. reduce postoperative bleeding from the surgical site.

27. After a laparoscopic cholecystectomy, the patient complains of shoulder pain. This pain is caused by: ***(1479)***
    1. positioning on the table during the surgical procedure.
    2. manipulation of the internal organs during surgery.
    3. residual carbon dioxide.
    4. irritation from the stones removed.

28. When caring for a patient with acute pancreatitis, which of the following laboratory reports may be anticipated? ***(1489-1490)***
    1. Hyperalbuminemia, hypocalcemia, elevated hematocrit, and hypoglycemia
    2. Hypoalbuminemia, hyperglycemia, elevated hematocrit, and leukocytosis
    3. Hyperglycemia, decreased hematocrit, leukocytosis, and hypercalcemia
    4. Hyperglycemia, decreased hematocrit, leukocytosis, and hypocalcemia

29. A patient voices concerns about contracting hepatitis E. What information should be provided to the patient? (Select all that apply) ***(1479)***
    1. Use caution when drinking water in locations with questionable filtration.
    2. Refrain from engaging in unprotected sex.
    3. Ensure proper disposal of needles.
    4. Do not eat uncooked seafood.

CRITICAL THINKING ACTIVITIES

Objectives

- Discuss two methods of surgical treatment for cholecystitis and cholelithiasis.
- Discuss the indicators for liver transplantation and the immunosuppressant drugs to reduce rejection.

Activity 1

30. A 34-year-old patient with a history of end-stage liver disease related to chronic hepatitis has been added to the waiting list to receive a liver transplant. During his preoperative education classes, he voices many questions and concerns. ***(1481-1482)***

    a. What are some common patient populations that may require liver transplants? ____________________

    ____

    ____

    ____

    ____

    b. What are the primary risks associated with the planned transplant? ____________________

    ____

    ____

    ____

    ____

c. What postoperative complications will the patient be at risk for?

d. How will the risk of organ rejection be handled?

e. Discuss the appropriate postoperative nursing care.

Activity 2

31. A 49-year-old patient comes to the emergency department complaining of right upper-quadrant pain. She reports that the pain began a few hours after eating at a local fast-food restaurant. Upon assessment, the abdomen is distended. The patient also has nausea and vomiting. ***(1484-1485)***

a. What does the nurse expect the patient to be diagnosed with?

b. What are some other signs and symptoms that may develop?

c. What diagnostic examinations may be used to help diagnose this patient? ______________________

____

____

____

____

d. The patient continues to complain of pain while awaiting confirmation of her diagnosis. She reports having had a positive experience with morphine for severe pain during a previous hospitalization. How will you respond to her request?

____

____

____

____

Student Name______________________________ Date______________

chapter **47**

Care of the Patient with a Blood or Lymphatic Disorder

Answer Key: Textbook page references are provided as a guide for answering these questions. A complete answer key was provided for your instructor.

COMPONENTS OF BLOOD

Objectives

- Describe the components of blood.
- Differentiate between the functions of erythrocytes, leukocytes, and thrombocytes.
- Discuss the several factors necessary for the formation of erythrocytes.
- Describe what the *leukocyte differential* means.

1. Complete the table below with information on the components of blood. ***(1499-1500)***

Component	Common Name	Normal Value	Function	Significance of Abnormality
a. Erythrocytes				
What are the factors necessary for the formation of erythrocytes?				
b. Leukocytes				
Describe what *differential* means.				
c. Neutrophils				
d. Eosinophils				
e. Basophils				
f. Monocytes				
g. Thrombocytes				

BLOOD CLOTTING

Objective

- Describe the blood clotting process.

2. Label each step of the blood clotting mechanism. ***(1501)***

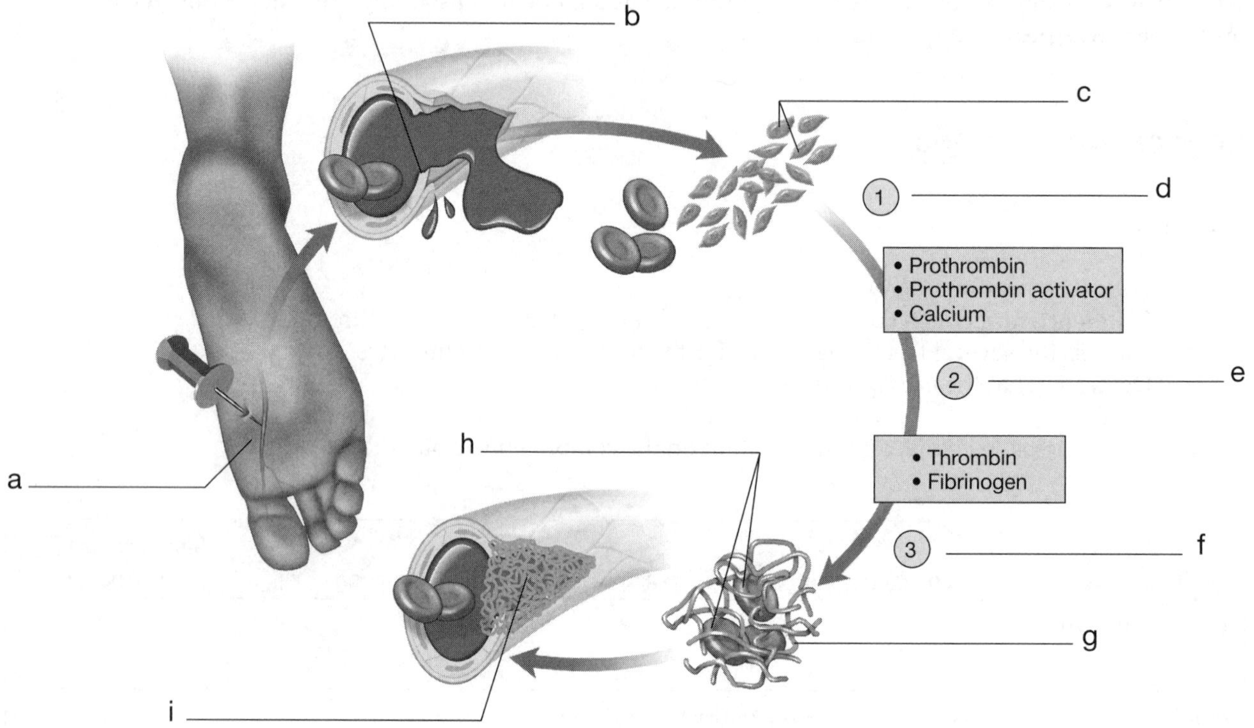

BLOOD GROUPS

Objective

- List the names of the basic blood groups.

3. List the names of the basic blood groups. Specify the types of antibodies and antigens contained in each group. Identify which one of the types can be a universal donor and which one is the universal recipient. ***(1502-1503)***

   a. ____

   ____

   b. ____

   ____

c. ______________________________

____

d. ______________________________

____

ORGANS OF THE LYMPHATIC SYSTEM

Objective

- Describe the generalized function of the lymphatic system and list the primary lymphatic structures.

4. Label each of the organs of the lymphatic system. ***(1504)***

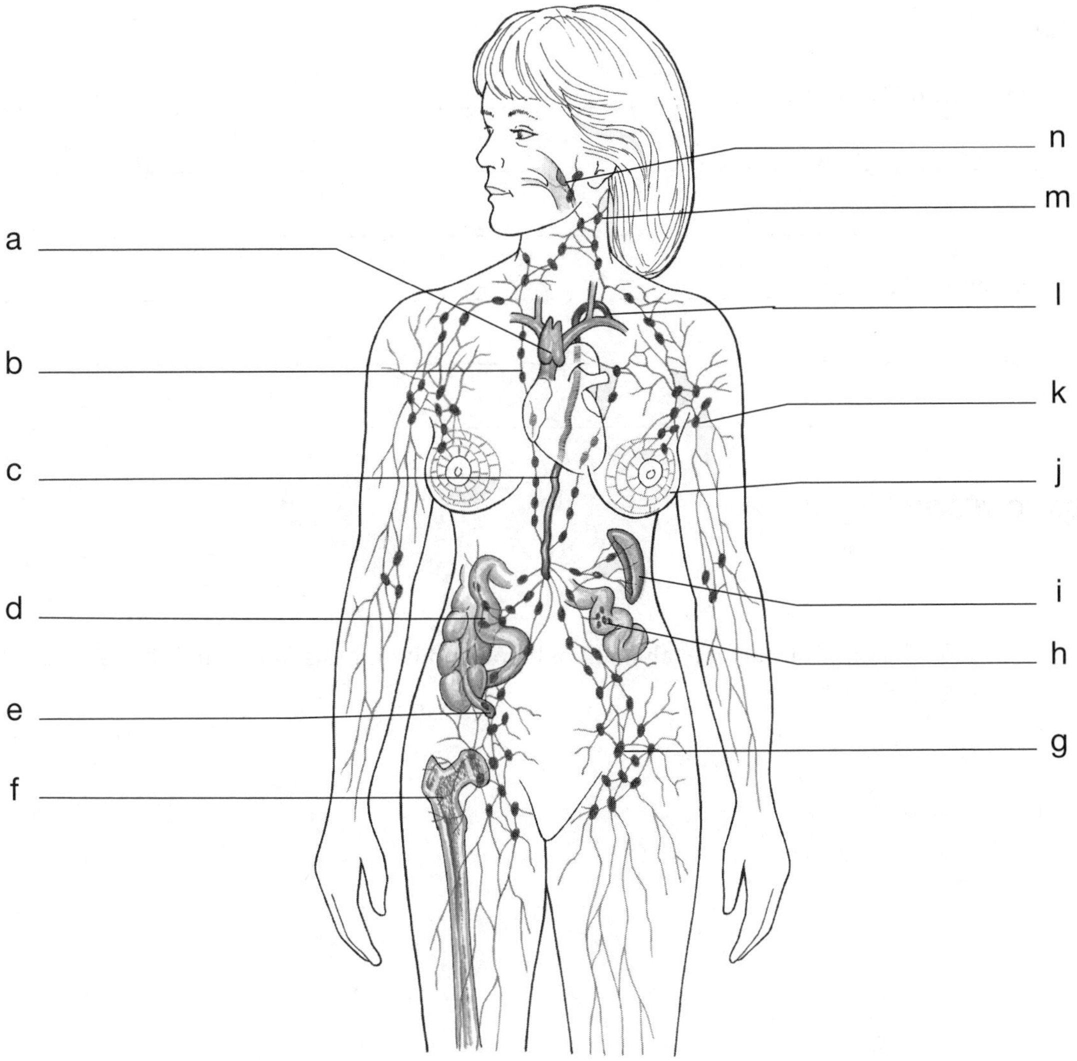

LYMPHATIC SYSTEM

Objective

- Describe the generalized functions of the lymphatic system and list the primary lymphatic structures.

5. The patient asked the nurse what the lymphatic system is and why it is important. How does the nurse explain its three functions to her? Also identify the function of each structure. Be sure to use terms the patient would understand. ***(1503-1504)***

   a. Functions

      i. ______________________________

      ii. ______________________________

      iii. ______________________________

   b. Structures

      i. Lymph and lymph vessels: ______________________________

      ____

      ____

      ii. Lymphatic tissues: ______________________________

      ____

      ____

DIAGNOSTIC TESTS

Objective

- List common diagnostic tests for evaluation of blood and lymph disorders, and discuss the significance of the results.

6. Explain, by completing the table below, each of the diagnostic tests that is usually done as an evaluation tool for patients with blood or lymphatic disorders. ***(1505)***

Diagnostic Test	Explanation of Procedure	Significance of Results
a. Complete blood count (CBC)		
b. Red cell indices		
c. Peripheral smear		
d. Schilling test		
e. Gastric analysis		
f. Lymphangiography		
g. Bone marrow aspiration or biopsy		

NURSING PROCESS

Objective

- Apply the nursing process to the care of the patient with disorders of the hematological and lymphatic systems.

7. Develop an index card that highlights the nursing process for patients with disorders of the hematological and lymphatic systems. ***(1534-1535)***

ANEMIA

Objectives

- Compare and contrast the different types of anemia in terms of etiology and pathophysiology, clinical manifestations, assessment, diagnostic tests, medical management, nursing interventions, and prognosis.
- Discuss important issues to cover in patient teaching and home care planning for the patient with pernicious anemia.

8. List and define the five types of anemia. ***(1505-1513)*** ______

9. Compare and contrast the two types of aplastic anemia. ***(1509-1510)*** ______

10. Review the clinical manifestations of aplastic anemia. ***(1510)*** ______

11. Why are blood transfusions avoided in cases of aplastic anemia? ***(1509-1510)*** ______

12. Which anemia is associated with abnormal, crescent-shaped red blood cells (RBCs)? ***(1512)*** ______

13. What special instructions should be given to the patient who is prescribed iron? ***(1513)*** ______

14. Discuss the primary symptom of sickle cell anemia. ***(1514)*** ______

15. Discuss the pain management strategies for sickle cell anemia. ***(1514-1515)*** ______

16. Why is the method of Z-track administration used for iron therapy? ***(1512)*** ______

17. The patient with pernicious anemia questions how people can get this disorder. What information should be provided to the patient? ***(1509)***

18. Describe the long-term therapy planned for the patient with pernicious anemia. ***(1509)*** ______

COAGULATION DISORDERS

Objective

- Compare and contrast the disorders of coagulation (thrombocytopenia, hemophilia, disseminated intravascular coagulation [DIC]) in terms of etiology and pathophysiology, clinical manifestations, assessment, diagnostic tests, medical management, nursing interventions, and prognosis.

19. List the common information about thrombocytopenia, hemophilia, and DIC. Then list the information that is specific to each disorder. ***(1520-1527)***

	Common Information
a. Pathophysiology	
b. Assessment	
c. Nursing interventions	

	Thrombocytopenia	Hemophilia	DIC
d. Pathophysiology			
e. Assessment			
f. Nursing interventions			

HEMOPHILIA AND DIC

Objective

- Discuss medical management of patients with hemophilia and DIC.

20. The patient wants to know the difference between hemophilia and DIC. Explain the medical management of hemophilia and DIC in terminology that she can understand. ***(1524-1525)***

____

____

HYPOVOLEMIC SHOCK

Objective

- List six signs and symptoms associated with hypovolemic shock.

Activity 1

21. The nurse is admitting a patient who has had a traumatic amputation of his right arm. What signs and symptoms of hypovolemic shock could the nurse expect the patient to exhibit? ***(1507)***

 a. ____

 b. ____

 c. ____

 d. ____

 e. ____

 f. ____

Activity 2

22. How is hypovolemic anemia diagnosed? ***(1507)*** ____

____

____

23. Discuss the medical management of hypovolemia. ***(1507)***____

____

____

24. Develop two nursing interventions for hypovolemia. ***(1507)*** ______________________________

____

____

25. List nursing interventions for the care of a patient experiencing hypovolemia. ***(1507)***______________

____

____

PROGNOSIS

Objective

- Discuss the etiology and pathophysiology, clinical manifestations, assessment, diagnostic tests, assessment, medical management, nursing interventions, patient teaching, and prognosis for patients with acute and chronic leukemia.

26. The nurse has a patient with chronic leukemia who wants to know the prognosis for her disorder. List the usual prognoses for both acute and chronic leukemia. ***(1520)***

____

____

MULTIPLE MYELOMA

Objective

- Discuss the etiology and pathophysiology, clinical manifestations, assessment, diagnostic tests, medical management, nursing interventions, patient teaching, and prognosis for the patient with multiple myeloma, malignant lymphoma, and Hodgkin's disease.

27. Develop an index card that will assist the nurse during nursing interventions and patient teaching for a patient with multiple myeloma. ***(1527-1528)***

HODGKIN'S OR NON-HODGKIN'S DISEASE

Objective

- Discuss the etiology and pathophysiology, clinical manifestations, assessment, diagnostic tests, medical management, nursing interventions, patient teaching, and prognosis for the patient with multiple myeloma, malignant lymphoma, and Hodgkin's lymphoma.

28. Identify the medical management and nursing interventions for Hodgkin's and non-Hodgkin's lymphomas. ***(1529-1534)***

	Medical Management	Nursing Interventions
a. Hodgkin's		
b. Non-Hodgkin's		

LYMPHEDEMA

Objective

- Discuss the primary goal of nursing interventions for the patient with lymphedema.

29. Using an index card, develop a short nursing care plan for the patient with lymphedema, including diagnosis, goal, and interventions. ***(1529)***

MULTIPLE CHOICE

30. When caring for a patient who is a Jehovah's Witness scheduled to undergo surgery, the nurse must be aware of which of the following? (Select all that apply) ***(1506)***
    1. Some Jehovah's Witnesses may permit the use of certain blood volume expanders.
    2. It is not legal for this patient to refuse transfusions if the bleeding is truly life-threatening.
    3. Some Jehovah's Witnesses may consent to certain types of autologous blood transfusions.
    4. It is a nursing responsibility to request the patient to clarify his specific intentions related to blood transfusions.

31. When the nurse is caring for a patient experiencing an initial sickle cell crisis, his mother asks what is causing the pain. Based on the nurse's knowledge, the best explanation is that: ***(1514)***
    1. the red blood cells are caught in the vessels and causing pain in the joints.
    2. the pain occurs as the red blood cells are hemolyzed.
    3. medical science is still unable to pinpoint the exact cause of the pain.
    4. the tissue ischemia is the cause of the pain.

32. The expected laboratory profile for the patient diagnosed with primary polycythemia includes: ***(1515-1516)***
    1. an increase in erythrocytes, platelets, and granulocytes.
    2. a decrease in erythrocytes, platelets, and granulocytes.
    3. an increase in erythrocytes and platelets, and a decrease in granulocytes.
    4. a decrease in erythrocytes, and an increase in platelets and granulocytes.

33. When caring for an older adult patient whose chief complaint is back pain and who has an elevated total serum protein, what potential disease should be considered? ***(1527)***
    1. Leukemia
    2. Sickle cell anemia
    3. Multiple myeloma
    4. Lymphangitis

CRITICAL THINKING ACTIVITIES

Activity 1

34. A 23-year-old patient is seen with complaints of her "heart racing," nausea, sore tongue, and difficulty swallowing. Upon oral examination, her tongue is smooth and erythematous. ***(1508)***

    a. What medical diagnosis would a nurse anticipate? ______________________

    ____

    ____

    b. What diagnostic tests will support this suspicion? ______________________

    ____

    ____

c. What treatment options are available for this patient? ___

d. After completing 2 months of treatment, the patient states she is feeling well and now plans to discontinue the treatments. How should the nurse respond to the patient?

___

Activity 2

35. A 32-year-old female patient comes for care with complaints of fatigue, dizziness, and pallor. Her past history includes childbirth 3 months ago, a subgastrectomy 3 years ago, and hernia repair 18 months ago. Her Hgb level is 10 g/dL. ***(1511-1512)***

a. Based on the nurse's knowledge, what is the anticipated medical diagnosis? ___

b. What risk factors does this patient have that support development of this disorder? ___

c. Identify other signs and symptoms that may accompany this disorder. ___

d. Discuss medical management of this disorder. ___

Student Name______________________________ Date______________

chapter **48**

Care of the Patient with a Cardiovascular or a Peripheral Vascular Disorder

Answer Key: Textbook page references are provided as a guide for answering these questions. A complete answer key was provided for your instructor.

TRACING A DROP OF BLOOD

Objectives

- Discuss the location, size, and position of the heart.
- Identify the chambers of the heart and their functions.
- Identify the valves of the heart and their locations.
- Explain what produces the two main heart sounds.

1. Trace a drop of blood in the aorta backward around the systemic circulatory system, ending with the drop of blood back at the aorta. *(1541)*
   a. List all of the chambers and valves of the heart and their functions.
   b. Indicate when the blood changes from oxygenated to deoxygenated.
   c. Insert the heart sounds and how they are produced.
   d. Name all vessels carrying the blood and what type of blood they carry.

Aorta → ____________________ → ____________________ →

____________________ → ____________________ →

____________________ → ____________________ →

____________________ → ____________________ →

____________________ → ____________________ →

____________________ → ____________________ →

____________________ → ____________________ →

____________________ → ____________________ →

____________________ → Aorta

IMPULSE PATTERN

Objective

- Discuss the electrical conduction system that causes the cardiac muscle fibers to contract.

2. Identify the impulse pattern of the electrical conduction system of the heart, inserting the normal electrocardiographic (ECG) deflections. ***(1543)***

_______________ → _______________ →

_______________ → _______________

CORONARY CIRCULATION

Objective

- Trace the path of blood through the coronary circulation.

3. Label each of the coronary vessels that supply blood to the heart. ***(1543)***

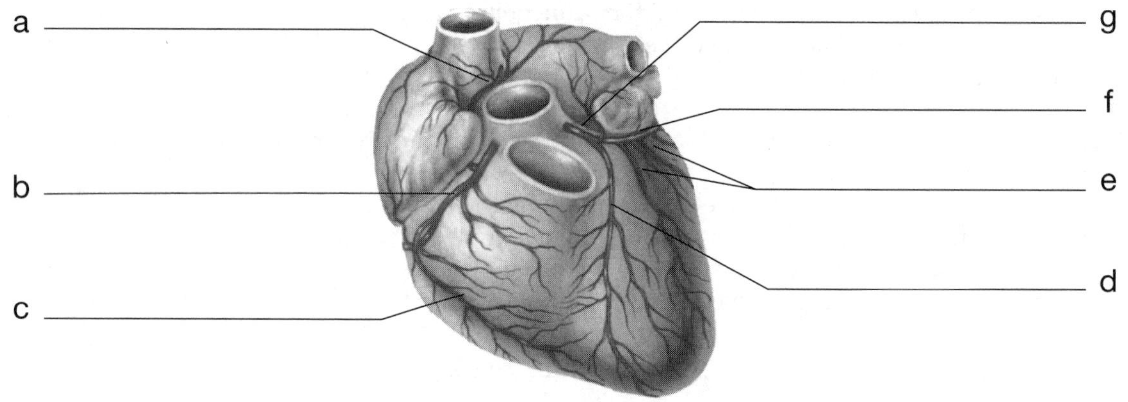

TERMS

Objective

- Define the key terms as listed.

4. Define the following using medical terminology. In the last column, indicate how the nurse could explain the meaning of that term to a patient. ***(1539-1605)***

Term	Medical Terminology	Patient Terminology
a. Aneurysm		
b. Angina pectoris		
c. Arteriosclerosis		

d. Atherosclerosis		
e. Bradycardia		
f. Cardioversion		
g. Coronary artery disease		
h. Defibrillation		
i. Dysrhythmia		
j. Embolus		
k. Endarterectomy		
l. Heart failure		
m. Hypoxemia		
n. Intermittent claudication		
o. Ischemia		
p. Myocardial infarction		
q. Occlusion		
r. Orthopnea		
s. Peripheral		
t. Pleural effusion		
u. Polycythemia		
v. Pulmonary edema		
w. Tachycardia		

RISK FACTORS

Objectives

- For coronary artery disease, compare nonmodifiable risk factors with factors that are modifiable in lifestyle and health management.
- Identify risk factors associated with peripheral vascular disorders.

5. Identify which risk factors can be modified, and what modification can be made by the patient to decrease cardiac disease. ***(1548-1550)***

Risk Factor	Nonmodifiable	Modifiable	Modification by Patients
a. Smoking			
b. Age			
c. Race			
d. Family history			
e. Hyperlipidemia			
f. Diabetes mellitus			
g. Sex			
h. Hypertension			
i. Obesity			
j. Sedentary lifestyle			
k. Stress			
l. Oral contraceptives			
m. Psychosocial factors			

ABNORMALITIES

Objective

- List diagnostic tests used to evaluate cardiovascular function.

6. Discuss the data significant to the diagnosis and management of a patient with a myocardial infarction that can be identified by a complete blood count (CBC). ***(1589)***

____

____

7. During the care of a patient on anticoagulant therapy, what laboratory values should be monitored? ***(1600)***

____

____

8. Discuss the significance of the sodium, potassium, calcium, and magnesium values in relation to the cardiac patient. ***(1571)***

____

____

9. What does an elevated CK-MB level signify? ***(1564)***_______________________

____

____

10. Discuss the usefulness of troponin-1 in the diagnosis of a myocardial infarction. ***(1564)***_______________

____

____

11. In what population may homocysteine screening be beneficial? ***(1547)***_______________________

____

____

12. Discuss creatine kinase assessment in the context of a myocardial infarction. ***(1562-1564)*** _______________

____

____

CARDIAC DYSRHYTHMIAS

Objective

- Describe five cardiac dysrhythmias.

13. Explain the difference in the rates and the causes of the dysrhythmias. ***(1550-1553)***

Dysrhythmias	Rate	Causes
a. Sinus rhythm		
b. Sinus bradycardia		
c. Sinus tachycardia		
d. Supraventricular tachycardia		
e. Atrial dysrhythmias		
f. Ventricular dysrhythmias		

ANGINA PECTORIS, MYOCARDIAL INFARCTION, AND HEART FAILURE

Objective

- Compare the etiology and pathophysiology, clinical manifestations, assessment, diagnostic tests, medical management, nursing interventions, and prognosis for patients with angina pectoris, myocardial Infarction, or heart failure.

14. Discuss the similarities and differences between the manifestations of angina pectoris and myocardial infarction. ***(1563)***

____

____

15. How is angina pectoris managed? ***(1563)*** ____

____

____

16. Identify the classifications of medications used in the medical management of heart failure. ***(1571)***

____

____

17. What are common signs and symptoms of heart failure? ***(1570)***______________________

____

____

PULMONARY EDEMA

Objective

- Discuss the etiology and pathophysiology, clinical manifestations, assessment, diagnostic tests, medical management, nursing interventions, and prognosis for the patient with pulmonary edema.

18. Describe nursing interventions for patients with pulmonary edema. ***(1576)***

    a. ____

    ____

    b. ____

    ____

    c. ____

    ____

    d. ____

    ____

    e. ____

    ____

RHEUMATIC HEART DISEASE, PERICARDITIS, AND ENDOCARDITIS

Objective

- Compare and contrast etiology and pathophysiology, clinical manifestations, assessment, diagnostic tests, medical management, nursing interventions, and prognosis for patients with rheumatic heart disease, pericarditis, and endocarditis.

19. What causes rheumatic heart disease? ***(1578)***

20. Discuss the onset of rheumatic heart disease. ***(1578)***

21. Review the signs and symptoms of rheumatic heart disease. ***(1578)***

22. Review the medical management of rheumatic heart disease. ***(1578)***

23. What is pericarditis? ***(1579-1580)***

24. Identify the causes of pericarditis. ***(1579-1580)***

25. Review the signs, symptoms, and medical management of pericarditis. ***(1579-1580)***

26. How do pericarditis and endocarditis differ? ***(1579-1580)***

27. Review the risk factors for endocarditis. ***(1579-1580)***

SECONDARY CARDIOMYOPATHY

Objective

- List the 10 conditions that can result in the complication of secondary cardiomyopathy.

28. There are 10 conditions that can result in the complication of secondary cardiomyopathy. What are they? ***(1582-1583)***

    a. ______________________________

    b. ______________________________

    c. ______________________________

    d. ______________________________

    e. ______________________________

    f. ______________________________

    g. ______________________________

    h. ______________________________

    i. ______________________________

    j. ______________________________

PATIENT TEACHING

Objective

- Specify patient teaching for patients with cardiac dysrhythmias, angina pectoris, myocardial infarction, heart failure, and valvular heart disease.

Activity 1

29. List common patient teaching that the nurse should provide to any patient who has cardiac dysrhythmias, angina pectoris, myocardial infarction, heart failure, or valvular heart disease. ***(1552-1553)***

    ____

    ____

    ____

    ____

Activity 2

30. In the table below, add the specific patient teaching that the nurse should provide for the patient with each disorder.

Disorder	Specific Patient Teaching
a. Cardiac dysrhythmias *(1553)*	
b. Angina pectoris *(1554)*	
c. Myocardial infarction *(1566)*	
d. Heart failure *(1567)*	
e. Valvular heart disease *(1578)*	

CARDIAC TRANSPLANTATION

Objective

- Discuss the indications and contraindications for cardiac transplant.

31. What condition is most commonly the underlying cause for cardiac transplantation? ***(1583)***__________

32. What types of evaluations are performed on a potential candidate for cardiac transplant? ***(1583)***__________

33. List factors that are used to determine donor matching. ***(1583)*** __________

ARTERIAL AND VENOUS DISORDERS

Objective

- Compare and contrast signs and symptoms associated with arterial and venous disorders.

34. Review each of the signs and symptoms listed. Place an "X" in the column of the disorder type that is best described. ***(1587)***

Sign or Symptom	Arterial Disorder	Venous Disorder
a. Pain onset with activity		
b. Aching to cramping pain		
c. Diminished pulses		
d. Cool skin		
e. Stasis ulcers		

AGING

Objective

- Describe the effects of aging on the peripheral vascular system.

35. List the changes that occur to the peripheral vascular system as the body ages. ***(1584)***

Vascular System Part	Changes	Effect of Change
a. Inner walls		
b. Middle walls		

NURSING INTERVENTIONS

Objective

- Discuss nursing interventions for arterial and venous disorders.

36. Place a check next to the nursing intervention that is usually done for patients with arterial or venous disorders. Use the last column to indicate whether the intervention can be done for both disorders. ***(1539-1605)***

Nursing Intervention	Arterial Disorders	Venous Disorders	Both
a. Monitor skin color and temperature			
b. Assess sensation and movement of extremity			
c. Assess peripheral pulses and capillary refill			
d. Monitor extremity for edema			
e. Promote circulation			
f. Avoid sharp flexion of extremities			
g. Administer prescribed nonsteroidal antiinflammatory drugs (NSAIDs)			
h. Measure calf or thigh circumference daily			
i. Have patient wear elastic stockings			
j. Avoid crossing the legs at the knee			
k. Elevate legs when sitting			
l. Assess level of discomfort			

HYPERTENSION

Objectives

- Compare essential (primary) hypertension, secondary hypertension, and malignant hypertension.
- Discuss the importance of patient education for hypertension.
- Discuss the etiology and pathophysiology, clinical manifestations, assessment, diagnostic tests, medical management, and nursing interventions for the patient with hypertension.

37. List the factors common to essential (primary) hypertension and secondary hypertension. ***(1587-1589)***

____

____

38. Explain why it is important to do patient education regarding hypertension. ***(1587-1589)*** ____________

____

____

39. Discuss what constitutes a diagnosis of hypertension. ***(1587-1589)*** ____________________

____

____

40. Review the causes of primary hypertension. ***(1587-1589)*** ______

41. List the potential clinical manifestations of hypertension. ***(1587-1589)*** ______

42. What diagnostic tests are associated with the medical diagnosis and the management of hypertension? ***(1587-1589)***

43. Identify nonpharmacologic measures used to aid in the management of hypertension. ***(1587-1589)***

ARTERIAL ANEURYSM, BUERGER'S DISEASE, AND RAYNAUD'S DISEASE

Objective

- Compare and contrast the etiology and pathophysiology, clinical manifestations, assessment, diagnostic tests, medical management, nursing interventions, and prognosis for patients with arterial aneurysm, Buerger's disease, and Raynaud's disease.

44. Review each of the disorders. Complete the chart by writing in the information requested for each disorder. ***(1595-1597)***

	Arterial Aneurysm	Buerger's Disease	Raynaud's Disease
a. At risk populations			
b. Areas of the body or vessels involved			
c. Clinical manifestations			
d. Medical management			

THROMBOPHLEBITIS

Objective

- Discuss appropriate patient education for thrombophlebitis.

45. From the list below, check patient education that is appropriate for a patient with thrombophlebitis and explain the rationale for adherence to the directions in a way that would be suitable to use with a patient. ***(1618-1619)***

Patient Education	Appropriate	Rationale for Adherence
a. Maintain diuretic therapy		
b. Restrict sodium in diet		
c. Stay in bed in acute phase		
d. Remove elastic stockings		
e. Elevate legs when sitting		
f. Massage extremities when painful		
g. Avoid flexion-extension exercise		
h. Avoid crossing legs at knee, tight stockings, or garters		
i. Encourage ambulation during acute phase		
j. Monitor calf or thigh circumference daily		

THROMBOPHLEBITIS, VARICOSE VEINS, AND STASIS ULCERS

Objective

- Discuss the etiology and pathology, clinical manifestations, assessment, diagnostic tests, medical management, nursing interventions, and prognosis for patients with thrombophlebitis, varicose veins, and stasis ulcers.

46. Compare and contrast the pathophysiology of thrombophlebitis, varicose veins, and stasis ulcers. ***(1618-1619)***

____

____

47. Identify potential causes of varicose veins. ***(1618-1619)*** ______________________________

____

____

48. List the signs and symptoms of varicose veins. ***(1618-1619)*** ______________________________

____

____

49. How are varicose veins treated? ***(1618-1619)*** ______________________________

____

____

50. Review the treatment options available for venous stasis ulcers. ***(1618-1619)*** ______________________________

____

____

51. Identify the signs and symptoms of venous stasis ulcers. ***(1618-1619)***______________________________

____

____

CARDIAC REHABILITATION

Objective

- Discuss the purposes of cardiac rehabilitation.

52. In the table below, add the specific patient teaching that a nurse should provide for the patient with each component of cardiac rehabilitation. ***(1567-1568)***

Component	Specific Patient Teaching
a. Exercise program	
b. Diet	
c. Medications	
d. Stress reduction	
e. Sexual activities	

MULTIPLE CHOICE

53. During a discharge teaching session, the patient voices concern about why her risk of heart disease is elevated simply because she has a history of diabetes mellitus. Based on the nurse's knowledge, a good explanation is that: ***(1585)***
    1. elevated insulin levels associated with diabetes cause vasoconstriction.
    2. elevated blood glucose levels promote arterial damage and contribute to arterial damage.
    3. diabetics are often obese and thus at higher risk.
    4. there must be some misunderstanding, since risk for heart disease is not higher for the patient who has diabetes.

54. For the patient receiving care for a myocardial infarction, the typical vital signs will display which of the following? ***(1562-1564)***
    1. Hypotension, tachycardia, weakened pulse, and temperature elevation
    2. Hypertension, tachycardia, weakened pulse, and temperature elevation
    3. Hypertension, bradycardia, weakened pulse, and temperature elevation
    4. Hypotension, bradycardia, weakened pulse, and temperature elevation

55. Which of the following is appropriate patient teaching for self-administration of nitrate medications? ***(1558)***
    1. Refrigerate medications until use.
    2. Apply patches in the morning and remove them at bedtime.
    3. A burning sensation on the tongue indicates an allergic reaction and requires immediate reporting.
    4. Pain relief should occur after a minimum of two administrations.

56. A 53-year-old patient presents with complaints of syncope, fatigue, and dyspnea with exertion. Based on the nurse's knowledge, a medical diagnosis can be anticipated of: ***(1557)***
    1. cardiomyopathy.
    2. angina.
    3. left-sided heart block.
    4. rheumatic heart disease.

CRITICAL THINKING ACTIVITIES

Activity 1

57. A 56-year-old man arrives in the emergency department seeking care. He is complaining of crushing chest pain. The pain is radiating down his left shoulder and arm. The patient, who has a history of angina, reports this pain as being more severe and lasting longer than a typical angina episode. ***(1562-1564)***

    a. What does the nurse anticipate this patient's medical diagnosis will be? ________________

    ____

    ____

    b. Discuss the potential causes of this type of occurrence. ________________

    ____

    ____

    c. During the medical diagnostic work-up of this patient, what tests are likely to be ordered? ________

    ____

    ____

    d. What are the goals of the medical management of this patient? ________________

    ____

    ____

    e. Identify four nursing interventions for this patient's care. ________________

    ____

    ____

Activity 2

58. A 43-year-old woman of American-Indian ethnicity presents with complaints of "heaviness in her chest." She reports that it radiates down her left inner arm. Her medical history includes childbirth, pancreatitis, and hypertension. The medical diagnosis of angina is made. ***(1557)***

    a. What risk factors for heart disease does the patient have? ____________________

    ____

    ____

    b. What medication is used to treat angina? ____________________

    ____

    ____

    c. During the diagnostic work-up, what tests may be ordered?____________________

    ____

    ____

    d. While caring for the patient, she asks the nurse, "What has caused this to happen?" How will the nurse respond to her inquiry?

    ____

    ____

Student Name________________________________ Date______________

Care of the Patient with a Respiratory Disorder

chapter **49**

Answer Key: Textbook page references are provided as a guide for answering these questions. A complete answer key was provided for your instructor.

EXTERNAL AND INTERNAL RESPIRATION AND GAS EXCHANGE

Objective

- Differentiate between external and internal respiration.

1. After being seen by his doctor, the patient voices questions about the respiratory system. Formulate an explanation of the difference between external and internal respiration in terms that the patient would understand. ***(1610)***

____

____

RESPIRATORY TRACT

Objectives

- Describe the purpose of the respiratory system.
- List and define the parts of the upper and lower respiratory tracts.
- List the ways in which oxygen and carbon dioxide are transported in the blood.

2. Describe the purpose of the respiratory system. ***(1610-1613)***____________________

____

____

3. Next to each part of the upper and lower respiratory system, describe the part and name its function. ***(1610-1614)***

Respiratory Tract Part	Description	Function
a. Nose		
b. Pharynx		
c. Larynx		
d. Trachea		
e. Bronchial tree		
f. Lungs		

4. The patient asks how oxygen and carbon dioxide are transported in the blood. Explain the answer in terms the patient will understand. ***(1614-1615)***

____

____

5. The adult patient asks the nurse, "What is a normal respiratory rate?" How would the nurse best answer this question? ***(1614)***

____

____

ALVEOLUS AND GAS EXCHANGE

Objective

- List the ways in which oxygen and carbon dioxide are transported in the blood.

6. Make a list of all of the areas of the body that are involved in gas exchange. ***(1614)*** ____________________

____

____

7. Briefly describe how oxygen and carbon dioxide are transported around the body. ***(1614-1615)*** __________

____

____

REGULATORS

Objective

- Discuss the mechanisms that regulate respirations.

8. The terms below are the parts of the human body that regulate respiration. Explain how the regulation occurs in each area. ***(1614)***

   a. Medulla oblongata and pons of the brain: ____

   ____

   ____

   b. Chemoreceptors located in the carotid and aortic bodies: ____________________________

   ____

   ____

HYPOXIA AND ADVENTITIOUS BREATH SOUNDS

Objectives

- Identify those signs and symptoms that indicate a patient is experiencing hypoxia.
- Differentiate among sonorous wheezes, sibilant wheezes, crackles, and pleural friction rub.

9. Create a list of all of the clinical manifestations associated with hypoxia. ***(1614-1615)*** __________________

____

____

10. Describe the differences between the following adventitious breath sounds: sonorous wheezes, sibilant wheezes, crackles, and pleural friction rub. What will the nurse hear? What may the specific sound indicate? ***(1614-1615)***

    a. Sonorous wheezes: ______________________________

    ____

    b. Sibilant wheezes: ______________________________

    ____

    c. Crackles: ______________________________

    ____

    d. Pleural friction rub: ______________________________

    ____

DIAGNOSTIC TESTS

Objectives

- Describe the purpose, significance of results, and nursing interventions related to diagnostic examinations of the respiratory system.
- Describe the significance of arterial blood gas values and differentiate between arterial oxygen tension (Pao_2) and arterial oxygen saturation (Sao_2).

11. Briefly describe how each diagnostic test is performed and how it can be used to assist in developing a medical diagnosis for a patient. Include appropriate nursing interventions related to each diagnostic test. ***(1615-1616)***

    a. Chest radiography: ______________________________

    ____

    ____

    b. Computed tomography: ______________________________

    ____

    ____

    c. Pulmonary function testing (PFT): ______________________________

    ____

    ____

d. Mediastinoscopy: ____

____

____

e. Laryngoscopy: ____

____

____

f. Pulmonary angiography: ____

____

____

g. Ventilation-perfusion scan (V/Q scan): ____

____

____

h. Bronchoscopy: ____

____

____

i. Thoracentesis: ____

____

____

j. Lung biopsy: ____

____

____

k. Pulse oximetry: ____

____

____

l. Arterial blood gases: ____

____

12. During preparation of a patient for a chest radiograph, why must any article of clothing or jewelry containing metal be removed? ***(1615-1616)***

13. How do inspiratory capacity and total lung capacity differ? ***(1616)***

14. How is the helical computed tomography (CT) scan different from the standard CT scan? ***(1616)***

15. Identify four nursing interventions for patients after bronchoscopy. ***(1617)***

16. Discuss the relevance of arterial blood gases. ***(1618-1619)***

17. What is the difference between arterial oxygen tension and arterial oxygen saturation? How is each measured? ***(1629)***

UPPER AIRWAY DISORDERS

Objective

- Discuss the etiology and pathophysiology, clinical manifestations, assessment, diagnostic tests, medical management, nursing interventions, and prognosis of the patient with disorders of the upper airway.

18. Identify potential causes of laryngitis. ***(1629)***

19. What signs and symptoms may accompany a diagnosis of laryngitis? ***(1629)*** ______

20. How is laryngitis managed? ***(1629)*** ______

21. Why does the prognosis for the adult with laryngitis differ from that for the infant or young child with the disorder? ***(1629)***

22. Discuss the signs and symptoms of pharyngitis. ***(1630)*** ______

23. Identify the categories of medications that may be prescribed to care for the patient diagnosed with pharyngitis. ***(1630)***

LARYNGECTOMY

Objective

- Discuss nursing interventions for the patient with a laryngectomy.

24. Listed below are four priority areas of care for the patient with a recent laryngectomy. Under each heading, identify two nursing interventions to support optimal patient outcomes. ***(1632)***

    a. Prevention of postoperative infection:

        i. ______

        ii. ______

    b. Patient education:

        i. ______

        ii. ______

c. Nutrition:

i. ______

ii. ______

d. Communication:

i. ______

ii. ______

LOWER AIRWAY DISORDERS

Objective

- Discuss the etiology and pathophysiology, clinical manifestations, assessment, diagnostic tests, medical management, nursing interventions, and prognosis of the patient with disorders of the lower airway.

25. List the clinical manifestations of acute bronchitis. ***(1632)*** ______

26. Describe how Legionnaire's disease is treated medically. ***(1632)*** ______

27. How is severe acute respiratory syndrome (SARS) diagnosed? ***(1633)*** ______

28. What are some common clinical manifestations associated with inhalational anthrax? ***(1634)*** ______

29. What are the four most common pathogens associated with bacterial pneumonia? ***(1640-1641)*** ______

30. What are some common clinical manifestations associated with pleurisy? ***(1643)***____________________

31. How are pleural effusions and empyemas medically managed? ***(1644)*** ____________________

32. How does the site and the degree of airway occlusion affect the severity of atelectasis? ***(1646)*** __________

33. What are some important nursing interventions to perform for a patient diagnosed with a pneumothorax? ***(1648-1649)***

34. What are some common signs and symptoms associated with lung cancer? ***(1649)*** ____________________

35. List the five causes of pulmonary edema listed in the text. ***(1651)*** ____________________

36. Describe how a pulmonary embolism can be diagnosed. ***(1652-1653)***____________________

37. What are two common nursing diagnoses associated with acute respiratory distress syndrome (ARDS)? ***(1655-1656)***

NURSING INTERVENTIONS

Objective

- List five nursing interventions to assist patients with retained pulmonary secretions.

38. The patient is having problems related to retention of pulmonary secretions. List five nursing interventions that the nurse can initiate to assist the patient to expel secretions. ***(1617-1618)***

    a. ____________________

    b. ____________________

    c. ____________________

    d. ____________________

    e. ____________________

TUBERCULOSIS

Objectives

- Differentiate between tuberculosis infection and tuberculosis disease.
- List four medications commonly prescribed for the patient with tuberculosis.

39. The nurse is caring for a patient who has recently been diagnosed with tuberculosis. He asks about each of the four medications he has been prescribed. List each of the four most common medications prescribed for tuberculosis. What teaching should be provided for this patient regarding his medications? ***(1636)***

    ____

    ____

    ____

    ____

40. The patient requests information regarding tuberculosis infection and tuberculosis disease. Accurately provide information about the differences between the two conditions in terms the patient would understand. ***(1637-1638)***

    ____

    ____

    ____

    ____

CLOSED CHEST DRAINAGE

Objective

- List five nursing assessments or interventions pertaining to the care of the patient with closed chest drainage.

41. The nurse has arrived on the nursing unit and found that the patient has a closed chest drainage system. ***(1646)***

    a. Discuss the level of the chest drainage system.______________________________

    b. What nursing assessments should be performed for this patient? ______________________________

    c. How should the tubing be positioned? ______________________________

    d. What is indicated if there is no tidaling (air bubbling) noted in the drainage collection bottles?

    e. What should be considered if there is constant bubbling? ______________________________

PULMONARY EMBOLI

Objective

- Discuss three risk factors associated with pulmonary emboli.

42. The patient has developed a pulmonary embolism and wants to know about why this condition occurred. Discuss all of the risk factors associated with the development of a pulmonary embolism. ***(1652-1653)***

43. What would the nurse expect to find during the physical assessment of a patient with a pulmonary embolism? ***(1653-1654)***

____

____

CHRONIC OBSTRUCTIVE PULMONARY DISEASE

Objective

- Compare and contrast the etiology and pathophysiology, clinical manifestations, assessment, diagnostic tests, medical management, nursing interventions, and prognosis for the patient with chronic obstructive pulmonary disease, including emphysema, chronic bronchitis, asthma, and bronchiectasis.

44. List the causes, the signs and symptoms, and the management for the following disorders. ***(1657-1666)***

Disorder	Causes	Signs and Symptoms	Nursing Interventions
a. Emphysema			
b. Asthma			
c. Bronchiectasis			

ASTHMA OR EMPHYSEMA

Objectives

- Differentiate between medical management of the patient with emphysema and the patient with asthma.
- Discuss why low-flow oxygen is required for patients with emphysema.

45. List the medical management of a patient with emphysema and of a patient with asthma. Include why low-flow oxygen is required for patient with emphysema. ***(1657-1666)***

Medical Management
a. Emphysema
b. Asthma
i. Rationale for low-flow oxygen for patients with emphysema:

NURSING DIAGNOSES

Objective

- State three possible nursing diagnoses for the patient with altered respiratory function.

46. List five nursing diagnoses that could be applied to a patient with altered respiratory function. ***(1665-1666)***

a. ______________________________

b. ______________________________

c. ______________________________

d. ______________________________

e. ______________________________

MULTIPLE CHOICE

47. A patient recently diagnosed with peripherally located lung cancer reports he is experiencing severe chest pain. Based on the nurse's knowledge, the reason for the pain is understood to be: ***(1625)***
    1. the tumor's compression of a nerve.
    2. pleural effusion.
    3. hypoxemia related to impaired air exchange.
    4. all of the above.

48. A patient being treated for atelectasis has been prescribed acetylcysteine. What is the purpose of this medication? ***(1637)***
    1. To prevent infection
    2. To dilate the bronchioles
    3. To enhance the cough reflex
    4. To reduce the viscosity of the secretions

49. Areas of concern when caring for a patient with a chest tube include which of the following? (Select all that apply) ***(1644-1646)***
    1. Proper system function
    2. Potential atelectasis resulting from hypoventilation
    3. Increased air in the pleural space
    4. Complication from infection

50. The primary manifestations of nasal septal deviations and polyps include ____________________ respirations, dyspnea, and possibly postnasal drip. ***(1621)***
    1. stertorous
    2. wheezing
    3. crackling
    4. rale-like

CRITICAL THINKING ACTIVITIES

Activity 1

51. A 34-year-old man comes to the physician's office seeking care. He is complaining of fatigue and headaches in the morning. The nurse's assessment reveals he is 5′9″ and weighs 293 pounds. His blood pressure is 155/92 mm Hg. His health history reveals a history of elevated blood pressure, hernia repair, appendectomy, and recent injuries suffered from a motor vehicle accident after falling asleep while driving. During the interview, his wife states he should never be tired, because he snores so loudly at night that she is the one who is kept awake. ***(1623-1624)***

    a. Based on the nurse's knowledge, what medical diagnosis is anticipated? ____________________

    ____

    ____

    ____

    ____

b. What does this diagnosis mean? ______

c. What risk factors and elements of the patient's personal history support this diagnosis? ______

d. What diagnostic examinations may be ordered by the physician to support the diagnosis? ______

e. Discuss the medical management of this condition. ______

Activity 2

52. A 72-year-old man is transferred from the nursing home to the hospital with a diagnosis of viral pneumonia. ***(1640-1642)***

a. What signs and symptoms are associated with this type of pneumonia? ______

b. What diagnostic tests can the nurse expect to be completed for this patient? ____________________

____

____

____

____

c. What types of medications may be prescribed for this patient?____________________

____

____

____

____

d. Identify critical nursing assessments that should be performed for this patient. ____________________

____

____

____

____

Student Name____________________ Date__________

chapter **50**

Care of the Patient with a Urinary Disorder

Answer Key: Textbook page references are provided as a guide for answering these questions. A complete answer key was provided for your instructor.

STRUCTURES

Objective

- Describe the structures of the urinary system, including functions.

1. Next to each structure, explain its function. ***(1670-1672)***

Structure	Function
a. Kidneys	
b. Renal capsule	
c. Medulla	
d. Pyramids	
e. Renal pelvis	
f. Nephron	
g. Glomeruli	
h. Bowman's capsule	
i. Renal tubule	
j. Juxtaglomerular apparatus	

HORMONES

Objective

- Name three hormones and their influence on nephron function.

2. What types of phenomena will cause a decrease in the amount of filtrate produced by the kidneys? ***(1673-1674)***

____

____

3. What role does antidiuretic hormone play on the nephron function? ***(1673-1674)*** ____________

____

____

4. Where are the adrenal glands located? What role do they play in renal function? ***(1673-1674)***______

____

____

URINE

Objectives

- List the three processes involved in urine formation.
- Compare the normal components of urine to the abnormal components.

Activity 1

5. Identify the phases of urine production. Complete the table below. ***(1673)***

Phase of Urine Formation	Activities	Location
a.		
b.		
c.		

Activity 2

6. The urinalysis of a patient experiencing a urinary tract infection will most likely reveal abnormal: ***(1684)***
   1. albumin.
   2. erythrocytes.
   3. leukocytes.
   4. protein.

7. The presence of __________ in the urine may be associated with diabetes, dietary intake, or medications. ***(1684)***
   1. ketones
   2. red blood cells
   3. white blood cells
   4. albumin

8. Casts in the urine are associated with: ***(1684)***
   1. type 1 diabetes mellitus.
   2. corticosteroid use.
   3. renal disease.
   4. urinary structure trauma.

9. The nurse is reviewing the specific gravity results of an assigned client. Which finding is within normal limits? ***(1684)***
   1. <1.003 g/mL
   2. 1.03 g/mL
   3. 1.10 g/mL
   4. 1.25 g/mL

RENAL TUBULES

Objective

- Describe the structures of the urinary system, including functions.

10. Label each part of the renal tubule. ***(1673)***

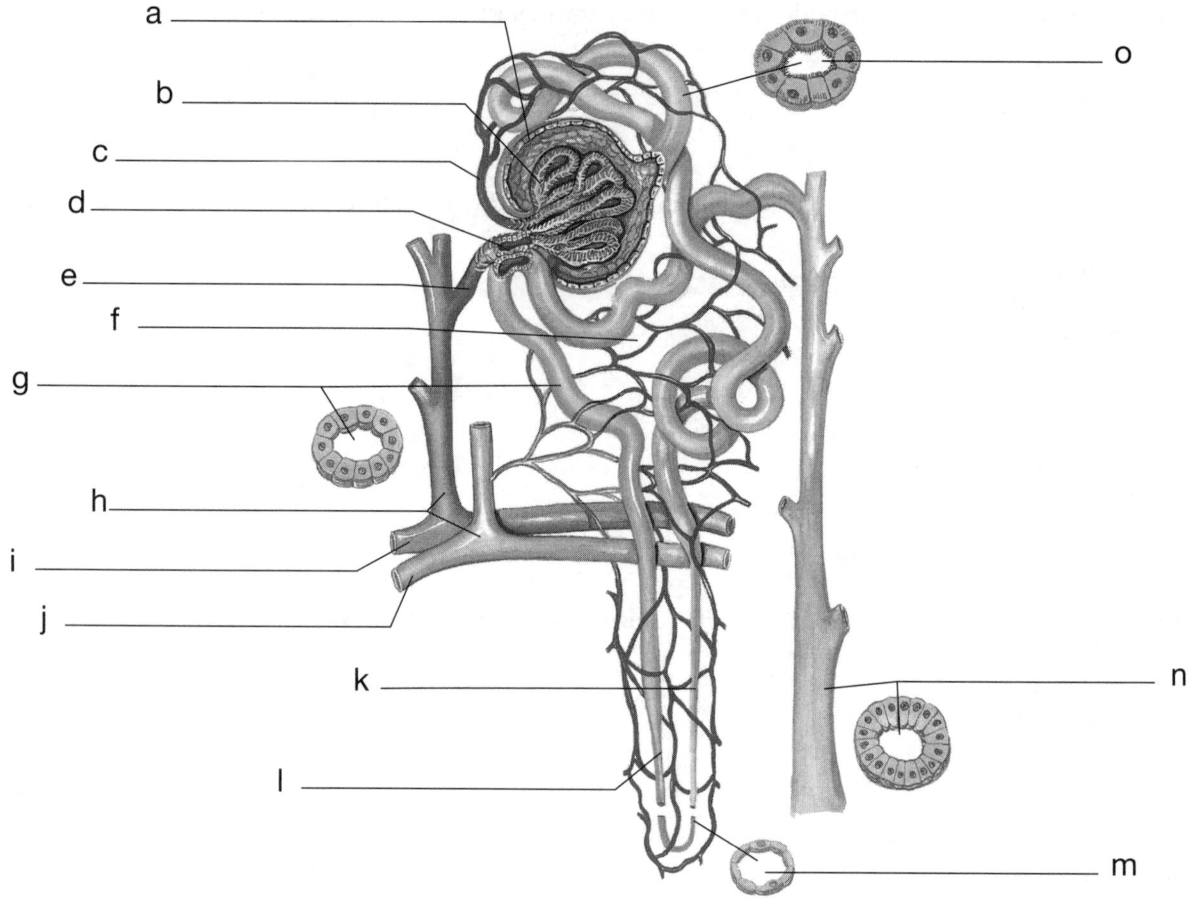

ALTERATIONS

Objective

- Describe the alterations in renal function associated with disorders of the urinary tract.

11. Identify the potential causes of urinary retention. ***(1684)***____

12. How can long-term urinary retention result in urinary incontinence? ***(1684)***________________________

13. During the evaluation of a patient with urinary retention, what objective data should be assessed? ***(1684)***

____

____

14. List potential causes of incontinence. ***(1684)*** _______________

____

____

15. List nursing interventions that may be used in the care of a patient with urinary incontinence. ***(1684)***

____

____

16. Discuss the progression and risk associated with hydronephrosis. ***(1684)*** _______________

____

____

17. What clinical manifestations are associated with hydronephrosis? ***(1693)*** _______________

____

____

18. What risk factors are associated with the development of renal tumors? ***(1693)*** _______________

____

____

19. What tests are used to diagnose renal tumors? ***(1695)*** _______________

____

____

NURSING DIAGNOSES

Objective

- Select nursing diagnoses related to alteration in urinary function.

20. Identify two nursing diagnoses for each of the disorders listed below. ***(1695)***

    a. Urinary tract infection:

    i. ______________________________

    ii. ______________________________

    b. Urinary incontinence:

    i. ______________________________

    ii. ______________________________

    c. Interstitial cystitis:

    i. ______________________________

    ii. ______________________________

    d. Pyelonephritis:

    i. ______________________________

    ii. ______________________________

    e. Hydronephrosis:

    i. ______________________________

    ii. ______________________________

    f. Renal tumors:

    i. ______________________________

    ii. ______________________________

    g. Cancer of the prostate:

    i. ______________________________

    ii. ______________________________

SPECIAL NEEDS

Objective

- Prioritize the special needs of the patient with urinary dysfunction.

21. List three special needs of the patient with urinary dysfunction. ***(1715)***

    a. ______________________________

    b. ______________________________

    c. ______________________________

BODY IMAGE

Objective

- Appraise the changes in body image created when the patient experiences an alteration in urinary function.

22. The patient had an ileal conduit inserted 3 days ago because of cancer of the bladder. List appropriate assessments that the nurse would do to determine if she is having body image changes. ***(1715)***

____

____

KOCK POUCH

Objective

- Prioritize the special needs of the patient with urinary dysfunction.

23. Label each part of the Kock pouch. ***(1715)***

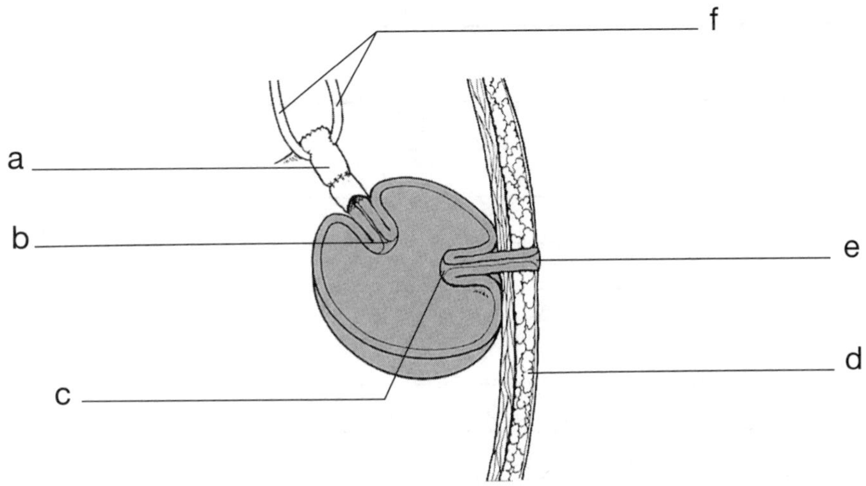

AGING

Objective

- Identify the effects of aging on urinary system function.

24. List seven effects of aging on the urinary system function. ***(1675)***

 a. ______________________________

 b. ______________________________

 c. ______________________________

 d. ______________________________

 e. ______________________________

 f. ______________________________

 g. ______________________________

DRUGS AND NUTRITION

Objective

- Incorporate pharmacotherapeutic and nutritional considerations into the nursing care plan of the patient with a urinary disorder.

25. Develop an index card that would assist the nurse to incorporate pharmacotherapeutic and nutritional considerations into the nursing care plan of the patient with a urinary disorder. ***(1681)***

PATIENT AND FAMILY SUPPORT

Objectives

- Discuss the effect of renal disease on family function.
- Investigate community resources for support for the patient with significant others as they face lifestyle changes from chronic urinary disorders and treatments.
- Address patient concerns in teaching about altered sexuality secondary to urinary disorders and treatments.
- Design culturally sensitive care of the patient with a urinary disorder.

26. Identify urinary disorders and/or treatment plans that may result in the changes to the sexuality of the patient. ***(1682, 1702)***

____

____

27. Identify two nursing diagnoses that may be appropriate for the patient who may be facing changes in sexuality related to a urinary disorder. ***(1682, 1702)***

____

____

28. Discuss the influence of culture on the patient being treated for a urinary disorder. ***(1682, 1702)***________

____

____

29. Identify two conditions of the urinary system that often make community resource referrals beneficial for the patient. ***(1711)***

____

____

MULTIPLE CHOICE

30. Identify the renal disorders associated with an abnormal elevation in creatinine. (Select all that apply) ***(1676)***
    1. Prostatitis
    2. Glomerulonephritis
    3. Pyelonephritis
    4. Acute tubular necrosis
    5. Urinary obstruction

31. A 49-year-old man's prostate-specific antigen (PSA) result is 9.5 ng/mL. Based on the nurse's knowledge, which of the following is understood to be true? (Select all that apply) ***(1676)***
    1. This is within the allowable range.
    2. This may indicate prostate cancer.
    3. This may indicate benign prostatic hypertrophy.
    4. This may indicate prostatitis.

32. During a urodynamic study, cholinergic and anticholinergic medications may be administered to: ***(1678-1679)***
    1. relax the patient.
    2. reduce urine production during the test.
    3. determine their effects on bladder function.
    4. increase uptake of dye administered during the examination.

33. _______________ is an example of a potassium-sparing diuretic. ***(1679)***
    1. Lasix
    2. Diuril
    3. Mannitol
    4. Aldactone

CRITICAL THINKING ACTIVITIES

Activity 1

34. A 42-year-old patient is admitted to the unit with a diagnosis of pyelonephritis. As the nurse collects data, she reveals a history of diabetes mellitus, femur fracture, frequent nosebleeds, and frequent urinary tract infections. ***(1691-1692)***

    a. What does the nurse answer when the patient asks for an explanation of pyelonephritis? __________

    ____

    ____

    b. What signs and symptoms would the nurse anticipate the patient to demonstrate? ______________

    ____

    ____

    c. Discuss the diagnostic tests that may be used in the treatment of the patient, and their probable results.

    ____

    ____

    d. Identify two nursing diagnoses for this patient. ______________________

    ____

    ____

Activity 2

35. A patient reports to the emergency department complaining of severe flank pain, nausea, and vomiting. The patient reports that the pain starts in the flank area and radiates to the groin and inner thigh. A urinalysis reveals the presence of hematuria. ***(1693-1694)***

    a. What medical diagnosis can the nurse anticipate?

    b. What diagnostic tests will be performed to support this diagnosis?

    c. How will the nurse explain these examinations to the patient?

    d. Discuss both the conservative and invasive techniques that may be used in the management of this condition.

    e. After successful treatment, the nurse is preparing the patient for discharge. Discuss long-term preventive management options. Include diet and medications.

Activity 3

36. A 53-year-old man has been diagnosed with acute renal failure. A nurse is assigned to his care. During the course of the shift, he voices many questions and concerns. ***(1706-1707)***

    a. He asks why this has happened to him. How will the nurse respond?

    b. He reports that his doctor told him he is in the oliguric phase. He asks the nurse to clarify this information.

c. What potential clinical manifestations should the nurse be aware of when completing the nursing assessment?

d. The patient's wife asks if she can bring him a hamburger and fries from a local fast-food restaurant. How will the nurse respond?

Activity 4

37. A 22-year-old woman seeks care at the doctor's office complaining of burning with urination, perineal pain, and blood-tinged urine. ***(1687-1689)***

a. What diagnosis does the nurse anticipate?

b. What other signs and symptoms may be present?

c. What tests may be used to provide a definitive diagnosis of the problem?

d. What medical treatments can be anticipated in the management of this patient?

e. The patient asks what other "natural" things she can do to treat her condition. What answer does the nurse give?

Student Name______________________________ Date______________

chapter

51

Care of the Patient with an Endocrine Disorder

Answer Key: Textbook page references are provided as a guide for answering these questions. A complete answer key was provided for your instructor.

GLANDS AND HORMONES

Objectives

- List and describe the endocrine glands and their hormones.
- Explain the action of the hormones on their target organs.

1. Complete the table below by listing the hormones that each gland produces and the action they have on their target organs. ***(1721-1725)***

Endocrine Gland	Hormone	Action on Target Organ
a. Anterior pituitary:		
i.		
ii.		
iii.		
iv.		
v.		
vi.		
b. Posterior pituitary:		
i.		
ii.		

(Continued next page)

Endocrine Gland	Hormone	Action on Target Organ
c. Thyroid:		
i.		
ii.		
iii.		
d. Parathyroid:		
i.		
e. Adrenal cortex:		
i.		
ii.		
iii.		
f. Adrenal medulla:		
i.		
ii.		
g. Pancreas:		
i.		
ii.		
h. Ovaries:		
i.		
ii.		
i. Testes:		
i.		
j. Thymus:		
i.		
k. Pineal:		
i.		

HORMONAL IMBALANCE

Objectives

- Define the negative feedback system.
- Discuss the etiology and pathophysiology, clinical manifestations, assessment, diagnostic tests, medical management, nursing interventions, patient teaching, and prognosis for patients with acromegaly, gigantism, dwarfism, diabetes insipidus, syndrome of inappropriate antidiuretic hormone (SIADH), hyperthyroidism, hypothyroidism, goiter, cancer of the thyroid, hyperparathyroidism, hypoparathyroidism, Cushing's syndrome, and Addison's disease.
- Differentiate between the clinical manifestations of Cushing's syndrome and those of Addison's disease.

Activity 1

2. Complete the chart below. ***(1725-1744)***

Disease	Cause	Clinical Manifestations	Treatment
a. Acromegaly			
b. Gigantism			
c. Dwarfism			
d. Diabetes insipidus			
e. Syndrome of inappropriate antidiuretic hormone			
f. Hyper-thyroidism			

(Continued next page)

Disease	Cause	Clinical Manifestations	Treatment
g. Hypo-thyroidism			
h. Goiter			
i. Hyperpara-thyroidism			
j. Hypopara-thyroidism			
k. Cushing's syndrome			
l. Addison's disease			

Activity 2

3. List the tests that may be used to diagnose acromegaly. ***(1725)***____________________________

____

____

4. Discuss why the patient with acromegaly may experience visual disturbances. ***(1725)*** ______________

____

____

5. List three nursing interventions for the care of a patient with acromegaly. ***(1725-1727)***

   a. ______

   b. ______

   c. ______

6. Identify two nursing diagnoses applicable for the patient with gigantism. ***(1727)***

   a. ______

   b. ______

7. How do acromegaly and gigantism differ? ***(1725-1727)*** ______

8. Discuss the diagnostic tests and the typical results for the patient with SIADH. ***(1729-1730)*** ______

9. Explain why the patient with SIADH does not experience peripheral edema. ***(1730-1731)*** ______

10. Review the dietary management for the patient with hyperthyroidism. ***(1733-1734)*** ______

11. Discuss the medical management of a patient diagnosed with hypothyroidism. ***(1732-1733)*** ______

12. What is the long-term prognosis for a patient with hypothyroidism? ***(1734)*** ______

13. Explain the negative feedback used by the endocrine system. ***(1721)*** ______________________________

____

____

14. What is the relationship between the hypothalamus and the pituitary gland? ***(1721)***______________

____

____

STRUCTURE OF THE ADRENAL GLANDS

Objective

- List and describe the endocrine glands and their hormones.

15. Label the parts of the adrenal gland. ***(1724)***

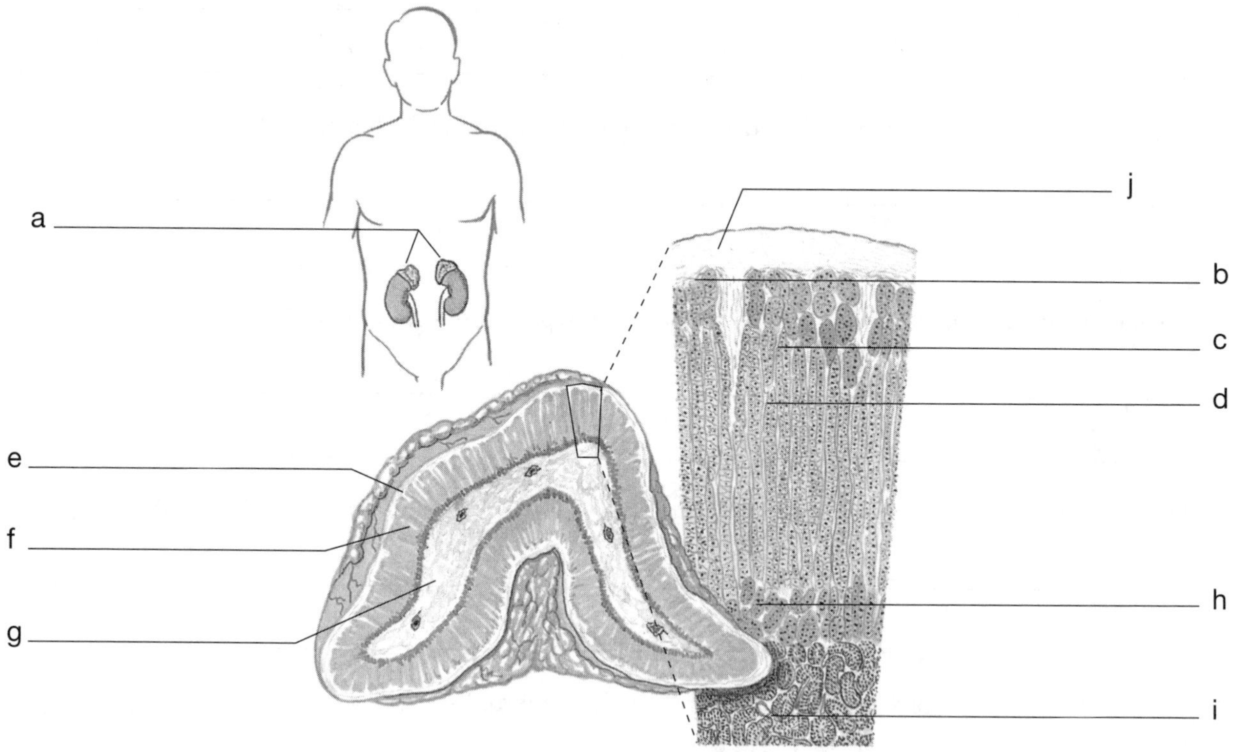

THYROID DISORDERS

Objectives

- List four tests used in the diagnosis of hyperthyroidism.
- Explain how to test for Chvostek's sign, Trousseau's sign, and carpopedal spasms.
- List two significant complications that may occur after thyroidectomy.
- Discuss the medications commonly used to treat hyperthyroidism and hypothyroidism.

Activity 1

16. When reviewing the laboratory results for a patient diagnosed with hyperthyroidism, which of the following may be anticipated? (Select all that apply) ***(1731-1732)***
    1. Elevation in thyroid-stimulating hormone (TSH) levels
    2. Decrease in TSH levels
    3. Radioactive iodine reuptake level of 30%
    4. Radioactive iodine reuptake level of 50%
    5. Decrease in free thyroxine (T_4) levels

17. The nurse is caring for a patient being treated for hyperthyroidism. The patient questions when she will likely begin to feel improvement. What response by the nurse is most correct? ***(1733-1734)***
    1. Within 2–4 weeks
    2. Within 4–6 weeks
    3. Within 6–8 weeks
    4. Within 3 months

18. When caring for a patient suspected of having complications as a result of removal of the thyroid gland, the nurse recognizes the need to assess for the presence of Trousseau's sign by inflating the sphygmomanometer cuff for a period of ____________. ***(1734)***
    1. 30 seconds
    2. 60 seconds
    3. 120 seconds
    4. 180 seconds

19. When monitoring the postoperative patient for the onset of a thyroid crisis, the nurse must be aware that the greatest risk of onset is within: ***(1733-1734)***
    1. 4 hours.
    2. 8 hours.
    3. 12 hours.
    4. 24 hours.

20. The postoperative patient should be monitored for the release of PTH in the blood stream; the patient with which of the following manifestations should be immediately reported? ***(1732)***
    1. Fatigue
    2. Nausea
    3. Tingling around the mouth
    4. Feelings of facial coolness

Activity 2

21. List two complications that may result after a thyroidectomy. ***(1733-1734)***

    a. ____________________

    b. ____________________

22. What medications may be prescribed to manage hypothyroidism? ***(1732)*** ____________________

    ____

    ____

ADRENAL DISORDERS

Objective

- Differentiate between the clinical manifestations of Cushing's syndrome and Addison's disease.

23. Obtain an index card. Label one side of the card "Cushing's Syndrome" and the other side "Addison's disease." On each side, write the signs and symptoms consistent with the relevant disorder. ***(1740-1744)***

DIABETES MELLITUS

Objective

- Describe the pathophysiology, clinical manifestations, assessment, diagnostic tests, medical management, nursing interventions, patient teaching, and prognosis for the patient with diabetes mellitus.

24. List the pathophysiology and the clinical manifestations of type 1 and type 2 diabetes mellitus. ***(1747)***

Type of Diabetes	Pathophysiology	Manifestations
a. Type I		
b. Type II		

INSULIN

Objectives

- Discuss the various types of insulin and their characteristics.
- Describe the proper way to draw up and administer insulin.
- Discuss the various classes of oral hypoglycemic medications to treat type 2 diabetes mellitus.
- Discuss how oral agents work to improve the mechanisms by which insulin and glucose are produced and used by the body.
- Discuss the two new subcutaneous insulin-enhancing drugs, exenatide (Byetta) and pramlintide (Symlin), and their mechanisms of action.

Activity 1

25. Complete the table below. ***(1750-1752)***

Insulin	Classification	Onset	Peak	Duration
a. Lispro (Humalog)				
b. Regular				
c. NPH or Lente				
d. Ultralente				
e. Lantus				

Activity 2

26. Where does most commercially used insulin come from? ***(1750)***

27. Through what route is insulin administered? ***(1750)***

28. Which type of insulin can be administered by intravenous (IV) route in cases of emergency? ***(1752)***

29. When planning to administer regular insulin, how long before a meal should it be administered? ***(1752-1753)***

30. What is the subcutaneous pocket? ***(1752-1753)***

31. What gauge of needle is used to administer insulin? ***(1753)***

32. How should insulin be stored? ***(1753)***

33. What body locations may be used for insulin administration? ***(1755)***

34. What must be present for oral hypoglycemic medications to be effective? ***(1756)***

35. What is the mode of action for sulfonylureas? ***(1756)*** ______________________________

____

____

36. Why are first-generation sulfonylureas such as Orinase and Tolinase rarely used today? ***(1756-1757)***

____

____

37. What is the mode of action for alpha-glucosidase inhibitors? ***(1756)*** ______________________________

____

____

38. Which classification of oral hypoglycemic agents works to increase the sensitivity at insulin receptor sites? ***(1757)***

____

____

39. How does pramlintide (Symlin) work in the management of diabetes mellitus? ***(1757)*** ______________________________

____

____

40. In what type of diabetes can exenatide (Byetta) be used? ***(1757)*** ______________________________

____

____

DIABETES MANAGEMENT

Objectives

- Explain the roles of nutrition, exercise, and medication in the control of diabetes mellitus.
- List five nursing interventions that foster self-care in the activities of daily living of the patient with diabetes mellitus.

41. Develop an index card that will prompt the nurse during patient teaching for the patient with diabetes mellitus. Include how nutrition, exercise, and medication will help control the disorder. List four nursing interventions that will foster self-care in the activities of daily living for this patient. ***(1745-1750)***

SIGNS OF PROBLEMS

Objectives

- Differentiate between the signs and symptoms of diabetic ketoacidosis, hyperglycemic hyperosmolar nonketotic coma, and hypoglycemic reaction.
- Differentiate between the signs and symptoms of hyperglycemia and hypoglycemia.

Activity 1

42. List the signs and symptoms of diabetic ketoacidosis, hyperglycemic reactions, hyperglycemic hyperosmolar nonketotic coma, and hypoglycemic reactions. ***(1747)***

Problem	Signs and Symptoms
a. Diabetic ketoacidosis	
b. Hyperglycemic reactions	
c. Hyperglycemic hyperosmolar nonketotic coma	
d. Hypoglycemic reactions	

Activity 2

43. Complete the table below. ***(1747, 1754)***

Reaction	Signs and Symptoms	Triggers	Management
Hypoglycemia			
Hyperglycemia			

COMPLICATIONS OF DIABETES

Objective

- Discuss the acute and long-term complications of diabetes mellitus.

44. Identify three acute complications of diabetes mellitus. ***(1759-1762)***

 a. ______________________________

 b. ______________________________

 c. ______________________________

45. What type of insulin administration is indicated in the management of hyperglycemic reaction? ***(1747)***

____

____

46. Why are patients with diabetes mellitus at a higher risk for the development of infection? ***(1750)*** ______

____

____

47. What chronic complications are associated with diabetes mellitus? ***(1762-1764)*** ______________

____

____

MULTIPLE CHOICE

48. Cortisol is responsible for what bodily function? ***(1722)***
    1. The regulation of sodium levels
    2. The regulation of potassium levels
    3. The provision of extra energy reserves during stress
    4. The conservation of glucagon

49. Urine excreted by a patient with diabetes insipidus will exhibit which of the following characteristics? ***(1728)***
    1. Dilute, with a specific gravity of 1.005–1.030 g/mL
    2. Dilute, with a specific gravity of 1.001–1.005 g/mL
    3. Concentrated, with a specific gravity of 1.005–1.030 g/mL
    4. Concentrated, with a specific gravity of 1.001–1.005 g/mL

50. Which of the following nursing interventions should be employed for a patient with diabetes insipidus? (Select all that apply) ***(1729)***
    1. Assessment of skin turgor
    2. Daily weight measurement
    3. Fluid restriction
    4. Monitor intake and output
    5. Encouraging intake of fluids containing caffeine

51. A patient asks what causes his unsightly goiter. Based on the nurse's knowledge, the nurse responds that: ***(1736)***
    1. the elevated levels of triiodothyronine (T_3) result in an inability of the body to respond to changing iodine levels.
    2. high levels of serum iodine cause hyperplasia.
    3. the increasing formation of thyroglobulin accumulates in the thyroid follicles.
    4. the body is attempting to compensate for reduced levels of T_5.

CRITICAL THINKING ACTIVITIES

Activity 1

52. A 19-year-old woman seeks care because of complaints of excessive thirst, hunger, and fatigue. She reports she has not been able to sleep all night for the past few weeks because of needing to go to the bathroom. ***(1728-1729)***

    a. Based on the nurse's knowledge, what medical diagnosis is anticipated? ____________________

    ____

    ____

    ____

    ____

b. What other clinical manifestations may occur in this patient? ______________________________

c. What are topics that should be discussed during the patient's education? ______________________________

d. The patient states she works with someone who "just has to take a pill" to control his diabetes. She asks if she will be able to do the same. How will the nurse respond?

e. Upon realizing this condition is not curable, the patient asks what long-term complications are associated with diabetes. How will the nurse respond to this inquiry?

Activity 2

53. The parents of a 6-year-old boy report to the doctor with concerns about their son's height. They report that he is the smallest child in the school. The parents are of normal stature. Assessment reveals that the child is indeed significantly small for his age. ***(1728)***

a. What diagnostic tests can be anticipated? ______________________________

b. Examinations confirm a diagnosis of dwarfism. The parents are tearful. They ask what caused this to happen. How will the nurse respond?

c. What other clinical manifestations may be exhibited by the child?

d. Another question voiced by the parents concern future implications for their child. How will the nurse respond?

e. What medical treatment will be prescribed for this patient?

Student Name______________________________ Date______________

chapter **52**

Care of the Patient with a Reproductive Disorder

Answer Key: Textbook page references are provided as a guide for answering these questions. A complete answer key was provided for your instructor.

FUNCTIONS

Objective

- List and describe the functions of the organs of the male and female reproductive tracts.

1. Complete the table below by filling in the functions of the organs of the male and female reproductive tracts. ***(1770-1773)***

Organ	Function
a. Male Reproductive Tract	
i. Testes	
ii. Epididymis	
iii. Ductus deferens (vas deferens)	
iv. Ejaculatory duct and urethra	
v. Accessory glands	
• Seminal vesicles	
• Prostate gland	
• Cowper's gland	
vi. Urethra and penis	

(Continued next page)

Organ	Function
b. Female Reproductive Tract	
i. Ovaries	
ii. Fallopian tubes (oviducts)	
iii. Uterus	
iv. Vagina	
v. External genitalia	
vi. Accessory glands	
vii. Mammary glands	

SEXUALITY

Objective

- Discuss the impact of illness on the patient's sexuality.

2. Develop an index card listing how illness may affect a patient's sexuality. ***(1774-1775, 1777)***

MENSTRUAL DISTURBANCES

Objectives

- Discuss menstruation and the hormones necessary for a complete menstrual cycle.
- List nursing interventions for patients with menstrual disturbances.

3. The nurse is preparing to discuss menstruation with a group of preteen girls. In preparation for the discussion, list on a note card information that has to be included concerning the following elements. *(1782)*

   a. At what age do girls typically begin menstruation? __________

   b. Approximately how much blood is lost during the average menstrual period? __________

   c. List the hormones involved in the menstrual cycle. __________

4. The nurse is caring for a 20-year-old patient who reports that her health care provider has diagnosed her condition as secondary dysmenorrhea. She asks what this means and requests clarification between primary dysmenorrhea and secondary dysmenorrhea. How should the nurse respond? *(1782)*

5. The patient in the above scenario asks what causes dysmenorrhea. What should the nurse tell her? *(1783)*

6. What are the symptoms of dysmenorrhea? *(1783)* __________

7. Identify two nursing diagnoses that would be applicable to the patient with dysmenorrhea. *(1783)*

8. What treatment options are available to a patient suffering from dysmenorrhea? ***(1783)***_______________

9. What diagnostic tests would be considered for a patient diagnosed with menorrhagia? ***(1783)***_______________

10. What elements should be incorporated into the interview and the plan of care for a patient experiencing increased vaginal bleeding? ***(1783)***

11. Discuss premenstrual syndrome (PMS). Include the population affected, the causes, the manifestations, and the treatment. ***(1786)***

Activity 1

12. Next to each disturbance of menstruation, list appropriate nursing interventions. ***(1783-1784)***

Disturbances	Nursing Interventions
a. Amenorrhea	
b. Dysmenorrhea	
c. Abnormal uterine bleeding	
i. Menorrhagia	
ii. Metrorrhagia	

SECTIONAL VIEW OF THE UTERUS

Objective

- List and describe the functions of the organs of the male and female reproductive tracts.

13. Label the parts of the female reproductive organs. ***(1772)***

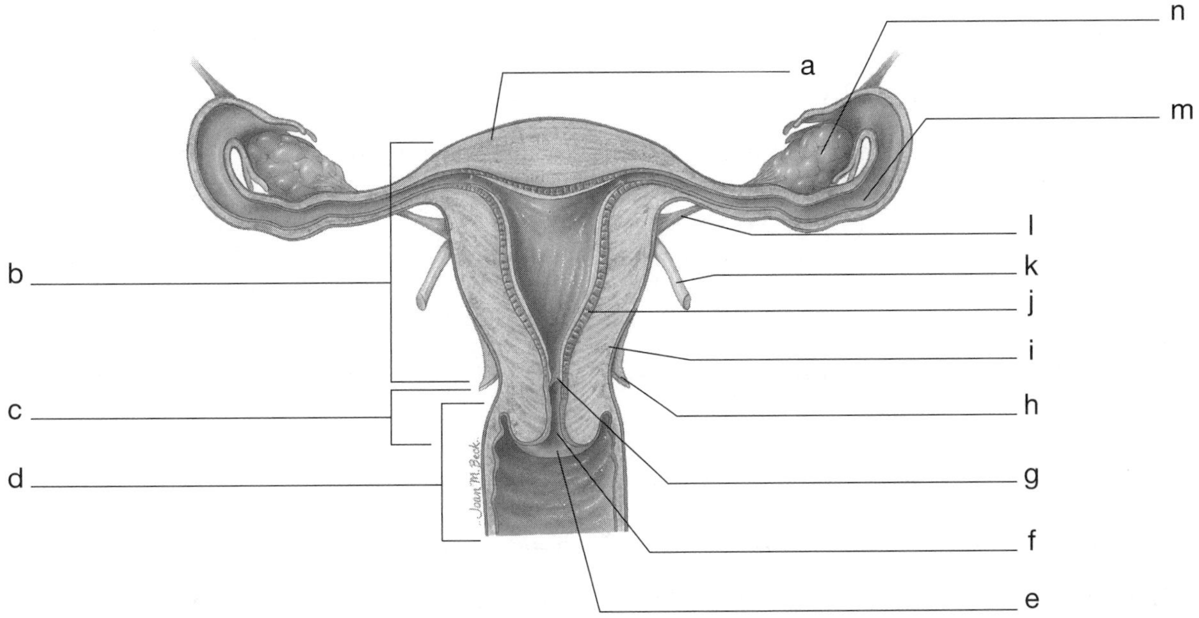

DIAGNOSTIC STUDIES

Objective

- Discuss nursing interventions for the patient undergoing diagnostic studies related to the reproductive system.

14. The nurse is caring for a patient who is undergoing a culdoscopy. What care should be provided to the patient after the procedure? ***(1778)***

____

____

15. The nurse is working on the medical-surgical unit and is assigned to care for a patient who has had a laparoscopic examination. After the procedure, the patient questions the presence of shoulder pain. What information can be provided to the patient concerning this manifestation? ***(1778)***

____

____

16. A patient has been scheduled for a conization to assess cervical tissue. What care will be necessary to provide to the patient after the procedure? Will the patient be hospitalized overnight? ***(1780)***

____

____

17. List the indications for a hysterosalpingogram. ***(1780)*** ____________________________________

____

____

18. A pelvic ultrasound has been ordered for a patient. What information concerning preparation and the test procedure is necessary to provide to the patient? ***(1781)***

____

____

19. A patient has had a CA-125 performed. The CA-125 level is elevated. What does an elevation in the CA-125 level indicate? ***(1781)***

____

____

20. The nurse is preparing to discharge a patient to home after a testicular biopsy. What information can be provided to the patient to promote comfort? ***(1781)***

____

____

21. A couple reporting difficulty conceiving a child has reported to the physician's office for evaluation. The physician has ordered a semen analysis. Discuss options available for the collection of the specimen. ***(1781)***

____

____

22. The physician has ordered a cystoscopy. What information concerning the procedure may be provided to the patient? ***(1781)***

____

____

PAP SMEAR

Objective

- Discuss the importance of the Papanicolaou smear test in early detection of cervical cancer and mammography as a screening procedure for breast cancer.

23. The patient, a teenager, is in for her first Papanicolaou (Pap) smear. How does the nurse explain to her what the American Cancer Society recommends for all women about early detection of cervical cancer and why? ***(1778)***

____

____

24. Discuss what a Pap smear entails. ***(1778)*** ____

____

____

25. The patient, age 38, asks the nurse to explain the guidelines for breast self-examination and mammogram. How will the nurse best respond? ***(1808-1809)***

____

____

INFECTIONS OF THE FEMALE REPRODUCTIVE TRACT

Objective

- Discuss etiology, pathophysiology, clinical manifestations, assessment, diagnostic tests, medical management, nursing interventions, patient teaching, and prognosis for infections of the female reproductive tract.

26. Identify the most common organisms that cause infections of the female reproductive tract. ***(1792)***

____

____

27. Identify ways by which infectious agents are potentially introduced into the reproductive tract. ***(1792-1793)***

____

____

28. When is the best time of day to administer a vaginal suppository, and why? ***(1793)*** ____________________

____

____

29. Discuss patient teaching that must accompany the use of medications to treat vaginal infections. ***(1793)***

____

____

PELVIC INFLAMMATORY DISEASE

Objective

- Discuss four important points to be addressed in discharge planning for the patient with pelvic inflammatory disease (PID).

30. Develop a short checklist of four important points to include in discharge planning for the patient with PID. ***(1794)***

 a. ____

 b. ____

 c. ____

 d. ____

ENDOMETRIOSIS

Objective

- List four nursing diagnoses pertinent to the patient with endometriosis.

31. Identify four nursing diagnoses pertinent to the patient who has endometriosis. ***(1796)***

 a. ____

 b. ____

 c. ____

 d. ____

FISTULA

Objective

- Identify the clinical manifestations of a vaginal fistula.

32. List the clinical manifestations for a patient with a vagina fistula. *(1797)* ______________________________

____

____

SURGERY

Objective

- Describe the preoperative and postoperative nursing interventions for the patient requiring major surgery of the female reproductive system.

33. Develop an index card to use to prompt the nurse during care of the patient who requires major surgery of the female reproductive system. *(1798)*

CYSTOCELE AND RECTOCELE

Objective

- Describe the common problems of cystocele and rectocele, and the related medical management and nursing interventions.

34. Fill in the chain of events below for the patient with a cystocele or rectocele. ***(1798)***

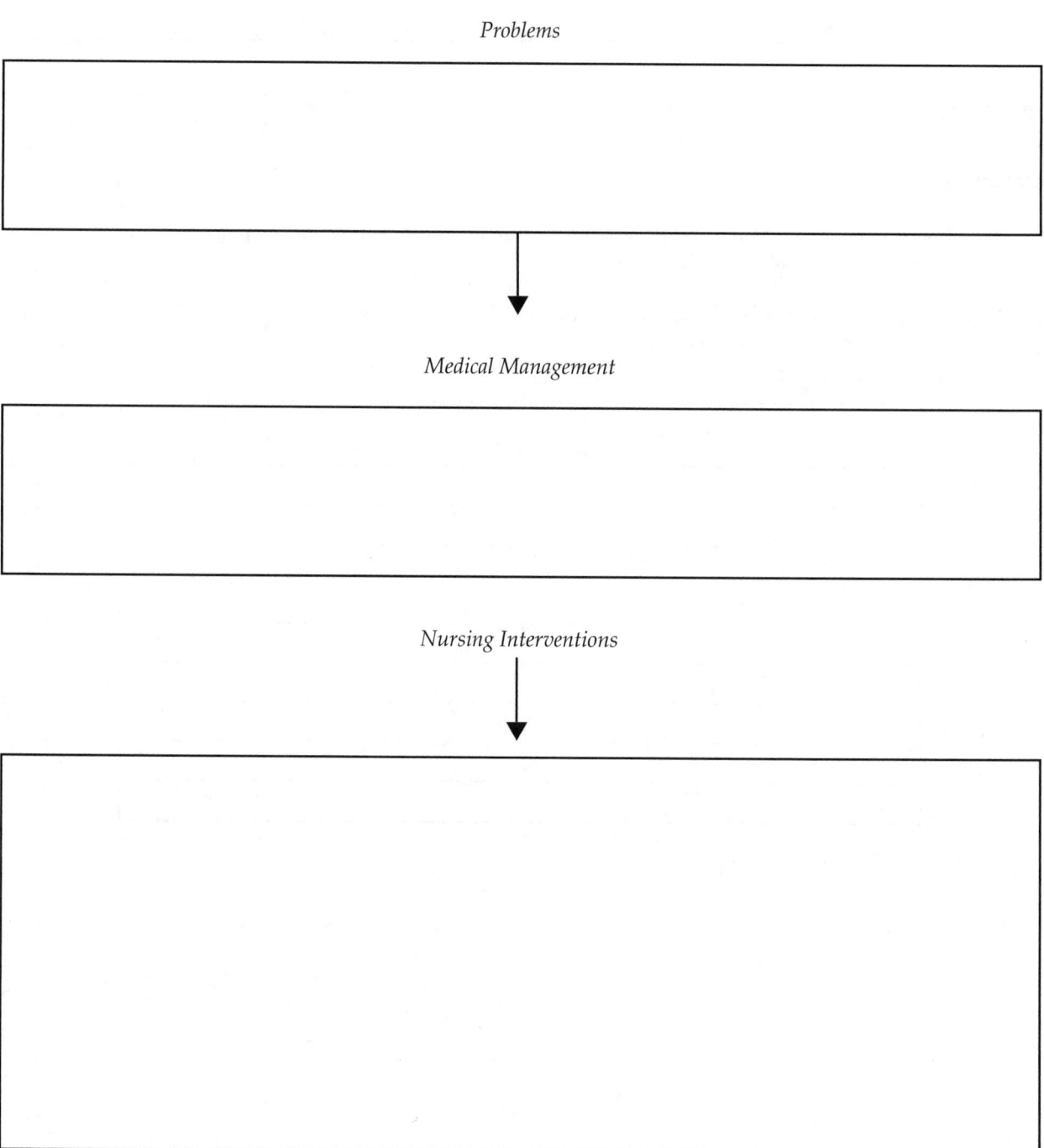

Problems

Medical Management

Nursing Interventions

CANCER OF THE REPRODUCTIVE SYSTEM

Objectives

- Discuss the etiology and pathophysiology, clinical manifestations, assessment, diagnostic tests, medical management, nursing interventions, patient teaching, and prognosis for cancers of the reproductive system.
- Identify four nursing diagnoses pertinent to ovarian cancer.

35. What populations are at the greatest risk for the development of cervical cancer? ***(1801)*** ______________

____

____

36. Discuss the progression of symptoms associated with cervical cancer. ***(1802)*** ______________

____

____

37. What population is most often affected by cancer of the endometrium? ***(1803)*** ______________

____

____

38. Discuss the treatment options available for the patient diagnosed with cancer of the endometrium. ***(1802)***

____

____

39. Identify four nursing diagnoses that are potentially applicable when assisting the registered nurse with the planning of care for a patient diagnosed with ovarian cancer. ***(1803)***

    a. ____

    b. ____

    c. ____

    d. ____

40. Compare and contrast the survival rate for patients diagnosed with cervical, ovarian, and endometrial cancer. ***(1801-1803)***

Cancer Type	General Prognosis	Rate of Growth	5-year Survival Rate
Cervical			
Endometrial			
Ovarian			

BREAST SELF-EXAMINATION

Objective

- Describe six important points to emphasize in teaching breast self-examination.

41. Develop an index card highlighting the important teaching points to include when teaching breast self-examination. ***(1808-1809)***

TREATING BREAST CANCER

Objectives

- Describe four surgical approaches for cancer of the breast.
- Discuss adjuvant therapies for breast cancer.

42. How do the simple mastectomy and the modified radical mastectomy differ? ***(1812)*** ______

43. List an advantage to a lumpectomy to manage breast cancer. *(1812)* ______________________________

____

____

44. List a disadvantage of a lumpectomy to manage breast cancer. *(1812)* ______________________________

____

____

45. Are there differences in survival rates between the lumpectomy with radiation and the modified radical mastectomy? *(1812)*

____

____

Multiple Choice

46. Radiation has been scheduled for a patient diagnosed with breast cancer. When developing the plan of care, when should the nurse anticipate radiation will take place? *(1812)*
    1. Radiation will begin within 72 hours after surgery.
    2. Radiation will begin within 2 weeks after surgery.
    3. Radiation will begin 3 to 4 weeks after surgery.
    4. Radiation will begin 4 to 6 weeks after surgery.

47. An advantage of brachytherapy over traditional radiation therapy is: *(1812)*
    1. brachytherapy is less expensive.
    2. the course of brachytherapy will likely take less time to complete.
    3. brachytherapy is associated with fewer side effects.
    4. brachytherapy uses a lower dosage of radiation.

48. Anemia is a side effect associated with chemotherapy. Which of the following medications may be ordered to manage this complication? *(1812)*
    1. Epoetin alfa (Procrit)
    2. Prochlorperazine (Compazine)
    3. RhoGAM
    4. Ondansetron (Zofran)

49. Tamoxifen has been ordered to manage a patient diagnosed with breast cancer. Which of the following is associated with tamoxifen? Select all that apply. *(1812)*
    1. Tamoxifen inhibits the growth effects of estrogen.
    2. Tamoxifen use is limited to individuals who are diagnosed as being in mid- to late-stage breast cancer.
    3. Tamoxifen is used to manage recurrent breast cancer.
    4. Tamoxifen is used to prevent the development of breast cancer in high-risk individuals.

50. A bone marrow transplant is planned for a patient with breast cancer. Which of the statements concerning this treatment is correct? ***(1812)***
    1. Radiation is administered before the transplant to reduce the cancerous growth.
    2. Bone marrow may be obtained from donors or from the actual patient.
    3. Chemotherapy administration reduces the likelihood of success for the bone marrow transplant.
    4. Plasmapheresis is performed on the donor stem cells before transplantation.

POSTOPERATIVE CARE

Objectives

- Discuss nursing interventions for the patient who has had a modified radical mastectomy.
- List several discharge planning instructions for the patient who has undergone a modified radical mastectomy.

Activity 1

51. Develop an index card listing five priority instructions for the patient who has had a modified radical mastectomy. ***(1813-1817)***

52. The nurse is assigned to care for a patient who has had a modified radical mastectomy. What position will be most therapeutic for this patient? ***(1813-1817)***

53. Identify two priority nursing diagnoses during the postoperative period after a modified radical mastectomy. ***(1813-1817)***

54. What can reduce the risk of lymphedema in the patient who has had a mastectomy? ***(1815)*** ____________

____

____

55. What treatments may be prescribed to manage prolonged edema in the surgical arm? ***(1815)*** ____________

____

____

56. Discuss the benefit of isometric exercises for the patient who has had a mastectomy. ***(1815)*** ____________

____

____

57. The spouse of a mastectomy patient voices concerns about the emotional state of his wife. He asks what can be expected in the coming months as she meets the challenges associated with her condition. What information can be provided? ***(1816)***

____

____

HYDROCELE AND VARICOCELE

Objective

- Distinguish between hydrocele and varicocele.

58. Complete the chart below. ***(1821)***

	Hydrocele	Varicocele
a. Pathophysiology		
b. Clinical manifestations		
c. Population at greatest risk		
d. Management		

TESTICULAR SELF-EXAMINATION

Objective

- Discuss the importance of monthly testicular self-examination beginning at 15 years of age.

59. The nurse has a 16-year-old male patient in the office for his annual examination. How would the nurse explain to him the need that he do a monthly testicular self-examination? ***(1821-1822)***

____

____

SEXUALLY TRANSMITTED INFECTIONS

Objective

- Discuss patient education related to prevention of sexually transmitted infections.

60. What actions can be taken to help reduce the risk of contracting a sexually transmitted oropharyngeal infection? ***(1822-1823)***

____

____

61. What types of lubricants can be used with condoms? ***(1822-1823)*** ____________________

____

____

62. Discuss the relationship between douching and contracting sexually transmitted infections. ***(1822-1823)***

____

____

63. List four actions a sexually active individual can take to help prevent contracting a sexually transmitted infection. ***(1822-1823)***

a. ____

b. ____

c. ____

d. ____

64. What special care should be given to individuals who are sexually active with more than one partner? ***(1822-1823)***

____

____

MULTIPLE CHOICE

65. A 22-year-old woman who has a history of cervical dysplasia is scheduled for a procedure to remove a small eroded area on her cervix. The procedure that will be performed will be a: ***(1783)***
    1. conization.
    2. coloscopy.
    3. culdoscopy.
    4. Pap smear.

66. When teaching a patient about the rationale for prescribing oral contraceptives to treat dysmenorrhea, the nurse's statement is based on the understanding that oral contraceptives will: ***(1783-1784)***
    1. suppress ovulation by increasing prostaglandin levels.
    2. suppress ovulation by increasing estrogen levels.
    3. suppress ovulation by inhibiting prostaglandin levels.
    4. promote ovulation by increasing estrogen levels.

67. What is the treatment of choice for primary syphilis? ***(1825)***
    1. Penicillin
    2. Acyclovir
    3. Valtrex
    4. Tetracycline

68. A 22-year-old man comes to the clinic with complaints of urethritis, dysuria, and purulent penile discharge. What medical diagnosis should be anticipated? ***(1825)***
    1. Genital herpes
    2. Syphilis
    3. Chlamydia
    4. Gonorrhea

CRITICAL THINKING ACTIVITIES

Activity 1

69. A 20-year-old patient reports to the family planning clinic complaining of painful, erythematous vesicles on her genitals. She is scared and voices many questions and concerns about her condition. ***(1823)***

    a. Based on the nurse's knowledge, what is anticipated to be her medical diagnosis? ______________

    ____

    ____

b. After being advised of her condition, the patient becomes tearful and asks what will be done to cure her. How should the nurse respond to her requests?

c. What treatment options and interventions are available to the patient?

d. What should be included in her patient education?

Activity 2

70. A 37-year-old patient reports to the office. She states her periods became irregular 4 or 5 months ago. She expresses questions and concerns about her condition. ***(1774)***

a. Given her age, could this condition be menopause?

b. Is the condition permanent?

c. Is contraception still necessary? ______________________________

d. What other signs and symptoms could she expect to experience? ______________________________

e. How will the condition be evaluated and diagnosed? ______________________________

Student Name________________________________ Date________________

Care of the Patient with a Visual or Auditory Disorder

chapter
53

Answer Key: Textbook page references are provided as a guide for answering these questions. A complete answer key was provided for your instructor.

SENSORY ORGANS

Objectives

- List the major sense organs and discuss their anatomical position.
- List the parts of the eye and define the function of each part.
- List the three divisions of the ear and discuss the function of each.

1. Next to each sensory organ, list its anatomical position and function. ***(1838-1839)***

Sensory Organ	Anatomical Position	Function
a. Eye		
i. Lacrimal apparatus		
ii. Conjunctiva		
iii. Extrinsic eye muscles		
iv. Sclera		
v. Cornea		
vi. Choroid		
vii. Pupil		
viii. Retina		
ix. Rods and cones		
x. Crystalline lens		

(Continued next page)

Sensory Organ	Anatomical Position	Function
xi. Aqueous humor		
xii. Vitreous humor		
b. Ear, External		
i. Tympanic membrane		
ii. Ceruminous glands		
c. Ear, Middle		
i. Eustachian tube		
ii. Ossicles		
d. Ear, Inner		
i. Labyrinth		
• Semicircular canal		
• Vestibule		
• Cochlea		
ii. Cochlear nerve		
iii. Vestibular nerve		

THE PHYSIOLOGY OF SIGHT AND VISION

Objective

- Describe the physiologic processes involved in normal vision and hearing.

Activity 1

2. Label the following events in the physiologic process of vision in sequence from 1 to 7. ***(1840)***

   ______ The light is transmitted to the cerebral cortex of the brain.

   ______ The light passes through the pupil.

______ The light passes arrives at the rods and the cones of the retina.

______ The light passes through the vitreous humor.

______ The light passes through the cornea.

______ The light passes through the aqueous humor.

______ The light passes through the crystalline lens.

Activity 2

3. The organ of hearing is the ______________. ***(1841)***

4. The message is carried to the brain by the eighth cranial nerve, called the ______________. ***(1841)***

5. The sensory hair cells of the ear are referred to as the ______________. ***(1841)***

6. The ______________ is the inner ear and is composed of a series of sacs and tubes containing fluids that carry the sound waves through the inner ear system. ***(1841)***

7. The ______________, the ______________, and the ______________ are three small bones in the middle hear that carry sound waves from the external ear to the inner ear. ***(1841)***

8. Sound vibrations are transmitted to the inner ear by the ______________. ***(1841)***

AGING

Objectives

- Describe two changes in the sensory system that occur as a result of the normal aging process.
- Describe age-related changes in the visual and auditory systems and differences in assessment findings.

Activity

9. Develop a patient teaching tool that highlights the changes in the sensory system that occur in connection with the normal aging process. ***(1842)***

____

____

____

____

____

DIAGNOSTIC STUDIES

Objective

- Describe the purpose, significance of results, and nursing responsibilities related to diagnostic studies of the visual and auditory systems.

10. Complete the following table of diagnostic studies by including the purpose, the significance of the abnormal results, and the nursing interventions for each. ***(1844-1845)***

Diagnostic Study	Purpose	Abnormal Results' Significance	Nursing Interventions
a. Snellen test			
b. Color vision test			
c. Refraction test			
d. Ophthalmoscopy			
e. Tonometry			
f. Amsler grid test			
g. Schirmer's tear test			
h. Otoscopy			
i. Tuning fork test			
j. Audiometry			
k. Vestibular testing			

LACRIMAL APPARATUS

Objective

- List the major sense organs and discuss their anatomical position.

11. Identify each part of the lacrimal apparatus. ***(1838)***

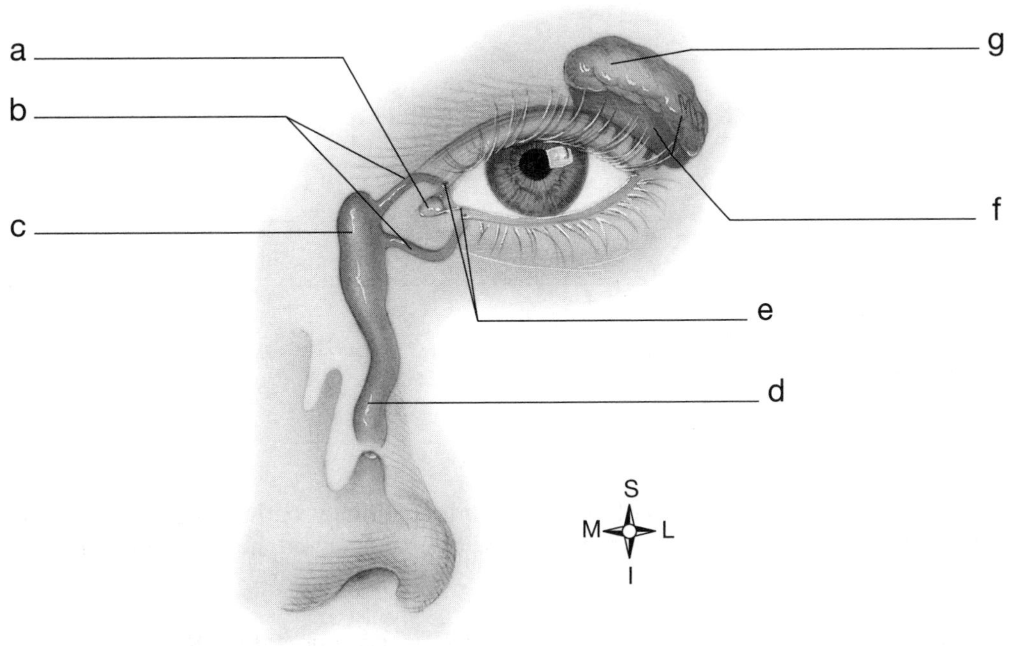

REFRACTORY EYE DISORDERS

Objective

- Discuss the refractory errors of astigmatism, strabismus, myopia, and hyperopia, including etiology, pathology, clinical manifestations, assessment, diagnostic tests, medical management, nursing interventions, and patient teaching.

12. What are the key differences between myopia and hyperopia? ***(1847-1848)***____________________

____

____

13. What causes astigmatism? ***(1847-1848)*** ______________________________

____

____

14. Identify the condition in which the eyeball position is not symmetrical. ***(1847)***______________________

____

____

15. A patient has reported to the health care provider with a reported inability to see objects at a distance. Diagnostic testing is planned. What tests can be anticipated? ***(1847)***

____

____

16. The health care provider has recommended Intacs to a patient. What are they? What conditions may be managed with their use? ***(1848)***

____

____

INFLAMMATORY EYE DISORDERS

Objective

- Describe inflammatory conditions of the eye including etiology, pathophysiology, clinical manifestations, assessment, diagnostic tests, medical management, nursing interventions, patient teaching, and prognosis.

17. What is the most common mode of transmission of bacterial conjunctivitis? ***(1850)***__________________

____

____

18. Identify the most common causative agents of bacterial conjunctivitis. ***(1850)*** ______________________

____

____

19. List the signs and symptoms of conjunctivitis. ***(1850)***______________________________________

____

____

20. How is conjunctivitis diagnosed? ***(1850)***____

____

____

21. How do a hordeolum and a chalazion differ? ***(1849)*** ______________________________

____

____

22. A patient reports dry, scaling eyelid. He also reports tearing and photophobia. What inflammatory condition of the eye manifests with these signs and symptoms? ***(1849)***

____

____

23. Discuss the management and treatment of a cyst. ***(1849-1850)*** ______________________________

____

____

24. When caring for a patient with an infectious or inflammatory process affecting the eye or lids, what should be a primary objective of care? ***(1849-1850)***

____

____

25. What should be included in the teaching plan for the patient experiencing an inflammatory condition of the eyes? ***(1850)***

____

____

26. Viruses of what two body systems may become secondary infections of the eye? How does this transmission take place? ***(1850)***

____

____

NONINFECTIOUS EYE DISORDERS

Objectives

- Compare the nature of cataracts, diabetic retinopathy, macular degeneration, retinal detachment, and glaucoma, including the etiology, pathophysiology, clinical manifestations, assessment, diagnostic tests, medical management, nursing interventions, patient teaching, and prognosis.
- Discuss Sjögren's syndrome, ectropion, and entropion, including etiology, pathophysiology, clinical manifestations, diagnostic tests, medical management, nursing interventions, and prognosis.

Activity 1

27. Complete the following table of noninfectious eye disorders by supplying the cause, the clinical manifestations, the diagnostic tests, and the treatment for each. ***(1853-1863)***

Disorder	Cause	Clinical Manifestations	Diagnostic Tests	Treatment
a. Cataracts				
b. Diabetic retinopathy				
c. Retinal detachment				
d. Glaucoma				
e. Macular degeneration				

Multiple Choice

28. A patient has recently been diagnosed with keratoconjunctivitis sicca. Based upon the nurse's understanding, this condition is believed to be caused by: ***(1851)***
    1. environmental humidity.
    2. cosmetics tainted with bacteria.
    3. an autoimmune disorder.
    4. a reduction in aqueous humor.

29. Patients with Sjögren's syndrome typically report: ***(1851-1852)***
    1. feeling that their eyes are gritty.
    2. blurred vision.
    3. feeling worse in the morning.
    4. seeing floaters in the field of vision.

30. Ectropion is often characterized by: (Select all that apply) ***(1852)***
    1. tearing.
    2. reddened eyes.
    3. thick eye discharge.
    4. corneal dryness.

31. What diagnostic tests are used to confirm the presence of entropion? ***(1852)***
    1. Amsler's grid
    2. Snellen's examination
    3. Ophthalmoscopic examination
    4. Pneumatic retinopexy

CORNEAL INJURIES

Objective

- Discuss corneal injuries, including etiology, pathophysiology, clinical manifestations, assessment, diagnostic tests, medical management, nursing interventions, patient teaching, and prognosis.

32. What is the most common cause of corneal injury? ***(1863-1864)*** ______________________________

____

____

33. Describe the clinical manifestations of a corneal abrasion. ***(1863-1864)*** ______________________

____

____

34. Review the diagnostic tests used to confirm, and to assess the degree of, a corneal injury. ***(1863-1864)***

____

____

35. Discuss the management of a corneal injury caused by foreign body. ***(1863-1864)*** ______________

____

____

CARE OF THE HEARING AID

Objective

- Describe the appropriate care of the hearing aid.

36. Using an index card, list five facts to include when planning education for a patient about the care of a hearing aid. ***(1870)***

COMMUNICATION

Objective

- List tips for communicating with hearing- and sight-impaired people.

37. Use an index card. Label one side of the card as "DOs." Label the other side of the card as "DON'Ts." List four "do's and don'ts" for communicating with the hearing- or sight-impaired person on the appropriate side. ***(1869)***

TREATMENT OF THE EYE AND THE EAR

Objectives

- Describe the various surgeries of the eye, including the nursing interventions and prognosis.
- Describe the various surgeries of the ear, including the nursing interventions, patient teaching, and prognosis.
- Describe appropriate nursing interventions for the patient having eye and ear surgery.

38. The patient had a car accident and is returning to your unit from vitrectomy surgery of the right eye and a myringotomy of the right ear. List the appropriate nursing interventions for this patient. ***(1869)***

____

____

HEARING LOSS

Objective

- Differentiate between conductive and sensorineural hearing loss.

39. List the common characteristics of conductive and sensorineural hearing loss in the center column below. In other columns, list information specific to conductive and sensorineural hearing loss. ***(1871)***

Conductive Hearing Loss	Common Characteristics	Sensorineural Hearing Loss

INFLAMMATORY AND INFECTIOUS EAR DISORDERS

Objective

- Describe major ear inflammatory and infectious disorders including etiology, pathophysiology, clinical manifestations, assessment, diagnostic tests, medical management, nursing interventions, and prognosis.

40. External otitis is sometimes known as what? ***(1871)*** ____

____

____

41. Identify the potential causes of external otitis. ***(1872)***

42. When interviewing the patient complaining of an inflammatory ear disorder, what subjective data should be collected? ***(1872)***

43. When interviewing the patient complaining of an inflammatory ear disorder, what objective data should be collected? ***(1871-1872)***

44. List the classifications of medications that may be used in the treatment of inflammatory ear disorders. ***(1871-1872)***

45. Identify the most common causes of otitis media. ***(1872)***

46. Why are children most susceptible to otitis media? ***(1872)***

47. Identify the clinical manifestations of otitis media. ***(1872)***

NONINFECTIOUS EAR DISORDERS

Objective

- Discuss noninfectious disorders of the ear including etiology, pathophysiology, clinical manifestations, assessment, diagnostic tests, medical management, nursing interventions, patient teaching, and prognosis.

48. Complete the following table of noninfectious ear disorders by including the cause, the clinical manifestations, the diagnostic tests, and the treatment for each. ***(1876-1877)***

Disorder	Cause	Clinical Manifestations	Diagnostic Tests	Treatment
a. Otosclerosis				
b. Ménière's disease				

CARING FOR PATIENTS WITH SENSORY IMPAIRMENTS

Objectives

- Identify communication resources for people with visual and/or hearing impairment.
- Describe home health considerations for people with eye or ear disorders or surgery or visual and hearing impairments.

49. Discuss the importance of meeting the communication needs of a patient with a vision or hearing disorder. ***(1881-1882)***

____

____

50. Where can patients obtain listings of agencies to assist them in locating services? ***(1846)*** ______________

____

____

51. Identify two primary concerns in the home environment for the patient with a visual or hearing impairment. ***(1846, 1865, 1879, 1882)***

____

____

PATIENT TEACHING

Objective

- Give patient instructions regarding care of the eye and ear in accordance with written protocol.

52. Develop an index card to use to prompt the nurse during patient teaching for care of the eye and ear in accordance with written protocol. ***(1236-1241, 1854-1859, 1864, 1870, 1871, 1875)***

MULTIPLE CHOICE

53. The typical type of visual distortions associated with diabetic retinopathy will include: ***(1854)***
    1. tunnel vision.
    2. a loss of visual acuity accompanied by "floaters."
    3. a sudden onset of peripheral vision.
    4. reddened eyes accompanied by a yellow discharge.

54. A 65-year-old patient reports to the office complaining of visual deficits, including disturbances in color vision and visual clarity, and a darkened area in the center of vision. What medical diagnosis does the nurse anticipate will be made? ***(1857)***
    1. Macular degeneration
    2. Glaucoma
    3. Herpetic keratitis
    4. Cataracts

55. Tonometry is used in the diagnosis of what condition? ***(1860)***
    1. Corneal abrasions
    2. Blepharitis
    3. Glaucoma
    4. Retinal detachment

56. The patient has been diagnosed with a visual disorder. Contact lenses have been prescribed. Which of the following statements indicates the need for further instruction? (Select all that apply) ***(1854)***
    1. "I will need to avoid exceeding the recommended time for leaving the lens in to prevent injury to my retina."
    2. "To save money, I can use a 50:50 tap water/saline solution to clean my lens.
    3. "I will need to be careful not to mix up my left and right lens."
    4. "I will carefully wash and dry my hands before handling my lens."

57. Which of the following should be incorporated when positioning the patient after a stapedectomy? ***(1877)***
    1. Keep the operative side facing upward.
    2. Elevate the head of the bed to at least 45 degrees.
    3. Turn, cough, and deep-breathe every 2 hours.
    4. Use a neck brace to ensure minimal movement for the first 2 hours.

CRITICAL THINKING ACTIVITIES

Activity 1

58. An 18-year-old patient has just returned from surgery for the enucleation of his right eye after injuries suffered in an automobile accident. ***(1865)***

    a. Discuss the nursing interventions that will be required over the next 24 hours.____________________

    ____

    ____

    ____

    ____

    b. What findings are indicative of complications and warrant an immediate report to the health care provider?

    ____

    ____

    ____

    ____

    c. The patient expresses concerns about his appearance. How will the nurse address his concerns?

    ____

    ____

    ____

    ____

Activity 2

59. A 20-year-old patient reports with complaints of a worsening ear pain. After completing his history, it is determined he had recently had an ear infection and he failed to take the full course of prescribed medications. His other complaints include earache, fever, headache, malaise, and purulent exudates. ***(1871)***

    a. What should the nurse anticipate the patient's medical diagnosis will be? ______________________

    ____

    b. How did this condition occur? ______________________

    ____

    ____

    ____

    ____

    c. Discuss the treatment and the prognosis of this condition. ______________________

    ____

    ____

    ____

    ____

Student Name______________________________ Date______________

Care of the Patient with a Neurologic Disorder

chapter **54**

Answer Key: Textbook page references are provided as a guide for answering these questions. A complete answer key was provided for your instructor.

DIVISIONS OF THE NERVOUS SYSTEM

Objective

- Name the two structural divisions of the nervous system and give the functions of each.

1. Identify the two structural divisions of the nervous system. *(1887)* ____________________

2. What is the primary role of the central nervous system (CNS)? *(1887)* ____________________

3. Identify the divisions and the roles of the two systems that make up the peripheral nervous system. *(1887)*

4. What is another name for the autonomic nervous system? *(1887)* ____________________

NEURON

Objective

- List the parts of the neuron and describe the function of each part.

Activity 1

5. a. Identify each part of the neuron. Next to each label, describe the function of that part. ***(1887-1888)***

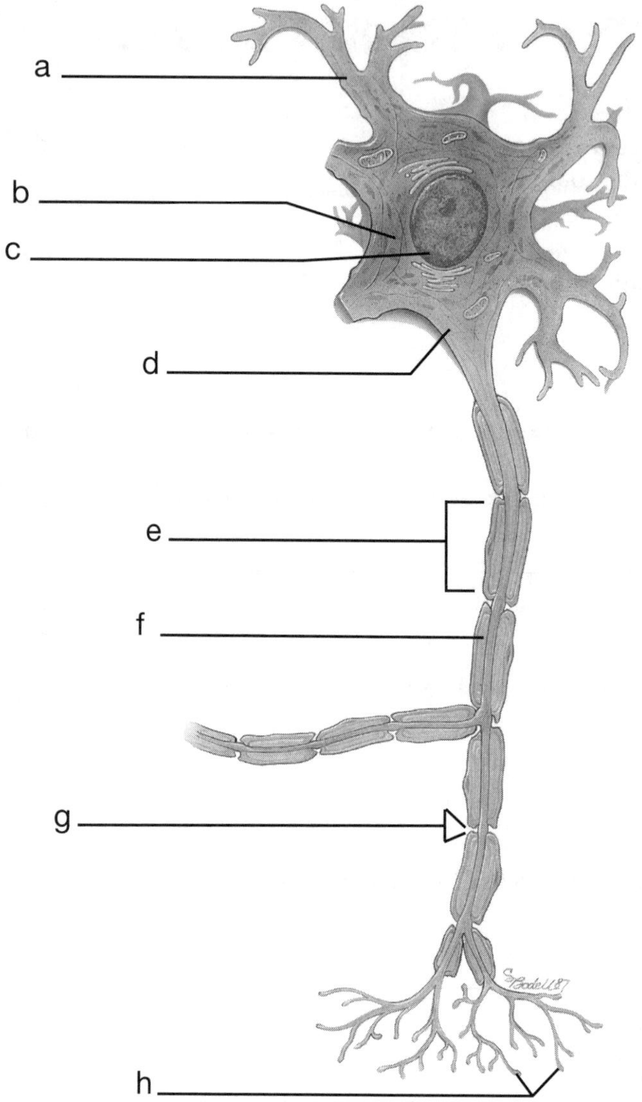

b. Describe the function of each part.

a. ______________________________

b. ______________________________

c. ______________________________

d. ______________________________

e. ______________________________

f. ______________________________

g. ____________________

h. ____________________

NERVOUS SYSTEM

Objectives

- Explain the anatomical location and functions of the cerebrum, brainstem, cerebellum, spinal cord, peripheral nerves, and cerebrospinal fluid.
- Discuss the parts of the peripheral nervous system and how the system works with the central nervous system (CNS).

Activity 1

6. Identify the parts of the brain. ***(1889)***

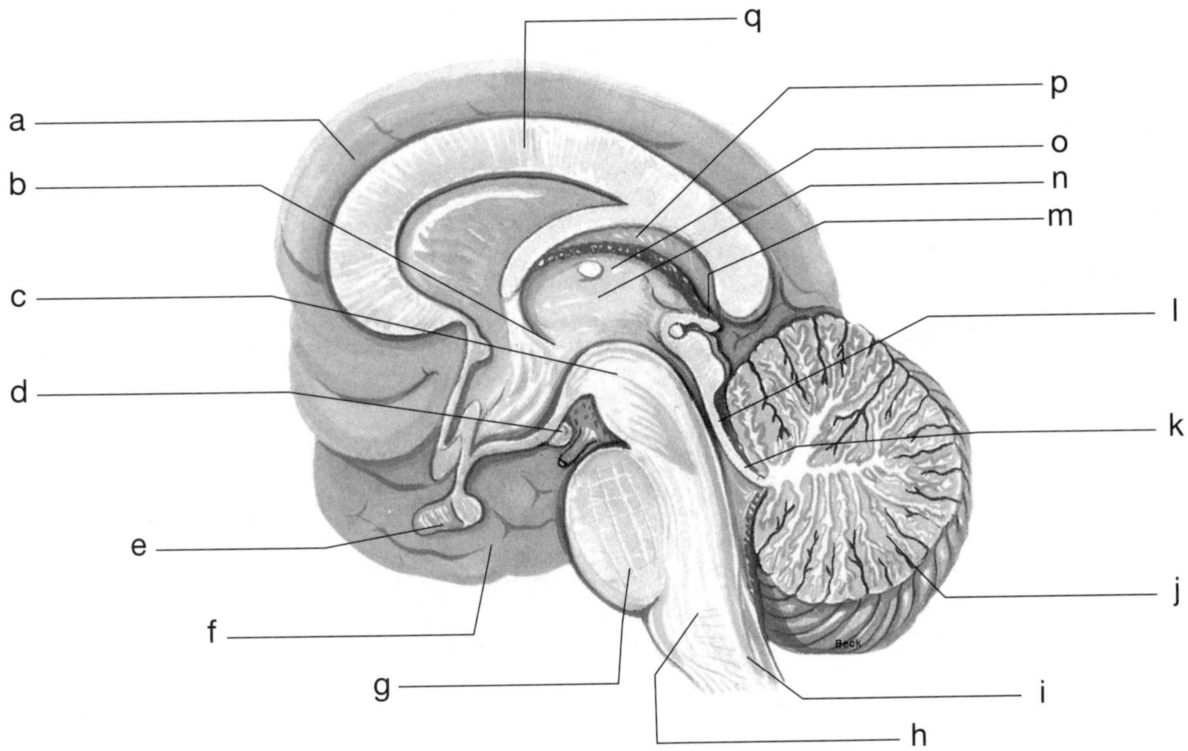

Activity 2

7. Complete the table below by listing the function of each part of the brain indicated. ***(1888-1890)***

Part	Function
a. Cerebrum	
b. Brainstem	
c. Cerebellum	
d. Spinal cord	
e. Peripheral nerves	

CRANIAL NERVES

Objective

- Name the 12 cranial nerves and list the areas they serve.

8. Read each of the following descriptive functions. Identify the cranial nerve that serves it by name and number. ***(1893)***

    a. Sensations of throat, taste, swallowing movements, secretion of saliva: ______________________

    ____

    b. Vision: ____

    ____

    c. Turning eyes outward: ____

    ____

    d. Sense of smell: ____

    ____

    e. Hearing; sense of balance: ____

    ____

f. Tongue movements: ______

g. Eye movements, pupillary control: ______

h. Shoulder movements and turning movements of head: ______

i. Eye movements: ______

j. Sense of taste; contraction of muscles of facial expression: ______

k. Sensations of face, scalp, and teeth; chewing movement: ______

l. Sensations of throat, larynx, and thoracic and abdominal organs; swallowing, voice production, slowing of heartbeat, acceleration of peristalsis:

______

AGING

Objective

- List the physiologic changes that occur in the nervous system with aging.

9. Develop a fact sheet about changes to the nervous system that occur with aging. ***(1891)***

   a. Brain weight: ______

   b. Structural changes: ______

   c. Neuron changes: ______

   d. Body function changes: ______

DIAGNOSTIC TESTS

Objectives

- List common laboratory and diagnostic examinations for evaluation of neurologic disorders.
- Give examples of six degenerative neurologic diseases and explain the etiology, pathophysiology, clinical manifestations, assessment, diagnostic tests, medical management, nursing interventions, and prognosis for each.

Activity 1

10. Write a brief description of each of the listed diagnostic tests. ***(1887-1891)***

    a. Magnetic resonance imaging (MRI) scan: ____________________

    ____

    ____

    b. Positron emission tomography (PET) scan: ____________________

    ____

    ____

    c. Lumbar puncture: ____________________

    ____

    ____

    d. Magnetic resonance angiography (MRA): ____________________

    ____

    ____

    e. Electroencephalogram (EEG): ____________________

    ____

    ____

    f. Myelogram: ____________________

    ____

    ____

g. Angiogram: ______________________________

h. Carotid duplex: ______________________________

i. Electromyogram (EMG): ______________________________

j. Echoencephalogram: ______________________________

Activity 2

11. For each of the disorders listed below, identify a diagnostic test that may be used to confirm it.

a. Multiple sclerosis: ***(1917)*** ______________________________

b. Parkinson's disease: ***(1921)*** ______________________________

c. Alzheimer's disease: ***(1934)*** ______________________________

d. Myasthenia gravis: ***(1928)*** ______________________________

e. Huntington's disease: ***(1930)*** ______________________________

GLASGOW COMA SCALE

Objective

- Discuss the Glasgow coma scale.

12. Complete the table below for the nurse to use as a guide when assessing a patient's level of consciousness. ***(1895)***

Response	Score
a. Eyes open	
b. Verbal	
c. Motor	
d. Total	

ASSESSMENT AND MANAGEMENT OF NEUROLOGIC DISORDERS

Objectives

- Identify the significant subjective and objective data related to the nervous system that should be obtained from a patient during assessment.
- Differentiate between normal and common abnormal findings of a physical assessment of the nervous system.
- Discuss various neurologic disturbances in motor function and sensory-perceptual function.
- Give examples of six degenerative neurologic diseases and explain the etiology, pathophysiology, clinical manifestations, assessment, diagnostic tests, medical management, nursing interventions, and prognosis for each.

Activity 1

13. When eliciting the history from a patient experiencing neurologic changes, what inquiries should be made concerning potential subjective changes? List five. ***(1893-1894)***

a. ______________________________

b. ______________________________

c. ______________________________

d. ______________________________

e. ______________________________

14. Neurologic changes may be obvious to family members of the patient. What inquiries may be made to the family members concerning changes in their loved one? ***(1894)***

____

____

15. What is the greatest indicator of neurologic status? ***(1894)*** _______________

____

____

16. When evaluating a patient, what components are used to assess awareness? ***(1894)*** _______________

____

____

17. What elements are assessed to determine motor functioning? ***(1896)*** _______________

____

____

18. What elements are assessed to determine sensory and perceptual status? ***(1897)*** _______________

____

____

Activity 2

19. The nurse has completed the data collection from the patient reporting to the clinic with complaints of weakness and numbness in the arms and legs. The patient reports having fallen three times recently. The patient's husband, who is present during this interaction, expresses concerns about his wife's constantly fluctuating emotions. Based upon this assessment, what degenerative neurologic condition might the nurse believe may be diagnosed? ***(1916)***

____

____

20. A patient with multiple sclerosis is being seen at the ambulatory care clinic with complaints of burning on urination. A urinary tract infection is diagnosed. In addition to the prescribed medications, what interventions can be encouraged to reduce future urinary tract infections? ***(1918)***

____

____

____

____

21. The nurse working in a long-term care facility is completing the intake assessment of a new resident; only a limited history is available. When performing the assessment, the nurse notes the patient has a flat facial expression, hand tremors, and bradykinesia. Based upon these findings, which degenerative neurologic conditions may be present? ***(1919)***

22. The primary care physician for the patient with Alzheimer's disease has added medications to manage the changes in the patient's condition. The new orders include lorazepam (Ativan) and sertraline (Zoloft). Based upon the nurse's understanding, what clinical manifestations of the disease will be managed by these medications? ***(1925)***

23. A patient has recently been diagnosed with myasthenia gravis. The patient is questioning the nurse about what physical changes will be occurring with this disease. What information can be provided to the patient? ***(1928)***

PREVENTION

Objective

- Explain the importance of prevention in problems of the nervous system, and give at least one example of prevention.

24. The patient has asked the nurse what she could do to reduce her risk factors that may contribute to a neurologic problem. Explain below what the nurse could tell her. Be sure to list at least one example. ***(1892)***

INTRACRANIAL PRESSURE (ICP)

Objectives

- List five signs and symptoms of increased intracranial pressure and why they occur, as well as nursing interventions that decrease intracranial pressure.
- Discuss various neurologic disturbances in motor function and sensory-perceptual function.

25. Identify five signs and symptoms of increased intracranial pressure (ICP) and why they occur. *(1905-1906)*

Signs and Symptoms	Rationale for Occurrence
a.	
b.	
c.	
d.	
e.	

SEIZURES

Objective

- List four classifications of seizures, their characteristics, clinical signs, aura, and postictal period.

26. How are seizures classified? *(1912)* ______________________________

____

____

27. List the four types of seizures. ***(1912)***

    a. ____

    b. ____

    c. ____

    d. ____

28. Define *epilepsy*. ***(1951)*** ____

29. Identify potential causes of nonepileptic seizures. ***(1912)*** ____

30. List and discuss the phases in a seizure. ***(1912-1913)*** ____

31. What is status epilepticus? Why is it a critical event? ***(1912)*** ____

32. How is status epilepticus managed? ***(1912)*** ____

33. What examination is used to evaluate seizures? ***(1914)*** ____

34. List three primary goals of the nursing care for a patient having a seizure. ***(1915)***

    a. ____

    b. ____

    c. ____

35. Identify nursing interventions used to care for a patient having a seizure. ***(1915)*** ____

STROKE AND TRAUMATIC BRAIN INJURY

Objectives

- Explain the mechanism of injury to the brain that occurs with a stroke and traumatic brain injury.
- Discuss the etiology, pathophysiology, clinical manifestations, assessment, diagnostic tests, medical management, and nursing interventions of a stroke patient.

36. Complete the chain of events for a patient who has suffered a stroke or a traumatic brain injury. ***(1930-1931)***

Mechanism of Injury

↓

Medical Management

Nursing Interventions

↓

Acute care
Rehabilitation care

SPINAL CORD TRAUMA

Objectives

- Discuss the etiology, pathophysiology, clinical manifestations, assessment, diagnostic tests, medical management, and nursing interventions for intracranial tumors, craniocerebral trauma, and spinal cord trauma.
- Identify the significant subjective and objective data related to the nervous system that should be obtained from a patient during assessment.
- Discuss various neurologic disturbances in motor function and sensory-perceptual function.

37. Differentiate between complete cord injury and incomplete cord injury. ***(1946)*** ____________________

____

____

38. A patient who experiences injury to the cervical segment of the spinal cord will face what degree of injury? ***(1946)***

____

____

39. At what level of the spinal cord have paraplegics experienced injury? ***(1946)*** ____________________

____

____

40. The period of flaccid paralysis and complete loss of reflexes during the initial period following injury is known as what? ***(1946)***

____

____

41. What is another term for autonomic dysreflexia? ***(1946)*** ____________________

____

____

42. Why does autonomic dysreflexia occur? ***(1946)*** ____________________

____

____

43. List the signs and symptoms of autonomic dysreflexia. ***(1946, 1948)*** ____________________

____

____

44. What stimuli can cause autonomic dysreflexia? ***(1948-1949)*** ______

______

______

45. Identify three potential complications related to paralysis. ***(1948-1949)*** ______

______

______

TRIGEMINAL NEURALGIA AND BELL'S PALSY

Objective

- Differentiate between trigeminal neuralgia and Bell's palsy.

46. Differentiate between trigeminal neuralgia and Bell's palsy. ***(1936-1938)*** ______

______

______

INFECTIOUS AND INFLAMMATORY DISORDERS OF THE NEUROLOGIC SYSTEM

Objective

- Discuss the etiology, pathophysiology, clinical manifestations, assessment, diagnostic tests, medical management, nursing interventions, and prognosis for GBS, meningitis, encephalitis, and AIDS.

47. A 35-year-old female patient has sought care at the physician's office for complaints of weakness in the lower extremities and marked fluctuations in blood pressure readings. The history includes a recent strep infection. The physician has made a tentative diagnosis of Guillain-Barré syndrome (GBS) and recommends hospitalization. ***(1939)***

    a. Stating she feels well enough to go home, the patient asks why hospitalization is necessary. What response by the nurse is indicated?

    ______

    ______

    b. The nurse in the hospital is completing the admission on the patient in the scenario. What diagnostic tests can be anticipated?

    ______

    ______

48. What is the prognosis for the patient diagnosed with GBS? ***(1939)*** ______

49. A patient has been admitted to the intensive care unit (ICU) with a diagnosis of insect-borne encephalitis. When planning the care that will be of the highest priority to the patient, what is necessary to include? ***(1940)***

50. The spouse of a patient hospitalized with encephalitis has asked what types of impairments patients with the disorder may experience after recovery from the disease. Based upon your understanding of the condition, what types of long-term complications may exist for this patient? ***(1941)***

51. The family of a patient diagnosed with encephalitis reports they have heard more about meningitis and question what difference is between the two diseases. What information can be provided? ***(1941)***

52. Discuss the incidence and type of neurologic complications frequently experienced by patients with acquired immunodeficiency virus (AIDS). ***(1942-1943)***

53. What are the priorities of care for the patient hospitalized with AIDS dementia complex (ADC)? ***(1943)***

54. What is the prognosis for the AIDS patient experiencing neurologic complications? ***(1943)*** ______

PATIENT EDUCATION

Objective

- Discuss patient teaching and home care planning for the patient with stroke, multiple sclerosis, Parkinson's disease, and myasthenia gravis.

55. Obtain two index cards. Label each side with one of the following: multiple sclerosis, myasthenia gravis, Parkinson's disease, and stroke. List four teaching points to discuss with patients diagnosed with each of the disorders. ***(1943)***

MULTIPLE CHOICE

56. A 35-year-old man who suffers from tension headaches asks for clarification concerning why he is not given narcotics for the pain even though he finds the headaches painful and debilitating. Based on the nurse's knowledge, a reason may be that: ***(1902)***
    1. narcotics are avoided because of the risk of abuse.
    2. tension headache pain is not bad enough to warrant narcotic use.
    3. the pain receptor sites associated with tension headaches respond best with the use of acetaminophen products.
    4. the pain associated with tension headaches will subside without narcotic use.

57. Foods and beverages attributed to causing or worsening migraine headaches include which of the following? ***(1902)***
    1. Italian foods
    2. Apples
    3. Dairy products
    4. Ripened cheese

58. Which of the following changes is a late sign of increased intracranial pressure? ***(1905)***
    1. Changes in level of consciousness
    2. Changes in muscle coordination
    3. A widened pulse pressure
    4. Diplopia

59. Select the measures that may be implemented to reduce venous volume in a patient experiencing increased intracranial pressure. (Select all that apply) ***(1907)***
    1. Restrict fluid intake.
    2. Elevate the head of the bed to 90 degrees.
    3. Avoid flexion of the hips.
    4. Administer enemas as needed (prn) to prevent constipation.
    5. Administer oxygen.

CRITICAL THINKING ACTIVITIES

Activity 1

60. A 21-year-old patient reports with complaints of frequent headaches. When asked, she describes the pain as viselike and throbbing. She states she frequently experiences numbness and tingling in her hands just before their onset. ***(1891-1892)***

    a. What type of headache is the patient experiencing? ________________________________

    ____

    ____

    ____

    ____

b. The patient asks about the significance of the numbness in her hands. What will the nurse tell her?

c. Discuss dietary management options to control the headaches.

d. What medications can be given to treat the headaches?

e. Discuss nonpharmacologic interventions to promote comfort.

Activity 2

61. A 58-year-old man reports he experienced numbness in his legs, a loss of sensation in his arms, and an inability to speak. Upon questioning, he reported that the entire event lasted only about 15 minutes. ***(1932)***

    a. Based on your knowledge, what has the patient experienced?

b. Since this event was short in duration, is it of any long-term significance? Why or why not?

____

____

____

____

c. What diagnostic examinations would you anticipate will be performed? ______________

____

____

____

____

Student Name______________________________ Date______________

chapter 55

Care of the Patient with an Immune Disorder

Answer Key: Textbook page references are provided as a guide for answering these questions. A complete answer key was provided for your instructor.

IMMUNITY

Objective

- Differentiate between natural and acquired immunity.

1. Describe how natural and acquired immunity work within the body. ***(1956)***

   a. Natural immunity:______________________________

   ____

   ____

   b. Acquired immunity: ______________________________

   ____

   ____

TYPES OF IMMUNITY

Objective

- Compare and contrast humoral and cell-mediated immunity.

2. How is cell-mediated immunity achieved? ***(1956)***______________________________

   ____

   ____

3. What happens to sensitized T cells? ***(1959)***______________________________

   ____

   ____

4. What is the significance of cell-mediated immunity? ***(1959, 1966)*** ______________________

5. What type of cells initiate antibody production? ***(1957)*** ______________________

6. What is active immunity? Include an example. ***(1957)*** ______________________

7. What is passive immunity? Include an example. ***(1957)*** ______________________

8. Which cells mediate humoral immunity? ***(1957)*** ______________________

9. What is released in an antigen-antibody reaction? ***(1957-1958)*** ______________________

10. What type of antigens does humoral immunity respond to? ***(1957-1958)*** ______________________

IMMUNITY DIFFERENCES

Objective

- Explain the concepts of immunocompetency, immunodeficiency, and autoimmunity.

11. The patient has asked the nurse to explain the differences among immunocompetency, immunodeficiency, and autoimmunity. She said that she had written these three words down, but does not have any idea what they mean. How will the nurse explain the differences to her in terms she can understand? ***(1956-1958)***

ORGANIZATION OF THE IMMUNE SYSTEM

Objective

- Review the mechanisms of immune response.

12. Describe how immunization and immunotherapy can be used to help the body develop immunity. ***(1959)***

    a. Immunizations:

    b. Immunotherapy:

HYPERSENSITIVITY DEVELOPMENT

Objective

- Discuss five factors that influence the development of hypersensitivity.

13. Identify common substances that can initiate a hypersensitivity disorder. ***(1960)***

14. Discuss the manner in which exposure to substances may occur. ***(1960)***

15. What is thought to be the primary cause of hypersensitivity disorders? ***(1960)***

16. How are hypersensitivity disorders diagnosed? ***(1961)*** ______________________________

____

____

17. What are common clinical manifestations of hypersensitivity disorders? ***(1961)***______________

____

____

18. List factors that can increase the symptoms of hypersensitivity. ***(1961)***____________________

____

____

19. List three nursing diagnoses applicable to a patient experiencing a hypersensitivity reaction. ***(1962)***

    a. ____

    b. ____

    c. ____

ANAPHYLAXIS

Objectives

- Identify the clinical manifestations of anaphylaxis.
- Outline the immediate aggressive treatment of systemic anaphylactic reaction.

20. List the body system and the sign or symptom that would indicate that the patient may be having an anaphylactic response. In the last row, outline the treatment of a systemic anaphylactic reaction. ***(1963)***

System	Sign or Symptom
a.	
b.	
c.	
d.	
e. Treatment:	

LATEX ALLERGIES

Objective

- Discuss the two types of latex allergies and recommendations for preventing allergic reactions to latex in the workplace.

21. Describe the differences between type IV allergic contact dermatitis and type I allergic reactions. ***(1964)***

____

____

22. List the eight recommendations from the National Institute for Occupational Safety and Health (NIOSH) that can be used to prevent allergic reactions to latex in the workplace. ***(1964-1965)***

    a. ____

    b. ____

    c. ____

    d. ____

    e. ____

    f. ____

    g. ____

    h. ____

TRANSFUSION REACTION

Objective

- Discuss selection of blood donors, typing and cross-matching, storage, and administration in preventing transfusion reaction.

23. List all of the ways that transfusion reactions can be prevented. ***(1965)*** ______________________

____

____

24. What is the best method for preventing transfusion reactions? ***(1965)***______________________

____

____

IMMUNODEFICIENCY DISEASE

Objective

- Explain an immunodeficiency disease.

25. Describe the following characteristics of an immunodeficiency disease. ***(1966)***

    a. First evidence: ______________________________

    ____

    ____

    b. Result of immunodeficient state: ______________________________

    ____

    ____

    c. Two types:

    i. ______________________________

    ii. ______________________________

    d. Factors that alter immune response:

    i. ______________________________

    ii ______________________________

    iii. ______________________________

    iv. ______________________________

AUTOIMMUNE DISORDERS

Objectives

- Discuss the cause of autoimmune disorders.
- Explain plasmapheresis in the treatment of autoimmune diseases.

26. The patient has an autoimmune disorder. How will the nurse explain to him what could be the possible causes of autoimmune disorders and how plasmapheresis treatment will be helpful? ***(1966)***

    ____

    ____

MULTIPLE CHOICE

27. Within 15 minutes of initiating a blood transfusion, the patient reports shortness of breath, chills, and urticaria. After stopping the transfusion and notifying the physician, which laboratory test must be completed? ***(1965)***
    1. Urinalysis
    2. Hematocrit
    3. Hemoglobin
    4. White blood cell count

28. The suppressed humoral immune response in older adults is associated with: ***(1966)***
    1. degeneration of the spleen.
    2. reduction in the production of white blood cells.
    3. reduction in effectiveness of white blood cells.
    4. decreased immunoglobulin levels.

29. During plasmapheresis, the plasma may be replaced with which of the following? (Select all that apply) ***(1967)***
    1. Normal saline
    2. Lactated Ringer's solution
    3. Albumin
    4. Fresh-frozen plasma

30. The treatment protocol for anaphylaxis includes which of the following? ***(1960)***
    1. 1:10,000 epinephrine hydrochloride intramuscularly
    2. 1:1000 epinephrine hydrochloride subcutaneously
    3. 1:1000 epinephrine hydrochloride intradermally
    4. 1:10,000 epinephrine hydrochloride subcutaneously

CRITICAL THINKING ACTIVITIES

Activity 1

31. A 22-year-old patient has just completed allergy testing. Her health care provider has prescribed a regimen of weekly allergy shots. ***(1960)***

    a. What special precautions should be taken with the patient after the injection? ____________________

    ____

    ____

    ____

    ____

b. What teaching should be provided for a patient who is receiving allergy shots at home? __________

c. After administering the shots at home for more than a month, the patient calls and reports she has been ill and unable to take the medications for the past 2 weeks. How should the nurse advise the patient?

Activity 2

32. A 67-year-old patient voices concern about his health status. He reports he never used to "get sick" but now has been hospitalized three times in the last month with a variety of illnesses. How will the nurse respond to the patient's concerns? ***(1966-1967)***

Student Name________________________________ Date________________

Care of the Patient with HIV/AIDS

chapter

56

Answer Key: Textbook page references are provided as a guide for answering these questions. A complete answer key was provided for your instructor.

THE CAUSE OF HIV

Objectives

- Describe the agent that causes HIV disease.
- Describe the definition of AIDS given in January 1993 by the Centers for Disease Control and Prevention.
- Explain the differences between HIV infection, HIV disease, and AIDS.
- Define the nurse's role in the prevention of HIV infection.

1. The nurse is instructing a young male patient about human immunodeficiency virus (HIV) disease and the differences among HIV infection, HIV disease, and acquired immunodeficiency syndrome (AIDS). Develop information that the nurse will be able to share with him about this disease, including the definition of AIDS that the Centers for Disease Control and Prevention gave in January 1993. After developing this information, describe the nurse's role in the prevention of HIV infection. ***(2005-2006)***

____

____

____

____

____

____

____

THE PATHOLOGY OF THE HIV INFECTION

Objectives

- Discuss the pathophysiology of HIV disease.
- List signs and symptoms that may be indicative of HIV disease.
- Describe the progression of HIV infection.

Activity 1

2. Label the significance of viral load in the blood and early time course (months) of the disease. ***(1975)***

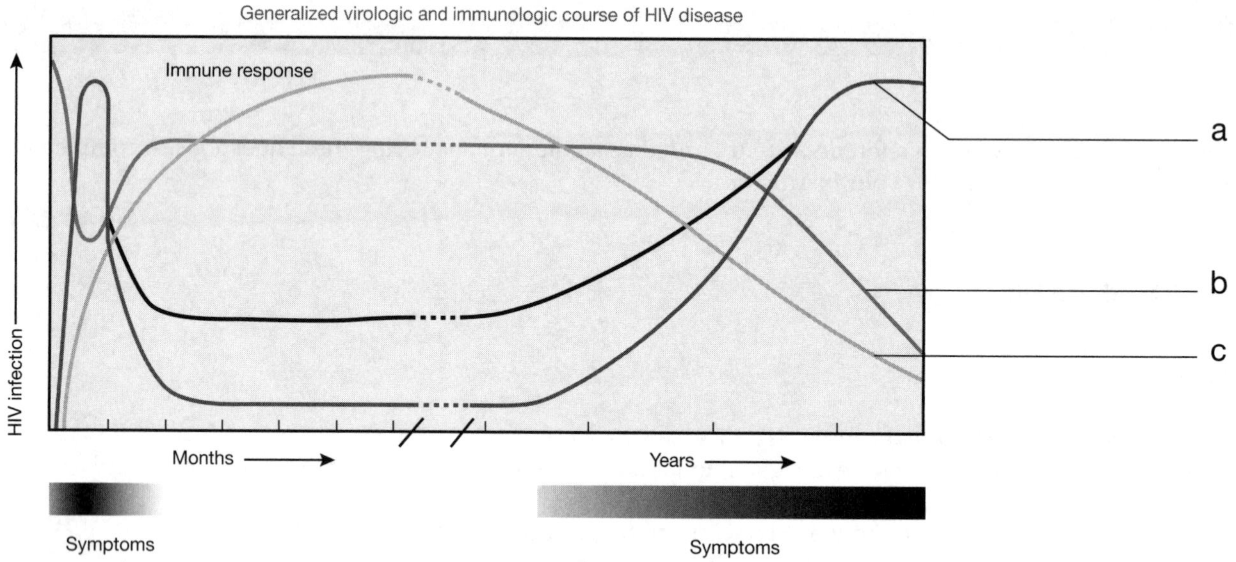

Activity 2

3. The course of HIV disease varies. Discuss factors that may influence the mortality and morbidity of the disease. ***(1978)***

____

____

4. Discuss the patterns of progression associated with HIV disease. ***(1978)*** ______________

____

____

5. When, in relation to exposure, does the process of seroconversion take place? ***(1981)*** ______________

____

____

6. Review the signs and symptoms that may occur during the period of seroconversion. ***(1981)*** ______________

____

____

7. How does a late diagnosis of HIV infection affect the progression of the disease? ***(1997)*** ______________

____

____

8. Discuss the relationship between viral set point and the HIV disease survival rate. ***(1981)***______________

____

____

DIAGNOSTIC TESTS

Objective

- Discuss the laboratory and diagnostic tests related to HIV disease.

9. Complete the following table about diagnostic tests used to determine the status of a patient with HIV disease. ***(1983-1985)***

Diagnostic Test	Implications and Process
a. HIV antibody testing	
i.	
ii.	
iii.	
iv.	
v.	
b. CD_4^+ cell monitoring	
c. Viral load monitoring	
d. Complete blood count (CBC)	
e. Liver function	
f. Syphilis	

RISK FOR HIV

Objectives

- Describe patients who are at risk for HIV infection.
- Discuss the use of effective prevention messages in counseling patients.
- Discuss how HIV is and is not transmitted.

Activity 1

10. Identify patients who are at risk for HIV infections in the column to the left. In the column on the right, describe effective prevention messages. ***(1974)***

Patients at Risk	Effective Prevention Messages

Activity 2

11. To what are nearly half of all new HIV infections in the United States attributed? ***(1973)*** ______________

____

____

12. What factors are believed to be responsible for the reduction in pediatric HIV cases? ***(1975)*** ___________

____

____

13. List the five factors that HIV transmission is dependent upon. ***(1975)***

    a. ____

    b. ____

    c. ____

    d. ____

    e. ____

14. Identify four methods of HIV transmission. ***(1975-1976)***

   a. ______________________________

   b. ______________________________

   c. ______________________________

   d. ______________________________

15. Identify populations associated with the highest rate of spread of HIV infection in the United States. ***(1974-1985)***

   ____

   ____

16. What are the three most common means of HIV infection transmission? ***(1974-1976)***

   a. ______________________________

   b. ______________________________

   c. ______________________________

17. Discuss underlying factors that may increase the risk of sexual transmission of the HIV virus. ***(1976-1977)***

   ____

   ____

18. Discuss the risk to health care providers with regard to HIV transmission. ***(1983-1985)*** ______________

   ____

   ____

19. Identify factors that increase the risk of transmission of HIV infection to a baby during labor and delivery. ***(1983-1985)***

   ____

   ____

ISSUES WITH TESTING

Objective

- Discuss the issues related to HIV antibody testing.

20. Prepare a short checklist of topics that the nurse should include when counseling a patient about HIV antibody testing. Include general guidelines and pretest and post-test counseling. ***(1983-1985)***

    a. General guidelines

        i. ______________________________

        ii. ______________________________

        iii. ______________________________

    b. Pretest counseling

        i. ______________________________

        ii. ______________________________

        iii. ______________________________

        iv. ______________________________

        v. ______________________________

        vi. ______________________________

        vii. ______________________________

        viii. ______________________________

        ix. ______________________________

        x. ______________________________

    c. Post-test counseling

        i. ______________________________

        ii. ______________________________

NURSE'S ROLE

Objective

- Discuss the nurse's role in assisting the HIV-infected patient with coping, grieving, reducing anxiety, and minimizing social isolation.

21. Make an index card of helpful information about coping, grieving, reducing anxiety, and minimizing social isolation to assist the nurse during care of an HIV-infected patient. ***(1998-1999)***

MULTIDISCIPLINARY CARE

Objective

- Describe the multidisciplinary approach in caring for a patient with HIV disease.

22. The patient wants to know why she has so many doctors and nurses in her room all the time. How might the nurse explain to her the multidisciplinary approach that is being utilized in her care? ***(1998-1999)***

____

____

____

____

OPPORTUNISTIC INFECTIONS

Objective

- List opportunistic infections associated with advanced HIV disease (AIDS).

23. List the opportunistic infections that the patient may develop because of advanced HIV disease. List the infections under each system, and then list common symptoms that would alert the nurse to the possibility that the patient had an opportunistic infection. ***(1986-1988)***

System	Opportunistic Infections
a. Respiratory	
b. Integumentary	
c. Eye	
d. Gastrointestinal	
e. Neurologic	

CARE PLAN

Objective

- Implement a care plan for the patient with AIDS.

24. The nurse has been assigned to a patient who has AIDS. Since nursing care is complex and constant, make a list of care that the nurse should give and goals that the nurse should promote. ***(1996, 2004)***

____

____

____

____

MULTIPLE CHOICE

25. A 32-year-old patient diagnosed with HIV reports she is looking into some alternative and complementary therapies to treat her disease. Which of the following is your best response? ***(1993)***
    1. "You should just use those medications prescribed by the doctor. Anything else might cause some type of reaction."
    2. "Be careful; there are so many unscrupulous people who are only after your money."
    3. "Many patients in your position also look into alternative treatments. Please let me know what you are considering."
    4. "I have heard several great things about these methods. Let me know how they work for you."

26. While caring for a known HIV-positive patient in the emergency department, the nurse notices the phlebotomist preparing to draw blood. What action by the nurse is correct? ***(1999)***
    1. Do nothing, because all patients should be treated with standard precautions.
    2. Ask the technician if the nurse can see him before he completes the procedure.
    3. Flag the chart to let all health care providers know the patient's status.
    4. Discretely hand a second pair of gloves to the technician as a signal.

27. An HIV-positive patient voices concern about his reoccurring bouts with diarrhea. He asks for clarification about the cause. Based on the nurse's knowledge, which of the following is recognized to be true? (Select all that apply) ***(1982)***
    1. Side effects from the medications
    2. Infections of the gastrointestinal tract
    3. Damage to the intestinal villi
    4. Caused by the fluctuating white blood cell (WBC) count

28. A 34-year-old patient has recently been diagnosed with HIV-associated cognitive motor complex. He asks questions about the complex. How does the nurse best respond? ***(2003)***
    1. "It is an unfortunate but expected complication of HIV."
    2. "The symptoms may be treatable if the cause can be identified."
    3. "It will fortunately be a short-term disorder."
    4. "It is associated with end-stage HIV."

CRITICAL THINKING ACTIVITIES

29. A nursing student has just been stuck by a needle while providing care for a patient whose lifestyle has placed him at high risk for HIV infection. After reporting to the clinic, she has questions. ***(1999-2000)***

    a. What course of action should be taken initially? ______________________________

    ____

    ____

    ____

    ____

b. What patient-based factors will affect her level of susceptibility? ____________________

____

____

____

____

c. Upon hearing the recommendation for her to begin prophylactic drug therapy, she asks to wait a few days before beginning the medication regimen. How would you advise her?

____

____

____

____

d. After a discussion of the need to begin the medications as soon as possible, she asks for an explanation concerning the pros and cons of taking the drugs.

____

____

____

____

e. List two nursing diagnoses for this patient.

i. ____________________

ii. ____________________

f. The patient voices concerns about having contact with her husband and child. How will the nurse respond to her concerns?

____

____

____

____

Student Name________________________ Date______________

Care of the Patient with Cancer

chapter **57**

Answer Key: Textbook page references are provided as a guide for answering these questions. A complete answer key was provided for your instructor.

EARLY CANCER DETECTION

Objectives

- Discuss the American Cancer Society's recommendations for preventive behaviors and seven screening tests for men and women.
- State seven warning signs of cancer.

1. A nurse is a member of a committee planning to hold an educational session discussing methods to promote early detection of cancer and the related warning signs to report. Prepare an index card to use as a prompt: on one side, identify recommendations for screening tests for both men and women. On the other side of the card, list seven "CAUTION" warning signs of cancer that warrant further assessment. ***(2017)***

RISK FACTORS

Objectives

- List seven risk factors for the development of cancer.
- Discuss the incidence of cancer as one of the leading causes of death in the United States.
- Compare the three most common sites for cancer in men and women.

2. List seven risk factors for the development of cancer. ***(2016-2017)***

   a. ______

   b. ______

   c. ______

   d. ______

   e. ______

   f. ______

   g. ______

3. Discuss the "5 a Day for Better Health" program. ***(2016)*** ______

4. For what cancers is obesity considered a risk factor? ***(2016)*** ______

5. Identify potential chemical carcinogens. ***(2017)*** ______

6. What populations are at higher risk for cancers related to chemical exposure? ***(2017)*** ______

7. Discuss the relationship of cancer development with aging. ***(2021)*** ______

8. In the United States, what population has the highest incidence of developing cancer? ***(2015)*** ______

9. On average, how many men and women can expect to be diagnosed with cancer? What is the current death rate? ***(2015)***

____

____

10. Compare and contrast the leading cancer types in men and women. ***(2015)*** ______________

____

____

PREVENTION AND DETECTION

Objectives

- Discuss development, prevention, and detection of cancer.
- Explain common reasons for delay in seeking medical care when a diagnosis of cancer is suspected.

11. Develop a chart below to explain how cancer develops, how it can be prevented and detected, and common reasons for delaying seeking medical care. Prepare this in such a way that a young adult would be interested in hearing your remarks. ***(2017)***

MALIGNANT CELLS

Objectives

- Define the terminology used to describe cellular changes, characteristics of malignant cells, and types of malignancies.
- Describe the pathophysiology of cancer, including the characteristics of malignant cells and the nature of metastasis.
- Describe the process of metastasis.

12. Describe cellular changes and pathophysiology and characteristics of malignant cells, and list the types of malignancies in the box below. In the bottom box, explain the process of metastasis. ***(2021)***

Explain the Process of Metastasis

TUMOR STAGING

Objective

- Define the systems of tumor classification: grading and staging.

Activity 1

13. Provide a brief description for each histopathologic level. *(2022)*

Level of Histopathologic Progression	Description
G_1	
G_2	
G_3	
G_4	

Activity 2

14. List the subclasses used in the classification of cancerous growths. *(2022)*

 a. ______________________________

 b. ______________________________

 c. ______________________________

CHEMOTHERAPEUTIC AGENTS

Objective

- Describe the major categories of chemotherapeutic agents.

Activity 1

15. Prepare a hint sheet of six major categories of chemotherapeutic agents. Include mode of action and common side effects that the nurse would need to know when taking care of a patient receiving this type of treatment. ***(2029)***

Categories	Mode of Action and Common Side Effects
a.	
b.	
c.	
d.	
e.	
f.	

Activity 2

16. Explain the dangers of leukopenia. ***(2027)*** ______________________________

____

____

17. Discuss special interventions for the patient with neutropenia. ***(2027)*** ______________

____

____

18. How is the risk of *Candida* infection managed? ***(2032)*** ______________________

____

____

19. Why is excess bleeding a problem for cancer patients? ***(2031)***______________________________

____

____

20. Review special precautions for the patient undergoing chemotherapy that help prevent respiratory complications. ***(2032)***

____

____

21. Identify two available treatment options for anemia related to chemotherapy. ***(2032)***

    a. ______________________________

    b. ______________________________

22. List four interventions to reduce the risk associated with thrombocytopenia. ***(2031)***

    a. ______________________________

    b. ______________________________

    c. ______________________________

    d. ______________________________

23. List two nursing diagnoses for the patient undergoing chemotherapy. ***(2034)***

    a. ______________________________

    b. ______________________________

DIAGNOSTIC TESTS

Objectives

- List common diagnostic tests used to identify the presence of cancer.
- Explain why biopsy is essential in confirming a diagnosis of cancer.

24. Complete the table below listing diagnostic tests by indicating the purpose of each. ***(2022-2025)***

Diagnostic Test	Purpose
a. Biopsy	
b. Endoscopy	
c. Bone scanning	
d. Computed tomography (CT)	
e. Ultrasonographic tests	
f. Magnetic resonance imaging (MRI)	
g. Alkaline phosphatase determination	
h. Serum calcitonin determination	
i. Carcinoembryonic antigen determination	
j. PSA and CA-125 determination	
k. Stool examination	

TYPES OF BIOPSY

Objective

- List common diagnostic tests used to identify the presence of cancer.

25. Label each type of biopsy. ***(2023)***

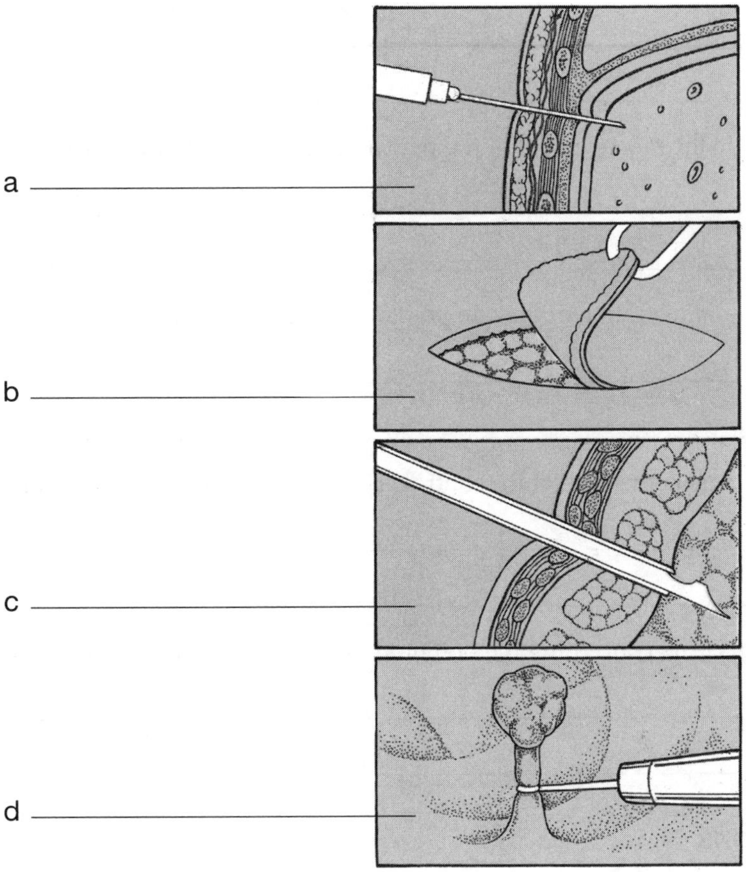

PAIN

Objective

- Discuss six general guidelines for the use of pain relief measures for the patient with advanced cancer.

Activity 1

26. List the six guidelines for use in pain relief. ***(2037)***

a. ______________________________

b. ______________________________

c. ______________________________

d. ______________________________

e. ______________________________

f. ______________________________

Activity 2

27. What causes pain in the patient with cancer? ***(2037)***

28. Identify opioids used in the management of the pain associated with cancer. ***(2037)***

29. Discuss the different administration options in pain management. ***(2037)***

30. List methods of pain management in which control is exerted primarily by the patient. ***(2037)***

31. How should a patient's fears concerning the potential for addiction be addressed? ***(2038)***

NURSING INTERVENTIONS

Objective

- Describe nursing interventions for the individual undergoing surgery, radiation therapy, chemotherapy, bone marrow, or peripheral stem cell transplantation.

32. Make an index card that you can use listing nursing interventions for the patient undergoing surgery, radiation therapy, chemotherapy, or bone marrow or peripheral stem cell transplantation. ***(2038-2039)***

TUMOR LYSIS SYNDROME

Objective

- Explain the etiology and pathophysiology of and medical management and nursing intervention for tumor lysis syndrome.

33. Complete the flow chart below, explaining the etiology and pathophysiology of, and the medical management and the nursing interventions for, tumor lysis syndrome. ***(2035)***

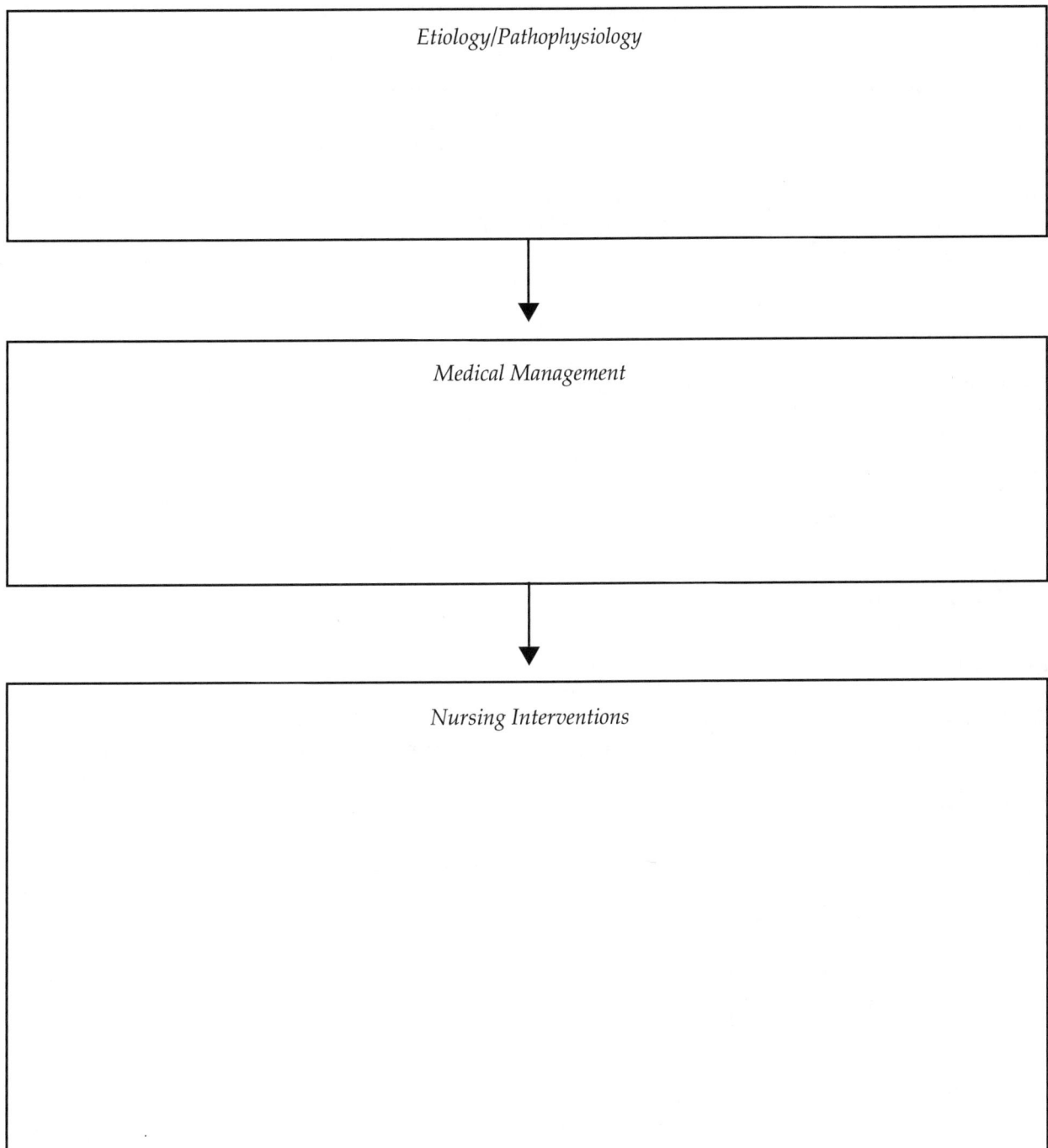

Etiology/Pathophysiology

↓

Medical Management

↓

Nursing Interventions

MULTIPLE CHOICE

34. While caring for a 23-year-old patient undergoing chemotherapy, she voices concerns about her hair loss. The nurse advises her that: ***(2032)***
    1. the loss of her hair will not be permanent.
    2. hair loss will only affect facial areas.
    3. the loss of hair occurs due to the destruction of the hair follicles.
    4. when the hair grows back, it will be thicker.

35. During meal planning for a cancer patient, the patient reports that things have a "strange" taste, which is affecting her appetite. Select those possible responses that accurately pertain to her inquiry. (Select all that apply) ***(2038)***
    1. This is a common occurrence and will get better after her treatments end.
    2. This phenomenon is a permanent and unfortunate consequence associated with cancer.
    3. Onion and ham may help to improve the taste of her vegetables.
    4. Lemon juice is frequently used with success to mask these taste alterations.

36. Select those factors which have been shown to have an impact on the determination of how well a patient will cope with a diagnosis of cancer. (Select all that apply) ***(2039)***
    1. Age at the time of the diagnosis
    2. Availability of significant others
    3. Presence of symptoms
    4. Type of cancer

37. When providing an educational program to a group of women in their 20s, the nurse should advise them to have a medical examination of their skin performed: ***(2018)***
    1. annually.
    2. every 3 years.
    3. every 2 years.
    4. annually beginning at age 30.

CRITICAL THINKING ACTIVITIES

Activity 1

38. During a routine check-up, a 40-year-old man voices questions about his potential for developing colon cancer. He relates his concerns to the recent death of his maternal grandfather from colon cancer. ***(2025)***

    a. Discuss the appropriate screening examinations for this patient. ______________________________

    ____

    ____

    ____

    ____

b. What preventive behaviors should be included in discussions with this patient? ____________

c. Develop two nursing diagnoses for this patient.

i. ____________

ii. ____________

Activity 2

39. A 32-year-old patient is undergoing radiation therapy for treatment of cervical cancer. ***(2025)***

a. The patient's mother asks for clarification concerning the differences between radiation therapy and chemotherapy.

____

b. After returning to her room after the first treatment, the patient asks if she can shower. Discuss this patient's request.

____

c. What precautions should be observed with this patient? ____________

d. The patient's husband asks about the visitation policy for the couple's 2-year-old daughter. How should the nurse respond?

____

____

____

____

e. Identify nursing interventions for the care of this patient. ______________________

____

____

____

____

Student Name________________________ Date____________

chapter **58**

Professional Roles and Leadership

Answer Key: Textbook page references are provided as a guide for answering these questions. A complete answer key was provided for your instructor.

TERMS

Objective

- Define the key terms as listed.

1. Define the following terms.

   a. Advancement: ***(2051)***________________________________

   b. Burnout: ***(2066)***________________________________

   c. Endorsement: ***(2056)***________________________________

   d. Nurse practice act: ***(2057)***________________________________

   e. Transcribe: ***(2069)***________________________________

CAREER PLANNING

Objectives

- Discuss the three methods of applying for a job.
- Describe what can be expected from an interview for a new job.
- Discuss career opportunities for the LPN/LVN.
- List the advantages of membership in professional organizations.
- Discuss the place and the nature of telephone manners in professionalism.
- Identify strategies for burnout prevention.

2. Identify the steps in career planning for the nurse. ***(2046)*** ____________________

3. What are the guidelines for preparing a letter of application for a position? ***(2046)*** ____________________

4. The purpose and components of a good resume are: ***(2047)*** ____________________

5. How can the applicant prepare for a successful interview? ***(2048)*** ____________________

6. What specific communication techniques should be employed for a successful interview? ***(2049)*** ____________________

7. Identify if the interviewer is allowed to ask the interviewee about the following. ***(2049)***
   a. Job-related criminal convictions _____
   b. Financial or credit status _____
   c. Marital status _____
   d. Age _____
   e. Educational background _____
   f. Reason for leaving prior employment _____

8. What is usually included in an employment contract? ***(2048, 2050)*** ____________________

9. Identify the organizations that represent LPN/LVNs and their major functions. ***(2053)*** ____________________

10. What is the purpose of continuing education, and what types are usually offered? ***(2053)*** ____________

____

____

11. The LPN/LVN who wants to continue his or her formal professional education should investigate ____________. ***(2054)***

12. What types of certification are available to the LPN/LVN? ***(2054)*** ____________

____

____

13. Appropriate telephone communication regarding physician's orders involves: ***(2068-2069)*** ____________

____

____

14. Identify possible career opportunities for the LPN/LVN. ***(2058-2062)*** ____________

____

____

BOARD OF NURSING

Objectives

- Describe the nurse practice act.
- Identify three important functions of a state board of nursing.
- List four reasons a state board of nursing could revoke a nursing license.
- Discuss the computerized adaptive testing (CAT) for the National Council Licensure Examination (NCLEX-PN® and -RN®).
- Discuss the chemically impaired nurse.

15. For the NCLEX-RN® and -PN® examinations, identify the following. ***(2055-2056)***

    a. Minimum number of questions: ____________

    b. Maximum number of questions: ____________

    c. Maximum time allowed: ____________

    d. Goal of CAT testing: ____________

    e. Average time to receive results: ____________

    f. Approval for candidate to take the test given by: ____________

    g. Examples of alternate-item format questions: ____________

16. Identify the role and functions of a state board of nursing. ***(2057-2058)*** ______________________

____

____

17. The state board of nursing may revoke a nurse's license for the following reasons: ***(2058)*** __________

____

____

18. What is the purpose of the Nurse Licensing Compact? ***(2057)*** ______________________

____

____

19. What is the Model Disciplinary Diversion Act? ***(2072)*** ______________________

____

____

WORK ISSUES

Objectives

- Describe the night shift survival guide.
- Discuss the future of computers in nursing.

20. Identify the type of nursing that the following LPNs/LVNs are involved in. ***(2060-2062)***

    a. Working in an auto manufacturing plant: ______________________

    b. Working with the terminally ill: ______________________

    c. Working in the community: ______________________

21. Identify the signs and symptoms of burnout and strategies that may be implemented to prevent this problem. ***(2066-2067)***

____

____

22. Identify how computers are used to aid nurses in their practice. ***(2068)*** ______________________

____

____

23. Identify an action that the nurse on the night shift should take for each of the following. ***(2051)***

    a. Staying alert at work: ______________________________

    b. Getting to sleep: ______________________________

    c. Balancing his or her life with work: ______________________________

LEADERSHIP

Objectives

- Explain the organizational position and the role of the charge nurse.
- Discuss the guidelines for being an effective leader.
- Discuss styles of leadership that may be used by nurses.
- Discuss the duties of a nurse team leader.
- Discuss mentoring.

24. Identify the type of leadership style that is being described. ***(2063-2064)***

    a. Leader relinquishes all control and delegates responsibility to the group: ______________________________

    b. People-centered approach that allows employees to have more control and participation in decision making: ______________________________

    c. Leader retains all authority and responsibility and has one-way communication with the group: ______________________________

    d. Takes into account the style of the leader and the characteristics of the group: ______________________________

25. What is the usual role of a team leader? ***(2064)*** ______________________________

26. Identify the guidelines for effective leadership. ***(2065)***

27. Principles of time management include: ***(2065)***

28. The LPN is working with another staff member who has not done what she was supposed to do for the patient. This is not the first time that this has occurred, and the LPN is becoming angry. What should this LPN do? ***(2066)***

29. What is the role of a nurse mentor? ***(2058)***

Multiple Choice

30. There has been an earthquake in the area, and the disaster victims are being brought into the emergency department. In this situation, the type of leadership that is the most effective for the nurse manager is: ***(2063-2064)***
    1. democratic.
    2. autocratic.
    3. situational.
    4. laissez-faire.

LEGAL ISSUES

Objectives

- Discuss confidentiality.
- List the three types of physician's orders and discuss the legal aspects of each.
- List three ways the nurse can ensure accuracy when transcribing physician's orders.
- List the pertinent data necessary to compile an effective end-of-shift report.
- Discuss the importance of malpractice insurance.

31. What precautions should be taken by the nurse when transcribing a physician's orders? ***(2068-2069)***

32. For the following, identify if the action is appropriate. ***(2068-2070)***
    a. The nurse is unsure of the order that is written, but believes that it is appropriate and transcribes it to the medication administration record. ______________________
    b. The nurse administers a preoperative treatment to a patient the afternoon following the surgery. ______________________
    c. A discontinued medication is crossed out with a highlighting marker. ______________________

33. For a change-of-shift report, identify the following. ***(2071)***
    a. Purpose: ____
    ____
    b. Methods: ____
    ____
    c. Information to include: ____
    ____

34. Why should the nurse have malpractice insurance? ***(2072)*** ______________________________
____
____

35. Identify all of the following actions that are appropriate and maintain patient confidentiality. ***(2052)***
    a. Discussing patient information in the cafeteria _____
    b. Copying patient information to review at home _____
    c. Providing information on patient status to the police _____
    d. Keeping information on the password-entry patient data system _____
    e. Giving updates on patient assessment during report _____

Multiple Choice

36. The nurse delegates the task of changing the surgical dressing to the certified nursing assistant (CNA). Which right of delegation is the nurse not following? (Select all that apply) ***(2068)***
    1. Task
    2. Direction
    3. Person
    4. Supervision

Skills Performance Checklists

These checklists were developed to assist in evaluating the competence of students in performing the nursing interventions presented in *Foundations and Adult Health Nursing*. The checklists are perforated for easy removal and reference. Students can be evaluated with a "Satisfactory (S)" or an "Unsatisfactory (U)" performance rating by putting a check in the appropriate column for each step. Specific instruction or feedback can be provided in the "Comments" column. All the checklists have been streamlined to include **only** the critical steps needed to satisfactorily master the skill. They are **not** intended to replace the text, which describes and illustrates each nursing skill in detail.

Student Name______________________________ Date______________

PERFORMANCE CHECKLIST 4-1

MEASURING BODY TEMPERATURE

	S	U	Comments
1. Introduce self to patient	❑	❑	________
2. Identify patient	❑	❑	________
3. Explain procedure to patient	❑	❑	________
4. Assess for signs and symptoms of temperature alterations and for factors that influence body temperature	❑	❑	________
5. Prepare for procedure			
a. Assemble the appropriate thermometer and other necessary supplies	❑	❑	________
b. Provide privacy	❑	❑	________
c. Determine whether patient has consumed hot or cold beverage or food or has been smoking	❑	❑	________
6. Obtaining an oral temperature: electronic thermometer			
a. Follow steps 1 through 5	❑	❑	________
b. Perform hand hygiene and don clean gloves	❑	❑	________
c. Remove thermometer pack from charging unit; remove probe from storage well of recording unit	❑	❑	________
d. Insert probe snugly into probe cover—red probe for rectal readings, blue probe for oral and axillary readings	❑	❑	________
e. Inspect digital display	❑	❑	________
f. Request that patient open mouth and gently insert probe correctly; request that patient hold thermometer in place with lips closed	❑	❑	________
g. Wait for audible signal	❑	❑	________

	S	U	Comments
h. Remove probe from patient's mouth and remove probe cover and dispose correctly	❑	❑	
i. Provide for patient comfort	❑	❑	
j. Read and write down reading; return thermometer to storage unit	❑	❑	
k. Perform hand hygiene	❑	❑	
l. Complete procedure by following step 10, a through d	❑	❑	
7. Obtaining rectal temperature: electronic thermometer			
a. Follow steps 1 through 5b	❑	❑	
b. Assist patient to the Sims' position	❑	❑	
c. Perform hand hygiene and don clean gloves	❑	❑	
d. Remove thermometer pack from charging unit; make certain correct rectal probe is attached to the unit and slide disposable plastic cover over thermometer probe	❑	❑	
e. Lubricate thermometer probe	❑	❑	
f. Gently spread buttocks and insert thermometer probe appropriately; hold on to thermometer throughout procedure	❑	❑	
g. Hold electronic probe until audible signal occurs; read temperature on digital display	❑	❑	
h. Carefully remove probe from rectum and dispose of plastic cover appropriately	❑	❑	
i. Return probe to storage unit and later return the unit to its charging device	❑	❑	
j. Clean anal area of lubricant and possible feces; remove and dispose of gloves and perform hand hygiene	❑	❑	
k. Assist patient to a position of comfort	❑	❑	
l. Write down reading	❑	❑	
m. Complete procedure by following step 10, a through d	❑	❑	

Student Name_______________________________ Date_______________

	S	U	Comments
8. Obtaining axillary temperature: electronic thermometer			
a. Follow steps 1 through 5b	❑	❑	________
b. Perform hand hygiene and don gloves	❑	❑	________
c. Assist patient to supine or sitting position	❑	❑	________
d. Expose axilla; make certain the area is clean and dry	❑	❑	________
e. Prepare electronic thermometer	❑	❑	________
f. Insert probe into the correct area and position body part correctly	❑	❑	________
g. Hold electronic probe until audible signal occurs and read digital display	❑	❑	________
h. Remove probe from patient's axilla; remove probe cover and dispose correctly	❑	❑	________
i. Return electronic probe to storage well	❑	❑	________
j. Assist patient to regown and position for comfort	❑	❑	________
k. Remove gloves and perform hand hygiene	❑	❑	________
l. Return thermometer to charger base	❑	❑	________
m. Write down reading	❑	❑	________
n. Complete procedure by following step 10, a through d	❑	❑	________
9. Obtaining tympanic temperature: electronic thermometer			
a. Follow steps 1 through 5b	❑	❑	________
b. Perform hand hygiene	❑	❑	________
c. Assist patient to an appropriate position	❑	❑	________
d. Remove hand-held thermometer unit from charging base	❑	❑	________
e. Slide disposable plastic speculum cover over otoscope-like tip	❑	❑	________
f. Follow manufacturer's instructions for tympanic probe positioning	❑	❑	________

	S	U	Comments
(1) Gently tug ear pinna up and back for an adult; down and back for a child	❑	❑	______
(2) Move thermometer gently in a figure-eight fashion	❑	❑	______
(3) Fit ear probe snugly into canal	❑	❑	______
(4) Point toward the nurse, following manufacturer's positioning recommendations	❑	❑	______
g. Depress scan button on hand-held unit and read assessment	❑	❑	______
h. Carefully remove sensor from ear and push release button to eject plastic speculum cover, discarding in proper receptacle	❑	❑	______
i. Return hand-held unit to charging base	❑	❑	______
j. Assist patient to a comfortable position	❑	❑	______
k. Perform hand hygiene	❑	❑	______
l. Write down reading	❑	❑	______
m. Complete procedure by following step 10, a through d	❑	❑	______
10. Postprocedure for measuring body temperature			
a. Compare temperature findings with baseline and normal temperature range for patient's age group	❑	❑	______
b. If temperature is abnormal, repeat procedure; if indicated, choose alternate site or instrument for second reading	❑	❑	______
c. Record temperature on vital sign flow sheet/graphic sheet/nurse's notes correctly and report abnormal findings to nurse in charge or physician	❑	❑	______
d. Do patient teaching	❑	❑	______

Student Name____________________ Date____________

PERFORMANCE CHECKLIST 4-2

Obtaining a Pulse Rate

	S	U	Comments
1. Introduce self	❏	❏	________
2. Identify patient	❏	❏	________
3. Explain procedure	❏	❏	________
4. Prepare for procedure			
a. Assemble all necessary supplies	❏	❏	________
b. Provide privacy	❏	❏	________
5. Perform hand hygiene and don clean gloves as necessary	❏	❏	________
6. Implement procedure			
Count pulse for 60 seconds	❏	❏	________
a. Palpate pulse			
(1) Radial pulse correctly	❏	❏	________
(2) Ulnar pulse correctly	❏	❏	________
(3) Brachial pulse correctly	❏	❏	________
(4) Femoral pulse correctly	❏	❏	________
(5) Popliteal pulse correctly	❏	❏	________
(6) Dorsalis pedis pulse correctly	❏	❏	________
(7) Posterior tibial pulse correctly	❏	❏	________
b. Determine strength of pulse	❏	❏	________
7. Write down rate	❏	❏	________
8. Perform hand hygiene	❏	❏	________
9. Document rate correctly	❏	❏	________
10. Follow up by reporting any abnormal pulse rates	❏	❏	________
11. Do patient teaching	❏	❏	________

Student Name______________________________ Date______________

PERFORMANCE CHECKLIST 4-3

Obtaining an Apical Pulse Rate

	S	U	Comments
1. Introduce self	❑	❑	______
2. Identify patient	❑	❑	______
3. Explain procedure	❑	❑	______
4. Prepare for procedure			
a. Assemble all necessary supplies	❑	❑	______
b. Provide privacy	❑	❑	______
5. Perform hand hygiene	❑	❑	______
6. Implement procedure			
a. Clean stethoscope as recommended	❑	❑	______
b. Position patient and expose patient's chest as necessary	❑	❑	______
c. Place stethoscope against patient's chest in correct position	❑	❑	______
d. Count pulse rate correctly; assist patient to dress	❑	❑	______
7. Write down pulse rate	❑	❑	______
8. Perform hand hygiene	❑	❑	______
9. Document rate correctly	❑	❑	______
10. Report any abnormal pulse rates	❑	❑	______
11. Do patient teaching	❑	❑	______

Student Name______________________________ Date______________

PERFORMANCE CHECKLIST 4-4

OBTAINING A RESPIRATORY RATE

	S	U	Comments
1. Introduce self	❑	❑	______
2. Identify patient	❑	❑	______
3. Explain procedure	❑	❑	______
4. Prepare for procedure			
a. Assemble all necessary supplies	❑	❑	______
b. Provide privacy	❑	❑	______
c. If patient has been active, wait the recommended time	❑	❑	______
d. Position patient comfortably	❑	❑	______
5. Perform hand hygiene	❑	❑	______
6. Implement procedure			
a. Place fingertip as if to obtain a radial pulse	❑	❑	______
b. Observe and count respiratory rate correctly	❑	❑	______
c. Provide comfort	❑	❑	______
7. Write down rate	❑	❑	______
8. Perform hand hygiene	❑	❑	______
9. Document rate correctly	❑	❑	______
10. Report abnormal rates	❑	❑	______
11. Do patient teaching	❑	❑	______

Student Name________________________________ Date______________

PERFORMANCE CHECKLIST 4-5

Obtaining a Blood Pressure Reading

	S	U	Comments
1. Introduce self	❑	❑	______
2. Identify patient	❑	❑	______
3. Explain procedure	❑	❑	______
4. Determine if patient has ingested caffeine or has been smoking and wait the suggested length of time	❑	❑	______
5. Prepare for procedure			
a. Assemble all necessary supplies; determine correct cuff size	❑	❑	______
b. Provide privacy	❑	❑	______
c. Position patient correctly	❑	❑	______
d. Determine site for blood pressure measurement	❑	❑	______
6. Perform hand hygiene	❑	❑	______
7. Implement procedure			
a. Apply cuff correctly	❑	❑	______
b. Palpate radial artery	❑	❑	______
c. Inflate cuff, determine approximate systolic pressure	❑	❑	______
d. Deflate the cuff correctly	❑	❑	______
e. Palpate the brachial artery and place the stethoscope bell/diaphragm correctly	❑	❑	______
f. Correctly reinflate cuff	❑	❑	______
g. Correctly deflate cuff	❑	❑	______
h. Accurately determine blood pressure reading while listening to Korotkoff sounds	❑	❑	______
i. Completely deflate and remove the cuff	❑	❑	______
j. Provide comfort	❑	❑	______

	S	U	Comments
8. Write down rate	❑	❑	______
9. Perform hand hygiene	❑	❑	______
10. Document reading correctly	❑	❑	______
11. Report abnormal readings	❑	❑	______
12. Do patient teaching	❑	❑	______

Student Name________________________ Date____________

PERFORMANCE CHECKLIST 4-6

MEASURING HEIGHT AND WEIGHT

	S	U	Comments
1. Introduce self	❑	❑	______
2. Identify patient	❑	❑	______
3. Explain procedure	❑	❑	______
4. Prepare for procedure			
a. Assemble supplies	❑	❑	______
b. Provide privacy	❑	❑	______
5. Perform hand hygiene	❑	❑	______
6. Implement procedure			
a. Balance scales at zero and place paper towel for patient to stand on	❑	❑	______
b. Place paper towel over base of scale where patient will stand, if patient is barefoot	❑	❑	______
c. Assist patient onto scales correctly	❑	❑	______
d. Measure height correctly	❑	❑	______
e. Measure weight correctly	❑	❑	______
f. Assist patient off scales correctly	❑	❑	______
g. Provide comfort	❑	❑	______
7. Write down measurements	❑	❑	______
8. Perform hand hygiene	❑	❑	______
9. Document measurements	❑	❑	______
10. Follow up by reporting measurement	❑	❑	______

Student Name____________________ Date____________

PERFORMANCE CHECKLIST 10-1

Care of the Body After Death

	S	U	Comments
1. Assemble appropriate equipment	❑	❑	____
2. Perform hand hygiene	❑	❑	____
3. Don clean gloves	❑	❑	____
4. Close patient's eyes and mouth as necessary	❑	❑	____
5. Remove all tubing and other devices from around patient's body unless contraindicated	❑	❑	____
6. Place patient in supine position (do not place one hand on top of the other); elevate head	❑	❑	____
7. Replace soiled dressings with clean ones	❑	❑	____
8. Bathe patient as necessary (place absorbent pad under buttocks)	❑	❑	____
9. Brush or comb hair	❑	❑	____
10. Apply clean gown	❑	❑	____
11. Care for valuables (jewelry) and personal belongings; if wedding band is to remain on the deceased, secure ring to finger with a small strip of tape over ring	❑	❑	____
12. Allow family to view body and remain in room if family wishes; a sheet or light blanket over the body with only the head and upper shoulders exposed will maintain dignity and respect for the deceased; remove unneeded equipment from the room; provide soft lighting and offer chairs	❑	❑	____
13. After the family has left the room, attach special label if patient had a contagious disease	❑	❑	____
14. Close door to room	❑	❑	____
15. Await arrival of ambulance or transfer to morgue	❑	❑	____

	S	U	Comments
Some agencies use a shroud to enclose the body before transfer to morgue. If shroud is to be used, enclose body into shroud at this time			
a. The body is in the dorsal recumbent position; arms are straight at the sides; there is a pillow under the head and shoulders	❑	❑	______
b. Place the body on the shroud	❑	❑	______
c. Bring the top of the shroud down over the head	❑	❑	______
d. Fold the bottom of the shroud over the feet	❑	❑	______
e. Fold the sides over the body, tape or pin the sides together, and attach the identification tag	❑	❑	______
16. Document procedure and disposition of patient's body as well as belongings and valuables	❑	❑	______

Student Name____________________ Date____________

PERFORMANCE CHECKLIST 11-1

Admitting a Patient

	S	U	Comments
1. Perform hand hygiene	❑	❑	____________
2. Prepare the room			
a. Care items in place	❑	❑	____________
b. Bed at proper height and opened	❑	❑	____________
c. Light on	❑	❑	____________
3. Greet the patient and family; introduce self, roommate; project interest and concern	❑	❑	____________
4. Check the ID band and verify its accuracy; in long-term care facilities, the residents do not wear ID bands; a picture of the resident is used for identification purposes	❑	❑	____________
5. Assess immediate needs	❑	❑	____________
6. Orient the patient to the unit: lounge and nurses' station	❑	❑	____________
7. Orient the patient to the room: explain the use of equipment, call light system, bed controls, telephone, and television	❑	❑	____________
8. Explain hospital routines such as visiting hours, meals, and morning wake-up	❑	❑	____________
9. Provide privacy, assist to undress as necessary	❑	❑	____________
10. Properly care for valuables, clothing, and medications	❑	❑	____________
11. Obtain the patient's health history, and do the initial nursing assessment correctly	❑	❑	____________
12. Provide for safety: bed in low position, side rails up, call light within easy reach	❑	❑	____________
13. Begin care as ordered by the physician	❑	❑	____________
14. Invite the family back into the room if they left earlier	❑	❑	____________
15. Perform hand hygiene	❑	❑	____________

	S	U	Comments
16. Record the information correctly on the patient's chart according to agency policy	❑	❑	______
17. Provide the patient and the family time for privacy	❑	❑	______
18. Do patient teaching	❑	❑	______

Student Name________________________________ Date________________

PERFORMANCE CHECKLIST 11-2

TRANSFERRING A PATIENT

	S	U	Comments
1. Perform hand hygiene	❑	❑	________
2. Check physician's order	❑	❑	________
3. Inform the patient and family of transfer	❑	❑	________
4. Notify receiving unit of patient transfer and when to be expected	❑	❑	________
5. Gather the patient's belongings and necessary care items to accompany the patient	❑	❑	________
6. Assist in transferring the patient, usually by wheelchair or stretcher	❑	❑	________
7. Properly introduce patient and family to new unit: nurses and roommate	❑	❑	________
8. Provide a brief summary of medical diagnoses, treatment care plan, and medications; review medical orders with nurse assuming care. If transfer is to another facility, complete an interagency transfer form correctly	❑	❑	________
9. Explain equipment, policies, and procedures that are different on the new unit	❑	❑	________
10. Perform hand hygiene	❑	❑	________
11. Record condition of patient and means of transfer; the nurse on the new unit should also record an assessment of the patient's condition on arrival	❑	❑	________
12. Notify other hospital departments of the transfer as necessary, such as diagnostic imaging, laboratory, switchboard, dietary, and business offices	❑	❑	________
13. For an interagency transfer, dress the patient appropriately; if oxygen is required, a small transport tank may be used; a nurse generally accompanies a critically ill patient who is being transferred	❑	❑	________

	S	U	Comments
14. If patient is a child, adjust procedure appropriately	❑	❑	______
15. Do patient teaching	❑	❑	______

Student Name________________________________ Date________________

PERFORMANCE CHECKLIST 11-3

DISCHARGING A PATIENT

	S	U	Comments
1. Perform hand hygiene	❑	❑	________
2. Verify written discharge order	❑	❑	________
3. Arrange for patient or family to visit business office as necessary	❑	❑	________
4. If no discharge order has been written, have patient sign appropriate AMA form	❑	❑	________
5. Notify the family or person who will be transporting the patient home	❑	❑	________
6. Make certain patient and family understand instructions for care (medications, special diet, exercise)	❑	❑	________
7. Gather equipment, supplies, and prescriptions that the patient is to take home	❑	❑	________
8. Check to see that business office has given a release	❑	❑	________
9. Assist the patient in dressing and packing items to go home	❑	❑	________
10. Check clothing and valuables list made on admission according to policy	❑	❑	________
11. Transfer the patient and belongings via wheelchair to the vehicle; assist patient into the vehicle if needed; as with all procedures, use good communication skills and wish the patient well	❑	❑	________
12. Perform hand hygiene	❑	❑	________
13. Chart entire discharge procedure; document the following: teaching, patient's condition, method of discharge	❑	❑	________
14. If patient is a child, adjust procedure as appropriate	❑	❑	________

Student Name______________________________ Date______________

PERFORMANCE CHECKLIST 12-1

Performing Hand Hygiene

	S	U	Comments
1. Inspect hands, observing for visible soiling, breaks, or cuts in the skin or cuticles	❑	❑	______
2. Determine contaminant of hands	❑	❑	______
3. Assess areas around the hands that are contaminated	❑	❑	______
4. Explain to the patient the importance of handwashing	❑	❑	______
5. Remove jewelry (except plain wedding band) and push watch and long sleeves above wrists	❑	❑	______
6. Adjust the water to appropriate temperature and force	❑	❑	______
7. Wet hands and wrists, keeping hands lower than elbows	❑	❑	______
8. Lather hands with liquid soap	❑	❑	______
9. Perform hand hygiene thoroughly, using a firm, circular motion and friction on back of hands, palms, and wrists; wash each finger individually, paying special attention to areas between fingers and knuckles by interlacing fingers and thumbs and moving hands back and forth, causing friction	❑	❑	______
10. Wash 1 minute thoroughly, rinse thoroughly, re-lather and wash another minute using a continuous amount of friction	❑	❑	______
11. Rinse wrists and hands completely, keeping hands lower than elbows	❑	❑	______
12. Clean fingernails carefully under running water, using fingernails of other hand or blunt end of an orange stick	❑	❑	______
13. Dry hands thoroughly with paper towels	❑	❑	______
14. Turn off faucets with a dry paper towel	❑	❑	______
15. Use hand lotion	❑	❑	______
16. Inspect hands and nails for cleanliness	❑	❑	______

	S	U	Comments
17. If hands are visibly soiled, use an alcohol-based waterless antiseptic for routine decontamination of hands in all clinical situations	❑	❑	______
18. Do patient teaching	❑	❑	______
19. If contamination continues, technique must be reassessed	❑	❑	______

Student Name________________________________ Date______________

PERFORMANCE CHECKLIST 12-2

GLOVING

	S	U	Comments
Donning Gloves			
1. Obtain gloves from dispenser	❑	❑	______________
2. Inspect gloves for perforation	❑	❑	______________
3. Don gloves as recommended	❑	❑	______________
4. Change gloves after direct handling of infectious material such as wound drainage	❑	❑	______________
5. Do not touch side rails, tables, or bed stands with contaminated gloves	❑	❑	______________
Removing Gloves			
6. Remove first glove by grasping outer surface at palm with other gloved hand and pulling glove off and inside out; place this glove in other hand	❑	❑	______________
7. Remove second glove by placing finger under cuff and turning glove inside out and over other glove; drop gloves into waste container	❑	❑	______________
8. Perform hand hygiene	❑	❑	______________
9. Do patient teaching	❑	❑	______________
10. If contamination continues, technique must be reassessed	❑	❑	______________

Student Name________________________________ Date____________

PERFORMANCE CHECKLIST 12-3

GOWNING FOR ISOLATION

	S	U	Comments
1. Remove watch and push up long sleeves	❑	❑	____________
2. Place watch on a paper towel or see-through baggie before taking vital signs	❑	❑	____________
3. Perform hand hygiene	❑	❑	____________
4. Don gown by securely tying gown at neck and waist	❑	❑	____________
5. When finished with patient care, remove gown appropriately	❑	❑	____________
6. Discard soiled gown appropriately	❑	❑	____________
7. Perform hand hygiene	❑	❑	____________
8. Record use of gown in isolation procedure if agency's policy (some agencies charge a daily rate for isolation precautions)	❑	❑	____________
9. Do patient teaching	❑	❑	____________
10. If contamination continues, technique must be reassessed	❑	❑	____________

Student Name________________________________ Date________________

PERFORMANCE CHECKLIST 12-4

DONNING A MASK

	S	U	Comments
1. Obtain a mask	❑	❑	________
2. Don mask when ready to begin patient care by covering the nose, mouth, and eyes (glasses) with the device; a mask with protective eye shield is worn when the risk of splashing is imminent; secure mask in place with elastic band or by tying the strings behind the head	❑	❑	________
3. Wear mask for recommended period of time, until it becomes moist but no longer than 20 to 30 minutes	❑	❑	________
4. Make certain patient feels comfortable and accepted by nurse	❑	❑	________
5. Remove mask by untying the strings or moving the elastic; make certain not to touch mask	❑	❑	________
6. Dispose of soiled mask appropriately	❑	❑	________
7. Perform hand hygiene thoroughly	❑	❑	________
8. Record use of mask during patient care (some agencies require documentation of specific barriers used)	❑	❑	________
9. Do patient teaching	❑	❑	________
10. If contamination continues, technique must be reassessed	❑	❑	________

Student Name________________________________ Date______________

PERFORMANCE CHECKLIST 12-5

ISOLATION TECHNIQUE

	S	U	Comments
1. Determine causative microorganism or effectiveness of patient's immune system	❑	❑	________
2. Recognize mode of transmission and how microorganism exits the body	❑	❑	________
3. Follow agency policy for specific type of isolation used	❑	❑	________
4. Provide an environment with adequate equipment and supplies			
a. Private room or isolation with anteroom	❑	❑	________
b. Place sign stating isolation category	❑	❑	________
c. Adequate handwashing facilities	❑	❑	________
d. Special containers for trash, soiled linen, and sharp instruments such as needles	❑	❑	________
5. Plan time to explain isolation technique to patient, family, and visitors	❑	❑	________
6. Post card on door of patient's room or wall outside room stating the protective measures in use for patient care	❑	❑	________
7. Supply the room with designated lined containers for soiled linens and for trash	❑	❑	________
8. Perform hand hygiene	❑	❑	________
9. Don gloves and appropriate apparel	❑	❑	________
10. Assess vital signs, administer medication, administer hygiene, and collect specimens all in the appropriate manner	❑	❑	________
11. When finished with patient care, remove gloves and apparel per correct protocol	❑	❑	________
12. Perform hand hygiene	❑	❑	________
13. Report changes in the patient's health status	❑	❑	________

	S	U	Comments
14. Record assessments and performance of protective asepsis	❑	❑	
15. Determine patient's level of understanding	❑	❑	
16. Do patient teaching	❑	❑	
17. If contamination continues, technique must be reassessed	❑	❑	
18. Additional techniques for acid-fast bacillus (AFB) isolation			
a. Before entering room, apply recommended mask; be sure it fits snugly	❑	❑	
b. Explain purpose of AFB to patient, family, and others	❑	❑	
c. Offer opportunity for questions	❑	❑	
d. Instruct patient to cover mouth with tissue when coughing and to wear disposable surgical mask when leaving room	❑	❑	
e. The particulate respirator that the health care worker wears is not to be placed on the patient; the added work of breathing through the respirator is an added stress on an already compromised pulmonary system; simply apply a regular surgical mask			
(1) Provide care	❑	❑	
(2) Leave the room and close the door	❑	❑	
(3) Remove respiratory protective device	❑	❑	
(4) Place reusable device in labeled paper bag for storage, being careful not to crush device (check agency policy for number of times it can be reused)	❑	❑	
(5) Perform hand hygiene	❑	❑	
(6) Record assessments and performance of patient care	❑	❑	

Student Name________________________________ Date______________

PERFORMANCE CHECKLIST 12-6

SURGICAL HAND HYGIENE

	S	U	Comments
1. Inspect hands for presence of abrasions, cuts, or open lesions	❑	❑	________
2. Apply surgical shoe covers, cap or hood, face mask, and protective eyewear	❑	❑	________
3. Surgical handwashing			
a. Turn on water using knee or foot control and adjust to comfortable temperature	❑	❑	________
b. Wet hands and arms under running lukewarm water and lather with detergent to 5 cm (2 inches) above elbows (hands need to be above elbows at all times)	❑	❑	________
c. Rinse hands and arms thoroughly under running water	❑	❑	________
d. Under running water, clean under nails of both hands with nail pick; discard after use	❑	❑	________
(1) Wet clean sponge and apply antimicrobial detergent; scrub nails of one hand with 15 strokes; holding sponge perpendicular, scrub palm, each side of thumb and fingers, and posterior side of hand with 10 strokes each	❑	❑	________
(2) Mentally divide arm into thirds; scrub each third 10 times; entire scrub should last 5 to 10 minutes; rinse sponge and repeat sequence for other arm; a two-sponge method may be substituted (check agency policy)	❑	❑	________
e. Discard sponge and rinse hands and arms thoroughly; turn off water with foot or knee control and back into room entrance with hands elevated in front of and away from the body	❑	❑	________

	S	U	Comments
(1) Walk up to sterile tray and lean forward slightly to pick up sterile towel	❑	❑	________
(2) Dry one hand thoroughly, moving from fingers to elbow; dry in a rotating motion, from cleanest to least clean area	❑	❑	________
f. Repeat drying method for other hand by carefully reversing towel or using a new sterile towel	❑	❑	________
g. Discard towel	❑	❑	________
h. Proceed with sterile gowning	❑	❑	________
4. Alternate method using alcohol-based antiseptic			
a. Perform hand hygiene with soap and water for 10 to 15 seconds to remove soil	❑	❑	________
b. Under running water, clean under nails of both hands with nail pick; discard after use and dry hands with a paper towel	❑	❑	________
c. Apply enough alcohol-based waterless antiseptic to one palm to cover both hands thoroughly; spread the antiseptic over all surfaces of the hands and fingernails; follow product instructions for length of time to rub over hand surfaces; allow to air-dry	❑	❑	________
d. Repeat process and allow hands to air-dry before applying sterile gloves	❑	❑	________

Student Name________________________________ Date______________

PERFORMANCE CHECKLIST 12-7

Preparing a Sterile Field

	S	U	Comments
1. Prepare sterile field just before planned procedure; supplies are to be used immediately	❑	❑	________
2. Select clean work surface above waist level	❑	❑	________
3. Assemble necessary equipment			
a. Sterile drape	❑	❑	________
b. Assorted sterile supplies	❑	❑	________
4. Check dates, labels, or condition of package for sterility of equipment	❑	❑	________
5. Perform hand hygiene thoroughly	❑	❑	________
6. Place pack containing sterile drape on work surface and open without contamination	❑	❑	________
7. With fingertips of one hand, pick up folded top edge of sterile drape	❑	❑	________
8. Gently lift drape up from its outer cover and let it unfold by itself without touching any object; discard outer cover with your other hand	❑	❑	________
9. With other hand, grasp adjacent corner of drape and hold it straight up and away from your body; now drape can be properly placed while using two hands; the drape must be held away from unsterile surfaces	❑	❑	________
10. Holding drape, first position the bottom half over intended work surface	❑	❑	________
11. Allow top half of drape to be placed over work surface last	❑	❑	________
12. Perform procedure using sterile technique	❑	❑	________

Student Name________________________________ Date______________

PERFORMANCE CHECKLIST 12-8

Donning a Sterile Gown

	S	U	Comments
1. Don surgical cap, shoe covers, protective eye wear, and mask	❑	❑	______________
2. Perform surgical hand hygiene	❑	❑	______________
2. Ask circulating nurse to open sterile gown and sterile glove packages	❑	❑	______________
3. Don the gown			
a. If available, the scrub nurse will assist by pulling the gown over your extended hands and arms. If there is no assistance from a scrub nurse:			
(1) Pick up the gown touching only the inner surface bellow the neck	❑	❑	______________
(2) Maintain constant control of the folded layers of the gown	❑	❑	______________
(3) While holding the gown at arm's length, allow the gown to unfold from top to bottom; be sure that the gown does not touch the floor	❑	❑	______________
(4) While holding the inside of the gown near the shoulders and below the neckband, slide hands and arms into the sleeves with your fingers stopping at the end of the cuffs	❑	❑	______________
(5) Ask another staff member to grasp the card that is attached to the ties of the gown in order to draw the ties around to the back with the gown overlapping itself; the staff member should now tie the gown, avoiding touching any part of the gown except the ties	❑	❑	______________

Student Name________________________________ Date______________

PERFORMANCE CHECKLIST 12-9

Performing Open Sterile Gloving

	S	U	Comments
1. Obtain proper-sized sterile gloves	❑	❑	________
2. Perform thorough handwashing	❑	❑	________
3. Remove outer glove package wrapper by carefully separating and peeling apart sides	❑	❑	________
4. Grasp inner package and lay it on clean, flat surface just above waist level; open package, keeping gloves on wrapper's inside surface	❑	❑	________
5. Identify right and left gloves; each glove has cuff approximately 2 inches (5 cm) wide; glove dominant hand first	❑	❑	________
6. With thumb and first two fingers of nondominant hand, grasp edge of glove cuff for dominant hand; touch only glove's inside surface	❑	❑	________
7. Carefully pull glove over dominant hand, leaving cuff and being sure cuff does not roll up wrist; be sure thumb and fingers are in proper spaces	❑	❑	________
8. With gloved dominant hand, slip fingers underneath second glove's cuff because the cuff will protect the gloved fingers	❑	❑	________
9. Carefully pull second glove over nondominant hand; do not allow fingers and thumb of gloved dominant hand to touch any part of exposed nondominant hand; keep thumb of dominant hand abducted back	❑	❑	________
10. After second glove is on, interlock hands together; cuffs usually fall down after application	❑	❑	________
Glove Disposal			
11. Grasp outside of one cuff with other gloved hand; avoid touching wrist	❑	❑	________

	S	U	Comments
12. Pull glove off, turning it inside out; discard in receptacle	❑	❑	______________
13. Take fingers of bare hand and tuck inside remaining glove cuff; peel glove off, inside out; discard in receptacle	❑	❑	______________

Student Name____ Date__________________

PERFORMANCE CHECKLIST 12-10

PREPARING FOR DISINFECTION AND STERILIZATION

	S	U	Comments
1. Prepare equipment and assemble supplies			
a. Disinfectant to use for cleansing	❑	❑	
b. Method of sterilization	❑	❑	
c. Gloves	❑	❑	
d. Running water	❑	❑	
e. Scrub brush	❑	❑	
f. Cloth wrapper	❑	❑	
2. Perform hand hygiene	❑	❑	
3. Don gloves	❑	❑	
4. Rinse article under cool running water	❑	❑	
5. Wash article with detergent	❑	❑	
6. Use scrub brush to remove material in grooves	❑	❑	
7. Dry article thoroughly	❑	❑	
8. Prepare article for sterilization by wrapping it in cloth wrapper	❑	❑	
9. Clean work area and put in order	❑	❑	
10. Perform hand hygiene	❑	❑	
11. Do patient teaching	❑	❑	

Student Name________________________ Date____________

PERFORMANCE CHECKLIST 13-1

Changing a Sterile Dry Dressing

	S	U	Comments
Prepare for procedure			
1. Refer to medical record, care plan, or Kardex	❑	❑	________
2. Introduce self	❑	❑	________
3. Identify patient	❑	❑	________
4. Explain the procedure	❑	❑	________
5. Assess need for and provide patient teaching	❑	❑	________
6. Assemble equipment and complete necessary charges	❑	❑	________
7. Perform hand hygiene	❑	❑	________
8. Assess patient	❑	❑	________
9. Prepare patient for intervention			
a. Close door/pull privacy curtain	❑	❑	________
b. Raise bed to comfortable working height; lower side rail on side nearest the nurse	❑	❑	________
c. Position and drape patient as necessary	❑	❑	________
During the skill			
10. Promote patient involvement as possible	❑	❑	________
11. Assess patient's tolerance	❑	❑	________
12. Place refuse container in convenient location away from sterile field	❑	❑	________
13. Set up sterile field correctly	❑	❑	________
14. Loosen tape appropriately	❑	❑	________
15. Don clean gloves	❑	❑	________
16. Remove dressing and discard correctly	❑	❑	________
17. Assess status of wound and wound drainage/exudate correctly	❑	❑	________
18. Remove and discard soiled gloves	❑	❑	________

	S	U	Comments
19. Perform hand hygiene and don sterile gloves	❑	❑	________
20. Cleanse wound and surrounding area correctly	❑	❑	________
21. Use sterile 4 x 4 dressing to dry in same manner or allow antiseptic to air-dry	❑	❑	________
22. Cleanse drain site appropriately if applicable	❑	❑	________
23. Apply antibiotic ointment, if ordered, using same techniques as for cleansing	❑	❑	________
24. Cover wound with appropriately sized dry sterile dressing and use drain dressing, if applicable	❑	❑	________
25. Secure dressing with appropriate tape, Montgomery straps, or binder	❑	❑	________
Postprocedure			
26. Assist patient to a position of comfort and place needed items within easy reach; be certain patient has a means to call for assistance and knows how to use it	❑	❑	________
27. Raise side rails and lower bed to lowest position	❑	❑	________
28. Remove gloves and all protective barriers; dispose of soiled supplies and equipment appropriately	❑	❑	________
29. Perform hand hygiene after patient contact and after wearing gloves	❑	❑	________
30. Document and do patient teaching	❑	❑	________
31. Report any unexpected appearance of wound or drainage or accidental removal of drain within an hour to physician	❑	❑	________

Student Name________________________ Date____________

PERFORMANCE CHECKLIST 13-2

CHANGING A WET-TO-DRY DRESSING

	S	U	Comments
Prepare for procedure			
1. Refer to medical record, care plan, or Kardex	❑	❑	________
2. Introduce self	❑	❑	________
3. Identify patient	❑	❑	________
4. Explain the procedure	❑	❑	________
5. Assess need for and provide patient teaching during procedure	❑	❑	________
6. Assemble equipment and complete necessary charges	❑	❑	________
7. Perform hand hygiene	❑	❑	________
8. Assess patient	❑	❑	________
9. Prepare patient for intervention			
a. Close door/pull privacy curtain	❑	❑	________
b. Raise bed to comfortable working height; lower side rail on side nearest the nurse	❑	❑	________
c. Position and drape patient as necessary	❑	❑	________
During the skill			
10. Promote patient involvement as possible	❑	❑	________
11. Assess patient's tolerance	❑	❑	________
12. Place waterproof pad appropriately	❑	❑	________
13. Place refuse container appropriately	❑	❑	________
14. Set up sterile field	❑	❑	________
15. Loosen tape correctly	❑	❑	________
16. Don clean gloves; remove dressing appropriately and discard	❑	❑	________
17. Assess status of wound and wound exudate/drainage	❑	❑	________

	S	U	Comments
18. Remove gloves and discard; perform hand hygiene and don sterile gloves	❑	❑	______
19. Cleanse wound correctly	❑	❑	______
20. Place 4 x 4 dressing into basin	❑	❑	______
21. Wring excess solution from dressing, leaving it slightly moist	❑	❑	______
22. Place dressing over open wound surfaces and press into depressed areas	❑	❑	______
23. Apply dry dressing over wet dressing	❑	❑	______
24. Cover with additional dressing as needed	❑	❑	______
25. Secure with tape or Montgomery straps	❑	❑	______

Postprocedure

26. Assist patient to a position of comfort and place needed items within easy reach; be certain patient has a means to call for assistance and knows how to use it	❑	❑	______
27. Raise side rails and lower bed to lowest position	❑	❑	______
28. Remove gloves and all protective barriers; dispose of soiled supplies and equipment appropriately	❑	❑	______
29. Perform hand hygiene after patient contact and after wearing gloves	❑	❑	______
30. Document and do patient teaching	❑	❑	______
31. Discuss change in dressing procedure with physician as wound surface becomes clean and granulation tissue is evident	❑	❑	______

Student Name______________________________ Date______________

PERFORMANCE CHECKLIST 13-3

APPLYING A TRANSPARENT DRESSING

	S	U	Comments
Prepare for procedure			
1. Refer to medical record, care plan, or Kardex	❏	❏	______
2. Introduce self	❏	❏	______
3. Identify patient	❏	❏	______
4. Explain procedure	❏	❏	______
5. Assess need for and provide patient teaching during procedure	❏	❏	______
6. Assemble equipment and complete necessary charges	❏	❏	______
7. Perform hand hygiene	❏	❏	______
8. Assess patient	❏	❏	______
9. Prepare patient for intervention			
a. Provide privacy	❏	❏	______
b. Raise bed to working height and lower nearest side rail	❏	❏	______
c. Position and drape patient as necessary	❏	❏	______
During the skill			
10. Promote patient involvement as possible	❏	❏	______
11. Assess patient's tolerance	❏	❏	______
12. Place refuse container in convenient location away from contamination	❏	❏	______
13. Set up sterile field	❏	❏	______
14. Don clean gloves	❏	❏	______
15. Loosen tape and remove old dressings	❏	❏	______
16. Remove soiled gloves and with soiled dressings dispose of in refuse container	❏	❏	______
17. Assess status of wound	❏	❏	______

	S	U	Comments
18. Don sterile gloves	❑	❑	______
19. Cleanse area gently	❑	❑	______
20. Allow skin surface to dry	❑	❑	______
21. Apply transparent dressings according to manufacturer's direction	❑	❑	______
22. Remove soiled gloves and discard; perform hand hygiene	❑	❑	______
Postprocedure			
23. Assist patient to a position of comfort and place needed items within easy reach	❑	❑	______
24. Raise side rails and lower bed to lowest position	❑	❑	______
25. Remove gloves and all protective barriers; dispose of soiled supplies and equipment appropriately	❑	❑	______
26. Perform hand hygiene after patient contact and after wearing gloves	❑	❑	______
27. Document	❑	❑	______
28. Report any unexpected appearance of the wound or exudate	❑	❑	______
29. Do patient teaching	❑	❑	______

Student Name______________________________ Date______________

PERFORMANCE CHECKLIST 13-4

PERFORMING A STERILE IRRIGATION

	S	U	Comments
Prepare for procedure			
1. Refer to medical record, care plan, or Kardex for special interventions	❑	❑	______
2. Introduce self	❑	❑	______
3. Identify patient	❑	❑	______
4. Explain the procedure	❑	❑	______
5. Assess need for and provide patient teaching during procedure	❑	❑	______
6. Assemble equipment and complete necessary charges	❑	❑	______
7. Perform hand hygiene	❑	❑	______
8. Assess patient	❑	❑	______
9. Prepare patient for intervention			
a. Close door/pull privacy curtain	❑	❑	______
b. Raise bed to comfortable working height; lower side rail on side nearest the nurse	❑	❑	______
c. Position and drape patient as necessary	❑	❑	______
During the skill			
10. Promote patient involvement as possible	❑	❑	______
11. Assess patient's tolerance	❑	❑	______
12. Position waterproof pad appropriately	❑	❑	______
13. Place refuse container in convenient location away from contamination	❑	❑	______
14. Set up sterile field	❑	❑	______
15. Don gown and goggles as appropriate	❑	❑	______
16. Don clean gloves, remove dressing, and discard appropriately	❑	❑	______
17. Remove gloves, dispose of in proper receptacle, and perform hand hygiene	❑	❑	______

	S	U	Comments
18. Assess status of wound and exudate/drainage	❑	❑	________
19. Place collection basin appropriately	❑	❑	________
20. Perform hand hygiene and don sterile gloves	❑	❑	________
21. Cleanse area around wound correctly	❑	❑	________
22. Fill irrigating syringe with solution; attach soft catheter if irrigating a deep wound with small opening	❑	❑	________
23. Instill solution gently into wound, holding syringe approximately 1 inch above wound; if using catheter, gently insert into wound opening until slight resistance is met, pull back, and gently instill solution	❑	❑	________
24. Allow solution to flow from clean area of wound to dirty area	❑	❑	________
25. Pinch off catheter during withdrawal from wound	❑	❑	________
26. Refill syringe and continue irrigation until solution returns clear	❑	❑	________
27. Blot wound edges with sterile dressing	❑	❑	________
28. Redress wound, if applicable	❑	❑	________
29. Remove and dispose of gloves	❑	❑	________
30. Perform hand hygiene	❑	❑	________
Postprocedure			
31. Assist patient to a position of comfort and place needed items within easy reach; be certain patient has a means to call for assistance and knows how to use it	❑	❑	________
32. Raise side rails and lower bed to lowest position	❑	❑	________
33. Remove gloves and all protective barriers; dispose of soiled supplies and equipment appropriately	❑	❑	________
34. Perform hand hygiene after patient contact and after wearing gloves	❑	❑	________
35. Document and do patient teaching	❑	❑	________
36. Report immediately any evidence of fresh bleeding, sharp increase in pain, retention of irrigant, or signs of shock to attending physician	❑	❑	________

Student Name________________________ Date____________

PERFORMANCE CHECKLIST 13-5

Removing Staples or Sutures (Applying Steri-Strips)

	S	U	Comments
Prepare for procedure			
1. Refer to medical record, care plan, or Kardex	❑	❑	________
2. Introduce self	❑	❑	________
3. Identify patient	❑	❑	________
4. Explain the procedure	❑	❑	________
5. Assess need for and provide patient teaching during procedure	❑	❑	________
6. Assemble equipment and complete necessary charges	❑	❑	________
7. Perform hand hygiene	❑	❑	________
8. Assess patient	❑	❑	________
9. Prepare patient for intervention			
a. Close door/pull privacy curtain	❑	❑	________
b. Raise bed to comfortable working height; lower side rail on side nearest the nurse	❑	❑	________
c. Position and drape patient as necessary	❑	❑	________
During the skill			
10. Promote patient involvement as possible	❑	❑	________
11. Assess patient's tolerance, being alert for signs and symptoms of discomfort and fatigue	❑	❑	________
12. Place refuse container in convenient location away from sterile field	❑	❑	________
13. Set up sterile field	❑	❑	________
14. Don clean gloves	❑	❑	________
15. Remove dressing and soiled gloves; discard appropriately	❑	❑	________
16. Assess status of wound and drainage on dressing correctly	❑	❑	________

	S	U	Comments
17. Perform hand hygiene and don sterile gloves	❑	❑	______
18. Cleanse area correctly	❑	❑	______
Staple removal			
19. Place staple remover under both sides of staple; squeeze handles together and gently remove staples from skin	❑	❑	______
20. Release handles and discard staple in refuse container	❑	❑	______
21. Repeat steps 19 and 20 until all staples have been removed	❑	❑	______
22. Count number of staples removed	❑	❑	______
23. Notify physician immediately if inadequate wound healing is noted; discontinue removal of all staples	❑	❑	______
Applying Steri-Strips			
24. It is common to see wounds closed with Steri-Strips; these interventions should be followed when applying Steri-Strips			
a. Gently cleanse suture line	❑	❑	______
b. Carefully inspect the incision	❑	❑	______
c. When skin is dry, apply Steri-Strips	❑	❑	______
d. Instruct patient to take showers rather than soak in bathtub according to physician's preference	❑	❑	______
e. Many physicians request upon removal of sutures that only 1–3 sutures be removed at a time; Steri-Strips are then applied, repeating this action until all sutures are removed and Steri-Strips applied	❑	❑	______
25. Assess healing status of wound	❑	❑	______
26. Cleanse area with antiseptic swabs	❑	❑	______
Removal of intermittent sutures			
27. Grasp and elevate knotted end of suture with hemostat or forceps	❑	❑	______

Student Name________________________________ Date______________

	S	U	Comments
28. Snip suture at skin level on opposite side, proximal to knot	❑	❑	________
29. Gently remove entire suture with forceps and discard on sterile gauze	❑	❑	________
30. Repeat steps 27 to 29 until all sutures have been removed	❑	❑	________
Removal of continuous sutures including blanket stitch sutures			
31. Cut first suture close to skin on side away from knot	❑	❑	________
32. Remove gently from knotted side with forceps and discard on sterile gauze	❑	❑	________
33. Snip second suture on same side	❑	❑	________
34. Repeat steps 31 to 33 until all sutures have been removed	❑	❑	________
35. Apply sterile dressing or leave open to air as ordered	❑	❑	________
36. Remove gloves and perform hand hygiene	❑	❑	________
Postprocedure			
37. Assist patient to a position of comfort and place needed items within easy reach; be certain patient has a means to call for assistance and knows how to use it	❑	❑	________
38. Raise side rails and lower bed to lowest position	❑	❑	________
39. Remove gloves and all protective barriers; dispose of soiled supplies and equipment appropriately	❑	❑	________
40. Perform hand hygiene after patient contact and after wearing gloves	❑	❑	________
41. Document and do patient teaching	❑	❑	________
42. Report any abnormalities	❑	❑	________

Student Name____ Date____________________

PERFORMANCE CHECKLIST 13-6

Maintaining Hemovac or Davol Suction and T-tube Drainage

	S	U	Comments
Prepare for procedure			
1. Refer to medical record, care plan, or Kardex	❑	❑	____________
2. Introduce self	❑	❑	____________
3. Identify patient	❑	❑	____________
4. Explain the procedure	❑	❑	____________
5. Assess need for and provide patient teaching	❑	❑	____________
6. Assemble equipment and complete necessary charges	❑	❑	____________
7. Perform hand hygiene	❑	❑	____________
8. Assess patient	❑	❑	____________
Prepare patient for intervention			
9. Close door/pull privacy curtain	❑	❑	____________
10. Raise bed to comfortable working height; lower side rail on side nearest the nurse	❑	❑	____________
11. Position and drape patient as necessary	❑	❑	____________
During the skill			
12. Promote patient involvement as possible	❑	❑	____________
13. Assess patient's tolerance	❑	❑	____________
14. Examine drainage system	❑	❑	____________
15. Don goggles as appropriate	❑	❑	____________
16. Don clean gloves	❑	❑	____________
17. Remove Hemovac/Davol plug labeled "pouring spout;" empty drainage into measuring device, handling device correctly	❑	❑	____________
18. Hold pump of Hemovac tightly compressed and reinsert plug; when caring for a Davol, repump to reestablish suction	❑	❑	____________
19. T-tube maintenance			
a. Remove plug, holding drainage spout over calibrated container	❑	❑	____________

	S	U	Comments
b. Empty drainage into measuring container and replace plug, maintaining sterility	❑	❑	______
c. Always keep drainage bag below the level of the common bile duct to prevent contamination from backflow; may be fastened to patient's gown. Be very careful to prevent tension on and displacement of T-tube	❑	❑	______
20. Observe the drainage	❑	❑	______
21. Measure and record amount of drainage; rinse measuring container	❑	❑	______
22. Position drainage system on bed and secure system	❑	❑	______
23. Dispose of drainage and rinse measuring container	❑	❑	______
Postprocedure			
24. Remove gloves and all protective barriers; dispose of soiled supplies and equipment appropriately	❑	❑	______
25. Perform hand hygiene after patient contact and after wearing gloves	❑	❑	______
26. Assist patient to a position of comfort and place needed items within easy reach; be certain patient has a means to call for assistance and knows how to use it	❑	❑	______
27. Raise side rails and lower bed to lowest position	❑	❑	______
28. If specimen is ordered, label and send to laboratory	❑	❑	______
29. Perform hand hygiene after patient contact	❑	❑	______
30. Observe Davol/Hemovac/T-tube every 2–4 hours; measure drainage	❑	❑	______
31. Document and do patient teaching	❑	❑	______
32. Report any abnormal characteristics of drainage. Normal amounts of bile drainage vary from 250–500 mL for 24 hours; normal characteristics are thick consistency with greenish-brown color, slightly blood-tinged in the first 24 hours (excessive bile leakage from wound can indicate an occluded system; notify physician)	❑	❑	______

Student Name____ Date________________

PERFORMANCE CHECKLIST 13-7

Wound Vacuum-Assisted Closure

	S	U	Comments
Prepare for procedure			
1. Refer to medical record, care plan, or Kardex	❑	❑	________
2. Introduce self	❑	❑	________
3. Identify patient	❑	❑	________
4. Explain procedure and the reason for it	❑	❑	________
5. Assess need for and provide patient teaching	❑	❑	________
6. Assemble equipment and complete necessary charges	❑	❑	________
7. Perform hand hygiene and don clean gloves	❑	❑	________
8. Assess patient	❑	❑	________
9. Prepare patient for intervention			
a. Close door and pull privacy curtain	❑	❑	________
b. Raise bed to a comfortable working height, lower side rail closest to nurse	❑	❑	________
c. Position and drape patient as necessary	❑	❑	________
During the skill			
10. Promote patient involvement as possible	❑	❑	________
11. Assess patient's tolerance	❑	❑	________
12. Place disposable waterproof bag within work area with top folded down to make a cuff	❑	❑	________
13. When VAC® is in place, begin by pushing therapy on/off button	❑	❑	________
a. Keeping tube connection with VAC® unit, disconnect tubes from each other to drain fluids into canister	❑	❑	________
b. Before lowering, tighten clamps on canister tube	❑	❑	________

	S	U	Comments
14. With dressing tube unclamped, introduce 10–30 mL of normal saline, if ordered, into tubing to soak underneath foam	❑	❑	______
15. Gently stretch transparent film horizontally and slowly pull up from the skin	❑	❑	______
16. Remove old VAC® dressing and observe; discard dressings and remove gloves; perform hand hygiene	❑	❑	______
17. Apply sterile or clean gloves (new surgical wound calls for sterile technique; chronic wound may use clean technique); irrigate wound with solution ordered by physician; gently blot dry	❑	❑	______
18. Measure wound as ordered; remove and discard gloves	❑	❑	______
19. Apply clean gloves or sterile gloves (depending on type of wound)	❑	❑	______
20. Prepare VAC® foam			
a. Select appropriate foam	❑	❑	______
b. Using sterile scissors, cut foam to wound size	❑	❑	______
21. Gently place foam into wound making certain that foam is in contact with entire wound base	❑	❑	______
22. Apply tubing to foam in the wound	❑	❑	______
a. For deep wounds, regularly reposition tubing to minimize pressure on wound edges	❑	❑	______
b. Patients with restricted mobility or sensation must be repositioned frequently so they do not lie on the tubing	❑	❑	______
23. Apply skin protectant to wound edges	❑	❑	______
24. Apply wound VAC® dressing			
a. Cover VAC® foam	❑	❑	______
b. Apply wrinkle-free transparent dressing	❑	❑	______
c. Secure tubing to transparent film; ensure occlusive seal	❑	❑	______
25. Secure tubing several centimeters away from dressings	❑	❑	______

Student Name____ Date____________________

	S	U	Comments
26. Once wound is completely covered, connect tubing from dressing to tubing from canister and VAC® unit			
a. Remove canister from sterile packaging and push into VAC® unit until a click is heard	❑	❑	________
b. Connect dressing tubing to canister tubing; make certain both clamps are opened	❑	❑	________
c. Place VAC® unit on level surface or hang from foot of bed	❑	❑	________
d. Press green-lit power button and set pressure as ordered	❑	❑	________
27. Discard all dressing material; remove gloves; perform hand hygiene	❑	❑	________
28. Inspect wound VAC® system to verify that negative pressure is achieved			
a. Verify that display screen reads "therapy on"	❑	❑	________
b. Be sure clamps are open and tubing is patent	❑	❑	________
c. Identify air leaks	❑	❑	________
d. If leak is present, seal with strips of transparent film	❑	❑	________
Postprocedure			
29. Assist patient to a position of comfort and place needed items within easy reach; be certain patient has a means to call for assistance and knows how to use it	❑	❑	________
30. Raise side rails and lower bed to lowest position	❑	❑	________
31. Remove gloves and all protective barriers; dispose of soiled supplies and equipment appropriately	❑	❑	________
32. Perform hand hygiene after patient contact and after wearing gloves	❑	❑	________
33. Document and do patient teaching	❑	❑	________
34. Report any unexpected appearance of wound or drainage	❑	❑	________

Student Name________________________ Date____________

PERFORMANCE CHECKLIST 13-8

APPLYING A BANDAGE

	S	U	Comments
Prepare for procedure			
1. Refer to medical record, care plan, or Kardex	❑	❑	________
2. Introduce self	❑	❑	________
3. Identify patient	❑	❑	________
4. Explain the procedure	❑	❑	________
5. Assess need for and provide patient teaching during procedure	❑	❑	________
6. Assemble equipment and complete necessary charges	❑	❑	________
7. Perform hand hygiene	❑	❑	________
8. Assess patient	❑	❑	________
9. Prepare patient for intervention			
a. Close door/pull privacy curtain	❑	❑	________
b. Raise bed to comfortable working height; lower side rail on side nearest the nurse	❑	❑	________
c. Position and drape patient as necessary	❑	❑	________
During the skill			
10. Promote patient involvement as possible	❑	❑	________
11. Assess patient's tolerance	❑	❑	________
12. Ensure that skin and/or dressing is clean and dry	❑	❑	________
13. Separate any adjacent skin surfaces	❑	❑	________
14. Don gloves as necessary	❑	❑	________
15. Align part to be bandaged appropriately	❑	❑	________
16. Apply bandage from distal to proximal part	❑	❑	________
17. Apply bandage correctly			
a. Circular bandage	❑	❑	________

	S	U	Comments
b. Spiral bandage	❑	❑	______
c. Spiral-reverse bandage	❑	❑	______
d. Recurrent (stump) bandage	❑	❑	______
e. Figure-eight bandage	❑	❑	______
18. Secure first bandage before applying additional rolls	❑	❑	______
19. Apply additional rolls without leaving any uncovered areas	❑	❑	______
20. Assess tension of bandage and circulation of extremity	❑	❑	______
Postprocedure			
21. Assist patient to a position of comfort and place needed items within easy reach; be certain patient has a means to call for assistance and knows how to use it	❑	❑	______
22. Raise side rails and lower bed to lowest position	❑	❑	______
23. Remove gloves and all protective barriers; dispose of soiled supplies and equipment appropriately	❑	❑	______
24. Perform hand hygiene after patient contact and after wearing gloves	❑	❑	______
25. Document and do patient teaching	❑	❑	______
26. Report any unexpected outcomes	❑	❑	______

Student Name________________________ Date____________

PERFORMANCE CHECKLIST 13-9

Applying a Binder, Arm Sling, and T-binder

	S	U	Comments
Prepare for procedure			
1. Refer to medical record, care plan, or Kardex	❏	❏	________
2. Introduce self	❏	❏	________
3. Identify patient	❏	❏	________
4. Explain the procedure	❏	❏	________
5. Assess need for and provide patient teaching during procedure	❏	❏	________
6. Assemble equipment and complete necessary charges	❏	❏	________
7. Perform hand hygiene	❏	❏	________
8. Assess patient	❏	❏	________
9. Prepare patient for intervention			
a. Close door/pull privacy curtain	❏	❏	________
b. Raise bed to comfortable working height; lower side rail on side nearest the nurse	❏	❏	________
c. Position and drape patient as necessary	❏	❏	________
During the skill			
10. Promote patient involvement as possible	❏	❏	________
11. Assess patient's tolerance	❏	❏	________
12. Don gloves as necessary	❏	❏	________
13. Change dressing if appropriate; cleanse skin if needed	❏	❏	________
14. Separate skin surfaces or pad bony prominences	❏	❏	________
15. Apply binder	❏	❏	________
a. Triangular binder (sling)			
(1) Have patient flex arm at approximately 80-degree angle, depending on purpose of binder	❏	❏	________

	S	U	Comments
(2) Place end of triangular binder over shoulder of the uninjured side	❑	❑	________
(3) Grasp other end of binder and bring it up and over injured arm to shoulder of injured arm	❑	❑	________
(4) Use square knot to tie two ends together at lateral area of neck on uninjured side	❑	❑	________
(5) Support wrist well with binder; do not allow it to extend over end of binder	❑	❑	________
(6) Fold third triangle end neatly around elbow and secure with safety pins	❑	❑	________
b. T-binder			
(1) Using appropriate binder, place the waistband smoothly under patient's waist; tail(s) should be under patient	❑	❑	________
(2) Secure two ends of waistband together with safety pin	❑	❑	________
(3) Single tail—bring the tail up between legs to secure dressing in place; two tails—bring tails up one on each side of penis or large dressing	❑	❑	________
(4) Bring tails under and over waistband; secure with safety pins	❑	❑	________
c. Elastic abdominal binder			
(1) Center binder smoothly under appropriate part of patient	❑	❑	________
(2) Bring ends around patient and overlap away from incision	❑	❑	________
(3) Secure binder with Velcro or safety pins placed horizontally on abdomen	❑	❑	________
d. For postsurgical application of scultetus abdominal binder, proceed upward from the bottom, attach each set of tails with safety pins away from incision	❑	❑	________
16. Note comfort level of patient and smooth binder to prevent wrinkles	❑	❑	________

Student Name____ Date____________________

	S	U	Comments
Postprocedure			
17. Assist patient to a position of comfort and place needed items within easy reach; be certain patient has a means to call for assistance and knows how to use it	❑	❑	________________
18. Raise side rails and lower bed to lowest position	❑	❑	________________
19. Remove gloves and all protective barriers; dispose of soiled supplies and equipment appropriately	❑	❑	________________
20. Perform hand hygiene after patient contact and after wearing gloves	❑	❑	________________
21. Document and do patient teaching	❑	❑	________________
22. Report any unexpected outcomes	❑	❑	________________

Student Name________________________________ Date____________

PERFORMANCE CHECKLIST 14-1

Applying Safety Reminder Devices

	S	U	Comments
1. Refer to medical record, care plans, and Kardex; review agency policy	❑	❑	____________
2. Perform hand hygiene	❑	❑	____________
3. Introduce self	❑	❑	____________
4. Identify patient	❑	❑	____________
5. Procedure			
a. Explain procedure	❑	❑	____________
b. Provide privacy and assemble necessary supplies	❑	❑	____________
c. Assess patient for need of SRD (a comprehensive nursing assessment of the patient's potential for injury / treatment related to need for SRD, is crucial before application of SRD)	❑	❑	____________
6. Obtain written permission for application of SRD	❑	❑	____________
7. Apply appropriate type of SRD			
a. Wrist or ankle (extremity) SRD			
(1) If using Kerlix gauze, make a clove hitch correctly (form a figure-eight and pick up loops)	❑	❑	____________
(2) Pad the extremity appropriately	❑	❑	____________
(3) Slip the wrist(s) or ankle(s) through loops directly over the padding; if using a commercially made SRD, wrap the padded portion of the device around affected extremity, thread tie through slit in SRD, and fasten to second tie with a secure knot correctly	❑	❑	____________

	S	U	Comments
(4) Secure ends of ties to movable portion of bed frame that moves with the patient when the bed is adjusted, *not to side rails*	❑	❑	________
(5) Leave as much slack as possible	❑	❑	________
(6) Palpate pulses below the SRD	❑	❑	________
b. Elbow SRD			
(1) Place SRD over the elbow(s)	❑	❑	________
(2) Wrap SRD snugly, tying the SRD at the top. For small infants, tie or pin SRDs to their shirts	❑	❑	________
c. Vest			
(1) Apply device over the patient's gown	❑	❑	________
(2) Put vest on patient with V-shaped opening in the front	❑	❑	________
(3) Pull tie at end of vest flap across the chest, and slip tie through slip on opposite side of vest	❑	❑	________
(4) Wrap the other end of the flap across patient and secure the straps to frame of bed or behind wheelchair; use the quick-release knot	❑	❑	________
(5) Allow enough space between the vest and the patient appropriately (there should be room for a fist in the space between the vest and the patient)	❑	❑	________
d. Gait or safety reminder belts			
(1) Apply belt over patient's gown	❑	❑	________
(2) If patient is ambulating, place belt around the patient's waist	❑	❑	________
(3) If the belt does not have a buckle, fasten in slip knot	❑	❑	________
8. A quick-release knot rather than a regular knot should be used to secure the safety reminder devices to the bed frame	❑	❑	________
9. Secure SRDs so that the patient cannot unfasten them	❑	❑	________

Student Name________________________________ Date________________

	S	U	Comments
10. Apply SRD with gentleness and compassion	❑	❑	________
11. Perform hand hygiene	❑	❑	________
12. Document procedure completely and accurately	❑	❑	________
13. Follow-up			
a. Monitor for skin impairment	❑	❑	________
b. With the use of extremity SRD, assess extremity distal to SRD at least every 30 minutes	❑	❑	________
(1) Remove SRD on one extremity at a time at least every 2 hours for 5 minutes	❑	❑	________
c. Monitor position of SRD, circulation, and skin condition	❑	❑	________
d. With the use of vest SRD, monitor respiratory status	❑	❑	________
e. SRD should be removed at least every 2 hours; patient should NOT be left unattended during this time	❑	❑	________
f. Massage skin beneath SRD; lotion or powder may be applied	❑	❑	________
g. SRD should be changed when soiled or wet	❑	❑	________
h. Check frequently for tangled ties or pressure points from knots; adjust SRD device(s) as needed	❑	❑	________
i. Monitor and document physical and mental status, circulation, and need for SRD; SRDs should be removed when they are no longer needed	❑	❑	________
j. If SRD use is necessary because of changes in the patient's condition, document the changes and efforts to calm or safeguard the patient without SRD use	❑	❑	________
k. Assess for any related problems	❑	❑	________
14. Evaluation			
a. The SRD is adequate and appropriate for the individual patient's condition	❑	❑	________

	S	U	Comments
b. SRDs are correctly applied	❑	❑	________
c. Quick-release knots are easily released	❑	❑	________
d. Related problems, such as to the skin or the musculoskeletal system, are identified	❑	❑	________
15. Do patient teaching	❑	❑	________
16. Mummy restraint for infants and children (person applying restraint should not be parent or guardian)			
a. Open a blanket and fold one corner toward center; place infant on blanket with shoulders at fold and feet toward opposite corner	❑	❑	________
b. With infant's arm straight down against the body, pull right side of blanket firmly across right shoulder and chest, and secure beneath left side of body	❑	❑	________
c. Place left arm straight against body, bring left side of blanket across shoulder and chest, and lock beneath infant's body on right side	❑	❑	________
d. Align infant's legs, pull corner of blanket near feet up toward body, and tuck snugly in place or fasten securely with safety pins	❑	❑	________
e. Remain with infant while restrained and remove restraint immediately after treatment is complete; if restraint is required for an extended period of time, remove at least every 2 hours and perform range of motion exercise on all extremities	❑	❑	________

Student Name______________________________ Date______________

PERFORMANCE CHECKLIST 15-1

POSITIONING PATIENTS

	S	U	Comments
1. Assess patient's body alignment and comfort level while patient is lying down	❑	❑	______
2. Assemble equipment and supplies	❑	❑	______
3. Request assistance as needed	❑	❑	______
4. Introduce self	❑	❑	______
5. Identify patient	❑	❑	______
6. Explain procedure	❑	❑	______
7. Perform hand hygiene	❑	❑	______
8. Prepare patient			
a. Close doors	❑	❑	______
b. Raise level of bed	❑	❑	______
c. Remove pillows and devices used in previous position	❑	❑	______
d. Position bed flat or as low as patient is able to tolerate and lower side rail closest to nurse	❑	❑	______
9. Position patient			
a. Dorsal supine position			
(1) Place patient on back with head flat	❑	❑	______
(2) Place small rolled towel under lumbar spine	❑	❑	______
(3) Place pillow under upper shoulders, neck, and head	❑	❑	______
(4) Place trochanter roll or sandbag along lateral surface of thighs	❑	❑	______
(5) Place small pillow or roll under back of ankles to elevate heels	❑	❑	______
(6) Support feet with firm pillows, footboard, or high-top sneakers	❑	❑	______

	S	U	Comments
(7) Place pillows under pronated forearms, keeping upper arms parallel to patient's body	❑	❑	______
(8) Place hand rolls in patient's hands	❑	❑	______
b. Dorsal recumbent			
(1) Lower head of bed	❑	❑	______
(2) Move patient and mattress to head of bed	❑	❑	______
(3) Turn patient onto back	❑	❑	______
(4) Assist patient to raise legs, bend knees, and allow legs to relax	❑	❑	______
(5) Replace pillow	❑	❑	______
c. Fowler's			
(1) Move patient and mattress to head of bed	❑	❑	______
(2) Raise head of bed to 45–60 degrees	❑	❑	______
(3) Replace pillow	❑	❑	______
(4) Use footboard	❑	❑	______
(5) Use pillows to support arms and hands if needed	❑	❑	______
(6) Place small pillow or roll under ankles	❑	❑	______
d. Semi-Fowler's			
(1) Move patient and mattress to head of bed and remove pillow	❑	❑	______
(2) Raise head of bed to 30 degrees	❑	❑	______
(3) Replace pillow	❑	❑	______
e. Orthopneic			
(1) Elevate head of bed to 90 degrees	❑	❑	______
(2) Place pillow between patient's back and mattress	❑	❑	______
(3) Place pillow on overbed table and assist patient to lean over, placing head on pillow	❑	❑	______

Student Name________________________ Date____________

	S	U	Comments
f. Sims' position			
(1) Place patient in supine position	❑	❑	______
(2) Place patient in left lateral position, lying partially on the abdomen	❑	❑	______
(3) Draw right knee and thigh up near abdomen and support with pillows	❑	❑	______
(4) Place patient's left arm along back	❑	❑	______
(5) Bring right arm up, flex elbow, and support with pillow	❑	❑	______
(6) Allow patient to lean forward to rest on chest	❑	❑	______
g. Prone			
(1) Assist patient onto abdomen with face to one side	❑	❑	______
(2) Flex arms toward the head	❑	❑	______
(3) Position pillows for comfort	❑	❑	______
h. Knee-chest (genupectoral)			
(1) Turn patient onto abdomen	❑	❑	______
(2) Assist patient to kneeling position; arms and head should rest on pillow while upper chest rests on bed	❑	❑	______
i. Lithotomy			
(1) Position patient to lie supine	❑	❑	______
(2) Request patient to slide buttocks to the edge at end of examining table	❑	❑	______
(3) Lift both legs, have patient bend knees, and place feet in stirrups	❑	❑	______
(4) Drape patient appropriately	❑	❑	______
(5) May need a small lumbar pillow	❑	❑	______

	S	U	Comments
j. Trendelenburg's			
(1) Place patient's head lower than body with body and legs elevated and on an incline (foot of bed may be elevated on blocks); Trendelenburg position is not used to treat shock because of pressure it causes on diaphragm by organs in the abdomen	❑	❑	______
10. Reassess patient for			
a. Proper body alignment	❑	❑	______
b. Comfort	❑	❑	______
c. Skin integrity	❑	❑	______
d. Respiratory difficulty	❑	❑	______
e. Tolerance of position	❑	❑	______
f. Reposition every 2 hours	❑	❑	______
11. Perform hand hygiene	❑	❑	______
12. Document appropriate alignment and position of patient	❑	❑	______
13. Do patient teaching	❑	❑	______

Student Name____ Date__________________

PERFORMANCE CHECKLIST 15-2

PERFORMING RANGE-OF-MOTION EXERCISES

	S	U	Comments
1. Refer to medical record, care plan, or Kardex for special interventions	❑	❑	____________
2. Assemble equipment	❑	❑	____________
3. Introduce self	❑	❑	____________
4. Identify patient	❑	❑	____________
5. Explain procedure	❑	❑	____________
6. Perform hand hygiene; don clean gloves according to agency policy and guidelines from CDC and OSHA	❑	❑	____________
7. Prepare for procedure by providing privacy and assembling necessary supplies	❑	❑	____________
8. Assist patient to a comfortable position, either sitting or lying down	❑	❑	____________
9. Medicate patient as needed	❑	❑	____________
10. Begin by following exercises in sequence; each movement should be repeated 5 times during exercise period; discontinue if patient complains of pain or if there is resistance or muscle spasm	❑	❑	____________
11. Assist patient in putting each joint through full ROM, appropriately supporting the body part being exercised	❑	❑	____________
a. Neck—Place palm of each hand against side of patient's face, or place one hand under patient's head and one hand on patient's chin; begin by following exercise in sequence; each movement should be repeated 5 times during the exercise period	❑	❑	____________
(1) Bring head forward until chin touches sternum	❑	❑	____________
(2) Return head to straight position and have patient look straight ahead	❑	❑	____________
(3) Bend head backward with chin positioned toward ceiling	❑	❑	____________
(4) Return head to extension	❑	❑	____________

	S	U	Comments
(5) Bend head laterally with ear toward shoulder, first toward right ear then left ear	❑	❑	________
b. Shoulder—Cup one hand beneath elbow, and grasp wrist with other hand			
(1) Bring arm away from body	❑	❑	________
(2) Return arm toward side of body	❑	❑	________
(3) Abduct the arm; continue movement until patient's hand is toward head of bed	❑	❑	________
(4) Abduct arm to shoulder level	❑	❑	________
c. Elbow—Support patient's arm by grasping center of forearm with one hand and just above elbow with other hand			
(1) Bend lower arm toward biceps	❑	❑	________
(2) Straighten lower arm	❑	❑	________
(3) Hold patient's hand as if to shake hands, and turn palm upward	❑	❑	________
(4) Continue holding patient's hand, and turn palm of hand downward	❑	❑	________
d. Wrist—Hold wrist joint with one hand, and hold palm of patient's hand with other hand			
(1) Bend wrist toward lower arm with fingers pointing downward	❑	❑	________
(2) Return wrist to a straight position	❑	❑	________
(3) Bend wrist with fingers pointing upward toward ceiling	❑	❑	________
(4) Extend wrist, and bend it laterally toward ulna side	❑	❑	________
e. Fingers—Place palm and fingers of one hand directly against back of patient's hand and fingers			
(1) Curve fingers with nurse's fingers to resemble a fist	❑	❑	________
(2) Straighten all fingers	❑	❑	________

Student Name____ Date________________

	S	U	Comments
(3) Using thumb and index finger of one hand, spread fingers apart by moving each one away from nearest finger	❑	❑	________
(4) Return fingers together until touching each other	❑	❑	________
f. Thumb—Hold patient's thumb with nurse's thumb and index finger			
(1) Manipulate thumb across the palm of hand to touch tip of each finger to tip of patient's thumb	❑	❑	________
(2) Move thumb away from index finger return thumb toward index finger	❑	❑	________
(3) Move thumb joint forward and backward	❑	❑	________
g. Hip—Support under knee joint with one hand, and grasp ankle joint with other hand			
(1) Raise leg with knee straight; return leg to bed in straight position	❑	❑	________
(2) Raise leg and bend knee toward chest to flex to 110–120 degrees; straighten knee and return to bed	❑	❑	________
(3) Move leg out away from midline	❑	❑	________
(4) Bring leg back toward other leg	❑	❑	________
(5) Position legs straight and roll leg outward, toes pointing outward	❑	❑	________
(6) Position legs straight and roll leg inward, toes pointing toward each other	❑	❑	________
h. Knee—Support under knee joint with one hand, and grasp ankle joint with the other hand	❑	❑	________
(1) Bend knee with calf touching thigh	❑	❑	________
(2) Straighten knee	❑	❑	________
(3) Extend knee beyond the normal point of extension	❑	❑	________
(4) Rotate knee and lower leg toward midline	❑	❑	________

	S	U	Comments
i. Ankle—Grasp heel in palm of one hand, touching inner aspect of the forearm to the sole of the foot; support top of foot just above ankle with other hand			
(1) Gently press against the sole of the foot with inner arm, toes pointing upward	❑	❑	______
(2) Press on top of foot to point toes downward	❑	❑	______
(3) Turn foot away from midline	❑	❑	______
(4) Turn foot inward	❑	❑	______
j. Toes—Place fingers over toes; support bottom of foot with hand and bottom of toes with other hand			
(1) Curl toes downward toward bottom of foot	❑	❑	______
(2) Raise toes to point upward	❑	❑	______
(3) Spread toes apart	❑	❑	______
(4) Return toes toward each other	❑	❑	______
12. Position patient for comfort	❑	❑	______
13. Adjust bed linens	❑	❑	______
14. Remove and dispose of gloves and perform hand hygiene	❑	❑	______
15. Documentation			
a. Report and record abnormal findings	❑	❑	______
b. Report and record normal findings	❑	❑	______

Student Name______________________________ Date______________

PERFORMANCE CHECKLIST 15-3

Moving the Patient

	S	U	Comments
1. Refer to medical record, care plan, or Kardex for special interventions	❑	❑	______
2. Assemble equipment	❑	❑	______
3. Introduce self	❑	❑	______
4. Identify patient	❑	❑	______
5. Explain procedure	❑	❑	______
6. Perform hand hygiene	❑	❑	______
7. Prepare patient for procedure; close doors; adjust the bed level; medicate patient as needed	❑	❑	______
8. Arrange for assistance as necessary	❑	❑	______
9. Lifting and moving patient up in bed			
a. Place patient supine with head flat	❑	❑	______
b. Face side of bed and provide base of support	❑	❑	______
c. Place one arm under axilla and opposite arm under shoulder and neck	❑	❑	______
d. Ask patient to flex knees and push up with feet on count of 3 while assisting	❑	❑	______
e. Nurses position selves on both sides of patient facing each other and support patient's back with one arm with the second arm under shoulder and neck	❑	❑	______
f. On count of 3, each nurse moves patient up to head of bed	❑	❑	______
(1) Roll patient from side to side placing a pull sheet under the patient	❑	❑	______
(2) One nurse on opposite side of the patient's bed grasps pull sheet firmly with hands near patient's upper arms and hips, rolling the sheet material until hands are close to the patient	❑	❑	______

	S	U	Comments
(3) Nurses' knees are flexed with body facing the direction of the move	❏	❏	______
(4) Instruct patient to rest arms on body and to lift head on the count of 3	❏	❏	______
10. Turning the patient			
a. Stand with feet slightly apart and flex knees	❏	❏	______
b. Place one arm under patient's neck and shoulders and other arm under waist	❏	❏	______
c. Move patient toward nurse	❏	❏	______
d. Turn patient on side facing raised side rail	❏	❏	______
e. Flex one leg over the other, place pad or pillow between legs	❏	❏	______
f. Align shoulders	❏	❏	______
g. Support back with pillows if necessary; a "tuck" pillow may be made folding pillow lengthwise	❏	❏	______
11. Dangling patient			
a. Assess pulse and respirations	❏	❏	______
b. Move patient to side of bed toward nurse	❏	❏	______
c. Lower bed to lowest position	❏	❏	______
d. Raise head of bed	❏	❏	______
e. Support patient's shoulders and help to swing legs around and off bed	❏	❏	______
f. This may also be accomplished by rolling the patient onto his/her side before sitting up	❏	❏	______
g. Help patient don slippers; cover legs	❏	❏	______
h. Assess patient's pulse and respirations	❏	❏	______
12. Logrolling the patient			
a. Enlist assistance of at least one other person	❏	❏	______
b. Lower head of bed as low as the patient can tolerate	❏	❏	______
c. Place a pillow between the patient's legs	❏	❏	______

Student Name____ Date____________________

	S	U	Comments
d. Extend patient's arm over patient's head unless shoulder movement is restricted	❑	❑	________________
e. Both nurses on the same side of the bed, one places one hand on the patient's shoulder and the other on the hip while the other nurse places one hand to supports the back and the other behind the knees. If a pull sheet is used, hands are placed alternately to provide even support for the length of the rolled sheet	❑	❑	________________
f. Using a count of 3, turn the patient with a continuous, smooth, coordinated effort	❑	❑	________________
g. Support the patient with pillows as previously discussed	❑	❑	________________
13. Transferring the patient from bed to straight chair or wheelchair			
a. Lower bed to lowest position	❑	❑	________________
b. Raise head of bed	❑	❑	________________
c. Support patient's shoulder, and help patient to sit up and to swing legs around and off of bed	❑	❑	________________
d. Assist patient to don robe and slippers	❑	❑	________________
e. Position chair beside bed with seat facing foot of bed			
(1) Lock wheels of wheelchair and place at right angle after bed is lowered	❑	❑	________________
(2) Place straight chair against wall	❑	❑	________________
f. Stand in front of patient, and place hands at waist level or below and allow patient to use arms and shoulders to facilitate the move	❑	❑	________________
g. Assist patient to stand and swing around with back toward seat of chair	❑	❑	________________
h. Help patient to sit down as nurse bends knees	❑	❑	________________
i. Apply blanket over legs for warmth	❑	❑	________________

	S	U	Comments
j. If a transfer belt is used, apply after patient is sitting on side of bed and follow these guidelines			
(1) Stand in front of the patient	❑	❑	______
(2) Request patient to hold onto mattress or to place fists on the bed by the thighs	❑	❑	______
(3) Place patient's feet flat on the floor	❑	❑	______
(4) Request patient to lean forward	❑	❑	______
(5) Instruct patient to place his hands on nurse's shoulder	❑	❑	______
(6) Grasp the transfer belt on each side	❑	❑	______
(7) Brace your knees against the patient's knees (block patient's feet with your feet)	❑	❑	______
(8) Request patient to push down on the mattress and to stand on the count of 3. At the same time, lift the patient into a standing position as you straighten your knees	❑	❑	______
(9) Pivot the patient so he can grasp the arm rest of the chair—the back of his legs should be touching the chair	❑	❑	______
(10) Continue to turn the patient until he can grasp the other arm rest	❑	❑	______
(11) As you bend your hips and knees, gradually lower the patient into the chair; the patient can assist by leaning forward and bending his elbows and knees.	❑	❑	______
(12) Make certain the patient's buttocks are up against the back of the chair	❑	❑	______
(13) Cover patient's lap and legs with a blanket	❑	❑	______
14. Transferring from bed to stretcher/gurney/back to bed			
a. Position bed flat and raise to the same height as gurney; lower side rails	❑	❑	______

Student Name______________________________________ Date__________________

	S	U	Comments
b. Cover patient with top sheet or blanket and remove linens without exposing patient	❑	❑	______________
c. Assess for IV line, Foley catheter, tubes, or surgical drains, and position them to avoid tension during the transfer	❑	❑	______________
d. Position the gurney as close to the bed as possible and lock the wheels of the bed and gurney (side rails should be lowered)	❑	❑	______________
e. When patient can assist, stand near side of gurney and instruct patient to move feet, then buttocks, and finally upper body to the gurney bringing cover along; be certain the patient's body is centered on the gurney	❑	❑	______________
f. When patient is unable to assist, place a folded sheet or bath blanket under patient so that it supports patient's head and extends to mid-thighs; roll the sheet or bath blanket close to the patient's body; assist patient to cross arms over chest; two caregivers reach over the bed to patient and two caregivers stand as close to the gurney as possible; a fifth caregiver stands at the foot to transfer the feet. Using a coordinating count of 3, all five caregivers lift the patient to the edge of the bed; with another effort, lift the patient from edge of bed to gurney (roller devices may be used)	❑	❑	______________
15. Perform hand hygiene	❑	❑	______________
16. Assess for appropriate body alignment	❑	❑	______________
17. Document procedure	❑	❑	______________

Student Name______________________ Date______________

PERFORMANCE CHECKLIST 15-4

USING LIFTS FOR MOVING PATIENTS

	S	U	Comments
1. Refer to medical record, care plan, or Kardex for special interventions	❑	❑	______
2. Assemble equipment	❑	❑	______
a. Hoyer lift			
b. Seat sling attachment			
c. Two cotton blankets			
3. Introduce self	❑	❑	______
4. Identify patient	❑	❑	______
5. Explain procedure	❑	❑	______
6. Perform hand hygiene	❑	❑	______
7. Prepare for procedure			
a. Close door/pull curtains	❑	❑	______
b. Adjust bed to working height	❑	❑	______
c. Medicate patient as needed	❑	❑	______
8. Secure appropriate number of personnel	❑	❑	______
9. Place chair near bed	❑	❑	______
10. Appropriately place canvas seat under patient	❑	❑	______
11. Slide horseshoe-shaped bar under bed on one side	❑	❑	______
12. Lower horizontal bar appropriately	❑	❑	______
13. Fasten hooks on chain to openings in sling	❑	❑	______
14. Raise head of bed	❑	❑	______
15. Fold patient's arms over chest	❑	❑	______
16. Pump lift handle until patient is raised off bed	❑	❑	______
17. With steering handle, pull lift off bed and down to chair	❑	❑	______
18. Release valve slowly to lower patient toward chair	❑	❑	______
19. Close off valve and release straps	❑	❑	______
20. Remove straps and hydraulic lift	❑	❑	______

	S	U	Comments
21. Perform hand hygiene	❑	❑	________
22. Document procedure	❑	❑	________
a. Evaluate body alignment	❑	❑	________
b. Evaluate patient's response to movement	❑	❑	________
23. Do patient teaching	❑	❑	________

Student Name________________________________ Date________________

PERFORMANCE CHECKLIST 18-1

BATHING THE PATIENT AND ADMINISTERING A BACKRUB

	S	U	Comments
1. Refer to medical record, care plan, or Kardex	❑	❑	________
2. Assemble supplies and complete necessary charges	❑	❑	________
3. Introduce self	❑	❑	________
4. Identify patient	❑	❑	________
5. Explain procedure to patient	❑	❑	________
6. Perform hand hygiene and don clean gloves as appropriate	❑	❑	________
7. Assess the patient	❑	❑	________
8. Prepare patient for intervention			
a. Close door/pull curtain	❑	❑	________
b. Drape for procedure as appropriate	❑	❑	________
c. Suggest use of bedpan/urinal/bathroom	❑	❑	________
d. Arrange supplies	❑	❑	________
e. Adjust room temperature	❑	❑	________
f. Raise bed to comfortable working position	❑	❑	________
9. Bed bath			
a. Lower side rail; position patient on side of bed closest to nurse	❑	❑	________
b. Loosen top linens from the foot of the bed; place bath blanket over the top linens; remove top linens appropriately	❑	❑	________
c. Place soiled laundry in laundry bag	❑	❑	________
d. Assist patient with oral hygiene	❑	❑	________
e. Remove patient's gown, all undergarments, and jewelry	❑	❑	________
f. Raise side rail and fill water basin correctly	❑	❑	________
g. Remove pillow and raise head of bed	❑	❑	________
h. Form mitt with bath cloth; dip mitt and hand into bath water	❑	❑	________

	S	U	Comments
i. Wash around patient's eyes correctly; dry gently	❑	❑	______
j. Rinse bath cloth and finish washing face, cleansing ears and neck	❑	❑	______
k. Expose arm farthest from nurse; place towel lengthwise under patient's arm; place wash basin on towel and place patient's hands in basin of water; bathe arm; supporting arm, raise it above patient's head to bathe the axilla; rinse and dry well	❑	❑	______
l. Do nail care; clean under nails and file smooth; dry thoroughly	❑	❑	______
m. Bathe arm closest to nurse as in steps k and l	❑	❑	______
n. Cover patient's chest with bath towel; fold bath blanket down to waist and wash chest with circular motion	❑	❑	______
o. Fold bath blanket down to pubic area, keeping chest covered with dry towel; wash abdomen, including umbilicus and skin folds; dry thoroughly	❑	❑	______
p. Raise side rail; empty basin in proper receptacle	❑	❑	______
q. Rinse basin and wash cloth; refill basin correctly	❑	❑	______
r. Expose leg farthest away from nurse, keeping perineum covered; place bath towel lengthwise on bed under patient's leg; place wash basin on towel, and place patient's foot in basin	❑	❑	______
s. Use long, firm strokes to bathe leg and foot; after soaking, do nail care	❑	❑	______
t. Bathe leg and foot closest to nurse as in steps r and s	❑	❑	______
u. Raise side rail; make sure patient is covered with bath blanket; change the water; lower side rail; if patient tolerates, position in prone or in Sims' position; place towel lengthwise on bed along back; wash and dry back from neckline down to buttocks	❑	❑	______
v. Reposition patient in supine position; provide basin of water, soap, wash cloth, and towel and instruct patient to cleanse perineal area, while providing privacy	❑	❑	______

Student Name____________________ Date____________

	S	U	Comments
w. Make certain patient is covered with blankets; raise side rail; empty basin, and wash and rinse basin; replace basin in bedside stand; place wash cloth in laundry bag for soiled linen	❑	❑	________
x. Position patient in Sims' or prone position close to nurse; place towel lengthwise along patient's back; give backrub	❑	❑	________
y. Assist patient into clean gown	❑	❑	________
z. Place all soiled linen into laundry bag; make certain all bath equipment is clean and replaced as necessary	❑	❑	________
aa. Place call light, overbed table, night stand, and telephone within easy reach	❑	❑	________
bb. Position patient for comfort and provide warmth	❑	❑	________
cc. Remove gloves; discard them in proper receptacle and perform hand hygiene	❑	❑	________
10. The partial bed bath differs from the bed bath only in that the patient does not need assistance bathing various anatomic regions. The nurse then helps bathe areas that the patient cannot reach. All steps of the bath are followed, and the same considerations prevail. Supplies are placed within easy reach. Water is changed as noted in the bed bath, and back care, skin care, nail care, and hair care are given. A partial bath, in which the face, neck, axilla, and perineum are washed, is practiced in some agencies	❑	❑	________
11. Towel bath			
a. Follow steps 1 to 7	❑	❑	________
b. Prepare patient			
(1) Remove patient's clothing and excess bedding; place patient on bath blanket, and cover patient with bath blanket	❑	❑	________
(2) Cover with plastic any surgical dressing, casts, or areas that should not be wet	❑	❑	________

	S	U	Comments
(3) Fan-fold a clean bath blanket at foot of the bed	❑	❑	______
(4) Place the patient in supine position	❑	❑	______
c. Prepare towel			
(1) Fold towel in half, top to bottom; fold in half again, side to side; then roll towel-bath towel with bath towel and wash cloth inside, beginning with folded edge	❑	❑	______
(2) Place rolled-up towel-bath towel in plastic bag with selvage edges toward open end of bag	❑	❑	______
(3) Draw 2000 mL of water at the correct temperature into plastic pitcher; measure 30 mL of concentrate with a pump; mix 2000 mL of water and concentrate	❑	❑	______
(4) Pour mixture over towel in plastic bag and close bag	❑	❑	______
(5) Knead the solution quickly into towel; position plastic bag with open end in sink and squeeze out excess water, giving added wringing twist to selvage edges of towel	❑	❑	______
d. Bathe patient			
(1) Fold bath blanket down to waist; remove large warm, moist towel from plastic bag and place on patient's right or left chest with open edges up and outward	❑	❑	______
(2) Open towel to cover entire body while removing top bath blanket; tuck towel-bath towel in and around body	❑	❑	______
(3) Begin bathing at feet, using gentle, massaging motion	❑	❑	______
(4) Fold lower part of towel upward away from feet as bathing continues	❑	❑	______
(5) Place clean bath blanket up over patient as nurse moves upward; leave 3 inches of exposed skin between towel and bath blanket; moisture evaporates quickly	❑	❑	______

Student Name________________________ Date____________

	S	U	Comments
(6) Wash face, neck, and ears with one of the prepared wash cloths	❑	❑	______
(7) Turn patient onto side	❑	❑	______
(8) Use smaller prepared bath towel for back care	❑	❑	______
(9) Use second wash cloth for perineal care; don disposable gloves (a basin of warm water, soap, wash cloth, and towel may be necessary)	❑	❑	______
(10) When bath is completed, remove towel and place with soiled linens in plastic laundry bag	❑	❑	______
(11) If top bath blanket is not soiled, fold for reuse	❑	❑	______
e. Make occupied bed	❑	❑	______
12. Tub bath or shower			
a. Follow steps 1 and 3 to 7	❑	❑	______
b. Determine whether activity is allowed	❑	❑	______
c. Make certain tub or shower appliance is clean; place nonskid mat on tub or shower floor and disposable mat outside of tub or shower	❑	❑	______
d. Assemble all items for bathing and complete necessary charges	❑	❑	______
e. Assist patient to tub or shower	❑	❑	______
f. Instruct patient on how to use call signal; place "in use" sign on tub or shower door if private bath is not being used	❑	❑	______
g. If tub is used, fill with warm water at correct temperature; have patient test water, then adjust temperature; instruct patient on use of faucets—which is hot and which is cold; if shower is used, turn water on and adjust temperature	❑	❑	______
h. Caution patient to use safety bars; discourage use of bath oil in water; check on patient every 5 minutes; do not allow to remain in tub more than 20 minutes	❑	❑	______
i. Return to room when patient signals and offer to wash the patient's back; knock before entering	❑	❑	______

	S	U	Comments
j. Assist patient out of tub and with drying; observe patient for signs and symptoms of weakness; if patient complains of weakness, vertigo, or syncope, drain tub before patient gets out and place towel over patient's shoulder	❑	❑	____________
k. Assist patient into clean gown, robe, and slippers; accompany to room, position for comfort	❑	❑	____________
l. Make unoccupied bed if patient can tolerate sitting in chair; perform back, hair, nail, and skin care	❑	❑	____________
m. Return to shower or tub; clean according to agency policy; wear gloves as appropriate; place all soiled linens in laundry bag and return all articles to patient's bedside	❑	❑	____________
n. Perform hand hygiene	❑	❑	____________
13. Tepid sponge bath for temperature reduction			
a. Follow steps 1 to 8	❑	❑	____________
b. Cover patient with bath blanket, remove gown, and close windows and doors	❑	❑	____________
c. Test water temperature; place wash cloths in water, then apply wet cloths to each axilla and groin; if patient is in tub, allow to stay in water for 20–30 minutes	❑	❑	____________
d. Gently sponge an extremity for about 5 minutes; if patient is in tub, gently sponge water over upper torso, chest, and back	❑	❑	____________
e. Continue sponge bath to other extremities, back, and buttocks for 3–5 minutes each; determine temperature and pulse every 15 minutes	❑	❑	____________
f. Change water and reapply freshly moistened wash cloths to axilla and groin as necessary	❑	❑	____________
g. Continue with sponge bath until body temperature falls to slightly above normal; keep body parts that are not being sponged covered; discontinue procedure according to agency policy	❑	❑	____________

Student Name______________________________ Date______________

	S	U	Comments
h. Dry patient thoroughly and cover with light blanket or sheet; avoid rubbing the skin too vigorously; leave patient in comfortable position	❑	❑	________
i. Return equipment to storage, clean area, and change bed linens as necessary; wash hands	❑	❑	________
14. Medicated bath			
a. Follow steps 1 to 7	❑	❑	________
b. Prepare tub bath	❑	❑	________
c. Add agent as ordered	❑	❑	________
d. Don gloves as necessary	❑	❑	________
e. Assist patient to tub	❑	❑	________
f. Allow patient to remain in tub for required time	❑	❑	________
g. Assist patient out of tub	❑	❑	________
h. Gently pat dry; teach patient not to scratch lesions to avoid further irritation and to prevent infection	❑	❑	________
i. Assist patient into gown or pajamas	❑	❑	________
j. Assist patient to return to bed, and position for comfort	❑	❑	________
k. Remove and dispose of gloves; perform hand hygiene	❑	❑	________
15. Backrub			
a. Prepare supplies	❑	❑	________
b. Follow steps 1 to 7 and provide quiet environment	❑	❑	________
c. Lower side rail; position patient with back toward nurse and drape patient with bath blanket after top linens have been fan-folded neatly to the foot of the bed	❑	❑	________
d. Warm hands if necessary; warm lotion by holding some in hands; explain that lotion may feel cool	❑	❑	________
e. Begin massage by starting in sacral area using circular motion; stroke upwards to shoulders	❑	❑	________
f. Use firm, smooth strokes to massage over scapulae; continue to upper arms with one smooth stroke and down along side of back to iliac crest	❑	❑	________

	S	U	Comments
g. Gently but firmly knead skin by grasping area between thumb and fingers; work across each shoulder and around nape of neck; continue downward along each side to sacrum to increase circulation. Do not break contact with patient's skin	❑	❑	______
h. With long, smooth strokes, end massage, remove excess lubricant from patient's back with towel, and retie gown; position for comfort; lower bed and raise side rail as needed and place call button within easy reach	❑	❑	______
i. Place soiled laundry in proper receptacle and perform hand hygiene	❑	❑	______
16. Assess patient for			
a. Tolerance of activity	❑	❑	______
b. Level of discomfort	❑	❑	______
c. Cognitive ability	❑	❑	______
d. Musculoskeletal function; extent of joint ROM	❑	❑	______
e. Risk for skin impairment	❑	❑	______
f. Knowledge of skin hygiene in terms of its importance	❑	❑	______
g. Vital signs	❑	❑	______
17. Document			
a. Type of bath	❑	❑	______
b. Duration of treatment	❑	❑	______
c. Level of assistance required	❑	❑	______
d. Condition of skin	❑	❑	______
e. Vital signs, if applicable	❑	❑	______
f. Patient's response	❑	❑	______
g. Patient teaching	❑	❑	______
18. Report alterations in skin integrity to nurse in charge or physician	❑	❑	______

Student Name________________________________ Date________________

PERFORMANCE CHECKLIST 18-2

Administering Oral Hygiene

	S	U	Comments
1. Refer to medical record, care plan, or Kardex	❑	❑	________
2. Assemble supplies and complete necessary charges	❑	❑	________
3. Introduce self	❑	❑	________
4. Identify patient	❑	❑	________
5. Explain procedure to patient	❑	❑	________
6. Perform hand hygiene; don clean gloves	❑	❑	________
7. Assess patient			
a. Integrity of lips, teeth, buccal mucosa, gums, palate, and tongue	❑	❑	________
b. Risk of dehydration	❑	❑	________
c. Presence of nasogastric or oxygen (O_2) tubes	❑	❑	________
d. Chemotherapeutic drugs or radiation therapy to head and neck	❑	❑	________
e. Presence of artificial airway	❑	❑	________
f. Oral surgery, trauma to mouth	❑	❑	________
g. Aging	❑	❑	________
h. Diabetes mellitus	❑	❑	________
i. Ability to perform own oral care	❑	❑	________
8. Prepare patient for intervention			
a. Close door/pull privacy curtain	❑	❑	________
b. Raise bed to comfortable working position	❑	❑	________
c. Arrange supplies	❑	❑	________
d. If patient can tolerate activity, provide supplies in bathroom and allow privacy	❑	❑	________

	S	U	Comments
e. If patient is on bed rest but can tolerate the activity while remaining in bed, arrange overbed table in front of patient; provide supplies and allow patient privacy	❑	❑	______
f. Position patient's head toward the nurse if patient is unconscious	❑	❑	______
9. Oral care			
a. Place towel under patient's face and emesis basin under patient's chin	❑	❑	______
b. Carefully separate patient's jaws	❑	❑	______
c. Cleanse mouth; clean inner and outer teeth surfaces; swab roof of mouth and inside cheeks; use flashlight for better visualization of oral cavity; gently swab tongue; rinse and repeat cleansing action as necessary	❑	❑	______
d. Apply lubricant to lips	❑	❑	______
10. Cleansing dentures			
a. Fill emesis basin half-full of tepid water	❑	❑	______
b. Ask patient to remove dentures and place in emesis basin; if patient is unable to remove own dentures, break suction that holds upper denture in place; with gauze apply gentle downward tug and carefully remove from patient's mouth; next remove lower denture	❑	❑	______
c. Cleanse biting surfaces; cleanse outer and inner teeth surfaces; be certain to cleanse under surface of dentures	❑	❑	______
d. Rinse dentures thoroughly with tepid water	❑	❑	______
e. Replace dentures either in patient's mouth or in container of solution placed in safe location	❑	❑	______
f. When reinserting the dentures, replace the upper denture first if patient has both dentures; moisten dentures for easier insertion; make certain that dentures are comfortably situated in patient's mouth before leaving the bedside	❑	❑	______

Student Name______________________________ **Date**______________

	S	U	Comments
g. Before replacing dentures in patient's mouth or after storing dentures properly, gently brush patient's gums, tongue, and inside of cheeks and rinse thoroughly	❑	❑	______
11. Dispose of gloves; clean and store supplies; perform hand hygiene	❑	❑	______
12. Position patient for comfort, raise side rail, and lower bed	❑	❑	______
13. Assess for patient comfort	❑	❑	______
14. Document			
a. Procedure	❑	❑	______
b. Pertinent observations	❑	❑	______
c. Most facilities have flow sheets for documenting ADLs, but condition of oral cavity should be noted in nurse's notes	❑	❑	______
d. Patient teaching	❑	❑	______
15. Report bleeding or presence of lesions to nurse in charge or physician	❑	❑	______

Student Name______________________________ Date______________

PERFORMANCE CHECKLIST 18-3

Care of the Hair, Nails, and Feet

	S	U	Comments
Prepare for procedure			
1. Refer to medical record, care plan, or Kardex	❑	❑	______
2. Assemble supplies and complete necessary charges			
a. Bed shampoo	❑	❑	______
b. Shaving	❑	❑	______
c. Nail and foot care	❑	❑	______
3. Introduce self	❑	❑	______
4. Identify patient	❑	❑	______
5. Explain procedure	❑	❑	______
6. Perform hand hygiene and don clean gloves, as appropriate	❑	❑	______
7. Assess patient			
a. Contraindications to shampooing, shaving, or nail care	❑	❑	______
b. Restrictions to positioning	❑	❑	______
c. Condition of scalp, hair, nails, or feet; color and temperature of toes, feet, and fingers	❑	❑	______
d. Ability to care for own hair, nails, and feet	❑	❑	______
e. Knowledge of foot and nail care practices	❑	❑	______
8. Prepare patient for intervention			
a. Close door/pull privacy curtain	❑	❑	______
b. Raise bed to a comfortable working height	❑	❑	______
c. Arrange supplies at bedside or, if patient is able to perform procedure, have supplies available in the bathroom and offer assistance as needed	❑	❑	______
9. Bed shampoo			
a. Position patient close to one side of bed; place shampoo board under patient's head and wash basin at end of spout; make sure spout extends over edge of mattress	❑	❑	______

	S	U	Comments
b. Position rolled-up bath towel under patient's neck	❑	❑	
c. Brush and comb patient's hair; if hair is matted with blood, hydrogen peroxide is effective as a cleansing agent	❑	❑	
d. Obtain water in pitcher at correct temperature	❑	❑	
e. If patient is able, instruct patient to hold wash cloth over eyes; completely wet hair and apply small amount of shampoo	❑	❑	
f. Massage scalp with fingertips, not nails; shampoo hairline, back of neck, and sides of hair	❑	❑	
g. Rinse thoroughly and apply more shampoo, repeating steps e and f; rinse and repeat, rinsing until hair is free from shampoo	❑	❑	
h. Wrap dry towel around patient's head; dry patient's face, neck, and shoulders; dry hair and scalp using second towel if necessary	❑	❑	
i. Comb hair and/or dry with blow dryer	❑	❑	
j. Complete styling hair and position patient for comfort	❑	❑	
10. Shaving the patient			
a. Assist patient to sitting position	❑	❑	
b. Observe face and neck	❑	❑	
c. Use shaving cream or soap	❑	❑	
d. Shave in direction hair grows; use short strokes; start with upper face and lips, and then extend to neck; if patient is able, it will help if he will hyperextend his head to help shave curved areas	❑	❑	
e. Pull skin taut with nondominant hand below the area being shaved	❑	❑	
f. Rinse razor after each stroke	❑	❑	
g. Rinse and dry face	❑	❑	
h. If patient desires, apply lotion or cologne	❑	❑	
i. Dispose of blades in sharps container	❑	❑	

Student Name____ Date____________________

	S	U	Comments
11. Hand and foot care			
a. Position patient in chair; place disposable mat under patient's feet	❑	❑	______________
b. Fill basin with water at correct temperature; place basin on disposable mat and assist patient to place feet into basin; allow to soak 10–20 minutes; rewarm water as necessary	❑	❑	______________
c. Place overbed table in low position in front of patient; fill emesis basin with water at 100°–110° F (43°–46° C); place basin on table and place patient's fingers in basin; allow fingernails to soak 10–20 minutes; rewarm water as necessary	❑	❑	______________
d. Using orangewood stick, gently clean under fingernails; with clippers, trim nails straight across and even with fingertips; with emery board, shape fingernails; push cuticles back gently with wash cloth or orangewood stick	❑	❑	______________
e. Don gloves and with wash cloth scrub areas of feet that are callused	❑	❑	______________
f. Trim and clean toenails following step d	❑	❑	______________
g. Apply lotion or cream to hands and feet; return patient to bed and position for comfort	❑	❑	______________
h. On completion of procedure, observe the nails and surrounding tissue for condition of skin and any remaining rough edges	❑	❑	______________
i. If the patient's nails are extremely hard or if the patient is unable to perform personal nail care, a podiatrist can provide nail care	❑	❑	______________
12. Dispose of gloves in proper receptacle; clean and store supplies; place soiled laundry in hamper; perform hand hygiene	❑	❑	______________
13. Assess for patient's comfort, lower bed level, raise side rails, and place call button within easy reach	❑	❑	______________
14. Document			
a. Procedure	❑	❑	______________

	S	U	Comments
b. Pertinent observations	❑	❑	______
c. Most facilities have flow sheets for ADLs; shaving and nail and foot care are usually not recorded in nurse's notes; know agency policy	❑	❑	______
d. Patient teaching	❑	❑	______
15. Report abnormal findings	❑	❑	______

Student Name________________________ Date____________

PERFORMANCE CHECKLIST 18-4

Perineal Care: Male and Female and the Catheterized Patient

	S	U	Comments
Prepare for procedure			
1. Refer to medical record, care plan, or Kardex	❑	❑	________
2. Assemble supplies and complete necessary charges			
a. Perineal care (uncatheterized patient)	❑	❑	________
b. Perineal care (catheterized patient)	❑	❑	________
3. Introduce self	❑	❑	________
4. Identify patient	❑	❑	________
5. Explain procedure	❑	❑	________
6. Perform hand hygiene and don gloves to assess patient for			
a. Accumulated secretions	❑	❑	________
b. Surgical incision	❑	❑	________
c. Lesions	❑	❑	________
d. Ability to perform self-care	❑	❑	________
e. Extent of care required by patient	❑	❑	________
f. Knowledge of importance of perineal care	❑	❑	________
7. Remove gloves, discard appropriately	❑	❑	________
8. Prepare patient for intervention			
a. Close door/pull privacy curtain	❑	❑	________
b. Raise bed to comfortable working height and lower side rail	❑	❑	________
c. Arrange supplies at bedside	❑	❑	________
d. OB patients are allowed to perform this procedure by themselves while sitting on the stool by using a plastic squeeze bottle	❑	❑	________

	S	U	Comments
e. Patients allowed tub/shower baths will do this by themselves; make certain supplies are close by			
(1) Assist patient to desired position in bed, supine for males or dorsal recumbent for females	❑	❑	______
(2) Drape for procedure	❑	❑	______
(3) When perineal care is given other than routinely during the bath, the nurse will need to fill the perineal bottle (peribottle) with cleansing solution and position the patient on the bedpan in bed	❑	❑	______
9. Perform hand hygiene and don clean gloves	❑	❑	______
10. Female perineal care			
a. Raise side rail and fill basin two-thirds full of water at correct temperature	❑	❑	______
b. Position patient in bed with knees aligned and slightly abducted, with waterproof pad/towel under buttocks; drape for privacy	❑	❑	______
c. Using a disposable wash cloth wrapped around one hand, wash and dry patient's upper thighs	❑	❑	______
d. Wash both labia majora and labia minora; cleanse in direction anterior to posterior; use separate corner of wash cloth for each skin fold	❑	❑	______
e. Separate labia to expose the urinary meatus and vaginal orifice; wash downward toward rectum with smooth strokes; use separate corner of wash cloth for each smooth stroke	❑	❑	______
f. Cleanse, rinse, and dry thoroughly (if patient is on bedpan and peribottle is used, direct flow of cleansing solution down over perineal area and dry thoroughly)	❑	❑	______
g. Assist patient to side-lying position and cleanse rectal area with toilet tissue; wash area by cleansing from perineal area toward anus (several wash cloths may be needed). (Many facilitates have disposable wipes; if so, use them.) Wash, rinse, and dry thoroughly	❑	❑	______

Student Name________________________ Date______________

	S	U	Comments
11. Male perineal care			
a. Raise side rail, fill basin two-thirds full of water at the correct temperature, and position patient supine in bed	❑	❑	______
b. Gently grasp shaft of penis; retract foreskin of uncircumcised patient	❑	❑	______
c. Wash tip of penis with circular motion	❑	❑	______
d. Cleanse from meatus outward; two wash cloths may be necessary; wash, rinse, and dry gently	❑	❑	______
e. Replace foreskin, and wash shaft of penis with a firm but gentle downward stroke	❑	❑	______
f. Rinse and dry thoroughly	❑	❑	______
g. Cleanse scrotum gently; cleanse carefully in underlying skin folds; rinse and dry gently	❑	❑	______
h. Assist patient to a side-lying position; cleanse anal area; follow step g of female perineal care	❑	❑	______
12. Catheter care			
a. Raise side rail and fill basin two-thirds full of water at the correct temperature	❑	❑	______
b. Position and drape the female patient in bed, supine as described in step 11	❑	❑	______
c. Cleanse around urethral meatus and adjacent catheter; cleanse entire catheter with soap and water	❑	❑	______
d. Repeat cleansing to remove all exudate from meatus and catheter	❑	❑	______
e. If ointment is ordered, open package of sterile cotton-tipped applicators; do not touch cotton tip; apply ointment to applicator; do not touch wrapper to cotton tip	❑	❑	______
f. Apply ointment to junction of catheter and urethral meatus	❑	❑	______
13. Remove gloves; clean and store equipment; dispose of contaminated supplies in proper receptacle; perform hand hygiene	❑	❑	______
14. Position patient for comfort	❑	❑	______

	S	U	Comments
15. Document			
a. Procedure	❑	❑	______
b. Pertinent observations such as			
(1) Character and amount of discharge and odor if present	❑	❑	______
(2) Condition of genitalia	❑	❑	______
(3) Patient's ability to perform own care	❑	❑	______
(4) Patient teaching	❑	❑	______
16. Report abnormal findings to nurse in charge or physician	❑	❑	______

Student Name______________________________ Date______________

PERFORMANCE CHECKLIST 18-5

BEDMAKING

	S	U	Comments
Prepare for procedure			
1. Refer to medical record, care plan, or Kardex	❑	❑	______
2. Assemble supplies and complete necessary charges	❑	❑	______
3. Introduce self	❑	❑	______
4. Identify patient	❑	❑	______
5. Explain procedure	❑	❑	______
6. Perform hand hygiene and don gloves as necessary	❑	❑	______
7. Prepare patient			
a. Close door/pull privacy curtain	❑	❑	______
b. Raise bed to appropriate height and lower side rail on the side closest to the nurse	❑	❑	______
c. Lower head of bed if patient can tolerate it	❑	❑	______
d. Assess patient's tolerance of procedure; be alert for signs of discomfort and fatigue	❑	❑	______
8. Occupied bed			
a. Remove spread and blanket separately and, if soiled, place in laundry bag; if linens will be reused, fold neatly and place over back of chair	❑	❑	______
b. Place bath blanket over patient on top of sheet	❑	❑	______
c. Request patient to hold onto bath blanket and remove top linens	❑	❑	______
d. Place soiled sheet in laundry bag	❑	❑	______
e. With assistance from coworker, slide mattress to top of bed	❑	❑	______
f. Position patient to far side of bed with the back toward nurse; adjust pillow for comfort; be sure side rail is up	❑	❑	______

	S	U	Comments
g. Beginning at head and moving toward foot, loosen bottom linens; fan-fold linen draw sheet, protective draw sheet, and bottom sheet, tucking edges of linens under patient	❑	❑	______
h. Apply clean linens to bed by first placing mattress pad (if used); fold lengthwise, making sure crease is in center of bed; likewise, unfold bottom sheet and place over mattress pad; hem of bottom sheet (if flat is used) should be placed with rough edge down and just even with bottom edge of mattress	❑	❑	______
i. Miter corners (if flat sheet) at head of bed; continue to tuck in sheet along side toward front, keeping linens smooth	❑	❑	______
j. Reach under the patient to pull out protective draw sheet (if used), and smooth out over clean bottom sheet; tuck in; unfold linen draw sheet and place center fold along middle of bed, smooth out over protective draw sheet and tuck in; tuck in folded linens in center of bed so they are under patient's buttocks and torso	❑	❑	______
k. Keep palms down as linens are tucked under mattress	❑	❑	______
l. Raise side rail and assist patient to roll slowly toward nurse over folds of linen; go to opposite side of bed and lower side rail	❑	❑	______
m. Loosen edges of all soiled linens; remove by folding into a bundle and place in laundry bag	❑	❑	______
n. Spread clean linens, including protective draw sheet, out over mattress and smooth out wrinkles; assist patient to supine position and position pillow for comfort	❑	❑	______
o. Miter top corner of bottom sheet, pulling sheet taut; tuck bottom sheet under mattress all the way to foot of bed	❑	❑	______
p. Smooth out draw sheets; pulling sheet taut, tuck in protective draw sheet and then tuck in linen draw sheet	❑	❑	______

Student Name________________________________ Date______________

	S	U	Comments
q. Place top sheet over bath blanket that is over patient; request patient to hold top sheet while nurse removes bath blanket; place blanket in laundry bag; if blanket is used, place over sheet and place spread over blanket; form cuff with top linens under patient's chin	❏	❏	________
r. Tuck in all linens at foot of bed, making modified miter corner; raise side rail and make opposite side of bed; make toe pleat by placing fold either lengthwise down center of bed or across foot of bed	❏	❏	________
s. Change pillow case; grasp closed end of pillow case, turning case inside out over hand; now grasp one end of pillow with hand in the case and smooth out wrinkles	❏	❏	________
9. Unoccupied bed			
a. Starting at head of bed, loosen linens all the way to foot; go to opposite side of bed, loosen linens, roll all linens up in ball, and place in soiled laundry bag; perform hand hygiene after handling soiled linens	❏	❏	________
b. If blanket and spread are to be reused, fold neatly and place over back of chair; remove soiled pillow case	❏	❏	________
c. Slide mattress to head of bed	❏	❏	________
d. If necessary, clean mattress with cloth moistened with antiseptic solution and dry thoroughly	❏	❏	________
e. Begin to make bed standing on side where lines are placed; unfold bottom sheet, placing fold lengthwise down center of bed; make certain rough edge of hem lies down away from patient's heels and even with edge of mattress; smooth out sheet over top edge of mattress and miter corners; tuck remaining sheet under mattress all the way to foot	❏	❏	________
f. Place draw sheet on bed so that center fold lies down middle of bed; if protective draw sheet is to be used, place it on first; smooth out over mattress and tuck in; keep palms down	❏	❏	________

	S	U	Comments
g. Place top sheet over bed and smooth out; place blanket over top sheet; smooth out; place spread over blanket and smooth out; make cuff with top linens	❑	❑	______
h. Allow for toe pleat; make modified mitered corner by not tucking tip of under mattress	❑	❑	______
i. Move to opposite side of bed and complete making bed as described in steps 9e to 9h; pull linens tight and keep taut as linens are tucked in	❑	❑	______
j. Put on clean pillow case (see step 8s); position pillow at head of bed; place call light within easy reach and lower bed level	❑	❑	______
k. If patient is to return to bed, fan-fold top linens down to foot of bed; make sure cuff at top of linens is easily accessible to patient	❑	❑	______
10. Arrange personal items on bed table or bedside stand and place within patient's easy reach	❑	❑	______
11. Leave area neat and clean	❑	❑	______
12. Place all soiled linens in proper receptacle; perform hand hygiene	❑	❑	______
13. Assist patient to bed and position for comfort	❑	❑	______
14. Documentation (Bedmaking does not need to be recorded. Record patient's vital signs, signs and symptoms only if there are changes.)	❑	❑	______
15. Report any abnormal findings to nurse in charge or physician	❑	❑	______

Student Name____________________ Date____________

PERFORMANCE CHECKLIST 18-6

Positioning the Bedpan

	S	U	Comments
Prepare for procedure			
1. Refer to medical record, care plan, or Kardex	❑	❑	______
2. Assemble supplies and complete necessary charges	❑	❑	______
3. Introduce self	❑	❑	______
4. Identify patient	❑	❑	______
5. Explain procedure	❑	❑	______
6. Perform hand hygiene and don clean gloves	❑	❑	______
7. Assess patient's needs	❑	❑	______
8. Prepare patient			
a. Close door/pull privacy curtain	❑	❑	______
b. Arrange supplies close to the bedside	❑	❑	______
c. Place protective pad under patient's buttocks	❑	❑	______
9. Warm metal bedpan under running warm water	❑	❑	______
10. Position patient in supine position with knees flexed and bottom of feet flat on bed surface; as patient raises hips, support patient's lower back with arm and position bedpan under patient; when patient has finished with elimination, remove bedpan in same manner	❑	❑	______
11. For patient unable to assist self on bedpan			
a. Turn patient away toward opposite side rail, moving linens out of way	❑	❑	______
b. Fit bedpan to patient's buttocks	❑	❑	______
c. Assist patient to turn over onto bedpan while nurse secures bedpan	❑	❑	______
d. Raise head of bed 30 degrees	❑	❑	______
e. Place toilet tissue and call light within easy reach	❑	❑	______

	S	U	Comments
12. For those patients who can be out of bed but are unable to ambulate far, there is the bedside commode; some are equipped with wheels that allow the patient to be moved to the bathroom	❑	❑	____________
13. When transferring a patient to the commode, assist the patient in the same manner as if assisting to a chair	❑	❑	____________
14. Document according to agency policy			
a. Amount	❑	❑	____________
b. Color	❑	❑	____________
c. Consistency	❑	❑	____________
d. Abnormal findings	❑	❑	____________
15. Report abnormal findings	❑	❑	____________

Student Name______________________________________ Date__________________

PERFORMANCE CHECKLIST 19-1

Preparing Patient for Diagnostic Examination

	S	U	Comments
1. Refer to medical record, care plan, or Kardex	❑	❑	____________
2. Ensure that informed consent has been obtained when necessary (most invasive diagnostic tests require informed consent)	❑	❑	____________
3. Assemble equipment and supplies	❑	❑	____________
4. Introduce self	❑	❑	____________
5. Identify patient	❑	❑	____________
6. Explain procedure; assess patient's understanding of procedure and purpose; assess patient for allergy to dye (if dye is to be used)	❑	❑	____________
7. Perform hand hygiene and don clean gloves	❑	❑	____________
8. Prepare patient for procedure			
a. Transfer to examining room; maintain safety precautions	❑	❑	____________
b. Close door and pull curtains	❑	❑	____________
c. Raise bed or arrange examination table to convenient height	❑	❑	____________
d. Drape for procedure if necessary	❑	❑	____________
9. Assist physician with procedure	❑	❑	____________
Postprocedure			
10. Answer patient's questions	❑	❑	____________
11. Deliver specimen to laboratory promptly, label specimen according to agency policy: patient's name, birth date, age, room number, physician, date and time, type of specimen, and collector's initials; CDC and OSHA recommend inserting specimen (in container) into another plastic bag for transport to laboratory	❑	❑	____________

	S	U	Comments
12. Document procedure			
a. Type of procedure	❑	❑	______
b. Time	❑	❑	______
c. Specimen obtained	❑	❑	______
d. Sent to laboratory with requisition	❑	❑	______
e. Patient's response	❑	❑	______
f. Patient teaching	❑	❑	______

Student Name________________________ Date____________

PERFORMANCE CHECKLIST 19-2

Collecting a Midstream Urine Specimen

	S	U	Comments
1. Refer to medical record, care plan, or Kardex	❑	❑	____
2. Assemble supplies	❑	❑	____
3. Introduce self	❑	❑	____
4. Identify patient	❑	❑	____
5. Explain procedure to patient; make certain patient understands how to perform procedure	❑	❑	____
6. Prepare patient for procedure	❑	❑	____
a. Close door/pull privacy curtain	❑	❑	____
b. Offer assistance if required	❑	❑	____
7. Perform hand hygiene and don clean gloves	❑	❑	____
8. If patient is able, allow patient to cleanse perineum from anterior to posterior with antiseptic solution. Separate the labia well on a female patient. Retract foreskin of an uncircumcised male. Use each cotton ball that is saturated with antiseptic solution one time only. If patient is unable to cleanse area, the nurse will don gloves and assist with procedure	❑	❑	____
9. Request that patient (1) begin to void into urine receptacle about 30 mL, then place the sterile specimen container so that sides of the labia of the female do not touch; (2) without stopping flow, void a small amount into specimen cup; and (3) without stopping flow, finish voiding into toilet	❑	❑	____
10. Secure lid on container	❑	❑	____
11. Cleanse and return toilet seat collector; empty and flush bedpan/urinal	❑	❑	____
12. Label specimen appropriately; enclose in plastic bag for transport	❑	❑	____
13. Remove gloves, discard in proper receptacle, and perform hand hygiene	❑	❑	____

	S	U	Comments
14. Ensure that specimen is taken to laboratory with proper requisition slip (many facilities mandate within 1 hour)	❏	❏	______________
15. Document procedure per protocol	❏	❏	______________

Student Name________________________________ Date______________

PERFORMANCE CHECKLIST 19-3

Collecting a Sterile Urine Specimen Via Catheter Port

	S	U	Comments
1. Refer to medical record, care plan, or Kardex	❑	❑	______
2. Assemble supplies	❑	❑	______
3. Introduce self	❑	❑	______
4. Identify patient	❑	❑	______
5. Explain procedure to patient	❑	❑	______
6. Perform hand hygiene and don clean gloves	❑	❑	______
7. Catheter port collection			
a. Clamp just below catheter port for about 30 minutes	❑	❑	______
b. Return in 30 minutes; don clean gloves; clean port with alcohol prep	❑	❑	______
c. Insert *needleless* adapter into port at 30-degree angle, and withdraw 5–10 mL of urine for a specimen	❑	❑	______
d. Place urine in sterile specimen cup	❑	❑	______
e. Unclamp catheter	❑	❑	______
f. Label specimen, enclose in plastic bag, and send to laboratory with requisition	❑	❑	______
8. Remove gloves and perform hand hygiene	❑	❑	______
9. Document procedure and observations	❑	❑	______

Student Name________________________________ Date________________

PERFORMANCE CHECKLIST 19-4

Collecting a 24-Hour Urine Specimen

	S	U	Comments
1. Refer to medical record, care plan, or Kardex	❑	❑	________
2. Assemble supplies and equipment	❑	❑	________
3. Introduce self	❑	❑	________
4. Identify patient	❑	❑	________
5. Explain procedure			
a. Instruct patient about the importance of collecting all urine for a period of 24 hours	❑	❑	________
b. Instruct patient not to place toilet tissue or fecal material in urine	❑	❑	________
6. Post signs in all appropriate places	❑	❑	________
7. Perform hand hygiene and don gloves	❑	❑	________
8. Have patient void when the 24-hour specimen collection is to begin; discard this voiding	❑	❑	________
9. Place labeled container on ice if required	❑	❑	________
10. Save all urine for the 24-hour period; place each voided specimen into the larger container with preservative; all urine must be saved or results will be altered	❑	❑	________
11. Instruct patient to void a few minutes before end of 24 hours; this urine is part of the 24-hour specimen	❑	❑	________
12. Send specimen to lab promptly; be certain label is complete with all pertinent information. If more than one container is necessary, make certain all are labeled and numbered	❑	❑	________
13. Remove gloves, perform hand hygiene	❑	❑	________
14. Document procedure and observations	❑	❑	________
15. Do patient teaching	❑	❑	________

Student Name______________________________ Date______________

PERFORMANCE CHECKLIST 19-5

MEASURING BLOOD GLUCOSE LEVELS

	S	U	Comments
1. Refer to medical record, care plan, or Kardex	❑	❑	______
2. Assemble supplies	❑	❑	______
3. Introduce self	❑	❑	______
4. Identify patient	❑	❑	______
5. Explain procedure to patient	❑	❑	______
6. Perform hand hygiene and don clean gloves	❑	❑	______
7. Remove cap from lancet using sterile technique	❑	❑	______
8. Place lancet into automatic lancing device according to instructions in operating manual	❑	❑	______
9. Select site on side of any fingertip (heel used for infant)	❑	❑	______
10. Wipe selected site with alcohol swab, and discard	❑	❑	______
11. Ask patient to hold arm at side for 30 seconds	❑	❑	______
12. Gently squeeze fingertip with thumb of same hand	❑	❑	______
13. Hold lancing device	❑	❑	______
14. Place trigger platform of lancing device on side of finger, and press	❑	❑	______
15. Squeeze finger in downward motion (wipe off first drop of blood)	❑	❑	______
16. While holding strip level, touch drop of blood to test pad (prevent skin from touching test pad)	❑	❑	______
17. Begin recommended timing. After 60 seconds, blot blood off test strip, place reagent strip into appropriate site on meter, and wait for numeric readout	❑	❑	______

	S	U	Comments
18. Remove lancet from device, and discard	❑	❑	________
19. Remove gloves and discard; perform hand hygiene	❑	❑	________
20. Document procedure and observations	❑	❑	________
21. Do patient teaching	❑	❑	________

Student Name________________________________ Date________________

PERFORMANCE CHECKLIST 19-6

COLLECTING A STOOL SPECIMEN

	S	U	Comments
1. Refer to medical record, care plan, or Kardex	❑	❑	________
2. Assemble supplies	❑	❑	________
3. Introduce self	❑	❑	________
4. Identify patient	❑	❑	________
5. Explain procedure to patient; make certain patient understands what is expected	❑	❑	________
6. Perform hand hygiene and don gloves	❑	❑	________
7. Assist to bathroom when necessary	❑	❑	________
8. Request that patient defecate into commode, specimen device, or bedpan, and prevent urine from entering specimen	❑	❑	________
9. Transfer stool to specimen cup with use of a tongue blade and close lid securely	❑	❑	________
10. Remove gloves and perform hand hygiene	❑	❑	________
11. Attach requisition slip, enclose in plastic bag, and send specimen to laboratory; specimens for ova and parasites must be taken to the laboratory stat; other stool specimens may be kept at room temperature	❑	❑	________
12. Assist patient to bed	❑	❑	________
13. Document procedure and observations	❑	❑	________
14. Do patient teaching	❑	❑	________

Student Name________________________ Date____________

PERFORMANCE CHECKLIST 19-7

DETERMINING THE PRESENCE OF OCCULT BLOOD IN STOOL

	S	U	Comments
1. Refer to medical record, care plan, or Kardex	❑	❑	________
2. Assemble supplies	❑	❑	________
3. Introduce self	❑	❑	________
4. Identify patient	❑	❑	________
5. Explain procedure	❑	❑	________
6. Perform hand hygiene, and don gloves	❑	❑	________
7. Collect stool specimen appropriately	❑	❑	________
8. Follow steps on Hemoccult slide test			
a. Open flap	❑	❑	________
b. Smear very small amount of stool with tongue blade in first box (A)	❑	❑	________
c. Smear very small amount of stool with tongue blade from another part of stool specimen, and transfer to box (B)	❑	❑	________
d. Close card, label (label before collecting specimen), and place in plastic bag	❑	❑	________
e. Send specimen to laboratory with requisition slip	❑	❑	________
9. Remove gloves and perform hand hygiene	❑	❑	________
10. Document procedure and observations	❑	❑	________
11. Do patient teaching	❑	❑	________

Student Name_______________________________ Date_______________

PERFORMANCE CHECKLIST 19-8

COLLECTING GASTRIC SECRETIONS OR EMESIS SPECIMEN

	S	U	Comments
1. Refer to medical record, care plan, or Kardex	❑	❑	________
2. Assemble supplies	❑	❑	________
3. Introduce self	❑	❑	________
4. Identify patient	❑	❑	________
5. Explain procedure	❑	❑	________
6. Perform hand hygiene and don gloves	❑	❑	________
7. To obtain specimen of gastric contents using NG or nasoenteral tube, position patient in high-Fowler's in bed or chair	❑	❑	________
8. Verify NG tube placement	❑	❑	________
9. Collect gastric contents via NG tube or nasoenteral tube			
a. Disconnect tube from suction or gravity drainage	❑	❑	________
b. Attach bulb- or cone-tipped syringe	❑	❑	________
c. Aspirate 5 to 10 mL	❑	❑	________
d. To obtain sample of emesis, use a 3-mL syringe or wooden applicator	❑	❑	________
e. Using applicator or syringe, apply 1 drop of gastric sample to Gastroccult blood test slide	❑	❑	________
f. Apply 2 drops of commercial developer solution over sample and 1 drop between positive and negative performance monitors	❑	❑	________
g. After 60 seconds, compare color of gastric sample with that of performance monitors	❑	❑	________
h. Verify that performance monitor turns blue in 30 seconds	❑	❑	________
10. Close card and label	❑	❑	________

	S	U	Comments
11. Enclose specimen in plastic bag and send to laboratory with requisition slip	❑	❑	__________
12. Reconnect NG tube to drainage system, suction, or clamp as ordered	❑	❑	__________
13. Dispose of equipment, remove gloves, and perform hand hygiene	❑	❑	__________
14. Document procedure and observations	❑	❑	__________
15. Do patient teaching (patients are usually informed of test results)	❑	❑	__________

Student Name______________________________ **Date**______________

PERFORMANCE CHECKLIST 19-9

Collecting a Sputum Specimen by Suction

	S	U	Comments
1. Refer to medical record, care plan, or Kardex	❑	❑	________
2. Assemble supplies	❑	❑	________
3. Introduce self	❑	❑	________
4. Identify patient	❑	❑	________
5. Explain procedure; encourage patient to breathe normally to prevent hyperventilation	❑	❑	________
6. Arrange equipment and prepare necessary charges	❑	❑	________
7. Perform hand hygiene	❑	❑	________
8. Assess patient			
a. Determine when patient last ate a meal	❑	❑	________
b. Respiratory status: rate, depth, pattern, lung sounds, and color	❑	❑	________
c. Anxiety level	❑	❑	________
9. Position patient for procedure			
a. Close door/pull curtains	❑	❑	________
b. The higher semi-Fowler's position is recommended	❑	❑	________
c. Prepare suction machine or device and make certain it is functioning properly	❑	❑	________
d. Drape patient as necessary	❑	❑	________
e. Adjust bed to appropriate height and lower side rail	❑	❑	________
10. Connect suction tube to adapter on sputum trap	❑	❑	________
11. Apply sterile glove to dominant hand	❑	❑	________
12. Preoxygenate the patient for 1 minute with 100% oxygen, if available	❑	❑	________
13. Using sterile gloved hand, connect sterile suction catheter tubing on sputum trap	❑	❑	________

	S	U	Comments
14. Gently insert tip of suction catheter prelubricated with sterile water through nasopharynx, endotracheal tube, or tracheostomy without applying suction	❑	❑	______
15. Warn patient to expect to cough and gently and quickly advance catheter into trachea	❑	❑	______
16. As patient coughs, apply suction for 5 to 10 seconds, collection 2 to 10 mL of sputum	❑	❑	______
17. Release suction and remove catheter, then turn off suction	❑	❑	______
18. Detach catheter from specimen trap, and dispose of catheter into appropriate receptacle; connect rubber tubing on sputum trap to plastic adapter	❑	❑	______
19. If any sputum is present on outside of container, wash it off with disinfectant	❑	❑	______
20. Offer patient tissues after suctioning; dispose of tissues in emesis basin or trash container; remove and dispose of gloves	❑	❑	______
21. Securely attach properly completed identification label and laboratory requisition to side of specimen container (not the lid)	❑	❑	______
22. Enclose specimen in a plastic bag; send specimen immediately to laboratory	❑	❑	______
23. Offer patient mouth care and assist to a comfortable position and place needed items within easy reach	❑	❑	______
24. Raise side rail and lower bed to lowest position	❑	❑	______
25. Store, remove, or dispose of supplies and equipment as appropriate	❑	❑	______
26. Document procedure			
a. Method used to obtain specimen	❑	❑	______
b. Date and time collected	❑	❑	______
c. Type of test ordered and how specimen was transported to the laboratory	❑	❑	______
d. Characteristics of sputum specimen	❑	❑	______
e. Patient's oxygenation and respiratory status	❑	❑	______

Student Name____ Date____________________

PERFORMANCE CHECKLIST 19-10

Collecting a Sputum Specimen by Expectoration

	S	U	Comments
1. Refer to medical record, care plan, or Kardex	❑	❑	____________
2. Assemble supplies	❑	❑	____________
3. Introduce self	❑	❑	____________
4. Identify patient	❑	❑	____________
5. Explain procedure to patient	❑	❑	____________
6. Perform hand hygiene and don gloves	❑	❑	____________
7. Position patient in Fowler's position	❑	❑	____________
8. Instruct patient to take three breaths, and force cough into sterile container	❑	❑	____________
9. Label specimen container (if any sputum is present on outside of container, wash it off with disinfectant)	❑	❑	____________
10. Attach laboratory requisition, place in plastic bag, and send specimen to laboratory; specimen should be analyzed promptly for accurate results	❑	❑	____________
11. Remove gloves and perform hand hygiene	❑	❑	____________
12. Document procedure and observations	❑	❑	____________
13. Do patient teaching	❑	❑	____________

Student Name________________________________ Date______________

PERFORMANCE CHECKLIST 19-11

OBTAINING A THROAT SPECIMEN

	S	U	Comments
1. Refer to medical record, care plan, or Kardex	❑	❑	________
2. Assemble supplies	❑	❑	________
3. Introduce self	❑	❑	________
4. Identify patient	❑	❑	________
5. Explain procedure	❑	❑	________
6. Perform hand hygiene and don gloves	❑	❑	________
7. Instruct patient to tilt head backward; for patients in bed, place pillow behind shoulders	❑	❑	________
8. Ask patient to open mouth and say "ah"	❑	❑	________
9. Have swab stick ready for use (you may want to loosen top so swab can be removed easily)	❑	❑	________
10. If pharynx is not visualized, depress tongue with tongue blade and note inflamed areas of pharynx of tonsils; depress anterior third tongue only (illuminate with penlight as needed)	❑	❑	________
11. Insert swab without touching lips, teeth, tongue, or cheeks	❑	❑	________
12. Gently but quickly swab tonsillar area side to side, making contact with inflamed or purulent sites	❑	❑	________
13. Carefully withdraw swab without striking oral structures; immediately place swab in culture tube, using a 2 x 2 gauze; cover end of tube and crush ampule at bottom of tube; push tip of swab into liquid medium	❑	❑	________
14. Securely attach properly completed label and requisition slip to side of specimen container (not the lid)	❑	❑	________
15. Enclose in a plastic bag	❑	❑	________

	S	U	Comments
16. Send specimen immediately to laboratory or refrigerate	❑	❑	____________
17. Discard gloves and perform hand hygiene	❑	❑	____________
18. Document procedure	❑	❑	____________

Student Name________________________________ Date______________

PERFORMANCE CHECKLIST 19-12

Obtaining a Nose Culture

	S	U	Comments
1. Refer to medical record, care plan, or Kardex	❑	❑	______
2. Assemble supplies	❑	❑	______
3. Introduce self	❑	❑	______
4. Identify patient	❑	❑	______
5. Explain procedure	❑	❑	______
6. Perform hand hygiene and don gloves	❑	❑	______
7. Ask patient to blow nose, and then check nostrils for patency with penlight; select nostril with greatest patency	❑	❑	______
8. Ask patient to tilt head back; patients in bed should have a pillow behind the shoulders	❑	❑	______
9. Gently insert nasal speculum in one nostril (optional); carefully pass swab into nostril until it reaches that portion of mucosa that is inflamed or containing exudate; rotate swab quickly (NOTE: If nasopharyngeal culture is to be obtained, use a special swab on a flexible wire that can be flexed downward to reach nasopharynx)	❑	❑	______
10. With dominant hand, remove swab without touching sides of speculum or nasal canal	❑	❑	______
11. With nondominant hand, carefully remove nasal speculum (if used) and place in basin; offer patient facial tissue	❑	❑	______
12. Immediately place swab in culture tube	❑	❑	______
13. Cover end of tube with 2 x 2 gauze, then crush ampule at bottom of tube to release culture medium; push tip of swab into liquid medium	❑	❑	______
14. Place top on tube securely	❑	❑	______
15. Discard supplies into trash	❑	❑	______

	S	U	Comments
16. Send to laboratory with completed requisition and attached label (not attached to the lid); enclose in a plastic bag	❑	❑	______
17. Remove and discard gloves, perform hand hygiene	❑	❑	______
18. Document procedure	❑	❑	______

Student Name______________________________ Date______________

PERFORMANCE CHECKLIST 19-13

PERFORMING THE VENIPUNCTURE

	S	U	Comments
1. Refer to medical record, care plan, or Kardex	❑	❑	______
2. Assemble supplies	❑	❑	______
3. Introduce self	❑	❑	______
4. Identify patient	❑	❑	______
5. Explain procedure	❑	❑	______
6. Arrange equipment and complete necessary charges	❑	❑	______
7. Perform hand hygiene and don clean gloves	❑	❑	______
8. Assess patient	❑	❑	______
9. Prepare patient for procedure			
a. Provide privacy; close door/pull curtain	❑	❑	______
b. Position supine or semi-Fowler's with arm extended to form straight line from shoulders to waist	❑	❑	______
c. Place small pillow or towel under upper arm	❑	❑	______
d. Adjust bed to appropriate height and lower nearest side rail	❑	❑	______
e. Drape patient	❑	❑	______
10. Apply tourniquet 3–4 inches above puncture site	❑	❑	______
11. Palpate distal pulse. If pulse is not palpable, reapply tourniquet more loosely	❑	❑	______
12. Keep tourniquet on patient no longer than 1–2 minutes. If tourniquet is left on too long, remove and assess other extremity or wait 60 seconds before reapplying	❑	❑	______
13. Request patient to open and close fist several times, finally leaving fist clenched; avoid vigorous opening and closing of fist, which may cause erroneous laboratory results	❑	❑	______
14. Quickly assess extremity for best venipuncture site, looking for straight, prominent vein without edema or hematoma	❑	❑	______

	S	U	Comments
15. Palpate selected vein with fingers; note if vein is firm and rebounds when palpated or if vein feels rigid and cordlike and rolls when palpated	❑	❑	______
16. Select venipuncture site	❑	❑	______
17. Obtain blood samples	❑	❑	______
a. Syringe method			
(1) Make certain syringe with appropriate needle is securely attached	❑	❑	______
(2) Cleanse venipuncture site with alcohol swab, moving in circular motion from site for approximately 2 inches (5 cm) and allow to dry	❑	❑	______
(3) Remove needle cover and inform patient a "stick" will be felt	❑	❑	______
(4) Place thumb and forefinger of nondominant hand 1 inch below site and pull skin taut. Stretch skin down until vein is stabilized	❑	❑	______
(5) Hold syringe and needle at 15- to 30-degree angle from patient's arm with bevel up	❑	❑	______
(6) Slowly insert needle into vein	❑	❑	______
(7) Hold syringe securely and pull back gently on plunger	❑	❑	______
(8) Look for blood return	❑	❑	______
(9) Obtain desired amount of blood, keeping needle stabilized	❑	❑	______
(10) After obtaining specimen, release tourniquet	❑	❑	______
(11) Apply a gauze pad or alcohol swab over needle site without applying pressure, quickly but carefully withdraw needle from vein, and apply pressure to puncture site	❑	❑	______
(12) Carefully transfer blood from syringe into vacuum tube	❑	❑	______
(13) Discard needle without recapping in proper receptacle	❑	❑	______
(14) Remove and discard gloves; perform hand hygiene	❑	❑	______

Student Name________________________ Date____________

	S	U	Comments
b. Vacuum tube method			
(1) Attach double-ended needle to vacuum tube	❑	❑	______
(2) Have proper blood specimen tube resting inside vacuum tube without puncturing rubber stopper	❑	❑	______
(3) Cleanse venipuncture site properly with alcohol swab	❑	❑	______
(4) Remove needle cover and inform patient "stick" will be felt	❑	❑	______
(5) Place thumb and forefinger of nondominant hand 1 inch below site and pull taut. Stretch skin down until vein is stabilized	❑	❑	______
(6) Hold vacuum tube at a 15- to 30-degree angle from arm with bevel up	❑	❑	______
(7) Slowly insert needle into vein	❑	❑	______
(8) Grasp vacuum tube securely and advance specimen tube into needle of holder	❑	❑	______
(9) Note flow of blood into tube	❑	❑	______
(10) After specimen tube is filled, grasp vacuum tube firmly and remove tube. Insert additional specimen tubes as needed	❑	❑	______
(11) After last tube is filled, release tourniquet	❑	❑	______
(12) Apply 2 x 2 gauze pad over needle site without applying pressure and quickly but carefully withdraw needle from vein, applying pressure over puncture site	❑	❑	______
(13) Remove and discard gloves; perform hand hygiene	❑	❑	______
18. For blood obtained by syringe, transfer specimen to tubes			
a. Using one-handed technique, insert needle through stopper of blood tube and allow vacuum to fill tube; do not force blood into tube	❑	❑	______
b. Alternative method is to remove needle from syringe and stopper to each test tube; gently inject required amount of blood into each tube; reapply stopper	❑	❑	______

	S	U	Comments
19. For blood obtained for culture			
a. Cleanse venipuncture site with providone-iodine or appropriate antiseptic; allow to dry	❑	❑	______
b. Clean bottle tops of vacuum tubes or culture bottles with appropriate antiseptic (check agency policy)	❑	❑	______
c. Collect 10 to 15 mL of venous blood by venipuncture from each venipuncture site	❑	❑	______
d. Discard needle on syringe; replace with new sterile needle before injecting blood sample into culture bottles	❑	❑	______
e. If both aerobic and anaerobic cultures are needed, inoculate anaerobic first	❑	❑	______
f. Mix medium gently after inoculation	❑	❑	______
g. After venipuncture, apply 2 x 2 gauze pad over puncture site without applying pressure, and quickly but carefully withdraw needle from vein	❑	❑	______
20. For blood tubes containing additives, gently rotate back and forth 8–10 times	❑	❑	______
21. Inspect puncture site for bleeding and apply adhesive tape with gauze	❑	❑	______
22. Check tubes for any sign of external contamination with blood; decontaminate with alcohol, if necessary; remove and discard gloves; perform hand hygiene	❑	❑	______
23. Securely attach properly completed ID label to each tube, affix proper requisition, and transfer to laboratory promptly	❑	❑	______
24. Remove and appropriately discard gloves; perform hand hygiene	❑	❑	______
25. Assist patient to a comfortable position and place needed items within easy reach	❑	❑	______
26. Raise side rail and lower bed to lowest position	❑	❑	______
27. Store, remove, and dispose of supplies and equipment as is appropriate	❑	❑	______
28. Document procedure	❑	❑	______

Student Name________________________ Date____________

PERFORMANCE CHECKLIST 19-14

PERFORMING AN ELECTROCARDIOGRAM (ECG)

	S	U	Comments
1. Refer to medical record, care plan, or Kardex	❑	❑	________
2. Assemble supplies	❑	❑	________
3. Introduce self	❑	❑	________
4. Identify patient	❑	❑	________
5. Explain procedure	❑	❑	________
6. Arrange equipment and complete necessary charges	❑	❑	________
7. Perform hand hygiene and don clean gloves	❑	❑	________
8. Assess patient for			
a. Chest pain	❑	❑	________
b. Dyspnea	❑	❑	________
c. Heart rate and rhythm	❑	❑	________
d. Blood pressure, pulse, respirations	❑	❑	________
9. Prepare patient for procedure			
a. Close door/pull curtain	❑	❑	________
b. Position patient supine and provide for comfort	❑	❑	________
c. Drape patient	❑	❑	________
d. Adjust bed to proper height and lower nearest side rail	❑	❑	________
10. Perform ECG			
a. Cleanse and wipe skin area with alcohol	❑	❑	________
b. Apply electrode paste and attach leads. For 12-lead ECG			
(1) Chest (precordial leads)			
• V_1—Fourth intercostal space (ICS) at right sternal border	❑	❑	________

	S	U	Comments
• V_2—Fourth ICS at left sternal border	❑	❑	______
• V_3—Midway between V_2 and V_4	❑	❑	______
• V_4—Fifth ICS at midclavicular line	❑	❑	______
• V_5—Left anterior axillary line at level of V_4 horizontally	❑	❑	______
• V_6—Left midaxillary line at level of V_4 horizontally	❑	❑	______
(2) Extremities—one at lower portion of each extremity			
• aVR—Right wrist	❑	❑	______
• aVL—Left wrist	❑	❑	______
• AVF—Left ankle	❑	❑	______
c. Obtain tracing	❑	❑	______
d. Disconnect leads, wipe excess paste from chest	❑	❑	______
e. Remove gloves, dispose of appropriately and perform hand hygiene	❑	❑	______
f. Deliver EGG tracing promptly to laboratory or nursing unit	❑	❑	______
11. Assist patient to position of comfort and place needed items within easy reach	❑	❑	______
12. Raise side rail and lower bed to lowest position	❑	❑	______
13. Store supplies and equipment as is appropriate	❑	❑	______
14. Document procedure	❑	❑	______

Student Name________________________________ Date________________

PERFORMANCE CHECKLIST 20-1

Eye Irrigation

	S	U	Comments
Prepare for procedure			
1. Refer to medical record, care plan, or Kardex	❏	❏	________
2. Introduce self	❏	❏	________
3. Identify patient	❏	❏	________
4. Explain procedure and reason it is to be done	❏	❏	________
5. Assess need for and provide patient teaching during procedure	❏	❏	________
6. Assemble equipment and complete necessary charges	❏	❏	________
7. Perform hand hygiene	❏	❏	________
8. Assess patient	❏	❏	________
9. Prepare patient for intervention			
a. Close door/pull privacy curtain	❏	❏	________
b. Raise bed to comfortable working height; lower side rail on side nearest the nurse	❏	❏	________
c. Position and drape patient as necessary	❏	❏	________
During the skill			
10. Promote patient involvement as possible	❏	❏	________
11. Assess patient's tolerance	❏	❏	________
12. Assess condition of both eyes	❏	❏	________
13. Place patient lying toward side to be irrigated	❏	❏	________
14. Place towel under patient's head	❏	❏	________
15. Use a sterile plastic squeeze bottle unless very large amounts of solution are needed (sometimes a medicine dropper is sufficient)	❏	❏	________
16. Don gloves	❏	❏	________
17. Place an emesis basin at side of face	❏	❏	________

	S	U	Comments
18. Using the thumb and index finger of the nondominant hand, separate the patient's eyelids	❑	❑	______
19. Gently direct the irrigating solution along the conjunctiva from the inner to the outer canthus	❑	❑	______
20. Avoid directing a forceful stream onto the eyeball	❑	❑	______
21. Avoid touching any parts of the eye with irrigation equipment	❑	❑	______
22. A piece of gauze may be wrapped around the gloved index finger to raise upper lid	❑	❑	______
23. Gently dry the eyelids	❑	❑	______
24. Remove gloves and perform hand hygiene	❑	❑	______
Postprocedure			
25. Assist patient to a position of comfort and place needed items within easy reach; be certain patient has a means to call for assistance and knows how to use it	❑	❑	______
26. Raise side rails and lower bed to lowest position	❑	❑	______
27. Store or remove and dispose of soiled supplies and equipment appropriately	❑	❑	______
28. Remove gloves and all protective barriers; dispose of soiled supplies and equipment appropriately	❑	❑	______
29. Perform hand hygiene after patient contact and after wearing gloves	❑	❑	______
30. Document and do patient teaching	❑	❑	______
31. Report any unexpected outcomes	❑	❑	______

Student Name________________________________ Date________________

PERFORMANCE CHECKLIST 20-2

WARM, MOIST EYE COMPRESSES

	S	U	Comments
Prepare for procedure			
1. Refer to medical record, care plan, or Kardex	❑	❑	________
2. Introduce self	❑	❑	________
3. Identify patient	❑	❑	________
4. Explain procedure and reason it is to be done	❑	❑	________
5. Assess need for and provide patient teaching during procedure	❑	❑	________
6. Assemble equipment and complete necessary charges	❑	❑	________
7. Perform hand hygiene	❑	❑	________
8. Assess patient	❑	❑	________
9. Prepare patient for intervention			
a. Close door/pull privacy curtain	❑	❑	________
b. Raise bed to comfortable working height; lower side rail on side nearest the nurse	❑	❑	________
c. Position and drape patient as necessary	❑	❑	________
During the skill			
10. Promote patient involvement as possible	❑	❑	________
11. Assess patient's tolerance	❑	❑	________
12. Don clean gloves	❑	❑	________
13. Assess condition of both eyes	❑	❑	________
14. Assist patient to a comfortable position; when applying warm compresses, have the patient sit if possible; support the head with a pillow and turn the head slightly to the unaffected side	❑	❑	________
15. Place the towel/waterproof pad under the patient's head	❑	❑	________
16. Use sterile technique when infection or ulceration is present; clean technique may be used for allergic reactions	❑	❑	________

	S	U	Comments
17. Change gloves, dispose of in proper receptacle, and perform hand hygiene before treating each eye	❑	❑	______
18. Temperature of compresses should not exceed 120° F (49° C); to heat solution, place the uncapped bottle of solution in a basin of hot water; pour the warmed solution into a sterile bowl, filling it halfway; place sterile gauze pads in the bowl	❑	❑	______
19. Take two 4 x 4 gauze pads from the basin; squeeze out excess moisture	❑	❑	______
20. Instruct the patient to close his or her eyes; gently apply the pads—one on top of the other—to the affected eye	❑	❑	______
21. Do not exert pressure on eyelids	❑	❑	______
22. Change compress every few minutes, as necessary, for the prescribed length of time	❑	❑	______
23. If sterility is not necessary, moist heat may be applied by means of a clean wash cloth	❑	❑	______
24. After removing each compress, assess the periorbital skin for signs that the compress solution is too hot	❑	❑	______
25. Cleanse patient's eye and dry with the remaining gauze pads	❑	❑	______
26. If ordered, apply ophthalmic ointment or eye patch	❑	❑	______
Postprocedure			
27. Assist patient to a position of comfort and place needed items within easy reach; be certain patient has a means to call for assistance and knows how to use it	❑	❑	______
28. Raise side rails and lower bed to lowest position	❑	❑	______
29. Remove gloves and all protective barriers; dispose of soiled supplies and equipment appropriately	❑	❑	______
30. Perform hand hygiene after patient contact and after wearing gloves	❑	❑	______
31. Document and do patient teaching	❑	❑	______
32. Report any unexpected outcomes	❑	❑	______

Student Name____ Date____________________

PERFORMANCE CHECKLIST 20-3

EAR IRRIGATION

	S	U	Comments
Prepare for procedure			
1. Refer to medical record, care plan, or Kardex	❑	❑	____________________
2. Introduce self	❑	❑	____________________
3. Identify patient	❑	❑	____________________
4. Explain procedure and reason it is to be done	❑	❑	____________________
5. Assess need for and provide patient teaching during procedure	❑	❑	____________________
6. Assemble equipment and complete necessary charges	❑	❑	____________________
7. Perform hand hygiene	❑	❑	____________________
8. Assess patient	❑	❑	____________________
9. Prepare patient for intervention			
a. Close door/pull privacy curtain	❑	❑	____________________
b. Raise bed to comfortable working height; lower side rail on side nearest the nurse	❑	❑	____________________
c. Position and drape patient as necessary	❑	❑	____________________
During the skill			
10. Promote patient involvement as possible	❑	❑	____________________
11. Assess patient's tolerance	❑	❑	____________________
12. Advise patient of sensations that might be experienced: vertigo, fullness, and warmth	❑	❑	____________________
13. Don gloves as necessary	❑	❑	____________________
14. Assess condition of external ear structures and canal for erythema, edema, and exudate	❑	❑	____________________
15. Assist patient to either a side-lying or sitting position with head tilted toward affected ear and position emesis basin under ear	❑	❑	____________________
16. Place towel under patient's shoulder just under ear and emesis basin	❑	❑	____________________

	S	U	Comments
17. Inspect auditory canal for any accumulation of cerumen or debris. Remove what you can see with the naked eye or the otoscope using cotton or the applicator and solution (do not force cerumen into the canal)	❑	❑	______
18. Assess irrigation solution for proper temperature; test temperature of solution by sprinkling a few drops of solution on inner wrist; fill bulb syringe with appropriate volume	❑	❑	______
19. Straighten auditory canal for introduction of solution correctly according to age	❑	❑	______
20. With tip of syringe just above canal, irrigate gently by creating steady flow of solution against roof of canal; do not occlude canal with tip of syringe	❑	❑	______
21. Continue irrigation until all debris has been removed or all solution has been used; reassess auditory canal with otoscope	❑	❑	______
22. Assess patient for vertigo or nausea; onset of symptoms may require temporary cessation of procedure	❑	❑	______
23. Dry off auricle and apply cotton ball loosely to auditory meatus	❑	❑	______
24. Position patient on side of affected ear for 10 minutes	❑	❑	______
25. Return to patient to assess character and amount of drainage and determine patient's level of comfort	❑	❑	______
Postprocedure			
26. Assist patient to a position of comfort and place needed items within easy reach; be certain patient has a means to call for assistance and knows how to use it	❑	❑	______
27. Raise side rails and lower bed to lowest position	❑	❑	______
28. Remove gloves and all protective barriers; dispose of soiled supplies and equipment appropriately	❑	❑	______
29. Perform hand hygiene after patient contact and after wearing gloves	❑	❑	______
30. Document and do patient teaching	❑	❑	______
31. Report any unexpected outcomes	❑	❑	______

Student Name______________________________ Date______________

PERFORMANCE CHECKLIST 20-4

PERFORMING A NASAL IRRIGATION

	S	U	Comments
Prepare for procedure			
1. Refer to medical record, care plan or Kardex	❑	❑	______
2. Introduce self	❑	❑	______
3. Identify patient	❑	❑	______
4. Explain procedure and reason it is to be done	❑	❑	______
5. Assess need for and provide patient teaching during procedure	❑	❑	______
6. Obtain equipment, assemble, and complete necessary charges	❑	❑	______
7. Perform hand hygiene; don clean gloves	❑	❑	______
8. Assess patient for comfort level and any nasal secretions	❑	❑	______
9. Prepare patient			
a. Close door/pull privacy curtain	❑	❑	______
b. Position patient sitting upright comfortably near equipment leaning over the basin or sink	❑	❑	______
10. Prepare equipment			
a. Mix solution as needed	❑	❑	______
b. Warm solution	❑	❑	______
c. Fill irrigating device	❑	❑	______
d. Place basin as collecting receptacle	❑	❑	______
During the skill			
11. Instruct patient to keep mouth open and breathe rhythmically during procedure	❑	❑	______
12. Teach patient neither to speak nor swallow during procedure	❑	❑	______

	S	U	Comments
13. Remove irrigating device tip from nose if patient reports the need to cough or sneeze	❑	❑	______
14. If using commercial kit, follow directions on package	❑	❑	______
15. Don clean gloves and perform procedure			
a. Electrical irrigating device			
(1) Insert tip about 1/2 to 1 inch into patient's nostril	❑	❑	______
(2) Begin with a low pressure setting	❑	❑	______
(3) Irrigate both nostrils	❑	❑	______
b. Bulb syringe			
(1) Fill bulb with warm saline solution	❑	❑	______
(2) Insert tip 1/2 inch into patient's nostril	❑	❑	______
(3) Squeeze bulb until a gentle stream of warm solution washes through the nose	❑	❑	______
(4) Avoid forceful squeezing	❑	❑	______
(5) Irrigate both nostrils until returns are clear	❑	❑	______
16. Assess returns and report any abnormalities			
a. Color	❑	❑	______
b. Viscosity	❑	❑	______
c. Volume	❑	❑	______
d. Blood	❑	❑	______
e. Necrotic material	❑	❑	______

Postprocedure

	S	U	Comments
17. Request patient to wait a few minutes before blowing nose	❑	❑	______
18. Instruct patient to gently blow both nostrils at the same time	❑	❑	______
19. Clean and store equipment	❑	❑	______

Student Name____ **Date**__________________

	S	U	Comments
20. Remove gloves and all protective barriers; dispose of soiled supplies and equipment appropriately	❑	❑	__________________
21. Assist patient to cleanse and dry self	❑	❑	__________________
22. Assist patient to a position of comfort and place needed items within easy reach; be certain patient has a means to call for assistance and knows how to use it	❑	❑	__________________
23. If in bed, raise side rail and lower bed to lowest position	❑	❑	__________________
24. Perform hand hygiene after patient contact and after wearing gloves	❑	❑	__________________
25. Document	❑	❑	__________________
26. Observe and assess patient for any adverse reactions	❑	❑	__________________
27. Do patient teaching	❑	❑	__________________

Student Name________________________ Date____________

PERFORMANCE CHECKLIST 20-5

APPLYING A HOT, MOIST COMPRESS TO AN OPEN WOUND

	S	U	Comments
Prepare for procedure			
1. Refer to medical record, care plan, or Kardex	❑	❑	________
2. Introduce self	❑	❑	________
3. Identify patient	❑	❑	________
4. Explain procedure and reason it is to be done	❑	❑	________
5. Assess need for and provide patient teaching during procedure	❑	❑	________
6. Assemble equipment and complete necessary charges	❑	❑	________
7. Perform hand hygiene; don clean gloves	❑	❑	________
8. Assess patient	❑	❑	________
9. Prepare patient for intervention			
a. Close door/pull privacy curtain	❑	❑	________
b. Raise bed to comfortable working height; lower side rail on side nearest the nurse	❑	❑	________
c. Position and drape patient as necessary	❑	❑	________
During the skill			
10. Promote patient involvement as possible	❑	❑	________
11. Assess patient's tolerance	❑	❑	________
12. Describe sensations to be felt; explain precautions to prevent burning	❑	❑	________
13. Assess condition of exposed skin and wound on which compress is to be applied	❑	❑	________
14. Place waterproof pad under area to be treated	❑	❑	________
15. Assemble equipment; pour warmed solution into sterile container	❑	❑	________

	S	U	Comments
16. Open sterile packages and drop gauze into container to immerse in solution; set Aquathermia pad (if used) to correct temperature and assess fluid level of unit	❑	❑	______
17. Don disposable gloves; remove any existing dressings covering wound; dispose of gloves and dressings in proper receptacle	❑	❑	______
18. Apply sterile gloves	❑	❑	______
19. Apply sterile petroleum jelly (optional) with cotton swab to skin surrounding wound; do not apply jelly on impaired skin	❑	❑	______
20. Pick up one layer of immersed gauze and squeeze out excess water	❑	❑	______
21. Apply gauze lightly to open wound; observe response and ask whether patient feels discomfort; in a few seconds, lift edge of gauze to assess for erythema	❑	❑	______
22. If patient tolerates compress, pack gauze snugly against wound; be certain all wound surfaces are covered by hot compress	❑	❑	______
23. Wrap or cover moist compress with dry bath towel; if necessary, pin or tie in place	❑	❑	______
24. Change hot compress frequently as ordered	❑	❑	______
25. Apply Aquathermia or waterproof heating pad over compress (optional); keep it in place for desired duration of application	❑	❑	______
26. Assess patient periodically for discomfort or burning sensation; observe area of skin not covered by compress	❑	❑	______
27. Remove pad, towel, and compress; again assess wound and condition of skin	❑	❑	______
28. Apply dry, sterile dressing as ordered	❑	❑	______
29. Ask patient if any unusual burning sensation is noticed that was not felt before	❑	❑	______

Student Name______________________________ **Date**______________

	S	U	Comments
Postprocedure			
30. Assist patient to a position of comfort and place needed items within easy reach; be certain patient has a means to call for assistance and knows how to use it	❑	❑	______________
31. Raise side rails and lower bed to lowest position	❑	❑	______________
32. Remove gloves and all protective barriers; dispose of soiled supplies and equipment appropriately	❑	❑	______________
33. Perform hand hygiene after patient contact and after wearing gloves	❑	❑	______________
34. Document and do patient teaching	❑	❑	______________
35. Report an unexpected outcomes	❑	❑	______________

Student Name________________________ Date______________

PERFORMANCE CHECKLIST 20-6

INITIATING INTRAVENOUS THERAPY

	S	U	Comments
Prepare for procedure			
1. Refer to medical record, care plan, or Kardex	❑	❑	________
2. Introduce self	❑	❑	________
3. Identify patient	❑	❑	________
4. Explain procedure and reason it is to be done	❑	❑	________
5. Assess need for and provide patient teaching during procedure	❑	❑	________
6. Assemble equipment and IV solution to be infused	❑	❑	________
7. Perform hand hygiene; don clean gloves	❑	❑	________
8. Assess patient	❑	❑	________
9. Prepare patient for intervention			
a. Close door/pull privacy curtain	❑	❑	________
b. Raise bed to comfortable working height; lower side rail on side nearest the nurse	❑	❑	________
c. Position and drape patient as necessary	❑	❑	________
During the skill			
10. Promote patient involvement as possible	❑	❑	________
11. Assess patient's tolerance	❑	❑	________
12. Identify venipuncture sites	❑	❑	________
13. Apply tourniquet	❑	❑	________
14. Select venipuncture site	❑	❑	________
15. Cleanse site with alcohol swab, or other special agent such as Betadine, using friction	❑	❑	________
16. Stretch skin taut and stabilize vein with nondominant hand	❑	❑	________
17. Holding angiocatheter bevel up, pierce skin above and slightly to side of vein at 45-degree angle	❑	❑	________

	S	U	Comments
18. When using a needleless over-the-needle catheter safety device (ONC)			
a. Insert ONC with bevel up at 10- to 30-degree angle, slightly distal to actual site of venipuncture in direction of vein	❑	❑	______
b. Look for blood return in flash back chamber on ONC; advance catheter off stylet into vein until head rests at venipuncture site; do not reinsert stylet once it is loosened; advance safety device by using push-off tab to thread catheter	❑	❑	______
c. Stabilize catheter; apply gentle but firm pressure above insertion site; release tourniquet and retract stylet from ONC; do not recap stylet; for safety device slide, catheter off stylet while guiding protective guard over stylet	❑	❑	______
19. Lower angle to 10 degrees and enter vein wall; slight resistance and "pop" accompany entry into vein	❑	❑	______
20. Follow vein lumen with tip of needle to ensure placement within vein, watching for blood return through angiocatheter backflow chamber	❑	❑	______
21. Release tourniquet	❑	❑	______
22. Holding guide needle in place, gently thread plastic catheter off needle and into vein	❑	❑	______
23. Applying gentle pressure over catheter in vein, remove guide needle, and attach sterile connection end of primed tubing into catheter hub	❑	❑	______
24. Stabilizing insertion site, slowly open flow valve to begin intravenous infusion	❑	❑	______
25. Following agency policy, secure and dress site with tape, medications, and dressings	❑	❑	______
26. Label site and tubing according to agency policy	❑	❑	______
27. Adjust fluid flow rate according to accurate drop-rate calculations or set infusion rate on infusion pump	❑	❑	______
28. If infusion pump is used, set milliliters to be infused (volume to be infused)	❑	❑	______

Student Name____ Date____________________

	S	U	Comments
Postprocedure			
29. Assist patient to a position of comfort and place needed items within easy reach; be certain patient has a means to call for assistance and knows how to use it	❑	❑	________________
30. Raise side rails and lower bed to lowest position	❑	❑	________________
31. Remove gloves and all protective barriers; dispose of soiled supplies and equipment appropriately	❑	❑	________________
32. Perform hand hygiene after patient contact and after wearing gloves	❑	❑	________________
33. Document and do patient teaching	❑	❑	________________
34. Report any unexpected outcomes	❑	❑	________________

Student Name________________________ Date____________

PERFORMANCE CHECKLIST 20-7A
MAINTAINING AN INTRAVENOUS SITE:

CHANGING A PERIPHERAL IV DRESSING

	S	U	Comments
Prepare for procedure			
1. Refer to medical record, care plan, or Kardex	❑	❑	________
2. Introduce self	❑	❑	________
3. Identify patient	❑	❑	________
4. Explain procedure and reason it is to be done	❑	❑	________
5. Assess need for dressing change and provide patient teaching	❑	❑	________
6. Assemble equipment and complete necessary charges	❑	❑	________
7. Perform hand hygiene; don clean gloves	❑	❑	________
8. Assess patient	❑	❑	________
9. Prepare patient for intervention			
a. Close door/pull privacy curtain	❑	❑	________
b. Raise bed to comfortable working height; lower side rail on side nearest the nurse	❑	❑	________
c. Position and drape patient as necessary	❑	❑	________
During the skill			
10. Promote patient involvement as possible	❑	❑	________
11. Assess patient's tolerance	❑	❑	________
12. Prepare equipment	❑	❑	________
13. Assess IV site			
a. When was dressing last changed	❑	❑	________
b. Assess present dressing	❑	❑	________
c. Observe present IV system for proper functioning or complications	❑	❑	________
d. Palpate catheter site through intact dressing	❑	❑	________

	S	U	Comments
e. Inspect exposed catheter site	❑	❑	______
f. Monitor body temperature	❑	❑	______
g. Determine patient's understanding of need for procedure	❑	❑	______
14. Remove any overlying tape, transparent membrane dressing, gauze dressing and tape; leave tape securing catheter to skin	❑	❑	______
15. Observe insertion site	❑	❑	______
16. If IV is infusing properly, remove tape securing catheter; stabilize catheter with one finger; remove adhesive residue if necessary	❑	❑	______
17. Cleanse peripheral insertion site properly; allow to dry; apply skin protectant solution if necessary	❑	❑	______
18. Transparent dressing			
a. Place transparent dressing over venipuncture site correctly	❑	❑	______
b. Taking a 1-inch piece of tape, place correctly over transparent dressing	❑	❑	______
19. Gauze dressing			
a. Apply single 4-inch strip of sterile nonallergic tape under catheter hub correctly	❑	❑	______
b. Place gauze over venipuncture site and catheter hub properly; secure edges	❑	❑	______
20. Secure dressing and tubing to arm at insertion site; place gauze under catheter tubing correctly; curl a loop of tubing as directed in skill; secure tubing in two places (Transparent dressings are also currently used.)	❑	❑	______

Postprocedure

	S	U	Comments
21. Label dressing completely and accurately	❑	❑	______
22. Secure arm or hand to board as necessary	❑	❑	______

Student Name________________________________ **Date**________________

	S	U	Comments
23. Assist patient to a position of comfort and place needed items within easy reach; be certain patient has a means to call for assistance and knows how to use it	❑	❑	________
24. Raise side rails and lower bed to lowest position	❑	❑	________
25. Remove gloves and all protective barriers; dispose of soiled supplies and equipment appropriately	❑	❑	________
26. Perform hand hygiene after patient contact and after wearing gloves	❑	❑	________
27. Document	❑	❑	________
28. Report any unexpected outcomes	❑	❑	________

Student Name________________________ Date____________

PERFORMANCE CHECKLIST 20-7B
MAINTAINING AN INTRAVENOUS SITE:

CHANGING INFUSION TUBING

	S	U	Comments
Prepare for procedure			
1. Refer to medical record, care plan, or Kardex	❑	❑	____________
2. Introduce self	❑	❑	____________
3. Identify patient	❑	❑	____________
4. Explain procedure and reason it is to be done	❑	❑	____________
5. Assess need for tubing change and provide patient teaching	❑	❑	____________
6. Assemble equipment and complete necessary charges	❑	❑	____________
7. Perform hand hygiene; don clean gloves	❑	❑	____________
8. Assess patient's IV setup	❑	❑	____________
9. Prepare patient for intervention			
a. Close door/pull privacy curtain	❑	❑	____________
b. Raise bed to comfortable working height; lower side rail on side nearest the nurse	❑	❑	____________
c. Position and drape patient as necessary	❑	❑	____________
During the skill			
10. Promote patient involvement as possible	❑	❑	____________
11. Assess patient's tolerance	❑	❑	____________
12. Prepare equipment	❑	❑	____________
13. Assess			
a. New infusion set necessary	❑	❑	____________
b. Observe tubing	❑	❑	____________
c. Determine patient's need for continued IV infusion	❑	❑	____________

	S	U	Comments
14. Open new infusion set, connect add-on pieces (keeping sterile where necessary); secure all junctions correctly; avoid use of tape	❑	❑	______
15. If necessary, remove IV dressing as catheter hub needs to be visible; maintain catheter securely to skin; if necessary, place small piece of sterile tape across hub	❑	❑	______
16. For existing continuous infusion			
a. Close roller clamp on new tubing	❑	❑	______
b. Slow rate of flow on existing IV properly	❑	❑	______
c. Compress and fill drip chamber of old tubing	❑	❑	______
17. a. Remove IV container from pole	❑	❑	______
b. Invert container	❑	❑	______
c. Remove old tubing from solution container	❑	❑	______
d. Hold container 36 inches above IV site	❑	❑	______
18. Place insertion spike of new tubing into old fluid container opening; hang container on IV pole and adjust correctly	❑	❑	______
19. a. Slowly open roller clamp	❑	❑	______
b. Remove protector cap from adapter	❑	❑	______
c. Flush new tubing with solution	❑	❑	______
d. Stop infusion and replace cap	❑	❑	______
20. Turn roller clamp on old tubing off	❑	❑	______
21. a. Stabilize hub of catheter and apply pressure appropriately	❑	❑	______
b. Disconnect old tubing and insert adapter of new tubing correctly	❑	❑	______
22. a. Open roller clamp and adjust correctly	❑	❑	______
b. Regulate per physician's order	❑	❑	______
c. Monitor hourly rate	❑	❑	______
23. Provide reference (label) to determine next time for tubing change	❑	❑	______
24. If necessary, apply new dressing to insertion site	❑	❑	______

Student Name____ **Date**__________________

	S	U	Comments
25. Secure tubing to patient's arm	❏	❏	________________

Postprocedure

	S	U	Comments
26. Assist patient to a position of comfort and place needed items within easy reach; be certain patient has a means to call for assistance and knows how to use it	❏	❏	________________
27. Raise side rails and lower bed to lowest position	❏	❏	________________
28. Remove gloves and all protective barriers; dispose of soiled supplies and equipment appropriately	❏	❏	________________
29. Perform hand hygiene after patient contact and after wearing gloves	❏	❏	________________
30. Document	❏	❏	________________
31. Report any unexpected outcomes	❏	❏	________________

Student Name________________________________ Date______________

PERFORMANCE CHECKLIST 20-7C
MAINTAINING AN INTRAVENOUS SITE:

CHANGING FLUID CONTAINER

	S	U	Comments
Prepare for procedure			
1. Refer to medical record, care plan, or Kardex	❑	❑	________
2. Introduce self	❑	❑	________
3. Identify patient	❑	❑	________
4. Explain procedure and reason it is to be done	❑	❑	________
5. Assess need for container change and provide patient teaching	❑	❑	________
6. Assemble equipment and complete necessary charges	❑	❑	________
7. Perform hand hygiene; don clean gloves	❑	❑	________
8. Prepare patient for intervention			
a. Close door/pull privacy curtain	❑	❑	________
b. Raise bed to comfortable working height; lower side rail on side nearest the nurse	❑	❑	________
c. Position and drape patient as necessary	❑	❑	________
During the skill			
9. Promote patient involvement as possible	❑	❑	________
10. Assess patient's tolerance	❑	❑	________
11. Prepare equipment	❑	❑	________
12. Determine compatibility of all IV fluids and additives	❑	❑	________
13. Assess patency of current IV site	❑	❑	________
14. a. Prepare next solution at least 1 hour before needed	❑	❑	________
b. Order up from pharmacy if necessary	❑	❑	________
c. Check that solution is correct and properly labeled	❑	❑	________

	S	U	Comments
d. Check solution expiration date	❑	❑	______
e. Observe for precipitate or discoloration	❑	❑	______
15. Change solution when fluid is in neck of container or when new type of solution has been ordered	❑	❑	______
16. Stop flow rate correctly and remove old IV fluid container from IV pole	❑	❑	______
17. a. Quickly remove spike from old container	❑	❑	______
b. Remove protective cover from new fluid container	❑	❑	______
c. Insert spike into new bag or bottle using sterile technique	❑	❑	______
18. Hang new bag or bottle of solution on pole	❑	❑	______
19. Check tubing for air; remove bubbles appropriately	❑	❑	______
20. Make certain drip chamber is 1/3 to 1/2 full	❑	❑	______
21. Regulate flow to prescribed rate	❑	❑	______
22. Place time label on side of container with appropriate information	❑	❑	______

Postprocedure

	S	U	Comments
23. Assist patient to a position of comfort and place needed items within easy reach; be certain patient has a means to call for assistance and knows how to use it	❑	❑	______
24. Raise side rails and lower bed to lowest position	❑	❑	______
25. Remove gloves and all protective barriers; dispose of soiled supplies and equipment appropriately	❑	❑	______
26. Perform hand hygiene after patient contact and after wearing gloves	❑	❑	______
27. Document correctly; do patient teaching	❑	❑	______
28. Report any unexpected outcomes	❑	❑	______

Student Name________________________________ Date________________

PERFORMANCE CHECKLIST 20-7D
MAINTAINING AN INTRAVENOUS SITE:

Discontinuing IV Medications

	S	U	Comments
Prepare for procedure			
1. Refer to medical record, care plan, or Kardex	❑	❑	________
2. Introduce self	❑	❑	________
3. Identify patient	❑	❑	________
4. Explain procedure and reason it is to be done	❑	❑	________
5. Assess need for discontinuation and provide patient teaching	❑	❑	________
6. Assemble equipment and complete necessary charges	❑	❑	________
7. Perform hand hygiene; don clean gloves	❑	❑	________
8. Prepare patient for intervention			
a. Close door/pull privacy curtain	❑	❑	________
b. Raise bed to comfortable working height; lower side rail on side nearest the nurse	❑	❑	________
c. Position and drape patient as necessary	❑	❑	________
During the skill			
9. Promote patient involvement as possible	❑	❑	________
10. Assess patient's tolerance	❑	❑	________
11. Prepare equipment	❑	❑	________
12. a. Observe for complete infusion of all medication	❑	❑	________
b. Review orders for any necessary blood samples	❑	❑	________
c. Continue to monitor patient's response to medication	❑	❑	________
13. Move roller clamp on infusion tubing to off	❑	❑	________

	S	U	Comments
14. Remove any clasping devices and discontinue medication delivery tubing from injection port	❑	❑	______
15. Remove needle or needleless adapter; discard appropriately; replace with sterile cap or cover as indicated	❑	❑	______
16. Swab injection port or adapter on main IV tubing	❑	❑	______
17. a. If medication is piggybacked into a continuous infusion, flush line appropriately but gently	❑	❑	______
b. Regulate fluid flow as ordered	❑	❑	______
18. If using a saline/heparin lock, flush catheter appropriately but gently; if necessary, attach sterile injection port cover	❑	❑	______
19. Prepare patient for blood samples if necessary after medication infusion	❑	❑	______

Postprocedure

	S	U	Comments
20. Assist patient to a position of comfort and place needed items within easy reach; be certain patient has a means to call for assistance and knows how to use it	❑	❑	______
21. Raise side rails and lower bed to lowest position	❑	❑	______
22. Remove gloves and all protective barriers; dispose of soiled supplies and equipment appropriately	❑	❑	______
23. Perform hand hygiene after patient contact and after wearing gloves	❑	❑	______
24. Document correctly; do patient teaching	❑	❑	______
25. Report any unexpected outcomes	❑	❑	______

Student Name______________________________ Date______________

PERFORMANCE CHECKLIST 20-7E
MAINTAINING AN INTRAVENOUS SITE:

Discontinuing Peripheral IV Access

	S	U	Comments
Prepare for procedure			
1. Refer to medical record, care plan, or Kardex	❑	❑	________
2. Introduce self	❑	❑	________
3. Identify patient	❑	❑	________
4. Explain procedure and reason it is to be done	❑	❑	________
5. Assess need for discontinuation and provide patient teaching	❑	❑	________
6. Assemble equipment and complete necessary charges	❑	❑	________
7. Perform hand hygiene; don clean gloves	❑	❑	________
8. Prepare patient for intervention			
a. Close door/pull privacy curtain	❑	❑	________
b. Raise bed to comfortable working height; lower side rail on side nearest the nurse	❑	❑	________
c. Position and drape patient as necessary	❑	❑	________
During the skill			
9. Promote patient involvement as possible	❑	❑	________
10. Assess patient's tolerance	❑	❑	________
11. Prepare equipment	❑	❑	________
12. a. Observe existing IV site for signs and symptoms of infection	❑	❑	________
b. Determine patient's understanding of procedure	❑	❑	________
13. Turn IV tubing roller clamp to "off" position; remove tape securing tubing	❑	❑	________
14. Remove IV site dressing and tape; stabilize catheter	❑	❑	________

	S	U	Comments
15. Hold dry gauze or alcohol swab over site; apply light pressure; withdraw catheter appropriately	❑	❑	______
16. Apply pressure to site for 2 to 3 minutes using a dry, sterile gauze pad; secure with tape	❑	❑	______
17. Inspect the removed catheter for intactness, noting tip integrity and length	❑	❑	______
18. Instruct patient to report any abnormal signs and symptoms	❑	❑	______
Postprocedure			
19. Assist patient to a position of comfort and place needed items within easy reach; be certain patient has a means to call for assistance and knows how to use it	❑	❑	______
20. Raise side rails and lower bed to lowest position	❑	❑	______
21. Remove gloves and all protective barriers; dispose of soiled supplies and equipment appropriately	❑	❑	______
22. Perform hand hygiene after patient contact and after wearing gloves	❑	❑	______
23. Document correctly; do patient teaching	❑	❑	______
24. Report any unexpected outcomes	❑	❑	______

Student Name______________________________ Date______________

PERFORMANCE CHECKLIST 20-8

Oxygen Administration

	S	U	Comments
Prepare for procedure			
1. Refer to medical record, care plan, or Kardex	❑	❑	________
2. Introduce self	❑	❑	________
3. Identify patient	❑	❑	________
4. Explain procedure and reason it is to be done	❑	❑	________
5. Assess need for (perform oximetry to obtain oxygen saturation) and provide patient teaching during procedure	❑	❑	________
6. Assemble equipment and complete necessary charges	❑	❑	________
7. Perform hand hygiene; don clean gloves	❑	❑	________
8. Assess patient	❑	❑	________
9. Prepare patient for intervention			
a. Close door/pull privacy curtain	❑	❑	________
b. Raise bed to comfortable working height; lower side rail on side nearest the nurse	❑	❑	________
c. Position and drape patient as necessary	❑	❑	________
During the skill			
10. Promote patient involvement as possible	❑	❑	________
11. Assess patient's tolerance	❑	❑	________
12. Explain necessary precautions during oxygen therapy	❑	❑	________
13. Place patient in Fowler's or semi-Fowler's position	❑	❑	________
14. Assess patient's airway	❑	❑	________
15. Consider laboratory reports	❑	❑	________
16. Suction any secretions obstructing the airway and reassess lung sounds with stethoscope	❑	❑	________

	S	U	Comments
17. Fill humidifier container to designated level, if used: use sterile, distilled water or as prescribed	❑	❑	____________
18. Attach flowmeter to humidifier and insert in proper oxygen source	❑	❑	____________
19. Administer oxygen therapy	❑	❑	____________
Nasal cannula			
a. Attach nasal cannula to oxygen tubing, then attach to flowmeter	❑	❑	____________
b. Place prongs in cup of water; adjust flow meter to 6–10 L to flush tubing and prongs with oxygen; wipe off water	❑	❑	____________
c. Adjust flow rate to the prescribed amount	❑	❑	____________
d. Place a nasal prong into each naris of the patient; adjust liter flow per physician's order or to maintain oxygen saturation at 91% or greater	❑	❑	____________
e. Adjust straps of the cannula over the ears and tighten under the chin	❑	❑	____________
f. Place padding between strap and ears	❑	❑	____________
g. Provide slack in tubing and secure to patient's garment	❑	❑	____________
h. Maintain regular assessment			
(1) Assess cannula frequently for possible obstruction	❑	❑	____________
(2) Observe external nasal area, nares, and superior surface of both ears for skin impairment every 6–8 hours	❑	❑	____________
(3) Assess nares and prongs and cleanse with cotton-tipped applicator as needed; apply water-soluble lubricant to nares to prevent from drying	❑	❑	____________
(4) Refer to physician's orders for any prescribed changes in flow rate	❑	❑	____________
(5) Auscultate lung sounds	❑	❑	____________
(6) Monitor oxygen saturation	❑	❑	____________

Student Name_______________________ Date_______________

	S	U	Comments
(7) Maintain solution in humidifier container at appropriate level at all times	❑	❑	________
Face masks			
i. Adjust flow rate of oxygen per physician's order; monitor oxygen saturation	❑	❑	________
j. Allow patient to hold mask and place your hand over patient's hand	❑	❑	________
k. Place mask over bridge of nose, then cover mouth	❑	❑	________
l. Adjust straps around patient's head and over ears; place cotton ball or gauze over ears under elastic straps	❑	❑	________
m. Observe reservoir bag if one is attached to mask	❑	❑	________
(1) Partial-rebreather mask: reservoir should fill on exhalation and almost collapse on inhalation	❑	❑	________
(2) Nonrebreathing mask: reservoir should fill on exhalation and should never totally collapse on inhalation	❑	❑	________
n. Maintain regular assessments			
(1) Remove mask and clean and dry skin regularly	❑	❑	________
(2) Refer to physician's orders for prescribed flow rate and any changes to maintain oxygen saturation of 91% or greater	❑	❑	________
(3) Maintain solution in humidifier container, if used, at appropriate level at all times	❑	❑	________
Postprocedure			
20. Assist patient to a position of comfort and place needed items within easy reach; be certain patient has a means to call for assistance and knows how to use it	❑	❑	________

	S	U	Comments
21. Raise side rails and lower bed to lowest position	❑	❑	______
22. Remove gloves and all protective barriers; dispose of soiled supplies and equipment appropriately	❑	❑	______
23. Perform hand hygiene after patient contact and after wearing gloves	❑	❑	______
24. Document, including oxygen saturation levels, and do patient teaching	❑	❑	______
25. Report any unexpected outcomes	❑	❑	______

Student Name______________________ Date______________

PERFORMANCE CHECKLIST 20-9

Tracheostomy Care and Suctioning

	S	U	Comments
Prepare for procedure			
1. Refer to medical record, care plan, or Kardex	❑	❑	________
2. Introduce self	❑	❑	________
3. Identify patient	❑	❑	________
4. Explain procedure and reason it is to be done	❑	❑	________
5. Assess need for and provide patient teaching during procedure	❑	❑	________
6. Assemble equipment and complete necessary charges	❑	❑	________
7. Perform hand hygiene; don clean gloves	❑	❑	________
8. Assess patient	❑	❑	________
9. Prepare patient for intervention			
a. Close door/pull privacy curtain	❑	❑	________
b. Raise bed to comfortable working height; lower side rail on side nearest the nurse	❑	❑	________
c. Position and drape patient as necessary	❑	❑	________
During the skill			
10. Promote patient involvement as possible	❑	❑	________
11. Assess patient's tolerance	❑	❑	________
12. Assess patient's tracheostomy	❑	❑	________
13. Position patient in semi-Fowler's position	❑	❑	________
14. Provide paper and pencil for patient	❑	❑	________
15. Position self at head of bed facing patient	❑	❑	________
16. Auscultate lungs; monitor oxygen saturation	❑	❑	________
17. Place towel or prepackaged drape under tracheostomy and across chest	❑	❑	________

	S	U	Comments
18. Prepare equipment and supplies on overbed table			
a. Open suction catheter, leaving it in its wrapper, and attach it to suction machine	❑	❑	______
b. Pour cleansing solution (hydrogen peroxide) in one basin and rinsing solution (normal saline) in another basin	❑	❑	______
c. Turn on suction machine (120 mm Hg in adults); apply sterile glove; keep dominant hand sterile	❑	❑	______
d. Apply another sterile glove, still keeping dominant hand sterile	❑	❑	______
19. Unlock and remove inner cannula; place in cleansing solution; place fingers on tabs of outer cannula	❑	❑	______
20. Suction inner aspect of outer cannula			
a. Aspirate sterile rinsing solution through catheter	❑	❑	______
b. Ask patient to take several deep breaths or if patient is receiving oxygen, remove oxygen immediately before suctioning	❑	❑	______
c. Remove thumb from suction control or pinch catheter with gloved thumb and index finger; insert catheter 5–6 inches	❑	❑	______
d. Apply intermittent suction	❑	❑	______
e. Suction for a maximum of 10 seconds	❑	❑	______
f. Allow patient to rest between each episode of suctioning	❑	❑	______
g. Rinse catheter with sterile normal saline and repeat suctioning if needed	❑	❑	______
h. Turn off suction and dispose of catheter appropriately	❑	❑	______
21. Apply second sterile glove, if one-glove technique is used, or apply new pair of sterile gloves; clean inner cannula			

Student Name____ Date__________________

	S	U	Comments
a. Use pipe cleaners and brush to clean inside and outside of inner cannula with hydrogen peroxide solution	❑	❑	______________________
b. Place inner cannula in sterile normal saline solution, rinse thoroughly	❑	❑	______________________
c. Inspect inner and outer areas of inner cannula; remove excess liquid	❑	❑	______________________
d. Insert inner cannula and lock in place	❑	❑	______________________
22. Clean skin around tracheostomy and tabs of outer cannula; use wipes that are free of lint around the tracheostomy opening	❑	❑	______________________
23. Thoroughly rinse cleansing solution from skin; place dry, sterile dressing around tracheostomy face plate	❑	❑	______________________
24. Change cotton tapes			
a. Untie one side of cotton tape from outer cannula and replace with clean one	❑	❑	______________________
b. Bring clean tape under back of neck	❑	❑	______________________
c. Untie other side from outer cannula and replace with clean tape	❑	❑	______________________
d. Tie ends of two clean cotton tapes together and position knot appropriately	❑	❑	______________________
25. Auscultate lung sounds; monitor oxygen saturation	❑	❑	______________________
26. Provide mouth care	❑	❑	______________________
27. Remove gloves and all protective barriers and/or remove and dispose of soiled supplies and equipment appropriately	❑	❑	______________________
28. Perform hand hygiene after patient contact and after wearing gloves	❑	❑	______________________

	S	U	Comments
Postprocedure			
29. Assist patient to a position of comfort and place needed items within easy reach; be certain patient has a means to call for assistance and knows how to use it	❑	❑	______
30. Raise side rails and lower bed to lowest position	❑	❑	______
31. Place call light, paper, and pencil within easy reach	❑	❑	______
32. Reassess patient's tracheostomy	❑	❑	______
33. Document and do patient teaching	❑	❑	______
34. Report any unexpected outcomes	❑	❑	______

Student Name________________________________ Date______________

PERFORMANCE CHECKLIST 20-10

Care of the Patient with a Cuffed Tracheostomy Tube

	S	U	Comments
Prepare for procedure			
1. Refer to medical record, care plan, or Kardex	❑	❑	______
2. Introduce self	❑	❑	______
3. Identify patient	❑	❑	______
4. Explain procedure and reason it is to be done	❑	❑	______
5. Assess need for and provide patient teaching during procedure	❑	❑	______
6. Assemble equipment and complete necessary charges	❑	❑	______
7. Perform hand hygiene; don clean gloves	❑	❑	______
8. Assess patient	❑	❑	______
9. Prepare patient for intervention			
a. Close door/pull privacy curtain	❑	❑	______
b. Raise bed to comfortable working height; lower side rail on side nearest the nurse	❑	❑	______
c. Position and drape patient as necessary	❑	❑	______
During the skill			
10. Promote patient involvement as possible	❑	❑	______
11. Assess patient's tolerance; monitor oxygen saturation	❑	❑	______
12. Suction patient as in Skill 20-8 steps 12 through 20h; connect syringe to pilot balloon valve	❑	❑	______
13. Position stethoscope in sternal notch or above tracheostomy tube and listen for minimal amount of air leak at end of inspiration	❑	❑	______
14. Remove all air from cuff if no air leak is auscultated	❑	❑	______

	S	U	Comments
15. While listening with stethoscope, slowly inflate cuff with 0.5–1 mL of air at a time; when no air leak is heard, stop injecting air and slowly withdraw up to 0.5 mL of air until air leak is auscultated with stethoscope	❑	❑	______
16. If excessive air leak is heard, slowly add air as in step 15	❑	❑	______
17. Remove stethoscope and cleanse diaphragm with alcohol swab	❑	❑	______
18. Do not leave syringe attached to pilot balloon valve; remove syringe and either discard in proper container or store per agency's policy	❑	❑	______
Postprocedure			
19. Assist patient to a position of comfort and place needed items within easy reach; be certain patient has a means to call for assistance and knows how to use it	❑	❑	______
20. Raise side rails and lower bed to lowest position	❑	❑	______
21. Remove gloves and all protective barriers; dispose of soiled supplies and equipment appropriately	❑	❑	______
22. Perform hand hygiene after patient contact and after wearing gloves	❑	❑	______
23. Document and do patient teaching	❑	❑	______
24. Report any unexpected outcomes	❑	❑	______

Student Name______________________________ Date______________

PERFORMANCE CHECKLIST 20-11

Clearing the Airway

	S	U	Comments
Prepare for procedure			
1. Refer to medical record, care plan, or Kardex	❑	❑	______
2. Introduce self	❑	❑	______
3. Identify patient	❑	❑	______
4. Explain procedure and reason it is to be done	❑	❑	______
5. Assess need for and provide patient teaching during procedure	❑	❑	______
6. Assemble equipment and complete necessary charges	❑	❑	______
7. Perform hand hygiene; don clean gloves	❑	❑	______
8. Assess patient	❑	❑	______
9. Prepare patient for intervention			
a. Close door/pull privacy curtain	❑	❑	______
b. Raise bed to comfortable working height; lower side rail on side nearest the nurse	❑	❑	______
c. Position and drape patient as necessary	❑	❑	______
During the skill			
10. Promote patient involvement as possible	❑	❑	______
11. Assess patient's tolerance; monitor oxygen saturation	❑	❑	______
12. Position patient			
a. If patient is alert and conscious, place in semi-Fowler's position with head to one side	❑	❑	______
b. If patient is unconscious, place in side-lying position facing nurse	❑	❑	______
(1) Place towel lengthwise under patient's chin and over pillow	❑	❑	______

	S	U	Comments
13. Pour sterile normal saline solution into sterile container	❑	❑	________
14. Turn on suction machine, and select appropriate suction pressure, usually 120 mm Hg for adults	❑	❑	________
15. Select appropriate catheter size	❑	❑	________
16. Aspirate solution through catheter	❑	❑	________
17. Remove thumb from Y-connector opening or pinch catheter with thumb and index finger; if using suction catheter with vent, remove thumb from vent opening	❑	❑	________
18. Insert catheter	❑	❑	________
Oropharyngeal suctioning			
a. Gently insert Yankauer into one side of mouth	❑	❑	________
b. Glide Yankauer toward oropharynx without suction	❑	❑	________
c. Apply suction and move Yankauer tonsillar tip catheter around mouth until secretions are cleared	❑	❑	________
d. Encourage patient to cough	❑	❑	________
e. Rinse Yankauer; turn off suction	❑	❑	________
f. Repeat procedure as necessary	❑	❑	________
Nasopharyngeal suctioning			
g. Holding catheter, assess for correct length of insertion	❑	❑	________
h. Lubricate catheter with water-soluble lubricant	❑	❑	________
i. Hold catheter to observe its natural curvature and gently insert catheter into one side of nasal passage	❑	❑	________
Nasotracheal suctioning			
j. Holding catheter, measure for correct length	❑	❑	________

Student Name________________________ Date____________

	S	U	Comments
k. Lubricate catheter with water-soluble lubricant	❏	❏	________
l. Ask patient if either side of nose is obstructed; use unobstructed side; hold catheter to observe its natural curvature and gently insert catheter into one side of nasal passage	❏	❏	________
m. Stimulate coughing reflex, or ask patient to cough to guide catheter into trachea; if no cough reflex is present or if patient cannot assist, insert catheter when patient inhales	❏	❏	________
19. Apply intermittent suction	❏	❏	________
20. Observe patient closely and limit suction for the appropriate time	❏	❏	________
21. Repeat suctioning if needed	❏	❏	________
22. Allow 1 to 2 minutes rest between suctioning if procedure must be repeated; if oxygen is administered by nasal cannula, mask, or other means, reapply oxygen during rest period	❏	❏	________
23. If patient is alert and can cooperate, request patient to breathe deeply and cough	❏	❏	________
24. When suctioning is complete, suction between cheeks and gum line and under tongue; suction mouth last	❏	❏	________
25. Place catheter in solution and supply suction	❏	❏	________
26. Discard catheter	❏	❏	________
27. Place sterile, unopened catheter at patient's bedside	❏	❏	________
28. Provide mouth care	❏	❏	________
29. Assess patient's breathing patterns	❏	❏	________
30. Monitor oxygen saturation	❏	❏	________

Postprocedure

	S	U	Comments
31. Assist patient to a position of comfort and place needed items within easy reach; be certain patient has a means to call for assistance and knows how to use it	❏	❏	________

	S	U	Comments
32. Raise side rails and lower bed to lowest position	❑	❑	________________
33. Remove gloves and all protective barriers; dispose of soiled supplies and equipment appropriately	❑	❑	________________
34. Perform hand hygiene after patient contact and after wearing gloves	❑	❑	________________
35. Document and do patient teaching	❑	❑	________________
36. Report any unexpected outcomes	❑	❑	________________

Student Name______________________________ Date______________

PERFORMANCE CHECKLIST 20-12

CATHETERIZATION: MALE AND FEMALE

	S	U	Comments
Prepare for procedure			
1. Refer to medical record, care plan, or Kardex	❑	❑	________
2. Introduce self	❑	❑	________
3. Identify patient	❑	❑	________
4. Explain procedure and reason it is to be done	❑	❑	________
5. Assess need for and provide patient teaching during procedure	❑	❑	________
6. Assemble equipment and complete necessary charges	❑	❑	________
7. Perform hand hygiene; don clean gloves	❑	❑	________
8. Assess patient	❑	❑	________
9. Prepare patient for intervention			
a. Close door/pull privacy curtain	❑	❑	________
b. Raise bed to comfortable working height; lower side rail on side nearest the nurse	❑	❑	________
c. Position and drape patient as necessary	❑	❑	________
During the skill			
10. Promote patient involvement as possible	❑	❑	________
11. Assess patient's tolerance	❑	❑	________
12. Arrange for extra nursing personnel to assist	❑	❑	________
13. Position patient			
a. Male: Supine position with thighs slightly abducted	❑	❑	________
b. Female: Dorsal recumbent position with knees flexed, soles of feet flat on bed, and feet about 2 feet apart	❑	❑	________
14. Drape patient with bath blanket	❑	❑	________

	S	U	Comments
15. Place waterproof, absorbent pad under patient's buttocks	❑	❑	______
16. Arrange supplies and equipment on bedside table; provide a good light	❑	❑	______
17. Don clean gloves and wash perineal area	❑	❑	______
18. Remove disposable gloves and place in proper receptacle	❑	❑	______
19. Facing patient, stand on left side of bed if right-handed (on right side if left-handed)	❑	❑	______
20. Open packaging using sterile technique; don sterile gloves	❑	❑	______
21. If indwelling catheter is used, test balloon appropriately	❑	❑	______
22. Add antiseptic to cotton balls; open lubricant container; lubricate catheter the appropriate length	❑	❑	______
23. Wrap edges of sterile drape around gloved hands and request patient to raise hips, then slide drape under patient's buttocks	❑	❑	______
24. Cleanse perineal area using forceps to hold cotton balls soaked in antiseptic solution			
a. Male: If male is not circumcised, retract foreskin with nondominant hand; if erection does occur, discontinue procedure momentarily			
(1) Grasp penis at shaft below glans with one hand; continue to hold throughout insertion of catheter	❑	❑	______
(2) With other hand, use forceps to hold cotton balls soaked in antiseptic solution	❑	❑	______
(3) Cleanse meatus in circular motion	❑	❑	______
(4) Repeat cleansing two more times using sterile cotton balls each time	❑	❑	______
b. Female			
(1) Have assistant hold pen light or flashlight to provide adequate lighting	❑	❑	______

Student Name__________________________ Date__________

	S	U	Comments
(2) Spread labia minora with thumb and index finger of nondominant hand and be prepared to hold throughout the insertion of the catheter	❑	❑	______
(3) With other hand, use forceps to hold cotton balls soaked in antiseptic solution	❑	❑	______
(4) Cleanse area from clitoris toward anus, using a different sterile cotton ball each time—first to the right of the meatus, then to the left of the meatus, then down the center over meatus	❑	❑	______
25. Pick up catheter with free sterile, gloved hand near the tip; hold remaining part of catheter coiled in hands; place distal end in basin	❑	❑	______
26. Insert catheter gently, 15–18 cm (6–7 inches) for male or 5–10 cm (2–4 inches) for female	❑	❑	______
27. Collect urine specimen, if needed	❑	❑	______
28. Type of catheter			
a. Indwelling catheter			
(1) Inflate balloon with required amount of normal saline or sterile water	❑	❑	______
(2) Pull gently to feel resistance	❑	❑	______
(3) Attach drainage bag below the level of bladder (most catheters are presealed to the collecting tube of the drainage system)	❑	❑	______
(4) Attach collection bag to side of bed	❑	❑	______
(5) Secure catheter to patient			
• Male: Tape catheter to top of thigh appropriately	❑	❑	______
• Female: Tape catheter to inner thigh appropriately	❑	❑	______
(6) Clip drainage tubing to bed linen appropriately	❑	❑	______

	S	U	Comments
b. Straight catheter			
(1) Hold coiled catheter in hand with opening draining into sterile basin or into presealed plastic drainage bag	❑	❑	______
(2) Empty bladder	❑	❑	______
(3) Withdraw catheter slowly	❑	❑	______
29. Dry perineal area	❑	❑	______
Postprocedure			
30. Assist patient to a position of comfort and place needed items within easy reach; be certain patient has a means to call for assistance and knows how to use it	❑	❑	______
31. Raise side rails and lower bed to lowest position	❑	❑	______
32. Assess flow of urine and drainage tubing setup	❑	❑	______
33. Remove gloves and all protective barriers; dispose of soiled supplies and equipment appropriately	❑	❑	______
34. Perform hand hygiene after patient contact and after wearing gloves	❑	❑	______
35. Document type of catheter used, amount and color of urine, and do patient teaching	❑	❑	______
36. Report any unexpected outcomes	❑	❑	______
37. Label urine specimen appropriately	❑	❑	______
38. Transport to laboratory immediately	❑	❑	______

Student Name________________________ Date____________

PERFORMANCE CHECKLIST 20-13

Performing Routine Catheter Care

	S	U	Comments
Prepare for procedure			
1. Refer to medical record, care plan, or Kardex	❏	❏	________
2. Introduce self	❏	❏	________
3. Identify patient	❏	❏	________
4. Explain procedure and reason it is to be done	❏	❏	________
5. Assess need for and provide patient teaching during procedure	❏	❏	________
6. Assemble equipment and complete necessary charges	❏	❏	________
7. Perform hand hygiene; don clean gloves	❏	❏	________
8. Assess patient	❏	❏	________
9. Prepare patient for intervention			
a. Close door/pull privacy curtain	❏	❏	________
b. Raise bed to comfortable working height; lower side rail on side nearest the nurse	❏	❏	________
c. Position and drape patient as necessary	❏	❏	________
During the skill			
10. Promote patient involvement as possible	❏	❏	________
11. Assess patient's tolerance	❏	❏	________
12. Position patient			
a. Male: In bed in supine position	❏	❏	________
b. Female: In bed in dorsal recumbent position	❏	❏	________
13. Place waterproof disposable pad under patient's buttocks and to the side from which catheter care will be given	❏	❏	________
14. Drape patient with bath blanket, exposing only perineal area	❏	❏	________

	S	U	Comments
15. If using sterile catheter care kit			
a. Open supplies using sterile technique and arrange on bedside table	❑	❑	______
b. Don sterile gloves	❑	❑	______
c. Place cotton balls in sterile basin and saturate with sterile solution	❑	❑	______
d. With one hand expose urethral meatus			
(1) **Male**: retract foreskin, then hold penis erect	❑	❑	______
(2) **Female**: gently retract labia minora away from urinary meatus and hold in position	❑	❑	______
e. Wash the area at the meatus and around the catheter with cotton balls saturated with sterile solution			
(1) **Male**			
• With one cotton ball, cleanse around meatus and catheter in a circular motion	❑	❑	______
• Repeat twice more, using different cotton balls each time	❑	❑	______
(2) **Female**			
• With one cotton ball, swab to one side of labia minora from anterior to posterior	❑	❑	______
• Repeat with second cotton ball on opposite side	❑	❑	______
• Repeat with third cotton ball down middle over meatus and around catheter	❑	❑	______
f. Discard soiled cotton balls in other basin in kit	❑	❑	______
g. With forceps, pick up cotton ball soaked in antiseptic solution or mild soap and water and cleanse around catheter from urethral opening	❑	❑	______
16. If using a collection of sterile supplies			
a. Open separate sterile packages observing sterile technique	❑	❑	______

Student Name____ **Date**__________________

	S	U	Comments
b. Don clean gloves	❑	❑	________________
c. Arrange refuse bag	❑	❑	________________
d. Cleanse the perineal area with mild soap and warm water; pat dry			
(1) Male: retract foreskin then hold the penis erect	❑	❑	________________
(2) Female: gently retract labia away from urinary meatus and hold in position	❑	❑	________________
e. Apply in appropriate amount of sterile antiinfective ointment (if used) on sterile cotton-tipped applicator and gently apply around catheter at site of insertion (this is seldom used now)	❑	❑	________________
f. Release labia of female patient; replace foreskin of male patient	❑	❑	________________
17. Observe meatus, catheter, and surrounding tissue to assess normal or abnormal condition; determine presence or absence of inflammation, edema, malodorous exudate, color of tissue, and burning sensation	❑	❑	________________
18. Dispose of equipment and linen; remove gloves and all protective barriers; dispose of soiled supplies and equipment appropriately	❑	❑	________________
19. Retape catheter to thigh	❑	❑	________________

Postprocedure

	S	U	Comments
20. Assist patient to a position of comfort and place needed items within easy reach; be certain patient has a means to call for assistance and knows how to use it	❑	❑	________________
21. Raise side rails and lower bed to lowest position	❑	❑	________________
22. Perform hand hygiene after patient contact and after wearing gloves	❑	❑	________________
23. Document and do patient teaching	❑	❑	________________
24. Report any unexpected outcomes	❑	❑	________________

Student Name________________________________ Date______________

PERFORMANCE CHECKLIST 20-14

Catheter Irrigation: Open, Intermittent, Continuous, and Bladder Instillation

	S	U	Comments
Prepare for procedure			
1. Refer to medical record, care plan, or Kardex	❑	❑	______
2. Introduce self	❑	❑	______
3. Identify patient	❑	❑	______
4. Explain procedure and reason it is to be done	❑	❑	______
5. Assess need for and provide patient teaching	❑	❑	______
6. Assemble equipment and complete necessary charges	❑	❑	______
7. Perform hand hygiene; don clean gloves	❑	❑	______
8. Assess patient	❑	❑	______
9. Prepare patient for intervention			
a. Close door/pull privacy curtain	❑	❑	______
b. Raise bed to comfortable working height; lower side rail on side nearest the nurse	❑	❑	______
c. Position and drape patient as necessary	❑	❑	______
During the skill			
10. Promote patient involvement as possible	❑	❑	______
11. Assess patient	❑	❑	______
12. Position patient			
a. **Male**: Supine in bed	❑	❑	______
b. **Female**: Dorsal recumbent in bed	❑	❑	______
13. Place waterproof absorbent pad under patient's buttocks and to the side from which bladder irrigation will be done	❑	❑	______
14. Arrange supplies and equipment at bedside on overbed table	❑	❑	______

	S	U	Comments
15. Open method			
a. Pour sterile irrigating solution (normal saline unless otherwise specified) into sterile graduated container and recap solution bottle; irrigating solution should be at room temperature	❑	❑	______
b. Don sterile gloves	❑	❑	______
c. Place sterile basin between patient's legs, close to perineal area	❑	❑	______
d. Disconnect catheter from drainage system and plug drainage tubing with sterile plug	❑	❑	______
e. Draw 30 mL of sterile solution into syringe	❑	❑	______
f. Cleanse catheter end with antiseptic swab	❑	❑	______
g. Place tip of syringe into end of catheter and gently insert solution	❑	❑	______
h. Withdraw syringe and allow solution to drain into basin by gravity	❑	❑	______
i. If solution does not return, turn patient on side facing nurse	❑	❑	______
j. Repeat injection of solution until amount ordered is injected and returned	❑	❑	______
k. Remove plug from drainage tubing, and connect tubing to catheter	❑	❑	______
l. Measure solution (to determine amount returned and amount of urine expelled)	❑	❑	______
16. Closed intermittent method (repeat steps 1 to 14)			
a. Pour sterile irrigating solution (normal saline unless otherwise specified) into graduated container	❑	❑	______
b. Draw up sterile solution into syringe	❑	❑	______
c. Clamp catheter below injection port	❑	❑	______
d. Cleanse port with antiseptic	❑	❑	______
e. Insert needle of syringe into port	❑	❑	______
f. Inject solution into catheter slowly	❑	❑	______
17. Closed continuous method or continuous bladder irrigation (CBI)			

Student Name_______________________________ Date______________

	S	U	Comments
a. Set up irrigating solution (normal saline unless otherwise specified) by attaching tubing to irrigation bag	❑	❑	____________
b. Clamp off tubing so no solution flows through	❑	❑	____________
c. Suspend bag on IV pole	❑	❑	____________
d. Open clamp and allow solution to flow through tubing	❑	❑	____________
e. Cleanse irrigating lumen on end of triple lumen catheter	❑	❑	____________
f. Connect irrigating solution tubing to catheter lumen	❑	❑	____________
g. Restore flow as ordered; run drip rate to keep drainage system clear	❑	❑	____________
h. Deduct solution from urine in drainage bag when emptying to compute true urine	❑	❑	____________
18. Bladder instillation			
a. Disconnect catheter from tubing—stabilize tubing to prevent touching the floor (triple lumen catheter does not require disconnection from drainage tubing)	❑	❑	____________
b. Cleanse end of catheter with antiseptic swab	❑	❑	____________
c. Draw medication or solution ordered into syringe	❑	❑	____________
d. Place tip of syringe into end of catheter and slowly inject medication or solution ordered	❑	❑	____________
e. Clamp off end of catheter for period of time necessary; then reconnect catheter and tubing, making certain the system is tightly connected	❑	❑	____________
f. Measure solution	❑	❑	____________

	S	U	Comments
Postprocedure			
19. Assist patient to a position of comfort and place needed items within easy reach; be certain patient has a means to call for assistance and knows how to use it	❑	❑	________
20. Raise side rails and lower bed to lowest position	❑	❑	________
21. Remove gloves and all protective barriers; dispose of soiled supplies and equipment appropriately	❑	❑	________
22. Perform hand hygiene after patient contact and after wearing gloves	❑	❑	________
23. Document and do patient teaching	❑	❑	________
24. Report any unexpected outcomes	❑	❑	________

Student Name______________________________ Date______________

PERFORMANCE CHECKLIST 20-15

Removing an Indwelling Catheter

	S	U	Comments
Prepare for procedure			
1. Refer to medical record, care plan, or Kardex	❑	❑	________
2. Introduce self	❑	❑	________
3. Identify patient	❑	❑	________
4. Explain procedure and reason it is to be done	❑	❑	________
5. Assess need for procedure and provide patient teaching	❑	❑	________
6. Assemble equipment and complete necessary charges	❑	❑	________
7. Perform hand hygiene; don clean gloves	❑	❑	________
8. Assess patient	❑	❑	________
9. Prepare patient for intervention			
a. Close door/pull privacy curtain	❑	❑	________
b. Raise bed to comfortable working height; lower side rail on side nearest the nurse	❑	❑	________
c. Position and drape patient as necessary	❑	❑	________
During the skill			
10. Position patient supine	❑	❑	________
11. a. Females: place waterproof pad under catheter; abduct legs and place drape between thighs	❑	❑	________
b. Males: lay drape on thighs	❑	❑	________
12. Insert hub of syringe into inflation valve (balloon port) and aspirate until tubing collapses	❑	❑	________
13. Remove catheter steadily and smoothly; do not use force	❑	❑	________
14. Wrap catheter in waterproof pad	❑	❑	________

	S	U	Comments
15. Unhook collection bag and drainage tubing from bed	❑	❑	______
16. Measure urine and empty drainage bag	❑	❑	______
17. Record output	❑	❑	______
18. Cleanse perineum; dry thoroughly	❑	❑	______
19. Do patient teaching	❑	❑	______
20. Place urine hat on toilet seat	❑	❑	______

Postprocedure

	S	U	Comments
21. Assist patient to a position of comfort and place needed items within easy reach; be certain patient has a means to call for assistance and knows how to use it	❑	❑	______
22. Raise side rails and lower bed to lowest position	❑	❑	______
23. Remove gloves and all protective barriers; dispose of soiled supplies and equipment appropriately	❑	❑	______
24. Perform hand hygiene after patient contact and after wearing gloves	❑	❑	______
25. Document and finish patient teaching	❑	❑	______
26. Report any unexpected outcomes	❑	❑	______

Student Name______________________________ Date______________

PERFORMANCE CHECKLIST 20-16

Performing a Vaginal Irrigation or Douche

	S	U	Comments
Prepare for procedure			
1. Refer to medical record, care plan, or Kardex	❑	❑	______
2. Introduce self	❑	❑	______
3. Identify patient	❑	❑	______
4. Explain procedure and reason it is to be done	❑	❑	______
5. Assess need for and provide patient teaching during procedure	❑	❑	______
6. Assemble equipment and complete necessary charges	❑	❑	______
7. Perform hand hygiene; don clean gloves	❑	❑	______
8. Assess patient	❑	❑	______
9. Prepare patient for intervention			
a. Close door/pull privacy curtain	❑	❑	______
b. Raise bed to comfortable working height; lower side rail on side nearest the nurse	❑	❑	______
c. Position and drape patient as necessary	❑	❑	______
During the skill			
10. Promote patient involvement as possible	❑	❑	______
11. Assess patient's tolerance	❑	❑	______
12. Prepare equipment			
a. Solution should be at body temperature	❑	❑	______
b. Allow some solution to drain down the tubing out through the nozzle into bedpan	❑	❑	______
13. Gently retract labial folds and direct nozzle toward the sacrum, following the floor of the vagina	❑	❑	______
14. Raise the container approximately 30–50 cm (12–20 in) above level of vagina	❑	❑	______

	S	U	Comments
15. Insert nozzle appropriately through vaginal meatus	❏	❏	______
16. Allow solution to flow while inserting and rotating nozzle	❏	❏	______
17. Instruct patient to tighten perineal muscles as if to suppress urination and then relax; repeat four to five times during procedure	❏	❏	______
18. Administer all of the solution while rotating nozzle gently during instillation	❏	❏	______
19. Withdraw nozzle and assist patient to a comfortable position while she remains on the bedpan	❏	❏	______
20. Allow patient to remain on bedpan a short time (10 minutes), then don clean gloves; remove bedpan, assessing results; dispose of remaining solution in proper manner	❏	❏	______
21. Cleanse and dry patient or allow her to cleanse and dry herself	❏	❏	______
Postprocedure			
22. Assist patient to a position of comfort and place needed items within easy reach; be certain patient has a means to call for assistance and knows how to use it	❏	❏	______
23. Raise side rails and lower bed to lowest position	❏	❏	______
24. Remove gloves and all protective barriers; dispose of soiled supplies and equipment appropriately	❏	❏	______
25. Perform hand hygiene after patient contact and after wearing gloves	❏	❏	______
26. Document and do patient teaching	❏	❏	______
27. Report any unexpected outcomes	❏	❏	______

Student Name____ Date________________

PERFORMANCE CHECKLIST 20-17

INSERTING A NASOGASTRIC TUBE

	S	U	Comments
Prepare for procedure			
1. Refer to medical record, care plan, or Kardex	❏	❏	________________
2. Introduce self	❏	❏	________________
3. Identify patient	❏	❏	________________
4. Explain procedure and reason it is to be done	❏	❏	________________
5. Assess need for and provide patient teaching during procedure	❏	❏	________________
6. Assemble equipment and complete necessary charges	❏	❏	________________
7. Perform hand hygiene; don clean gloves	❏	❏	________________
8. Assess patient	❏	❏	________________
9. Prepare patient for intervention			
a. Close door/pull privacy curtain	❏	❏	________________
b. Raise bed to comfortable working height; lower side rail on side nearest the nurse	❏	❏	________________
c. Position and drape patient as necessary	❏	❏	________________
During the skill			
10. Promote patient involvement as possible	❏	❏	________________
11. Assess patient's tolerance	❏	❏	________________
12. Assess patient for condition of nares and oral cavity	❏	❏	________________
13. Assess patient's oral cavity	❏	❏	________________
14. Position patient in high Fowler's position with pillow behind head and shoulders	❏	❏	________________
15. Stand at right side of bed if right-handed and left side if left-handed	❏	❏	________________
16. Place bath towel over patient's chest; give tissues to patient	❏	❏	________________

	S	U	Comments
17. Instruct patient to relax and breathe normally while occluding one naris; repeat this action for other naris	❑	❑	________
18. Measure distance to insert tube correctly (measure distance from tip of nose to earlobe to xiphoid process)	❑	❑	________
19. Mark length of tube to be inserted with piece of tape or note distance from next tube marking	❑	❑	________
20. Curve end of tube tightly around index finger; release	❑	❑	________
21. Lubricate end of tube generously with water-soluble lubricating jelly	❑	❑	________
22. Initially instruct patient to extend neck back against pillow; insert tube slowly through naris with curved end pointing downward	❑	❑	________
23. Continue to pass tube along floor of nasal passage, aiming down toward ear; when resistance is felt, apply gentle downward pressure to advance tube (do not force past resistance)	❑	❑	________
24. If resistance continues, withdraw tube, allow patient to rest, relubricate tube, and insert into other naris	❑	❑	________
25. Continue insertion of tube until just past nasopharynx by gently rotating tube toward opposite naris			
a. Stop tube advancement, allow patient to relax, and provide tissues	❑	❑	________
b. Explain that the next step requires swallowing	❑	❑	________
26. With tube just above oropharynx, instruct patient to flex head forward and dry swallow or suck in air through straw; advance with each swallow; if patient has trouble swallowing and is allowed fluids, offer glass of water; advance tube with each swallow of water; while advancing the tube in an unconscious patient (or in a patient who cannot swallow), stroke the patient's neck	❑	❑	________
27. If patient begins to cough, gag, or choke, stop tube advancement; instruct patient to breathe easily and take sips of water	❑	❑	________

Student Name________________________ Date____________

	S	U	Comments
28. If patient continues to cough, pull tube back slightly	❑	❑	________
29. If patient continues to gag, assess back of oral pharynx using flashlight and tongue blade	❑	❑	________
30. After patient relaxes, continue to advance tube desired distance	❑	❑	________
31. Ask patient to talk	❑	❑	________
32. Assess posterior pharynx for presence of coiled tube	❑	❑	________
33. Attach cone-tipped syringe to end of tube; aspirate gently back on syringe to obtain gastric contents	❑	❑	________
34. Measure pH of aspirate with color-coded pH paper	❑	❑	________
35. If tube is not in the stomach, advance another 2.5–5 cm (1–2 in) and repeat step 33	❑	❑	________
36. After tube is properly inserted, clamp end or connect it to suction	❑	❑	________
37. Cleanse nose with alcohol and Skin Prep for better adherence of nasal guard	❑	❑	________
38. Secure tube to nose with a nasal guard; avoid putting pressure on nares	❑	❑	________
39. Fasten end of tube to gown by looping rubber band around tube in slip knot; pin rubber band to gown	❑	❑	________
40. Unless physician orders otherwise, head of bed should be elevated 30 degrees	❑	❑	________

Postprocedure

	S	U	Comments
41. Assist patient to a position of comfort and place needed items within easy reach; be certain patient has a means to call for assistance and knows how to use it	❑	❑	________
42. Raise side rails and lower bed to lowest position	❑	❑	________
43. Remove gloves and all protective barriers; dispose of soiled supplies and equipment appropriately	❑	❑	________

	S	U	Comments
44. Perform hand hygiene after patient contact and after wearing gloves	❏	❏	__________
45. Document and do patient teaching	❏	❏	__________
46. Report any unexpected outcomes	❏	❏	__________

Student Name________________________________ Date________________

PERFORMANCE CHECKLIST 20-18

Nasogastric Tube Irrigation

	S	U	Comments
Prepare for procedure			
1. Refer to medical record, care plan, or Kardex	❑	❑	______________
2. Introduce self	❑	❑	______________
3. Identify patient	❑	❑	______________
4. Explain procedure and reason it is to be done	❑	❑	______________
5. Assess need for and provide patient teaching during procedure	❑	❑	______________
6. Assemble equipment and complete necessary charges	❑	❑	______________
7. Perform hand hygiene; don clean gloves	❑	❑	______________
8. Assess patient	❑	❑	______________
9. Prepare patient for intervention			
a. Close door/pull privacy curtain	❑	❑	______________
b. Raise bed to comfortable working height; lower side rail on side nearest the nurse	❑	❑	______________
c. Position and drape patient as necessary	❑	❑	______________
During the skill			
10. Promote patient involvement as possible	❑	❑	______________
11. Assess patient's tolerance	❑	❑	______________
12. Place patient in semi-Fowler's position	❑	❑	______________
13. Verify that tube is in right place by attaching syringe to end of tube and aspirating for stomach content	❑	❑	______________
14. Assess abdomen	❑	❑	______________
15. Pour normal saline into container; draw up 30 mL (or amount ordered) into piston syringe	❑	❑	______________

	S	U	Comments
16. Clamp connection tubing distal to connection site for drainage or suction apparatus; disconnect tubing and lay end on a towel or waterproof pad	❑	❑	______
17. Insert tip of irrigating syringe into end of NG tube; hold syringe with tip pointed toward the floor and instill 30 mL or ordered amount saline slowly and evenly **(do not force solution)**	❑	❑	______
18. If resistance is met, assess tubing for kinks, change patient's position, and repeat attempt; if resistance continues, confer with RN or physician	❑	❑	______
19. Withdraw fluid into syringe and measure; continue irrigating with ordered amount of saline until purpose of irrigation has been accomplished	❑	❑	______
20. Reconnect NG tube to suction, introduce 30 mL of air into blue air vent lumen to clear air vent tubing; do not put liquid irrigant into blue airway lumen; secure airway lumen above level of stomach	❑	❑	______
21. Note amount of saline instilled and withdrawn; subtract amount instilled from amount withdrawn and record difference as output	❑	❑	______
Postprocedure			
22. Assist patient to a position of comfort and place needed items within easy reach; be certain patient has a means to call for assistance and knows how to use it	❑	❑	______
23. Raise side rails and lower bed to lowest position	❑	❑	______
24. Remove gloves and all protective barriers; dispose of soiled supplies and equipment appropriately	❑	❑	______
25. Perform hand hygiene after patient contact and after wearing gloves	❑	❑	______
26. Document and do patient teaching	❑	❑	______
27. Report any unexpected outcomes	❑	❑	______

Student Name________________________ Date______________

PERFORMANCE CHECKLIST 20-19

Gastric and Intestinal Suctioning Care

	S	U	Comments
Prepare for procedure			
1. Refer to medical record, care plan, or Kardex	❑	❑	________
2. Introduce self	❑	❑	________
3. Identify patient	❑	❑	________
4. Explain procedure and reason it is to be done	❑	❑	________
5. Assess need for and provide patient teaching during procedure	❑	❑	________
6. Assemble equipment and complete necessary charges	❑	❑	________
7. Perform hand hygiene; don clean gloves	❑	❑	________
8. Assess patient	❑	❑	________
9. Prepare patient for intervention			
a. Close door / pull privacy curtain	❑	❑	________
b. Raise bed to comfortable working height; lower side rail on side nearest the nurse	❑	❑	________
c. Position and drape patient as necessary	❑	❑	________
During the skill			
10. Promote patient involvement as possible	❑	❑	________
11. Assess patient's tolerance	❑	❑	________
12. Assess suction apparatus	❑	❑	________
a. For suction machine (Gomco)			
(1) Make certain machine is plugged in securely	❑	❑	________
(2) Make certain light is blinking on and off	❑	❑	________
(3) Make certain tubing connections are secure	❑	❑	________
(4) Make certain setting is correct	❑	❑	________

	S	U	Comments
b. For wall suction			
(1) Make certain pressure gauge connections are tight	❑	❑	____
(2) Make certain pressure indicated on gauge is as ordered or according to agency policy, 80–100 mm Hg; pressure above 120 mm Hg results in gastric bleeding	❑	❑	____
(3) Suction is set on intermittent or continuous as ordered	❑	❑	____
13. Assess patient			
a. Oral/nasal cavities	❑	❑	____
b. Abdomen for bowel sounds and extent of distention (be certain to turn off wall suctioning during assessment to prevent hearing Salem sump sounds)	❑	❑	____
c. NPO status	❑	❑	____
d. Lips and oral mucosa	❑	❑	____
14. Ensure that tubing is not kinked and that patient is not lying on tubing	❑	❑	____
15. Pin NG tube to patient's gown with enough slack to allow movement	❑	❑	____
16. Verify that drainage is moving through tubing to drainage collection bottle	❑	❑	____
17. For Salem sump tube see that vent is pointing upward; listen at opening of blue air vent; if no hissing sounds are heard, instruct patient to cough or reposition to the right or left Sims' or supine position; it may be necessary to momentarily disconnect the NG tube from the suction tubing; be certain to reconnect immediately	❑	❑	____
18. Measure amount of drainage in bottle, noting color; empty when becoming full and at end of each shift	❑	❑	____

Student Name____ Date______________

	S	U	Comments
Postprocedure			
19. Assist patient to a position of comfort and place needed items within easy reach; be certain patient has a means to call for assistance and knows how to use it	❑	❑	________________
20. Raise side rails and lower bed to lowest position	❑	❑	________________
21. Remove gloves and all protective barriers; dispose of soiled supplies and equipment appropriately	❑	❑	________________
22. Perform hand hygiene after patient contact and after wearing gloves	❑	❑	________________
23. Document and do patient teaching	❑	❑	________________
24. Report any unexpected outcomes	❑	❑	________________

Student Name________________________________ Date________________

PERFORMANCE CHECKLIST 20-20

NASOGASTRIC TUBE REMOVAL

	S	U	Comments
Prepare for procedure			
1. Refer to medical record, care plan, or Kardex	❑	❑	________
2. Introduce self	❑	❑	________
3. Identify patient	❑	❑	________
4. Explain procedure and reason it is to be done	❑	❑	________
5. Assess need for and provide patient teaching during procedure	❑	❑	________
6. Assemble equipment and complete necessary charges	❑	❑	________
7. Perform hand hygiene; don clean gloves	❑	❑	________
8. Assess patient	❑	❑	________
9. Prepare patient for intervention			
a. Close door / pull privacy curtain	❑	❑	________
b. Raise bed to comfortable working height; lower side rail on side nearest the nurse	❑	❑	________
c. Position and drape patient as necessary	❑	❑	________
During the skill			
10. Promote patient involvement as possible	❑	❑	________
11. Assess patient's tolerance	❑	❑	________
12. Reassure that removal is less distressing than insertion	❑	❑	________
13. Assess			
a. Patient's abdomen for bowel sounds (turn off wall suction during assessment to prevent misinterpreting Salem sump sounds for peristalsis)	❑	❑	________
b. Patient's nasal and oral cavity	❑	❑	________

	S	U	Comments
14. If tube is attached to suction, turn off suction machine and disconnect tubing, remove nose guard, and unfasten pin from gown	❑	❑	______
15. Place towel or waterproof pad across patient's chest	❑	❑	______
16. Instruct patient to take deep breath and hold it; pinch tube with fingers or clamp; quickly and smoothly remove tube while patient is holding breath	❑	❑	______
17. Provide patient with tissues to cleanse nasal passage	❑	❑	______
18. Place tubing in plastic bag or towel	❑	❑	______
19. Cleanse nose with alcohol to remove residue from nasal guard placement	❑	❑	______
20. Provide oral and nasal care; make patient comfortable	❑	❑	______
21. Dispose of tube and equipment; measure drainage; note color and write down for documentation	❑	❑	______
22. Inspect condition of nares and oral cavity	❑	❑	______
Postprocedure			
23. Assist patient to a position of comfort and place needed items within easy reach; be certain patient has a means to call for assistance and knows how to use it	❑	❑	______
24. Raise side rails and lower bed to lowest position	❑	❑	______
25. Palpate abdomen periodically, noting any distention, pain, and rigidity; auscultate abdomen for bowel sounds	❑	❑	______
26. Remove gloves and all protective barriers; dispose of soiled supplies and equipment appropriately	❑	❑	______
27. Perform hand hygiene after patient contact and after wearing gloves	❑	❑	______
28. Document and do patient teaching	❑	❑	______
29. Report any unexpected outcomes	❑	❑	______

Student Name______________________________ Date______________

PERFORMANCE CHECKLIST 20-21

INSERTING A RECTAL TUBE

	S	U	Comments
Prepare for procedure			
1. Refer to medical record, care plan, or Kardex	❑	❑	________
2. Introduce self	❑	❑	________
3. Identify patient	❑	❑	________
4. Explain procedure and reason it is to be done	❑	❑	________
5. Assess need for and provide patient teaching	❑	❑	________
6. Assemble equipment and complete necessary charges	❑	❑	________
7. Perform hand hygiene; don clean gloves	❑	❑	________
8. Assess patient	❑	❑	________
9. Prepare patient for intervention			
a. Close door/pull privacy curtain	❑	❑	________
b. Raise bed to comfortable working height; lower side rail on side nearest the nurse	❑	❑	________
c. Position and drape patient as necessary	❑	❑	________
During the skill			
10. Promote patient involvement as possible	❑	❑	________
11. Assess bowel sounds	❑	❑	________
12. Request patient to assume Sims' position	❑	❑	________
13. Arrange gown and top sheet to prevent soiling	❑	❑	________
14. Place waterproof pad under buttocks	❑	❑	________
15. Don gloves	❑	❑	________
16. Lubricate tube well	❑	❑	________
17. Expose anus	❑	❑	________
18. Insert tube appropriately	❑	❑	________

	S	U	Comments
19. Insert drainage end into receptacle or use commercially prepared set	❑	❑	______
20. Instruct patient to lie quietly	❑	❑	______
21. Leave tube in place the allotted time	❑	❑	______
22. Notify physician as necessary	❑	❑	______
23. Remove tube and assist patient to bedpan/toilet or commode	❑	❑	______
24. Assess for bowel movement	❑	❑	______
25. Provide for hygiene	❑	❑	______
26. Assess for bowel sounds	❑	❑	______

Postprocedure

	S	U	Comments
27. Assist patient to a position of comfort and place needed items within easy reach; be certain patient has a means to call for assistance and knows how to use it	❑	❑	______
28. Raise side rails and lower bed to lowest position	❑	❑	______
29. Remove gloves and all protective barriers; dispose of soiled supplies and equipment appropriately	❑	❑	______
30. Perform hand hygiene after patient contact and after wearing gloves	❑	❑	______
31. Document and do patient teaching	❑	❑	______
32. Report any unexpected outcomes	❑	❑	______

Student Name____________________ Date__________

PERFORMANCE CHECKLIST 20-22

Administering an Enema

	S	U	Comments
Prepare for procedure			
1. Refer to medical record, care plan, or Kardex	❑	❑	______
2. Introduce self	❑	❑	______
3. Identify patient	❑	❑	______
4. Explain procedure and reason it is to be done	❑	❑	______
5. Assess need for and provide patient teaching during procedure	❑	❑	______
6. Assemble equipment and complete necessary charges	❑	❑	______
7. Perform hand hygiene; don clean gloves	❑	❑	______
8. Assess patient	❑	❑	______
9. Prepare patient for intervention			
a. Close door/pull privacy curtain	❑	❑	______
b. Raise bed to comfortable working height; lower side rail on side nearest the nurse	❑	❑	______
c. Position and drape patient as necessary	❑	❑	______
During the skill			
10. Promote patient involvement as possible	❑	❑	______
11. Assess patient's tolerance	❑	❑	______
12. Prepare solution	❑	❑	______
13. Arrange equipment at bedside	❑	❑	______
14. Assist patient to Sims' position; when giving an enema to a patient who is unable to contract the external sphincter, position the patient on the bedpan	❑	❑	______
15. Place waterproof pad under patient	❑	❑	______
16. Place bath blanket over patient and fan-fold linen to foot of bed; adjust patient's gown	❑	❑	______
17. Clamp tubing 28 cm (7 in) from end; fill container with correctly warmed solution (usually 1000 mL at 105° F for adults) and any additives; allow solution to fill tubing to prevent air in colon	❑	❑	______

	S	U	Comments
18. Lubricate tubing; spread patient's buttocks to expose anus; while rotating tube, gently insert it 7–10 cm (3–4 in); instruct patient to breathe out slowly through mouth (for commercially prepared enemas, remove cover from tip of enema device; add additional lubricant and insert entire tip into anus, squeeze container until it is empty; continue to squeeze container and remove and discard device appropriately)	❏	❏	______
19. Elevate container 30–45 cm (12–18 in) above level of anus	❏	❏	______
20. Release clamp; allow more solution to flow slowly while holding clamp	❏	❏	______
21. Lower container or clamp tubing if patient complains of cramping; encourage slow, deep breathing (when severe cramping, bleeding, or sudden abdominal pain occurs that is unrelieved by temporarily stopping or slowing flow of solution, stop enema and notify physician)	❏	❏	______
22. Clamp and remove tube when all of the solution has been administered; encourage patient to retain solution at least 5 minutes	❏	❏	______
23. When patient can no longer retain solution, assist to bedpan, bedside commode, or bathroom	❏	❏	______
24. Instruct patient to call for nurse to inspect results before flushing stool; observe characteristics of feces/solution	❏	❏	______
25. Provide for patient hygiene	❏	❏	______
Postprocedure			
26. Assist patient to a position of comfort and place needed items within easy reach; be certain patient has a means to call for assistance and knows how to use it	❏	❏	______
27. Raise side rails and lower bed to lowest position	❏	❏	______
28. Remove gloves and all protective barriers; dispose of soiled supplies and equipment appropriately	❏	❏	______

Student Name____ Date____________________

	S	U	Comments
29. Perform hand hygiene after patient contact and after wearing gloves; provide for patient hygiene and assist patient to the bed or to the chair	❑	❑	____________________
30. Document and do patient teaching	❑	❑	____________________
31. Report any unexpected outcomes	❑	❑	____________________

Student Name______________________________ Date______________

PERFORMANCE CHECKLIST 20-23

Digital Examination with Removal of Fecal Impaction

	S	U	Comments
Prepare for procedure			
1. Refer to medical record, care plan, or Kardex	❑	❑	______
2. Introduce self	❑	❑	______
3. Identify patient	❑	❑	______
4. Explain procedure and reason it is to be done	❑	❑	______
5. Assess need for and provide patient teaching during procedure	❑	❑	______
6. Assemble equipment and complete necessary charges	❑	❑	______
7. Perform hand hygiene; don clean gloves	❑	❑	______
8. Assess patient	❑	❑	______
9. Prepare patient for intervention			
a. Close door/pull privacy curtain	❑	❑	______
b. Raise bed to comfortable working height; lower side rail on side nearest the nurse	❑	❑	______
c. Position and drape patient as necessary	❑	❑	______
During the skill			
10. Promote patient involvement as possible	❑	❑	______
11. Assess patient's tolerance	❑	❑	______
12. Assist patient to assume the Sims' position and place waterproof pad under patient's buttocks	❑	❑	______
13. Place the bedpan on the bed close to the patient's buttocks	❑	❑	______
14. Don gloves; lubricate forefinger well with petroleum or water-soluble lubricant; use the index finger of your dominant hand	❑	❑	______

	S	U	Comments
15. Insert finger gently; slowly but gently move finger into and around the fecal mass; as pieces of the mass are broken off, remove them to bedpan	❑	❑	______
16. Instruct patient to take slow, deep breaths	❑	❑	______
17. Continue procedure until impaction is removed	❑	❑	______
18. Stop procedure for a few minutes if patient complains of severe discomfort; give patient opportunity to rest; be alert for complications such as adverse vagal response	❑	❑	______
19. After removal is complete, wash and dry perineal area	❑	❑	______
20. Assist the patient to toilet or position on the bedpan if urge to defecate develops	❑	❑	______
Postprocedure			
21. Assist patient to a position of comfort and place needed items within easy reach; be certain patient has a means to call for assistance and knows how to use it	❑	❑	______
22. Raise side rails and lower bed to lowest position	❑	❑	______
23. Remove gloves and all protective barriers; dispose of soiled supplies and equipment appropriately	❑	❑	______
24. Perform hand hygiene after patient contact and after wearing gloves	❑	❑	______
25. Document and do patient teaching	❑	❑	______
26. Report any unexpected outcomes	❑	❑	______

Student Name________________________ Date____________

PERFORMANCE CHECKLIST 20-24

Performing Colostomy, Ileostomy, and Urostomy Care

	S	U	Comments
Prepare for procedure			
1. Refer to medical record, care plan, or Kardex	❑	❑	________
2. Introduce self	❑	❑	________
3. Identify patient	❑	❑	________
4. Explain procedure and reason it is to be done	❑	❑	________
5. Assess need for and provide patient teaching during procedure	❑	❑	________
6. Assemble equipment and complete necessary charges	❑	❑	________
7. Perform hand hygiene; don clean gloves	❑	❑	________
8. Assess patient	❑	❑	________
9. Prepare patient for intervention			
a. Close door/pull privacy curtain	❑	❑	________
b. Raise bed to comfortable working height; lower side rail on side nearest the nurse	❑	❑	________
c. Position and drape patient as necessary	❑	❑	________
During the skill			
10. Promote patient involvement as possible	❑	❑	________
11. Assess patient's tolerance	❑	❑	________
12. Arrange supplies/equipment at bedside or in bathroom	❑	❑	________
13. Position patient supine and make comfortable	❑	❑	________
14. Unfasten and remove belt, if worn; carefully remove wafer seal from skin	❑	❑	________
15. Place reusable pouch in bedpan or disposable pouch in plastic bag. Place bag away from patient to prevent unpleasant odors	❑	❑	________
16. Cleanse skin with warm water; pat dry	❑	❑	________

	S	U	Comments
17. Measure stoma using measuring device	❏	❏	
18. Place toilet tissue or disposable wash cloth over stoma; use gauze for ileostomy; if using Skin Prep, apply to skin and allow to dry	❏	❏	
19. Apply protective skin barrier about 1/16 inch from stoma; assess stoma to determine color and viability	❏	❏	
20. Apply protective wafer with flange, cutting an opening in the center of wafer to 1/16 inch larger than stoma	❏	❏	
21. Gently attach pouch to flange by compressing the two together (a device is available called Autolok which snaps into place with a smooth lock, thus eliminating the need to compress the flange to the pouch)	❏	❏	
22. Remove tissue or gauze from stoma and backing from protectant; center opening over stoma and press against skin for 1–2 minutes	❏	❏	
23. Fold bottom edges of pouch over one time to fit clamp	❏	❏	
24. Secure clamp	❏	❏	
25. If belt is used, attach properly	❏	❏	
26. Assist patient to comfortable position in bed or chair; remove equipment from bedside	❏	❏	
27. Empty, wash, and dry reusable pouch	❏	❏	
Urostomy care			
28. Follow steps 1 to 13 of ostomy care procedure	❏	❏	
29. Empty urine into graduated pitcher; write down amount and characteristics of urine for later documentation (mucus will be present in urine from shedding of mucus by mucous membrane of intestine as urine passes over the intestinal conduit)	❏	❏	
30. Carefully remove water seal from skin and place pouch in plastic bag	❏	❏	
31. Cleanse skin with warm water and pat dry	❏	❏	
32. Measure stoma using measuring device	❏	❏	

Student Name____ **Date**____________________

	S	U	Comments
33. Place gauze over stoma	❏	❏	____________________
34. If using Skin Prep, apply to skin and allow to dry; apply protective stoma paste about 1/16 inch from the stoma	❏	❏	____________________
35. Apply protective wafer with flange, cutting an opening in the center of wafer 1/16 inch larger than stoma; assess stoma to determine color and viability	❏	❏	____________________

Postprocedure

	S	U	Comments
36. Assist patient to a position of comfort and place needed items within easy reach; be certain patient has a means to call for assistance and knows how to use it	❏	❏	____________________
37. Raise side rails and lower bed to lowest position	❏	❏	____________________
38. Remove gloves and all protective barriers; dispose of soiled supplies and equipment appropriately	❏	❏	____________________
39. Perform hand hygiene after patient contact and after wearing gloves	❏	❏	____________________
40. Document and do patient teaching	❏	❏	____________________
41. Report any unexpected outcomes	❏	❏	____________________

Student Name________________________________ Date______________

PERFORMANCE CHECKLIST 20-25

Performing a Colostomy Irrigation

	S	U	Comments
Prepare for procedure			
1. Refer to medical record, care plan, or Kardex	❑	❑	______
2. Introduce self	❑	❑	______
3. Identify patient	❑	❑	______
4. Explain procedure and reason it is to be done	❑	❑	______
5. Assess need for and provide patient teaching during procedure	❑	❑	______
6. Assemble equipment and complete necessary charges	❑	❑	______
7. Perform hand hygiene; don clean gloves	❑	❑	______
8. Assess patient	❑	❑	______
9. Prepare patient for intervention			
a. Close door/pull privacy curtain	❑	❑	______
b. Raise bed to comfortable working height; lower side rail on side nearest the nurse	❑	❑	______
c. Position and drape patient as necessary	❑	❑	______
During the skill			
10. Promote patient involvement as possible	❑	❑	______
11. Assess patient's tolerance	❑	❑	______
12. Position patient			
a. Bathroom: instruct patient to sit on toilet or on a chair in front of the toilet	❑	❑	______
b. Bed: have patient lie comfortably with head of bed slightly elevated	❑	❑	______

	S	U	Comments
13. Remove pouch, cleanse skin, and place irrigation sleeve over stoma; attach belt if using; place end of sleeve in toilet	❑	❑	________
14. Close clamp on irrigating tubing; fill irrigating container with 1000 mL tepid water (or as otherwise ordered); container may be hung on a hook at patient's shoulder level	❑	❑	________
15. Allow a small amount of water to flow through tubing	❑	❑	________
16. Attach cone to tubing; lubricate cone; gently insert cone into stoma through top of sleeve	❑	❑	________
17. While holding cone in place, allow solution to flow slowly into colon (500–1000 mL over 15 minutes)	❑	❑	________
18. After all solution is instilled, remove cone and close top of sleeve	❑	❑	________
19. Instruct patient to sit about 15–20 minutes while returns flow into toilet	❑	❑	________
20. Drain sleeve; remove and rinse it	❑	❑	________
21. Observe patient and results of irrigation; flush toilet	❑	❑	________
22. Perform colostomy care	❑	❑	________
Postprocedure			
23. Assist patient to a position of comfort and place needed items within easy reach; be certain patient has a means to call for assistance and knows how to use it	❑	❑	________
24. Raise side rails and lower bed to lowest position	❑	❑	________
25. Remove gloves and all protective barriers; dispose of soiled supplies and equipment appropriately	❑	❑	________
26. Perform hand hygiene after patient contact and after wearing gloves	❑	❑	________
27. Document and do patient teaching	❑	❑	________
28. Report any unexpected outcomes	❑	❑	________

Student Name________________________ Date____________

PERFORMANCE CHECKLIST 21-1

ADMINISTERING NASOGASTRIC TUBE FEEDINGS

	S	U	Comments
1. Refer to medical record, care plan, or Kardex for special interventions; physician's order will state formula, rate, route, and frequency of feeding	❑	❑	____________
2. Introduce self	❑	❑	____________
3. Identify patient	❑	❑	____________
4. Explain procedure	❑	❑	____________
5. Assess need for patient teaching	❑	❑	____________
6. Assemble equipment and complete necessary charges; organize procedure	❑	❑	____________
7. Perform hand hygiene; don clean gloves	❑	❑	____________
8. Assess patient, auscultate for active bowel sounds to assess abdomen for distention or tenderness	❑	❑	____________
9. Prepare patient for intervention			
a. Close door / pull privacy curtain	❑	❑	____________
b. Raise bed to a comfortable working height	❑	❑	____________
c. Elevate level of bed to Fowler's, at least 30 degrees, or reverse Trendelenburg if spinal injury present	❑	❑	____________
10. Check for placement of feeding tube			
a. Aspirate gastric or intestinal contents with appropriate cone-tipped syringe inserted into end of tube	❑	❑	____________
b. Place drop of GI contents on pH test paper (gastric content should have a pH of 0–4, tracheobronchial and pleural secretions should have a pH > 6 and intestinal contents usually have a pH of 7 or greater)	❑	❑	____________
c. Inspect oral cavity for tube kinking or curling in back of pharynx	❑	❑	____________
d. If unable to aspirate, consider tube is occluded or kinked, and attempt to flush with 30 mL of warm water	❑	❑	____________

	S	U	Comments
11. Readminister residual volume to patient slowly	❑	❑	________
a. If residual amounts are greater than last infusion or 150 mL, hold feeding for one hour and reassess residual	❑	❑	________
12. Prepare formula for administration	❑	❑	________
13. Bolus or intermittent feedings			
a. Administer tube feeding with 60 mL bulb or plunger syringe	❑	❑	________
b. Remove cap or plug from end of feeding tube and pinch closed	❑	❑	________
c. Attach syringe by removing bulb or plunger and inserting tip into end of tube; elevate to no more than 18 inches above insertion site	❑	❑	________
d. Fill syringe with formula, release tube, and allow syringe to empty gradually, refilling until prescribed ordered amount has been administered	❑	❑	________
e. Flush tube with 30–60 mL tap water	❑	❑	________
f. Recap/plug tube	❑	❑	________
14. Continuous drip method			
a. Administer tube feeding with gavage bag	❑	❑	________
b. Prepare administration set: clamp tubing, prepare gavage bag with prescribed type and amount of formula, unclamp and prime tubing to remove air, then reclamp tubing	❑	❑	________
c. Label bag with tube feeding type, strength, and amount. Include date, time, and initials	❑	❑	________
d. Pinch end of feeding tube. Remove plug/cap and securely attach gavage tubing to end of feeding tube	❑	❑	________
e. Set rate by adjusting roller clamp on tubing	❑	❑	________
f. Flush tube with 30–60 mL tap water	❑	❑	________
g. Recap/plug tube	❑	❑	________
15. Feeding via infusion pump			
a. Administer tube feeding as a continuous drip via infusion pump	❑	❑	________

Student Name____________________ Date__________

	S	U	Comments
b. Prepare administration set. Clamp tubing, spike bag, unclamp and prime tubing. Reclamp tubing	❑	❑	________
c. Label bag with tube feeding type, strength, and amount. Include date, time, and initials	❑	❑	________
d. Hang tube feeding set on IV pole with infusion pump. Connect tubing to pump and set rate	❑	❑	________
e. Pinch end of feeding tube. Remove plug/cap. Connect infusion tubing to patient feeding tube	❑	❑	________
f. Open roller clamp on infusion tubing	❑	❑	________
g. Check residual volumes every 4 hours	❑	❑	________
16. Fill a 60 mL syringe with ordered volume of water (30–50 mL). Inject into feeding tube to flush after bolus or as ordered with continuous drip	❑	❑	________
17. Flush tube with water every 4–8 hours, clamp it when no feedings are infusing	❑	❑	________
18. Rinse syringe or bag and tubing with warm water. Remove and discard gloves and wash hands	❑	❑	________
19. Ask if patient is comfortable while infusion is continuing; diarrhea should be reported to physician	❑	❑	________
20. Assist patient to a position of comfort and place needed items within reach	❑	❑	________
21. Raise side rails and lower bed to lowest position	❑	❑	________
22. Remove gloves, dispose of used supplies and perform hand hygiene	❑	❑	________
23. Document	❑	❑	________
24. Monitor weight and laboratory values daily	❑	❑	________
25. Observe and assess patient for any adverse reactions, such as shortness of breath, low oxygenation saturation, and presence of feeding from airway	❑	❑	________

Student Name____ Date____________________

PERFORMANCE CHECKLIST 21-2

ADMINISTERING ENTERAL FEEDINGS VIA GASTROSTOMY OR JEJUNOSTOMY TUBE

	S	U	Comments
Observe all guidelines for nasal gastric tube feedings and follow steps 1 to 9 of Skill 21-1 and then continue with the steps below.			
1. Verify tube placement—see Skill 21-1, step 10			
a. Gastrostomy tube: aspirate gastric secretions, check pH; return aspirated contents to stomach unless volume exceeds 150 mL	❑	❑	______
b. Jejunostomy tube: aspirate intestinal secretions, check pH	❑	❑	______
2. Flush with 30 mL water	❑	❑	______
3. Initiate feedings. Usually gastrostomy and jejunostomy feedings are given continuously to ensure proper absorption. However, initial feedings may be given by bolus to assess patient's tolerance to formula			
a. Syringe feedings			
(1) Pinch proximal end of gastrostomy tube	❑	❑	______
(2) Remove plunger and attach barrel of syringe to end of tube, then fill syringe with formula	❑	❑	______
(3) Allow syringe to empty gradually. Refill until prescribed amount has been delivered to patient	❑	❑	______
(4) Flush with ordered volume of water (30-50 mL)	❑	❑	______
b. Continuous drip method			
(1) Fill feeding container with enough formula for 4 hours of feeding	❑	❑	______
(2) Hang container on IV pole, and clear tubing of air	❑	❑	______
(3) Thread tubing on pump according to manufacturer's directions	❑	❑	______

	S	U	Comments
(4) Connect tubing to end of feeding tube	❑	❑	________
(5) Begin infusion at prescribed rate	❑	❑	________
4. Assess skin around tube exit site; skin around tube should be cleansed daily with warm water and mild soap	❑	❑	________
5. Dispose of supplies and perform hand hygiene	❑	❑	________
6. Monitor finger-stick blood glucose every 6 hrs until maximum administration rate is reached and maintained for 24 hours	❑	❑	________
7. Monitor intake and output	❑	❑	________
8. Weigh patient daily	❑	❑	________
9. Observe laboratory values	❑	❑	________
10. Inspect enteral site for signs of pressure	❑	❑	________
11. Document	❑	❑	________
12. Observe for any adverse reactions	❑	❑	________

Student Name________________________ Date____________

PERFORMANCE CHECKLIST 21-3

ASSISTING PATIENTS WITH EATING

	S	U	Comments
1. Complete or delay care that will interfere with eating	❑	❑	________
2. Provide period of rest or quiet before meals; offer patient a bedpan or urinal before mealtime	❑	❑	________
3. Provide patient with opportunity for hand-washing; offer mouth care before eating	❑	❑	________
4. Remove any soiled articles or clutter from room	❑	❑	________
5. Make patient comfortable for eating; use pain relief techniques if needed	❑	❑	________
6. Raise head of bed to sitting position if possible	❑	❑	________
7. Cover patient's upper chest with napkin or towel	❑	❑	________
8. Sit beside patient; avoid appearing hurried	❑	❑	________
9. Encourage patients to take part in their eating as much as possible and to extent that their condition permits	❑	❑	________
10. Provide flexible straw for patients who are unable to use a cup or glass (unless contraindicated)	❑	❑	________
11. Serve manageable amounts of food with each bite	❑	❑	________
12. For a stroke patient, direct food toward side of mouth that is not paralyzed	❑	❑	________
13. Serve food in order of patient's preference	❑	❑	________
14. Give patient time to chew thoroughly and swallow food	❑	❑	________
15. Modify utensils and texture of food if patient must remain flat while eating; use child's training cup or large syringe with flexible rubber tube; puree or grind foods if necessary	❑	❑	________
16. If you have begun to feed a patient, do not leave until he or she has finished eating; a meal should not be interrupted	❑	❑	________

	S	U	Comments
17. Talk with patient about pleasant subjects; eating is a social occasion	❑	❑	__________
18. Use suggested actions that involve removing a tray (see Skill 21-4)	❑	❑	__________

Student Name______________________________ Date______________

PERFORMANCE CHECKLIST 21-4

SERVING AND REMOVING TRAYS

	S	U	Comments
1. Be available when trays arrive from dietary department	❑	❑	______
2. Clear area where patient will eat	❑	❑	______
3. Check general appearance of tray for spilled liquids, missing items, or ordered food that is missing	❑	❑	______
4. Compare name on tray with name on patient's identification bracelet	❑	❑	______
5. Ensure that patients who are undergoing special tests have food withheld or provided according to test directions	❑	❑	______
6. Check to see that patient is not being served foods to which he or she is allergic, or that he or she cannot tolerate	❑	❑	______
7. Place tray so that it faces patient; remove food covers	❑	❑	______
8. Open milk cartons and cereal boxes, butter toast, cut up meat, and otherwise assist as necessary	❑	❑	______
9. Serve trays that have been kept warm last to those patients who need help with eating	❑	❑	______
10. Note kinds and amounts of food that patient is not eating	❑	❑	______
11. Observe whether patient feels satisfied with amounts of food served; serving sizes need to match appetite	❑	❑	______
12. Follow agency policies about serving food brought from home; ensure that food is covered, labeled, refrigerated, or stored properly	❑	❑	______
13. Be considerate and visit with patients who are on special diets and may be denied food they like because of a health problem	❑	❑	______
14. Encourage patients to eat, but do not scold those who feel they cannot	❑	❑	______

	S	U	Comments
15. Remove trays as soon as possible, and restore cleanliness of the eating area	❑	❑	______
16. Assist or offer patient an opportunity to brush and floss teeth	❑	❑	______
17. Record how patient ate and enter amounts of fluid consumed if appropriate	❑	❑	______
18. Always assess patient's appetite during first assessment of the day; ask how he or she ate breakfast, etc.	❑	❑	______
19. Use fractions (such as 1/4, 1/3, 1/2) or percentages (such as 35%, 50%, 100%) when documenting food eaten, or follow agency policy	❑	❑	______

Student Name____ Date__________________

PERFORMANCE CHECKLIST 22-1

MEASURING INTAKE AND OUTPUT (I&O)

	S	U	Comments
1. Identify patient	❏	❏	____________
2. Explain procedure	❏	❏	____________
3. Instruct patient to inform staff of all oral intake; provide a marked I&O container	❏	❏	____________
4. Instruct patient not to empty any output collection receptacles and to notify the nurse after elimination	❏	❏	____________
5. Alert all staff and remind patient of need to measure I&O	❏	❏	____________
6. Measure and record all fluids taken orally or per feeding tube, and all fluids administered parenterally	❏	❏	____________
7. Perform hand hygiene and don gloves	❏	❏	____________
8. Measure and record output in urinary drainage system, diarrhea stools, nasogastric suction, emesis, ileostomy, and output in surgical wound receptacles such as Davol, Jackson-Pratt, and Hemovac	❏	❏	____________
9. Remove gloves and perform hand hygiene	❏	❏	____________
10. Compute and document I&O on patient's record	❏	❏	____________
11. Be vigilant to maintain accurate I&O when ordered	❏	❏	____________

Student Name______________________________ Date______________

PERFORMANCE CHECKLIST 23-1

Administering Tablets, Pills, and Capsules

	S	U	Comments
1. Follow the six rights	❏	❏	______
2. Perform the three label checks	❏	❏	______
3. Follow standard precautions	❏	❏	______
4. Perform hand hygiene	❏	❏	______
5. Check for allergies	❏	❏	______
6. If using unit dose package, place unopened package in medicine cup	❏	❏	______
7. If using a multidose bottle, pour tablet (without touching it) into cap of bottle appropriately	❏	❏	______
8. Pour tablet from cap into medicine cup	❏	❏	______
9. If using medicine tray (for several patients), set it up from left to right, front to back with patient's name and room number	❏	❏	______
10. If pouring from multidose bottle and patient is to receive several tablets, use separate cup for medications such as digitalis. If the patient's pulse is less than 60/BPM, withhold the medication and report this to the RN. Place digitalis in a separate cup marked with a red heart to allow for easy identification	❏	❏	______
11. Do not use pills, tablets, or capsules that come from multidose bottles if they have been handled or dropped on the floor	❏	❏	______
12. Take medication to patient's room	❏	❏	______
13. Identify room, bed, patient, and patient's birthdate	❏	❏	______
14. Check again for allergies	❏	❏	______
15. Explain procedure to patient	❏	❏	______

	S	U	Comments
16. Document administration of medication in Medex or computer with initials, date, and time	❑	❑	____________
17. Return to assess patient's response to medication	❑	❑	____________
18. Document assessment	❑	❑	____________

Student Name________________________________ Date________________

PERFORMANCE CHECKLIST 23-2

ADMINISTERING LIQUID MEDICATIONS

	S	U	Comments
1. Follow the six rights	❏	❏	______
2. Perform the three label checks	❏	❏	______
3. Follow standard precautions	❏	❏	______
4. Perform hand hygiene	❏	❏	______
5. Check for allergies	❏	❏	______
6. Remove liquid preparation from patient's drug box/bin (or from medication cabinet or refrigerator)	❏	❏	______
7. Check dosage/mL and total volume of medication in container	❏	❏	______
8. Calculate dosage; if the dosage ordered is different from the dosage/mL stated on the label, calculate correct dose; if ordered medication is labeled in a different measurement system, convert by using appropriate equivalent. Work problem on paper correctly	❏	❏	______
9. Check calculations with another nurse	❏	❏	______
10. Obtain graduated medicine cup or appropriate syringe	❏	❏	______
11. Face label of bottle toward palm of hand to avoid soiling label; if label becomes soiled, return the bottle to the pharmacy; do not give medication if label is unreadable	❏	❏	______
12. Place medicine cup on flat surface, or hold at eye level while pouring	❏	❏	______
13. Place cap of bottle with inner rim up	❏	❏	______
14. Read dosage amount at lower level of meniscus	❏	❏	______
15. Transport medication to patient's room	❏	❏	______
16. Identify room, bed, patient, and patient's birthdate	❏	❏	______

	S	U	Comments
17. Check for allergies	❏	❏	______
18. Explain procedure to patient	❏	❏	______
19. Document administration of medication in Medex or computer with initials, date, and time	❏	❏	______
20. Return to assess patient's response to medication	❏	❏	______
21. Document assessment	❏	❏	______

Student Name____________________ Date__________

PERFORMANCE CHECKLIST 23-3

ADMINISTERING TUBAL MEDICATIONS

	S	U	Comments
1. Follow the six rights	❑	❑	________
2. Perform the three label checks	❑	❑	________
3. Follow standard precautions	❑	❑	________
4. Perform hand hygiene	❑	❑	________
5. Check for allergies	❑	❑	________
6. Prepare medication using the same procedure as for liquid medications	❑	❑	________
7. If tablet, crush pill, dissolve in 15-20 mL warm water. For capsules, open and dissolve powder in 15-30 mL warm water. For gelatin capsules, aspirate with syringe or capsule may be dissolved in warm water and remove gelatin outer layer	❑	❑	________
8. Gather equipment: 10 mL syringe, towel, stethoscope, bulb or Asepto syringe, tap water	❑	❑	________
9. Take equipment and medication to patient's room	❑	❑	________
10. Identify room, bed, patient, and patient's birthdate	❑	❑	________
11. Recheck for allergies	❑	❑	________
12. Explain procedure; answer questions patient may have about the procedure	❑	❑	________
13. Place patient in high Fowler's position	❑	❑	________
14. Put towel over patient's chest	❑	❑	________
15. Don disposable, unsterile gloves	❑	❑	________
16. Check and recheck placement and patency of tube with the appropriate procedure			
a. Method A: Attach bulb or Asepto syringe to end of NG tube; pull plunger back or release suction of bulb syringe to aspirate stomach contents; if stomach contents are seen, instill 10 to 20 mL of water before medication administration to clear tube; proceed with medication	❑	❑	________

	S	U	Comments
b. Method B: Place stethoscope over stomach; push 10 mL of air through NG tube with syringe	❑	❑	______
c. Method C: Many authorities now recommend the litmus test instead of the auscultatory (air-instillation) method: measure pH of aspirate with color-coded pH paper with range of whole numbers from 1 to 11; gastric aspirates have decidedly acidic pH values (preferably 4 or less); proceed with medication	❑	❑	______
17. Clamp tube with rubber-tipped hemostat or other clamping device	❑	❑	______
18. Attach syringe to end of tube correctly (with plunger out of syringe)	❑	❑	______
19. Pour medication into syringe	❑	❑	______
20. Unclamp tubing to allow medication to slowly flow by gravity	❑	❑	______
21. Follow medication with 30–50 mL of water	❑	❑	______
22. Clamp tubing; secure tube after medication is given	❑	❑	______
23. If NG tube is attached to suction, do not reconnect suction for 30 minutes	❑	❑	______
24. Remove towel from patient	❑	❑	______
25. Remove gloves and dispose of properly	❑	❑	______
26. Leave patient in comfortable position	❑	❑	______
27. Gather equipment; clean up patient and area appropriately	❑	❑	______
28. Perform hand hygiene	❑	❑	______
29. Document administration of NG medication in Medex or computer with initials, date, and time	❑	❑	______
30. Return to assess patient's response to medication	❑	❑	______
31. Document assessment	❑	❑	______

Student Name________________________ Date____________

PERFORMANCE CHECKLIST 23-4

ADMINISTERING RECTAL SUPPOSITORIES

	S	U	Comments
1. Follow the six rights	❑	❑	______
2. Perform the three label checks	❑	❑	______
3. Follow standard precautions	❑	❑	______
4. Perform hand hygiene	❑	❑	______
5. Check for allergies	❑	❑	______
6. Obtain water-soluble lubricant	❑	❑	______
7. Obtain suppository from refrigerator or from patient's medication bin	❑	❑	______
8. Place unopened suppository into medicine cup or souffle cup	❑	❑	______
9. Take disposable, unsterile gloves or finger cot to patient's room	❑	❑	______
10. Identify room, bed, patient, and patient's birthdate	❑	❑	______
11. Explain procedure to patient	❑	❑	______
12. Gain patient's cooperation	❑	❑	______
13. Provide privacy	❑	❑	______
14. Position patient appropriately in Sims' position (on left side with upper leg flexed at knee)	❑	❑	______
15. Unwrap suppository	❑	❑	______
16. Maintain privacy; expose buttocks	❑	❑	______
17. Don gloves	❑	❑	______
18. Apply lubricant, such as KY jelly, to tapered end of suppository	❑	❑	______
19. Ask patient to take deep breath; insert beyond internal anal sphincter; insert suppository as patient exhales to relax anal sphincter	❑	❑	______
20. Ask patient to retain suppository as long as possible; hold the buttocks together to help patient to retain suppository	❑	❑	______

	S	U	Comments
21. Discard gloves correctly	❑	❑	________
22. Help patient assume comfortable position	❑	❑	________
23. Perform hand hygiene	❑	❑	________
24. Document administration of suppository in Medex or computer with initials, date, and time	❑	❑	________
25. Return to assess patient's response to medication	❑	❑	________
26. Document assessment	❑	❑	________

Student Name________________________________ Date____________________

PERFORMANCE CHECKLIST 23-5

Applying Topical Agents

	S	U	Comments
1. Follow the six rights	❏	❏	____________
2. Perform the three label checks	❏	❏	____________
3. Follow standard precautions	❏	❏	____________
4. Perform hand hygiene	❏	❏	____________
5. Check for allergies	❏	❏	____________
6. Transport medication to patient's room	❏	❏	____________
7. Identify room, bed, patient, and patient's birthdate	❏	❏	____________
8. Recheck for allergies	❏	❏	____________
9. Introduce self; explain procedure to patient	❏	❏	____________
10. Provide privacy; place patient in comfortable position that allows exposure to selected site	❏	❏	____________
11. Don gloves	❏	❏	____________
12. Cleanse site with appropriate materials, removing debris, encrustations, and previous medications	❏	❏	____________
13. Read prescription instructions carefully	❏	❏	____________
14. Prepare medicinal agent (ointments, creams, and lotions may have to be squeezed or removed with a tongue blade, depending on preparation)	❏	❏	____________
15. Apply paper applicator, disk, lotion, ointment, or cream	❏	❏	____________
16. Remove gloves	❏	❏	____________
17. Leave patient properly draped or clothed in comfortable position	❏	❏	____________
18. Answer patient's questions, and teach patient to perform self-applications if appropriate	❏	❏	____________
19. Clean work area	❏	❏	____________

	S	U	Comments
20. Perform hand hygiene	❏	❏	______
21. Document administration of medication in Medex or computer with initials, date, and time	❏	❏	______
22. Return to assess patient's response to medication	❏	❏	______
23. Document assessment	❏	❏	______

Student Name____ **Date**__________________

PERFORMANCE CHECKLIST 23-6

ADMINISTERING EYEDROPS AND EYE OINTMENTS

	S	U	Comments
1. Follow the six rights	❑	❑	__________
2. Perform the three label checks	❑	❑	__________
3. Follow standard precautions	❑	❑	__________
4. Perform hand hygiene	❑	❑	__________
5. Check for allergies	❑	❑	__________
6. Transport medications to patient's room	❑	❑	__________
7. Identify medications as ophthalmic	❑	❑	__________
8. Identify room, bed, patient, and patient's birthdate	❑	❑	__________
9. Recheck for allergies	❑	❑	__________
10. Introduce self; explain procedure	❑	❑	__________
11. Provide privacy, position back of patient's head on pillow; direct patient's face upward toward ceiling. Review which eye or eyes to receive the medication; left eye, right eye, or both eyes	❑	❑	__________
12. Recheck for allergies	❑	❑	__________
13. Don gloves	❑	❑	__________
14. Remove exudate; clean eye as needed using sterile solution of saline; use cotton balls to wipe away exudate; use one cotton ball per stroke, wiping from inner canthus outward	❑	❑	__________
15. To apply drops, expose lower conjunctival sac by having patient look upward while gentle traction is applied to lower eyelid	❑	❑	__________
16. Put prescribed number of drops into conjunctival sac, not onto eyeball; conjunctival sac normally holds one or two drops	❑	❑	__________
17. Using a cotton ball or tissue, apply gentle pressure above bone at inner corner of eyelid for 1–2 minutes	❑	❑	__________
18. Apply sterile dressing if ordered	❑	❑	__________

	S	U	Comments
19. To apply ointment, expose lower conjunctival sac by having patient look upward while gentle traction is applied to lower eyelid	❑	❑	______
20. Squeeze ointment into lower conjunctival sac	❑	❑	______
21. Ask patient to close eye and to move it around in circular motion to spread medication	❑	❑	______
22. Apply sterile dressing if ordered	❑	❑	______
23. After applying drops or ointment to an eye, leave patient in comfortable position; clean up the work area	❑	❑	______
24. Remove gloves and perform hand hygiene	❑	❑	______
25. Answer patient's questions and if appropriate, teach patient to perform self-care	❑	❑	______
26. Document administration of medications in Medex or computer with initials, date, and time	❑	❑	______
27. Return to assess patient's response to medication	❑	❑	______
28. Document assessment in nurse's notes	❑	❑	______

Student Name________________________________ Date______________

PERFORMANCE CHECKLIST 23-7

ADMINISTERING EARDROPS

	S	U	Comments
1. Follow the six rights	❑	❑	______
2. Perform the three label checks	❑	❑	______
3. Follow standard precautions	❑	❑	______
4. Perform hand hygiene	❑	❑	______
5. Check for allergies	❑	❑	______
6. Transport medication to patient's room	❑	❑	______
7. Identify medications as otic	❑	❑	______
8. Identify room, bed, patient, and patient's birthdate	❑	❑	______
9. Recheck for allergies	❑	❑	______
10. Introduce self; explain procedure	❑	❑	______
11. Provide privacy; position patient with affected ear upward	❑	❑	______
12. Don gloves	❑	❑	______
13. Remove external exudate from ear; an order must be obtained before irrigating the ear	❑	❑	______
14. Draw medication into dropper	❑	❑	______
15. For adults and for children over 3 years old, turn head with affected side up; pull earlobe upward and back to straighten external auditory canal; give drops without touching ear with dropper	❑	❑	______
16. For children under 3 years old, turn head with affected side up; pull earlobe downward and back; instill drops without touching ear with dropper	❑	❑	______
17. Tell patient to remain in same position for a few minutes to allow medication to drain into ear by gravity	❑	❑	______

	S	U	Comments
18. A cotton ball may be placed loosely into ear as needed	❑	❑	______
19. Remove gloves	❑	❑	______
20. Leave patient in comfortable position; clean work area	❑	❑	______
21. Answer patient's questions and if appropriate, teach patient self-care	❑	❑	______
22. Perform hand hygiene	❑	❑	______
23. Document administration of medication in Medex or computer with initials, date, and time	❑	❑	______
24. Return to assess patient's response to medication	❑	❑	______
25. Document assessment in nurse's notes	❑	❑	______

Student Name______________________________ Date______________

PERFORMANCE CHECKLIST 23-8

ADMINISTERING NOSE DROPS

	S	U	Comments
1. Follow the six rights	❑	❑	______
2. Perform the three label checks	❑	❑	______
3. Follow standard precautions	❑	❑	______
4. Perform hand hygiene	❑	❑	______
5. Check for allergies	❑	❑	______
6. Transport medication to patient's room	❑	❑	______
7. Identify room, bed, patient, and patient's birthdate	❑	❑	______
8. Recheck for allergies	❑	❑	______
9. Introduce self; explain procedure	❑	❑	______
10. Provide privacy	❑	❑	______
11. Don gloves	❑	❑	______
12. Ask adult or older child to clear nose of accumulations by blowing gently into tissue	❑	❑	______
13. Determine which nostril (or both) is to receive the medication	❑	❑	______
14. Have patient lie down, hanging head backward over edge of bed or with pillow under shoulders to hyperextend the neck if patient can tolerate it	❑	❑	______
15. After drawing medication into dropper, instill medication while holding dropper above nostril being treated	❑	❑	______
16. If ordered, repeat procedure to instill drops in other nostril	❑	❑	______
17. Tell patient to hold position for a few minutes to allow medication to remain in place	❑	❑	______
18. Administer nosedrops to a younger child after positioning child on bed with head backward and downward, or to an infant while holding his head backward and downward	❑	❑	______

	S	U	Comments
19. Administer drops in same way as to an adult	❑	❑	
20. Remove gloves	❑	❑	
21. Tell patient to refrain from blowing nose immediately after instillation	❑	❑	
22. Offer tissues for later use	❑	❑	
23. Leave patient in comfortable position; clean work area	❑	❑	
24. Answer patient's questions and if appropriate, teach patient self-care	❑	❑	
25. Perform hand hygiene	❑	❑	
26. Document administration of medication in Medex or computer with initials, date, and time	❑	❑	
27. Return to assess patient's response to medication	❑	❑	
28. Document assessment in nurse's notes	❑	❑	

Student Name______________________________________ Date____________________

PERFORMANCE CHECKLIST 23-9

ADMINISTERING NASAL SPRAYS

	S	U	Comments
1. Follow the six rights	❑	❑	__________
2. Perform the three label checks	❑	❑	__________
3. Follow standard precautions	❑	❑	__________
4. Perform hand hygiene	❑	❑	__________
5. Check for allergies	❑	❑	__________
6. Transport medication to patient's room	❑	❑	__________
7. Identify room, bed, patient, and patient's birthdate	❑	❑	__________
8. Recheck for allergies	❑	❑	__________
9. Introduce self; explain procedure	❑	❑	__________
10. Provide privacy; position patient upright	❑	❑	__________
11. Don gloves	❑	❑	__________
12. Determine which nostril (or both) is to receive medication	❑	❑	__________
13. Have patient gently blow nose to clear nasal passages of accumulations	❑	❑	__________
14. Compress one nostril	❑	❑	__________
15. Shake bottle while holding it upright	❑	❑	__________
16. Insert tip of spray bottle into patient's patent nostril	❑	❑	__________
17. Instruct patient to inhale; while he inhales, squeeze bottle	❑	❑	__________
18. If ordered, repeat procedure for other nostril	❑	❑	__________
19. Tell patient to refrain from blowing nose for a few minutes; offer tissues for later use	❑	❑	__________
20. Answer patient's questions and if appropriate, teach self-administration	❑	❑	__________
21. Remove gloves and perform hand hygiene	❑	❑	__________

	S	U	Comments
22. Document administration of medication in Medex or computer with initials, date, and time	❑	❑	______
23. Return to assess patient's response to medication	❑	❑	______
24. Document assessment in nurse's notes	❑	❑	______

Student Name______________________________ Date______________

PERFORMANCE CHECKLIST 23-10

Administering Inhalants

	S	U	Comments
1. Follow the six rights	❑	❑	______
2. Perform the three label checks	❑	❑	______
3. Follow standard precautions	❑	❑	______
4. Perform hand hygiene	❑	❑	______
5. Check for allergies	❑	❑	______
6. Transport medication to patient's room	❑	❑	______
7. Identify room, bed, patient, and patient's birthdate	❑	❑	______
8. Recheck for allergies	❑	❑	______
9. Introduce self; explain procedure	❑	❑	______
10. Provide privacy	❑	❑	______
11. Allow patient opportunity to manipulate inhaler, canister, and spacer device (aerochamber); explain and demonstrate how canister fits into inhaler	❑	❑	______
12. Explain what metered dose is and warn patient about overuse of inhaler, including drug side effects	❑	❑	______
13. Remove mouthpiece cover from inhaler; shake inhaler well	❑	❑	______
14. Without aerochamber (spacer): Open lips and place inhaler 1–2 cm (1/2 to 1 inch) from mouth with opening toward back of pharynx. Lips should not touch inhaler. Avoid rapid influx of inhaled medication and subsequent airway irritation	❑	❑	______
15. With aerochamber (spacer): Exhale fully, then grasp mouthpiece with teeth and lips while holding inhaler with thumb at the mouthpiece and fingers at the top	❑	❑	______
16. Press down on inhaler to release medication while inhaling slowly and deeply through mouth	❑	❑	______

	S	U	Comments
17. Breathe in slowly for 2–3 seconds; hold breath for approximately 10 seconds	❑	❑	____________
18. Exhale through pursed lips	❑	❑	____________
19. Instruct patient to wait 2 to 5 minutes between puffs; more than one puff is usually prescribed	❑	❑	____________
20. If more than one type of inhaled medications are prescribed, wait 5–10 minutes between inhalations or as ordered by physician	❑	❑	____________
21. Explain that patient may feel gagging sensation in throat caused by droplets of medication on pharynx or tongue	❑	❑	____________
22. Instruct patient in removing medication canister and cleaning inhaler in warm water	❑	❑	____________
23. Teach patient to measure the amount of medication remaining in the canister by immersing it in a large bowl or pan of water	❑	❑	____________
24. Record administration in Medex or computer with initials, date, and time	❑	❑	____________
25. Return to assess patient's response to medication	❑	❑	____________
26. Document assessment in nurse's notes	❑	❑	____________

Student Name________________________________ Date__________________

PERFORMANCE CHECKLIST 23-11

Administering Sublingual Medications

	S	U	Comments
1. Follow the six rights	❑	❑	____________
2. Perform the three label checks	❑	❑	____________
3. Follow standard precautions	❑	❑	____________
4. Perform hand hygiene	❑	❑	____________
5. Check for allergies	❑	❑	____________
6. Identify room, bed, patient, and patient's birthdate	❑	❑	____________
7. Recheck for allergies	❑	❑	____________
8. Wear gloves to place tablet under patient's tongue	❑	❑	____________
9. Do not follow with water	❑	❑	____________
10. Instruct patient not to swallow tablet	❑	❑	____________
11. Explain to patient how to place medication under tongue; instruct patient to let it dissolve	❑	❑	____________
12. Remove gloves and perform hand hygiene	❑	❑	____________
13. Document sublingual administration in Medex or computer with initials, date, and time	❑	❑	____________
14. Return to assess patient's response to medication	❑	❑	____________
15. Document assessment in nurse's notes	❑	❑	____________

Student Name____ Date____________________

PERFORMANCE CHECKLIST 23-12

Administering Buccal Medications

	S	U	Comments
1. Follow the six rights	❑	❑	____________
2. Perform the three label checks	❑	❑	____________
3. Follow standard precautions	❑	❑	____________
4. Perform hand hygiene	❑	❑	____________
5. Check for allergies	❑	❑	____________
6. Identify room, bed, patient, and patient's birthdate	❑	❑	____________
7. Recheck for allergies	❑	❑	____________
8. Wear gloves to place tablet between patient's cheek and gum	❑	❑	____________
9. Do not follow with water	❑	❑	____________
10. Instruct patient not to swallow tablet; let it dissolve	❑	❑	____________
11. Explain to patient how to place medication between cheek and gum	❑	❑	____________
12. Remove gloves and perform hand hygiene	❑	❑	____________
13. Document buccal administration in Medex or computer with initials, date, and time	❑	❑	____________
14. Return to assess patient's response to medication	❑	❑	____________
15. Document assessment in nurse's notes	❑	❑	____________

Student Name_______________________________ Date_______________

PERFORMANCE CHECKLIST 23-13A
PREPARING PARENTERAL MEDICATIONS:

WITHDRAWING MEDICATION FROM A VIAL

	S	U	Comments
1. Follow the six rights	❑	❑	________
2. Perform the three label checks	❑	❑	________
3. Follow standard precautions	❑	❑	________
4. Check for allergies	❑	❑	________
5. Perform hand hygiene before handling equipment; prepare medication in clean area; reduce distractions	❑	❑	________
6. Keep sterile parts of syringe and needle sterile; use aseptic technique throughout preparation	❑	❑	________
7. Compare drug and dosage ordered with drug and dosage on hand; check expiration date, dosage per milliliter, total volume of solution in vial; look for contaminants or defects in vial	❑	❑	________
8. Calculate drug dosage and check calculations with another nurse	❑	❑	________
9. Check compatibility chart or consult pharmacy if mixing two medications	❑	❑	________
10. Remove metal cap from top of vial; wipe rubber diaphragm briskly with alcohol sponge	❑	❑	________
11. Pull plunger of syringe back to aspirate air into syringe equal to amount of drug to be withdrawn	❑	❑	________
12. Insert needle into inverted vial; inject air and withdraw volume of solution to be given; keep needle under solution to prevent aspiration of air into syringe	❑	❑	________
13. Push plunger gently to disperse solution to tip of needle; remove air bubbles by gently tapping syringe	❑	❑	________

Student Name________________________________ Date________________

PERFORMANCE CHECKLIST 23-13B
PREPARING PARENTERAL MEDICATIONS:

WITHDRAWING MEDICATION FROM AN AMPULE

	S	U	Comments
1. Follow the six rights	❑	❑	________
2. Perform the three label checks	❑	❑	________
3. Follow standard precautions	❑	❑	________
4. Check for allergies	❑	❑	________
5. Perform hand hygiene before handling equipment; prepare medication in clean area; reduce distractions	❑	❑	________
6. Keep sterile parts of syringe and needle sterile; use aseptic technique throughout preparation	❑	❑	________
7. Compare drug and dosage ordered with drug and dosage on hand; check expiration date, dosage per milliliter, total volume of solution in ampule; look for contaminants or defects in ampule	❑	❑	________
8. Calculate drug dosage and check calculations with another nurse	❑	❑	________
9. Check compatibility chart or consult pharmacy if mixing two medications	❑	❑	________
10. Tap the top of ampule to move solution from top of ampule to bottom of ampule	❑	❑	________
11. Cover neck of ampule with an alcohol sponge, break off top of ampule; deposit top of glass ampule in sharps container	❑	❑	________
12. Use a filter needle to aspirate medication from ampule. Filter or aspiration needles catch particles of glass that may be in the solution from the broken ampule	❑	❑	________
13. Insert filter needle into open neck of ampule, invert ampule to withdraw correct dose	❑	❑	________
14. Replace filter needle with needle appropriate for purpose of solution and viscosity of solution	❑	❑	________
15. Push plunger gently until the plunger measures the correct dose	❑	❑	________

Student Name______________________________ Date______________

PERFORMANCE CHECKLIST 23-13C
PREPARING PARENTERAL MEDICATIONS:

RECONSTITUTING A POWDERED DOSAGE FORM

	S	U	Comments
1. Follow the six rights	❑	❑	____________
2. Perform the three label checks	❑	❑	____________
3. Follow standard precautions	❑	❑	____________
4. Check for allergies	❑	❑	____________
5. Perform hand hygiene before handling equipment; prepare medication in clean area; reduce distractions	❑	❑	____________
6. Keep sterile parts of syringe and needle sterile; use aseptic technique throughout preparation	❑	❑	____________
7. Compare drug and dosage ordered with drug and dosage on hand; check expiration date, dosage per milliliter, total volume of solution in vial; look for contaminants or defects in vial	❑	❑	____________
8. Calculate drug dosage and check calculations with another nurse	❑	❑	____________
9. Check compatibility chart or consult pharmacy if mixing two medications	❑	❑	____________
10. Follow instructions on manufacturer's box and drug insert; the instructions will specify the type and amount of diluent to use (for example, add 10 mL bacteriostatic normal saline to prepare a ratio of 500 mg/mL)	❑	❑	____________
11. Remove the protective cap from diluent and cleanse with alcohol pad; withdraw diluent using sterile technique	❑	❑	____________
12. Withdraw needle from diluent vial	❑	❑	____________
13. Inject diluent into vial of powdered drug; remove syringe and needle; gently shake and tap vial to dissolve powder into solution	❑	❑	____________
14. If solution is multidose vial, label solution with			
a. Date and time mixed	❑	❑	____________

	S	U	Comments
b. Name of person who mixed drug and diluent	❑	❑	______
c. Dosage per milliliter obtained (concentration)	❑	❑	______
d. Amount and type of diluent used	❑	❑	______
15. Withdraw correct dose; change needle with a new needle; select appropriate needle gauge and length for patient	❑	❑	______

Student Name______________________ Date______________

PERFORMANCE CHECKLIST 23-13D
PREPARING PARENTERAL MEDICATIONS:

PLACING TWO MEDICATIONS INTO ONE SYRINGE (INSULIN EXAMPLE USED)

	S	U	Comments
1. Follow the six rights	❏	❏	____________
2. Perform the three label checks	❏	❏	____________
3. Follow standard precautions	❏	❏	____________
4. Check for allergies	❏	❏	____________
5. Perform hand hygiene before handling equipment; prepare medication in clean area; reduce distractions	❏	❏	____________
6. Keep sterile parts of syringe and needle sterile; use aseptic technique throughout preparation	❏	❏	____________
7. Compare drug and dosage ordered with drug and dosage on hand; check expiration date, dosage per milliliter, total volume of solution in vial; look for contaminants	❏	❏	____________
8. Calculate drug dosage and check calculations with another nurse	❏	❏	____________
9. Check compatibility of two drugs with a compatibility chart or call pharmacy	❏	❏	____________
10. Check and compare label of each drug ordered with label of each drug on hand	❏	❏	____________
11. Compare each label with medication order	❏	❏	____________
12. Roll long- and intermediate-acting insulin between the palms; do not shake any insulin [note: do not mix long-acting glargine insulin (Lantus) with regular insulin; Lantus insulin is clear and does not need to be rolled to mix]	❏	❏	____________
13. Briskly wipe tops of both vials with separate alcohol swab	❏	❏	____________
14. Pull back plunger of syringe to amount equal to volume of longer-acting insulin to be given	❏	❏	____________
15. Insert needle and inject air into vial of longer-acting insulin	❏	❏	____________

	S	U	Comments
16. Withdraw needle from vial; do not remove insulin	❑	❑	______
17. Pull back plunger of syringe to amount equal to volume of shorter-acting (regular) insulin to be given	❑	❑	______
18. Insert needle through rubber stopper of second vial; inject air into vial	❑	❑	______
19. Invert vial; withdraw volume of shorter-acting (regular) insulin first	❑	❑	______
20. Check and verify dosage in syringe with second nurse against medication order	❑	❑	______
21. Wipe rubber stopper of longer-acting insulin; insert needle of the syringe containing shorter-acting insulin and withdraw ordered dose of longer-acting insulin. Verify dosage with second nurse	❑	❑	______
22. Remove needle/syringe from vial	❑	❑	______
23. Check labels of both vials against medication order	❑	❑	______
24. Pull plunger back far enough to allow space in barrel of syringe for insulin to be gently mixed; mix by tilting syringe back and forth; remove air	❑	❑	______
25. Administer mixture of insulin within 5 minutes of preparation; regular insulin binds with NPH and the action of regular insulin is reduced	❑	❑	______
26. Identify room, bed, patient, and patient's birthdate	❑	❑	______
27. Don gloves	❑	❑	______
28. Inject subcutaneously	❑	❑	______
29. Record administration in Medex or computer with site, initials, date, and time including witness of second nurse	❑	❑	______
30. Return to assess patient's response to medication	❑	❑	______
31. Document assessment in nurse's notes	❑	❑	______

Student Name____________________ Date____________

PERFORMANCE CHECKLIST 23-14

Giving an Intramuscular Injection

	S	U	Comments
1. Follow the six rights	❑	❑	______
2. Perform the three label checks	❑	❑	______
3. Follow standard precautions	❑	❑	______
4. Perform hand hygiene	❑	❑	______
5. Check for allergies	❑	❑	______
6. Prepare medication according to standard procedure for injectables	❑	❑	______
7. Identify room, bed, patient, and patient's birthdate	❑	❑	______
8. Recheck for allergies	❑	❑	______
9. Don gloves	❑	❑	______
10. Explain procedure			
11. Select and expose site (according to IM site selection procedure); provide privacy	❑	❑	______
12. Clean skin with alcohol swab (from center outward), spread skin tight with thumb and index finger, and let dry	❑	❑	______
13. Ask patient to take a deep breath and exhale slowly to relax muscle as needle is inserted (lessens pain from injection)	❑	❑	______
14. Insert needle at a 90-degree angle quickly in a dartlike motion; quickness reduces discomfort	❑	❑	______
15. Maintain needle in muscle; gently aspirate (pull back plunger) to be certain needle is in muscle and not in a vein or an artery	❑	❑	______
16. If blood is seen, needle is in a vein or artery; withdraw needle; discard solution; prepare new medication; select another site	❑	❑	______
17. Slowly inject medication into muscle to lessen discomfort	❑	❑	______

	S	U	Comments
18. Withdraw needle quickly without bending or twisting it	❑	❑	______
19. Use pressure and gauze (2 x 2) or Band-Aid to stop any bleeding	❑	❑	______
20. Do not recap needle (if safety glide needle used, advance protective glide); dispose directly into sharps container	❑	❑	______
21. Remove gloves and perform hand hygiene	❑	❑	______
22. Document administration in Medex or computer including site used and amount and type of medication (for example, meperidine [Demerol] 50 mg given IM left ventrogluteal); record initials, date, and time. Remember, a quick, dartlike insertion followed by slow injection of the medication is much less painful to the patient	❑	❑	______
23. Return to assess patient's response to medication	❑	❑	______
24. Document assessment in nurse's notes	❑	❑	______

Student Name____________________ Date____________

PERFORMANCE CHECKLIST 23-15

GIVING A Z-TRACK INJECTION

	S	U	Comments
1. Follow the six rights	❑	❑	________
2. Perform the three label checks	❑	❑	________
3. Follow standard precautions	❑	❑	________
4. Perform hand hygiene	❑	❑	________
5. Check for allergies	❑	❑	________
6. Prepare medication according to standard procedure for injectables	❑	❑	________
7. Use one needle to withdraw dose from container; use another needle (1½ to 2 inches) to inject medication so that no solution remains on the outside of needle shaft	❑	❑	________
8. Draw up to 0.2 mL of air to create an air lock	❑	❑	________
9. Identify room, bed, patient, and patient's birthdate	❑	❑	________
10. Recheck for allergies	❑	❑	________
11. Don gloves	❑	❑	________
12. Expose and locate dorsogluteal or ventrogluteal site according to IM site selection procedure; provide privacy	❑	❑	________
13. Clean site with an alcohol swab	❑	❑	________
14. Ask the patient to take a deep breath and to slowly exhale (to relax the muscle); pull skin tightly in a lateral direction (move skin at least 1 to 1½ inch laterally) to one side; hold the skin taut with the nondominant hand	❑	❑	________
15. Insert needle at a 90-degree angle; aspirate; if no blood is seen, inject medication and air slowly; wait 10 seconds to allow the medication to disperse slowly	❑	❑	________

	S	U	Comments
16. Withdraw needle quickly; allow skin to return to its normal position, which leaves a zigzag path that seals the needle track wherever tissue planes slide across each other. The drug cannot escape from the muscle tissue	❑	❑	______________
17. Use a 2 x 2 gauze pad or Band-Aid as needed	❑	❑	______________
18. Do not massage site	❑	❑	______________
19. Do not recap needle (if safety glide needle used, advance protective glide); dispose directly into sharps container	❑	❑	______________
20. Remove gloves and perform hand hygiene	❑	❑	______________
21. Document administration in Medex or computer, including site used, Z-track method used, and amount and type of medication given; record initials, date, and time	❑	❑	______________
22. Return to assess patient's response to medication	❑	❑	______________
23. Document assessment in nurse's notes	❑	❑	______________

Student Name______________________________ Date______________

PERFORMANCE CHECKLIST 23-16

GIVING AN INTRADERMAL INJECTION

	S	U	Comments
1. Follow the six rights	❑	❑	______
2. Perform the three label checks	❑	❑	______
3. Follow standard precautions	❑	❑	______
4. Perform hand hygiene	❑	❑	______
5. Check for allergies	❑	❑	______
6. Prepare medication according to standard procedure for injectables	❑	❑	______
7. Identify room, bed, patient, and patient's birthdate; explain procedure	❑	❑	______
8. Recheck for allergies	❑	❑	______
9. Don gloves	❑	❑	______
10. Select and expose inner aspect of lower arm	❑	❑	______
11. Clean site gently with alcohol swab from center outward; let dry	❑	❑	______
12. Two injections are made if test is for sensitivity. One injection is a control using sterile water or bacteriostatic normal saline; the other is the substance that is to be tested	❑	❑	______
13. Advance needle through epidermis to approximately 1/8 inch (3 mm) below skin surface using a 25-gauge needle at approximately a 15-degree angle with bevel up directly under skin to make a small bleb (wheal) with test solution; needle can be seen through skin. Do not inject into subcutaneous tissue. Inject control of normal saline into another site for comparison with test substance at designated time interval	❑	❑	______
14. Do not massage site	❑	❑	______
15. Draw a circle around skin test with a marker; label area with date, time, and name of test. Another method is to make a diagram in patient's chart to indicate location of site	❑	❑	______

	S	U	Comments
16. Do not recap needle (if safety glide needle used, advance protective glide); dispose directly into sharps container	❑	❑	________
17. Remove gloves and perform hand hygiene	❑	❑	________
18. Chart site; intradermal; record initials, date, and time	❑	❑	________
19. If an indurated (hardened), erythematous area is observed, measure and record results in millimeters with metric ruler	❑	❑	________
20. Return to assess patient's response to medication	❑	❑	________
21. Document assessment in nurse's notes	❑	❑	________
22. At designated time, compare control with agent; document results in chart	❑	❑	________

Student Name________________________ Date____________

PERFORMANCE CHECKLIST 23-17

Giving a Subcutaneous Injection

	S	U	Comments
1. Follow the six rights	❑	❑	______
2. Perform the three label checks	❑	❑	______
3. Follow standard precautions	❑	❑	______
4. Perform hand hygiene	❑	❑	______
5. Check for allergies	❑	❑	______
6. Prepare medication according to standard procedure for injectables	❑	❑	______
7. Identify room, bed, patient, and patient's birthdate; explain procedure	❑	❑	______
8. Don gloves	❑	❑	______
9. Recheck for allergies	❑	❑	______
10. Select and expose site (check which site was used previously and rotate site); the abdomen is the usual preferred site when administering heparin or Lovenox	❑	❑	______
11. Clean site with alcohol swab from center outward using circular motion; let dry	❑	❑	______
12. **Method A (thin patient or child):** Spread skin of selected site taut and hold firmly; insert needle at 45-degree angle and aspirate; inject medication slowly; do not aspirate if heparin or Lovenox is being administered	❑	❑	______
Method B (average-size or obese patient): Grasp and press together skin of selected site so that it forms roll between fingers; insert needle at a 90-degree angle and aspirate; do not aspirate if heparin or Lovenox is being given; inject medication slowly	❑	❑	______
13. Withdraw needle quickly and apply an antiseptic swab or a 2 x 2 gauze sponge; do not massage the site if heparin or Lovenox is administered because this will increase local bleeding and ecchymosis will occur	❑	❑	______

	S	U	Comments
14. Do not recap needle (if safety glide needle used, advance protective glide); dispose directly into sharps container	❑	❑	________
15. Remove gloves and perform hand hygiene	❑	❑	________
16. Chart site used and amount and type of medication; subcutaneous; record initials, date, and time	❑	❑	________
17. Return to assess patient's response to medication	❑	❑	________
18. Document assessment in nurse's notes	❑	❑	________

Student Name________________________________ Date________________

PERFORMANCE CHECKLIST 24-1

APPLYING A TOURNIQUET

	S	U	Comments
1. Use a strong, wide, flat piece of material if possible (for example, towel, necktie, wide belt)	❑	❑	______________
2. Place pressure on the nearest pressure point to control bleeding while applying the tourniquet	❑	❑	______________
3. Apply a pad (piece of cloth, handkerchief, dressing) over the artery to be compressed to prevent impairment of skin integrity	❑	❑	______________
4. Place the tourniquet between the wound and the heart: allow some uninjured skin between the wound and the tourniquet; wrap the material around the limb twice, and tie a half-knot on the upper surface of the limb	❑	❑	______________
5. Place a stick or rod (approximately 6 inches long) over the knot, and secure it in place	❑	❑	______________
6. Twist the stick enough times to stop the bleeding	❑	❑	______________
7. Secure the stick firmly with the free ends of the tourniquet; do not cover the tourniquet	❑	❑	______________
8. Write "T" or "TK" (meaning tourniquet) on the victim's forehead and the time it was applied; attach a note to the victim's clothing describing the time and location of the tourniquet	❑	❑	______________
9. Treat for shock, and transport to the nearest medical facility	❑	❑	______________
10. Never loosen a tourniquet once it has been applied; always seek medical attention once tourniquet has been applied	❑	❑	______________

Student Name______________________________ Date______________

PERFORMANCE CHECKLIST 24-2

Applying an Arm Sling Using a Triangular (Sling and Swathe) Bandage

	S	U	Comments
1. Place one end of the base of the open triangle over the uninjured shoulder	❑	❑	______________
2. Place the apex of the triangle behind the elbow of the injured arm	❑	❑	______________
3. Bend the arm at the elbow with the hand elevated slightly (4–5 inches)	❑	❑	______________
4. Bring the forearm across the chest and over the bandage	❑	❑	______________
5. Take the lower end of the triangle, and bring it over the shoulder of the injured side; tie the bandage on the neck at the uninjured side so that the knot is on the side of the neck	❑	❑	______________
6. Twist the remaining end of the bandage, and tuck it in at the elbow	❑	❑	______________
7. Remember to keep fingertips exposed to assess circulation	❑	❑	______________

Student Name______________________ Date______________

PERFORMANCE CHECKLIST 24-3

MOVING THE VICTIM WITH A SUSPECTED SPINAL CORD INJURY

	S	U	Comments
1. Carefully roll the victim, supporting the entire length of the body, just enough to slip a solid board underneath the victim for support; this board must extend beyond the victim's head and feet	❑	❑	______
2. While another person steadies the victim's head, place a towel or padding in the space underneath the victim's neck (never put the head on a pillow)	❑	❑	______
3. Place additional padding (rolled up blankets, towels, sandbags, etc.) around the head and neck to hold the head in place, keeping the neck in line with the body; a cervical collar may be used	❑	❑	______
4. Secure the victim to the backboard with bandages, or improvise these so that the entire body is immobilized; tape the head in place	❑	❑	______
5. In the event of an emergency situation in which the victim is wearing a helmet, the nurse should immobilize the victim with the helmet left in place	❑	❑	______

Student Name_______________________ Date_______________

PERFORMANCE CHECKLIST 42-1

Performing a Surgical Skin Preparation

	S	U	Comments
1. Refer to medical record, care plan, or Kardex for special interventions	❑	❑	______
2. Refer to procedure manual to verify anatomical area to be shaved according to surgery to be performed	❑	❑	______
3. Obtain equipment	❑	❑	______
4. Introduce self	❑	❑	______
5. Identify patient	❑	❑	______
6. Close door, pull curtains	❑	❑	______
7. Explain procedure to patient	❑	❑	______
8. Wash hands and don clean gloves	❑	❑	______
9. Position bed and patient, raise bed to comfortable working level	❑	❑	______
10. Place towel or waterproof pad under area to be shaved	❑	❑	______
11. Fill basin with warm water	❑	❑	______
12. Use bath blanket to drape patient appropriately to limit exposure	❑	❑	______
13. Adjust lighting	❑	❑	______
14. Lather skin well with antiseptic soap and warm water	❑	❑	______
15. Hold razor at a 30- to 45-degree angle to skin	❑	❑	______
a. Shave small area at a time while holding skin taut	❑	❑	______
b. Use short, smooth strokes	❑	❑	______
c. Shave hair in direction it grows	❑	❑	______

	S	U	Comments
16. Provide washcloth and warm water for washing hands and face, provide oral hygiene, and return patient to comfortable position	❑	❑	______________
17. Remove and dispose of soiled gloves and wash hands	❑	❑	______________
18. Document exercises performed and patient's ability to perform them independently	❑	❑	______________
19. Do patient teaching	❑	❑	______________

Student Name________________________ Date____________

PERFORMANCE CHECKLIST 42-2

INCENTIVE SPIROMETRY/POSITIVE EXPIRATORY PRESSURE THERAPY AND "HUFF" COUGHING

	S	U	Comments
1. Refer to the physician's orders, care plan, or Kardex	❑	❑	________
2. Assess patient's respiratory status and lung sounds. Indicators for spirometry are: a. asymmetrical chest wall movement b. increased respiratory rate c. increased production of sputum d. diminished lung expansion postoperatively e. decreased oxygen saturation f. prevention of postoperative pneumonia g. prevention of atelectasis	❑	❑	________
3. Explain procedure, and instruct patient in the correct use of the spirometer. Frequently this is initially done by the respiratory therapist. However, it may be the nurse's responsibility to follow up and promote proper technique.	❑	❑	________
4. Obtain supplies and equipment	❑	❑	________
5. Wash hands and don gloves (if soiling is likely)	❑	❑	________
6. Place prescribed incentive spirometer at the bedside within easy reach of patient	❑	❑	________
7. Place patient in semi-Fowler's or full Fowler's position	❑	❑	________
8. Place tissues, emesis basin, and bedside trash bag within easy reach	❑	❑	________
Incentive spirometry			
a. Instruct patient to completely cover mouthpiece with lips and (a) inhale slowly until maximum inspiration is reached, (b) hold breath 2 or 3 seconds, and (c) slowly exhale	❑	❑	________
b. Instruct patient to relax and breathe normally for a short time	❑	❑	________

	S	U	Comments
c. Instruct and encourage patient to gradually increase depth of inspiration	❑	❑	________
d. Offer oral hygiene after spirometry is completed	❑	❑	________
e. Store spirometer in an appropriate place such as on the bedside table until next scheduled time. Make certain spirometer is within easy reach of patient	❑	❑	________
f. Encourage patient to perform procedure 10 times every hour while awake	❑	❑	________
g. Assess respiratory status and evaluate patient's response to spirometry	❑	❑	________
h. Document in nurse's notes: patient's respiratory status before and after incentive spirometry (the maximum of inspirations obtained in mL) and any adverse effects from the procedure	❑	❑	________
Positive expiratory pressure (PEP) therapy and "huff" coughing			
a. Wash hands	❑	❑	________
b. Set PEP device for setting ordered	❑	❑	________
c. Instruct the patient to assume semi-Fowler's or high Fowler's position, and place noseclip on patient's nose	❑	❑	________
d. Have patient place lips around mouthpiece. Patient should take a full breath and then exhale two or three times longer than inhalation. Pattern should be repeated for 10 to 20 breaths	❑	❑	________
e. Remove device from mouth, and have patient take a slow, deep breath and hold for 3 seconds	❑	❑	________
f. Instruct patient to exhale in quick, short, forced "huffs"	❑	❑	________
9. Position patient as desired or ordered	❑	❑	________

Student Name____ **Date**____________________

	S	U	Comments
10. Place call light within easy reach	❑	❑	____________________
11. Wash hands	❑	❑	____________________
12. Document	❑	❑	____________________

Student Name_______________________ Date_______________

PERFORMANCE CHECKLIST 42-3

Teaching Controlled Coughing

	S	U	Comments
1. Refer to medical record, care plan, or Kardex for special interventions	❑	❑	________
2. Obtain equipment	❑	❑	________
3. Introduce self	❑	❑	________
4. Identify patient	❑	❑	________
5. Explain procedure	❑	❑	________
6. Wash hands and don clean gloves	❑	❑	________
7. Assist patient to upright position; place pillow between bed or chair and patient	❑	❑	________
8. Demonstrate coughing exercise for patient			
a. Take several deep breaths	❑	❑	________
b. Inhale through nose	❑	❑	________
c. Exhale through mouth with pursed lips	❑	❑	________
d. Inhale deeply again and hold breath for a count of 3	❑	❑	________
e. Cough two or three consecutive times without inhaling between coughs	❑	❑	________
9. Caution patient against just clearing throat instead of coughing	❑	❑	________
10. Abdominal or thoracic incision can be splinted before coughing with hands, pillow, towel, or rolled bath blanket	❑	❑	________
11. Encourage patient to practice coughing while splinting the incisional area once or twice an hour during waking hours; assist patient as indicated	❑	❑	________

	S	U	Comments
12. Remind patient to use tissues and emesis basin for any mucus expectorated	❑	❑	________
13. Teach patient to examine sputum for consistency, amount, and color change	❑	❑	________
14. Provide washcloth and warm water for washing hands and face, provide oral hygiene, and return patient to comfortable position	❑	❑	________
15. Remove and dispose of soiled gloves and wash hands	❑	❑	________
16. Document exercises performed and patient's ability to perform them independently	❑	❑	________

Student Name______________________________ Date________________

PERFORMANCE CHECKLIST 42-4

Teaching Postoperative Breathing Techniques, Turning, and Leg Exercises

	S	U	Comments
1. Refer to medical record, care plan, or Kardex for special interventions	❑	❑	________
2. Obtain equipment	❑	❑	________
3. Introduce yourself	❑	❑	________
4. Identify patient	❑	❑	________
5. Explain procedure to patient	❑	❑	________
6. Wash hands and don clean gloves	❑	❑	________
7. Prepare patient for intervention			
a. Close door to room or pull curtain	❑	❑	________
b. Drape for procedure if necessary	❑	❑	________
8. Raise bed to comfortable working level	❑	❑	________
9. Premedicate with analgesic if indicated	❑	❑	________
Postoperative breathing techniques			
10. Place pillow between patient and bed or chair	❑	❑	________
11. Sit or stand facing patient	❑	❑	________
12. Demonstrate taking slow, deep breaths; avoid using shoulders and chest while inhaling; inhale through nose	❑	❑	________
13. Hold breath for a count of 3 and slowly exhale through pursed lips	❑	❑	________
14. Repeat exercise 3 to 5 times; have patient practice exercise	❑	❑	________
15. Instruct patient to take 10 slow, deep breaths every 2 hours until ambulatory	❑	❑	________

	S	U	Comments
16. If there is an abdominal or chest incision, instruct patient to splint incisional area using pillow or bath blanket, if desired, during breathing exercises	❑	❑	______
Leg exercises			
17. Lifting one leg at a time and supporting joints, gently flex and extend leg 5 to 10 times	❑	❑	______
18. Repeat exercise with opposite extremity; lifting leg while supporting joints, gently flex and extend leg 5 to 10 times	❑	❑	______
19. Alternately point toes toward the chin and toward the foot of the bed four to five times	❑	❑	______
20. Make a circle with ankles of both feet 4 to 5 times to the left and 4 or 5 times to the right	❑	❑	______
21. Assess pulse, respiration, and blood pressure	❑	❑	______
Turning exercises			
22. Instruct patient to assume supine position to right side of bed; side rails on both sides of bed should be in up position	❑	❑	______
23. Instruct patient to place left hand over incisional area to splint it	❑	❑	______
24. Instruct patient to keep left leg straight and flex right knee up and over left leg	❑	❑	______
25. Instruct patient to turn every 2 hours while awake	❑	❑	______
26. Remove and dispose of soiled gloves and wash hands	❑	❑	______
27. Document	❑	❑	______

Student Name________________________________ Date______________

PERFORMANCE CHECKLIST 42-5

Applying Thromboembolic Deterrent Stockings (TEDS)/Sequential Compression Devices (SCD)

	S	U	Comments
1. Refer to medical record, care plan, or Kardex for special interventions	❑	❑	______________
2. Obtain equipment	❑	❑	______________
3. Introduce yourself	❑	❑	______________
4. Identify patient	❑	❑	______________
5. Explain procedure	❑	❑	______________
6. Wash hands and, if appropriate, don clean gloves	❑	❑	______________
7. Prepare patient; close door to room, pull privacy curtain, and drape for procedure if necessary	❑	❑	______________
8. Raise bed to comfortable working level	❑	❑	______________
9. Examine legs and assess risk for conditions	❑	❑	______________
10. Assess patient for calf pain or positive Homans' sign	❑	❑	______________
11. Measure legs for stockings according to agency policy and order stockings	❑	❑	______________
Thromboembolic deterrent stockings			
12. Assist patient to supine position to apply stockings before patient rises	❑	❑	______________
13. Turn stockings inside out as far as heel; place thumbs inside foot part, and slip stocking on until heel is correctly aligned	❑	❑	______________
14. Gather fabric and ease it over ankle and up the leg	❑	❑	______________

	S	U	Comments
15. Pull leg portion of stocking over foot and up as far as it will go, making certain that gusset lies over femoral artery; adjust stocking to fit evenly and smoothly with no wrinkles	❑	❑	______
16. Repeat Steps 12 to 15 for opposite extremity	❑	❑	______
Sequential compression devices (SCD)			
17. Place sleeve under patient's leg, with fuller portion at top of thigh. Some SCDs are knee-high	❑	❑	______
18. Apply sleeve with opening at front of knee and closed portion behind knee. Some SCDs have a circular plastic inflatable sleeve	❑	❑	______
19. When in place, make sure there are no wrinkles or creases in stockings; fold Velcro strips over to secure stockings when appropriate	❑	❑	______
20. Attach tubing to SCD after both sleeves are applied; align arrows for correct connection and appropriate effect; plug in and turn on unit	❑	❑	______
21. Assess patient periodically	❑	❑	______
22. Assess stocking at regular intervals	❑	❑	______
23. Remove and dispose of soiled gloves and wash hands	❑	❑	______
24. Document	❑	❑	______
25. Do patient teaching	❑	❑	______

Student Name________________________________ Date____________

PERFORMANCE CHECKLIST 44-1

Care of the Patient in a Cast

	S	U	Comments
1. Patient teaching			
a. Explain why the cast is being applied and how it will be applied	❑	❑	________
b. Advise the patient that the plaster cast will feel warm as it dries	❑	❑	________
c. Explain the extent of immobilization	❑	❑	________
d. Explain care of the cast and expectations after discharge	❑	❑	________
e. Instruct patient not to insert sharp objects (coat hangers or pencils) under the cast	❑	❑	________
2. Handling the new cast			
a. Support wet cast with the flat of the hands or on pillows	❑	❑	________
b. Place cotton blankets or other absorbent material under the cast	❑	❑	________
c. Expose the cast to air as much as possible	❑	❑	________
d. Turn the patient frequently to aid drying	❑	❑	________
e. Use a cast dryer or hair dryer on warm (not hot) setting to circulate air over cast	❑	❑	________
f. Do not apply paint, varnish, or shellac to the cast; plaster is a porous material that allows air to circulate to the skin	❑	❑	________
3. Skin care			
a. Inspect skin at edges of cast and underlying cast for erythema and skin impairment	❑	❑	________
b. Remove plaster crumbs from skin with a washcloth moistened with warm water	❑	❑	________

	S	U	Comments
c. Use creams and lotions sparingly	❑	❑	______
d. Apply waterproof material around perineal area	❑	❑	______
e. Attend to patient's complaint of pain under the cast, particularly over bony prominences; if discomfort is not relieved by repositioning, report to physician; cast pressure may need to be relieved by windowing or bivalving	❑	❑	______
4. Turning to any position is generally permitted as long as the integrity of the cast is not compromised and the patient is comfortable; do not turn by grasping the abductor bar	❑	❑	______
5. Toileting—for a long leg or hip spica cast			
a. Use a fracture pan with blanket roll or padding	❑	❑	______
b. Elevate the head of the bed, if permitted, or place the bed in reverse Trendelenburg's position	❑	❑	______
6. Abdominal discomfort			
a. Cast may be "windowed" (an opening cut into it) to provide relief of abdominal distention or a port for checking bladder distention	❑	❑	______
7. Mobilization			
a. Weight-bearing is at the discretion of the physician, and the amount of weight-bearing will be prescribed	❑	❑	______
b. A cast shoe or a walking heel incorporated into a lower extremity cast will permit weight-bearing without damaging the cast	❑	❑	______

Student Name______________________________ Date______________

	S	U	Comments
8. Prevention of neurovascular problems (establish baseline measurements and assess neurovascular status before cast application; palpate distal pulses before cast application; assess color, temperature, and capillary refill of the appropriate fingers or toes; and assess neurologic function, including sensation and motion in the affected and unaffected extremity)			
a. Perform neurovascular checks every hour for at least 24 hours after cast application; notify physician of color changes, alterations in sensation, or motion unrelieved by position change; cast may need to be bivalved (cut in two) to relieve pressure	❑	❑	______________
b. Elevate affected extremity on pillows until danger of edema is over (usually 24 to 48 hours)	❑	❑	______________
c. After mobilization of patient with lower extremity or upper extremity cast, avoid keeping extremity in dependent position for prolonged periods	❑	❑	______________
d. After lower extremity cast is removed, encourage patient to wear elastic stocking and elevate affected leg at rest until full mobility is regained	❑	❑	______________

Notes

Notes

Notes

Notes

Notes

By the same author

FICTION

The Shadow of the Sun

The Game

The Virgin in the Garden

Still Life

Sugar and Other Stories

Possession: A Romance

Angels and Insects

The Matisse Stories

CRITICISM

Passions of the Mind: Selected Writings

BABEL TOWER

BABEL TOWER

A. S. BYATT

RANDOM HOUSE NEW YORK

Published in the United States by Random House, Inc., New York.

Published in Great Britain by Chatto & Windus Limited,
a division of Random House UK, London, in 1996.

Grateful acknowledgment is made to the following for permission to reprint previously published material: Harcourt Brace and Company: Excerpt from "Burnt Norton" in *Four Quartets* by T. S. Eliot. Copyright © 1943 by T. S. Eliot and renewed 1971 by Esme Valerie Eliot. Reprinted by permission of Harcourt Brace and Company. Houghton Mifflin Company and HarperCollins Publishers Ltd.: Excerpt from *The Hobbitt* by J.R.R. Tolkein. Copyright © 1966 by J.R.R. Tolkein. Rights outside the United States are controlled by HarperCollins Publishers Ltd., London. All rights reserved. Reprinted by permission of Houghton Mifflin Company and HarperCollins Publishers Ltd. Alfred A. Knopf, Inc.: Three lines from "Peter Quince at the Clavier," from *Collected Poems* by Wallace Stevens. Copyright © 1923 and renewed 1951 by Wallace Stevens. Reprinted by permission of Alfred A. Knopf, Inc. *The Observer*: Article by Maurice Richardson from the May 8, 1966, issue of *The Observer.* Copyright © 1966 by The Observer. Reprinted by permission. Random House, Inc.: Eight lines from "Death's Echo" and twenty lines from "Circe," from *W. H. Auden: Collected Poems* by W. H. Auden. "Death's Echo" copyright © 1936 by W. H. Auden. "Circe" copyright © 1969 by W. H. Auden. Reprinted by permission of Random House, Inc. Ronin Publishing: Copyright 1990P: Timothy Leary, from *Politics of Ecstasy* by Timothy Leary, Ph.D. Permission to reprint herein given by Ronin Publishing, Inc., Berkeley, CA. University Press of New England: Excerpt from *Life Against Death* by Norman O. Brown. Copyright © 1959 by Wesleyan University. Reprinted by permission of University Press of New England.

Library of Congress Cataloging-in-Publication Data
Byatt, A. S. (Antonia Susan)
Babel Tower / A.S. Byatt. — 1st ed.
p. cm.
ISBN 0-679-40513-5
1. Married women—England—London—Fiction. 2. Trials (Obscenity)—England—Fiction. 3. Family violence—England—Fiction. 4. Young women—England—Fiction. 5. Divorce—England—Fiction. I. Title.
PR6052.Y2B33 1996b
823'.914—dc20 95-53210

Manufactured in the United States of America on acid-free paper

24689753

For David Royle

A NOTE FOR AMERICAN READERS

The Profumo scandal and the Moors Murders were important public events which helped to define the moral atmosphere of "swinging London" and the "permissive society" in England in the 1960s. Other important events were the prosecution and acquittal of the publishers of *Lady Chatterley's Lover* in 1960 and the prosecution and conviction of the publishers of *Last Exit to Brooklyn* in 1967. The *Last Exit* decision was reversed on appeal. I have taken some legal details from that trial, particularly the unusual decision by the judge to hear the defence witnesses before those for the prosecution, and also the fact that it was tape-recorded in full on behalf of the publishers, who later used their transcript to prepare the appeal.

John Profumo was Secretary of State for War in Harold Macmillan's government. In 1963 there were rumours that he had slept with a prostitute, Christine Keeler, who had also slept with a Soviet naval attaché, Eugene Ivanov. National security was thought to be threatened by this. Profumo made a personal statement to the House of Commons in March, denying the allegations, but resigned in June, confessing that his statement had been a lie. Also in June Christine Keeler and another young woman, Marilyn (Mandy) Rice-Davis, were involved in the trial of Dr. Stephen Ward, osteopath and artist, who was convicted in August of living on their immoral earnings, but killed himself on the day of the verdict. The trial made public figures of the two composed and attractive young women, and aroused a swarm of rumours of sleaze and corruption in high places, which contributed to the fall of the Conservative government. Lord Denning, an eminent judge, wrote a report on the "Profumo Affair" dealing solemnly with, among other things, rumours that a government minister had attended sadistic orgies at Stephen Ward's house in "a black leather mask which laces up at the back," and that there were parties where "the man who serves dinner is nearly naked except for a small square lace apron round his waist such as a waitress might wear."

Ian Brady was found guilty in 1966 of the murders of Edward Evans, Lesley Ann Downey, and John Kilbride. Myra Hindley was found guilty of murdering Evans and Downey, not guilty of murdering Kilbride, but guilty of abetting Brady in that murder. The murders were particularly horrific because they seemed to have been committed for the pleasure of murdering. Brady did have the works of de Sade, amongst others, in his library. The victims were buried on the Moors, and Hindley later confessed that further victims were still hidden there. Both Brady and Hindley are still in prison.

Her Telepathic-Station transmits thought-waves
the second-rate, the bored, the disappointed,
and any of us when tired or uneasy
are tuned to receive.

So, though unlisted in atlas or phone-book,
Her Garden is easy to find. In no time
one reaches the gate over which is written
large: MAKE LOVE NOT WAR

. . .

She does not brutalise Her victims (beasts could
bite or bolt), She simplifies them to flowers,
sessile fatalists who don't mind and only
can talk to themselves.

All but a privileged Few, the elite She
guides to Her secret citadel, the Tower
where a laugh is forbidden and DO HARM AS
THOU WILT *is the Law.*

Dear little not-so-innocents, beware of
Old Grandmother Spider; rump Her endearments.
She's not quite as nice as She looks, nor you quite
as tough as you think.

W. H. Auden, "Circe"

La Nature n'a qu'une voix, dîtes-vous, qui parle à tous les hommes. Pourquoi donc que ces hommes pensent différemment? Tout, d'après cela, devait être unanime et d'accord, et cet accord ne sera jamais pour l'anthropophagie.

Mme. de Sade, Letter to her husband

I fear we are not getting rid of God because we still believe in grammar.

Nietzsche

BABEL TOWER

It might begin:

The thrush has his anvil or altar on one fallen stone in a heap, gold and grey, roughly squared and shaped, hot in the sun and mossy in the shade. The massive rubble is in a clearing on a high hill. Below is the canopy of the forest. There is a spring, of course, and a little river flowing from it.

The thrush appears to be listening to the earth. In fact he is looking, with his sideways stare, for his secret prey in the grass, in the fallen leaves. He stabs, he pierces, he carries the shell with its soft centre to his stone. He lifts the shell, he cracks it down. He repeats. He repeats. He extracts the bruised flesh, he sips, he juggles, he swallows. His throat ripples. He sings. His song is liquid syllables, short cries, serial trills. His feathers gleam, creamy and brown-spotted. He repeats. He repeats.

Characters are carved on the stones. Maybe runes, maybe cuneiform, maybe ideograms of a bird's eye or a creature walking, or pricking spears and hatchets. Here are broken alphabets, α and ∞, C and T, A and G. Round the stones are the broken shells, helical whorls like empty ears in which no hammer beats on no anvil. They nestle. Their sound is brittle. Their lips are pure white (*Helix hortensis*) and shining black (*Helix nemoralis*). They are striped and coiled, gold, rose, chalk, umber; they rattle together as the quick bird steps among them. In the stones are the coiled remains of their congeners, millions of years old.

The thrush sings his limited lovely notes. He stands on the stone, which we call his anvil or altar, and repeats his song. Why does his song give us such pleasure?

I

Or it might begin with Hugh Pink, walking in Laidley Woods in Herefordshire in the autumn of 1964. The woods are mostly virgin woodland, crowded between mountainsides, but Hugh Pink is walking along an avenue of ancient yews, stretched darkly over hills and across valleys.

His thoughts buzz round him like a cloud of insects, of varying colours, sizes and liveliness. He thinks about the poem he is writing, a rich red honeycomb of a poem about a pomegranate, and he thinks about how to make a living. He does not like teaching in schools, but that is how he has recently made some sort of living, and he reconstructs the smells of chalk and ink and boys, the noise of corridors and tumult, amongst the dark trees. The wood floor smells pungent and rotting. He thinks of Rupert Parrott, the publisher, who might pay him to read manuscripts. He does not think he will pay much, but it might be enough. He thinks of the blooded pink jelly of pomegranates, of the word "pomegranate," round and spicy. He thinks of Persephone and is moved by the automatic power of the myth and then repelled by caution. The myth is too big, too easy, too much for his pomegranate. He must be oblique. Why is there this necessity, now, to be oblique? He thinks of Persephone as he used to imagine her when he was a boy, a young white girl in a dark cavern, before a black table, with a gold plate containing a heap of seeds. He had supposed the six seeds she ate were dry seeds, when he was a boy and had never seen a pomegranate. Her head is bowed, her hair is pale gold. She knows she should not eat, and eats. Why? It is not a question you can ask. The story compels her to eat. As he thinks, his eyes take in the woods, brambles and saplings, flaming spindle-berries and gleaming holly leaves. He thinks that he will remember Persephone and holly, and suddenly sees that the soft quadruple rosy seed of the spindle is not unlike the packed seeds of the pomegranate. He thinks about spindles, touches on Sleeping Beauty and her pricked finger, goes back to Persephone, dreaming girls who have eaten forbidden bloody seeds. Not the poem he is writing. His poem is about fruit flesh. His feet make a regular rhythm on fallen needles and the blanket of soft decay. He will remember the trees for the images in his mind's eye, and the images for the trees. The brain does all sorts of work, Hugh Pink thinks. Why does it do this sort so well, so luxuriously?

At the end of the ride, when he comes to it, is a stile. Beyond the stile are rough fields and hedges. On the other side of the stile are a woman and a child, standing quietly. The woman is wearing country clothes, jodhpurs, boots, a hacking jacket. She has a green headsquare knotted under her chin, in the style of the Queen and her royal sister. She leans on the fence, without putting her weight on it, looking into the wood. The child, partly obscured by the steps of the stile, appears to be clinging to the leg of the woman, both of whose arms are on the top bar of the fence.

They do not move as Hugh Pink approaches. He decides to strike off himself, into a shady path on his left. Then she calls his name.

"Hugh Pink? Hugh Pink. Hugh—"

He does not recognise her. She is in the wrong clothes, in the wrong place, at the wrong time. She is helping the child on to the stile. Her movements are brisk and awkward, and this reminds him. The child stands on the top step, balancing with one hand on her shoulder.

"Frederica—" says Hugh Pink.

He is about to add her old surname, and stops. He knows she is married. He remembers the buzz of furious gossip and chatter at the time of this marriage. Someone nobody *knew,* they had said, they had complained, none of her old friends, a stranger, a dark horse. No one was invited to the wedding, none of her university lovers or gossips, they had found out purely by chance, she had suddenly vanished, or so they told each other, with variants, with embellishments. It was put about that this man kept her more or less locked up, more or less incommunicado, in a moated grange, would you believe, in the country, in outer darkness. There had been something else, some disaster, a death, a death in the family, more or less at the same time, which was said to have changed Frederica, utterly changed her, they said. She is very changed, everyone was saying, you would hardly know her. Hugh was on his way to Madrid at this time, trying to see if poetry and making a living could be done in that city. He had once been in love with Frederica, and in Madrid had fallen in love with a silent Swedish girl. Also he had liked Frederica, but had lost her, had lost touch, because love always came before and confounded liking, which is regrettable. His memories of Frederica are confused by memories of his own embarrassment and memories of Sigrid, and of that embarrassment.

It is true that she is changed. She is dressed for hunting. But she no longer looks like a huntress.

"Frederica," says Hugh Pink.

"This is Leo," says Frederica. "My son."

The boy's look, inside his blue hood, is unsmiling. He has Frederica's red hair, two or three shades darker. He has large dark brown eyes, under heavy dark brows.

"This is Hugh Pink. One of my old friends."

Leo continues to stare at Hugh, at the wood. He does not speak.

Or it might begin in the crypt of St. Simeon's Church, not far from King's Cross, at the same time on the same day.

Daniel Orton sits on a slowly rotating black chair, constrained by a twisted telephone wire. Round and back. His ear is hot with electric words that filter through the black shell he holds to his head. He listens, frowning.

"I say I'm completely shut in you know I say I say I say I don't get up off my butt and go out of this room any more I can't seem to get up the force I ought to try it's silly really but what's the point I say I say I say I say if I did get out there they'd all stomp on me I'd be underfoot in no time it isn't *safe* I say I say I say are you there are you listening do you give a damn is there anyone at all on the end of this line I say I say."

"Yes, there's someone. Tell me where you want to go. Tell me why you're afraid to go out."

"I don't need to go nowhere no one needs me there's no need that's why oh what's the point? Are you still *there*?"

"I'm here."

The crypt is dark and solid. There are three telephones, set round the base of a pillar, in plywood cubicles soundproofed with a honeycomb of egg-boxes. The other two telephones are unmanned. There is a small blue-and-white jug of anemones in Daniel's cubicle. Two are open, a white and a dark crimson with a centre full of soft black spikes and black powder. There are unopened blue and red ones, bright inside colours hidden under fur, steel-blue and soft pink-grey, above the ruffs of leaves. Over each telephone is a text, done in good amateur calligraphy. Daniel's says:

So likewise ye, except ye utter by the tongue words easy to be understood, how shall it be known what is spoken? For ye shall speak into the air.
There are, it may be, so many kinds of voices in the world, and none of them is without signification.
Therefore if I know not the meaning of the voice, I shall be unto him that speaketh a barbarian, and he that speaketh shall be a barbarian unto me. I Corinthians 14:9–11.

The second phone rings. Daniel has to decide to disengage from the first caller. Someone else should be there, but even saints can be tardy.

"Help me."

"If I can."

"Help me."

"I hope I can."

"I've done wrong."

"Tell me, I'll listen."

Silence.

"I'm here simply to listen. You can tell me anything. That's what I'm for."

"I can't. I don't think I can. I made a mistake, I'm sorry, I'll go."

"Don't go. It might help you to tell me."

He is a man playing a hooked creature in the dark depths on a long dark line. It gasps and twists.

"I had to get out, you see. I had to get out. I thought *I had to get out*. Every day that was what I thought."

"Many of us do."

"But we don't—but we don't—do what I did."

"Tell me. I'll simply listen."

"I've not told anybody. Not for a whole year, a whole year is probably what it is, I've lost count. It might kill me to tell anyone, I might just be—nothing, I am nothing."

"No. You are not nothing. Tell me how you got out."

"I was making the kiddies' tea. They were lovely kids, they were—"

Tears, hectic gulps.

"Your own kids?"

"Yes." In a whisper. "I was just making bread and butter. I had this big knife. This sharp big knife."

Daniel's spine stiffens. He has taught himself not to make imaginary faces or places for the voices; that has led to errors; he unmakes a cramped kitchen, a tight-lipped face.

"And?" he says.

"I don't know what come over me. I stood and just looked at everything, the bread, and the butter, and the cooker, and the dirty dishes, and that knife, and I just became *someone else.*"

"And?"

"And I put down the knife, and I didn't say anything, I just went and got my coat and my handbag, I didn't even say, 'I'm just going out for a minute or two,' I just went out of the front door quietly and shut it behind me. And I went on walking a long time. And. And I never went back. The little one was in his high-chair. He might have fallen over or anything might have happened. I just never went back."

"Did you get in touch after? With your husband? Do you have a husband?"

"I did, yes. I do have a husband, I suppose. I didn't get in touch. No. I couldn't. You see I couldn't."

"Do you want me to help you to get in touch?"

"No." Quickly. "No, no, no, no, no. I'd die, I'd die. I've done wrong. I've done terrible wrong."

"Yes," says Daniel. "But I wouldn't say it couldn't be helped."

"I've said it now. Thank you. I think I'll go now."

"I think I can help, I think you need help—"

"I don't know. I've done wrong. I'll go."

St. Simeon's is not in use as a parish church. It stands in a grimy courtyard, and has a heavy, square mediaeval tower, now surrounded by a bristling cage of scaffolding. The old church was enlarged in the eighteenth century and again in the nineteenth century, and was partly demolished by bombing in the Second World War. The Victorian nave was always too high and gaunt for its width, and this effect is emphasised by the fact that it has been only partly rebuilt, inside its old shell. It once had gaudy nineteenth-century stained glass, of no particular merit, depicting Noah's Ark and the story of the Flood on one side, and the stories of the raising of Lazarus, the appearance of the risen Christ at Emmaus and the tongues of fire descending at Whitsuntide, on the other. All these windows were sucked in by bomb blasts, leaving heaps of brilliant blackened fragments strewn in the aisles. A devout glazier in the congregation undertook to rebuild the windows, after the war, using the broken lights, but he was not able, or even willing, to reconstitute the narratives as they had been. What he made was a coloured mosaic of purple and gold constellations, of rivers of grass green and blood red, of hummocks of burned amber and clouded, smoke-stained, once-clear glass. It was too sad, he told the Vicar, to put the pictures together all smashed, with gaping holes. He thought it should all be bright and cheerful, and added modern glass here and there, making something abstract yet suggestive, with faces of giraffes and peacocks and leopards staring at odd angels out of red drapery, with white wings divided by sea blue and sky blue, angels and antediluvian storks and doves mingling with pentecostal flames. The peaks of Mount Ararat balance on a heap of smoky rubble, amongst which are planks of the Ark at all angles. Dead Lazarus's bound jaw has survived and one of his stiff white hands; both make a kind of wheel with the hand breaking bread at Emmaus and a hammering Ark-builder's hand. Parts of the primal rainbow flash amongst blue-and-white wave-crests.

Virginia (Ginnie) Greenhill clatters down on high heels. She explains about late buses and bad-tempered queues. No problem, says Daniel. She offers him tea, shortbread, comfort. She has a sweet face, round, with round glasses resting on round pink cheeks and a mouth arched upwards. She settles in her own armchair—hers does not spin—and spreads out an expanse of complicated Fair Isle, oatmeal and emerald. Her needles click. Daniel is drowsy. His telephone rings.

"Remember there is no God."

"So you have said before."

"And because there is no God, do as thou wilt shall be the whole of the law."

"So you have also said before."

"If you knew what that meant. If you really knew. You would not sound so complacent."

"I hope that is not how I sound."

"You sound stolid, you sound blinkered, you sound one-dimensional."

"You never let me say much, to sound anything."

"You are not supposed to mind that. You are supposed to listen to what I have to say to you."

"I do listen."

"I abuse you. You don't respond. I can hear you turning your other cheek. You are a Christian parson or person. I waste your time. You waste your own time, since there is no God. *Homo homini deus est, homo homini lupus est* and you are the dog in the fable with his neck worn bare by the dog-collar, wouldn't you agree?"

"You want me to dislike you," says Daniel, carefully.

"You do dislike me. I can hear it in your voice. I have heard it before. I tell you that God is dead, and you dislike me."

"I listen to you, God or no God."

"And you haven't once told me I must be very unhappy, which is very clever of you, since I am not."

"I am reserving judgement," says Daniel grimly.

"So just, so restrained, not a fool."

"The fool hath said in his heart, there is no God."

"So I am a fool?"

"No. I just said that, because it seemed to fit. I couldn't resist it. Count it unsaid, if you like."

"*Do* you wear a dog-collar?"

"Under a thick jumper. Like many these days."

"Bonhomie. Anomie. I waste your time. I *am* a waste of time. I occupy your line with God when other fools stuffed with Seconal or dripping gore may be trying to get through."

"Just so."

"They are nothing, if there is no God."

"I'll be the judge of that."

"It is my calling to call you and tell you there is no God. One day you will hear me, and understand what I say."

"You don't know what I understand. You are making me up."

"I've riled you. You will learn—slowly, because you aren't very bright—I go on until I have riled you, because it is your *job,* your calling, not to be riled, but in the end I can rile you. Aren't you going to ask me why I need to rile you?"

"No. I can ask myself. And I'm too riled. Satisfied?"

"You think I am childish. I am not."

"I'm no expert in childishness."

"Ah, you *are* riled. I'll go. Until next time."

"As you will," says Daniel, who is indeed riled.

"Steelwire," says Ginny Greenhill. She has given this name to the death-of-god-monger, because of his voice, a clear BBC twang, a produced voice, plangent and metallic.

"Steelwire," says Daniel. "He says he wants to *rile* me and he does. I can't work out why he goes on calling."

"He won't usually talk to me. It's you he likes. He just tells me there is no God and rings off. I say, yes dear, or something inane, and he rings off. I've no idea if he's upset, or malicious, or what. Down here, I suppose, we are likely to over-react, to suspect someone who merely wants to *rile* you, of being desperate, even if he isn't. We see the underside of the world, I suppose."

Her needles tap. Her voice is comfortable, like honey and toast. She is in her fifties, and unmarried. She does not invite questions about her private life. She once managed a corset shop, Daniel knows, and now lives perhaps off a small private income and a pension. She is a devout Christian and finds Steelwire harder to take than masturbators in phone-booths.

Canon Holly comes down the stairs as Ginnie Greenhill answers another call.

"No, we're here to help, *whatever* the problem, you *might* shock me of course, but I do doubt it—"

Canon Holly takes the third chair and watches Daniel write in the log.

4.15–4.45. Steelwire. There is no God, as usual. Daniel.

"Any idea what he's up to?" The Canon inserts a cigarette into a cracked amber holder and puffs smoke towards Daniel. He moves around in a cloud of smoke-scent, like a bloater.

"No," says Daniel. "Same message, same style. He set out to irritate, and did. It's possible he's really upset because there's no God, or God is dead."

"Theological despair as a motive for suicide."

"It's been known."

"Indeed."

"But I think he's too gabby to be suicidal. I wonder what he does all day and night. He rings at all times."

"Time will reveal," says the Canon.

"It doesn't always," says Daniel, who has had one or two nasty experiences, hearing desperate voices subside into meaningless babble and the burring of an empty telephone, or rise more and more shrilly before the sudden severing of the link across the air.

Or it might begin with the beginning of the book that was to cause so much trouble, but was then only scribbled heaps of notes, and a swarm of scenes, imagined and re-imagined.

Chapter I *Of the Foundation of Babbletower*

When the blissful dawn of the Revolution had darkened to the red light of Terror, when the paving-stones of the city shifted on flesh and oozed blood in their interstices, when the streaming blade rose and fell busily all day and the thick sweet smell of butchery flared in all men's nostrils, a small band of free spirits left the City separately, at night, in haste and secrecy. They wore various well-studied disguises, and had made their preparations well in advance, sending supplies secretly and ordering horses and carriages to be made ready at lonely farms, by those they could trust—for there was trust in some, even in those dark days. When they were gathered in the farmyard they seemed a ramshackle crew of rusty surgeons and filthy beggars, stolid peasants and milkmaids. In the farmyard those who seemed to be the leaders, or at least in charge of the plan of action, described the coming journey, across plains and through forests, always skirting large towns and villages, as far as the border of the land, where they would cross into a neighbouring mountainous country and make their way to the hidden valley, beyond the white-capped fangs of the mountains, where one of their number, Culvert, had a sequestered property, La Tour Bruyarde, which could be reached only across a narrow wooden bridge between two lines of peaks, across a dark and lifeless chasm.

They must travel fast, and circumspectly, never trusting anyone they met on the road, save certain helpers at posting stages, and in certain lonely inns and hamlets, who could be recognised by certain secret signs, a blue flower at a certain angle in the hatband, an eagle feather in a tuft of cock feathers. If they all came safely to their destination—as it was most vigorously to be hoped they would—they would be able to set up their own small society in true freedom, far from rhetoric, fanaticism and Terror.

So they travelled, through a press of dangers and menaces which will not be recounted here, but left to the imagination, for this story concerns itself not with the troubled world they left behind, but with the new world they meant so hopefully to build, if not for all men, since that hope had failed, then for these select few.

They did not all arrive. Two young men were caught by the military and pressed into the Army, from which they had much ado to escape a year later. One old man was knifed by an older woman as he rested in his sweat in a ditch and closed his eyes for sheer weariness. Three young women were caught and raped by a rabble of peasants, though they were well disguised as pox-ridden crones. When their young, smooth flesh was discovered under their artfully tattered clothing, they were raped again for their deceitfulness, and again for their sweetness and softness, and yet again, upon compulsion, so that they no longer had force to beg for mercy or tears to run down their blubbered cheeks, and then again, and so they died, of suffocation, of fear, of despair, who knows, or who knows if they thought it a merciful release. Their fate was never known by those more fortunate who came to the hidden tower, though rumours of it were rife on the roads. But in those days, so many were undone, these deaths were not remarkable.

The group who gathered on the crest of Mount Clytie, before making the crossing on the wooden bridge, might fairly have been thought remarkable. They were mud-stained and dishevelled, thinner after the privations of their journey, but full of vigour, their blood beating fiercely with renewed hope. They could not see La Tour Bruyarde (only one of the names of the place) from where they stood, but they were assured by their leader that once across the bridge and over the last natural bastion, they would behold a possible site for an earthly Paradise, a plain watered by swift streams and meandering brooks, in which was a wooded Mount or Mound on which stood their new home, on a site where his own family, throughout the ages, had always had a fortress-retreat.

This leader, though of noble birth, went by the name of Culvert, since it was a condition of their society that their names should be newly chosen, to signify relinquishment of the old world, and new beginnings in the new. His chief companion was the Lady Roseace. They were a beautiful pair, in the first strength of confident manhood and womanhood. Culvert was above the common height,. broad-shouldered but lithe; he wore his hair, which was black and gleaming, longer than was fashionable, and it fell in great negligent tresses on his shoulders. His face was strong and smiling, with a full red mouth, both firm and sensuous, and dark eyes under decisive brows. Roseace was slender but full-breasted, and pressed her saddle with firm but ample buttocks. Her hair was also worn freely over her shoulders, though she had only considered it safe to release it from her hood since they came to the summit of Mount Clytie, and she now tossed her head a little from sheer pleasure at the breezy clarity of the air and the empty spaces of rock, snow and green vegetation spread below her. Her face was thoughtful and imperious, her lips firmly arched and her winged brows drawn in a habitual questioning frown. She had in her young life been destined by her parents for an uncongenial husband, and by the Revolutionary Powers for denunciation, summary trial and rapid execution, but she had escaped both parents and gaolers with equal resourcefulness and ruthlessness. On the day when this narrative begins her golden hair was curling and tangled and her skin lightly veiled with a powdering of dust, amongst which glistened diamond drops of sweat.

Other members of the assembled company were the young Narcisse, pale, gentle and hardly more than a boy, full of tremulous self-doubt and sudden starts of eagerness; the careful Fabian, who had shared Culvert's student freedoms and had been a voice of caution in his wilder enterprises; and an older man, who called himself Turdus Cantor, and was wrapped in a heavy cloak, appearing to find the mountain air, even in the fresh sunlight, chill. Fabian's brave wife, Mavis, was there, and with them were their three children, newly named Florian, Florizel and Felicitas. More children had set out, two families with their own young and orphaned cousins, but these were not expected to reach the bridge for a few days, since their journey was necessarily slower. Three younger women, clustered together and speaking in low voices, were the raven-haired Mariamne and the palely glimmering twin girls, Coelia and Cynthia. There were also the servants in charge of carts and pack animals—of these, who were appointed to become companions with the rest, once their destination was reached, more will be told at a later date.

Culvert looked around him, and laughed, and said:

"So far we have come, through risk and dread, and now we shall enter into the possession of our own lives and our own ways of living. La Tour Bruyarde, where you will be received, had lapsed into disuse in my grandfather's time. Its stones were plundered for the walls of barns and chapels, its halls were empty and the vines were creeping through the broken windows. But much work has been done, many suites and chambers have been restored, the necessary offices are in order, although as you will soon see, the building work will continue above our heads, to make all more secure and harmonious.

"All of you, I think, know something of my plans in making our retreat here. I wish our new lives to be an experiment in freedom—freedom in large things, in education, in government of our society, in shared labour, in the life of the mind and the life of the passions. Attention will be paid to things that may appear to be lesser things—art, dress, food, the decoration of our living quarters, the cultivation of our plants and trees. These will all be debated amongst us and made new in ways now only partly to be imagined, as we live our passionate and reasonable lives with goodwill. Petty restrictions will be done away with. New combinations will be instituted. Those who desire one thing greatly shall be satisfied, and so shall those who wish to flutter like butterflies from flower to flower.

"When we and our fellow labourers have crossed this bridge, and when Damian and Samuel have waited here another seven days in hope of the wagon with the children, and other straggling companions, we shall take axes and cut the supports away from the bridge, which will render us unassailable from this direction, from where our danger comes."

"Will it," asked Fabian, "render us also unable to escape from this valley?"

"We hope no one will ever wish to escape. But also of course no one should be prevented—we are designing a community of entire freedom—and to the south there are narrow passes through the mountains and ways in which, with difficulties no greater than we have just faced, anyone might come out. But I hope we shall all be living in such pleasure, and delight, and mutual usefulness, that such wishes would be far indeed from your thoughts."

"Far indeed," said Roseace, smiling, and spurring on her horse to be the first to set foot on the bridge. So they passed over in safety, some averting their eyes from the giddy chasm below, in which a sullen torrent roared over sharp black basalt, dimmed by stream and spray, forever out of reach of the direct warmth of the sun. Fabian clasped his young son to his breast so that the boy should not look down, but the boy's sister gazed about her in all directions fearless and laughing. And so, talking animatedly of the haven they were so soon to see and enter, the company entered the rocky defile which would open on the Valley of Faisans.

Frederica seems set on coming into the wood, where Hugh is, rather than inviting him over to her side. She hands the boy into Hugh's hands and comes down quickly herself, rejecting assistance. She is as thin as ever, her sharp face still bony.

They wander along the paths between the trees. They do not know how to talk to each other. Once they met daily and discussed everything, Plato, the tanks in Budapest, Mallarmé, Suez, metre. This makes it harder, not easier, to ask for narratives of the six years that have passed. They mention old friends. Alan is teaching art history at the Samuel Palmer School of Art, Hugh says. He thinks he is also writing a few articles. He travels to Italy. Tony is doing rather well as a freelance journalist. He even does some television. Hugh himself is still writing, yes, he is still writing, it is the poetry that matters, he tells Frederica, who makes an affirmative noise, nodding her scarfed head, staring down at beech mast. He makes his living teaching, he says, but he would like not to. A publisher has offered him some reading, but it would only be for a pittance. Poets can only expect pittances, says Hugh Pink to Frederica, who makes the same, slightly suffocated, affirmative noise. She does not ask about Raphael Faber, whose poetry-reading group they once both attended. Hugh tells her that Raphael's poem "Lübeck Bells" has been published. He says it is much admired by those who can see what it is.

"I know," says Frederica.

"Do you still see Raphael?" asks Hugh innocently. Hugh was in love with Frederica and Frederica was in love with Raphael, but that was in what seems to him in this wood another country, another time, his youth, which is already gone.

"Oh no," says Frederica. "I've lost touch with everyone from that time."

"You were writing for *Vogue,*" says Hugh, who had found that almost as odd as this manifestation in jodhpurs and jacket. Frederica was intellectually stylish but hardly part of the world of consumer delights and chic gossip.

"I did for a bit. Before I married."

Hugh waits. He waits for an account of Frederica's marriage.

She says, "My sister was killed. I don't know if you knew. And I married Nigel not long after, and Leo was born, and I was quite ill, for a bit. You don't realise at first, Hugh, what a death is going to do to you."

Hugh asks about the death. He did not know Frederica's sister, who was older than Frederica, had also been at Cambridge, he believed, but had lived in Yorkshire, where Frederica came from. He could not remember Frederica talking much about a sister. She had always seemed to be a kind of solitary, one-off creature, fierce and striving.

Frederica tells him about her sister's death. He realises that this narrative is practised, this is the way she has found it convenient—possible—to tell it. Her sister, she says, was married to a vicar and had two small children. And the cat brought in a bird, a sparrow, which took refuge under the refrigerator, and her sister had pulled it out and reached under it, and the fridge was not properly earthed. She was very young, says Frederica. Afterwards, she says wryly, we all suffered from shock. Shock waves, she says grimly. Waves and waves of shock. How terrible, says Hugh Pink, prevented from imagining by Frederica's matter-of-fact tone.

"And Nigel looked after me. I'd never needed looking after before, but Nigel looked after me."

"I didn't know Nigel."

"He was around. He wasn't *at* Cambridge, he just visited. His name's Reiver, the family have a house, an old house, Bran House, just over those fields, those are their fields, over that stile."

They walk on. The boy holds Frederica's hand. He shuffles dead leaves with quick kicks.

"Look, Leo," says Frederica. "Conkers. Over there."

One or two gleam, polished ruddy-brown, through split spiked green balls lined with creamy-white. They lie in a drift of chestnut leaves, in a hollow.

"Go and get them," says Frederica. "We always used to be so excited when we found any. We didn't often, local boys had always combed the ground first. They threw stones at the branches, to bring them down. They were a great event. Every year. I never used to make holes and fight with them. Boys did, but I just kept them until they were dull and shrivelled, and then I threw them out. Every year."

The boy pulls at Frederica's hand. He will not gather the conkers without her. He pulls, and she follows, picking them up amongst the dead leaves and offering them to him—"humbly" is the word that comes to Hugh Pink.

Hugh says to Leo, "Do you like to put strings through them?"

The boy does not answer.

"He's like his father," says Frederica. "He doesn't talk much."

"*You* don't," says the boy. "*You* don't talk much."

"When your mother and I were friends, before," says Hugh Pink, "when we were younger, she never stopped talking."

Frederica straightens herself jerkily and begins to walk again, leaving the other two amongst the conkers. Hugh's foot uncovers a monster, a solid glistening globe, bursting its cape. He offers it to Leo, who hands him Frederica's offerings, in order to inspect this. Hugh says, "I've got a little bag here I had sandwiches in. You could put them all in there, to carry them."

"I could," says Leo. "Thanks."

He drops the chestnuts solemnly into Hugh's bag, hands it back to Hugh, and puts up his hand to be held. Hugh takes it. He cannot think of anything else to say. Leo says, "Come to tea in my house, now."

"Your mummy hasn't asked me."

"Come to tea."

They catch up with Frederica.

"This man," says Leo. "This man is coming to tea, in my house."

"That would be nice," says Frederica. "Come to tea, Hugh. It isn't far."

Once this is agreed, the boy suddenly appears to feel free to run about, and begins to make little journeys into the undergrowth, pocketing feathers, shells, and a tuft of fur. Hugh says, "You've done a lot of living, Frederica. Real things have happened to you."

"Having things happen to you and living" says Frederica. She begins again. "They aren't the same thing. I suppose they must be the same thing. I used to be so sure about living. I wanted."

The sentence has no object and no end, apparently.

They climb the stile, and cross into the afternoon fields, where a heavy white horse is grazing, where a bird is singing in a thorn bush, where Hugh trips on a molehill and rights himself. He has a feeling he can't find words for, although it is to do with his poetry. It is a feeling he thinks of as the *English* feeling, though in fact it may be simply a human feeling about death. It is a brief knowledge of his own temporary body, all the soft slippery dark organs, all the minute interlocking bones, all the snaking, fizzing, prickling veins and nerves. It is the knowledge that he is *inside* this skin, and it is intensely pleasurable because it always goes with a sense of the huge sweep and intricacy and age of what is *outside* hair, skin, eyeballs, nostrils, lips and the helix of the ear. It is the irrational pleasure of a creature in the fact that its surroundings were there long before its own appearance, and will be there long after. It was not a possible pleasure, Hugh thinks, before he had lived a certain time, before the repeated crossings of local earth, in his case England, had become part of the form of the soft pale mass in his skull, part of the active knowledge of his sight and smell and taste. You cannot have this particular pleasure in living, Hugh tells himself, before you have begun to know you are dying. He thinks it tends to come in this sort of landscape—bitten grass, exposed stones, bush, tree, hill, horizon—because generations of his ancestors, thousands and millions of years before towns and cities, and still after, have had this sense in this sort of place. The cells remember it, Hugh thinks. Every inch of this turf has absorbed, he supposes, knuckle-bones and heart-strings, fur and nails, blood and lymph. There are equally strong feelings in cities, which also turn the mind like whirlpools, but not this one, which is essentially green, and blue, and grey. The thing which can flash into the brain a memory of *this* thing is the repeated reading of words which, like turf and stones, are part of the matter of the mind: the Immortality Ode, say, the Nightingale, Shakespeare's sonnets. There again the pleasure of the sense of one's own vanishing briefness—Hugh stumbles—is part of the pleasure in the durable words.

Sometimes he fears this feeling is no longer general, that few in his world would recognise it, and those who did would be suspicious, would call it stock response, silly pastoral. But still the smell of the earth, the moving lips of the horse in the grass, the tree's black twigs on the grey air, move him, living and dying.

He says none of this. He picks himself up and walks onwards. He watches Frederica's son, trudging sturdily across the pasture. He tries to remember what it was like to be so small, to have the sense that years are very nearly infinite, other seasons unimaginably far away, as they would be to a man on a planet that took half a lifetime to circle its sun.

. . .

Beyond the next gate, over the brow of the meadow, is Bran House. Hugh Pink sees that it does indeed have a moat, not metaphorical, behind which is a high encircling wall, inside which are a tiled roof and Tudor chimney pots. The wall is both blank and beautiful, made of old, soft red bricks, crumbling here and there, encrusted with mosses and lichens, stonecrop and houseleeks, ivy-leaved toadflax and wild snapdragons. Branches—fruit trees, a cedar in the distance—rear above the wall.

"How beautiful," says Hugh.

"It is," says Frederica.

"What a place for Leo to grow up," says Hugh, still thinking of his "English" feeling.

"I know," says Frederica. "I know it is a wonderful place."

"We go in through the orchard," says the child, running on ahead. Round a corner is a humped wooden bridge, over the moat, and a door in the wall.

As they go through the trees, Hugh says, "I never thought of you as the mistress of a country house."

"Nor did I," says Frederica.

"Only connect," says Hugh vaguely, thinking of Margaret Schlegel at Howards End. The phrase itself produces a renewed wash or swoop of English feeling.

"*Don't say that,*" says Frederica, sounding more like the woman he once knew than she has done all afternoon. Leo is busy wiping his boots on a bootscraper. A door opens, and a woman appears, middle-aged, in woollen stockings and tongued brogues, who takes him in, an arm around his shoulder, telling him it is tea-time.

"This is Pippy Mammott," says Frederica. "Pippy, this is my friend Hugh Pink. We were at university together. Leo invited him to tea."

"I'll put out more cups," says Pippy Mammott. She strides off, holding Leo's hand. Hugh and Frederica cross a tiled hall, past a turning square staircase, into a drawing-room, with window-seats and comfy sofas.

"They'll bring tea," says Frederica. "They'll bring Leo. Nigel isn't here. He's working, I suppose. He works for his uncle's shipping business, he goes off for days or weeks and comes back."

"And you," says Hugh. "What do you do?"

"What does it look as though I do?"

"I don't know, Frederica. When I last saw you you were all flaming and ferocious. You were going to be the first woman Fellow of King's and have your own TV programme and write something—in some new form—"

They have not sat down. Frederica is staring out of the window. Two women come into the room and are introduced to Hugh as Olive and Rosalind Reiver, Nigel's sisters. The tea is brought on a trolley, and handed about by Pippy Mammott. Olive and Rosalind sit side by side on a sofa covered with pink and silver-green blowsy blooms printed on linen. They are square, dark women, with strong bones, and shadows on their upper lips. They wear comfortable jumpers, one oatmeal, one olive, tweed skirts and opaque stockings over strong, shapely legs. Their eyes are like Leo's, large, dark and lustrous, under heavy dark brows. They ask Hugh Pink all the questions Frederica has not asked. What does he do, where does he live, is he married, doesn't he love their beautiful part of the country, how can he bear to live in a city with the stench and the crowds and the machines, would he like to see the grounds, the home farm? Hugh says he is on a walking holiday and is a long way from his next stopping place. Olive and Rosalind say they can run him over in no time in the Land Rover, and Hugh says, no, that is not the point of a walking-tour, and he must be on his way soon, now, before the light goes. They accept this without demur. They say he is very right to stick to his project, they approve of that, they say, there is no way as good as walking to see the real country. Pippy Mammott hands out scones, slices of cake, tea, more tea. The boy ferries between his mother and his aunts, showing things first to one, then the other. Pippy Mammott takes his hand and says it is time to go, now. Leo says, "I want to stay here," but is led away. "Say good-bye to Mr. Pink," says Pippy Mammott. "Good-bye," says the boy, not bashfully.

Hugh decides he ought to go. It is true about the light and he feels he ought to go. Frederica sees him to the door, and then walks out with him down the long drive to the front gate, to set him on his way.

"Do you come to London, ever?"

"Not really. I used to. It didn't work out."

"You should come and see us all. Alan and Tony. Me. We miss you."

"You could write. You could write about poetry."

"Try and come. You seem to have lots of help—"

"It isn't *help*."

She stands awkwardly, helpless. He wonders if he can kiss her. He doesn't exactly want to. Her old restless energy is in abeyance and with it her sexual sharpness. He puts his arms rather suddenly round her and brushes his face with hers. She flinches and stiffens and then hugs him fiercely.

"I'm glad you were there in that wood. *You will keep in touch,* Hugh—"

"Of course," says Hugh.

The telephone babbles and quacks and purrs. Ginnie Greenhill tells, "Sex is so much a matter of how you feel about *yourself.* Oh, I know there are ideas about what is *normally* attractive, normal proportions as you put it, of course, yes, I do know—"

Babble, quack, purr, babble, a series of plosives inside the black shell.

"No, I'm not underestimating repulsion, of course it exists, it would be silly to underestimate it. But on the other hand there's such a *variety* of people around, such curiosity and goodwill—"

Canon Holly examines Daniel's log.

3.00–3.30. Woman who dare not go out of her room. No name, London voice, said she will call again. Daniel.

3.30–4.05. Unnamed caller, left home and children on impulse a year ago, she says. Northern voice. "I have done wrong." Reacted strongly against suggestion we might get in touch with family. Daniel.

4.15–4.45. Steelwire. There is no God, as usual. Daniel.

Canon Holly lights another cigarette. He is in his late fifties, handsome in a lean, long-faced, lined way, like a well-bred horse, with deepset eyes and long strong teeth, nicotine-stained. He is interested in Steelwire but has never picked up one of his calls. He himself is an expert on God. He has written a successful and controversial book called *Within God Without God* and has been seen on the television, supporting the Bishop of Woolwich and *Honest to God. Within God Without God* argues in a riddling and witty way that to lose the comfortable Old Man Up There, or for that matter the Friend of Little Children wandering amiably in the pastures beyond the stars, was to discover a Force which made all men Incarnate Words, Incarnate Souls, as Christ had shown. Godwithin, the Canon wrote, had not made us fearfully and wonderfully as a craftsman might pinch and poke a ball of inanimate dirt or clay. He made us much more fearfully and wonderfully because He was the inherent Intelligence in the first protozoa clinging together in the primal broth, because He had grown with us and still grew with us, He grew and divided in every cell of our growing and dividing body from egg to fertile parents. He was and is as Dylan Thomas has so beautifully put it, "the force that through the green fuse drives the flower."

Daniel is not sure how far Canon Holly's theological position differs from atheism or pantheism. He himself is temperamentally no theologian, only an instinctively religious man who is no longer sure what that word, "religious," means. He suspects also that his own position does not differ from that of Canon Holly. He sees that the Canon's thought works in a Christian framework of prayer, biblical references, ritual and theology, and that these things are part of the Canon's liveliness, his personal history, his self. Daniel is a watchful man. He thinks the Canon would shrivel if he were obliged to follow his own reasoning, his own metaphors, outside the walls, so to speak, of the Church, the singing, the ritual, the imposed duties. Daniel thinks also that he himself would *not* shrivel. Perhaps, given his very shaky assent to almost all the doctrines of his Church, he ought to go and live and work outside it. He stays, partly, because he needs the impersonality of the absolute requirement of virtue. He needs to be required, for instance, to be patient with Steelwire. This kind of work—without the impersonal sanction—becomes something different, more self-indulgent, something unnatural and perhaps unwholesome.

Within the walls, Canon Holly's sense of God working in all his cells like yeast gives him a bounding energy, at once touching and irritating. He is a founder-member of a group called Psychoanalysts in Christ, and has written a second book, *Our Passions Christ's Passion,* on sexuality and religion, drawing extensively on Freud and Jung, anthropologists and religious historians, William Blake, William James, St. Teresa of Avila, and St. John of the Cross. This book has had an even greater success than *Within God Without God* and has raised questions amongst the Church hierarchy, who wisely diverted him, along with Daniel, who was then recovering from a kind of breakdown, to the counselling centre, combined with a branch of the Listeners, in St. Simeon's. Canon Holly loves the work, he loves the callers, he loves Daniel and Ginnie and all the others. He listens to the incoming calls with an open-mouthed total attention, alert, shining-eyed, every sinew straining to leap into help, participation, communion. It is the sort of enthusiasm of which the Listeners have to be shrewdly suspicious. But it works. Daniel sees it at work, he hears the Canon's slightly husky voice urge on the hesitant:

"Go on, you needn't be afraid. Tell me, *tell me,* I cannot be shocked, I do assure you." Daniel sees that help is given and received. But he would not bring his own problems to Canon Holly. He would sooner set them out before Ginnie Greenhill's bland smile and comfortable nod. Ginnie Greenhill does not *need,* as far as he can see, to be told anyone's troubles, and yet she comes to listen. He has no idea why she does. He has not asked. He believes that a certain distance between them makes their work easier.

Ginnie Greenhill puts down the telephone with a little sigh.

"Another masturbator?" enquires Canon Holly.

"Not exactly. I didn't like this one. He's taken to following a girl from his work everywhere she goes. He says he's full right up of her, he's bursting with her, he doesn't sleep for the idea of her. He wants her to notice him but he knows he repels her."

"Does he?" asks Canon Holly.

"I could answer, How do I know? Judging from my own reactions I'd say I imagine he *does,* yes. People usually do if they think they do, don't they? You get more mistakes in the other direction. Though I remember one man who came here after *weeks* of going on about his awfulness and he was a big handsome brute who only needed to lose a few pounds and hold his head up. Odd how people see themselves."

"You handled him well," says the Canon, savouring the handling. "Real warmth, no false promises."

He brings out a letter from the Bishop in answer to an idea of his own for a sexual therapy workshop in St. Simeon's. Problems could be pooled, and professional advice given to unprofessional helpers. Ginnie Greenhill makes tea for all of them, and observes that in her view a money-management workshop would be just as helpful to a large number of callers.

"To listen to you, Ginnie dear," says the Canon, "one would think you were a frightful prude, ready to shy away from the first hint of bodily passion or misery. And one would be quite wrong, because I've *heard* you dispensing perfect acceptance and common sense to the most hurting and hurtful people."

Ginnie's knitting needles tap rhythmically. She bends her head over her wool. She says, "I do think, Canon, that the modern Church does somehow seem to be about sex, that does seem to be what it *cares* about, if I may say so."

The Canon is bright with glee. He lights another cigarette and sucks greedily.

"The Church has *always* been about sex, dear, that's what the problem is. Religion has always been about sex. Mostly about denying sex and rooting it out, and people who are trained to deny something and root it out become obsessed with it, it becomes unnaturally monstrous, that's why current moves to be more *accepting* and *celebratory* about our sexuality are so *exciting*—we may work *with* this force and not *against* it—"

"I thought," says Ginnie Greenhill, "that religion was about God, and about death. About how to live with the idea of death, that's what I thought it was."

And death too, the Canon begins on a run, what is death but part of sex, the germ cell is immortal but the sexually divided individual is doomed, it is sex that brought death into the world . . .

The telephone rings. The Canon leans forward.

"This is the Listeners. Can I help you?

"Yes, he's here. I'll fetch him. One moment. Don't go away."

He hands the receiver to Daniel, his hand cupped over the mouthpiece, holding in wisps of bitter smoke. "One of yours."

"Yes. This is Daniel. Who is that?"

"This is Ruth. Do you remember me, I used to come to the Young Christians, with Jacqueline, when you were up here, in Yorkshire?"

He has a vision of her, pale oval clear-cut face, heavy-lidded eyes, the long solid plait of pale hair falling between her shoulders.

"Of course I remember you. Can I help?"

"I rang to say I think you ought to come. Mary's had an accident, she's unconscious in Calverley Hospital. Her grandmother's with her, she's by the bed. I work in the Children's Ward, I think you know that, I said I'd find you."

Daniel is without words. He sees dancing mounds and hollows of egg-boxes humping like earthquakes.

"Are you there, Daniel?"

"Yes." His mouth is dry. "What happened to her?"

"She has a head injury. She was found in the playground. Some other little girl may have run into her, we don't know, she couldn't have fallen off anything, from where she was.

"Are you there, Daniel?"

He cannot speak. Ruth's little voice, as used as his own to dispensing comfort, says, "She'll almost certainly be all right, the wound's in the front of the head, not the back, and that's good. The skull's stronger there. But I thought you'd want to know, you'd want to be here."

"Yes," says Daniel. "Yes of course. I'll come right away. I'll get a train and come straight there, tell them all I'll come straight there. Thank you, Ruth."

"She's in the best place," says the far-away voice. "She'll be cared for as well as possible, you know."

"I know. I'll see you soon."

He puts down the phone and sits staring into the cubicle, a heavy man, shaking.

"Can we help?" says Canon Holly.

"My child's been hurt. In Yorkshire. I've got to go."

"You need hot sweet tea," says Ginnie. "Which you shall have. And the Canon will get King's Cross about trains, won't you? Do you know what happened, Daniel?"

"No. They don't seem to know. She was found in the playground. I must go."

The Canon has dialled and is listening to the burring tone.

"How old is she?"

"Eight," says Daniel.

He never talks about his children, and Holly and Ginnie never ask. They know his wife was killed accidentally and that he has children in Yorkshire, living with grandparents. He visits them, they know that, but he does not talk about these visits. Ginnie brings more tea and sweet biscuits—sugar for shock is one of their stocks-in-trade. The Canon suddenly begins to write down train times. At least, Ginnie says, Daniel has only a few minutes' walk to King's Cross, he can buy a toothbrush somewhere on the way. She asks practically about the child's state.

"She's not conscious. They say she'll almost certainly be all right, I expect they mean that, they'd be careful what they say, wouldn't they?"

"They would have to, yes."

"She's only a little thing," says Daniel.

But he cannot see Mary's face, conscious or unconscious. He sees Stephanie, his wife, lying on the kitchen floor, with her lip pulled back over damp teeth. This is who he is, the man who looked at that face. This is what she is, a terrible face; this sight persists in his brain. This is her after-life. He is hunted through his waking life by that face, he has developed the cunning of a hunted creature who twists and darts to avoid anything in the passages of the brain that might trigger, might switch on, that remembered face. There are words, there are innocent, pleasant memories, there are smells, there are whole people, whom he avoids with ferocity in case they call up that dead face. He even paints his dreams with black ink, he clamps his dreaming head with a vice of will, he never slips into dreaming that face and waking with the memory.

He has told himself that survivors, like himself, quite commonly feel they are dangerous to others, to other survivors. He does indeed feel that he is dangerous to Will and Mary, his children, though that is not the whole story, is not the whole reason why they are in Yorkshire and he is here in St. Simeon's, under the tower.

And now it is as though he has hurled a rock at his small daughter, or pushed her from a high place.

"There's a train in fourteen minutes," says Canon Holly, "and another in an hour and fourteen minutes. You can't make it in fourteen minutes."

"I can try," says Daniel. "I can run."

He sets off up the steps.

La Tour Bruyarde must have been almost invulnerable in its great days, long ago. As the company approached it across the plain and the mountain meadows that surrounded it, they saw how thick and frowning was its outer wall, crumbled and breached in many places, here rising proudly, there lying in a dense arrested fall of mossy blocks crusted on the hillside. Men could be seen on the ramparts and in the clefts, repairing the structure. They wore brightly coloured singlets, cerise, royal blue, scarlet, which gave their labours an appearance of cheerfulness. The Lady Roseace imagined she heard them singing, that a faint hum of musical noise was borne to them on the air.

Within the confine of the wall could be seen not one but many towers, and of all shapes and sizes, as though this citadel had been put up at random over the ages, all made of the same stone hewn from the same mountainside, but otherwise startling in their variety, square and conical, simply stolid and highly decorated, with turrets, with slate cones, with small lancet windows glinting like eyes, with galleries and turrets, with encrustations of ivy and other creeping life-forms. Many of these turrets appeared to be either unfinished or partly demolished, it was not always easy to say which, and the bright patches of colour of the workers' vests could be seen moving along these high ledges and opened rooftops. As they rode up the causeway which ascended the Mount or Mound a thin sound of cheering and welcome could be heard from high above them, and fruit and flowers were jubilantly thrown under their advancing feet.

They rode in between two great gate-towers, not, as the Lady Roseace had prefigured it to herself, into a central courtyard, but into a kind of dark tunnel, between walls which might be the sides of buildings or might be solid rocks, and which wound its way onward into the dark bowels of the place, lit occasionally by shafts of light in the gloom from high loopholes, and occasionally, at the darkest points, by lanterns hanging on smoke-blackened hooks from the stone. When they finally emerged they were in a well-like confine, with layer upon layer of dwellings towering above them, one corridor upon another, a Baroque balcony abutting a Gothic cloister, a series of classical windows, in elegantly diminishing proportions as they rose higher, under an unfinished thatched roof that might have suited a mediaeval byre. Some of the windows shone with myriad coloured lights, and some were gaping sockets with cracked arches. The sky was far, far away, it seemed to the Lady Roseace at that moment of arrival, and an intense blue, as the sky is when it is far, far away, scratched and scribbled on by the fingers and teeth, the stumps and domed skulls of the roofline.

The Living Quarters

Culvert led the Lady Roseace into the living quarters prepared for her. They travelled along many passages, through many doors and arches, up many flights of stairs and down almost as many, it seemed, so that she was quite amazed by their intricacy. Her door was hidden behind an embroidered hanging on a wall in a long gallery. She could not see what was depicted on the hanging, for the light was flickering and fitful, but had the impression of many heaped limbs energetically writhing, of spherical breasts pointing skywards and of watermelons, it seemed, bursting open on greensward.

Inside, all was rosy light. At first the Lady Roseace believed that she was in an internal chamber bathed in firelight, and then she saw that she was in a boudoir whose elegant windows were covered with a veil of translucent rosy silk, through which the sunlight poured. The room was sparsely furnished—there was an inlaid escritoire in rosewood, and a prie-dieu in the same wood upholstered in rose-coloured velvet, the most softly comfortable kneeling place possible to imagine. The rest of the furnishings were in a more oriental style, low divans, inlaid with ivory, spread with silk cushions of every size and shape, soft silken carpets woven with Persian roses and pinks and crimson-tipped daisies, huge soft floating daybeds, inviting languor, and hung with what appeared in that light to be flesh-coloured sealskins and cashmere shawls and rosy fox-furs. She ran through into the bedchamber, which had a high huge bed like a galleon, hung about with richly embroidered silken curtains and floating with muslins and nets. Everywhere on little tables and chests were fantastically luminous bottles and flasks, breathing soft perfumes of flowers and musks. A body—many bodies—might vanish entirely in the soft cushionings and quiltings of that secret bed.

The Lady Roseace walked from room to room, exclaiming and touching, fingering silks and ivories, tortoise-shells and lustres, satins and furs and feathers. When she drew back the silk curtain from the window and let in the daylight, the rosy fire died away in many of the fabrics and artefacts, revealing a new subtlety of snow-whites and creams and ivories, of northern furs and southern bones and tusks, of silvery threadwork and palest gold silk quilting.

A close inspection would reveal, in time, that this richness was a light covering over stony coldness and crumbling, that the flagstones were stained and chipped, and the walls flaking away. But they were covered for now with bravely stiff tapestries and draperies, all white and rose-red in honour of the Lady Roseace. There was a most exquisite depiction, all in reds and whites, roses and flesh tints, of the chaste Diana bathing under snowy branches by a silver spring, and of the lovely young Actaeon, part ruddy youth, part milk-white stag, and all laced and interlaced with gouts of brilliant crimson blood, which dripped also from the bright white teeth of the pale hounds, as they reached elegantly for his extended, panting throat . . .

The Coming of the Children

Towards mid-afternoon on the third day the company were gathered on a great balcony, drinking and discussing what was next to be done towards increasing the pleasure and fruitfulness of their life together. Serving men and women poured foaming ale and crimson and golden wine, constantly replenishing beakers and glasses. It had been decided that there should be no more servants and masters—decided, that was, by the masters, for the servants had not as yet been informed or consulted about this project—but no agreement had been reached about the time and manner of this great change in the relations of the population of the Tower. All that was agreed was that it should be debated fully when the whole company was gathered together and what had been set in motion could be deemed to be truly begun.

The Lady Roseace and Culvert, Turdus Cantor and Narcisse were all looking out over the meadows and the plain when the keen-eyed Narcisse detected a movement amongst the trees at the rim of the bowl of the valley. From that height what emerged from the dark woody shadows appeared at first to be a slow worm attended by dancing ants, but as it made its slow way across the meadows it could be seen to be a series of covered carts and carriages, attended by pricking outriders, and as it came still nearer, all could see that there were three great covered wagons, each drawn by two bullocks, and, as they came nearer still, that the bullocks were fantastically decked with garlands and the tips of their horns were gilded. A cry went up from the courtyards below, "The children, the children are coming," and the company waited to glimpse them from above as they paced towards the gatehouse, before hurrying down flight after flight of staircases to greet them in the inner fastness where their journey ended.

From above, no one could be seen in the swaying wagons, save their drivers, all of whom were cowled in heavy hooded cloaks, and carried stubby whips with long lashes, such as were usual in that country to urge on the blundering slow creatures. And indeed the labouring white flanks were blooded here and there, were scored by encouraging strokes, which appeared to have no effect on the steady, deliberate pace of the flower-decked beasts. There was trouble enough getting these ungainly vehicles through the passages to the centre, if it was the centre, of the Tower, and strange stifled sounds, pitiful lowings and nervous bellowings reached the ears of the company before the carts finally emerged into the dark courtyard.

And then the joyful moment, so eagerly awaited, was there. From every side, the coverings of the carts were pushed back, rolled up, burst open, and the small faces and the soft hair, the bright eyes and the tender fists of the children were seen. Some were sleepy, stretching their little limbs to rouse from the abandonment of sleep. Some were alert and mischievous, smiling eagerly at the adventures to be undertaken. Some were more timid, hanging their heads bashfully, flickering their silky lashes on their plump cheeks. Some were whimpering—there are always some who whimper in any group of children; no group of children, however generally cheerful and playful, but has some little whimperers among them—but these were quickly silenced in the general excitement as the children were welcomed and lifted down from the sides of the wagons on to the flagstones of their new abode. They were handed from loving arms to loving arms, they were softly kissed and their little clothes tenderly set to rights, and there was much laughter and general cheerfulness in the shadow of the high roofs.

The drivers too of the wagons were urged to come down from their perches and join the throng. This they did, pushing back their hoods from their dusty faces, coiling the lashes of their whips and tucking them away. The first was an old friend of all, Merkurius, lithe and muscular, with a fine face like a knife and a quizzical smile that quivered the gutstrings of Cynthia and Coelia. There was great rejoicing at the safe arrival of Merkurius, for rumours had been rife that he had been cut off by troops, that he had been taken naked as he made love to a whore in a city brothel, that he had died on the scaffold as a secret substitute for his great friend Armin, that he had drowned in an attempt to swim across a river in full spate. The fantasies of the company had been most fearfully exercised by all these contradictory reports. The sensitive, Narcisse as well as Cynthia and Coelia, had undergone drowning and decapitation, naked apprehension and coitus interruptus, the chase, the flight, the whipping branches, the strangling thickets. Indeed the only consolation for these sensitive souls had been the plethoric variety of these narrations, which could not all be true, so might all be false, as they were now joyfully proved to be.

The second driver had a round red face like a burning flower, and jet-black cropped hair like one a week or two away from escaping from prison or the army. It was only when this personage threw back the cloak with a rich, round peal of laughter that it could be seen that the cloak concealed a billowy female body, that this jovial gaol-bird was the Lady Paeony, heroine of many amorous adventures, and of more anecdotes of intrigue, false and true. Culvert and Roseace hastened to embrace this solid person, who gave her whip a last crack in the courtyard and declared that all her little charges had been golden-good and deserved sweetmeats, that they had been quiet as mice as they passed the pickets, and sung as sweetly as larks, to her great delectation, as they crossed the mountain meadows, and that she loved them all, she could crush them in her arms for love and happiness.

And now the third driver came forward, and pushed back his cowl slowly and deliberately and revealed a grizzled head and a grizzled beard, and a leathery skin wrinkling round pale-blue eyes. There was a hush in the courtyard, and a thrill of whispering ran through the company, for no one knew him, and all enquired of others, if they did, or had seen him before.

And the Lady Roseace said, quick as a flash and unthinking, "This man smells of blood."

And the man took a step or two forward, fingering his whip and perhaps smiling a little amongst his beard, and perhaps not—different impressions were formed by different persons.

"Who are you?" said Culvert.

"You know me well enough, by name at least, and some of you by more than name," said the man. "To my sorrow," he added, but not in a sorrowful tone.

"If it were not impossible," said Fabian thoughtfully, "I should say your name was Grim, that you are Colonel Grim of the National Army."

"I have been Colonel in the National Army," said Grim, "and Colonel in the Royal Army before that, and a professional soldier all my life. And now I am here, and wish to join you, if you will have me."

At this acknowledgement, a great murmuring and even hissing began amongst the people gathered round the carts, and several people repeated what Roseace had said, "This man smells of blood."

And Colonel Grim stood there easily amongst them all, looking from faces of hatred to faces of fear, and said, "That I smell of blood is true. I smell myself daily and the smell disgusts me. I have had enough of blood. The gutters of the city are running with blood, there are flecks of blood in the loaves of bread, blood feeds the roots of the apple trees where stinking dead men hang among the apples. You may not believe me now, but a killer by trade who has had enough of blood is a good founding member for a community based on kindness and freedom, as yours is to be."

"How can that be?" cried Coelia. "We know what you have done, we have heard the stories, the tortures, the punishments, the killing, the killing—how can such a creature be a fit companion for the gentle and the harmonious?"

"We should rather kill him," cried a young man, "we should put him to the sword for the sufferings of our families and our friends; we should cement our social bonds with his foul blood."

Colonel Grim said, "A man of blood can smell bloodthirstiness in any household, any society, any family. It is my business to smell bloodthirstiness. I am a wolf who can detect a rogue sheepdog, Monsieur Culvert. I am an instrument of control and have been an instrument of terror, and I can tell you much of the nature of control, and terror, and control by terror, which you do not now think you need to know. But it is what all men need to know, you will find, even if you expel or kill me. I bear the mark of Cain in your household, Monsieur Culvert. I have red hands, and most of you, all of you it may be, have not. But Cain was marked so that the children of Adam should not harm him. A man is not only the history of his deeds, I suppose, according to your philosophy, if not to that of my previous masters. You owe it to me to see how I can live peaceably."

"I do not understand how you have come here," said Culvert, frowning.

"I persuaded Merkurius and the Lady Paeony that I was another, that I was your old friend Vertumnus, who died, I am sad to have to tell you, in the oubliettes of the Tower. I had forged letters from yourself with which I convinced them. You must not blame them, sir. I am a sufficiently clever man."

"He will bring the national armies in his train," said Mavis.

"And how should that be?" asked Grim. "And why should I come, thus openly and alone, saying who I am, and leaving my fate to you, if the armies were following in secret. No, if I wished, I could have had the armies here to greet you. But I did not wish—your hopes are mine, my good friends—I hope you will be my good friends. The armies will not bother you here, and I am no longer Colonel Grim, but plain Grim, grey and grizzled and making a new start in the evening of his days, if you will have me."

"Turn him away," said the Lady Roseace, wrinkling her nostrils.

But Culvert said, "What he says is just. He may stay, until any of us detect him casting any baleful influence on our family. For all men are capable of change and redemption, as he says, though he must be watched, to see whether he says so with guile, or with honest intention."

So they all went into the citadel together, discussing the day's events.

II

Frederica reads to Leo. Inside his green and white room, which was Nigel's room, with its Beatrix Potter frieze, she sits on the edge of his fluffy eiderdown and reads to him about the Hobbit, setting out on his adventure. The curtains are drawn against the dark; they are lit by a bedside lamp inside a creamy glass shade, a creamy light.

"At first they passed through hobbit-lands," Frederica tells him, "a wide respectable country inhabited by decent folk, with good roads, an inn or two, and now and then a dwarf or a farmer ambling by on business. Then they came to lands where people spoke strangely and sang songs Bilbo had never heard before. Now they had gone on far into the Lone-lands, where there were no people left, no inns, and the roads grew steadily worse. Not far ahead were dreary hills, rising higher and higher, dark with trees. On some of them were old castles with an evil look, as if they had been built by wicked people. Everything seemed gloomy, for the weather that day had taken a nasty turn."

"A bit frightening," says Leo.

"A bit, yes," says Frederica, who believes there is pleasure in fear.

"Only a bit," says Leo.

"It gets more frightening later. More exciting."

"Go on reading."

"It was after tea-time; it was pouring with rain, and had been all day; his hood was dripping into his eyes, his cloak was full of water; the pony was tired and stumbled on stones; the others were too grumpy to talk."

"Poor pony. We don't let Sooty get too tired, do we? We look after him. He doesn't mind a bit of rain, Auntie Olive says. He's a tough little thing, Auntie Olive says."

"Yes, he is. Very tough. Shall I go on?"

"Go on."

" 'I wish I was at home in my nice hole by the fire, with the kettle just beginning to sing,' thought Bilbo. It was not the last time that he wished that!"

Leo rubs his eyes. He pushes his little fists into his eye-sockets and winds them energetically, so that Frederica's own eyeballs wince sympathetically.

"Be careful, Leo. You'll hurt your eyes."

"I won't. Those are *my* eyes. I don't hurt them. They itch."

"You're sleepy."

"I'm *not.* Go on reading."

"Still the dwarves jogged on," says Frederica, "never turning round or taking any notice of the Hobbit." Leo has settled into his bed: his head is in the hollow of his pillow, his cheek on his hand. She looks at him with appalled love. She knows every hair on his head, every inch of his body, every word, she thinks, of his vocabulary, even though he is constantly proving her wrong. And he has ruined her life, she thinks, for inside the new docile Frederica the old Frederica still has her histrionic passion-fits. I would walk out tomorrow if it were not for Leo, she tells herself hundreds of times each day, with contempt and puzzlement. She looks at his red hair, such a beautiful red, richer than hers, with the shine of those chestnuts he gathered with Hugh Pink. He is a very male child. He has strong shoulders and an aggressive jut to his chin. She is surprised by her passion for his small body as she was surprised by her passion for his father's, which it will no doubt grow to resemble; she thinks of Leo always as his father's child. She loves to see him straddle Sooty, his small legs at odds with the heavy straps and buckles and irons of the stirrups, his head, in its black velvet helmet, too important for his body, like a beetle, like a goblin. But Leo on Sooty is his father's son, in his father's world, where she doesn't belong, and isn't welcome. Nor does she want to belong or be welcome, she tells herself, with her usual mixture of honesty and fury, she has made a terrible mistake. Her voice goes on peacefully, dry and lively, telling about dwarves and wizard, Hobbit and trolls, things going bump in the dark, terror and mayhem, and Leo shudders agreeably. Inside her head she goes over and over what she has done, how she could have done it, how it cannot be undone, how she can live. Only connect, she thinks contemptuously, only connect, the prose and the passion, the beast and the monk. It can't be done and isn't worth doing, she thinks on a long repetitive whine, she has been here so often before. She thinks of Mr. Wilcox in *Howards End*, thinks of him with hatred, that stuffed man, that painted scarecrow. Margaret Schlegel was a fool in ways Forster had no idea of, because he wasn't a woman, because he supposed connecting was desirable, because he had no idea what it meant.

" 'Dawn take you all and be stone to you!' said a voice that sounded like William's. But it wasn't. For just at that moment the light came over the hill, and there was a mighty twitter in the branches. William never spoke for he stood turned to stone as he stooped—"

The door opens. Mother and son look up, and there is the man, the father, his return, as usual, unannounced. The sleepy boy is awake in a flash and sits up to be embraced. Nigel Reiver hugs his son and puts his arm round his wife. His cheek is cold from the outdoors—he has come straight up, he is even a little breathless, he is eager to see his family. He is a dark man in a dark suit, a soft armour, with the blue shadow of a dark beard on his solid cheek.

"Don't stop," he says. "Go on reading, I'll listen, it's my absolutely favourite book, *The Hobbit*."

"It's a bit frightening," says Leo. "Only a bit. Mummy says it gets more exciting than this, even more."

"Oh, it does," says the dark man, stretching himself on the bed beside his son, both heads on the pillow, looking up at Frederica, perched on the edge with the book.

He has nothing at all to do with Mr. Wilcox.

There is something to do with sex, which he is good at, and which Forster perhaps wanted Mr. Wilcox to be good at, but couldn't quite imagine, couldn't give life to.

The two pairs of dark eyes watch Frederica.

The room is full of slumberous warmth and watchful sharpness.

"And there they stand to this day, all alone, unless the birds perch on them; for trolls, as you probably know, must be underground before dawn, or they go back to the stuff of the mountains they are made of, and never move again. That is what had happened to Bert and Tom and William."

"I meant to stop there, it's a good stopping place, and Leo was nearly asleep, weren't you?"

"I *wasn't,* I was waiting for my Daddy to come."

"No you weren't. We didn't know he was coming."

"I did. I knew *in my bones* he would come this evening, I *knew* and I was right. Go on reading."

"Go on," says the man, lying on his back like a knight on a tombstone, his shiny dark shoes overhanging the bedfoot. So she goes on, for they are all happy, to the discovery of the treasure in the cave, and the end of the chapter.

"Have you been a good boy?" asks Nigel. "What has happened while I was away?"

"A man came to see Mummy, he was a very nice man with a funny name, his name was Pink, he found us in the woods and we asked him to tea."

"That was nice," says Nigel smoothly. He kisses his son good night, and Frederica kisses him, and the light is put out, and the little boy stirs his blankets into a containing nest.

Pippy Mammott has made supper for them to eat by the fire. She has made supper Nigel likes, shepherd's pie and baked apples with honey and raisins. She does not eat with Nigel and Frederica, but she does come in and out whilst they eat, offering second helpings, which Nigel accepts, refilling wineglasses, solicitously asking them to be careful of the apples, which are piping hot—"As they should be," says Nigel, detaining her to be congratulated on both pie and apples. He and Frederica sit in large armchairs each side of the wood fire, and Pippy Mammott stands between them with her back to the flames, warming her bottom. She tells him what Leo has been doing and saying, how well he is learning to ride Sooty, what a dauntless little boy he is, how they had an unexpected visitor, a friend of Frederica's apparently passing by quite accidentally on a walking tour.

"That was nice," says Nigel, smoothly, again. When Pippy has gone away with the trolley and the debris of the meal, he says, as Frederica is expecting him to say, "Who is this Hugh Pink?"

"An old friend from Cambridge. He writes poetry. Rather good poetry, I think. He was in Madrid for a year or two, and now he's back."

"You didn't say he was coming."

"I didn't know. He was on a walking holiday. Leo and I happened to bump into him, we gave him tea—it was Leo who invited him to tea—not me—"

"Why didn't you, if he was your friend?"

"Well, I would have, I expect, I would have got round to it—"

"Funny he just turned up—"

"Not really. He'd no idea this was where we lived. He was just walking. In the woods, like Leo says."

"I expect it was nice for you, to see an old friend?"

Frederica looks up, to see what is meant by this placid query. She calculates her answer.

"Of course it was. I don't seem to have seen any of my old friends for a long time."

"You miss them," states Nigel, in the same placid voice.

"Naturally," says Frederica.

"You should invite them," says Nigel. "You should feel free to invite them. You should ask them to stay."

Frederica chooses, after a moment, not to answer this remark. She stares, frowning, into the fire. She says, as placidly as he has been talking, "Are you back for long this time?"

"Does that make any difference? Why don't you just invite them? Maybe I'll be here, maybe I won't. I don't suppose my presence will affect your reunion."

"I didn't mean that. I just wanted to know how long will you be here this time?"

"I don't know. A few days. A few weeks. Why does it matter?"

"It doesn't. I just want to *know.*"

"Well, I don't know myself. There may be phone calls. Things may come up."

Frederica, looking into the logs, sees in her mind's eye a woman stepping barefoot across a bed of cinders, trying to find a path between little smouldering hot places, ready to break out into flames.

"When you go back, I'd like to come with you."

"Why?"

"Well. We used to do a lot of things together. Dancing, you know, things in town. And I would like to see some old friends, it's true, I would. I'm thinking, I might look for another job. I need something to *do.*"

This sentence comes out more tense, less casual, than she meant it to be.

"I would have thought you had a lot of things to do. A child needs his mother near him. There is a great deal here to occupy anyone."

"Don't talk to me like that, Nigel. That isn't the sort of thing *you* can say to *me.* You knew what I was when you married me—you knew I was clever and independent and—and ambitious—you seemed to *like* that. God knows I had nothing *else* someone like you might be interested in, no money, no connections, I'm not *beautiful*—all I was was bright and you can't marry someone for their brains and their—resourcefulness—and then expect them to behave like—"

"Like—"

"Like the sort of girl you might have been expected to marry—*but didn't*—one who has always gone hunting and shooting and likes just *being* in the country."

"I don't see why any girl would marry if she can't put up with being a wife. And a mother. If a girl becomes a wife and a mother, she must expect a few changes, I should think. I would have understood if you hadn't wanted to take the step. I don't think I more than half expected you would when I asked you—but you did. I thought you were a resourceful sort of girl. And now all you do is whinge. You have a lovely boy like Leo, and you whinge. It's not very pleasant."

Frederica stands up and begins to pace.

"Nigel, please listen to me. Please listen. I don't see very much of *you*—you don't tell me very much about where you are or what you do—"

"It wouldn't be of any interest to you."

"That may be. I don't know. But I *have to have something to do.*"

"You were always a great one for reading."

"But reading was *work*—"

"I see. You don't do it if you don't have to."

"I don't mean that. You know I don't. I know I don't *need* to earn my living—don't need, that is, in terms of money, don't *need*—"

Her need is so terrible, she is almost in tears.

"We aren't enough for you, Leo and me."

"You aren't ever here. And Leo has all sorts of people besides me, he's *rich* in people, Pippy and Olive and Rosalind, they adore him. He doesn't live in a nuclear family. All your friends, you and all your friends, were brought up by nannies."

"You know why in my case. My mother bolted, you know that. Bolted when I was two, you know that, I've told you. I've told you often enough. She had no strength of character, no resources. I thought you could look after Leo and be resourceful. I told you that."

He is rueful, charming, and bullying.

"Please," says Frederica. "Please let me come to London with you and see someone about some work. I could get some reading for publishers, I'm sure I could, and do almost all the work at home with Leo. Or I could go back to university and do a doctorate—I could work on that partly at home—and then, when Leo grows up, I could be ready, I could do something."

"You could see your friends. All your friends are men. I noticed. I can't take you this time, I'm going straight on to Tunis, I have to see my uncle, it isn't possible."

The little smouldering places are flaming here and there, like gas jets. Frederica takes fire.

"Then I shall just go. I shall just get up and go, myself, by myself. You don't care about me, you only care about your house and yourself—"

"And Leo."

"And *yourself.* You can't see *me,* you've no idea who I am, I am someone, I *was* someone. I am someone, someone nobody ever sees any more—"

She is less sure of this, that she is someone, than she passionately sounds. No one in Bran House sees what she thinks of as Frederica, not Pippy, not Olive, not Rosalind, not Leo, not even Nigel.

"Cambridge spoils girls," says Nigel, to provoke. "It's a sort of hothouse. It gives them ideas."

"I want to go back there," says Frederica.

"No, you don't," says Nigel. "You're too old."

Frederica goes to the door. She has some vague idea of throwing clothes into a suitcase and beginning to walk away down the road, in the night. She does not know where a suitcase is, and she is aware that such a plan is absurd. She feels that someone as clever as she is *must* be able to think of a way out of a situation—not a situation, a *life*—she should never have got into. Her nerve-endings hurt, in her hands, in her teeth, in her spine. Nigel stands between her and the door. He says in a small voice, a small, sad, honey voice, "I'm sorry, Frederica. I love you. I only get angry because I love you. You are here because I do love you, Frederica."

He has learned what a surprising number of men never learn, the strategic importance of those words. He is not a verbal animal. Much of what he says, Frederica has noticed without yet thinking about it, is dictated by the glaze of language that slides over and obscures the surface of the world he moves in, a language that is quite sure what certain things are, a man, a woman, a girl, a mother, a duty. Language in this world is for keeping things safe in their places. You must be brave, this kind of language says, and ordinary panic-struck human beings hear the imperative and perform extraordinary feats of tearless, uncomplaining stolidity. You might think that those who handle this solid currency with its few words would be able to add those other simple ringing ones, "I love you, I love you." They have clear meanings in this world, and women everywhere wait for them as dogs wait for titbits and sustenance, panting and slavering. And yet these words are withheld, for the most part, whether because their utterance renders the speaker vulnerable to rejection, or whether emotion embarrasses, is not usually clear. It is not a question of class. Working men and businessmen and owners of country houses do not say, "I love you," and women in council flats and women in town houses say constantly, "He never says he loves me."

Nigel Reiver has never put this generalisation to himself as a proposition. But if he does not think about language, he does think, and has thought, about women, and has discovered the force of these words as troublers of wrath, promoters of indecision, softeners of eyeballs and mucous membranes. If you say "I love you" to a woman, it makes her wet, his body knows. He stands between fierce Frederica and the door and watches her mouth soften slightly, watches the blood in her neck, watches her fists unclench a very little.

He concentrates on her. He wants her. He wishes to keep her. He chose her for the mother of his child. At this moment she is all he can see, all his senses are alert for her next movement, of repulsion, of uncertainty, of reconciliation. He watches as a cat might watch a frozen rabbit that cannot now jump this way or that; will it gain strength, will it look away, will it bow its head with beating heart? He loves her, that is what love is. He moves nearer, he puts his hand and his weight on the door, so that she cannot pull it open, so that her body is between his body and the hard wood. He knows without needing to think that if she smells his skin, if she touches his greed for her, she can move two ways, she can scratch with hatred, with the will to break free, she can want him to touch her, as she has before, she can do both together, scratch and want, want and scratch. When his body is in range he changes the verb.

"I want you, Frederica."

He names her so that she knows what he wants is *her,* is Frederica, not a woman, not Woman, not mindless relief, but Frederica. This is the language of courtly love, by instinct.

Her face is hot with rage, her blood is fizzing in her nostrils and ears. She moves her head this way and that to avoid his kiss, like the ritual dancing movements of gulls and grebes. He moves his head in rhythm with hers, he kisses her neck, her ear, with closed lips. She thinks, I am desperate, she feels desire, she is angry that she feels desire, she suppresses it, it recurs, it is like being electrocuted in parts and in small bursts, it is painful.

"I want you, I love you. I want you" go the small words. She is ready to sink to the floor, she cannot run away and will not respond. So he takes hold of her and takes her upstairs. Propels, lifts, supports, embraces, the verbs could go on for longer than the journey takes. From the swinging door to the kitchen quarters Pippy Mammott watches them go, and then removes the plates. She has seen this before. Frederica looks drunk, Pippy thinks, perhaps she is, Pippy thinks, she would like to think Frederica is drunk. Frederica has got a grip on Nigel, Pippy thinks, contrary to the evidence of her eyes.

Afterwards, he lies with his eyes shut, one heavy arm gently holding her to him. Frederica's body is warm and happy. The skin of her belly is glowing red with use and relaxation and happiness. Inside, also, she can hear her blood coursing, she thinks of it as "hearing" though this word is inaccurate, it is not to do with her ears. She wonders lazily why she thinks of it as "hearing" and decides that it is to do with the thrumming of one's own blood one hears in a shell and calls the sound of the sea. Frederica thinks in words, not exactly during lovemaking, or fucking, or whatever word custom and nicety choose for that activity, but before and after. She thinks now, looking at Nigel's damp heavy eyelids, at the droop of his mouth as though it had slackened after pain, that she loves him because he takes her beyond words, effortlessly and with skill. She thinks of Blake, the lineaments of gratified desire, and moves her sharp nose along his shoulder, sniffing his sweat, which belongs to her, which she knows, which she *knows* with her body. She thinks of the elaborate conceit of Donne, the pure and eloquent blood that spoke in the cheeks of the dead woman. Frederica's busy mind, in her skull under her skin and the tangled red hair on the moist pillow, casts about for the accurate quotation.

Her pure and eloquent blood
Spoke in her cheekes, and so distinctly wrought,
That one might almost say, her body thought.

"Her body thought," thinks Frederica. "Eloquent blood." Nigel wouldn't understand a word of all that, if she were suddenly to start talking in the night about lineaments of gratified desire and eloquent blood. It is only that his body thinks. She chose him for that, she thinks, and everything else goes with it. It ought to be possible to connect, she thinks, it ought, only connect, she thinks, and has an image of herself like a mermaid combing not only her hair but the fibres of her brain into harmony and alignment with damp, rosy fingers. Nigel utters words of his secret, sleepy speech. "Mn," he says, "hmn? a-hmn," and other such syllables. She breathes in his scent, their two breaths mix on the pillow, he answers tentatively "hmn, hmn," and their feet and hands communicate.

Mary's bed is curtained off at the end of the long ward. It is evening, and quiet, apart from the steady whimpering of one small child, his face muffled in his pillow. Mary lies on her back, quite still, her white face lit by a green-shaded lamp clipped to the metal bars of her bedhead. Daniel sits beside her, still hot and sweating, too heavy for the spindly visitor's chair. He has been there an hour, but his heart is still hammering, his collar is tight. Winifred, the grandmother, sits on the other side of the bed, peacefully knitting. She knows how to keep still, as her daughter did too, Daniel remembers, wanting not to remember. Mary's eyes are closed. Her breaths are regular and shallow. There is a neat narrow bandage round her brow, like a Greek princess's fillet. Her skin is white and cool, and spattered with freckles like brown seeds. Her hair is silky above the bandage, red-gold, gold-red. Her mouth is slightly open: he can see her teeth, baby-teeth and half-grown woman's teeth, together.

She does not move. Daniel sweats. Winifred knits. She breathes. Daniel shifts on his small seat, touches her cheek with a finger, draws back. Winifred says, "She has not changed since I got here. So still."

"They said the doctor would come."

"I suppose he will. He's bound to. We just have to wait."

Her knitting needles move steadily. Daniel resumes his study of his daughter's face.

After some time Ruth comes in, bends over the still face, and flicks up the eyelids with practised fingers, one, two, and looks into the unseeing eyes. "Good," she says professionally. She lays a palm on Mary's brow and says again, "Good." She is grave and beautiful in a grape-purple uniform, belted with a wide black elastic belt, under a white apron, with a pocket full of scissors and other implements. Her long pale plait is doubled up under her cap, which has a starched crown and a frilled fantail, like a dove displaying. She puts her cool little hand over Daniel's heavy ones and he is quite sure that outside the hospital she would never have touched him, but this is her place. She asks if he would like tea, and he says no, and asks when the doctor will come. "Soon," says Ruth, "soon, there have been other emergencies, he is on his way." She slips away, on black, rubber-soled feet. Daniel says to Winifred, "Marcus was taken with her, at one point."

"He still sees her, I think," says Winifred. "He's not given to discussing his life with us. As you know."

Daniel thinks about Ruth, and about Marcus. None of his thoughts are fit to tell Winifred, so he lapses into silence.

When the doctor comes, he is already on one foot, ready to go again, as doctors always are. Daniel knows doctors. He has been a hospital chaplain. Indeed, he has been a hospital chaplain in this hospital, in this ward, and knows why doctors do not meet the eyes of those to whom he now belongs, the anxious, the waiting, the helpless. Those *human gestures* were his own job, then. The doctor says to Daniel and to Winifred that the X-rays have shown no obvious damage—no fracture—and the child's condition seems stable, so that all that can be done is to watch and wait. She must be monitored for possible effects of internal bleeding. Time is most likely to heal. He is very young, and very pink, the doctor. He holds up the X-ray photographs of Mary's head, directing the light through them, and suddenly Daniel sees his child under the shadowy, cavernous image of her own skull, the nasal pits, the hollow eye-sockets, what appear to be superimposed layers of teeth and are suddenly seen to be the adult molars, buried in the jawbone, surging up under the rootless infant crowns. All in order, says the doctor, folding these images briskly away again.

Later still, it is the end of visiting hours, and Mary still has not moved. Ruth reappears and says that they ought to leave, now.

Winifred says she doesn't like to think of Mary being alone—waking alone, is how she puts it. She is folding her knitting as she speaks. Daniel says he will stay with his daughter.

"We'll look after her," says Ruth. "She'll be all right. We can get you in a moment, if—"

"I can sit here," says Daniel, "and upset nobody. I know, I've sat here in the past, from time to time, I know how to keep out of the way."

Winifred says, "Don't you want to see Will? He's with his grandfather—I expect he knows by now you are here—"

"Tomorrow," says Daniel. "Tomorrow, I'll see Will. Now, I'm staying here. In case she wakes."

He knows, and Winifred knows, that if Mary wakes, it will be Winifred she will look for. It is Winifred's *right* to be there when she wakes, he knows, he knows Winifred knows. But he repeats, "I want to stay. I know it can be managed, I remember. I want to stay with her."

"Of course," says Winifred. "When you've come so far. You can see Will tomorrow."

He listens vaguely for sharpness or irony and detects none: he is too taken up with his daughter. It is also true that he has come to love Winifred and knows that Winifred feels something like love for him. His own mother died not long after his wife, angry and rambling in a geriatric ward, and had never, that he could remember, felt out his feelings as Winifred is doing now. If she is being sharp and ironic, she is within her rights. He stands up—the shape of the seat is impressed into his buttocks—and shambles forward and hugs his mother-in-law. She is thinner and smaller than he remembered. He says, "Thank you. I do know, you—I do know *you*—I owe you, Winifred."

"You watch her," says Winifred. She cannot bring herself to say meaninglessly, She'll be all right, in case she is not, and so casts around for words. "I'll go and see to Bill and Will and come back tomorrow. You know you can ring us up any time, if—"

"Aye," says Daniel.

Ruth says, "There's a kind of folding bed you can put down by her. Try and get some sleep. I'll be round every fifteen minutes to check her pupils. I'll keep an eye on both of you."

Night comes early in children's wards. Night comes early, but not complete darkness—angled lamps here and there illuminate tangled hair, spread-eagled monkey-forms attached to tubing and pulleys, a passionate toddler snuffling hotly into a pillow. Ruth produces a toothbrush and a towel from a cupboard, and Daniel tidies himself in a carbolic-drenched lavatory. He pads back through the ward to his daughter. The walls are painted with cheerful pictures, mostly of sheep. The artist seems to have found sheep either fascinating, or easy, or both. Little Bo-Peep, in her hooped skirt and with her crook, stands under a large tree and peers one way, whilst behind her quite a large flock of multi-coloured sheep scamper and bound over a green hummock in the opposite direction, into a blue sky. They are composed mostly of squarish masses of circular brush strokes, out of which poke black ears, black faces and thin, stick-like black legs. Some attempt, not very successful, has been made to foreshorten the fleeing ones. The blue sky is full of solid sheepish clouds. Bo-Peep is drawn from the back, her face hidden by a bonnet, which suggests a failure of confidence in the artist. On the wall facing her, Mary with her little lamb is proceeding along a fence towards a small-windowed hut labelled SCHOOL. Mary is dressed in a crimson jumper and a green skirt. She wears a school beret on fluffy (sheep-like) blond curls, and carries a square brown satchel which seems to weigh nothing. There is something not quite right about the lamb. Perhaps its legs are too short, perhaps its face is too big for its body, perhaps its fixed smile is too human. Mary's face, on the other hand, is round and empty, apart from smily lips and round pale blue eyes. Some sheep are looking over the fence and staring down on the trotting lamb. Black faces, white faces, horned, woolly.

Daniel sits beside his daughter. The night flows past. Ruth comes from time to time and turns back the eyelids, with their reddish lashes. "Good," she says, "good," and whisks away again.

Mary's mouth is a little open. Her teeth are wet. Daniel thinks of Stephanie's dead face, suddenly, with the full violence of the unprepared—the staring eyes, the raised lip, the wet teeth. He feels—it is no exaggeration—his heart willing itself to stop beating, juddering in his body like an engine in trouble. He feels waves of nausea. He waits for the image to fade as he might wait for the touch of hot metal to stop throbbing. He waits till it is gone, the face in the mind's eye, and then puts out a heavy finger and closes his daughter's lip over her teeth. Her lip is warm, warm and soft. He remembers the energy of the bursting teeth in her bony jaw. He touches her cheek, her little shoulder, he takes hold, in the dark, of her cool hand, he says, "Mary—," he says again, "Mary—"

Mary wanders in dark blue caverns. She does not walk, she weaves, or floats, or flies, between muscular fanning trunks of huge plants, or veined rocks. It is dark blue, and there is purple, and slate-grey, and there is a kind of dark light in and on it, given off by the pillars, the boughs themselves. She weaves her way and pain runs beside her like a shining wire, it traces her intricate path, but it does not exactly touch her—its light hurts her if she shifts her attention in its direction, its edge, its razor-blade edge, its needle-point, its flames about to break—but she dances with it slowly, she moves as it moves, it moves as she moves, they bow together, they curve and recurve, they keep a distance, in which there is nothing at all, no blue light, nothing, no visible dark, nothing.

Ruth returns every half-hour. "Good," she says, peering under the eyelids. "Good." Daniel sits stolidly, holding his daughter's hand. Ruth says, "Try and get a little sleep."

"I don't want sleep."

"You need it. I don't think she'll wake now. They don't wake—in the deep night—on the whole. You'll find she'll wake with the daylight. Shall I bring you a cup of Ovaltine?"

"I'll come and get it. Thank you. I need to stretch my legs. I'm all pins and needles, I'm numb."

Ruth makes him a cup of Ovaltine in a little kitchen, and they sit by the night nurses' desk, their faces in shadow, the desk lit by a pool of contained light from a green-shaded desk lamp.

"We can see her from here," says Ruth. "It's designed so we can see everyone from here."

Daniel asks Ruth how she is, what she has been doing. He expects some placid, nondescript answer as she sits there, sipping tea, her pale oval face turned down. She says, "If it were not for my spiritual life, this place—this work—would be quite unbearable."

He remembers he is a clergyman. This both makes it incumbent on him to answer this remark seriously and provides a way to answer it chattily, which is not the way it was said.

"I remember you were a very regular member of the Young Christians. Do you still go to St. Bartholomew's?"

"Sometimes I do. It is not the same, of course, since Gideon and Clemency went away. The new vicar is not a very spiritual man. He goes through the motions. I shouldn't say that. How can one know another person's soul? But—anyway—he doesn't speak to *me.* I suppose you are still in touch with Gideon, now, where you are. He is doing such wonderful work."

"I'm afraid I live an odd life, very shut away, I don't see old friends," says Daniel blandly, his professional voice coming back to him. What he feels for Gideon Farrar, his ex-vicar, is hatred and contempt, which he tries to mitigate with some kind of charitable mental effort, from time to time.

"I belong to Gideon's flock, so to speak," says Ruth. "I am a Child of Joy. I can't get to many of the main meetings in London, you know, and York, I work such terrible hours here. But he has his Family Gatherings up here on the moors too—the movement has taken on such wonderful life—miracles happen, everyone is—is full of awareness and life. I wish he came more often himself, but Clemency comes, and other family heads, we are all constantly in touch—it is a great joy."

"I am very glad," says Daniel cautiously.

"I went into this work," says Ruth, "because I wanted to do some good, to help little children, the innocent who suffer. No one tells children's nurses, when they go into training, you know, that this is the *worst* kind of nursing—the worst. You might be glad when the old—slip away—but these little ones—and those who stay here—a long time—are even worse than those who die. You can't talk about it, of course. I can, to you, because you understand how it is changed—it seems different—if the suffering can be offered to Jesus, can be part of His suffering for us—now and then I really *feel* that, though I don't *understand* it, of course—but then, we do not have to understand—"

Another voice, ecstatic, confident, is speaking inside her placid, stolid, small notes. Daniel says, "I was hospital chaplain here, you know. I've worked here. Not like you, but I have seen what you're telling me."

"You must have been so *needed,*" says Ruth. "So few understand or can hear—"

This is not how Daniel remembers it.

He goes back to his child, who has not moved. Ruth looks again into the unseeing eyes and repeats, "Good."

Mary wanders among gentian-dark currents, through the lips of caverns, down falls and along conduits. The inky world swells and sways. There is a far, faint booming in the silence. Someone somewhere feels nausea.

Daniel dozes uneasily on the truckle bed. He is below the level of Mary's sleeping form, lifted up above him. His springs creak and groan. She turns, she moves, she flings an arm wide, a small hand touches him. He calls Ruth, who says, "Good," and checks the pupils again. Dawn comes, and with the dawn the day shift, busy with trolleys, with sponges, with thermometers. Ruth brings Daniel a cup of tea, and tells him she has to go now, but will be there in the evening. Daniel gulps the hot tea and feels it spread in his belly. Mary's lips move.

"Look," he says to Ruth. "Look there—look at her lips."

Mary is somewhere in a chalky cavernous mouth. She is being sucked up, blown up, she wishes to float and settle, like sediment, but the medium in which she is suspended is in turmoil, she will be ejected. Her grape-dark world, her gentian caverns, are shot with angry orange, she sees blood, she sees hot veils, she twists her head this way and that as pain takes hold of it. She sees flat, orange. She opens her eyes.

"Mary," he says. "Mary. There you are—"

She struggles furiously to sit up. She puts hot arms round his neck, she buries her face in his beard, he puts his nose to her living skin, her hot hair, the pulse in her thin neck. All her arms and legs are in turmoil, she worms her way out of the sheets and propels her whole body against him, anyhow. Her arms close in a stranglehold round his neck.

"My daddy, my daddy," says Mary, and Daniel kisses her hair, and his eyes are hot.

"I'm sorry," says Mary, "I'm sick, I'm sorry," and Daniel holds a dish for her to vomit. It is all a miracle, her voice, her struggling quickness, the heaving of her small stomach, the sounds of her retching, it is life, she is alive. Daniel wipes her mouth with his own clean handkerchief, he smooths her hair on her brow. He thinks, There are people who would always have known—if they were me, now—that she was alive, that she would wake. But I belong always to those who know she could not have done. He avoids, this time, calling up the dead face.

Mary is better. The family are at breakfast. Daniel is still in Yorkshire. Canon Holly has told him he has bloody got to stay there for the present, now he is there. His telephone is manned by a new volunteer, a successful trainee, just the ticket. Mary is at home, but not at school. She is resting. She cannot remember anything at all about how she came to be lying there, in the playground. She has said once, she seemed to be in a huge space and something was coming down very fast out of the sky—a big *bird,* says Mary uncertainly, a shiny dark bird . . .

They are all at breakfast. Bill Potter, Winifred, Daniel, Mary, and Will. They are no longer in the graceless house in Masters' Row where Bill spent his working life, and Winifred brought up her children, and then her small grandchildren. Bill is now sixty-seven and has been retired for two years. For five years before his retirement Winifred dreaded it daily. He was a man whose work was his life. When he was presented with his leaving presents—a small carving done by an ex-pupil, in granite, a recalcitrant material, of a group of stony sheep, the complete Oxford Dictionary and a very large book token—the headmaster, Mr. Thone, had said that to many, Bill Potter *was* Blesford Ride School, and there had been groans, whistles, cheers, tears, and a violent fit of clapping. Winifred had had a vision of Bill torn out of Blesford Ride like a live tooth with bleeding roots. Also, she feared for herself. Bill was a man to whom it was possible to be married only if he was mostly not there. He expanded like volatile gas, he roared, he flamed, he hammered. She had her own quiet ways, which depended on his absence.

Bill had revealed in his speech of thanks that he did not intend to stay in Masters' Row. He had the right to do so, for three years at least, and the school had supposed that he would help out, as his predecessors had, would mark exams, coach university entrants, detach himself bit by bit. It was characteristic of Bill that he had said nothing of his plans to anyone before this speech: there were those in the audience who thought he had made up his mind then and there, in the Hall, listening to the valedictory cheering.

"I do not intend," said Bill, "to stick around, getting cross at the way things are done, or contemplating my own mistakes. I am going off in search of beauty. You can laugh. Blesford Ride is a decent enough place, and its gardeners do a decent job, but nobody could call it beautiful. The only God in the Pantheon who has got any good looks to mention is Balder, and he's dead and gone. I'm going to buy a house up on the moors—I've got my eye on one—and it will be a seemly house, and a well-proportioned house—with a garden, which

I shall cultivate when I'm not busy—but I shall be busy, I intend to be *very busy,* those who are not alive are dead, I've always said, and I'm not dying, by no means."

He was almost in tears, Winifred saw, and one more time she forgave him for excluding her, for rushing at things. He had not asked her if she wanted to move, but she did not want to stay, and perhaps he had known that without needing to ask. She thought the idea of a moorland cottage was folly, and said so. Everyone knew that it was not a good idea to isolate oneself suddenly on retirement, and there were Will and Mary, then eight and six, to consider, what about their schooling, had Bill *thought*?

Bill had thought, it turned out. He had found an eighteenth-century grey stone house, in Freyasgarth, a village in a fold of the moors between Pickering and Goathland. Behind the house, with its climbing roses, white and gold, the garden stretched to a dry-stone wall, behind which grazed sheep, on the moorside. In the village was a primary school run by a head teacher called Margaret Godden, who was, Bill explained to Winifred, a *real* teacher, he had sat in on her classes, the woman had the essence of the matter in her. Miss Godden was large and blond and fortyish and smiling. She had a passion for imparting knowledge, and a patient perfectionism. There were only two other teachers, Mr. Hebble, who took the middle class, and Miss Chick, who took Reception. Mr. Hebble lived in the village, was married, and had four children in the school himself. Miss Chick lived next-door to Miss Godden, and was Miss Godden's pupil and *semblable,* also running to fat, and also a perfectionist. Winifred liked both teachers, and was overcome by the yellow and white roses. The inside of the house was graceful and solid; the kitchen had an Aga and a stone larder, there was an outhouse with an ancient pump. Winifred had a vision of living—as Bill had so suddenly said—with beautiful things. With subtle colours, and changing lights, and old wood, and yellow and white roses. She and Bill took to travelling to country auctions, buying chairs, tables, chests, a dresser—it became a shared passion; they talked to each other as in some ways they had never done. Winifred said, "It is like that game you play with yourself, travelling on the top of buses, looking in at windows, thinking, Who would I be if I lived *there,* what sort of life would I have in that house—"

"That's how I found it," said Bill. "From a bus, coming back from an extra-mural class. You always get that feeling most in the early evening—about houses—when there's still light in the sky but there's light inside, too—"

For a year or two Winifred had a not unpleasant feeling, sitting by an open fire in the evening, polishing an oval table, watering window-boxes, looking down from a wide landing to a stone-flagged hall, its wide step worn by centuries of the dead, going in and out, busy with other lives, that she was a kind of ghost on a kind of stage set, making the appropriate movements for the beauty of the place. And then it became more part of herself—the place where Will's knee had bled on the stone, the curtains she had sewn sitting in that window and hung in this one, white sprigged with lavender and broom yellow, blowing in when she opened the window. Most surprisingly, Bill does not roar in this house, he does not crowd, he is neither bored nor sulky, he is, as he said he was to be, *busy.* He has expanded his extra-mural teaching. He makes long journeys up and down the Yorkshire coast, he has classes in Scarborough and Whitby, Calverley and Pickering, talking away about D. H. Lawrence and George Eliot as though their lives depended on it. He has developed an interest in the old itinerant Methodists, who came and spoke fire in these very houses. He is writing a book. It is called, at different times, *English and the Community of Culture; Culture in the Community and English; English, Culture, Community.* He is away quite enough for Winifred's peace of mind, and when he comes home, he talks to her about where he has been, what has been said. Miss Godden, Mr. and Mrs. Hebble, Miss Chick, come to dinner, and so do various members of the staff of the University of North Yorkshire, who have bought weekend houses in the hill villages, who tramp past in seasoned boots and woolly socks and admire the roses.

They have breakfast in the kitchen looking directly out over the garden to the moors. Bill sits at one end of the table and Winifred at the other. Daniel and Mary are side by side, their two heads bent over bowls of porridge with spirals of treacle, melting gold into mealy-grey. On the other side of the table sits Will, who is now ten, a stocky, dark boy with black eyes under thick black brows. It is absurdly clear who his father is, and it is equally clear that he is not looking at his father, he is not talking to his father. He is eating rather fast and noisily, toast and boiled eggs, ready for school. Bill has unwisely embarked on a discussion of Will's schooling. He could sit the Scholarship Entrance to Blesford Ride, where, as Bill's grandson, he would pay much reduced fees, or he could go on to the local state schools and continue to live in Blithe House. Bill says, "Perhaps you would like to visit the school, Daniel, while you're here."

"It depends on Will," says Daniel.

"I shouldn't think there's much point," says Will. "Anyway, I want to go to Overbrow Comprehensive. Everyone else is. My friends."

"There are things to be said for and against comprehensive schools," says Bill sententiously. "And things to be said for and against the old establishment. Boys do *learn* something in the old place, and that matters."

"So they do in the comprehensive."

"I don't say they don't. Perhaps you and your father should go and look at it, together."

"You're the school expert, Grandpa. You come."

"We should at least discuss whether you are entered for the exam, Will," says Bill. He says to Daniel, "He's very bright, Will is, you must talk to his head teacher, she thinks very highly of him, very."

"We can't discuss it now," says Will. "I've got to go to school."

Daniel, who is not stupid, can see his son deliberating over whether to forbid him to talk to the head teacher, and is glad when Will draws back from the blow. Will pushes his chair back with a scrape, puts on his anorak, gathers up his heavy bookbag. Winifred hands him an apple, a shortbread, a flask. He kisses her on the cheek, includes Bill and Mary in a "good-bye" and nods curtly to Daniel. "See you," he mutters, "later." Both knit their black brows, tense and puzzled. Will goes.

Daniel looks down and sees Mary's wrist, her little fist closed round her busy spoon. Every movement of every muscle pleases him. Mary says, "Will wants to go to Overbrow with Keith and Micky and that girl with the funny hair." She thinks a little, and adds inconsequentially, "You won't go just yet, will you, Daddy? You've only just come. *I* wouldn't mind if you came to the school, I wouldn't."

"I can stay a bit longer," he tells her.

"A bit," she says. "A bit longer."

Two people are coming over the brow of the moor and making their way by sheep tracks down to the back gate. Winifred gets up to make more coffee. "It is Marcus and Jacqueline," she tells Daniel. "They have been up doing something or other with Jacqueline's snails. She's finishing a Ph.D on those snails. They get up at four o'clock to go and count them, and so on."

"She comes and talks to our class about snails," says Mary. "We have a *colony* of those snails we look after for her, we do real experiments, we see what they eat and what colour the babies are. We have a big snail book, we measure them, we write it all down, it's useful."

"If you think snails are useful," says Bill, not unamiably.

The figures are so small, it is at first only just possible to make out which is which. Both are wearing anoraks and rubber boots; it is damp, good snail weather; both are thin, and walk springingly. Daniel does not want to see Marcus. Marcus is Stephanie's brother, and was in the room when the sparrow fled under the refrigerator and the refrigerator struck. Daniel has never asked whether, if Marcus had shown more presence of mind, he could have saved her. He is afraid of his own rage. Marcus was in his house, in a state of complicated nervous withdrawal, all that year, upsetting Stephanie, invading privacy, *brooding.* A creature so nervous and futile, Daniel supposed, would be cast again into the stupor from which he was vaguely emerging. Marcus was part of his memory of his own terrible return to that house, a stick-like creature with a face like bad cheese, waxy and sweating, standing close, close to the refrigerator plug in the wall and shaking. Marcus was not, he decided then, a *possible* concern for himself. He could not help Marcus, because he was who he was. Neither of them could hope or expect he could help Marcus. Let him suffer, he saw he had thought, and now here is this young man, with the young woman, striding down the moorside and, he can hear, laughing as he comes to the gate in the garden wall. How can he laugh, says the demon that squats in Daniel. It is 1964, Daniel replies scrupulously. She died in 1958. We are all alive. Marcus is a young man. He has a degree now, Daniel does not know exactly in what; Winifred has just told him that Marcus has a doctorate, he is now Dr. Potter, he does some teaching at the North Yorkshire University and has just joined an important research team. We are all alive, Daniel tells himself again, knowing that he himself is not. Not exactly, not all, not. Mary tugs at his sweater. "Come and see the snails, come on."

Marcus and Jacqueline take off their coats and are given hot coffee and toast and bacon and eggs. These things are delicious after the hunting in the damp and dark, the peaty breath of the moorland air, the cold, the sunrise, the movement, all of which were also delicious. Jacqueline is monitoring two colonies of *Helix hortensis* and two of *Helix nemoralis,* studying the genetic changes in the populations, which can be read in the varied bands on the creatures' shells. She has brought back some snails for the captive colonies and NYU, and Mary exclaims over these—"Look at their lovely horns, look at their little mouths, they have *thousands* of teeth, Daddy, did you know, Jacqueline told me . . ."

Jacqueline has become a handsome young woman, with dark brown hair, worn long to the shoulders, with its own wiry curl. She has an outdoor skin, sunbrowned and supple, and bright brown eyes. In the old days, she used to come to the Young Christians, with Ruth. Daniel wonders if she too is a member of Gideon Farrar's Children of Joy. He tells her that Ruth has looked after Mary really well, and she replies that she doesn't know how Ruth can do that job, day after day, it is so hard. Her face is naturally smiling, even as she says this. Marcus says, "Hello, Daniel," and sits down to his breakfast. He says, "Hello, Mary, how is the head?" Mary says, "I still don't remember how I got hit, it's really funny not to know something—so important to *me—me* not to know." Marcus, who is now working on the neuroscience of the brain, and on memory particularly, agrees that it is interesting. "It might come back," he says. "You might remember without knowing you remember. And then one day, it will suddenly come clear, you will know."

Marcus does not want to see Daniel. Partly for Daniel's reasons. As Daniel remembers Marcus by the electric plug, Marcus remembers Daniel's face, Daniel coming in through the door, Daniel seeing *that.* Like Daniel, he supposed he himself could not survive the shock. That he did, he thinks, when he thinks of it, he owes to the care given to him by Jacqueline and Ruth. Ruth held his body, and waited until he could cry, and wiped his tears. Jacqueline, robustly, ruthlessly, required him to be interested in things not himself. She dragged him to lectures, which after a time he heard; she bombarded him with her own problems, which his curiously apt mathematical mind solved ingeniously without his emotions needing to uncoil from their shell; she made him go on field studies trips when he could hardly drag one foot after the other; she involved him in her own passion for what was beginning to be generally known as ecological studies. When in spite of his pain he found he was interested, Jacqueline made him know he was interested, made him see he was alive. He sat with her once in a cave in a storm up on Saddle Moor: it was a cave with stony walls and a roof of dark earth, through which poked wiry roots of things clinging to the surface somewhere above. They made their way through air and nosed back into earth. They hung and twisted, out of their elements. As the storm raged, water began to soak through into the cave, streaking the earth with dark rivulets, shining in sudden drops and splinter-shapes on the rock face, dripping down the blind roots. He often dreamed of those dark patches, those few bright drops. That was how it was. It was Jacqueline's tough exactitude that make him recognise that that was how it was, that the water was making its way in.

Marcus knows he is guilty of Stephanie's death. He does not know what to do with this knowledge. He knows that the one person—apart from the dead—whom he has mortally hurt is Daniel, though he knows also that irremediable harm has been done to Will and Mary, and, beyond them, to Bill and Winifred. He does not think of Frederica as someone wounded by what happened. He knows that for him to sink into grief and guilt will do no good, so he does not, but this does not help. He thinks Daniel should not have rushed abruptly off to London, and thinks he should not blame Daniel for things, but think of his own blame. At the same time, he does his work well, very well, and is interested in his colleagues. He lives, and somewhere else he stays, as Daniel does, but differently, in that terrible place with that terrible knowledge.

Bill opens his letters, which have just arrived. One, in a brown envelope, he leaves till last, and then laughs when he reads it. It is palely typed, on official writing paper. Bill says, "This is from Alexander Wedderburn. They have put him on a government committee to study the teaching of English. It is to be called the Steerforth Committee, after its chairman, who is Philip Steerforth, you know, the anthropologist; they wouldn't put an *English* specialist in charge of an English enquiry, not bloody likely. Our grammatical Vice-Chancellor is on the list, old Wijnnobel, I see, but not chairing it. Alexander was never more than a hit-and-miss teacher—well, he says as much here—he wants me to submit evidence to the committee because, he is kind enough to say, I am the best teacher he knows. He says he will be visiting schools and hopes to come by; he says he can pick the parts of the country he visits, and hopes to spend some time up here. I shall write to him about the wonders of Miss Godden's Top Class writing projects. I may well write some evidence for him. It won't do any good—I've never known one of these things *do any good*—but some good ideas, some sound principles, lying about in the Education Ministry, who knows?"

Daniel says he has seen Alexander, and Jacqueline asks if Alexander is writing any more plays. Nobody knows. Daniel asks Jacqueline about Christopher Cobb, the naturalist who runs the field station, and Jacqueline says he is away, at a pesticide conference in Leeds. Bill remarks that Cobb has become very vociferous about crop-spraying and seed-dressings, and Jacqueline says he has had to be, nobody understands what is being done to the earth. Only Marcus knows—and Marcus only partly—what happened to Jacqueline in 1961 and 1962, when they both began their research careers at NYU, Jacqueline working with a Dane called Luk Lysgaard-Peacock on the population genetics of snails, and he himself, at that stage, working on the mathematics of a model of consciousness with the mathematician Jacob Scrope, under the direction of the micro-biologist Abraham Calder-Fluss. Nineteen sixty-two, Marcus's second postgraduate year, was the year of the Cuban missile crisis. Marcus's generation, including Marcus, are haunted by nuclear fear, a millenarian anxiety that the ultimate weapon will be—hurled, deployed, unleashed?—leaving a world of winter and emptiness and sickness, a world imaginatively constituted by film of Hiroshima and Nagasaki, whose emblem is the upsurge of the mushroom cloud over Bikini atoll. When Cuba came, Jacob Scrope packed his books and clothes ready to depart for Ireland, out of range of a possible London bomb, or bomb on the Fylingdales Early Warning System, with its white globes resting on the moors. Marcus was rattled by Scrope's assessment of the risks, but Jacqueline was solidly unmoved—"They cannot be such *fools,*" she said, "they are just male creatures puffing themselves up like gannets and geese, they will back down and look the other way, you'll see, *they've got to,* they're human." Her confidence came out of her own good sense, which had been Marcus's life-line, but he could not quite share it. In his experience, good sense was not so strong in human beings as people like Jacqueline supposed, as the society they lived in was built on supposing. In effect, like gannets or geese, Khrushchev and Kennedy deflated their swollen breasts and stepped aside. In the interim, Jacqueline had begun to notice that thrush-anvils where she and Christopher Cobb had counted shells were deserted, that eggs were not hatching in nest-boxes, that dead owls were appearing in barns and farmyards. In the spring of 1961, tens of thousands of birds were found dead in the British countryside. Cobb's activities began to include the delivery of boxes of tiny corpses to the laboratories of NYU for analysis, where they were found to contain mercury, benzene hexachloride, and other poisons. In 1963 Rachel Carson's *Silent Spring* was published in England, and Jacqueline gave a copy to Marcus. On the royal estate in Sandringham, Jacqueline told him, the dead birds included: pheasants, red-legged partridges, wood-pigeons and stock-doves, green-finches, chaffinches, blackbirds, song-thrushes, skylarks, moorhens, bramblings, tree sparrows, house-sparrows, jays, yellowhammers, hedge sparrows, carrion crows, hooded crows, goldfinches and sparrow hawks.

She said to Marcus, "We shall kill the planet. We are a species that *has gone wrong* somewhere. We shall kill everything."

"We've all been saying that about the Bomb. I think we probably shall kill everything."

"We shall kill everything because we're too intelligent, and not intelligent enough to control our own intelligence. Nobody *meant* to kill these birds—they were just trying to improve something else—the wheat, the potatoes, a lot of this is owing to *seed-dressings*—trying to make things grow. I think—I do think—we might learn not to be so aggressive, when it's not just another man or another *army* that's at stake. But I think we're just too *stupid* not to destroy the planet."

Marcus said, "Fallout changes genes. Chemical mutagens change genes. Something that has taken millions and millions of years to make forms that *work*—we can just destroy—or turn into monstrosities—in a twinkling."

Jacqueline said, "There's so little one person can do. Collect dead birds."

"Make sure the evidence is watertight. For politicians who are short-sighted and won't care."

They were young and healthy, they were full of the huge, energetic despair of the young and healthy confronted with rational fear. Their waking dreams were haunted by the idea of sumps, and desert wastes, and rotted tree trunks, and lifeless lakes where no birds sing. Every pleasurable walk on the moors, looking for snails, listening to larks climbing and plovers calling, was as surely accompanied by the vision of all this rotting and vanishing as their ancestors' ramblings might have been by the vision of hell-fire, red-hot pincers, and eternal thirst.

Daniel asks Bill, watching him tidy away his post, what news he has of Frederica.

"None," says her father. "She doesn't deign to communicate. If I didn't know her better I'd say she'd cast us off as vulgar relations, but

I do know her better—she was properly brought up, as far as *that* goes, she may be an intellectual snob but she's no social snob and *I absolutely refuse to believe* she married that man out of any desire to rise in the world of saddle-thumping bottoms and hunt balls. Now and then she sends a packet of snaps of the little boy. I notice she isn't on them. We've got lots of pictures of him *on his pony* and *boating on lakes*—"

"Nothing wrong with ponies—"

"You know very well what I mean, Daniel. Very well. She's bitten off more than she can chew. I can't say I liked him—that *Nigel*—when we did meet, and I can't say I'd choose to spend any more time in his company even if I was asked, which I won't be. No, no good will come of it. She's closed off from us, like Beauty and the Beast, like Gwendolen and Grandcourt, and one of these days she'll turn up with bag and baggage, I wouldn't be surprised. She's not a patient creature, our Frederica, she might have been knocked sideways, but she'll stand up again one of these days, and look around, and—"

"I don't see how you can state all that, Bill," says his wife. "You've no evidence for any of it. She may be very happy."

"Do you think so? Do you think so?"

"No. But I don't know. And there's the little boy."

"She's my daughter. I know her. Something got into her. Something was always getting into her. She needed someone like you, Daniel, someone like us."

Daniel says, "You wouldn't even come to my wedding, you monster. You made everyone's life a misery. You can't just say we're alike, now."

"Well, we are. That was a battle of like with like. This isn't. I should think the attraction of that *Nigel* was exactly that he wasn't like us, that he had nothing to do with us. Well, there are lots of people who have nothing to do with us who would make better husbands for Frederica is all I can say—"

"You don't *know,* Bill. You're just hurt," Winifred says.

"No, I'm not hurt. I've learned a few things. I've learned that if one of your daughters is dead, you just have to feel glad the other's *alive,* even if she won't come to see you, that's what. You get things in perspective. What's alive is alive, and kicking, I suppose. Frederica was always kicking. I've upset Daniel. I didn't mean to. I'll take myself off and write to Alexander. Daniel, you *know* how things are between us, don't pucker up."

"I know," says Daniel. "Give my best to Alexander. He's a good man."

Marcus says he must go, and Jacqueline goes with him. Daniel shakes Marcus's hand, which is no longer, he notices, limp like a dead fish. Marcus is a perfectly ordinary intellectual-looking thin young man, with longish pale brown hair, and glasses. Daniel asks Jacqueline if she still sees Gideon Farrar.

"No. I gave all that up. It suddenly seemed not to mean anything. I'm sorry."

"Don't say that. I never liked it, myself."

"It does Ruth good. And it does her *no good,* too, in some ways, I think."

"Indeed."

Mary goes to bed, for a regulation prescribed rest, and Daniel is left alone with Winifred, in the quiet kitchen of Bill's beautiful house. Winifred says, "Honestly, Bill is *too much.* He worries a lot about Frederica. He misses her—and then, with Stephanie gone—he feels it more, that she seems to have abandoned us. I hope you think it's funny that he's decided you're like him. I hope it doesn't seem a final insult."

"No, no. The fire's gone out in that chimney. We should shake hands. Anyway, it's half-time. It's our duty to acknowledge truths. Half-truths included."

"And Will will come round," says Winifred, who wants everything to be calm, to be good, to be well.

"Why should he? What I did to him—what I did—was wicked, was preposterous. Look at it coldly, look at it straight: a woman dies, a man is left with two kids, so he walks out one day and *just leaves them*—so they've lost two at a stroke—how can that be forgiven?"

"But you can't look at it coldly, Daniel—you have to see how it was *then*—you were half-mad, and were doing them no good—and you can't say we haven't looked after them well."

"I don't. You've done wonders. They are *safe* kids. They have a home. A family. I'm not a family. I know all that."

"And for Bill. It has been important to him to have Will—he *plays* with Will—he couldn't play with Marcus, you know—he was awful—these things can't be redeemed—but he has done well, and it makes him happy."

"I didn't abandon my kids to make Bill happy."

"I know that."

"Before I met her—Stephanie—I had this idea of my life. At the edge, just over the edge. Where people weren't managing. When we were married—I tried ordinary happiness—I were lucky, we were happy—some of the time—and both of us knew what a *chance* it was, what the odds were against it—and what we'd—abandoned for it—her work, her books, her friends—my—my need to live where it's dangerous. Yes, that's it. Where it's dangerous. And when she died—I were pushed back, into *that* world—as though I shouldn't have tried to hoist myself out of it into a sunny shelf, wi' her—but a life, wi'out her—I couldn't—I thought."

"Daniel. I know. Don't hurt yourself."

"There's more. *Then* I felt—I were dangerous to *them*—Will and Mary. That I could do them no good, that they'd got to be got away from what were happening to me—for their own good—I really thought that—"

"It may have been true."

"Yes, but now. But *now.* Now there's Marcus—looking like—like an ordinary being, *laughing* with that girl, Jacqueline—and here's me—with my son hating me—how can I tell you? The world's changed, and Will and Mary have changed—disaster is my job, Winifred, I know what—the living look like, as opposed to the walking dead. They're the living."

"And you're the walking dead."

"That's it. I'm not. Not exactly. Only some of the time. Only *really.* Hell. I can do what the living do, I can eat my breakfast, I can think how lovely Mary looks, eating hers, I can find Bill funny, going on about Frederica, I can *smile*—I've got out of that—that *clear black state*—you see the world through a veil of coal, you know—"

"I know."

"And now I don't. How can I go back to what I do in London and leave Mary, when she were so nearly dead, and I wasn't there? How can I let Will hate me so? I can tell you—it's still truer that I'm the walking dead than that I'm so to speak resurrected. I love the smell of your toast, but it's only because I remember it, not because I notice it. You know? I don't know if you know. I think almost all human beings walk about over the crust of some *pit* they know is yawning for them—almost everyone has things they'd rather not see in their mind's eye—*daren't* let their thoughts start up—I'm no different from anyone."

"You're different because you say it. Because you see it in other people. Because you look at it, and work with it, instead of sidling away or looking in another direction. Those people in London need someone. There aren't many around like you. You can't be all things to all men."

Every morning the company in La Tour Bruyarde were awoken by delightful sounds of pipes and cymbals and fresh young voices. The Lady Paeony had formed the children into an enthusiastic choir, who sang their *aubades* in corridors and courtyards. No one was irritated by these dulcet sounds, which were most carefully kept sweet and low, so that pillowed heads only turned and lifted to hear more clearly. The assembled company broke their fast together in the Great Hall, and were served with bread freshly baked in the great ovens of the castle, with honey, and currant jellies, and little dishes of clotted cream and jugs of foaming milk from the cows who grazed on the grassy slopes below the fortress. The Lady Roseace had discovered the cowsheds, where the heavy gentle beasts were milked, and the dairy, where their milk was churned and sieved and skimmed and whipped, quite by accident, as she daily discovered new regions of their sequestered realm. She had cried out with delight upon entering the dairy thus unawares, and indeed from a rather dank and mouldering passage, which she had believed to be a shortcut to the latrines. It was a place of order and beauty, cool and glimmering, with earthenware tiles on its floor, and many varieties of tiles on its walls and working surfaces, tiles darkly green and richest lapis-blue, tiles sprigged with forget-me-nots, and decorated with blue milkmaids on white glaze, with windmills and weathercocks and other innocent country creatures. A large young woman with round red forearms was patting butter, and another was pouring a great flood of sweet, warm, foaming milk into an earthenware pancheon. The Lady Roseace had wandered delightedly round this quiet place, touching cool surfaces, tasting cheeses with a pink finger, and had finally walked from the dairy down a flagged passage into a byre where a young man and a young woman were milking two creamy-golden cows, in that smell of straw and mild piss and animal heat which is unforgettable as rose gardens. She watched entranced as the ten fingers pressed and coaxed and squeezed and tickled and stripped, and the two large udders softly shuddered and contracted under the finger-tips, and the teats sprang and started, and the white liquid spurted and hissed into the pails. The young man's face was pressed into the hairy groin of the cow, and both were softly beaded with sweat.

The Lady Roseace thought no employment could be more delightful, and said as much to Culvert, when he came into her rosy boudoir that morning, as he always came, to discuss the day's doings. She asked him who the delicious people were who inhabited the dairy and the byre, and he replied that they were the dairymaids and the cowman, those who had always had charge of those places. Inspired by the idea of the skimmer, and the butter-pats, and perhaps also by the memory of the warm, fragrant flank of the cow, the Lady Roseace said that this was a trade she would like to learn, and that it was their intention, was it not, to abolish the status of servants and masters, so that ideally there should surely be no dairymaid and no cowman?

Indeed, that was so, replied Culvert, and no one was more conscious of the urgent need to proceed with that project than he himself. Indeed, since their arrival in the Tower, he had busied himself with the writing of a Memorandum which should form the basis for a discussion of the best way to set about the division of labour in the community and in the economic circumstances in which they found themselves. And he had found, he went on, abstractedly inserting his hand in its customary place between Roseace's full breasts, and playing elegantly with her right nipple, that the consideration of the division of labour had entailed the consideration of all sorts of diverse other things, such as the system of education that might prove most fruitful, and ideas about desirable modes of dress, and new forms of language. His brain was in a turmoil, protested Culvert, transferring his delicate fingering to the left nipple and leaving the right one straining upright. The Lady Roseace stared dreamily out of the window, and shuddered agreeably, and said again that she would like to work in the dairy, she was very attracted to the idea of the dairy. She said also, as she sank dreamily to her knees on the goatskin rugs, and felt Culvert parting her moist thighs with his hard hand, that perhaps he should discuss division of labour with the whole company before his complex Memorandum was entirely complete. Otherwise they might think, she said, her voice frilling and shivering with bliss as he opened her lower lips, that he believed himself to be the master and architect, and not only one of a free and equal society, as they had agreed, she said, getting out the word "agreed" before a long wordless moan of bliss overtook it.

. . .

Culvert addressed the assembled company in the place he called sometimes the Theatre of Tongues and sometimes, though less often, simply the Theatre of Speech. There were other theatres, as we shall see, the Theatre of Mime, for instance, the Theatre also of Cruelty, in other parts of the citadel. The Theatre of Tongues had once been a chapel, like some of the other theatres, the Theatre of Sacrifice, for instance, and there were of course also other chapels in the Tower, some of them disused, some of them no more than an anchorite's cell, some of them adapted to other purposes, garderobes maybe, or wine-stores, or places for the strict examination of souls and bodies. No count of the chapels had ever come up with exactly the same number as any other, and so it was also, with even more exorbitant margins of error, with the other rooms in that place.

The Theatre of Tongues was so called partly at least because in the gloom of its upper vaulting could still be seen an ancient frieze depicting tongues of flame, boiling upwards like pyres or faggots and descending also like crowns. The walls were crumbling and the fresco damaged. Some believed the tongues of flame to be part of a lively depiction of hell-fire, and their case was partly borne out by the presence of a soot-black demon over the south door, brandishing eight arms, each holding a wailing infant, with his mouth, full of gnashing white fangs, ready to ingest them. But others believed that the flames were the relics of a depiction of the Pentecostal descent of the Spirit, and explained the shadowy stick-like figures barely visible beneath the tongues as the Apostles waiting in the Upper Room. They too had visual proofs, of a kind, for there was a faded frieze of bishops' mitres that ran beneath all.

The Theatre of Tongues was still lit dimly by Gothic windows along its two flanking walls, but where the altar would have been a new stage had been constructed, with midnight-blue velvet curtains spangled with golden stars, and everything necessary to raise and lower stage-sets, plinths, thrones, plaster walls, and other such useful adjuncts. The seats in this building were carved, high-backed benches, pews you might have called them, if in a church, not a theatre. They were not uncomfortable but gave the company, perforce, the rigid attentive posture of a jury.

Culvert made an entry from the rear of the stage, looking modest and dynamic, as he knew well how to look. He was beautifully dressed in green breeches and white stockings, with a simple but intricately tied cravat, and his glistening hair tied back. He spoke fluently, with wit and passion, for an hour and a half at least, reading from time to time from his unfinished Memorandum when his ideas became too intricate.

The main matters he touched on are listed below, for the convenience of the present reader. The truly curious may find his theory of the human passions and velleities set out in exhaustive detail in Appendix A2 of the present work—though it must be stressed here that his ideas at the time of his appearance in the Theatre of Tongues were in a very early stage of their formulation, and had by no means even begun to resemble their final carbuncular multi-faceted brilliance or their intricately systematised web of correspondences and cross-referred psychopolitical acuities. Indeed at that time the genius of Culvert was only instinctively *reaching towards* his visionary understanding that a community of bodies and minds could be forged by the general will and the general confluence of desires into One Being acting simply for its own self-preservation and its own entire delectation. To this end he was to elaborate his understanding, his taxonomy, of the co-operal passions, great and small, of human creatures, of the ways to release their energies as flowers release sweet smells and puff out pollen, all natural as breathing and bleeding.

These are the substantive headings of Culvert's speech. Whilst he delivered it, the Lady Roseace, and not only she, took intense pleasure in observing the decision and flexibility of his upper lip, the energetic pulse in his white throat, the muscular swell of his buttocks in his shining breeches and, not least, as his rhetorical urgency increased, the harder and rounder pressure of his virile member in its satin casing. By the end of the speech the Lady Roseace was positively aching to touch and release him, and relieved herself in a wild frenzy of clapping.

1 The community must strive towards complete freedom for each and every member to live and express himself—or herself—to the utmost.

2 To this end all false distinctions of the corrupt world from which they had fled must be abolished. There must be no masters and no servants, no payment and no debt, but a common consent about the work to be done, the delights to be enjoyed, the just sharing of these, and the proper remuneration of all from the common fund of goods and talents. Professions must be abolished, along with privileges, all

must turn their hands to all that was possible, as their desires led them, for work desired to be done is work well done, and slave labour is always ill done.

3 "It will be found," Culvert said, "I believe, upon just reflection, that many of the evil distinctions and oppressions in our world come from institutions we have not dared to question. Most of us have already questioned and rejected the religions of our forefathers and compatriots, seeing to what evils they have led, but we have not sufficiently studied how those *unnatural* institutions—marriage, the family, the patriarchy, the pedagogic authoritarian relation between teacher and pupil—have also harmed our natural impulses and inclinations. I believe I may be able to demonstrate how much harm has been done to female affections, as well as to male vigour, by the institution of monogamy, as I believe I may be able to show that both rationally and emotionally a child may be stunted by being left only to the attentions of its progenitors, however amiable and well-meaning."

He discussed also:

4 How it might be possible to fit work to the natural inclinations of all—men, women, and children—as they varied from home to home and from age to age.

5 How a more beautiful and less restrictive form of dress might be devised, doing away with false modesty, which in the new order would be unnecessary, and with harmful bones and laces, unless there were those—as he believed there would be found to be—who took pleasure in the constraints of such things on the flesh.

6 How language might in the end need to be reforged and reinvented, for there were no words in the language for many of the pleasurable exercises and human relations he proposed, and such words as there were were pejorative and harsh, carrying with them associations from the old prohibitions and pruriences of priests, patriarchs, and pedagogues. "Language," cried Culvert, throwing open the damp cavern of his mouth, with its hot quivering tongue and gleaming teeth, "language is a bodily product, a product of our earliest intimacies and desires, from the babble of the infant at the breast to the impassioned discourse of the visionary who tries to speak what is yet unformulated and unshaped. We will remake language in our own images," cried Culvert, "with our own kissings and sippings will we

make new names for what we will do and be, for the relations between ourselves, and the relations between ourselves and the world."

7 He proposed also that the whole community should take part in various theatrical performances from time to time, and on a regular schedule to be mutually agreed. There should be dance, mime, music, debate, choral singing, gymnastic displays, tumbling, juggling—

"Sword swallowing and fire-breathing," interjected a voice from the hinder pews.

"Those too if there can be found amongst our number persons whose sensuality inclines towards the taste of cold steel, or the thrill of scorched gullets.

"There shall also be dramatic presentations, and not only of old plays about old things, the ambitions of kings and generals, the moanings of monogamous lovers, but of new plays about new social forms, new encounters, new desires, new resolutions of new conflicts. And after the plays there shall be debates concerning the meanings and the value and the excellence and demerits of the performances, and these debates shall be no less full of energy and passion than the plays themselves.

"Also I propose that we regularly meet for story-telling. There may be those among you who suppose story-telling to be primitive and childish, but I say that story-telling is the primal human converse, since we are the only animals who look before and after, referring to past events and wisdom, and envisaging the future in the light of these things. I propose that we tell each other, one by one, the true stories of our lives, and this with several ends in view, viz., the greater understanding and friendship this will bring about for each of the other, and equally the greater understanding these narratives will give of the true patterns of passions and desires that rule each of our lives. And when these passions and desires are in this way made manifest, the community will the more easily be able to see how these energies may be cunningly put to use for the common good and the common delight. And as the narrators become more skilled and trusting, and as the listeners become more subtle in questioning and probing, so shall the stories become more and more truthful, as hidden things, shameful secrets, desires suppressed with violence in the harsh old days, are brought out into a clear and reasonable, friendly, and accepting light and warmth. For it is also my belief that what is kept secret and separate festers in body and brain, to the detriment of the individual and the community.

Sunlight cures suppurating diseases of the skin, and friendly contemplation may cure many boils and carbuncles on the psyche.

"Later we may even wish to *enact* these stories together, to enact them even with beneficent and healing differences, restoring losses, fulfilling desperate needs, who knows? I should hope that the tale-telling may become the central, the sacramental activity, so to speak, of our union.

"But these are only thoughts, and only *my* thoughts. We must all think long and deeply as to how to proceed, and skilfully and quickly about the immediately pressing problems."

Not only the Lady Roseace, but all the assembled company, including the little children and infants who could not have understood a word, applauded vigorously after this speech. Various questions were raised, in a spirit of co-operation and enthusiasm. Turdus Cantor, for instance, asked whether the proposal for autobiographical narrations—which he believed might be both instructive and amusing—did not smack in some way of the confessional practices of the old Church, and might not be, as the confessional had been, manipulated by unscrupulous men to instil fear and obedience in the weak. To which Culvert replied that that might be so in a *secret* confessional, as the Church's was, but not in the frank and open and sympathetic group of loving supporters he envisaged.

The Lady Mavis, clutching her infant Florizel to her breast, asked how soon Culvert proposed to institute communal care of the young, and whether it would be done without further thought being given to providing for all the needs of the smallest members of the community, including mother's milk and the lalling of the maternal voice. For speaking of her own desires, she said, she felt a passionate need to feed and cradle and comfort her own infants, and so she was sure did every woman. To which Culvert replied that nothing would be done without full debate, and that her confessed proclivities seemed to suggest, *prima facie*, her suitability for employment in the nurseries, but that this too, would need looking into, considering also the passional needs of the infants themselves, and of other possible nurses and wetnurses.

As for Lady Mavis's naïve view that all women had a natural inclination to caring for infants, specifically their own infants, he had only to call on history to prove her wrong. He had only to refer to the habit of exposing unwanted infants, usually females, in jars outside the walls of civilised Athens, or the Chinese habit of regular infanticide of unwanted female young, whom they suffocated with affection, or punished too captiously.

A young woman called Dora, who was, or had until that moment been, a lady's maid—if indeed that moment was the moment of emancipation, or unshackling, or evolution desiderated by Culvert—this young woman asked, in a pretty and languid voice, which the Lady Roseace prevented herself from characterising as "insolent," whether her own natural passional need to live the life of a lady, and drink tea, and lie on a couch, and flirt with gentlemen, could now be put to good use, in the new order. Culvert answered this flippancy with a most beaming gravity, saying that he hoped that from now on, from time to time, to be regulated and ordered by the organism of the community, everyone who so desired might lie on a couch and sip tea, for these were not insignificant pleasures by any means. And that also flirting with gentlemen, fulfilling the desires of gentlemen, and indeed sharing mutual pleasures with them, would be part of the rights and duties of all women in the Tower. And that also productive work must be done, the community must be fed, agriculture, cooking and so on must happen, and those unable to carry out any duties in the fields or kitchens must find other ways of benefiting the common wealth. The questioner could hardly be employed as a whore in the new order, he supposed, for pleasuring should be by mutual consent and freely given—unless particular passions felt an irreducible need to be paid for their services—for he had noticed that to some, coins of the realm in the palm of the hand, or the stocking under the bed, were a greater delight than any number of ejaculations or embraces, and he was not yet firm in his own mind as to whether this proclivity would disappear in a harmonious world, or persist ineradicably. The young woman appeared to be taking some time to think out the implications of this last observation—her pretty brow was knit and her mouth pouted thoughtfully.

From the back of the theatre, in the shadows, the dark voice of Colonel Grim could be heard, breaking into the momentary silence.

"And who will be responsible for cleaning the latrines?"

A further silence ensued. Colonel Grim said, brisk and conversational, "I ask again, who will be responsible for cleaning the latrines? And I offer you the observation that many previous attempts to found ideal societies or just commonwealths have foundered on just this question, which is not trivial but, if you will forgive a little wordplay, of *fundamental* importance."

No one could think of an answer to this question, though Narcisse proposed that the task be shared by the whole community, by rota, everyone working with a partner for so many days of the month or year. He added, with a graceful smile, that he would be only too happy himself to purchase his release from this duty with anything it might be in his power to offer anyone, after the institution of the new order. Merkurius said that the best way would be to find someone whose natural passion was ingenious invention, and who, with a system of pulleys and funnels, runnels and pumps, might perhaps make the latrines self-sufficient, might construct a self-perpetuating, self-evacuating, self-purifying *system*. Turdus Cantor said that if they were to work on the assumption that everyone had a set of passional inclinations that contributed to the good of a society, perhaps they should ask if anyone here had a passional inclination to the clearing of excrement. He had seen Bedlam lunatics happily at play with the substance, but he thought there were not yet any Bedlam lunatics amongst them. Culvert said that the persons in question might only have been restrained in Bedlam because their natural desire to handle turds was disapproved by society, and that such persons might indeed be usefully employed in latrines in a reasonable community. Another silence ensued which was broken by Marius, a twelve-year-old boy, who remarked that cleaning latrines could be a form of punishing offenders here, as in schools and military camps he had seen. The Lady Paeony said she hoped that no form of punishment would be thought desirable in the new world they intended to build, and the discussion moved away from Colonel Grim's question to the question of the desirability, or otherwise, of punishments and sanctions, which took up several sage, delightful and exhausting hours.

After the debate, Turdus Cantor said to Grim: "No answer was found to your question."

"No. And things are thereby already worse, for those who *did* clean the latrines will hardly continue to do so."

"Some leaders would have set an example by setting themselves at the head of the first rotating cohort of shit-shifters."

"That is not his style. But I believe he will find a solution to the shit-shifting. I do not think shit-shifting will be his downfall."

"Yet finding volunteers will not be easy."

"All men can be coerced into voluntary acts against their instincts. You will see."

"You are not sanguine about our success, Grim, I think."

"I do not say that. I say, I am not a young man, and if there is success, it will be so much delayed that I shall not live to see it. Whereas if there is failure at the outset, I shall be here, to take a hand. I can be relied upon for some things."

That evening, Culvert in his chamber was visited by Damian, who was, or who had been, his valet. Damian knocked as usual, discreetly and respectfully, and Culvert as usual answered negligently, "Come," and lay back on his couch with his booted legs extended. It was, or had been, Damian's duty to draw off these boots, kneeling solicitously at Culvert's side, and to carry them away, pushing his long arms into their warm sheaths, fingering and massaging the supple leather on to the tall boot-trees, before returning to tuck his master's toes into their embroidered velvet slippers. Around this minor ritual, over the years, master and man had arranged many solicitous little games. Sometimes, for instance, Damian would brush his lips over every inch of the damp silk stockings, one after the other. Sometimes he would strip them off gently, and kiss Culvert's beautiful naked feet, inserting his tongue precisely between every pair of toes, whilst the master lay back on the cushions with all sorts of smiles, voluntary and involuntary, playing over his sensuous lips. Damian was a thickset man, shorter than Culvert, and in all probability a few years older. He had a cap of very straight black hair, cut like a pudding-basin helmet, large, sad, deep-set dark eyes, and a luxuriant but well-dressed moustache, whose fronds aroused particularly delightful sensations in Culvert's toes, and not only his toes. Sometimes his attentions were spread upwards to the knees and the thighs, and sometimes he would respectfully unlace the breeches and nose and caress with his tongue the magnificent rod which sprang to view. He had a straight Norman nose, this Damian, with which he produced very particular shivers and frissons in Culvert's groin, and in the soft pouch which contained his balls. These games were for the most part wordless, and Damian had a very nice understanding of how far he might go—in the direction, that is, of the upwards exploration of his master's body, of which the full lips were the most sacred, most infrequently conceded treasure, and in the direction of vigorous manipulation or even attack. For there were certain days when the little ritual ended with the master spread-eagled naked among the cushions, and the man throwing himself upon him, with sinewy force, opening his own clothing as he did so, so that here and there skin met skin. If Damian, in these games misjudged the pressure required, caused too much, or too little pain, the master would kick out with his considerable muscular power, and tumble the man to the ground. Once he had cracked Damian's collar-bone with one sharp, well-placed impact of the elegant white foot.

Tonight, Damian came into the room and stood loosely inside the door, all his muscles relaxed.

"Come, come," said Culvert, kindly enough.

"I do not know what I should do," said Damian.

Culvert lounged against his cushions. His face was particularly beautiful in the light of a candle in a golden-rose Venetian glass shade, which stood on a shelf above him. After a moment's thought he saw what Damian seemed to be thinking, and said lazily, "You must do what you want, now, of course. You must do what gives you pleasure."

He added, with a singularly sweet smile, swinging his foot from the edge of the couch, "Perhaps you should take my place here. When we have played that game, when you have taken the place of the master, and I have been your slave, that has made you happy, I think. I have given you satisfaction in that capacity, have I not? Perhaps tonight we should play that game?"

Damian stood in the shadow of the doorway, stolid and hunched.

"That game is over for ever. You must see that. We cannot play that game any more, monseigneur, or should I say 'my friend,' after what you said today in the Theatre of Tongues."

"But I said also, we must all do what gives us pleasure. We must find out the subtle secrets of what most pleases us, and perform the acts we desire to perform. What we have done together has pleased you, Damian, I think. Your sweat was the sweat of an excited man, and your sperm has spurted into these cushions in joy. There is no reason why this should cease. Come and lie down here, and I will take off your boots and your breeches, and lick your feet and blow into your maidenhair."

"You understand nothing, I see," said Damian steadily. "The pleasure I felt then was in the pleasure of my independent thoughts whilst my body, like my life, was at your command. My livelihood depended on being able to please you, in this as in other things, the preparation of cravats, the service of wine and sweetmeats, the ready presentation of whips and cigarillos. If I was able to discharge my seed on your body or your cushions, my lord, it was because inside my head I watched, like a voluptuous sultan, a scene in which you were bound, ankles to neck, with cords that cut your fine flesh, whilst black girls whipped you with bull pizzles. I could come at will at the imaginary sight of those imaginary runnels of blood, sir, my friend, and so I was able to fulfil my duty. Of which I am now absolved."

Culvert sat upright, and the shadows chased each other like clouds across his ivory brow.

"Perhaps," he said doubtfully, "that is how we should proceed. I cannot, I fear, provide black girls or bull pizzles, but cords there are in plenty, and perhaps you should bind and hurt me, and thus fulfil your desires."

"You still do not understand," said the other. "Those too were the desires of a servant, a bondsman, a *man* with a master. Those are the desires of a man whose desires are secret, not his own, at another's command. Now I am a free man, or so you seemed to say, and I must learn the desires of a free man. And what I desire is perhaps not to do with you at all, but to lie in the arms of the Lady Roseace, and hear her sweet voice call me my love, my heart's desire, my dear darling, and other such tendernesses of which I know nothing, and to feel her fair fingers touch me with fear, and gentleness, and tenderness. And perhaps that may never be, for I do not know that she could ever desire me, bound or free. Unreciprocated desires, my lord, my friend, may prove to be as troublesome as latrines in your new economy."

It was then that Culvert felt the first movement of the invention that was to bring so much pleasure and so much terror to La Tour Bruyarde. It came to him that these problems—the regrettable desuetude of his pleasant games with Damian, the problem of Damian's desire for the Lady Roseace, and whether she could return it, were susceptible to a solution involving Art, involving Narrative, involving Theatre, as he had dimly adumbrated it earlier in that long day. For if the members of the community no longer had fixed identities or functions, but were all in need of finding themselves in the new flux of their beings, then a way, the way, the best way, for this self-discovery might be enactment of what had been and what might be in the future, or in the imagination, before the company, for the benefit of all. And in the Theatre he and Damian could again be, box and cox, master and man, and in the Theatre Roseace could safely simulate or feel desire for Damian that might be unforthcoming or unapparent if the man presented himself, requiring it simply for his own good, at her chamber door.

But he was unready to propound this new scheme of the universal benefit, so instead he said to Damian, "I propose, then, since I feel myself in urgent need of release and relief, that we find some strictly equal and balanced way of pleasuring each other, so that we may both go our own ways and sleep soundly. I propose that we lie here, face to face, cock to cock, naked on this carpet and perform upon each other only those acts which are the mirror-image of what the other performs. A kiss for a kiss, a handle for a handle, and so to satisfaction, and this shall be a seal of the new equality and respect between us, whatever we may subsequently choose to do, or not to do. What do you say to this, my friend?"

"I say," said Damian, "that it is an elegant solution, and one I shall accept with the intention of taking direct and not mendacious pleasure in your embrace."

So they stripped, and lay down together, mouth to mouth, cock to cock, awkward as two virgin boys, and Damian kissed Culvert long and hard upon the forbidden lips, which at first flinched away, and then opened deliciously and returned the kiss with good measure. And so matters went on, a little awkwardly at first, but then with more heat and animation, spurred on in inventiveness by the artifice of every embrace being exactly reciprocated. The details I well leave you to imagine for yourselves, for I know your imaginations will prove more fertile of quick breaths and jissom than my pen and ink shadows of desire. But I can assure you that they came together to a most triumphant and arching climax, and cried out, both together, in honest delight in their shared exploit. And Culvert thought to himself the Commonwealth had commenced well and inventively, as he meant it to proceed.

III

Dear Frederica,

You said you would like a letter, so I am writing one. It was so strange, seeing you in that wood, like a creature from another time, or another world, and with your beautiful son. It was a great shock to me to see him, because I had not even known of his existence, and this made me realise how far apart we had grown, which I am sorry about. I doubt if you ever knew how much you meant to me, and it is only since I saw you that I have come to realise just how much I miss your uncompromising intelligence and the sense I always had that you knew why reading and writing *mattered* in the world. We all thought we knew that, then, but that was why it was such an unreal, such an isolated, Paradisal time—that we should all be there *to read poetry,* that that was what we were *for.* I suppose if we had stayed on, this might have been possible to perpetuate—as Raphael has done—but I would feel uneasy about that, even if I were academically good enough, which I am not. I don't feel that I would be quite *real* if I spent the rest of my life inside the walls of a College—like Tennyson's soul in the Tower in "The Palace of Art"—although I do see that there is a perfectly tenable intellectual position from which this view is absurd. Raphael's life is a good, rich, exacting, complicated life—and just as *real* as the lives and deaths of his family in Auschwitz, though I completely see how, for him, *that* reality drains life from his own. Anyway, I think I will tell you a little about the reality I have made for myself—and its elements of unreality—and hope you will reply.

The most important thing to me is still writing poetry. I say that first because often I don't do it for days and weeks together and I *do* spend long hours either teaching or reading for the Papagallo Press, which makes defining myself as a poet rather absurd, and sometimes depressing. Some of the time I tell everyone I meet "I am a poet" and the rest of the time I never mention it at all, I say, "I am a temporary teacher," or, "I have a part-time job in publishing." I've written one or two things I'm quite pleased with, but I know I don't have my own voice yet, and this worries me, since for a poet I'm no longer young, really. If I get up the courage, I'll send you the pomegranate poem I was working out in my head when we met, and you will think how strange it is that those images came out of your yew trees—tho' yewberries are not unlike miniature pomegranates—an image I couldn't fit in. All poems trail behind them images that are part of them but can't be fitted in. Everything connects to everything, despite you being so *furious* when I quoted "Only connect" about your present life.

Monday to Thursday lunchtime I do supply teaching. This varies enormously from school to school. Sometimes I have eager sixth-formers doing *The Winter's Tale* or *Hamlet* and sometimes I have kids of thirteen and fourteen who cannot keep still or quiet or speak in words of more than one syllable and who do from time to time *frighten* me. I have had a pair of scissors pushed into my ribs and spent a week or two with one eye closed up by a blow with the corner of the Bible. There is something peculiarly *horrible* about going back into the atmosphere of school, which I can't say I ever enjoyed or liked (an understatement) and despite the violence, the stupidity and the philistinism (all of wch. you might think of as "real"). School has its own closed, tower-of-ivory reality with its own rules and language quite as much as Cambridge colleges. I'm lucky I think because I didn't *expect* to find it rewarding or exciting—colleagues with high ideals about sharing D. H. Lawrence or Hardy with London teenagers inevitably come to grief—one colleague who spent hours of his own time compiling an anthology of writings about Fire for a group of teenage girls had his classroom set alight amongst witchy shrieks of glee. There is a lot of educational idealism around but I think *Lord of the Flies* got it triumphantly right, and find that most children think so too, in schools where I am allowed to teach it. I hope this doesn't mean I shall find my head on a sacrificial stake in the playground, on the analogy with my fiery colleague.

Every now and then I meet surprising children—there is a boy called Boris in my present comprehensive with a perfect *ear,* the poetic version of perfect pitch, who gives me great pleasure and *savours* Hamlet's throwaway rhythms—but I do not want to get attached to any of them, that would make me A Teacher, and I am not. I teach for the books I teach—what I have discovered in *Hamlet* over the last year in Stepney and Tooting Bec and Morden would stagger even you, Frederica. And if I am any good as a teacher it is because I care more about the books than about the kids and some of the kids respect that, and I have a knack of frightening them wch. I think you may be born with or not, so sometimes they listen. I think it's because they know I don't love them and don't care what they think of me. I thought I'd be a hopeless disciplinarian, but I'm not. I say, "Shut up," and sometimes *they do* and that gives me pleasure. Who would have thought it?

And then for a day and a half I work for Rupert Parrott. The Papagallo Press is an offshoot of Bowers and Eden, a kind of loss-making highbrow branch where Rupert does things he considers worthwhile—poetry, a few literary novels, even essays. He wants very much to start a monthly journal under the Papagallo imprint, and if he ever does there is a slim chance I may get to be the first editor. But old Gimson Bowers is not too keen, and he controls the lucrative bit of it, the textbooks and the religious books, these days. Bowers is making a lot of money out of a curious theological tome called *Within God Without God* which everyone seems to need. The Papagallo Press is in Elderflower Court, a Covent Garden cul-de-sac, and consists of two dingy offices up a rickety staircase and a basement full of packaging. I love it. I even love all the very bad poems that come in, and I have to send back, because it makes you see how much poetry matters, even to people with no ear, no vocabulary and no thoughts to put together. When the schoolkids say, "Wot's it *for,* then," I tell them about how people pick up the pen when their baby's born or their gran dies or they see a wind in a wood.

Perhaps I will try to describe Parrott. He's curly, and plump, and not very tall, and public school. Late 30s early 40s. He wears waistcoats, sometimes red or mustard-yellow wool, sometimes sort of brocaded. He has a sweet, pursed-up little mouth, and a slightly high-pitched voice, which makes everyone think he's more limited than he is, because he fits easily to a stereotype. But he's actually very bright, and can tell a hawk from a handsaw, and is doing good things. He likes my poetry, but he has reservations, which I accept and respect. I don't think you'll imagine him *right* from this description, but it'll do to start with—you must come and meet him.

I had better stop writing this long letter and go back to marking essays on *Goblin Market*. I have seen both Alan and Tony recently and told them I had seen you and they were delighted—they miss you, they say, and send their love, and hope, as I do, to see you soon. We were callow creatures then and you had so many of us half or altogether in love with you—but that was then—and now we are older and wiser, I suppose.

I think I will include my pomegranate poem, if I work up the courage. Perhaps I will dedicate it to you, if it finds a home. I wonder sometimes if it is still *possible* to write poems about Greek myths—are they not dead, should we not be thinking about quite other things now? But poems about the classrooms and bits of the quotidian seem just as conventional and just as dead-alive to my eye, to my mind, as Demeter and Persephone. Who have been

Powers, Frederica, for much longer than the 1944 Education Act, or Canon Holly and his Inside-Out God. I don't know what I'm saying. They don't *feel dead* though of course the poem—I see as I write—is about Death in that sense too. You will see it doesn't really have an end and that's because I still don't know why it got written—I'll let you know if I find out. Do write back now I've found you again.

Lots of love,
Hugh

Pomegranate

Puzzle-fruit, skinny globe, parchment-tough,
Packed with jelly-cubes stained with
Blood and brown water, containing
Soot-black spheres like fine shot
Containing orchards.

Sherbet in the dark and black-skinned boys
Bring moonsilver plates with melons
Like crimson moons in snakeskins.
Bring burst pomegranates and curled segments
Of orange light with teardrops of tissue
Fat with sweet juice. Bring silver pins
For the seeds, and silver spoons
For the sirops and goblets
For blood-black wine. They sing
Sweet and low in the dark, they sing
Of deserts in moonlight.

She sits in a silver chair
His velvet-dark pupils
Stare, take her in and in
Do not reflect her. Such dark eyes
Are not seen elsewhere. This dim light only
Shines mildly, shines soft black
Blue-white teeth smiling
Between soft black lips.
He is large, he is comely.
His gaze is fixed on her.

She sits in a silver chair.
Picks with pink fingers, listless.
For politesse eats a few seeds.
Pomegranate-taste is almost
No taste, and so surprising. She savours
The absence, she swallows
The dark little spheres in their jelly.
Her throat ripples. Her palate
Considers, remembers

The taste of earth and water, faintly sweet.

He smiles in his darkness.

In the air the old woman ramps.
She is angry, she is dry, there is no moisture in her.
Her breasts are leather, they are dry as her shoesoles.
She has whirlwind and salt in her skirts.
She tramps on, she peers in fissures where hair roots
Shrivel and fail to grip. Bony birds
Peep and cheep. Their eggs are husks
With no flesh in them, no coiled lizard
With damp down, no nubs
To spring into pinions. She stumps
Through dry fields, leaving cracked clay
And dust. She will make earth's surface dust
All dust. The old woman's anger
Is single and fearful. Dust blows
And drags in her skirts. She stirs it
With horrible pleasure, extracting
Damp from soil and bones and soft seeds

Pippy Mammott brings this letter to Frederica at breakfast in Bran House. They are all round the breakfast table, looking out over the lawn to the moat and the fields and the woods. Leo is eating a boiled egg with toast soldiers, Olive and Rosalind are eating bacon and egg and fresh mushrooms, which they are praising as they eat. Nigel is helping himself to more mushrooms from the hotplate on the sideboard when Pippy Mammott comes in with the post. She puts his letters by his plate, and gives two each to Rosalind and Olive and one to Frederica. Then she goes back to her porridge.

The letter is fat and Frederica does not at first recognise the handwriting; she only knows she knows it well. Then she sees what the letter is, and puts the folded poem beside her plate, and considers putting the whole letter away until later, to read in private. She looks up, and sees eyes on her, Pippy's eyes, Olive's eyes, so she unfolds the letter and starts to read, smiling to herself a little. Nigel, returning from the sideboard, sees this smile.

"You've got a long letter. Who's it from?"

"An old friend." She does not look up, she reads. Nigel opens his letters with an unused butter-knife, rip, slash, rip.

"A Cambridge friend?"

"Yes."

"A good friend, a particular friend?"

"Yes, yes. Let me read my letter, Nigel."

"It seems a particularly *juicy* letter. Tell us what you're grinning at."

"I'm not grinning. It's a description of teaching in London schools. Read your own letters, Nigel."

He gets up, and goes back to the sideboard. Olive says the mushrooms are moreish. Nigel ignores this diversionary move. He says, "Share it with us, the joke, Frederica."

"There isn't one. Let me finish my letter."

"It must be a love letter," says Nigel, silkily, standing behind her. "What's this you've put aside?"

"None of your business."

Nigel leans over and picks up the folded paper.

"A poem. Nothing to do with you."

"The young man who came to tea wrote poems," says Rosalind, mildly enough.

"The young man who came all the way from London to get lost in the Old Forest," says Nigel. "I wish I'd been here to meet him. I do really. What does he say now he's found you, Frederica?"

He leans forward, and snatches the letter. His movements are quick and clean; Frederica's grip is loosed and her letter lost before she can think. He gives a little jump like a fencer and is out of reach, with the table between them. He holds up the letter. He reads:

"Dear Frederica, You said you would like a letter so I am writing one. It was so strange, seeing you in that wood, like a creature from another time, or another world, and with your beautiful son."

He reads in a clipped, childish voice. He says, "Etcetera etcetera etcetera here it is. 'I doubt if you even knew how much you meant to me, and it is only since I saw you that I have come to realise just how much I miss your uncompromising intelligence blah blah blah.' "

Pippy Mammott says, "Don't be *naughty,* Nigel." There is no expectation in her voice of being heard, or heeded.

Frederica says, "Give me that letter."

Nigel goes on reading out sentences in a faintly silly voice. No one reacts, so after a time he gives up and finishes reading the letter to himself, frowning darkly. Then he opens the poem, and starts on that, with a new mocking edge:

"She sits in a silver chair
Picks with pink fingers, listless.
For politesse eats a few seeds."

Frederica, rage rising in her, nevertheless notices that, even in the mock-sobbing voice he has now resorted to, he has put the stresses where they should be.

"What kind of nonsense is this?" he asks, bold and confident. "Why can't it say what it's about?"

"It does."

He reads a few more lines, again getting the stresses automatically right, and then gives up.

"Give me back my letter and my poem."

He cannot quite think what to say next or do next, and looks darkly about, threatening and ruffled. He is quite possibly about to give the papers back to Frederica when she says unwisely, "Where I come from, it is quite unforgivable to take away people's private papers."

"You aren't where you come from. You're here. Here I don't like you getting letters from soppy poets, here it isn't done to keep up with old boyfriends once you're married with a child."

"Your beautiful son," says Leo, in a musing voice, reminding them of his presence.

"Little boys aren't beautiful, dear," says Pippy Mammott. "A better word is 'handsome' or 'good-looking.' "

Leo repeats mulishly, "Like a creature from another time or another world and with your beautiful son, that's what it said. Like elves perhaps I thought or hobbits I think he means, you see, we surprised him, he was nice, I liked him."

Frederica, who has been working up to a roar of rage as full throated as ever her father uttered, stares dumbly.

Leo says, "I don't like you reading in that silly voice I don't like it. I myself asked him to tea, I *liked* him, I told you."

"It's easy to see he twisted *you* around his little finger," says Nigel, less dangerous already.

"I don't know what that means," says Leo. He looks from one of his parents to the other, trying to think what next to say or to perform to avert disaster.

Nigel says, "Here. Take your letter, then. I hope you mean to write a poem back."

"I can't write poems."

Frederica folds the violated letter, and watches Nigel eat his mushrooms. He stares down at his plate, black, black eyes under long black lashes. Such dark eyes / Are not seen elsewhere. I hate you, Frederica's head says, I hate you, I hate you, I should never have come here, I cannot *live* here, I have been a fool, a fool, a fool. She holds tight to her letter under the table and chews a little bread, thoughtfully, and thinks of Hugh and Frederica-then, another person. Frederica-then could tell immediately whether a man was or was not attractive to her, whether or not she could bear him to touch her. It had nothing to do with loving the same poems, or finding it easy to tell someone a grief, a success, an idea. There were men she felt potentially *connected to,* and men she did not. She thought about this for a moment, without understanding it. She liked, indeed she loved, Hugh Pink, *much* more than Nigel, she told herself crossly and in panic. But Nigel's body stirred hers as he angrily dissected mushrooms, and Hugh, whom she had been so pleased to see, gave her the pleasure of an old well-loved book, lost and found again. Not this appalling sense of connection, of being-to-do-with-*her,* which endures. Nigel munches mushrooms.

Hugh Pink's letter has changed Frederica's marriage. She is accustomed to telling herself her marriage is unhappy, but she is also accustomed to blaming herself for this. She made a wrong decision, she did not take account of the circumstances, wise little remarks of this kind she makes constantly to herself, mixed with more shapeless moanings of boredom or frustration. She does not blame Nigel yet for her unhappiness, although she is constantly angry at his long absences, and at his failure to see what she needs, by which she means *work,* not too well defined, but *work*. She is ready to explain that she loved him because he was different, but that this has not transformed her. She is still Frederica. She is ready to explain this, but the conversation never happens, for Nigel is not a talking man. She tells herself that she should have known this. Poor Frederica is so desirous of being responsible for her own fate. Human beings invented Original Sin because the alternative hypothesis was worse. Better to be at the centre of a universe whose terrors are all a direct result of our own failings, than to be helpless victims of random and largely malevolent forces. This is bad because I didn't think hard enough, says Frederica to herself. She is distressed by Nigel's letter-snatching, both because it is his first real act of aggression against her—not listening is not always aggression—and because it makes him look ridiculous. She is upset by how silly he looked, reciting Hugh Pink's words in that childish, finicking voice. She needs to love and want him, even if she does not like his friends, his family, his life. She likes him to look secret and dangerous. Not silly.

Hugh Pink's letter brings about other changes. Just when Nigel is for once at home and watchful, Frederica receives a spate of letters from old friends. These are unsolicited—she has written to no one—but she fears that Nigel may imagine they are all responses to desperate, or affectionate, messages from her. He watches her read them. He snatches no more, but he asks who they are from. She tells him. All your friends are men, he observes again, truthfully. Once he says, "You wouldn't like it if all my friends were women." "I wouldn't mind," says Frederica staunchly, but her imagination works for a moment on his absences, and she sees that she would mind. "It's just a peculiarity of my education," she says, placating. Nigel does not answer.

One letter is from Alan Melville.

Dearest Frederica,

Hugh Pink says you would like to hear from us, and told us all where you were. We all drank your health in the Lamb and Flag, Tony and Hugh and I, and one or two others. Hugh says you are living in a Country House, with woods and fields. I cannot see you doing this, but should like to, as I'm sure you do it very spectacularly, as you did everything. Do you have a collection of paintings in your house? I am thinking of writing a book on early Venetian art, and there are some surprising faces and places from those perpetual golden worlds hidden away in the corridors and the grey northern light of the English

House. I don't earn a living by this kind of thing, yet, so I teach—not in a school, like Hugh, but in the Samuel Palmer School of Art, in Covent Garden. I teach Art History to painters and potters and industrial designers and weavers who think they don't want to know about Giotto or Titian in case I make little dents in their Originality—they are all Sons of God, of course, even the most slavishly derivative. You would like to see this place, it would interest you.

Hugh isn't very good at describing buildings and people. He *noticed* some yew trees, a staircase, a ha-ha and some teacups but gave me no real idea of your surroundings or of you. He did mention your very beautiful son. Why didn't you send a card with a stork, or a silver basket of dragées? I am good at Country House sort of people nowadays—shall I come and see you?

Another is from Alan's close friend Tony Watson. In the old days, when they were room-mates, Frederica used to call them the chameleon and the fake, for Alan, a child of the Glasgow slums, had a blond, agile, classless social charm, and Tony, the progressively educated son of a distinguished Marxist man of letters, had a whole repertoire of working-class tastes and mannerisms, and an assiduously cultivated accent, part-Birmingham, part-Cockney. Tony's letter is longer than Alan's, and more affectionate, although it is Alan to whom Frederica feels more attached. It is with Alan that she has best negotiated real friendship, she considers, without any danger of falling into sexual abjection, instability or bullying. She has wondered from time to time if he is queer.

Dear Frederica [says Tony],

I gather you are in need of amusement. There is plenty here, what with the Election hotting up, and lots of dancing—twist, shout, shake, everyone's got dislocated spines or ankles, it's an epidemic. I wrote a piece on the Mod Clubs for the *Statesman*—you wd. appreciate my Leavisite analysis of the Lyrics of the Who—as you would appreciate my Italian trousers—tho' come to think of it, you never had any musical sense, and then again maybe you are twisting away somewhere in some swish night club and don't need me to report on the latest sounds. I wish we hadn't lost touch.

Seriously, though, the Election's the thing. I'm working hard in Belsize Park, leaflets, doorsteps, the lot. The atmosphere is electric—in *places,* honesty leads me to add—there are whole reaches of the Labour Party quite as staid and stuffy as the Shire Tories you seem madly to have decided to settle amongst. I shall have to rely on you to be the *agente provocateuse* of a one-woman Revolution amongst the bulls and the milk churns and the saddle-soap and all the braying. Tread carefully, Watson, you idiot. I go up and down promising a New Morality and a New Technology and no more nasty scandals with call-girls, trousersdown ministers, no Masked Men in frilly aprons with horsewhips, but good honest Liverpudlian economists and clean men in white overalls making *useful classless things* to bring about equality quicker and quicker (the washing-up machine as an agent of revolution goes down a treat on the North London doorstep, esp. to the larger part of the workers, i.e. women, trapped in unpaid sloggery and dirty dishwater).

I've got quite a bit of political reporting into the papers—two pieces in the *Mirror,* three in the *Statesman,* one in the *Manchester Guardian.* Witty breakdowns of long dull speeches, résumés of election meetings in unvisited places, that kind of thing—I'm making a name for myself, I think—but the real place to be these days is Television, you know—this is the first Election where it will play a major part—poor Lord Home (well, Sir Alec, but it sticks in my throat or ballpoint) has a face like a skull and ill-fitting teeth and you can see these trivial matters nailing down the coffin-lid tighter and tighter on every doorstep, which of course delights me, but I don't like the mindless malice. They call him Skullface and say he glares at them—like the Evil Eye. The TV's a Magic Box, Frederica, and its power is only just beginning to stir. I must get into it, I must get on it. Words are wonderful but *passé—that's where the power is,* girl, and I'm going there. Your heavy friend from the Socialist Club, Owen Griffiths, has got in on the Labour Party Press Relations, and can be seen from time to time grinning obsequiously on the silver screen—do you watch the box, my dear, or are you above such vulgar amusements in your pre-industrial Retreat? I'll say for Griffiths he's understood the essential thing, which is that the box is *small*—he's teaching people with the instincts and training of rabble-rousers to be urbane, and intimate, and say things quickly and not repetitively—a lot of them find it *so hard*—no Great Rally rhetoric for yr. fly Welsh boyo—he gets to tell the big nobs where they go wrong and what they do best—he'll go far, I predict—but I'm not sure how serious his *principles* are—

Hugh says you've produced a sprog. Difficult to imagine, frankly, but I suppose you handle it with your usual mix of frowning determination and *nerve.* I meet all sorts of people these days. Old friends were made slower and deeper. We love you, Frederica, come and visit us, come and play, come and *work* for Victory if you're allowed. (I suspect you're not. Now then, Watson, watch it!)

Do you remember *Comus*? Do you remember the brilliant person who organised *all* your admirers to come and see you perform—always resourcefully—a débacle? Well, the same extraordinary skill has set in motion a kind of leaflet-dropping-campaign amongst the cows, to show you're appreciated. Chin up, and imagine a big, hot kiss from

Tony

My dear Frederica,

It is not often I write a letter, but I gather one is in order. So here speaks a voice from the past, and I very much hope from the future, to say, *very* discreetly now you are a married lady of substance, do you remember a motorbike, and a quite *bloody* hotel in Scarborough, and my willingness to help out with your more esoteric problems? And a beach in the Camargue, and the terrace at Long Royston, and the smiles of a summer night, and your clear young voice (well, *I* remember your voice, *you* can only hear from inside your head, it is the one voice you *will never hear,* I can tell you professionally). "I will be still as stone, I will not bleed." The *timbre* of that voice is gone, inevitably, along with the lights in the trees, and I very much fear the renaissance of the Verse Drama, and will not come back, which is sad.

What are you doing? I am still riding two horses—both aimed at the stars—it cannot go on, I tell myself, I shall tumble in all my pink frills into the sawdust in the ring, to change the metaphor—I work as hard as two men, and have two lives. I have my lab. at North Yorkshire, in the Evolution Tower, where we are doing some very interesting work on the construction of vision, the perception of shapes, visual memory from birth, and that sort of thing. I see yr. brother from time to time, who is involved both with the microbiologists and the new neuroscientists, whose work of course impinges on my own psychological experiments on *active* brains—they think very highly of Marcus, do Abraham Calder-Fluss and Jacob Scrope, you will be glad to hear. Our idealistic Vice-Chancellor still holds to his vision that all Knowledge is One, and we do talk to each other across institutional boundaries, more than in most places of research. So I tell them that my Other Life—my secret, shameful flirtation with the magic Box—is really One with my serious analysis of how the human brain constructs and recognises faces and boxes, and they more or less buy it, because I do good work, and have good assistants.

I have been making one or two rather elegant little Arts programmes about art and perception, recently. Do you ever watch? You can hardly begin to imagine what *will* be possible to the screen—to the Box—of art and thought in the next ten or twenty years. We have a cultural instrument in our hands wch. can—which will—transfigure the way we see the world, and so the way we live, for good or ill. Probably for ill—knowing the deep human need for inertia, for ease, for non-thought, but the moment I write that, I see that the opposite is also true—it is human to *need* complexity, difficulty, thought, and the Box provides it, in its way. This is a more serious conversation than we have ever had, do you realise—because I can't see you, I'm not distracted by your face and your presence, so I say what I think. Written culture, not Box Culture, sweet Frederica, soon to be relegated to museums and dusty bookshelves. I will tell you a secret—you can't think in language in the Box. It *has to be* thought with images, associations, quick flickerings of form. The public fear is that the Box will be used by powerful manipulators to control the Masses—like Huxley's Soma—but that's not what interests me. It *could* be done, but anyone ingenious enough to do it would get bored with wanting to—I mean the scientists, of course, not the politicians, who are simple souls. What interests me is that these new thought-forms will change the *molecules in our minds* and what they do and can or can't do—and Shakespeare, and Kant, and Goethe and even Wittgenstein will be just too creaky and hard to bother with—*for better for worse,* Frederica, I make no judgement.

I didn't mean to embark on all that. I meant to write a ponderously gallant letter to a vanished flame, and to say, come back to us, come and see us, come and *talk*. There's a pilot programme of a TV game guessing literary quotations being made—and as always, they're desperately short of any women who know any quotations—now you aren't a famous writer or anything but you *are* quick-witted and presentable and you know a hell of a lot of quotations—so if you find yourself in London for a bit—give me a ring, I know the producer.

I am told you have a son. What a responsibility. I'm not sure I shall ever be fit to undertake it.

Look after yourself. Write to me. Whilst language is still a valid means of communication.

My love and homage,
Wilkie

Dear Frederica,

I have only just learned that you have a son, so am writing belatedly to congratulate you, and hope you are happy—you vanished rather suddenly from our midst. I think of you often, and do hope you are happy.

As for me, I work in educational television, producing little scenes from various plays and analyses of them. It's not wholly satisfactory, because one never gets to grips with a complete play, and even as teaching it isn't satisfactory because I never see the children I am addressing, but it is a pleasant enough life, and my colleagues and the actors I meet are agreeable, and so it goes on. I am not writing at present, though I have one or two ideas, both for television plays and for the theatre.

The most interesting thing that has happened to me is an invitation to be part of a Government Enquiry into the teaching of Language. We have had our first Meeting—we are chaired by an anthropologist who seems reasonable enough so far, and are a mixed bag of well-meaning persons—teachers, linguists, writers, broadcasters, a forensic psychologist and a physicist. We have a heavy programme planned of visits to schools and colleges, and huge heaps of Evidence are already coming in to be studied with care. I have written to yr. father asking him to give his views. He is the best teacher I have ever worked with, or met, and his mixture of down-to-earth practicality and high ideals is what we need, I think. Professor Wijnnobel, the NYU Vice-Chancellor, is one of us, tho' he is not the Chairman—as he is a grammarian, it was felt he might be too *parti-pris* I suppose to weave conflicting views together.

It would make me happy to hear how you are, and your husband and son, of course, also. I think this letter may be rather stilted, but you will read it with yr. usual acumen.

All best wishes,

Alexander

Dear Frederica,

Forgive a word out of the blue, or black, after so long. I was recently in the north—you may have heard that Mary had an accident, quite a serious accident, but is now well and back at school and seemingly happy. Perhaps you didn't hear, as you seem to have lost touch, as I did. That is why I am writing to you. I have been talking to your father, and I think he would very much appreciate a word from you. That is clergyman-talk for he's hurt, he's upset, he wants to hear from you and is too proud to say so. I'm not good at writing letters, and certainly not to you, to whom writing is second nature. Your father did me the honour to tell me he thought we resembled each other (him and me)—there is only you in the world now who would see the full humour and irony of that, so I am telling you. I did *not* hit him with anything, but agreed with him with Christian mildness, for there's a bit of truth in it. But the one who is really like him is you, Frederica, and he knows that too, and is not getting any younger. Forgive me for saying so—put it down to professional habits of meddling for God's sake—but he has already lost one daughter. I don't know why I don't mention your mother—she's a more patient and secret soul—but it was him I talked to. Much to both our surprises.

You don't need my news. I am still working in the crypt. Holding people back from the edge—sounds melodramatic and often is—who might or might not be better if they just plunged over. It's a funny specialisation. It suits me, but I see people singing in the streets, and they look queer, which makes me realise I am.

Look after your beautiful son, Frederica. (I saw the pictures you sent them.) I didn't do well by my son, and I see already I shall regret it for the rest of my life. I expect we shall see each other again, and I hope I know you well enough to be right in thinking you'll forgive me for interfering—whether or not you do as I suggest. Clergyman-talk again. God bless you.

Love,
Daniel

Nigel watches Frederica open these letters, one after the other. As she reads them she looks up at him, and watches him watch her. She reads Alan's words, and Tony's, and Edmund Wilkie's, and Alexander's and Daniel's, with his still, dark silence charged with watchfulness at the other side of the table. There is autumn sunlight on the white tablecloth and the silver spoons, and the dark man watches intently. The letters bring with them vivid ghostly images of friends, Alan's quiet smile, Alexander's fading beauty, Tony's curly humour, the improbable conjunction of Daniel and her father. They remind her of herself as she was, argumentative, passionate, silly, clever. When she rereads them in private—which means her bathroom, which has a window scratched by trailing jasmine fronds and dotted with the advancing suckers of Virginia creeper—the life of the words, and the quick ghosts of the writers, bring with them the presence of the dark watcher. He is more real than they are. She knows his shoulder-blades and his belly, his throat and his dark cock. She thinks of his cock, reading Wilkie's letter, Alan's letter, Tony's letter, and she licks up tears. He is more real than they are, and she is less real than she was.

She does not know if she dare answer all these letters, and put all the answers in the Chinese bowl in the hall, from which the letters are taken. She writes answers, tears them up, and writes other answers, and tears them up. She is afraid. She arranges to go into Spessendborough on market day with Olive and Rosalind, and there she buys a heap of postcards, addresses them, and writes brief notes on all of them saying, "Wonderful to have your letter. Answer coming soon. F." She has no address for Daniel, but remembers the name of the church and addresses it to the crypt. Olive and Rosalind watch her post these pictures of hills and riverbanks, and summer fields. She fans out the postcards so they can see how little she has written. She does not know why she does this.

Nigel stays at Bran House for a long time. They have good days. They picnic in the hills with Leo, they show him the tracks of deer and badgers. They discuss Leo. Later, Frederica will not remember what they talked about. She remembers his hand on hers in bracken, and a kind of happiness, she remembers two lazy bodies stretched on rugs, and frantic secret mental activity in her own head. She puts off answering all the letters until he goes again, and he does not go.

The next letter he takes is an innocuous brown one, with a typed label, addressed to Mrs. Nigel Reiver. He reaches across as she is about to open it, and says, "Give me that." She gives it to him; he reads it, and hands it back; it is a routine invitation to a Commemoration Dinner at her old college in Cambridge. "Please indicate the names of any other Old Students you may wish to sit near."

"Why did you do that?" she asks him.

"I thought you might be planning something. I thought maybe you were going on with what you once said about going back to that place. I got it wrong." He does not add, I'm sorry, but it is grudgingly in the air.

"Perhaps I shall."

"I don't see how you could."

"I could if—if I really wanted to. I could go up and down. Some time there, some time here. With ingenuity. *You* come and go."

"That's one reason why you can't."

"You can't just *say* that. It isn't *fair.*"

"I don't see why. You made a commitment. You knew what you were doing."

"No one ever knows exactly what they are doing—"

"I thought you were so clever. You don't get married and just go on as though you hadn't."

"You don't change your nature overnight if you get married."

"Perhaps not. But you change, all the same. I don't want you to go off here or there as though Leo and I don't exist. You've no need."

"You *can't* think it's as simple as that."

"I don't see why not."

In the end he is summoned again. Uncle Hubert telephones from Tunis. Nigel prepares to set off for Amsterdam. Frederica finds herself, to her annoyance, hurt and upset that he is going. She does not really know if this is because she will miss him, or because she is angry that he has autonomy and she does not, or because he can leave her so cheerfully. Marriage has its emotions that are part of its elastic cage, that don't exactly belong to the individual people who happen to be *in* that marriage. She thinks, I won't ever be so silly as to get married again, and then thinks how silly that thought is. Since she is married.

She finds Nigel, in their bedroom, reading her letters. It is the day before he is to go. He is sitting on their bed, with Wilkie's letter in one hand, and Tony's in the other.

"I was just making sure," he says, with his gathered, energetic calm, "that you weren't up to anything."

Frederica stands still in the doorway.

"And am I?" she says, with the ridiculous heavy irony of such situations.

"I don't like your friends," he says. "I don't like these people."

"They weren't writing to *you,*" says Frederica, studying his face.

"You are just a bitch, really," he says, in the same collected voice. "Just a silly bitch."

Frederica once had her father's capacity for rage. She stands for another moment in the door, tingling with anger in fingers and guts, and then begins to roar. She advances on Nigel and retrieves her letters—Daniel's is a little torn. She says what is always said in these scenes, that she will not be treated like this, that she will not stay another moment, that she is going, *now.* She opens wardrobes and flings clothes on the carpet. She finds an old suitcase and begins to throw things into it, weeping and screaming. Her letters, a nightdress, a toothbrush, a bra, a sweater; she can hardly see for tears; the things that *must* come, books, letters, are too heavy, are too many, the idea of their *weight* provokes a fresh spout of tears. "I'm going, I'm going, I'm not staying another minute," she screams, throwing things, any things, some black silk panties Nigel bought her that she has never worn, higgledy-piggledy into the suitcase. The release of adrenaline is a relief and an excitement. Nigel comes up behind her and takes hold of the red hair in the nape of her neck, and gives it a sharp professional twist. The pain is excruciating. Frederica hears various bones in her neck crack and shift. She thinks, "He has killed her," stops to marvel at the pronoun, and sees that she is still alive, in possession of her senses, and in pain.

"Silly bitch," says Nigel again, and gives her some sort of blow—with a knee? with the other elbow?—in the small of the back, again causing major pain with minimal effort. Frederica has never been in a physical fight. Her siblings were both almost uncannily gentle; her father's rages led to devastated furniture and burned books, but not to hurt flesh. Her schooling was respectable and her tongue caustic; she was not the sort of child to be victimised. This is new. Nigel's arm is across her face. He is breathing heavily. She opens her mouth and inhales hot cloth. Her tongue touches fuzz. She twists her head and her nose slides past cotton of shirt-cuff, and then skin, skin intimately known, skin acrid with anger. She sinks her teeth into it as best she can. She tastes blood. She cannot turn off some mocking self-censor in her brain that despises her, Frederica, for having to do such vulgar things.

"Bitch," says Nigel again, crashing his free fist into her ribs. Frederica is winded. She moves her head again from side to side, moans in pain and disbelief, grips with her teeth and more or less *chews,* producing rather a lot of blood, filling her mouth. "Bitches bite," she thinks in a suffocated way, and finds half a moment to wonder about vampires, as the blood runs between her teeth. Then she falls forward, limp, completely inert, dead meat. The oldest trick in the book, the commentating brain thinks. It works. Nigel lets go, stands up to look at the body, and Frederica kicks nastily at his legs with her full force, catching him off balance. He falls, half on the bed, half on the floor, and Frederica, counting the cost to her battered spine, stumbles to her own feet, and flings herself past him into the bathroom, locking the door.

There is a little pile of poetry books by the lavatory. Frederica likes to sit in there and learn things by heart, keeping something essential alive. There is Yeats, there is Mallarmé, there is Raphael Faber, there is a Shakespeare. Frederica sits on the lavatory lid and opens the Shakespeare. She finds she cannot see the words at all—the air is *simmering* and her sight seems veiled with a lucid poppy-scarlet. She licks blood meditatively from her lips and her teeth—salt, metal, and something else, she thinks, the taste of *life* and salt and metal. She is shaking too much to get up and rinse her mouth. Her teeth hurt, too. They are loose in their sockets. She sits there in a studious position, holding the Shakespeare, and breathes bathroom-air—body-smells, watery-smells, ghosts of perfume, a remote tang of bleach. Blood.

There is a silence. Then there is a shuffling. Nigel is moving about in the bedroom. She waits. There is a sudden explosion of terrible sound: he is battering the bathroom door with something heavy and howling imprecations. The door is solid. The house is solid. It is a house which once did not have many bathrooms, but those that have been added have solid doors. Frederica sits inside, holding Shakespeare, and says nothing. She cannot think what to do. She is a creature to whom impotence and indecision are painful. After this has gone on some time Frederica thinks of the other inhabitants of the house and wonders what they will think, what, if anything, they will do. She thinks Olive and Rosalind and Pippy Mammott will put their heads under the bedclothes and shut their ears. She thinks of Leo, which she has been trying not to do. Will he hear, will he be afraid, who will he blame? Now she feels both guilt, for the first time, and real hatred of Nigel, for the first time.

The barrage stops as suddenly as it started. She waits for a questing "Frederica?" but there is nothing. The door is so thick she cannot hear exactly what is happening out there. Shufflings, draggings, a crash. Silence. Silence. She looks at Shakespeare, and finds she has got him open at *Much Ado about Nothing.*

Benedick: I do love nothing in the world so well as you. Is not that strange?

Beatrice: As strange as the thing I know not. It were as possible for me to say I love nothing so well as you, but believe me not, and yet I lie not.

Frederica, skinny and freckled at twelve, Frederica angular and noisy at seventeen, Frederica surrounded by young men in Cambridge at twenty, has always had in her mind, as the image of love, this contented prosaic recognition of inevitability. What is love, what is love, is it just a dangerous *idea*? There is a kind of twang, and the room goes dark. There is also no line of light under the bathroom door. It is black, black. She cannot see Shakespeare or her own feet. It is the country, there are no street lamps, the window is black, too. She hears her own hot breath, and a drip of water, somewhere. Outside the bathroom door a thick voice asks, with desperate satisfaction, "And *now* what will you do?"

She doesn't answer.

"You can't stay in there for hours and read *now,* can you? Come out."

She cannot answer. She draws her knees up to her chin, enfolding Shakespeare in her body.

"I can wait. I can sit here and wait," says the voice.

She tiptoes to the door, and says through the keyhole, "You'll frighten Leo."

"And whose fault is that, you bitch, *who* wishes he'd never been born?"

There is a renewed battery on the door. Frederica retreats again. Her eyes have got used to the dark. The window is a small, smoky square, midnight-blue-black. She can see the shadows of the jasmine fronds and the creeper leaves. She can see a star or two, bright pinholes behind the glass, stars without identity, isolated from the spread of the sky.

A long time passes in the dark. Frederica reflects on Daniel's letter, and his interesting revelation that Bill thinks that Bill and Daniel resemble each other. She recognises the situation she is in, because all her childhood was passed amongst howls of rage, amongst tempests of invective and maudlin reconciliation. She thinks that she married Nigel at least in part because his composed silence appeared to be the opposite of Bill's wrath, and here she is, now as then, locked in the bathroom, waiting for the storm to subside. Stephanie too married Bill's opposite against Bill's wishes. And it is true what Daniel says, he resembles Bill. Fate comes up and hits you behind the head, Frederica thinks ruefully, probing her sore neck, her lumbar ganglion. *Mutatis mutandis*—Bill talked a lot, and did not hurt. Nigel repeated one word over and over, and hurt a great deal. Leo is an articulate child; perhaps he will not need to hurt people. At the thought of Leo, she begins to snivel again. Her mind puts it to her in a small way. "She is snivelling." A good, almost onomatopoeic word. Tears run down her nose.

"Can I come in, Frederica? I won't hurt you, I'm sorry. I won't hurt you."

If this were Bill, this would be the turning point. Anyway, she is tired out, and fatalistic. She creeps in the gloom and turns the key and retreats again. He comes in very slowly, feeling his way blindly along the wall. He has wrapped one of her cotton petticoats round his damaged hand, his left hand. He puts his other hand on her breast, hot on hot, heavy on pricking.

"You *are* a bitch, though," he says, his voice thick with indescribable things, but no longer aggressive. "Aren't you? A real bitch, I should have known. Look what you've done to my hand."

"I can't see. You ought to put the lights back on, whether you took out the fuse or interfered with the mains. In case—anyone else—wakes."

She is whispering.

"Come with me, then. I don't want you to do anything silly."

"I'm not in a state to."

"Come with me."

He puts his hand round her wrist. They negotiate the dark house, sidling along walls, padding across landings, taking courage on known staircases. The fusebox is in a kind of safe in the scullery. Nigel lets go of Frederica in order to be able to reach the master switch, which he pulls down with a kind of iron groan or twang. A streak of light appears in the doorway from a light left on in a dim corridor. There is no sound in the house. Nigel pats Frederica's buttocks, a man encouraging a mare. "There," he says.

They make their way more quickly back to their bedroom, lit as it was before only by table lamps and reading lights. It is a horrid scene. The bed is full of emptied bottles of Frederica's lotions and powders—mostly presents, since Frederica's favourite perfume is still Johnson's Baby Powder. The floor is scattered with broken chair legs. The broken chairs lie around like dead animals, amputated limbs in the air. The mirror is monstrously cracked. The curtains are bloodstained, and so, spectacularly, are the sheets and the bedspread. Frederica thinks of Wilkie's letter, reminding her of her unforgettable defloration, and speaks quickly, in case Nigel too is remembering this.

"It looks like the scene of a murder."

"It does look pretty bad." He seems rather proud, as well as moderately abashed.

"I'm not sleeping in here. I'm going to find somewhere else to sleep. Do you think we ought to clear all this up?"

"No. Why? *They* can, they're paid to clear up. Let's go somewhere else then. We could sleep in your old bed, where you used to stay. Where I came creeping in the night."

Frederica thinks of saying she wants to sleep alone. But she is tired and desperate for sleep, and afraid, more than she cares to admit to herself, so afraid that she is prepared, like many women at many times, to take comfort from the man she is afraid of. So they creep quietly along corridors to the guest room in which she used to sleep, and find the bed made up under a dust sheet, which Nigel pulls to the ground, leaving traces of blood in it. They make love. He is clever and gentle, and leaves the pillows bloodstained, she sees in the morning. The pain in her spine makes it hard for her to come, and once or twice she tries to give up, or to fake, but Nigel insists, he waits, he touches her most secret places, he sings his speechless song in her ear, and in the end, there it is, bliss, she comes, she cries out, her voice and her body shake, and Nigel says, "There you are. That's all right," meaningless phrases loaded with many meanings.

In the dark, lying with him, Frederica says, "You hurt me, badly."

"I could have killed you. I learned unarmed combat in the Commandos, doing my National Service. I could kill you any time, just like that, you would hardly notice."

Frederica cogitates.

"Are you saying I'm lucky you didn't kill me by accident?"

"Something like that. No, don't be silly. Just, I've been taught how to find where it hurts."

"And is that a warning or an apology?"

"Both, don't you think? I think it's better not to talk, talking makes it worse. Sleep on it, let it pass, you *liked* just now, what we did just now, didn't you, you were happy, weren't you?"

"Yes. But—"

"I said, don't talk. You are a talkative silly bitch, Frederica. Talking *hurts.*" He puts a hand, warm, hard, friendly, over the triangle between her legs. "Trust me. Go to sleep now."

The next day, there is a woman washing bloodstains from the wallpaper on the landing. Pippy Mammott is seen with a man in a van, who carries away the broken chairs. There are new sheets, the curtains are replaced, the depleted bottles restored to their places. Nigel goes away again. He kisses Frederica, and Leo, who wraps himself like a great squid around his neck. "Be good," he says to both of them. "I'll ring you. Be good."

Olive and Rosalind do not talk to Frederica. That is, conversation of a repetitive kind takes place at mealtimes, which take place regularly. Breakfast is quiet, lunch is administrative—"I think I need to go into Hereford for some stuff for the roses, and to get my hair cut, do you want to come?" Tea is rather more determinedly social, which means that the sisters and Pippy Mammott do try to talk to Frederica, which means in practice that they always all talk about Leo, who is always present for tea—lunch he sometimes, usually, has in the nursery. They discuss his achievements, his sayings, Sooty. They always end by saying he will get a big head if this goes on, and the child always puts his hands to the sides of his brow. The first time he did this, it was with genuine alarm because, Frederica could see, he feared his skull was swelling outwards, but now he does it for effect, because his aunts and Pippy Mammott always laugh so much. They sometimes also compare his doings with those of his father at his age. Tumbles are compared, also fear of the dark, "sharpness" and growth. In the early days there was some attempt to tell Frederica about Nigel's childhood, as though she was full of distress at having been shut out of this golden age, as though she needed, in order to be fully alive, to acquire their knowledge by proxy. This kind of talk happens rarely now, and nothing has succeeded it. Frederica wonders sometimes if Pippy was always there, if she was present during the growing up of Nigel, or if she has assimilated her knowledge from the house and its inhabitants. It would be simple to ask, but Frederica does not ask, just as no one in that house ever asks anything about Frederica's own past, her parents, her sister, her brother, her sister's children. She mentions these children from time to time by way of comparison with Leo—she plays the Leo conversations like a board game with herself, scoring increasing points for each repetition of certain clichés, and jackpots for a cliché that can be got to include Nigel, Marcus, Leo and Will in one banal generalisation. The sisters and Pippy know something is wrong with what observations she offers, but they do not know what, and do not, she supposes, greatly care.

She thinks they talk to each other quite differently when she is not there. Sometimes she hears a passionate buzz of talk behind a closed door, notes of urgency, notes of insistence, notes of pain, notes of laughter, none of which she ever hears face to face.

She does not want to know. She is not Olive's kind of person, nor Rosalind's, nor Pippy Mammott's. They let her know this, with no cruel intention, seeing no need for kindness, simply making certain things clear. She happens to be there, Nigel happens to want her, she is a necessary part of Leo's wonderful existence, the house is big, there is room for all of them, she doesn't say much, she is a bit feeble, really, a bit wet, they all go their own ways, and if she wants an errand done, or a doctor fetched, or a letter posted, they are only too ready to help. Only too happy to help. *Helping* her integrates her into the way of things. Helping her pleases Nigel and Leo. There is nothing she can do to help them. Except, possibly, keep out of the way, which indeed she does, though they don't wholly like the *manner* of her keeping out of the way.

. . .

In the early days of her marriage, she and Nigel treated the house as though it was a honeymoon retreat. They climbed the stairs hand in hand towards the bedroom, at all hours, coffee-time, noon, tea-time and evening. They touched each other, Frederica remembers, handing teacups, pouring wine. They passed the sisters, Pippy, on the stairs, and were unseen, as though they were not there. Frederica, alone and vulnerable, is now retrospectively embarrassed by this bad behaviour, or what she supposes was taken for bad behaviour, since nothing is, or was, said. Nigel is like a Pasha in his palace, she thinks, but cannot say. Leo is a male child in a harem. Leo will be sent away to school when he is eight or so. He will go to the school his father went to.

Frederica thinks she cannot bear Leo to be sent away to sleep in a dorm with boys. She has seen them cry. It is not good.

Frederica thinks that when Leo has gone, she can go.

Frederica thinks that when Leo is eight, she will be thirty-two and her life will be almost over.

She encounters Olive and Rosalind as one being, but they are not twins. Olive is older than Rosalind, but not by much, and both are older than Nigel, by five or six years, maybe seven—again, Frederica has not asked and is not told. This means they are well into their thirties, and must have thought about marriage themselves, though there is no sign of it. They are married to Bran House. They do not quarrel, they do not even have sisterly spats, which Frederica finds odd and baffling. She tells herself, without conviction, a long story in which they once fought to the death—over a man, over one of them's passionate desire to leave, to do something else, drive a rally car, nurse in a hospital, take a degree in poultry keeping, go on a Hellenic Cruise—Frederica's invention fails rapidly—and in her story, after this fight, they were both so battered and afraid that they agreed never to differ again. There is no evidence for this fantasy other than the tendency of their faces to set into masks of mild sullenness when they are unobserved. Like Nigel, they have large dark eyes sunk fairly deep under very definite, solid bars of dark brows. Nigel's beard is heavy and he shaves twice daily—the mussel-blue shadow from jaw to cheekbone, along the long face, is one of his attractions. All three have darkly shadowed upper lips. The hair on Olive and Rosalind's heads is neatly cut and solidly controlled. The rest of them is hairy—their tweeds, their handsome, dark-haired legs, their lips. It is not certain that they are unhappy because they look unhappy. Nigel can look intensely gloomy when he is most enjoying himself. It is the set of their faces. Leo has their solemn eyes in a much more volatile geometry.

They do have their own social life, in which they do not include Frederica. She has gone to one or two County Shows, and has enjoyed the drama of the jump-off, the smell of the horsehair and leather. She has learned to ride, which she does, in her way, enjoy—riding is the nearest she comes to being part of the alien world she thought would be full of surprises. She likes to ride with Nigel, she likes to canter over grassland with dew on it, she likes to see his neat body bent over the mane of the horse in front of her—*this* has an immediacy that excites her. She likes to strike out for the horizon. But riding with Olive and Rosalind is not like that. They like a companionable pottering trot, or they like to hunt, which Frederica will not attempt to do, for which they almost invisibly—What do *we* care what *you* think is right?—despise her. But riding friends come and go, other families come and go in Land Rovers. One woman, Peggy Gollisinger, an elegant nervous woman smelling overpoweringly of Ma Griffe, did try to make a friend of Frederica. She came once or twice and sat in the drawing-room with the new Mrs. Reiver, launching immediately into an intimate account of her husband's infidelities, soaking up gin and tonic like a hot bouquet reviving in water with aspirin. Then she fell asleep on the sofa, and Pippy Mammott showed in her chauffeur, who picked her up and carried her away. "That always happens, I'm afraid," said Pippy to Frederica. "There are those who just don't get out the gin, no matter what. She doesn't react too well to that treatment either. A lost soul, poor Peggy, I'm sad to say." Frederica wondered if she herself had been diagnosed as another potential lost soul.

Olive and Rosalind's most substantial friend, most frequently invited, most frequently invoked, is a woman a little younger than themselves, Alice English, petite, energetic, with a floppy mass of silvery-fair corkscrew curls, and a round face with a sharply pointed chin at the bottom of it, and widely spaced, very blue eyes in the top half. Alice is livelier than the Reiver sisters, and tells Frederica several times in the first weeks of their acquaintance, "We must be *great friends.*" Frederica comes to see that this is because Alice had hopes of Nigel, though she is far indeed from knowing whether these hopes had any justification.

Nigel has never mentioned Alice English, but this is no use as evidence in either direction. Alice English occasionally says with determined jauntiness, "I *know* Nigel thinks" this or that about things, such as the dangers of comprehensive education, or the wrongness of lying to the House, or the importance of an incorruptible judiciary, or the punishments to be inflicted on Communist spies. She comes round more frequently now the battle-lines for the election are drawn—she is something to do with the local Conservative Party Committee—and invokes Nigel's putative views more and more firmly and frequently. Frederica took a certain pleasure in Alice's earlier half-confessions. It is pleasant to be in possession of what someone else desires—or at the least reassuring to know that someone desires what you have got. But she cannot sympathise with this new bred-in-the-blood Tory Nigel who would, if he were there, be rousing the shire to fight in the back streets of Worcester for fear of letting in that nasty, sneaky little man Harold Wilson. Alice *knows* that Nigel thinks Wilson completely unprincipled, completely vicious, completely incompetent. Alice *knows* that Nigel thinks that Wilson wants to give everyone's hard-earned savings to scroungers who delight in milking the State to live in luxury in flats they pay next to nothing for, with cars parked outside, and tellys inside, oh yes. Alice even *knows* Nigel would want Frederica to come and help dissuade the shopkeepers from listening to that twisted man's blandishments. Nigel has never mentioned politics to Frederica. Frederica assumes he votes Tory—it is part of his illicit attraction, like Don Juan, like Byron, an ultimate, inadmissible *sinfulness.* She assumes he must know she can't and won't vote Tory, though lately she has begun to wonder. If he had ever said anything to her remotely resembling what Alice says she knows he thinks, Frederica might have thought twice about marrying him, for his class would have become—as Alice's is—aesthetically completely unacceptable. But he has appeared uninterested. And Frederica's Puritan upbringing has so far had a curious effect on her politics. For whereas both Bill and Winifred are wholehearted members of the Labour Party, by class origin, by instinct and by thoughtful conviction, they have brought up their daughter in that tolerant, non-conformist, cautiously sceptical tradition that requires you to look twice at everything, to look for the good and bad in everything. Bill has his fanaticisms, one of which is a fanatical rejection of fanaticism. So Frederica knows that her gut reaction against the Conservative Party is as questionable, on the face of it, as a gut reaction against homosexuals or Negroes. Homosexuals, Negroes, and Conservative Ladies are human beings, Frederica knows, and believes. Nevertheless when Alice English says, "You *must* give a hand, Frederica, you must support our people," Frederica feels ill with instinctive loathing, and replies, in a voice much more her own than is usually heard in that house, "They are *not my people.*" She thinks. She says, "And I am very glad they are not, I have to say."

She goes upstairs. Treading heavily. Bang, bang. She closes her bedroom door. Bang. What use is any of it?

She looks for Tony's letter, to comfort her. She has not looked at her clutch of letters since she put them away; they are contaminated by rage and bloodshed, which would horrify the writers. She finds Tony's letter, idealistic and canny, and also finds Daniel's, with a momentary surge of guilt. He is right. She should write to Bill and Winifred. She cannot. She is afraid of reliving in any way the days of the death of Stephanie. She wishes with part of her that *everything* had ceased to exist with her sister, her past, her home, *everything,* for good memories are more painful than bad. The violent ending makes the whole story appalling; Stephanie's smile, Stephanie's wisdom, Stephanie's lazy peacefulness all become ghouls, phantoms, terrible shapeless figures flailing in empty air. What Daniel says is of course right. Bill has lost one daughter and should not therefore lose two.

She thinks she *will* write a real letter to Bill, not now, not quite yet. She looks for Edmund Wilkie's letter and cannot find it. She goes through everything again. It is not there. It was the most personal and the most surprising of the letters—for Wilkie is less her true friend than Hugh, or Alan, or Tony, never loved, as Alexander was. It was also the only sexy letter, the only real provocation to an unauthorised reader. She turns out her drawer—her sweater drawer—where the letters had been hidden. She goes through her desk. Nothing. She becomes very rapidly convinced that Nigel has taken Wilkie's letter. Wilkie's letter flares in her mind into something hugely important, the lost object sought in dreams whose discovery will put everything right. She sees the scenes it evoked: the bed full of blood in Scarborough, the Evolution Tower in NYU. Also she begins to relive the pain of the blow in the spine, the torn hair. She feels hatred. Frederica is a fierce woman, but hatred terrifies her. She thinks of Nigel as something dangerous and repulsive, and she feels herself degraded by these feelings, herself sickens her.

When it is night, she begins to search Nigel's secret places. She has never opened his drawers, never touched the heaps of paper he leaves lying around. His papers are papers which are inert and a little dusty, not touched with life, as her own are. Now she goes through a heap—on the top of a chest of drawers—a futile and silly thing to do, since he would hardly take Wilkie's letter and leave it lying around amongst bills and bank statements. She then goes through his sock drawer, an apple-tray of tidy black balls, his shirt drawer, his underpants—so very neatly folded, so clean, so anonymous. She runs through the jackets in the wardrobe, looking inside envelopes crumpled in inside pockets with NIGEL on the outside, scrupulously reading *nothing,* as though her own lack of prying might protect her from his. She puts things back where she found them, even a sealed condom tucked in a brown envelope. Inside his wardrobe are various locked cases and briefcases. She looks at these, and then, still possessed by the black swollen hatred, she goes back to where she found a cigar box full of little keys at the back of the underwear drawer. This has the appearance of a place where a tidy man puts keys to things which may be lost, vanished or forgotten, keys which may be useful if other keys are lost. Keys which are the male equivalent of the sewing-machine key, the old jewel-box key, the key to the five-year diary that got finished and thrown away in embarrassment. She takes the cigar box over to the deep wardrobe and tries various of the keys on various of the boxes and cases. One largish suitcase gives off, when opened with a very simple key, an odour of decay like ripe cheese. It turns out to contain a wad of clearly unwashed rugger clothing, in various colours—tangerine and black, a sumptuous purple and crimson. There are socks with what she supposes to be ancient mud, liquid in the 1950s, even, caked dust since then—she has never known Nigel to play rugger. She locks it again quickly. The fitting of this key is encouraging, and so she persists through several failures, with a delicious sense of committing an outrage, a justified outrage. She opens another case—a kind of document folder—and finds a mass of school photographs, Nigel at five, Nigel at nine, Nigel in boater and blazer, Nigel black-a-vised amongst rows of staring young men with starting eyes and solid, fleshy mouths. Then a very small, rather complicated, not at all flimsy key—a key which is not one of an endless series randomly distributed, but a special key, with a barrel and fierce little teeth, opens a large rather battered document box not unlike the box brandished by the Chancellor of the Exchequer on Budget Day.

She has not found Wilkie's letters. She has found a collection of magazines and photographs. "*You* know the kind of thing," one man might say to another, or one woman to another. And nod, with sophisticated understanding. So much flesh, so very stretched over such muscles, such globes, so much clean, silky, peachy *skin* with a high gloss on it. Such damp holes laid bare, such glistening prongs, such pearly teeth approaching, ingesting, such purple sprouting veins. Such things, such trusses, such tresses, such improbable contortions of such essentially incompressible rubbery flesh. Such glossy pouts, such gouts of blood, such tears, such fear, such good fun, a bit of all sorts. Such inventive angles, a clitoris, an anus, a glans, an uvula, a cascade of this or that or the other liquid or solid. One was called *My Bad Little Bedside Book*. And another *Naughty Girls Well and Truly Punished*. The human body is not infinitely various but it is much more various than the range of poses and postures and parts in these pictures. The human erotic imagination appears to have strictly limited matter to work on. Padlocks, chains, thongs, spikes, cages, boots—nothing much has changed since the mediaeval torture-chamber was furnished, apart from the invention of rubber, which has produced some odd embellishments and habits. If you had asked Frederica whether these things did harm, or whether they should be suppressed, she would have given you an orthodox answer, an answer soon to be orthodox in advice columns everywhere, no, they do good, they are simply amusing, if people like them, they're good. She is quite unprepared for the effect on her own body of *seeing* these exposed buttocks, these sow breasts, these globular mouths. She thinks quickly of herself, of her own pleasure in the dark—to what extent her response to the pictures is erotic—and she thinks, whilst he is . . . whilst I am . . . whilst we are . . . in his mind he sees . . . And she is sick, and knows you cannot unsee what you have seen, and that this is *of no importance* and that it has changed everything in the flickering half-light of her erotic imagination. It is like finding trunks of butchered limbs, she tells herself wildly, hands and feet under the floorboards, I cannot manage to pretend I haven't seen. One is attracted or repelled and I am repelled, and it is not as Freud says, that attraction underlies repulsion, as with certain ambiguous smells, which I *do* understand—no, all this, it is simply horribly *simple,* like fairground dollies, and degrading, however my good liberal mind tries to avoid that judgemental word, degrading, and dirty, for all the pink and orange spanking cleanness of that overblown flesh.

She thinks of making a bonfire, and this causes her to remember her father making a bonfire in her childhood of her carefully concealed cache of *Girls' Crystals.* Poor Bill, how would he compare this with the sickly narratives and *Schwärmerei* of the *Crystals*? She can't tell. Her own erotic imagination works after words, in the not-said; before she knew precisely what men and women did together she imagined Elizabeth Bennet and Darcy naked at last, she imagined Mr. Rochester, but what he brought was a comfortable enfolding containing excitement, and a look of love, of love of *her,* Jane-Frederica, Frederica-Jane, the beloved.

If you put your finger on one of these fat breasts, she says to herself, it would spring back at you like a balloon, with a kind of a whine and a kind of a *ping.*

She locks up the box and puts it back where she found it.

In her dressing-gown pocket she finds Wilkie's letter.

It is of course possible that it was not herself who put that letter there. She certainly has no memory of doing so.

Frederica goes into Spessendborough in the Land Rover with Olive, Rosalind, Pippy and Leo. She says she wants to come for the ride, which is partly true—she needs to get out of Bran House—but she also wants to make private telephone calls, she is not sure to whom; she is almost too cast down to be in need of Wilkie's sharpness. Spessendborough is a small market town, one end of which is taken up with covered cattle pens and stained concrete yards. The other end is pretty, with an inn—the Red Dragon—a wide High Street along which run old-fashioned shops, a baker, a butcher, a sweetshop, a haberdashery with thick wavery glass windows, and more modern shops, selling more old-fashioned things—local craft pottery, home-made jams and preserves, a chemist's with coloured bottles. There are side streets of red-brick Georgian houses, and streets beyond them of low cottages with little gardens full of flowers, polished brass knockers, and spick-and-span lace curtains. There are two cafés, the Spinning Wheel and the Copper Kettle, full of dark spindle-legged armchairs with Jacobean chintz cushions and slightly rocky tables, oval and round. For some reason the Reivers always go to the Spinning Wheel, and never to the Copper Kettle. They like to have cream teas in the Spinning Wheel, scones and raspberry jam and Cornish clotted cream. The teapots have knitted teacosies with fluted panels and woolly bows on top. Frederica waits until Pippy has lifted the teapot and then says she has forgotten something at the chemist's and will be back shortly. There is a phone box just beyond the chemist's, out of the sight-line of anyone in the Spinning Wheel.

She has a large collection of pennies, and sixpences, and shillings. She stands in the red box and deploys all these on top of the directories, which are torn and mangled. There is the usual smell—stale tobacco, faint urine, airless dustiness, Bakelite and stone. She picks up the receiver and dials the operator, to whom she recites—making her decision at the last moment—Alan Melville's number. In the distance she hears the bellow of a protesting cow. She waits and hears clickings and hummings and vacancy and burring, and then suddenly a clear Scots voice.

"Hullo. Hullo?"

"Alan?"

"Yes. Can I help?"

"Alan, it's me. Frederica."

"Frederica," he says, in a pleased voice. "What do I say after so long? Are you well? Where are you? Are you ringing for any particular reason?"

He was always, even when closest, rather agreeably courteous and detached.

"No. Yes. I needed someone to talk to. I was so glad to have your letter. I feel you're a long way away—in all sorts of ways, not only miles. It's lovely to hear your voice, it really is. Damn, the money's running out. Hang on. That's better. I've put in a shilling, that'll keep us going."

"Can I ring you back? Where is your phone box?"

"Spessendborough. No, it's OK. I've saved lots of change. I'm ringing from a phone box because—I'm ringing because—I feel I can talk more *freely*—"

"Frederica, you don't sound happy. Is something wrong?"

"No. Not exactly. No. I'm a bit lonely. That's what it is."

There is a tapping on the glass walls of the box. It is Leo, whose white nose is pressed against the pane, at the level of Frederica's knees. She looks round. They are all staring in at her from different sides, Olive and Rosalind and Pippy Mammott. They look rather severe, but when they see her looking, they wave and smile, encouragingly.

"I've got to go now, Alan."

"But you haven't *said* anything, darling, you haven't even begun."

"I've got to go. They're all round the box."

"Let them wait a bit."

"I *can't* talk to you with them watching. I can't. I'll go. Give my love to the others. Tell them their letters were—were—"

"Frederica. Can I ring you back?"

"No. Yes. I don't know. I'll try again."

"You sound really *bothered,* Frederica."

"I've got to go. I've got to go."

"Frederica—"

"Good-bye. Give my love to Tony and the others. Good-bye—"

They do not need to criticise, they do not need to ask whom she is calling, they do not need to say, "You said you were going to the chemist's, and we find you in a phone box," because all these things are perfectly clear to all of them, immediately. Frederica says, "I'm sorry to keep you waiting," and they say, "Not at all, you weren't, we just happened to come by," and so they all pile into the Land Rover, Frederica between Pippy and Olive, with Leo on Pippy's knees.

Frederica thinks, The idea that I am *trapped* here is an illusion. I could just get up and go, tomorrow, I could. If I just said "I'm going now," it is quite likely these three would be *glad of it,* that's how it is.

Leo says, "Your tea was cold. We just wondered where you were." He puts a small hand into hers, and grips. She is kept rigid by the solid bottoms of Olive and Pippy, pressing against hers.

Leo develops a passion for the story of Tommy Brock and Mr. Tod. Frederica tries to read him other things, *Thomas the Tank Engine,* more Hobbits, but night after night he insists on coming back to this rather unsavoury tale. He can recite large parts of it, and particularly enjoys the dénouement, when the fox believes he has killed the badger with a trap.

"I will bury that nasty person in the hole which he has dug. I will bring my bedding out, and dry it in the sun," said Mr. Tod.

"I will get soft soap, and monkey soap, and all sorts of soap; and soda and scrubbing brushes; and persian powder; and carbolic to remove the smell. I must have a disinfecting. Perhaps I may have to burn sulphur."

"What is sulphur, Mummy? What is persian powder?"

"Sulphur is yellow and has a disagreeable smell," says Frederica, whose style is infected by Beatrix Potter's own idiom. "Matches have sulphur in them, and fireworks, and so does the smell of bad eggs, which you probably don't know—eggs don't seem to go bad these days. It's a nasty smell."

"Tommy Brock must have smelt *very* nasty if you need a bad-egg smell to get rid of his smell," says Leo. "What do you think he smelt of?"

"Like people's dirty feet when they haven't washed for *months,*" says Frederica. "You probably don't know what that smells like, either."

"I've smelt Mr. Wigg's shirt when he's been gardening," says Leo. "What a *pong,* Daddy says, Mr. Wigg makes. Do you think Tommy Brock smelled like Mr. Wigg, Mummy?"

"*Much worse,* Leo. And you ought not to say people pong, it's an ugly word, and you might hurt their feelings."

"I like it. Pong. Pong. Ping-pong-ping-pong. Ping is like needles and pong is like Sooty's piles and pools."

"That's enough of pongs. Let's get on with the story."

"You haven't told me what persian powder is."

"I haven't, have I? That's because I don't know. I told you yesterday I didn't know."

"You could have *found out.*"

"I could. How was I to know you would want Tommy Brock and Mr. Tod for a fourth time running?"

"You could have known. I *love* Tommy Brock and Mr. Tod. We will have them tomorrow too. I love it when they do horrible things to each other. They are horrible people and they do horrible things and everything is *horrible* and the little rabbits are all safe after all. Only a bit frightened, they were, the little rabbits. Their mummy *wringed* her ears, she was worried. How do you wring your ears?"

"You can't, if you aren't a rabbit. Something like this."

Frederica puts her hands to her head and more or less wrings her red hair. Leo laughs shrilly—the story overexcites him.

"Go on reading, now. Go on." He prompts. "Mr. Tod opened the door . . ."

"Tommy Brock was sitting at Mr. Tod's kitchen table, pouring out tea from Mr. Tod's tea-pot into Mr. Tod's teacup. He was quite dry himself and grinning; and he threw the cup of scalding tea all over Mr. Tod."

Leo shrieks with laughter and rolls about on his pillows, damp-skinned and catching his breath. Frederica touches his hair, and then buries her face in his chest. He clutches at her hair and kicks, convulsed with laughter.

One day, a week or so later, they are all having tea, Olive, Rosalind, Pippy Mammott, Frederica and Leo, when the sound of wheels is heard on the gravel outside. Rosalind says, "That must be Alice," and

Pippy Mammott, her mouth full of fruit cake says, "Not Alice's car. Land Rover." "Not our Land Rover," says Olive. "No shuddering noise." "Don't recognise it," says Rosalind. Pippy goes to the window. "Three men," she says. "No one we know. Getting out. Coming to the door." "Conservative canvassers?" says Olive. Pippy has gone to the door. There is a male murmur, which ends distinctly with "Frederica." Frederica stands up and goes herself to the door. There is Pippy Mammott, and there on the flight of steps leading up to the front door, where they have no right to be, where in some sense they do not exist, are Tony and Alan and Hugh Pink. The Land Rover is new and shiny. Hugh says, "Good afternoon, Mrs. Mammott. We happened to be passing—"

"And thought we would look up our old friend Frederica," says Tony.

Alan says, "Frederica. We aren't intruding, I hope?"

Frederica is afraid she will cry. She runs down the steps and puts her arms round Alan's neck. He hugs her. Tony hugs her. Hugh Pink gives her a peck of a kiss on a cheek. Pippy Mammott stands in the doorway and observes these indiscriminate embraces.

"Tea?" says Frederica with a slightly hysterical laugh. "Would you like to come in for some tea?"

"That's what we *hoped* you would say," says Tony, advancing on Pippy Mammott. "So kind," he says, though Pippy Mammott's expression is not exactly kind. "We've come such a long way, tea is just what we want, isn't it, Alan, isn't it, Hugh?"

They come in, a body of energy, they look around themselves curiously, they advance on Olive and Rosalind and shake their hands.

"You found your way back, I see," says Olive to Hugh Pink.

"It wasn't difficult. We happened to be passing. We thought we'd look up Frederica. On the off chance."

"The tea's cold," says Pippy Mammott. "I'll make fresh."

She goes off with the trolley. Frederica performs introductions: Tony, Alan, Hugh, Olive, Rosalind, Leo.

Everyone sits down and considers everyone else, watchfully. Alan says one or two polite things to Olive and Rosalind about the architecture of Bran House, to which they reply briefly, at a loss.

Tony says, "And you, dearest Frederica, how are you keeping? What are you doing with yourself, tell us how things are?"

"I have Leo," says Frederica, and stops. "Tell me—*you tell me*—about everyone—about what you are doing—"

Tony says, "Everyone's got election fever."

Alan says, "I've got some lectures to do at the Tate, on Turner, I've suddenly got interested in Turner, romanticism was never my thing, but I've got interested—"

Hugh says, "I actually sold my pomegranate poem, the one I sent you, to the *New Statesman.* I've written quite a lot, there might be a book, almost. Can't call it 'Bells and Pomegranates,' that's spoken for, but I'm having a go at bells. No competition with 'Lübeck Bells,' of course. More of a relation of 'Mary, Mary, Quite Contrary.' "

"With silver bells and cockle shells," says Leo.

"*Exactly,*" says Hugh to Leo. "A garden full of shiny things—"

"But a silver nutmeg. *And* a golden pear."

"Your son is a poet, Frederica."

"He likes words," says Frederica.

"He could hardly not," says Tony, looking at the dark aunts on their sofa. They do not speak. Pippy Mammott returns with the trolley, and fresh tea. Tony eats three slices of fruit cake and Alan eats a sandwich with cucumber and Gentleman's Relish.

"And Wilkie?" says Frederica. "You must have seen Wilkie?"

"He's full of his television game. He's made a pilot, he says it's hilarious, literary knights and theatrical ladies getting everything *deliciously* wrong, mistaking Auden for Byron, he says, and Dickens for Oscar Wilde, and Shakespeare for C. S. Forester, he told us to tell you you've got to come and play, everyone is playing, even *Alexander* is playing, you have to come and play . . ."

"You'd leave them all standing at the starting post, Frederica," says Alan.

"No one wants to see *me,*" says Frederica.

"No, but you will make them want to. You always did."

They take the tea, and smile vaguely at the denizens of the house who offer it, they talk in a trio, lightly and brightly, they reminisce, they cross-refer, they are not impenetrably rude and private, but they speak Frederica's shop, Frederica's staple chatter and gossip and thoughts, for which she is dry and thirsty. She begins to speak. She tells Hugh why she loved his poem. She discusses Persephone in the dark with the fruit and seeds, and furious dry Demeter in the air. They quote lines at each other, Hugh and Frederica, companionably.

Leo says suddenly, "Picks with pink fingers, listless."

Hugh smiles at him. "I didn't know your mother had read it to you too."

"She didn't," says Leo. "Daddy did."

The two dark women narrow their mouths and look at each other. Frederica puts out a hand towards Leo. Hugh, thinking of his poem, notices none of this. He says, "Did he like it?"

"I don't think so," says Leo.

"Poetry isn't his—" begins Frederica.

"He likes hobbits," says Leo. "*I* liked it," he says kindly.

Alan Melville says, "I should very much like to take a walk in your woods, Frederica, if we may? Do you think we could go on a walk? Being from the grey north I don't know this country. It's very beautiful."

Frederica stands up. "Let's walk," she says. "Yes, that would be wonderful, just what I need, a walk, let's *walk*."

Alan says to Olive and Rosalind, "Would you like to come with us?"

"Well, that would be—" says Rosalind.

"No thank you," says Olive.

"No thank you," says Rosalind.

It is the first time Frederica has seen them disagree, Frederica thinks; then she thinks she *must* be exaggerating, she just feels she is herself again, dangerously happy and observant.

"We won't be long," she says, going into the hall, getting a jacket. "I don't suppose we'll be all that long and anyway it doesn't matter, does it?"

"I'm coming," says Leo. "Wait for me."

"Better not, dear," says Pippy Mammott. "You might miss your supper. Lovely Welsh rarebit, you like that, and treacle tart, you like that, too."

"I'll get my coat too," says Leo, making for the door.

"Your mummy doesn't want you," says Pippy Mammott. "She'd like to see her friends she hasn't seen. We will all just stay here quietly until she comes back. We'll play Happy Families. You like that."

"She *does* want me," says Leo. He stands stiffly, near tears, full of force, Bill Potter's grandson, Nigel Reiver's son, a small figure by the chimney-piece. "She *doesn't want to see them* without me. She doesn't."

Frederica stands and looks at him. She doesn't speak, but she does meet his eye. It is Tony Watson who says, "Where's this coat then?" and Alan who says to Pippy, "We'll take *very* good care of him, we'll bring him back in plenty of time for his supper."

Frederica holds his coat for him, and he shrugs himself into it. They set off through the orchard and across the meadows, with Leo at first swinging between Hugh and Alan, and then riding on Tony's strong shoulders, clutching his curly head, and pointing things out, things rapidly becoming invisible in the thickening autumn evening, a crow, a jump, a trough, a gate with dead stoats and magpies nailed to it.

Because he is there, nobody asks Frederica about her life. It occurs to Alan that the child, however small, has come out with precisely that intention, conscious or unconscious, of preventing Frederica from talking to her friends about her life. If there is a reflective pause in the conversation the boy rushes in, with lots of bright, showy, slightly shrill chatter, *in case,* Alan thinks, *in case.* The three friends accommodate themselves to the situation. They are real friends, they came to help as best they can. It is quite dark in the woods, the smoky light lingers after sunset.

They come back companionably, discussing words for twilight: dusk, gloaming, *crépuscule, Dämmerung.* Hugh quotes Heine—"Im Dämmergrau, in das Liebeland / Tief in den Busch hinein." Alan says to Frederica, as they prolong the walk by coming back to the front door round the outskirt of the moat, "You really do live in a moated grange."

"When Hugh came, he kept quoting 'Only connect.' I got quite cross, but he was right, of course."

"Did you connect?"

"Look, Alan, how can one say one thing is more *real* than another, here and London, people with their heads full of books and people with their heads full of figures? But I got a bit sick of all the Cambridge literary intensity. I am half sick of shadows, I said to myself, I will Connect, and found myself in a moated grange."

"Complete with Mrs. Danvers."

"Don't. You can do *awful damage* with inappropriate comparisons."

Leo says, "Im Dämmergrau in das Liebeland."

Hugh says, "You can twist your tongue round anything."

Alan takes Frederica's hand.

They come round the corner, across the bridge over the opaque green water, and crunch across the gravel. There is another car beside the Land Rover, a shimmering silver Triumph, not Nigel's green Aston Martin. On the top step, looking down from a height, are three men, one of whom, much the smallest, is Nigel. The other two are both dressed in blazers and flannel trousers, formally informal. One has dark skin and a large curling white beard, elegantly trimmed. The other is bald, with horn-rimmed glasses. Alan drops Frederica's hand, and Tony lifts down Leo, who looks around him, and then makes a little rush across the gravel, and toils up the staircase to his father.

Frederica apologises for her friends, although she knows she should not. She introduces them, says they are old friends, explains that she had no idea they were in the neighbourhood. Whilst she says all this, falling over her words, Nigel and his companions remain stolidly in possession of the centre of the top step, in front of the door. He nods quickly and silently in the direction of Alan, Tony and Hugh, as they are introduced, neat, unsmiling, economical nods. He introduces his own companions, Govinder Shah and Gijsbert Pijnakker. Both these persons hold out their hands formally to Alan, Tony and Hugh, who have to take them on a slant, like courtiers.

"And my wife," says Nigel. "Delighted," says Shah. "So glad to meet you," says Pijnakker. Frederica has a sensation of being summed up and judged, by both at once, in different ways. Shah has soft full lips inside his beard, and deepset dark eyes, under curly white brows, with smile-lines set round them. He is wearing an Indian silk scarf inside an ivory silk shirt inside his dark blue blazer: it is flame and gold, with little flowers in crimson and black. Pijnakker is egg-shaped, a shining egg-head on a solid egg-body, neat and hairless. His shirt is striped butcher-blue and white, and he wears a navy scarf tied extremely neatly. Nigel is wearing a dark sweater and dark trousers. Alan, Tony and Hugh are all in corduroy jackets and trousers, over polo-necked sweaters. Nigel's friends make Frederica's friends look flimsy and insubstantial. Frederica's friends, on their own ground, might make Nigel's friends look pompous, but they are not on their own ground. The two groups might join and talk animatedly and fuse, but that is not going to happen. Nigel explains to Frederica's friends that he has important things to discuss with Pijnakker and Shah. He then offers the friends a drink, which they refuse, retreating towards their Land Rover. Tony says, "Why don't you lend us Frederica to have dinner with us in Spessendborough, whilst you talk?" There is an effort of pure will behind this casual invitation which everyone can feel. Nigel says, "Oh, I don't think so, I don't think she'd want to do that. We've only just arrived."

Frederica says, "You won't really need *me,* if you have things to discuss—"

She knows rationally that there is no reason why she should not say this.

She knows she will pay for saying it.

"We'll be around a bit," says Tony. "Staying in the Red Dragon. Perhaps we'll see you again."

"Perhaps," says Nigel. "Who knows?"

It is quite clear to everybody that he hopes never to see them again.

Frederica dines with Pijnakker, Shah and Nigel. She does not often meet Nigel's friends, and when she does, they do not much talk to her. Nigel's social life seems to be spent in a very male society, a society of clubs, bars, cigars and complicated intrigue. When he is at home, this world rings his moated grange invisibly, airy voices, guttural voices, suave voices, excitable voices, thick-cream voices, European voices, Asian voices, American voices, call him to the telephone, and he sits all evening, lying back in a leather armchair, talking to the wide world. Frederica supposes that if her friends had not come, she would not have been asked to sit through dinner with Pijnakker and Shah. On the rare occasions when people from out there do come to Bran House, she is somehow relegated to Leo's nursery supper, or Pippy Mammott puts her up something delicious on a tray by the fire. But tonight she sits through dinner and nobody has much to say to her. Pijnakker addresses her more or less in the third person, through Nigel. "Your lady wife is very comfortable here in the country," he says, including them both in a pleasant enough smile. "In Holland we have no such variety of landscape. It is all flat. Has your lady wife ever visited Holland, I wonder?" "No," says Frederica. "I should like to see the Rijksmuseum. I should like to see the Van Gogh paintings." "You must bring her, once, Reiver," says Pijnakker. "Rotterdam is not beautiful, but she would like Delft and Leiden, she would be interested in tulips." These are not words that interest Pijnakker, but his intentions are kindly. Shah says, "So you are interested in paintings, Mrs. Reiver." He, unlike Pijnakker, does look *at* Frederica. When her eyes meet his, he gives her a little private smile, which may or may not be automatic. He says, "I do admire your brown dress, Mrs. Reiver. It is *just* the brown for your lovely hair. What kind of pictures do you like particularly?"

Frederica is fond of the dress she has on, a jersey tube with a high neck and long thin sleeves in a dark brown, between coffee and chocolate. It makes the most of her long thin body, her long thin arms. Dresses are becoming shorter. It makes the most also of her long thin legs. Govinder Shah is considering her small breasts inside this tube. His look is kindly, but Frederica knows he does not find her attractive. He believes strongly that she *wants* him to find her attractive, and so his eyes linger where they can, politely.

She says, "I don't know a lot about pictures, I'm afraid. I know quite a lot about Van Gogh. I have a great friend who wrote a play about him. Literature is my subject."

"I believe there have been many plays about Van Gogh," says Pijnakker. "People find him very interesting, he was religious and mad, very Dutch. He sold only one painting in his lifetime. I admire his persistence, to go on against such odds. What normal man would paint hundreds and thousands of pictures no one wanted to buy? I ask myself, did he *know* they would come to be wanted, or was it pure chance?"

"Hundreds of people make things nobody wants," says Shah. "But I agree with you also, there are those with the courage of their convictions who make things they know people *will* want, those who are ahead of their time. Some of these appear to be madmen, and some of them are. I believe Van Gogh's brother was a dealer. He may have seen more clearly that people would some day want those pictures. Or he may not. I believe he bought them all, stored them all. Maybe he was merely kind. Maybe he was merely exercising family loyalty."

"He too died mad," says Pijnakker. "The Dutch are much given to melancholy-madness. It is the grey rain on our coasts. That is why we voyage, to escape the grey rain and the melancholy-madness."

"Whereas we in the sub-continent," says Shah, "we voyage if we must to escape the extreme poverty and mess we have made of our daily lives. We have made a world in which enterprise is impossible, because we are not orderly beings, but lazy and corrupt beings, and if we have any enterprise we brave your grey rain and your melancholy-madness in order to earn our daily bread and if we are lucky some butter and jam and perhaps eventually foie gras and caviare to put on our bread. But we do not like your grey mists and your miserable cold wet winds, we get sunsick, we like to go back and forth and cannot."

All three men laugh at this speech, as though it says more than it appears to say.

"Happy the man," says Shah, "with an office in Rotterdam, and an office in London, and a house on a hill in Kashmir, and a villa in Antibes, and a yacht in the Mediterranean and an ocean-going boat too in the North Sea, a free man."

Pijnakker says, "Vincent Van Gogh was melancholy-mad in the south, too. The sun did him no good, I think. I like the sun myself, I am partial to a week or two in North Africa or Italy or southern France, I protect my eyes and my skin, and do not expose myself excessively."

"You are presenting yourself as a cautious and moderate person, Gijsbert."

"Only in some ways, Govinder. Only in some personal ways. I take risks when I must. You cannot do business without taking risks."

"That is so. The important thing is, to be clever about *which* risks."

They laugh again. Frederica in her brown tube, is not there, not for those two, not even as a pair of female eyes to observe their male liveliness, for they do not exactly see her as female. Nigel does. He watches her, as well as watching Shah and Pijnakker; he fills their glasses often and hers not at all. She thinks perhaps he is not speaking much because he is partly thinking about the appearance of Alan and Tony and Hugh. But perhaps he never speaks, she wonders. Even his telephone world consists mostly of listening, his head cocked on one side, his lips and brows thoughtful.

The three friends are eating steak and kidney pie in the Red Dragon. They started with tomato soup, and went on to the pie, which is really very good. The dining-room has low beams, which may or may not be old, and a bar at one end. There is also a real wood fire, in a chimney. A wood fire is a cheering thing.

Tony says, "She can't stay there, she'll go mad."

"You can't just *say* that," says Hugh. "She went there. Perhaps she really likes it. Perhaps she had a hankering for country life. I do, from time to time."

"Do you think she likes it?"

"No. No. I don't."

"*Why* did she go there?" says Tony, as though a good analytic explanation could immediately be produced.

Alan says, "I have noticed that all sorts of people, who are perfectly sensible when offering opinions about Shakespeare, or Claude Lorrain, or even Harold Wilson, simply go off their rockers when deciding about getting married. Tough people get pressured by weak people and vice versa. People marry their *ideas* of what they wanted. I know a girl whose ideal was a man with coal-black hair and she found one, and much good it did her. He is the most *boring* man and keeps a model railway in the attic. And then I've noticed people marry to spite their parents, or to repeat the mistakes or the successes of their parents, or quite often both. People marry to get away from their mothers, and hundreds of people marry one lover in order to get away from another, and what they're really thinking about isn't the one they *are* marrying but the one they aren't. Or they marry to spite someone who didn't want them."

"Or for money," says Tony.

"Or for money," says Alan. "I would have thought it was built into Frederica's scheme of things *not* to do that, but of course she might have been in revolt against her scheme of things, temporarily at least."

"She said she got married because her sister died," says Hugh. "That is, that isn't *exactly* what she said, but she intimated that that changed her, her sister dying, and she was changed."

"I don't see," says Tony, "how the death of a sister could turn you into a country lady; it seems an odd reaction, to say the least."

"You could imagine a scenario," says Alan, "where a completely new beginning in a completely new place—a new life . . . She couldn't be so *silly*."

"She was always silly," says Tony. "That was what made her bearable. Silly and clever at once, and so sure she was right, poor dear. There's a certain *Schadenfreude* in seeing her in this mess."

"No, there isn't," says Hugh. "It's just *awful*. And that amazing little boy. He wasn't going to let her say a word to us. He didn't."

"*That* is the daftest thing of all," says Tony. "*That* makes the whole mess irretrievable."

There is an element of enjoyment in Tony's contemplation of Frederica's predicament. Alan and Hugh are more perturbed, but also less disposed to interfere. Hugh says, "You can't *tell*, of course. The most surprising couples are happy in the most surprising ways."

Alan says, "You can tell. She's miserable. She's lost and miserable and ashamed."

Tony says, "Well. What are we going to do?"

"Can we do anything?"

The waitress brings lemon meringue pie.

Alan says, "We can't just leave her."

Hugh says, "I don't think we'll find it easy to see her again."

The firelight flickers. The pub is comfortable. They order coffee and whisky, and talk about Harold Wilson and Rupert Parrott. Outside a wind gets up, with rain in it.

Frederica goes to bed early, and Nigel goes into the study, with Pijnakker and Shah. Frederica lies and reads Durrell's *Justine,* which she has picked up because she thinks its narrative is strong enough to be gripping even in the state she is in. She thinks, I could just get up and go to Alexandria, and then she thinks that those who *will* go to Alexandria are in fact Pijnakker and Shah and Nigel Reiver. None of them would probably give more than ten minutes to Durrell's mannered prose but they would be more at home in his world than she would. She does not want Durrell's Alexandria in her bedroom and turns out the light. Lying rigid in the dark, willing sleep to come, shakes the brain and causes bone-ache. She puts the light on again and takes up Rilke. She is reading *The Sonnets to Orpheus* in bed in a side-by-side translation, to keep her mind exercised. This goes better. A little grammatical wrestling is wonderfully soothing, and she finds two lines which shiver her flesh and which she thinks she must show Hugh.

Geht ihr zu Bette, so lasst auf dem Tische
Brot nicht und Milch nicht: die Toten ziehts.—

(If you go to bed, leave on the table
No bread, no milk: they draw the Dead.)

And then she thinks she will find it hard to show Hugh anything again.

When Nigel comes to bed, late, late, she pretends to be asleep. He crashes around, putting on lights: a quantity of malt whisky has been consumed. Frederica lies like an angry needle along one edge of the bed. He gets in, switches off the light, and reaches for her with a heavy arm. She wriggles away. He pulls at her. She has a sudden vision of the buttocks and breasts and mouths in the briefcase. She slips out of bed like an eel, snatching up Rilke, and retreats into the bathroom.

She hears his voice, "What were you holding his hand for?"

She tries to remember. The Moated Grange. There is no answer. She thinks of slamming the door, restrains herself, shuts it very quietly, and waits.

Ist er ein Hiesiger? Nein, aus beiden
Reichen erwuchs seine weite Natur . . .

(Is he from this world? No, from both kingdoms
Sprang his wide nature . . .)

She waits for the explosion. It does not come. Nigel has gone to sleep. Whisky is beautiful, sleep is beautiful, silence is blissful. Frederica's eye-rims are sore with suppressed tears.

The next day is Sunday. Frederica breakfasts with Shah and Pijnakker, who then set off in the Triumph. She finds herself walking. Along landings, along staircases, through rooms, back. She thinks of going out for a walk, but thinks also that the friends might come. And indeed, at about ten, she hears the telephone. Pippy is there to answer it in the hall. Frederica is on the landing.

"Hullo? Oh yes. I don't know where she is at the moment, or what her plans are. I'll go and see."

Frederica begins to come downstairs.

Nigel comes out of the drawing-room, and nods to Pippy. Pippy says to the telephone, after a decent moment's rest, "I'm so sorry, I find she's busy all morning, I'm afraid that won't be possible."

The telephone speaks gallantly. Frederica comes down the stairs. Nigel nods again at Pippy, who says with a cluck of sympathy, "I'm so sorry, she can't come to the telephone, she's gone out."

And before Frederica can move, she has put the phone down.

Frederica says, "You could see I *wasn't* out, Pippy. What is this?"

Pippy looks at her, drops her gaze, and trots away. Frederica says to Nigel, "So I am not to go anywhere, ever?"

"Don't be ridiculous."

"I'm not being. You have just told a lie to my friends, to my *old friends,* you have said I wasn't there when I was."

"I'm sorry," says Nigel, with the flexibility that is always disarming. "I'm sorry, that was bad. I just can't stand those people."

"You don't know them."

"They don't like me, and I don't like them. And you are married to *me.*"

They stare at each other. Frederica says, "I am going to call them and say I am here."

"I don't want you to. I want you, just this once, to stay here, to please me. We'll go out with Leo. We'll go for a drive. It will be good for Leo to have both his parents."

" 'Just this once,' " says Frederica, picking on the operative phrase. "What do you mean, 'Just this once'? I *never* go anywhere, I *never* see anyone, I have no life, and when my friends come, you have the gall to say 'Just this once, don't go.' "

"You have to understand," says Nigel, "I don't feel sure of you. You aren't the sort of girl I was accustomed to. In a sort of a way I was a bit scared of you. I'm frightened you might find me boring, me and Leo, and want to go off, or something. You can understand that?"

"Oh yes," says Frederica. "I can understand that. But I can't live with it, any more. If you keep me shut up here because I might go off, I *will* go off, you can see that?"

"Leo—" says Nigel.

"Don't blackmail me with Leo. I am myself, as well as Leo's mother. *I want to see my friends.*"

"Just this once—" Nigel begins doggedly, and then laughs, sharp and unhappy. "Look, we'll start again, we'll go to London, I'll take you to Amsterdam with Pijnakker and you can look at your pictures, we'll go on a holiday—we could go to the West Indies—"

"I don't *want* to go to the West Indies, I want to go where I can talk about books—where I can *think*—I have to *think,* the way you have to do whatever you do do, with Pijnakker and Shah—"

"You can think here. It isn't thinking you want, it's men. You need lots of men."

"*No,* Nigel. I need—"

"He was holding your hand."

"Is that so terrible?"

"Yes. Yes, it is. To me, it is."

"I'm sorry. It wasn't anything. Leo was even there. They are just my friends."

"Just this once—stay with me. I'm sorry. Stay with me."

She stays, because she sees only too well that if she *does* attempt to telephone the Red Dragon, all that will result will be hideous embarrassment and violence. They go out in the car, Frederica and Leo and Nigel, and they have what might be called a good day. Both of them talk to Leo, who chatters to both of them. Leo does not mention

Alan and Tony and Hugh, though Frederica is waiting for him to do so. It is as though they had never come, never existed.

When they come back, Nigel says, "There, that was a good day."

Pippy carries Leo off to bed. She brings supper for Nigel and Frederica. She does not meet Frederica's eye. Frederica is tired. She has got through another day, and finds this consoling, until, when relaxation dribbles a livelier blood into her veins, she starts thinking again: Getting through another day, and another day, what sort of a life is that? "Most people's lives," some cynical Good Fairy mutters in her head. "Most people's lives." Frederica stabs carrots, savagely, with her fork. She thinks, Today is Sunday, they all have jobs, they will have gone home.

Rifts are closed, but also sprung open, in bedrooms. Frederica sees that Nigel has a scenario for this night, a scenario of long, subtle, complex love-making, of gentleness and closeness, of pleasure and loss of self and exhausted sleep. She tries, because she is tired, and because in some ways she is in despair, to school herself to accept this, because it is what he has to give, and because she needs sleep and unconsciousness, and because of Leo. She watches Nigel undress—he likes to sleep naked—and she thinks to herself that his body is more real to her than those of Tony and Alan and Hugh added together—and Alexander and Wilkie and Raphael Faber, she tells herself rather wildly. She even sits quietly on the edge of her side of the bed, in a white lawn nightdress with long sleeves and a yoke and collar, and wonders whether women in previous centuries would even recognise her despair, given that she does not want to go away and make love to Tony, Alan and Hugh, but merely to talk to them, merely to feel a little mental space for freedom. The bedroom is dark, and Nigel has drawn the curtains, which are dark red, a kind of damask, with red trees and red blooms on a red ground. When Frederica is alone she leaves the curtains open and sees stars or clouds. She imagines Alan and Tony and Hugh in a large room with white walls and pale blue curtains, with open windows blowing the blue curtains, and sunlight coming in. She hunches her shoulders and stares at her knees. The naked man pads, strutting a little, as naked men do, in and out of the bathroom, making tap noises, spitting noises, flushing noises. Frederica sits and waits, and thinks. She thinks, I am a woman, and thinks what a silly pretentious thought *that* is. She thinks, I thought that, because the kind of woman I am is not quite sure she *is* a woman, she likes to be reassured about that. I am a thin woman, a sharp woman, a wordy woman, not the sort of animal men think of at all when they think of a woman. Cambridge obscured this, temporarily, there were so few women, we were all treated as though we were real ones, like nurses in prisons, like secretaries in barracks.

The man carries his penis in front of him, neither erect nor quiescent, but stirring with life, but solidifying. He says, "Darling." He approaches the motionless woman and pulls at her nightdress, intending to lift it romantically over her head.

Frederica sees in her head, with total clarity, the succession of images in the locked case, the screwed-up bodies, the blown-up flesh, the carmines and roses, the slippery rubbery masses. She twists away, clutching her garment, and says, "It's no use. None of it is any use. You know as well as I do that this is over, that I can't stay, that it hasn't worked. Tomorrow I will put some things together and get a taxi or something from Spessendborough and just *go* in a civilised sort of way. And then we can be friends and it will not be so awful."

She had not expected to say any of this, and is uncomfortably aware that her tone is that of a nanny talking to a child. Nigel stops a moment, and then continues his advance. The penis has not shrunk, it has become an angry club, wavering in front of him. His face is flushed. He takes hold of Frederica's hair, pulls her head back on to the bed—she lets herself fall quickly, remembering the commando grips—pushes up the nightdress and takes her. He does not try to hurt her, he does not kiss or caress her. He bangs away, and explodes, and sits back on the floor, swaying slightly. Frederica says, in a thin voice, frightened and furious, "*That* has nothing to say to it. I am going to go, tomorrow."

"No," says Nigel. His eyes are full of tears. They run on to his cheeks. Frederica wipes her legs with the sheet and the nightdress.

"It isn't *me* you want," says Frederica. "You just want to hold on to what you've got, like all possessive males, you're like one of the stags when one of the females tries to trot off, you bellow and rush. It's nothing to do with *me*."

"How do you know? You don't know my thoughts, you don't know *much,* I often think. You don't notice much. How do you know what I feel?"

"I don't think I care any more what you feel. I'm going to go and sleep in that other room. Good night."

She goes into the spare bedroom and sits on the edge of the bed, in the dark, and shakes. She waits. She is not thinking, she is simply afraid. She waits. When she hears footsteps along the corridor, she gets behind the door. She is still shaking. Perhaps she will faint. The door opens violently and the man comes into the room. He stands, accustoming his eyes to the dark, and Frederica whips round the door, and runs along the corridor and down the stairs. She runs into the kitchen and out into the scullery, and pulls at bolts, and chains, and goes out into the quiet damp night. She goes on running, across the back yard, through a gate into the stable-yard. She listens. At first there is no sound of pursuit and then she hears a door open. That is all. He is not crashing. He is coming quietly. Frederica opens the door to the saddle-room, quietly, quietly, slips in and shuts it. She does not like to be shut in. She wants to be out in the air, to run all the way to London, but that is silly, she needs to be very clever. She gets behind a rack of saddles and waits. She thinks, when he opens the door, if he opens the door, this nightdress will shimmer. She finds a horseblanket, drapes it over a chair and crouches under. Every hiding place is also more dangerous, because she cannot run. She can hear her own blood, banging in her head and her heart. Her mouth is dry. She crouches.

After what seems a long time, the door is thrown open with a crash. She can hear him breathing. She sees his bare feet, and the bottoms of his pyjama trousers, striped blue and white. She breathes shallow, shallow, just enough air to keep alive. He says, "Frederica?" She keeps still. He walks in and looks around. She thinks he must have a hunting animal's instinct for warm flesh and breath, but he listens, and does not come towards her. He says, "I'll find you," and she can tell from his voice that he does not know she is there, not really, he is a bit embarrassed, for all his heaving rage, to be talking to an empty room. He goes out, leaving the door open. She still cannot hear his feet on the paving stones, which makes her feel hysterical. She hears a door, another further door, a sudden movement of a horse in a stall, the scrape of a metal shoe. She hears the second door close. Then for a long time she hears nothing. She crouches in the cold in her damp nightdress and says to herself, "Come on, you are clever, intelligence can be used for *anything,* what are you going to do?" But she can think of nothing at all, except going back into the house, and hiding, and waiting until morning, and running on to the road, once she has some sensible clothes—and the road is some two and a half miles away, and unfrequented—and hitching a lift. And there is Leo. How can she run away when he is awake?

After perhaps two hours, she comes out, and stretches her cramped body. There is silence. He will be waiting for her in the house. Perhaps, she thinks, it will all get out of hand and he will kill me with his commando tricks. She does not *really* think he will do that. No human being in full possession of life and thought *really* supposes they are about to die. She thinks if she can just manage to hide *in* the house until breakfast time—until light—

She flickers back barefoot and silent round the edge of the stable-yard, across the back yard, to the back door. The air is cold and damp. The sky is overcast. The door is locked and bolted. She stands on the doorstep and thinks what to do next. She feels curiously relaxed. She will have to be let in bedraggled and cold, at dawn, but what will that matter? She breathes a deep sigh.

"And *now* what will you do?" he says, behind her, stepping out of the house-corner. He has put on a shirt and a pair of plimsolls. He is holding an axe. Frederica screams at the sight of the axe, as he meant her to. It is not a very big axe, as axes go, a neat, portable, shining little axe.

"Don't be ridiculous," says Frederica, doubtfully.

"I'll get you," he says thickly and moves towards her.

Frederica runs.

She runs like fury, through the yards, into the orchard, across the orchard, out into the field. He runs after her. He runs better, but she is madder, she runs quite extraordinarily fast, her mouth is wide and fills with cold night air, and drags at it in great gulps. She runs across the field. He laughs, he stands at the top of the slope of the field as she is stumbling down it, he gives a great whoop of laughter, and throws the axe at her.

She ducks and twists. She cannot see, she will never know how good or bad his aim is or was meant to be. The flat of the axe catches her on her ribs and winds her. She and the axe fall together, its blade bites the flesh of her hip, cuts at her calf. The nightdress reddens very fast, with blood. Frederica lies on her side and stares dumbly at the grass, at a molehill, at the skyline, at the black and grey clouded sky. She is winded. Her eyes hurt. She feels blood and blood, her blood, great hot puddles of it. It has a finality. She stares.

He runs to her side, he kneels beside her. He is beside himself, he is crying, he tears up her nightdress and makes an efficient bandage to stanch the blood. He says, "I didn't mean it, I didn't mean it, you know I didn't mean it."

"What's mean?" says Frederica incoherently, and lapses into blissful unconsciousness. She comes round in his arms: he is carrying her up the hillside, back into the house. She thinks, I might get some sleep.

He bandages her up very successfully. He straps her up in sticking plaster and lint, he swabs and stanches. He says, "They're only superficial cuts, you really don't need a doctor, I do know what I'm talking about—"

"Because of the commandos."

"It comes in useful. I am *terribly sorry.* What can I say? I don't know how I . . . I do love you . . . I don't want to hurt you."

"That's not what it looks like."

"I know. Oh, God, *I'm sorry.* You have to understand—"

"I understand."

"I don't like the way you say that."

"You aren't meant to."

"Please, Frederica."

"Go away. I need sleep."

"You need sleep."

He goes away, obediently. She lies in her bed, and Pippy Mammott brings her breakfast. Pippy Mammott says, "I gather you fell over something in the night."

"Something like that."

"I'd be more careful, if I was you."

"What do you mean by that, Pippy?"

"What I say. I'd be more careful, rushing around in the night."

She pretends to be worse than she believes she is. This gives her a kind of space for manoeuvre, though she does not know *what* she will manoeuvre. Leo comes to see her, and strokes her face.

"Poor thing. You're ill."

"I fell over. I was silly."

"You'll get better, Daddy says so."

"I just need a lot of sleep, Leo, that's all, I need to keep very very still. I can't walk very well."

"Poor thing. Poor thing."

"Leo, don't cry. I'll get better. I promise."

He weeps and weeps. She sits up and holds him. All this is not good for him.

"Your face is all bashed, it's horrible, you must have had a *horrible* fall."

"It was. It was quite horrible. But I'm getting better, you can see. No harm done."

"No harm done," says Leo in a little voice. "No harm."

Nigel and Leo go out riding. Olive and Rosalind have gone out too, to help Alice English with her leaflets. Frederica does not know where Pippy is—she might be anywhere—but she is desperate. She gets up, puts on a pair of slacks and a sweater, and goes down the stairs. She can walk perfectly well, although it hurts to do so. She is bruised by the fall, as well as cut by the axe. She stands in the hall, thinking, and then opens the front door and sets out over the gravel. If Pippy is there and is going to stop her, it will be now. There is no sign of Pippy. She crosses the moat, at the bridge, and starts to walk down the drive. She has half an idea that if she can get as far as the road, she will flag down a passing motorist. She does get to the end of the drive, and sits down on a bit of wall, at the edge of the empty road, which is very empty. She hears a sound of bicycle wheels and a creaking chain. She stares at her feet. A voice says, "Frederica!" She jumps. She cries out. It is Hugh Pink, on a very large, very old bicycle. They look at each other.

"What on earth have you done to yourself?"

"Do I look awful?"

"You look horrible. Black and blue and yellow and scraped."

"I fell over."

Hugh puts his bicycle down in the roadside. He gets out a handkerchief and wipes his face.

"And how did you fall over, Frederica?"

"Well," says Frederica. "It was in the course of a marital dispute."

"Go on."

"I can't. I shall cry. I don't want to cry, I want to think what to do. Why are you still here?"

"I wanted to see you. To see if you were all right. We thought we were making things worse, and we thought we hadn't any right to interfere, and we thought—we were worried about you."

"Thank you," says Frederica gravely. They sit side by side. She says, "Where are the others?"

"In the woods, in case you came that way. We rang once or twice, but you weren't there, they said you couldn't speak."

"I was there."

"We knew you were. That's why we stayed. It seemed rather feeble just to keep patrolling, but you see it worked."

"It did. Here we are. They might come any minute. What am I going to do?"

"Come back to London with us?"

"How can I? What about Leo?"

"Well," says Hugh, "we could bring the Land Rover to the track in the wood, at night. Can you get out? We could be in London before they saw you'd gone. I suppose you can't just walk out yourself?"

"I can't drive."

"That's remiss of you. You'd better learn. I mean it, we could whisk you away tonight, if you want. You look as though you *ought* to be whisked away, if I may say so. I never took you for a masochist."

"I'm not."

There is a long silence. Hugh says, "I'm sorry. I expect I spoke out of turn. Forget it."

"No, you didn't. Of course you didn't. I ought to get out. I've made a terrible mess of my life. There's Leo."

"Bring Leo."

"How can I? He's a happy little boy, or would be, if I was happy, he has a good life, he's loved, he has his *ways*—I'm not the most—not the central—"

"No?"

"No. I don't think so. I can't bring a little boy who doesn't know anything about all this—in the middle of the night—"

"I'm not saying you're coming *for ever,* Frederica. Just offering a lift to get away and think. You can arrange for Leo later. To see him, to have him, I don't know, to make a better arrangement—just coming away with us now can't be the *end,* you know."

"No."

There is another long silence. Hugh says, "You can't be that good for him, the state you're in, now."

Wounds have their uses. Frederica stays in the spare bedroom, claiming that hers will rest better in solitude. She goes to bed early, undresses and gets into bed with a book. She has no idea what she will do: the idea of a midnight escape is in one way absurd, romantic, ridiculous, and in another appalling. For how can Leo be left? And yet, how can she will her own annihilation, what will she be to Leo, if she is not Frederica? Mummy. It is a word she hates. Why do the English have the same word for a swaddled corpse and cuddly maternity? She thinks for a moment of her sister, Stephanie, like and unlike, mummy in both senses, Frederica thinks grimly. Stephanie too married for sex. It seems improbable, looking at fat Daniel, but Frederica knows it to be true. There they were, the children of a passionate liberal intellectual, and one married the Church and one the Shires, and for what, for sex. She thinks Stephanie was happy. No one is wholly happy, but Stephanie loved Daniel and loved Will and Mary, there was no doubt of that. Stephanie had some capacity to will her own annihilation. Frederica thinks she perhaps married Nigel because Stephanie had married Daniel, and was dead, is dead, will be dead. Stephanie had stepped outside the Cambridge circle of talk and endless discriminations, moral and aesthetic; she had grasped at sensuous happiness. Like Lady Chatterley, walking into the woods to be annihilated, trailing little threads of quotations from Milton's blindness and Swinburne's pale Galilean and Keats's unravished bride of quietness, and Shakespeare's Proserpina, willing them all to go away, so as to lose herself and find herself in the body, in the spring. And that was our myth, Frederica thinks, carrying on her conversation with Hugh, in her head, that the body is truth. Lady Chatterley hated *words,* and Nigel has no words, and I cannot do without them.

I came here, because Stephanie's death annihilated me, at least temporarily, so I was able to live in my body.

Leo lived in my body, a temporary visitor, part, not part, separate now.

Not altogether.

Who matters to him, "Mummy" here, Frederica there, somewhere where Frederica *is* Frederica?

I always resented my own mother's passive quietness. It was not a life. It was what I do not want. It was what I did not want. It is what I have got.

Leo. I could *steal* Leo. But here he is someone, here everyone loves him, here he has a real life, even if I don't.

Leo would have a better life here.

If Leo met me, met Frederica, *somewhere else,* where Frederica was Frederica, at least there would be some truthfulness. He would be angry, but we would talk.

Do you *really* think that?

No. No. I think if I go I might never see him again. I think if I stay we may both be destroyed. I think that's melodramatic. I think, even if it's melodramatic, it's *true.* Melodrama happens. Axes are thrown. Commando tricks are used.

You're just trying to talk yourself into anger, Frederica. Or fear, enough to leave. You *want to leave,* that is what you want, *even if Leo stays,* but you would like to think you *ought* to leave, too, you would like permission.

You won't get it. Leo is your son. You must stay with him or go. You must choose.

"*Now* what will you do?" says the melodramatic sneering voice in her head.

She gets up and begins to dress. The house is dark, the voices are silent, the doors are closed. She is about to commit a crime. She packs nothing; she wants nothing of this life. She is still discussing with herself whether she should go as she goes down the stairs. But her body has taken charge and is creeping with efficient stealth, like a cat burglar, through the kitchens, out of the house.

It is a very misty night. Frederica sees great grey veils moving in the stable yard, in the yard lights. She stops to pick up a torch from the saddle-room, and then sets off cautious, quick, picking her way in shadows of walls, back where she so frantically ran, into the walled orchard. The mist is mobile: it swirls around, apple trees, cherry trees, bare now, are suddenly silhouetted against it, and then suddenly clear in the light of the moon against a patch of blue-black sky with stars sprinkled on it. There is quite a lot of wind, in sudden gusts. Twigs rattle and creak. She hears her heart in the soles of her feet. She stays at the edge of the orchard, where it is darkest, amongst gooseberry bushes and espaliered pears and apricots. She thinks she hears footsteps padding after her, and stops suddenly to listen, and hears nothing but silence. She is jumpy. A man might spring out with an axe, or a sword or a gun. Or just with quick, efficient, chopping hands. The moon, when it is now and then uncovered, is almost full. The sky is in turmoil. Ribbons and rags and heaps of vapour race and coil.

She hears another sound in the bushes, a kind of blundering sound, and stops dead, against the wall, crouching. She thinks perhaps it is a badger: there are badgers in the woods which have been known to come into the orchard, that human place between the house and the wild. There is another very small crunching, and then silence. Some creature, foraging.

She reaches the orchard door, and turns the key, and opens it. Beyond, the field is dark and clammy and open. Behind her there is a sudden rush of running feet and she swings round in fury and turns the blinding light of the torch towards her pursuer. "And what will you do *now,*" she hears in her head. But there is no face in her torch-beam, only a flurry of sound and then arms clasping her damaged leg like a serpent coil tightening, strong, small arms, and a face buried in her wound and butting it.

"Leo. Let go. You're hurting my hurt. My love, let go."

"*No.*"

"I won't go anywhere. Come here."

There is a kind of exchange of grips in the dark. Frederica lifts her son, who clutches at every part of her as he rises, with wiry hands and almost prehensile feet. Then he is up, his arms in a stranglehold round her neck, his face driven into her collar-bone, the whole of his body glued to hers with furious determination. He is in his pyjamas. His feet are bare. His face is wet. His teeth are clenched.

"Leo. Leo."

He cannot speak. They stand there, then she sits down, the boy still knotted round her neck.

Many years later, somewhere on the Río Negro, an Indian called Nazareno will bring to Frederica a sloth he has detached from a tree. The sloth is covered with grey hairs and moves slowly, slowly, unable to move really, on the grass in front of the hotel in the clearing. She has three long crescent-shaped nails, and her bowed arms gesture feebly. She stares with round, dark, small, other eyes, without thought or expression. Frederica thinks the creature has a goitre on her neck, a swelling, and then sees it is not so: round the neck of the sloth is wound the child of the sloth, so tight that its lineaments can hardly be discerned, there are simply figures of eight in the strange grey fur and what might be a head lost in what might be a collar-bone. Frederica sees the strangeness of the sloth, and remembers suddenly with total clarity this moment at the gate of the orchard, when her son grips, grips, and tries to burrow back into her body. And she thinks, then, what she cannot think now, standing at the gate: That was the worst moment of my life. That was the worst.

Leo gets out, "I'm. Coming. With."

"It's all right. I'll take you back to bed. We'll go in."

"No. I'm. Coming."

"You don't understand."

"I'm tired," he says. "I'm tired of thinking and thinking what to do, I'm just *tired*. I want to come. You couldn't. You can't. Go without. You can't."

"Leo. Let go a bit. You're like the Old Man of the Sea. Strangling Sinbad."

"Go on," he says. "Go on. That's what he said, the Old Man."

And Frederica ceases to think at all, but sets off again, hurrying and limping, across the field, with the hot child clutched to her breast, clutching with hands and feet. And so, somehow or other, they get over the stile without his hold being relaxed, and set off through the wood, keeping to the ride between the yew trees. Frederica says from time to time, timidly, "Are you all right? Are you comfortable, my darling?" and he does not answer, only grips, heavy and sullen now, inert as if he were asleep, or dead, except that he grips. She sees the dark bulks of the tree trunks, and the clouds racing above the stiff and soughing branches, and she moves in pain, imagining another, younger Frederica, springing along for the joy of freedom. She will remember no man's body as she will remember this hot, angry, grasping boy: she will remember no pleasure of the flesh, and no pain, as she will remember the touch of these arms, the smell of this hair, the shudder of this effort of breath. Both of us know I meant to leave him, she thinks, as she stumbles on; this will be between us. Her grip on him is as tight as his on her: she can hear their two hearts thud, their breaths are mixed. And when Alan Melville steps out of the trees to meet her, his wavering torch lighting her path on the earth, he thinks for a moment of the lion in Stubb's absurd and wonderful picture of the great cat clawing for purchase on the shoulders of its white-maned mount and prey, he thinks of demons, before he sees what she is clutching, a small boy, at the end of his resources. Both woman and child have bared teeth and look not quite human.

"Hullo, Leo," says Alan, gravely. "Are you coming with us?"

The boy cannot answer.

Frederica says, "He took matters into his own hands. Can he come?"

"I don't think you can be separated," says Alan judiciously.

IV

. . . and it was also about that time, the time of the first flourish of the theatrical presentations in the Theatre of Tongues, but before the ceremonies instituted in the Lady Chapel and the Chapel of the Holy Innocents, that the Lady Roseace took to slipping away from La Tour Bruyarde to take solitary rides and rambles in the forest. She would have been hard put to it to explain why she did this, if asked, and thus sought a certain secrecy, in order to evade being asked, and perhaps also in order not to have to clarify to herself why she went. If challenged, she intended to say that her fancy chose solitary riding, as others' fancies or fantasies chose the actions and rituals now being acted out with much ruddiness of skin and much expenditure of hot pantings and licking of lips in the Theatre of Tongues. But she had a heartfelt wish not to be asked, for the desire of solitude—at least in others—was not a desire upon which Culvert smiled freely. There were still many discussions to be held on how to accommodate the incompatible desires of Damian, Culvert and the Lady Roseace. Culvert was hopeful of the outcome of these debates. The Lady Roseace, contrariwise, prided herself on being no man's creature. That was still in the springtime of the enterprise.

At that time it was also the springtime of the year, or just before. She still rode in a quilted jacket, but had laid aside her fur wraps and her furred hat, and went covered only in a light hood. She had discovered many wide rides, which, as they penetrated deeper under the cover of the trees, became little twisting paths which opened on pretty glades in some of which the first flowers were springing on the green turf, aconites and hellebores, primroses and shy violets. And she would dismount and wander distractedly amongst the dark trunks, seeing how the bright little buds advanced each week, and appropriating these secret places in her mind, saying, My primroses are further on than I had supposed, or, My thrush is making a great song and dance in my hazel coppice. She began to think of herself as the dryad of those trees, tending them, though she did nothing but stare and smile and walk to and fro. And she would get bolder and explore a little more and a little more, extending her domain, savouring the scents and the singing in the thickets, thinking sometimes of how she would pass the rest of her days in La Tour Bruyarde and sometimes more vaguely of what might be taking place in the world beyond the valley, in cities and harbours, on roads and highways, along rivers and on the open sea. A hen pheasant led a procession of little chicks across her path, and she bent to cup one of the soft little things in her hands, but they cried out, cheeping, and scattered and she followed, clutching her skirts and pushing back brambles and thorny branches from her face, seeing the burnished bronze of the female feathers flash amongst dead bracken, and so going onwards, until she came to another clearing where the trees were higher and blacker and not in bud, though they bore strange fruit. The clearing was circular and the trees held out their black stiff arms, and at their arms' length swung swaying and creaking things that she took at first for suits of clothing, or scarecrows, and then saw clearly to be the thing itself, human creatures whose faces were black, whose eyes were plucked by beaks, whose bellies were swollen and stank.

They turned and creaked, and the trees stood stiffly and rattled and creaked. And a voice behind Roseace said, so that her heart stopped, "The fruit of the forest, eh, my lady?"

Roseace turned, trembling with fear or outrage, and there close behind her was Colonel Grim, who must have crept up whilst she was preoccupied with brambles, and come close, close, whilst she stared at dead men.

"Et ego in Arcadia, is it not so, my lady? I am sorry if I gave you a fright. May I escort you away from these danglers, back to your pastoral hiding place?"

"I did not hear you."

"That is natural. You were preoccupied and I am a trained tracker of beasts and men. Allow me to hold back these branches for you."

"I came here to be alone."

"That is evident, and so you shall be. But it would be less than chivalrous in me to leave you quite immediately, quite suddenly, after you have had the shock of coming upon our fellow creatures in the state they are in."

"Who are they?"

"That I do not know. Such gatherings are alas not uncommon in these reaches of the forest. The usual explanation is that they are the victims of the Krebs, though the Krebs, like all bloody tribes, are made responsible for many foul things done by others."

"I do not know of the Krebs," said the Lady Roseace, standing stock-still and reluctant to turn back, for to turn back would be to touch in some way the bulky body of Colonel Grim. Like most if not all the inhabitants of La Tour Bruyarde, she felt a strong aversion to the idea of touching the Colonel. Whether or not he was aware of this, the Colonel took her by the arm and led her back through the branches to the previous clearing, where he invited her to sit on a mossy stump and recover her senses. The Lady Roseace had seen worse sights in the Revolutionary wars from which she had so decisively fled, and would have returned haughtily to her horse, if it were not for an uneasy sense that it would do her no good to make an enemy of Grim. So she sat, toying with her whip, and accepted a silver cannikin of aquavit from his flask.

"The Krebs," said Grim, "are a people, or tribe, who inhabit, or infest, the deep forests and the caves under the mountains. They are short and swarthy, and their bodies are hairy. They have an odour which is offensive to delicate nostrils, and an incomprehensible speech of grunts and spitting. They are not often seen—they hunt in packs, wearing furs and carrying leather bucklers. There is much dispute amongst the learned as to whether they are or are not human creatures. They have a reluctance to leave even their dead in human hands, with the result that we have been unable to examine even a corpse. No one has ever seen a female Krebs, unless it is that the two sexes are indistinguishable and fight side by side, fur-wrapped. They take no prisoners and destroy those who have seen them, it is said, either by blinding, or more often by the punishment of death. It is not good to have come even so close to their trails as to have seen those danglers, my lady. As far as I could see, the peculiar nooses of leather from which they dangle are the work of the Krebs, but I know—it is my business to know—that there are also roaming gangs of more ordinary villains and outlaws who imitate their styles, to safeguard, with fear, their own hiding places."

"You know a great deal," said the Lady Roseace.

"I patrol the bounds of Culvert's kingdom, my child," said the old soldier. "It is more vulnerable on this south side than he thinks, and the outside world has not ceased to exist because he has closed it off and turned away from it. I advise you to ride no more in these glades if you do not wish to become scattered bones and a skull picked clean."

He looked at her lovely face, with its full lips and wide, clear eyes suffused with sparkling liquid, and under the fine flesh of her face the Lady Roseace felt he saw her bone-cage, with staring sockets, dark nasal pits, and rattling pearly teeth in a gaunt jawbone. She bent her head in silence, and her interlocutor continued.

"And I should like to ask, if it is not impertinent, why you ride out so frequently into these woods, and always alone? It might be thought by prurient minds that you have assignations of some kind, but I have been your invisible companion on these wanderings from the first, and can vouch for your innocence of outside intrigues."

The Lady Roseace's breasts and throat were flooded with sudden heat as she answered, with her prepared answer:

"Culvert wishes to provide for the full exercise of all human passions, which he believes to be intrinsically valuable because they are human. And I have a newly discovered passion for solitude and secrecy, solitude, secrecy and wild nature, a not uncommon, indeed a banal, human passion, which I indulge. Or thought I indulged, until you revealed to me a moment ago that my solitude was an illusion, a most displeasing revelation."

"I could say I feared you might need sudden protection from the Krebs," Grim replied, seating himself on an adjacent stump and settling, it appeared, for a long conversation. "Or I could say I feared you were betraying the community, though that explanation does, I agree, lack plausibility. Or I could say, with truth, ma'am, that I have a long-standing passion for information, for knowing exactly the doings and comings and goings of everyone else. I have been a spy in my time, my lady, and it is an avocation that gives intense passional pleasure to men of my type. Here such passions can be freely acknowledged. Here they do no harm. If you take my advice, and wander no longer in these woods, you will never know from what horrors my inconvenient passion may have saved you."

The Lady Roseace compressed her lovely lips, for she saw both the sense and the chafing inconvenience of what he said.

"You take no pleasure in Culvert's popular discussions of pleasure?" the grim man asked, more conversationally. "I have noticed you are frequently absent from these delightful consortiums, into which the majority of our fellow citizens throw themselves with such passion."

"They repeat themselves somewhat tediously," replied the lady. "Their discussions are circular and rambling, and return again and again to the same assertions, which are not greatly elaborated from their first appearance. I agree with you that our fellow inhabitants do indeed take intense pleasure in these contests and concords of debate, but a passion for discussion, like the more usual female passion for gossip and scandal, appears to have been left out of my make-up. Indeed," she went on, interested enough in herself to forget her mistrust of her companion, "those aspects of my nature which caused me to seek this retreat, a desire for solitude, for retirement from the hurly-burly of meaningless, or alternatively dangerous, social activity, make me peculiarly unfitted for the incessant and almost feverish social activity which has, very naturally, it appears, sprung to life in our midst. I admire—I have always admired, even adored—the force, and charm, and powerful intelligence of Culvert. I see the logic of his endeavours to reform—or restore—human nature. But I am not prepared—not ready—not sufficiently convinced of the inevitability of his analysis—to submit myself to all his projects."

"I believe," said the Colonel, "that this morning's debate was to be on the pleasures and pains of micturition and evacuation, on the interest taken by certain persons, including some in our company, in the products thereof, liquids and solids both, and the relations, in the experience again of certain persons, of these processes with the intimate—or solitary—processes of love and desire. Do I have it pat?"

"More or less," said the lady, her mind straying to her own mild pleasures in these matters. A blush then spread over her whole body as she realised that if, as he said, the Colonel had been present unseen during all her wanderings, he must have seen her squatting amongst celandines and sighing with relief and delight as she loosed a streaming puddle into the mossy earth. Had he looked away, did he take pleasure in watching? She had held her skirts bunched high and had felt the balmy air circulating around those white and shapely buttocks, that warm and clinging slit which Culvert wished to offer on stage to the admiring gaze of the whole community. Had Grim seen her with pleasure, and if so, with what kind of pleasure? The idea of his secret eyes was more unpleasant, more interesting and more disturbing to the peace of her inner passages than Culvert's public project.

"If he can excite the community to excite themselves about these matters," the Colonel continued imperturbably, "he will have achieved a subtle political coup, and will be well on the way to solving his urgent housekeeping problem. For we positively must solve the problem of equitable shit-shifting, madame, companion, our very existence depends on it. I have seen fevers run riot in gaols and military camps with festering sanitation."

Roseace had no answer to this, so sat quietly, toying still with her whip.

"He must have foreseen," said the Colonel, "that point still to come when the discussion of the liberation of passions brings us to the liberation of those passions which take pleasure in the hurt of others. I do not speak of a manacle a little too tight, or a whipping that raises a man's member in protesting bliss, such things can be accommodated for our delectation and instruction, on stage or in the bedchambers and dungeons. No, I am curious about the point at which your Culvert will come to consider the pleasures felt by crowds in their Sunday best who watch the heads fall under the axe, or the lion's teeth sever the gladiator's jugular. Can he stage a public hanging and stop short of death? For he may find one suicide amongst us who will offer himself once—and once only—to those whose delight is to make meat of others. It may be that he can find more who have discovered, deliberately or inadvertently, the unsurpassable excitement of spending themselves, of dying in the poets' metaphysical sense, at the precise moment of giving up the ghost with the spurting seed, as the noose tightens, as those poor danglers must have done with no one to cut them down. A dangerous game, Madame Roseace, and still no real satisfaction to the meat-makers."

"Culvert would never countenance making one man happy at another's expense," retorted the lady, though she was inwardly troubled about adjustments of happiness to be made between herself, Culvert and Damian. "And your interest in bloodthirstiness, Colonel Grim, must stem from your own bloody nature, which you have acknowledged, and renounced, I believe."

"My pleasures, in part," he answered, "derive from the strategies of warfare, which have no place in our sealed and separate world, but may yet be needed to defend it. But I see that I have distressed you with my idle and perhaps wholly unfounded speculations, and I can assure you that I take no pleasure at all in torturing the imagination of the fairer and gentler sex. Shall we return to La Tour Bruyarde?"

"I am reluctant to do so," she answered, courteously enough. "The air is so balmy, the flowers and trees so soothing, despite the terrible fruit on the thorn trees in the next clearing. I feel well, out here, and would like to journey farther."

"I do counsel you most strongly not to do so," said he. "This is not a good place, not friendly to innocent humans, however it may wear a spring smile. Let me show you something, madame."

"I do not wish to go back to the danglers," said the lady, using the Colonel's word to disguise her nausea at the thought of them.

"There is no need, madame. Break off a twig from a thorn tree in *this* clearing—a young twig, not a dead one."

"Why should I?"

"Do it."

So she put out her hand and broke off a green twig, with tight, energetic little buds. And from the severed end came a slow dark gout of blood, a clot of thick blood like a liver-coloured slug humping its way free, and behind it gushed a freshet of red blood, which sprayed her habit with fine scarlet drops. She drew back in horror, crying out, brushing her hand against her skirt so that her fingers in turn were blooded. She begged the Colonel earnestly to tell her the reason and meaning of this phenomenon.

"I do not know for certain," he replied. "Various explanations have been put forth, all of them hypothetical, not to say, in certain cases, metaphysical. You will be aware, as a lady of culture, that the divine poet, Dante Alighieri, ascribes this phenomenon to the Wood of the Suicides in his journey through the Inferno, and the association of hanged men and this bloody sap persists also in the popular imagination in these parts. More vaguely, it is said that this is a place where so many men have been slaughtered, by the Krebs, or by others of their own kind, that the earth is drunk with blood and bonemeal; which bubbles up so prevalently that the trees cannot convert it to innocent green ichor, or phloem, or sap, but must regurgitate it in horror and disgust. And then there is a contrary legend, which asserts that the earth and the trees here hate men—like the Krebs, who are in some sense their foresters and *semblables*—and take pleasure in consuming the dead or the unwary who lie against their roots or under their shade. And there is also a tale, such as you will find all over the world, but without the attestation of bloody sap, that the trees are transfigured men and women, or maybe transfigured Krebs, that the Krebs may be trees that walk, or that these trees and the Krebs may bear the same relation to each other as do the caterpillar and the butterfly—men's ingenuity, and men's dreaming, make reasons for everything, as bees make honey, or trees make fruit. I only know that to me the place gives off a scent of hatred and pain. I am not welcome here. Nor are you."

The Lady Roseace shuddered with a primitive fear and disgust at these words, and allowed herself finally to be led back to her horse, and mounted by the Colonel.

They rode back over the plain to the Tower together; Roseace turned over many things in her mind. The sky was full of great full-bellied clouds, like flying clippers, like rolling drunkards, like racing steeds, fleeing before the wind. The Tower was above them, alternately in deep shadow, and bathed in brilliant golden light. It was not a shapely building, seen in this aspect. Its decaying ledges and terraces ran into one another, so that certain aspects appeared like a heap of rubble, or a rocky chaos, or an accidental heap. But under the sunlight, even from a distance, its inhabitants could be seen rushing zestfully about their business along couloirs and arcades, so that the huge mass pullulated with human life like an antheap. And the Lady Roseace, as she rode on, with the man of blood ambling quietly at her side, did not know if it was a longed-for home and haven, or voluntarily chosen *In-pace,* that is to say, dungeon.

"We are a Society for the Protection of Frederica," says Tony Watson.

"A Society for the Promotion of the Fortunes of Frederica," says Alan Melville.

They are meeting in Alexander Wedderburn's flat in Great Ormond Street, where, it had been agreed, she would be most comfortable and least likely to be immediately discovered. Alexander, surprised by various dawn telephone calls, has given up his bed to Frederica and her son, whom it is difficult to separate from her. His bed is large and comfortable. Frederica, after a fitful sleep, woke in it in one of his shirts and thought grimly of the irony of finally coming where she had for so many years hopelessly desired to be. She has even left two or three token smears of blood on Alexander's sheets, from the inflamed wound in her haunch. Alexander himself has passed a perfectly comfortable night in his spare bedroom, but he is apprehensive. The three friends have given him a colourful and alarming account of the vengeful and violent nature of Nigel, whom Tony, perhaps unfortunately, has labelled the Axeman.

Their discussion of the future is horribly complicated by the presence of Leo, who sits beside Frederica on Alexander's linen sofa and leans his body into hers, as though two could become one. Frederica looks ill. Tony says she must see a doctor. He is already thinking in terms of divorce: he thinks there must be a medical record of the wound, *now,* but cannot say so.

"It isn't too bad," says Frederica.

"It's bad enough," says Tony. "I can see you are in pain."

Alexander pours coffee for everyone from his blue coffee-pot. He remembers pouring coffee for Daniel Orton from this pot on his arrival in London after his flight from Blesford. He thinks: I am a person to whom people persist in coming for help, despite the fact that I am not helpful, I am not useful, I am not kind and concerned.

It is Hugh Pink who says directly to Frederica, "What do you want to do?"

Frederica puts an arm round Leo's head, an embrace which also half-muffles his ears.

"I can't go back. That's certain and might as well be said."

Leo's lips tighten. He does not speak.

"I need a place to be quiet, and think. I need work. I must be independent."

Everyone looks at Leo.

"We shall have to think it out step by step," says Frederica. "I need somewhere now where I can be with Leo. Later—Leo must think—"

"I do think," says Leo. "I want to come. You want me to come, you do. I know you do. You do want me to come."

"*Of course I do,*" says Frederica. "Only—"

She thinks of his pony, his settled journeys from kitchen and paddock, his little world. She thinks of starting her "career" with a small and anxious boy to look after.

"Only—" repeats Leo, his face quivering.

"Only nothing. We'll find somewhere. Something."

Alexander says, "I have an idea. It might even be a very good idea. What about Thomas Poole? He is living by himself—well, by himself with his children—in the Bloomsbury flat I used to lodge in. His wife left him. She went off with the actor, Paul Greenaway, who was Van Gogh in my play. He has two teenage boys and a girl who is about twelve, and a little boy, Simon, who is eight, who is bigger than Leo. He runs the Crabb Robinson Institute for Adult Education—he could almost certainly find some classes for Frederica to teach—it's a way of making part-time money that many women find helpful—he's got space in that huge flat—he might help out. No one would think of looking for anyone there."

"I liked him." Frederica remembers Poole, a colleague of Alexander and her father at Blesford Ride School. "He was good as Spenser in your play." Both Frederica and Alexander remember, and do not mention, Thomas Poole's affair with the beautiful Anthea Warburton, herself then, like Frederica, only a schoolgirl, which had ended in pregnancy, abortion, and grief. The grief, Frederica remembers, had seemed to be more Thomas Poole's. But appearances can be deceptive.

"If part-time teaching is a good thing," says Alan Melville, "I can find you a few hours immediately at the Samuel Palmer School. Now the artists have a degree course, they have to study things other than art, and we teach them literature. It's quite interesting."

"And I could ask Rupert Parrott about proof-reading and writing reports on books," says Hugh. "It's dog's-bodying, but it can be done at home. It's a way in, to that world."

"And there's Wilkie's television game," says Tony. "And you could try to get some reviewing. That isn't easy, but you could do it—"

"Work," says Frederica, "I need *work*."

"And then," says Tony. "We can think out the rest. What you will do. In the long run."

"We can," says Frederica.

Alexander, Frederica and Leo arrive at Thomas Poole's flat. This is a large, Edwardian mansion flat in Bloomsbury, on the sixth floor. Alexander lodged here in the late fifties when he was working on *The Yellow Chair.* Poole's wife, Elinor, left suddenly in 1961 to join Paul Greenaway, who was playing in a revival of *Pygmalion* in New York. The Pooles' four children, Chris, Jonathan, Lizzie and Simon were then fourteen, twelve, nine and five. They are now seventeen, fifteen, twelve and eight. The two elder boys are at Blesford Ride, where Alexander and Thomas met as teachers under Frederica's father. Alexander still thinks of them as little boys, but Chris is already working for university entrance. He asks after them as Poole shows them into his living-room, which was once Alexander's bedroom. It has a big, corner bay-window, out of which can be seen, like a rocket landed from another world, the discs, dishes, turrets and antennae sprouting from the column of the new Post Office Tower.

It is not possible to discuss Frederica's future in front of Leo, and it is still impossible, it seems, to detach Leo from Frederica's side. He sits beside her on a pale Swedish sofa and twists his hand into the fold of her skirt. A young Austrian woman appears, Waltraut Röhde, with brown curls, a sweet petal face and weightless bird-bones. Her smile is confidently shy. She tells them Lizzie is swimming, and Simon is in his room. She tells Leo she is bringing tea and chocolate torte. "Torte?" says Leo. "Keck," says Waltraut. "Cake. I made it. It is good."

Frederica looks round her. The walls are lined with books. She gives a little sigh. Thomas asks after her father; Frederica says she has not heard from him; Alexander says he has had several communications, because of the Steerforth Committee. "He is in his element," says Alexander. "He has his grandchildren, his house on the moors, his evening classes. We were all afraid for him, when his occupation was gone. And he is in his element."

Waltraut returns with a tray of teacups, and again with the chocolate torte. The chocolate torte attracts Simon Poole, who is a leggy boy with a delicate neck and shining straight brown hair flopping over his brow. He is shy, but courteous, and greets everyone. Waltraut tells Leo that Simon wishes to show him his railway. Simon agrees to this in a friendly mutter. Waltraut, whose English is more resourceful than her accent might suggest, tells Leo it has three separate tracks, a turntable, two stations and a Pullman coach. Simon says, "I'm making a new points system." Maybe because both Waltraut and Simon are so patently gentle and harmless, maybe because he is tired of gripping, maybe because the chocolate has soothed his brain, Leo allows himself to be led away. Frederica finds her hands are shaking. She tells the two friends in a rush that she can't talk in front of Leo, that she can't ever go back to Leo's father, that she must have work, she must start her life again, that she cannot think what should happen to Leo. "I can't go back, I can't keep him, I can't send him back. *I can't think,*" says Frederica to Thomas and Alexander, who look at her with concern and affection.

Thomas proposes, as Alexander had hoped, that Frederica should for the time being come to live in the flat. There is room, at least whilst the big boys are away at school. He, Waltraut and Frederica can look after Lizzie and Simon and Leo, and also do their own work. He can, in fact, offer her at least one evening class at the Crabb Robinson Institute, since one of his teachers is having a difficult pregnancy and has been ordered to rest. It is on "The Development of the Novel Form" or something like that. "I think I know you well enough to know you could make a go of it," says Thomas Poole, adding, perhaps unfortunately, "It must run in the blood, I should think."

"I always said I would never teach," says Frederica.

"We all said that," says Alexander.

"It is only a suggestion," says Poole.

Frederica looks round at the books.

"No," she says, "I'm not turning it down. I feel like Simon and Leo with that chocolate cake. Greed. Pure greed."

But her face, when she says that, does not, Alexander thinks, have quite the old rapacity.

Thomas asks Alexander how his work on the Steerforth Committee is going. Alexander says that he is absorbed by it and that everyone else appears to feel the same. They are worried that if there is a change of government at the Election, now imminent, they might be disbanded. He finds it interesting, he says, partly because he likes to watch the group at work as a group—the formation of alliances and conflicts, the little eddies of passion and incomprehension. The committee is very thorough: he has visited, or will visit, schools in villages and city centres, prosperous suburbs and agricultural fens, schools for infants and schools for teenagers. Anyone's idea of teaching and learning, he says, looking for confirmation at Poole's thoughtful face and Frederica's drawn one, comes from his own early experience of being taught. "And I suppose we all thought life was somewhere else, not in the classroom, that was the essence of it." He remembers, he summons up, a pervasive smell of trapped boredom, of brown linoleum and dusty windows, of slow, slow-ticking clocks and scratches and splutters of intransigent ink. And within this sea of brown air and chalky ennui a few moments of vision: a theorem coming out just so, a chorus ending from Euripides, Hamlet saying "Words, words, words." He can still catch that feeling, he says, on the visits to secondary schools. But in the primary schools there has been nothing less than an explosion of a *new* sense of what children are and can do. He has a sense sometimes, he says, that he and his fellows are like Alice, travelling in a brighter world Underground or through the Looking Glass. He has seen such things—such brilliant paper forests hung with poems and painted birds, such cardboard towers, such purposive hurrying and constructing and experimenting . . . He has talked to the experts in language acquisition and learning psychology on the committee and now knows that small children are miracle-workers of sentence-construction *ex nihilo,* and that once we understand this we need not drill, or force . . .

"It is all very exciting, certainly," says Thomas. "But there may be sufferers for all this ferment of activity. Simon, for instance, my own son, Simon. I think he's a natural quiet boy in a corner. But they are always saying he doesn't *relate* to other children . . ."

"He seems a bright boy, to me," says Alexander guardedly.

"I think so. But maybe he is emotionally disturbed, more than I think. I've tried to compensate for his mother's absence—"

Alexander's crest falls. He is almost sure that Simon, Simon Vincent Poole, is his son, and not Thomas Poole's son. Simon's mother, Elinor, was also almost sure, and took some pleasure, at the time of Simon's birth, in explaining to Alexander the exact degree of her almost-certainty. Since then, Simon's existence has been a constant preoccupation of Alexander's. When Simon was very small, and Elinor was still at home with the children, Alexander experienced him as a threatening problem, an extension of Elinor's emotional raids on his peace, which were alternately seductive and more or less sneering. He feared for his friendship with Thomas, which mattered to him, and which he had managed to sustain. Then, after Elinor's departure, he had had a bad few months *thinking,* as a moral conundrum, about Simon's hypothetical position, with a father who was not his father, and a mother departed. He had not experienced any wish to get to know Simon. He did not like small children. Simon was in a family, with his own siblings (or half-siblings) and a settled existence. Any claim of Alexander's was in a sense ludicrous, since it was a claim based on a moment of pleasure and the accident of genes. If genes were an accident. He avoided meeting Simon.

The major problem was Thomas. Alexander has not the slightest idea whether Thomas Poole knows, or suspects, any of this difficult history. He does not see how Thomas can know, and continue his amiable trust in Alexander. He does not see how he cannot know, given Elinor's fits of emotional teasing and taunting, which appear to be part of her nature. He thinks that if Thomas *did* suspect that Simon was Alexander's son, his present behaviour would be exactly as it is, if he could sustain it. And so every conversation between the two friends is ambiguous, for Thomas either is, or is not, partly trying to needle and wound Alexander with his obsessive accounts of Simon's problems and his assertions of his, Thomas's, Simon's father's, single-handed and single-minded care for the boy.

Things have taken another turn since the Steerforth Committee began to sit. For Alexander is now able to imagine eight-year-old boys. He has seen what they write, he has discussed what they feel and know. He would like to speak to Simon. And dare not. Sex is a short thing, thinks Alexander, looking at Frederica, whom he once desired, who once desired him, and its consequences are long.

Leo and Simon come back into the room.

"We are going to stay here for a bit," Frederica tells Leo. "With Waltraut and Simon. Will that be all right?"

"I think so," says Leo.

Alexander looks at Simon. His nose has no real form yet, but his mouth, his mouth surely . . . Thomas Poole puts an arm round the boy and draws him close.

"OK, Simon?" says Thomas.

Simon rests his brow on Thomas's shoulder.

"OK," says Simon. "I don't mind."

Much later that evening, Thomas Poole and Frederica sit together, on either side of the hearth. Poole remembers the Frederica of the play, awkward, incandescent, full of ambition. He has made an appointment for her to see his doctor, and cannot bear to see her so damaged. He says none of this. He says, "I like your Leo."

Frederica frowns and gulps.

"So do I. He is . . . I would have left him. But he came, he *would come*—"

"If you had left him, you would have gone back?"

"Would I? I suppose I would. It's like still being attached by a rope, by a cord, that stretches for ever. I can't bear to go back. Not only because—because things have gone wrong. Because I shouldn't have gone there." She looks round. "There's a room that's called the library, but there isn't a book in the house that anyone *reads,* except children's books, of course."

"Why did you go there?" asks Thomas, quietly, neutrally.

Frederica looks round at the books.

"It's like my parents' home here, the same things matter. And I wanted to get out of that, then. When Alexander was talking about his education, that was how I remember my childhood—*brown air,* he said, that's how it felt, stifling. I thought people were *really living* somewhere else, not just doing everything at second hand. Well, that was part of the reason. There was Stephanie. She made all the past, all my world—a way into death. And then there was Nigel. He *was* more alive than—nice, clever, second-hand Cambridge people. I thought he was the opposite of everything—so *faded,* so—so *discussy* and not *doing*—but he wasn't really. I was a total fool. It would be simply a ghastly lesson, if it wasn't for Leo."

"A child needs his mother," says Thomas Poole. "Conventional wisdom. But true, as I know to my cost."

Frederica says, "There, he has everything. He has two devoted aunts and a kind of super-nanny, he has a pony, and a house with a moat, and stables, and an orchard and the earth—don't tell me all these are simply material things, for they aren't, he loves them, he belongs there—I don't, I only love them out of the glamour they have because they *aren't* what I am or want—but he—I ought not to take him away."

"You didn't, as I understand it. He came."

"How can he know *anything* about how we should have to live, how can he make any sort of anything anyone can call a *decision*—he just *came*—he probably supposes if we're together we shall go back together—"

"He may suppose that. Has he said that?"

Frederica considers. "No. But children don't say what they really think, almost ever, do they? They can't say what they hope, in case it's gone, like a flash, if anyone truly says no."

"Nevertheless, he is a clever boy, and he came. And children need their mother."

"Nigel might let *me* go without too much terrible fighting. I don't know anything about divorce; I'll think that out next. But he'll never let *him* go, and he'll be right not to, a child needs two parents, and Nigel loves Leo—"

"Then, in time, a *modus vivendi*—"

"I don't think so. He's like my father. An absolute master of the will. No, he won't let me go and see Leo at all, I know that, inside myself. I don't want to *use* Leo, in a battle of wills—"

"Nothing you have said leads me to suppose you have any idea of the sort. You love Leo. Leo came. Take it gently. Your instinct was right. A boy needs his mother. I don't know why Elinor left as she did. That is, I can see she was in love, and all that sort of thing, and perhaps she wanted a different sort of life, that's understandable, too. But to leave like that—to go out one evening—when I was teaching—and leave a note with the baby-sitter—and simply never—never voluntarily—speak to any of us again. She took *nothing,* not a photograph, not any of their writing. Can you understand that?"

"In a way. It may have been the only way. To be able to go at all."

"But she cannot have imagined—or let herself imagine—them, the next morning—in a month—in a year—"

Thomas Poole is full of passion. He is reliving the next morning, the next month, the next year.

Frederica says, "She can't have permitted herself to imagine—"

Thomas says, "A child needs—"

Frederica begins to weep, hoarsely, desperately, racked by great sobs. Thomas puts an arm round her. The door opens. It is Leo. He looks at Thomas to see if Thomas is responsible for the tears, works out that he is not, and launches himself, like a bolt, into Frederica's lap.

"Don't," he says. "Don't, don't, don't."

Frederica obediently dries her tears.

"I don't know what you'll make of him," Hugh Pink says, more than once, on the way to see Rupert Parrott at Bowers and Eden. "He isn't quite what he appears to be."

Frederica is getting into her stride. Bookshops. Vegetable litter from the market. Election posters. London. Life. She is wearing a kind of shift dress in a sacking-like cloth, with a black bow at the neck, cut just above the knee. I shall have to get my hair cut, she thinks, looking keenly at the passers-by. Will it work, has it enough weight, my hair?

"You keep saying that," she says to Hugh. "As though he's a magician. Or shady."

"No, no, it's nothing like that. On the contrary. It's just that he appears to be so *typical* of something, and isn't quite. You'll see."

It is Hugh's day off supply teaching. He is giving it up to take Frederica to meet Parrott, who might give her some manuscripts to read. This is kind of him, as he needs that sort of work himself, in order to write his poetry. He has become obsessed with Orpheus, is reading

Rilke, is afraid that this is banal and is overwhelmed by the vision of the dead head still singing. He tries lines in his own head:

The dead
Head
  Eddies, is held
Briefly by a crag, the blood
Reddens the river briefly
Becomes watery, water
  The song
  Runs on
The dead eyes
Are wet with the water

"Do *you* like him?" says Frederica.

"Parrott? Oh yes. Very much." He thinks. "He's religious. That's what you don't see at first."

"Is that bad?"

"No, why should it be? Just surprising." The poem is no good, it sounds *soft,* it should be cut and clear but running on.

Number 2, Elderflower Court, does not feel quite safe on its joists. It is a tall, thin house, which is in fact joined back to back to other tall, thin houses, by makeshift doors in walls and bridging corridors across shafts of dim courtyard. The entrance hall is minute, and contains a schoolmistressy table in oak and two armchairs with dusty padded seats and oak arms. There is a rather faded display of books, front-on, on a shelf in the wall. *Within God Without God* and *Our Passions Christ's Passion* by Adelbert Holly. *Within God Without God* has a kind of Op Art black-and-white spiral, swirling into a vanishing black hole which is also the O in Holly. *Our Passions Christ's Passion* has the same spiral, in blood-red and a flaming orange. They are elegant, and evidence of energy.

Inside a cubby-hole opening out of the entrance hall is a lift, with a creaking iron trellis door, and a jerking, whining, ramshackle method of hoisting itself. Frederica and Hugh go up to the fourth floor and, almost ducking, travel round three sides of an uneven rectangle in dusty corridors painted bottle-green. Parrott's office is in what must once, in Dickensian times, have been a servant's attic. It has a sloping mansard ceiling and is painted in a colour resembling tobacco-stained onion skin. The floor is heaped with dusty books; there are shelves of dusty books; there is a desk piled high with dusty paper, on which are two photographs, a posed bride in veil and train, and a row of smiling babies in suits with frilly collars.

Rupert Parrott is a small man, with a lot of tight dark reddish-blond curls, which are kept from being a mop only by rigorous training with scissors. His face and body show the same effects of discipline. He should be plump-cheeked but is not, quite. He should have a double chin, but it is barely perceptible, and the little paunch which should be beneath his lilac shirt and his pink-and-silver-spotted purple tie is also not really there, though the eye stubbornly tries to sketch it in. His mouth is, as Hugh has told Frederica, round, a little puckered, with soft lips drawn in. His eyes are blue and his nose nondescript. His voice has a public school drawl, which, with the impression of now-you-see-it-now-you-don't fleshiness, should make him seem slow. But the overall impression is of quickness, of energy, of an ease perturbed only by his own need to get going.

Hugh introduces Frederica and explains her urgent need for work. Parrott asks her what her interests are, and she replies that they are rather narrowly literary, but that she is quick at learning and interested in everything, really. Parrott says that they pay a number of readers, almost all of them women, to work their way through the slush heap—that is, the unsolicited manuscripts that arrive in dozens every morning.

"We pay them, I say, but *not very much,*" says Parrott, looking at Frederica, "because we haven't got very much, and because there are so many intelligent women sitting at home with children, desperate for bits of work to do, you see."

"I see," says Frederica.

"The firm in the past," says Parrott, "has concentrated on politics, standard thirties left-wing politics, Fabian analyses of leisure, that sort of thing. It was me that persuaded Gimson Bowers that religion could be a big seller. He's an old-style socialist, takes a simplistic line, religion's not true, it's nonsense, why bother. I said I thought there *was* an interest, a definite interest—the established Church is in a sort of ferment, look at *Honest to God,* a quiet SCM pamphlet by a quiet bishop, a national bestseller, and *what a furore.* And there's much more extreme stuff than the Bishop of Woolwich, much sexier, *literally*—sex and religion, both in the Church, and amongst all these new youth cultures. Death of God theology, exciting stuff. Charisma.

Studies of charisma. The breaking up of our moral structure as we know it. All the trouble about Christine Keeler and Profumo and the Establishment—it's all cracking up, the *conventional visions* we were happy to live by even if we didn't believe them. And now it isn't possible, and people want to read about it all, they want to know what to think. We're moving into a period of moral ferment, moral re-alignment, fruitful chaos, people want to know what's going on.

"I thought of a series called something like *Touchstones of Modern Thought.* I really need a word like 'beacons,' but you can't call anything beacons because it sounds like primary-school readers. And perhaps beacons are out of date anyway; they sound Napoleonic and we want to be in the white heat of spiritual energy, so to speak. Torches? Spearheads?"

"Arrows of desire," says Hugh. "Or warheads."

"Burning issues," says Frederica.

Rupert Parrott considers this.

"*Al*most," he says. "Not bad. Burning Issues in Religion. Burning Issues in Psychiatry. Burning Issues in Sociology. It isn't quite right."

"Burning Issues in Witchcraft," says Hugh.

"Don't mock. Witchcraft is a real issue. It's on the increase. There's a lot of interest in *wicca,* the Old Religion. I don't share it—I'm tied up in Christianity—but readers do. They write in. It's a serious interest."

He hands Frederica a book with a cover depicting a cross-legged prisoner in a padded cell in a dunce's cap.

LANGUAGE OUR STRAITJACKET
BY ELVET GANDER

Frederica opens the book. All the pages are blank.

"It's a dummy," says Parrott. "Though he'd like that joke, that you opened up his anti-language book and found pure, pristine white space. He's another of my discoveries. I discovered Canon Holly, I personally discovered Canon Holly, and I had the idea of writing to Gander, after I heard him talk at the Round House on the anti-psychiatry movement—very powerful stuff, the idea that it is the psychiatric institutions themselves that are disabling, that if we label people as schizophrenic and psychotic we *reify* these descriptions, we make people into madmen by calling them that. We published his first book, *Am I My Brother's Keeper?,* you may have seen that, it had a considerable *succès d'estime* and sold a lot of copies."

Frederica studies the jacket. Elvet Gander is apparently a gnome-like person with deepset eyes, a long, thin nose, a curly mouth, not much hair and a deep suntan, though that may be the effect of the photograph, in which he is cut off at the waist, but is clearly sitting in a high, winged, throne-like chair, although he is wearing an open-necked shirt. The jacket copy says that *Language Our Straitjacket* is part of a whole new intellectual movement which questions the constricting forms of our civilisation, and asks if they may even be a function of our language, of the printed word more especially. It quotes Marshall McLuhan:

"A state of collective awareness may have been the preverbal condition of men. Language as the technology of human extension, whose powers of division and separation we know so well, may have been the 'Tower of Babel' by which men sought to scale the highest heavens. Today computers hold out the promise of a means of instant translation of any code or language into any other code or language. The computer, in short, promises by technology a Pentecostal condition of universal understanding and unity.

"Elvet Gander," the jacket copy concludes, "accepts McLuhan's premise that language divides, but questions his hope that Pentecostal understanding will be found in technology, or primarily in technology. He has his own daring ideas about how such understanding may be re-created and renewed."

"Interesting," says Frederica.

"You must go and hear him speak," says Parrott. "He is charismatic. Truly charismatic."

"Charismatic" is a word he savours.

He finds four manuscripts from the slush heap for Frederica to read, all novels, one neatly typed with large spacing, one messily typed and dog-eared, one a single-spaced carbon and one handwritten. The neatly typed one is *The Voyage of the Silver Ship* by Richmond Bly. The dog-eared one is *Mad Dogs and Englishmen* by Bob Gully. The carbon is *A Thing Apart* by Margot Cherry. The handwritten one is *Daily Bread* by Phyllis K. Pratt and has an attached letter. "I am sorry to send you my book in a handwritten state. There is in fact a typewriter in this house, but it is not in a state that will produce anything more legible than my manuscript. I hope you will be able to read it, and look forward to hearing your opinion of it."

Frederica agrees to write brief reports on all these works. As they go home, Hugh says, "It would be better, really, to *write* a novel, Frederica."

She looks stricken.

"I know. I don't have any ideas. I've been educated out of it. Have you noticed people who write novels never studied English literature? They did philosophy, or classics, or history . . . or nothing. Even thinking of it brings on a kind of panic. The only kind of novel I could write is the sensitive-student-at-Cambridge kind of stuff I know enough to flinch at and *despise*—"

(Oh, but the bliss of talking about books, all the same, and not about houses, and things, and possessions.)

She is limping along at great speed. Her limp is more pronounced. Hugh says, "Does your leg hurt?"

"Yes. It won't heal. Thomas is sending me to his doctor."

Frederica sits down in the evening in the Bloomsbury flat—in fact, at the same desk at which Alexander wrote *The Yellow Chair*—and begins work on these manuscripts. She reads. She cooks supper with Thomas Poole, and she, Lizzie, Leo, Simon and Thomas eat stuffed pancakes and fruit salad (Waltraut is at her English class). Leo is more relaxed: Simon is a kindly boy, and has taken him under his wing. Alan Melville telephones: tomorrow he has arranged an interview for her at the Samuel Palmer School. There are two part-time courses to be taught, on metaphysical poetry and the nineteenth-century novel.

Frederica takes pleasure in writing her reports on the four novels.

The Voyage of the Silver Ship by Richmond Bly

> The plot of this work, if it can be called a plot, concerns the determination of a group of misfits and magical beings to rediscover the land of their origins, Eled-Durad-Or, which is believed to be the home of ancestral beings able to live for ever, to communicate without speech, and to change the material world by the power of thought. The world in which the group live (Bonodor) has been enslaved by a dark Enchanter (Miltan) who has covered it with disfiguring mills (nineteenth-century mills, to judge from the architecture), tall chimneys and fastnesses with drawbridges, fire-throwers etc. operated by grinding technology. On the outskirts of the industrial wasteland are a few stunted woods and some sooty rivers. The friends are summoned by mysterious messages to a gathering at a hill of dust and ashes. They are mostly known by descrip-

tions: the Tattered Man, the Hairy One, the Brownie, the Fool, the Half-Man (who is also half-goat), the Stone Spirit and Frog. This last is suspected throughout of being an emissary of the Enemy but turns out to be a sacrificial hero, whose grisly death in a stone doorway prevents the door from closing and makes it possible for the rest of the crew to enter Eled-Durad-Or.

It is hard to differentiate between these beings, since they all speak in the same high style and find much—possibly most—of their experience inept for putting into words, e.g.:

"Then was the Fool carried away into another sphere, where his spirit moved amongst the dark roots of the world like a blind being, and his whole body communicated with unutterable powers, so that he was nigh fainting because of his extreme apprehensions."

Many "adventures" are embarked on. There is a good scene where the crew are being hunted across an almost non-visionary i.e. almost concrete moorland by a pack of black dogs with red glittering eyes, and there is also a good scene, when, having managed to find the mooring place of the Silver Ship, they embark on the Utmost Sea and are becalmed amongst ice-floes and are attacked by a pod, or posse, or herd of dangerous narwhals which advance in gleaming and serried ranks, waving their horny lances. Mr. Bly is possibly more at home with herds of inarticulate creatures than with thinking human, or semi-human beings, or Frogs. There is little, even no, sexual interest in this tale. All the women (or female spirits) are inhabitants of, or visitants from, Eled-Durad-Or and are tall silvery figures with very beautiful belts who raise their arms frequently in interesting gestures I feel resemble the Dalcroze movements executed by Ursula and Gudrun by the lakeside in *Women in Love.* But nothing ever really *happens* to any of these characters. Every threat, even the great Borg on the Ice Mountain, dissolves into a visionary experience of the ineffable, and causes most of the characters to make long rhapsodic speeches. These could almost, but not quite, be scanned as blank verse, which makes them unpleasant to the inner ear.

This story obviously has ambitions to be like Tolkien—because of genuine admiration, I should guess, and not out of a desire to emulate his sales. But it entirely lacks his narrative urgency, physical weather, real earth. It also lacks his merry humour, which might be thought to be a good thing, but is not, I assure you. The story also has all sorts of echoes (unintentional, I imagine) of *The Wizard of Oz.* It is a curiously vacant work, whose driving force appears paradoxically to be the desire to create and people an imaginary world.

Mad Dogs and Englishmen by Bob Gully

I cannot believe there is not already a book with this title. If I were asked to imagine one, I might imagine this one, in a gloomy mood. It is, I suppose, a picaresque narrative and describes the adventures of a sour-tempered Englishman in his twenties called Johnny Hipp who is hitch-hiking his way round the south of France. He is being relentlessly pursued by an unfortunate girl from his home town (Preston, Lancs.) called Deanna, who has hairy legs, spots, mild halitosis, dirndl skirts, greasy hair and a wart on her chin which is the object of some would-be Joycean paragraphs of execration. From Deanna's handbag Johnny Hipp occasionally steals wads of currency. ("She does nothing to earn it and gets no pleasure from it and doesn't need it, whereas I am in urgent need, and know how to get pleasure from life with only a minimum of dough.") These thefts appear to be his only means of support, since he appears never to have worked, or done anything at all except bumming around and autostop. He is fed and housed by beautiful French and Italian women who stop their sports cars and take him up, apparently deducing from his unsavoury external appearance the rigour and dimensions of his "todger." They come in several colours, "silky raven," "shimmering platinum," "flaming *rousse,*" but have identical globular breasts, honey-pots, and sweet-smelling pubic hair. He tends to leave them because he has seen an even better one out of the window of a restaurant or Ferrari waiting at a petrol station.

There is a lot of food in this novel—mountainous cassoulets, wonderfully glistening aïolis, "brandad de morrue" (sic), "boullabaise" (sic) and so on. The meals are only a prelude to ravenous couplings, however, and the food is nothing beside the drink—mostly beer, oddly, considering the surrounding vineyards. But Johnny Hipp is also not averse to Pernod, Martini, white port, muscat, vin rosé (*faute de mieux*), cognac, armagnac, crème de menthe, Cointreau, Chartreuse and so on, all of which he regurgitates along with the food wherever convenient (or inconvenient). I have not done a page count but I think it is a damned close-run thing between copulation and vomiting. Any satire or irony is buried too deep beneath a sickly affection for Johnny Hipp and his stamina to be discerned. There is little dialogue. ("There was no need for mere words. I threw myself upon her and she opened wetly and the dialogue of bodies, disrupted by some mumblings and gruntings from my out-of-synch gut, began its rhythmic wallop.")

Johnny Hipp's own appearance is probably, to a dispassionate outsider, at least as repulsive as Deanna's is to him. He spends a lot of time lingering on the smells of his crotch, armpits and toenails, on his dirt-encrusted underwear, his filthy shoes, his stained shirts, his beard-stubble, as though these were all evidence of some goat-like virility mixed with honesty and lack of affectation which attract women as honey attracts flies (one of his own comparisons).

His geography is insecure. He would need a jet plane to get from Cannes to Nîmes in the time he allots to the journey; Vence is nowhere near Montpellier as far as I can remember, and much of the Camargue is not open to road-users.

The book, as you might suppose, ends exactly where it began, with Johnny Hipp, blear-eyed, hungover, belching and full of self-admiration waiting outside the gate of Aigues-Mortes (as he is when the book opens) to be picked up. Anyone in his senses (or her senses) would drive past quickly.

A Thing Apart by Margot Cherry

This novel is the history of a sensitive young working-class girl called Laura (she would not be called Laura if she were working class, and I suspect she is anyway lower-middle-class which everyone finds the least interesting origin, though it is what very many, perhaps most? people are). Laura gets a scholarship to Oxford to read English, and falls in love with a young man called Sebastian, who does not fall in love with her, and may even be in love with his best friend Hugh; they were at school together, in the army together, and are now very brilliantly reading English together, and acting at OUDS.

Laura spends several chapters agonising over whether or not to go to bed with various young men, and spends various *nuits blanches* with one or another. Her virginity is finally taken, not by Sebastian, but by Hugh (who is naturally smaller, stronger, more muscular, less dreamy than his willowy friend). We have here the beginning of a faintly interesting triangular relationship, of which Margot Cherry makes nothing, as she is interested in diagnosing who is "in love" with whom. Some narrative satisfaction might be gained if we were told whether Laura married Sebastian or Hugh or no one or someone else altogether, but we are not told: Oxford days come to an end, and everything is vague and shadowy and in the air.

This is the sort of novel every young woman at university reading English imagines she can write—though most ["most of us" Frederica writes honestly, and then crosses it out in the interest of impartiality and objectivity]—most don't have the stamina or determination actually to write all these hundreds of pages. There is something peculiarly touching about the details of daily life that Margot Cherry includes, even if her characters are stereotypes and sticks. She describes the bathtubs in Somerville College, water running down her arms when she punts, college gardens, electric kettles, coffee bars, the Bodleian library, as though these things had never been seen or described before. This has a curious effect on the reader, for they have in fact been described *so often* that they have a kind of banal mythic force, into which Margot Cherry's pale narrative drives suckers, and soaks up a kind of energy. This applies also, to a certain extent, to the emotions of the books, the empty *longing,* the clumsy negotiation of sexual decisions. I think on balance Margot Cherry can write, and might write well if she had something to write about.

And why is not Oxford, and young love, and Shakespeare *something,* I do ask myself. Because it fills me with a kind of nausea I suspect would not be peculiar to me. It is déjà vu in its youth and newness. It is a reason why sensitive young women should refrain from writing sensitive young novels about Oxbridge. All the same, having done these pages, she might do something else?

Daily Bread by Phyllis K. Pratt

This novel opens with a woman making bread. It describes the action of the living yeast, and the dough, which is beaten down and swells up. It describes the patience of waiting for dough to prove, it describes buns and loaves and hot cross buns in the oven.

The heroine of this book is a clergyman's wife in a Warwickshire village, who has thirteen children and is obsessed with bread-making. Her name is Peggy Crump. Her husband is the Reverend Evelyn Crump. She met him when they were both volunteers in refugee camps, and was converted to Christianity by the strength of his faith and its obvious useful life in the world. He was not advanced as he hoped—he is very irascible when not labouring in extreme situations—and they are now living in genteel near poverty in a backwater. Various incidents (a death from leukaemia, a pompous bishop, capital punishment, a vision of "*delightful emptiness*") cause Peggy to lose her faith in God, but Evelyn forces her to continue "as if" and indeed with all those children she has little choice.

The drama of this novel—and although it appears at first to be a storm in a teacup, it is a real drama—occurs when Evelyn himself has a dark night of the soul, and has a vision of the devil, who tells him a) that he himself, the devil, is a fiction and b) that Christianity is also a fiction, and that Evelyn must learn to live without fiction, in the world of death.

This vision reduces Evelyn to extremes of pessimism, sleep-walking, self-starvation, histrionic riddling sermonising and deliberately incompetent suicide bids. Peggy tells him, as he told her, that he should live "as if" and when he tells her that a consecrated priest can do no such thing, although it is quite all right for a housewife to do so, she attacks him, after premeditation, with a bread-knife, and there is a great deal of blood everywhere.

This novel is not a tragedy, and not a melodrama, but a peculiarly poised black comedy. There is a most wonderful comic jumble sale (an image of cosmic and social disorder and pointlessness), some sanely and rigorously observed teenagers, a sweet curate, a pugnacious donkey, a menacing baby and all sorts of other good things.

The book turns on the image of bread, in a completely satisfying way. The bulging life and expanding energy of Peggy's bread is contrasted with the communion wafer which is no longer the Host for the body of the Lord. It is almost (but not quite, not *tidily,* symbolic) as though the yeast cells were the true God, sustaining everything. The metaphor threads its way through the text, bobbing up in cucumber sandwiches, brioches at the bishop's palace, mould and penicillin.

I think you should read this book and consider it carefully. It made me laugh and it made my hair stand on end. Also, it made me feel that the English language can *say* things, deep, funny, difficult things—something in which I was beginning to lose faith after reading the other three books.

When Frederica has finished writing these reports she feels a kind of complicated glee. It has many components: she has enjoyed the act of writing, of watching language run black out of the end of her pen; this has in turn made her feel that she is herself again, and has made her body real to her, because her mind is alive. And then there is the idea of money, however little, money earned, which is independence. And then there is pleasure, not only in Phyllis K. Pratt's handwritten bombshell, but also in the industry of Bly, Gully and Cherry, who have felt writing to be important enough to sit down day after day or night after night and invent imagined worlds as though it mattered. And this pleasure in turn makes her feel more tolerant towards Olive and Rosalind and Pippy Mammott, now they are no longer the bounds of her world—because of them she recognises Peggy Crump's imprisonment with a strong savouring, whereas Margot Cherry's Laura seems infinitely far away.

Thomas Poole knocks at her door and tells her supper is ready. He has cooked it: it is gammon and spinach and béchamel. Frederica tries to describe to him her pleasure in writing the reports. She says, "I love having something to do I *can do.* And I love it that all these people have done all this work even if it's hopeless. Is that silly?"

"Oh no," says Poole. "Pleasure in use of energy, I know that so well. Like when a rather stolid boy at school would suddenly write twelve pages instead of one, and you saw his mind was *going.* It was enough."

"I must *work,*" says Frederica. "It kills you, unused energy, it turns against you."

She thinks of the yeast.

"I like to see you smiling," says Poole. He hesitates. "I am so glad you have come here. It seems odd, when I remember you—such a cross girl, such a wayward girl, such a puzzle to your father. And now a woman, with Leo, and here."

Frederica smiles with a little constraint, pleased and bothered by the word "woman."

They have a good supper together. They talk about Phyllis K. Pratt, and Elvet Gander, and about why sensitive young women should not write novels. They do not talk about Nigel. But soon they must.

Bill Potter is rewriting his lecture on *Mansfield Park.* He has been giving extra-mural classes on *Mansfield Park* now for thirty years, not every year, but most, and he always rewrites his lecture, partly out of courtesy to the new students, who deserve more than stale repetition, partly because his relations with this secret and sad text change constantly and slowly, like a man's relations with his own family. He is thinking about Sir Thomas Bertram, who paid insufficient attention to his daughters' moral upbringing, but is able to make a satisfactory substitute family from his wife's sister's son and daughters, the Prices. He thinks with love of his grandchildren who live with him.

Outside, the village is quiet. A car purrs in the distance, expands its roar, and does not pass, but stops. The door bell sounds. Bill supposes Winifred will answer, but she appears not to be there. It rings again, and he goes to open the door.

It takes him a moment to recognise his son-in-law, Nigel Reiver. He sees a stocky man in a scarlet polo neck and a tweed jacket over cavalry twill trousers. Nigel sees a gnome-like old man, with a few strands of flyaway grey-and-ginger hair and sharp, faded blue eyes.

"I want to speak to Frederica."

"Well, you've come to the wrong place. She isn't here."

"I think she is. I've come instead of using the telephone, because I worked out you'd say she wasn't there, or she might not want to speak to me. I have to speak to her."

"Young man, you have written yourself a story in your head that bears no relation to fact. I didn't know she wasn't with you until you just told me. I'm sorry she hasn't come here, if she's seen fit to go away, but she hasn't."

"I don't believe you," says Nigel. Bill sees he is what he thinks of as "all worked up." "I'm coming in, to look for her. She's got to talk to me. And I want Leo."

"I can't help you," says Bill. "And if I could, I wouldn't. What sort of a life are you making her lead?"

"A very comfortable life," says Nigel. "Would you mind getting out of the way? I'm coming in, to look for my wife and son."

"I don't tell lies," says Bill. "They aren't here."

He tries to shut the door. Nigel's face works. He pushes the door open with such force that Bill's head is crushed against the rough wall behind it. Bill, grazed, bleeding and dizzy, falls to his knees in the hall before Nigel, who immediately puts his arms round him, murmuring frantic and inarticulate apologies, touching the grazed scalp with horrified fingers. They stagger, in a kind of embrace, into the kitchen, where Nigel, curiously efficient, finds a clean tea-towel and begins to bathe his father-in-law's head.

Bill says, with quavering sharpness, "Look about you. Do you see any sign of them? Go through the house if you must, now you've forced your way in. You won't find them."

Nigel is indeed staring round the kitchen, almost *smelling,* it appears, for traces of the lost. He does make a dash into the hall, at this invitation, and Bill hears him crashing doors on the upper landings. Blood trickles into Bill's eyes. Nigel reappears, carrying a green, full-skirted dress.

"This is hers."

"It is. It's been here since she went off to be married. Cast-off. We've got a cupboardful. Think if you've seen her in it."

"I'll take it."

"As you please. Shouldn't think she wants to see it again."

"I'm sorry I hurt you."

"It's easy to be sorry after the event," says Bill, and stops short. It is a sentence often said to Bill by others. He looks more closely at Nigel, and dabs blood with a dirty handkerchief from his brows.

"No—use mine—it's clean," says Nigel. He sits down on a stool, at the corner of the table, next to Bill.

"She ran away in the night. With Leo. I hadn't been too nice to her. I'm going to be better. I get, I get carried away. *You know,*" says Nigel, recognising that Bill, *mutatis mutandis,* does in a way, know. Bill does not reply. He dabs busily with Nigel's handkerchief.

"I was sure she'd have come up here. That's what women do. They go back to their mothers. I waited a bit—I was so furious, I felt I needed to calm down and think—I thought it out."

"Frederica doesn't do what 'most women' do."

"I don't know how to start finding her friends. I'll kill them. I'll kill them all—"

"She won't thank you for *that*."

"I love her. She knows I love her. And how can she have taken Leo? He was happy. He had a happy time. He'll be all bewildered and upset. Children need homes, and routines. He *belongs in my house.* She can't just take him from me, in the middle of the night, with no discussion, no warning, no message, no—"

"You don't appear to be very good at *discussion,*" says Bill.

Nigel glowers at him.

"I'll go now." He looks anxious. "Will you be all right? Should I stay till someone comes? Do you feel faint?"

"No," says Bill, who does feel faint. "I shall be very glad if you do go. Now, if you will."

"Will you let me know if you hear—if they are all right, if they need money or anything, if—"

"I will do as Frederica wishes," says Bill. "As you should know."

Marcus, coming home for lunch, sees a man outside his house arranging a green party-dress like a fainted woman in the back seat of a green Aston Martin. He watches it drive off, skilful but far too fast, back through the village.

The General Election finally comes on October 15th. Frederica and Thomas Poole watch the results together on the television, along with Hugh and Alan, who have no televisions, and Alexander, who has taken to dropping in more frequently since the arrival of Frederica and Leo. Poole himself is a literary man not naturally inclined to want a television in his house—he fears it as self-indulgence, he is puritanically inclined to regard it as a waste of time. But he has been talked into it by his children, who claim to be social pariahs at school because they cannot discuss *Batman* and *Top of the Pops.* Tony Watson is in Huyton for Harold Wilson's count; he is writing an in-depth analysis of the effects of television on elections, and is full of exasperated admiration for Wilson's ability to adjust his television appearances, his shape, his message, to what the opinion polls tell him. The election is very close, and it is not clear until the next afternoon that the Labour Party has in fact achieved an effective overall majority of five. The friends eat chilli con carne and drink a great deal of red wine. Frederica thinks often, but does not speak, of Olive and Rosalind and Pippy Mammott watching with bated breaths the fluctuations in the fate of "our people" as the balance sways. They are the enemy; the Conservative Government is somehow involved in sleaze and failure and ridicule, in the prancing of Christine Keeler and Mandy Rice-Davies, in a huge gap between public and private fronts, in deceit and humiliation. She is ready to like Wilson, suddenly seen at midnight waving his arms wildly, in the crowded hall at Huyton. He has trebled his majority. He kisses his wife for the cameras. Behind him can be seen the large, gleeful face of Owen Williams.

"He wanted to marry me," Frederica announces. "I wonder what would have happened if I—"

"I should think it would have been horrible," says Alan, placidly. "He's wedded to his politics, you'd have had to be a Hostess, you'd have hated it."

Hugh says, uncharacteristically sharply, "It was just Cambridge. Everybody felt they had to snap up somebody. A lot of misery was caused, a lot of silly misery. There were too few women, everyone was silly."

Frederica is vaguely hurt. Harold Wilson beams manically at the camera. It is at this point still quite possible that he has lost the election.

Alexander says, "If he wins, I wonder if he will disband my committee. I was beginning to think we were doing something useful. We have become, so to speak, bonded. We are a Group, I am interested. I want to go on. We're visiting primary schools all next week. Like Brobdingnagians. I'm learning things."

Nobody has any thoughts to offer on this. They separate in the small hours, mildly drunk, mildly contented. Thomas and Frederica see them out at the door of the flat, like a married couple. Thomas puts an arm round Frederica's shoulder. She does not break free, but does not respond to the gesture.

"Do you think Hugh Pink is in love with you?" Thomas asks Frederica.

"No," she says. "He was once, I think, but as he says, everyone was in love with everyone, especially women. We thought we were special and we were only scarce."

"Were you in love with him?"

"Oh no. I was in love with Raphael Faber. Or with the idea of Raphael Faber. The unattainable, you know, the teacher, the tabu, the monastic. I could *feel* a lot and nothing happened. It's far away."

"You've changed," says Thomas Poole. He thinks a moment, and then pulls her towards him and kisses the top of her hair, softly. He releases her.

"Good night. Sleep well."

"And you. Tomorrow we shall be in the new white-hot technological world. Or not."

They are.

On the steps of the Samuel Palmer School of Art and Craft, the word "portal" comes into Frederica's mind, seeming odd and bristling, as words do when they detach themselves and insist. The School does indeed have an imposing portal, which has a whole paragraph to itself in Pevsner's architectural guide to London. It is a long stone building which takes up the whole of one side of Lucy Square, which is next to Queen's Square beyond Russell Square and Southampton Row. The front is adorned with bas-reliefs by Eric Gill and the portal, reached by a flight of wide, shallow steps, is set deep in a round stone arch, at either side of which stand Adam and Eve, life-size, also carved by Gill, both holding apples and both smiling as though the Fall were a matter of little or no consequence. The arch above them is composed of serried ranks of flying figures, though whether these are angels, genii or fairies is not wholly clear. The handles of the two heavy dark doors are brass castings of a sphinx and a mermaid, both with golden breasts rubbed bright by constant touching.

"Portal," says Frederica to Alan Melville. "This qualifies as a portal. It's a queer word, portal."

"'Beauty is momentary in the mind—/The fitful tracing of a portal;/But in the flesh it is immortal,'" says Alan, grasping the brass breast of the sphinx.

"I may have been thinking of Lady Chatterley quoting Swinburne," says Frederica. "She goes on about 'Pale beyond porch and portal' and how she has to go through them. Something to do with Proserpina coming up from the earth."

They are in the building, which is, and is not, like any teaching institution. There are long corridors and staircases—all solid and stony, made to endure—and a faint whiff of the institutional smell of polish and disinfectant. But the corridors are also lined with paintings, bright abstracts, Pop portraits of singers and filmstars, Blake-like clouds of flying bodies, collages of masks. And the smell of disinfectant is drowned by the smells of the work itself—oil, turpentine, putty, hot metal. Alan is telling her about Liberal Studies.

"I always said I would never teach," says Frederica. "But it will be nice to be working with you."

The Head of Liberal Studies has a panelled office, with bright colour-spattered linen curtains (made by the textiles students). He offers Frederica coffee in a tomato-red cup (made by the ceramics students) and looks through her CV, which she and Thomas Poole have expertly put together. He is a large and handsome man, with what Frederica's mother would have called a sweet face, bright blue eyes, great wings of groomed black-and-white-streaked hair, and a soft, smiling mouth. He is wearing a blue corduroy suit and a red knitted silk tie. Round the room, three deep, are paintings and prints with beautifully lettered verses and quotations underneath them, all of which Frederica sees are from Blake. An abstract of splashes: "Exuberance is Beauty." A rather childlike face on a blue starry ground: "He whose face gives no light, shall never become a star." Trees, a huge collage: "A fool sees not the same tree that a wise man sees." An eye: "One thought fills immensity." "The tygers of wrath are wiser than the horses of instruction." There is also a large, Piranesi-derived etching, with the verse

Such are Cathedron's golden Halls in the City of Golgonooza.
And Los's Furnaces howl loud, living, self-moving, lamenting
With fury and despair, and they stretch from South to North
Thro' all the Four Points. Lo! The Labourers at the Furnaces
Rintrah and Palambron, Theotormon and Bromion, loud lab'ring
With the innumerable multitudes of Golgonooza round the Anvils of Death!

"Golgonooza" is a word that has always annoyed Frederica. It is infant-babble, not true language-forging. It is unintentionally comic. The Head of Liberal Studies murmurs "Impressive" as he reads the CV, and looks up to see her studying the varied images.

"I make Blake the centre of my teaching here. He is the greatest English poet and the greatest English painter. He draws the mind out of itself. The students find him inspirational. Over the years I have made this collection of their tributes to his genius—as you can see, the styles are diverse, but the source is One. I like to employ creative people. Do you write yourself, Miss Potter?"

(Frederica has decided to return to her maiden name.)

"No, I'm afraid not. Studying English literature knocks the desire out of you. But it might be different here—where everyone is making things."

"There is a special atmosphere. I try to write myself. I think if one is entrusted with the minds of creative people one should at least try to create oneself, don't you think?"

"Oh, yes."

"I have been inspired by the Prophetic Books."

Frederica, unguarded, begins, "I could never stomach the Prophetic Books because the language is ugly—whereas the Songs of Innocence—"

He smiles forgivingly. "I think you will find upon closer attention that the language does have a beauty all of its own, a peculiar beauty. A *free* beauty—free, as he said, of the monotonous Cadence—the *bondage*—the fetters of rhyme and blank verse. 'Poetry Fetter'd Fetters the Human Race.' You need an ear made new. It is visionary—the vision of Albion and the Druids as the foundation and source for the Hebrew religion—"

"It's an interesting myth," says Frederica, trying to read the dedication of a rather wistful water-colour of the invisible worm in the heart of the Rose.

"Or truth, or true myth," he says smilingly, as she deciphers the dedication.

"To Richmond Bly, who taught me to understand the infinite nature of Desire, with admiration and love from Marigold Topping."

Frederica whitens momentarily as her gleeful dissection of *The Voyage of the Silver Ship* rises in total recall to her mind. She swallows nervously. Richmond Bly does not notice. He is offering Frederica a year's part-time employment, on probation, and an office in which to see students and write lectures. Alan will take her to see it.

Up, up, up. The solid, shallow-stepped staircase hugs the wall of the Samuel Palmer School. It is wide—large objects are regularly carried up and down it. It has an elegant wrought-iron balustrade and its steps are worn in the centres, reminding Frederica of external processional staircases for monks. The staircase is dark, but at the top are the studios, roofed with glass, full of light. Alan takes Frederica through these, to the end of the building, past flashes of colour, past pools of dark and light, in the smell of oil and acrylic and turpentine and spirits. In the last airy space, in the centre, stands a strange object, surrounded by a swarm of students in black, tight clothes, and two men in jeans with what seem to be projectors of some kind. The object is a huge flask, or retort, or diving bell, with rounded sides rising to a kind of funnel into which one of the projectors appears to be pouring coloured light. As Frederica watches, this light changes from red-gold to cyan blue, and then to indigo, and then to acid yellow, and then to rose-pink. The walls of the retort or cask are painted matt black with variegated shapes and sizes of portholes out of which shimmer ribbons and flashes of changing coloured light. The light has a thick, liquid quality. The students are armed with black cardboard tubes, or periscopes, and drawing pads, and are peering in where they can, some crouched at low portholes, some perched on high stools. The operations are being directed by a burly man with not much hair, in a paint-streaked and unravelling mariner's sweater in oiled wool. Alan introduces this person, who seems to know and like Alan, as Desmond Bull, who is a painter, in charge of the Foundation Year. "This is Frederica Reiver—Potter—" says Alan. "She's going to teach literature."

"Good luck to her," says Desmond Bull.

"Can I look at what you are doing?"

"Please. Go up to the top, the view's best from there. Matthew here invented these coloured lights—he's got all sorts of oils inside jars and frames—it's a kind of instructive colour-happening. Come up this ladder."

Frederica climbs up, and peers in. The diving bell appears to be full of liquid light, but it is only air, somehow dense with colour. The background colour changes and is traversed by shoals of green spots, or golden streaks or waving lines of crimson and emerald. So delightful, so mesmerising, is the play of energy, light and colour that it takes Frederica some time to see that something is coiled below the imaginary depths, a wavering trousse of hair, or seaweed, a smooth succession of stones, or limbs, hard to fix, hard to discern, as it shifts from gold to green to sky blue.

"Is it a sculpture?" she asks, delighted, and is answered by a voice from the depths, plangent and twanging. "No. It is a living creature. The Human Form Divine, precisely. Any movement is illusory. I am a professional."

"You can come out now," says Desmond Bull. "Coffee-break time."

Frederica retreats from the brim of the flask. Whoever is inside gives a little jump, and clasps the edge of the tank with long greyish fingers, distinctly grey, once out of the coloured light, though whether intrinsically grey or by contrast is hard to say. A head then appears above the rim, a head long, long, with a long, fine nose, hooded eyes and a thin mouth, a head clothed and veiled in long, iron-grey hair, dead-straight, smooth, long, iron-grey hair that cloaks the shoulders and bust as they rise, so that it is impossible to see whether this is a man or a woman. A long, grey leg, sinewy and thin, is then hoist over the edge of its prison, also cloaked in the long, grey threads, and then the strange figure, all blue-grey in the daylight, is perched briefly on the edge, jumps down, and advances towards Frederica on tall, thin legs moving amongst its tent of hair. Frederica's eyes focus on the genitals, which a swing of the hair-curtain, accidental or deliberate, reveals to be male, rather small, clouded by iron-grey pubic hair. The creature holds out a bony hand.

"Jude," he says.

"Frederica," says Frederica, registering a not very nice smell, a smell of fish, of old frying pans, of rancid oils.

"A very ancient, fish-like smell," says Jude, in his high-pitched, cultivated voice. Frederica feels a frisson of distaste, and catches him looking at her, waiting for just such a frisson. When he has noted it, he turns away, and moves towards the folding chair by the studio heater, three roses of red elements on a metal stalk. He extends his grey hands into the red light, turns a thin grey shank in the rose. The skin on his ribs, the skin on his buttocks, hangs in sculpted folds, not flapping, but folded, like the plated armour of a rhinoceros. Students bring him coffee in plastic cups and offer him biscuits, which he refuses. A whole group gather at his feet.

Alan takes Frederica into her little office, which is a partitioned-off corner of the high studio, still under the studio lights, and with a white table and a good anglepoise, not a desk. The chair is pink moulded plastic, with hands, feet, and a microcephalic head for her own head to rest against, its long-lashed eyelids closed, its red mouth pursed to kiss.

"Who was *that*?" says Frederica to Alan.

"Jude. Jude Mason. Not his real name, I suspect. He's a bit of a mystery man, a bit of a poseur. No one knows where he lives or where he comes from. He doesn't say much, but occasionally he lectures the students on Nietzsche. They like him. They listen to him. He turns up for some sessions and asks for modelling work, and then he vanishes, and then he returns. Art school models are hard to come by, and he's reliable."

"He looks like Gollum. Or Blake's Nebuchadnezzar only thinner."

"He's not very pro-Blake. He gets into arguments with Richmond Bly's Blake-clique or -claque. He prefers Nietzsche."

"Which reminds me of something awful." Frederica recounts the story of *The Voyage of the Silver Ship.* She cannot resist making it funny. It is funny, funny and sad. She says, "When I saw the mills of Golgonooza I knew. I should have listened to you telling me his *name,* but I obviously couldn't bear to hear it. What can I *do*?"

"Keep very quiet," says Alan. "Tell nobody else, no matter how tempting—you always talked too much, my dear, and I'm glad to see it coming back to you, but resist, resist. Forget the Silver Ship and all who sail in her."

"You never talk too much," says Frederica, turning her attention to her friend. All the way through Cambridge, she would ask herself, and occasionally him, who he loved, what he loved, and never came up with an answer. He is neat, and fair, and kindly, and she is sure of his friendship, and sure she does not know him. She likes this state of affairs.

"What is it like," she asks him, beglamourised by her surroundings, by the other-side-of-the-mirror world beyond the portals. "What is it like, teaching art history to artists?"

"Horrible," says Alan. "They think the dead are dead, and irrelevant to their own problems, or worse, threatening to their *originality.* Well, not all of them. Most. You'll see. It's quite testing. It tests your own reasons for caring about Raphael. Or Giotto, or Piero della Francesca. But they tend to vote with their feet, so you don't always have the pleasure of arguing the toss with them. That's one thing. Another is that places like this are run on the energies of part-timers, paid low rates for piece-work. If they don't come, you've got no class, no course and *no money.*"

"All the same," says Frederica. "It's alive, here."

V

Alexander's fears that the new Labour Government might disband the Steerforth Committee prove to be unnecessary. What happens is that two new members are added, to give it a more popular aspect. Like all committees, this one is a mixture of the relevant Great and Good from some perennial Civil Service list, and judiciously balanced professionals in its field. The original list was as follows:

Professor Sir Philip Steerforth	Chairman, holder of a personal Chair in Anthropology in Glasgow University
Professor Gerard Wijnnobel	Vice-Chancellor of the University of North Yorkshire, grammarian and polymath
Dr. Naomi Lurie	Reader in English at Oxford, author of *Various Traditions of Meditational Verse* (1955) and of *Dissociated Sensibility, Myth or History?* (1960)
Alexander Wedderburn	Playwright, Producer, BBC Educational Television
Malcolm Friend	Journalist and broadcaster
Hans Richter	Physicist, now employed by Eurobore Oil Company
Arthur Beaver	Head of Child Development, Institute of Education, Chester University
Emily (Milly) Perfitt	Children's book writer
Auriol Worth	Headmistress, St. Clare's School for Girls, Dorking

Guy Croom	Headmaster, Botton Grammar School, Derbyshire
Alex Swinburn	Head of English, Goldengrove Comprehensive School, Croydon
Louis Roussel	Psychologist
Walter Priest	Devonshire LEA English adviser
Walter Bishop	Acting Head, Conisborough Teacher Training College

To these the new government had added:

Mickey Impey	Liverpool poet and performer
Roger Magog	Freelance writer and teacher, author of twenty-seven books, including *The Sacramental Calling* (1956), an account of the transformation of a secondary modern school English group after being encouraged to write "freely"

There are also Civil Servants in attendance: Aubrey Wace, the Secretary of the Committee, and his assistant, Agatha Mond.

The brief of the committee is to make recommendations for the teaching of English language in both primary and secondary schools. This brief included attention to areas where small wars are raging: the teaching of reading—sound or sight?; the usefulness or harm of teaching grammar; freedom of expression against correctness and conformity to rules. In his preliminary speech to the committee, sitting uneasy and inhibited round a board table in the Ministry of Education, Philip Steerforth said:

"Language and children are two things we might say previous generations in our culture took for granted. We have made both problematic, and made them objects of intense study. Between us we bring to bear a formidable array of expertise and talent in both fields, that is, child development and education, and the study of the nature and behaviour of language itself. We must be philosophically rigorous, and we must also be intensely *practical;* otherwise we shall be sitting here in another twenty years, for both subjects are young, are in transition and flux, and our work may be *helpful* but cannot hope to be definitive. Let us also remember that we are, many of us, parents, and consult our hopes and fears and understandings from that source."

The work of the committee is divided into two kinds: the gathering of evidence and consultation with teachers, and the debates in the Ministry. There is also the evidence, which pours in by the sackful, passionately written pleas for grammar, for the abolition of grammar, for learning poetry, for learning nothing ever again "by rote," for "look and say," for sonics, for mixed-ability teaching, for remedial teaching, for the gifted child, for the non–native speaker. There is a brief moment when Alexander surveys this mass of passionate paper like a cool human observer, knowing that he is about to become part of it, that he is about to join the battle and the battlefield.

He does not wholly know why he agreed to join the committee. Partly, he was flattered to be asked. Partly, he is interested in language; it is the medium of what he still thinks of as his art. Partly, his art is not going well. He wants to write differently, and does not know how. There is a new life in the theatre, and it is not one that bears any relation to the lyrical richness of his one great success, the 1953 verse-drama, *Astraea*. The new theatre is based on Artaud's Theatre of Cruelty. It believes, not in measured verse, but in "shattering language in order to shatter life." It is a theatre of blood, of screams, of bodily extremity. It is iconoclastic in a mannered way. Glenda Jackson has appeared as Christine Keeler, stripped, bathed, and ritually clothed as a convict to the recitation of the words of the Keeler court case. She has then appeared, to the same chanted words, as Jacqueline Kennedy, preparing herself for the funeral of the President. This has been followed by *The Persecution and Assassination of Marat as Performed by the Inmates of Charenton under the Direction of the Marquis de Sade.*

Alexander, the man, was moved and appalled by the production, by the writhings and moanings and ritual head-bangings of the impersonators of the insane: by the concatenation of the artist-Marquis and the tormented revolutionary, by Jackson again, a wildly erotic Charlotte Corday beating de Sade with her long hair. He also feels that *it is not good* to release such violence as spectacle. And beyond that, secretly, he thinks "childish." But what is "childish"? The child is wiser than the man, in the thought of this time. He is old, he is out of date, he once believed in contemplation, in singing rhythms, in thinking things out, and all this is swept away by this new bleeding, and howling. It may sound bathetic to say that he joined the committee also to observe the drama of the politics of groups, but it is so; there may be an idea there.

The consultation process is wide-ranging. The committee is too large to crowd into any classroom or staffroom, so it divides itself into platoons, which make local forays, north, south, east and west, visiting schools in Wales and the Fens, in Cumberland and Dumfriesshire, in Devon and in Belfast. Alexander manages to attach himself to a group which is to be based for two nights in York, and will visit primary schools in Leeds and Freyasgarth, grammar schools and comprehensive schools in Calverley and Northallerton. He has chosen this group partly because it will enable him to see Bill Potter, whose grandchildren's primary school, at Alexander's suggestion, is one of the chosen ones. He has also chosen it because it will be organised and accompanied by Agatha Mond, the young Principal from the Ministry of Education.

The rest of the group are Professor Wijnnobel, Hans Richter, Louis Roussel, Auriol Worth and the two new members, Mickey Impey and Roger Magog.

Alexander manages to travel from London to York with Agatha Mond. She is a darkly beautiful woman, around thirty, he thinks. She says little, and keeps her head down, studying the papers in front of her. Her hair is long and straight and worn in a loose bun. Her eyelashes are long and black. Her hands are fine. She is perhaps a little thin, and looks perhaps a little sad and withdrawn. She is Alexander's type; he recognises her; a woman reluctantly self-sufficient with a secret anxiety, or fear, under her cool look. All the women he has loved have been like this, quick dark women with potential passion. Except Frederica. He does not like to think about the very brief period when Frederica enforced love from him. He sits opposite Agatha Mond and watches her arrange her papers, as the London suburbs go past, and the edge of the Midlands. He fetches her a cup of coffee and observes that early rising is tiring. He asks if she has far to come.

"I live in Kennington. It isn't too bad. I get claustrophobic in the Tube."

"I can walk to King's Cross. I am fortunate. I live alone."

"I live with my daughter," says Agatha, answering his question precisely. "She is four. I have to make arrangements for her when I go on these visits, and of course I worry about her. She has just started at a local nursery school."

"Her father?" says Alexander, who has already observed that there is no wedding ring.

"She has no father," says Agatha Mond. She does not elaborate. After a moment she says, "Careers for women are not easy in this country. One of the odder and more humane provisions of the British Civil Service is that women may have up to three illegitimate children, with maternity leave, and no questions asked. It is unexpected. And useful."

"Indeed. But your life must be very strenuous."

"It is not easy. But it is quite manageable. I am very fortunate to have this job."

They ride on in companionable silence. Alexander says, "What are our new recruits like?"

"You must form your own judgement. Mickey Impey did begin a degree course at Liverpool, but dropped out. He performs at the Cavern and the teachers and children get very excited to hear he is coming. They ask for him to recite his poetry. I suppose no harm can come of that."

"And Magog?"

"Don't ask. He writes to the department every week, with new ideas for educational initiatives. When this committee was first mooted, he wrote suggesting himself as an obvious member. Civil servants react badly to that kind of thing. He may be quite all right. He just seemed—overwhelming. But it was not felt that we could—at the present juncture—resist any suggestion of the new Minister. It was thought better to absorb him."

"Now you look very official."

"I love the impersonal verbs. 'It was not felt.' So useful."

"Elegant and stuffy."

"Exactly."

"I don't think you are stuffy."

"Oh, I have to be. I have to be. Actually, I like it."

When they get to Doncaster, he says, "It must be very interesting for you, to do this work, with a four-year-old child."

"I talk to her like a watermill. I hear so much about the need to talk, and *how* to talk. I exhaust her with talking." She laughs, and then frowns. "I love her too much, because I'm on my own. I try not to talk about her but I think about her all the time."

Alexander thinks of saying: I have a son who thinks he is another man's son. But he does not say it. He thinks: Here is someone to whom I might say it, one day. But maybe she thinks I am an old buffer, a has-been. Maybe she is being kind to me. He has never had to worry about this before.

Just before York, she says, "I've been wanting to tell you. I once acted in a production of *Astraea.* It was OUDS, at Oxford. I was doing research at the time. I was Bess Throckmorton. I married Walter Raleigh. I loved it."

"When it was first put on," says Alexander, "I was in love with the woman who played Bess Throckmorton."

She too was his type, dark, secret, smouldering.

"I fell in love with Edmund Spenser, but it came to nothing," says Agatha Mond. "Short and sweet, a midsummer's night."

They are at York. They step out into the station. Alexander takes Agatha's bag. As they get into the taxi, he says, "What is your daughter's name?"

"Saskia. She doesn't look like her, like Rembrandt's Saskia. She looks like me. But I always think of Saskia as *complete,* somehow. It's a name of good omen."

They are becoming friends, Alexander feels. He is alive. Yes, he is alive.

Their first visit is to the Star Primary School in a Leeds suburb. They are driven there from the Dean Court Hotel in York. Alexander is not able to sit next to Agatha Mond, who is having a serious discussion in the front seat with Professor Wijnnobel about the grammar evidence. Wijnnobel is too tall to fit comfortably into a minibus seat: he stoops, and inclines his large face gravely. Hans Richter sits behind Alexander, who is one of the few people he talks voluntarily to. He wears a business suit, and has well-cut grizzled grey hair and a neat, unremarkable face, with glasses. Louis Roussel sits at the back of the bus, away from Wijnnobel, to whom he is ideologically opposed. He is a little man, dark and birdlike, energetic and short-tempered. The two new members sit apart from each other and everyone else, as new members usually do. Roger Magog looks suspiciously around at the others, sussing them out, summing them up, at once self-conscious about their probable attitudes to him, and vaguely believing that his scrutinising self is invisible. Alexander wonders how he himself knows all this. Magog wears a shabby off-white polo neck under a shapeless tweed jacket, the garments of a slightly passé authenticity. His thinning hair is pale red, and his fat curly beard is dark russet.

The Liverpool poet is very pretty, with a mane of buttercup-coloured curls, a sweet full mouth, and huge innocent blue eyes. He is wearing a collarless jacket over a bright blue shirt that intensifies his eyes. He has been very pleasant to everyone so far, helping the women up the bus step, standing aside for the older men. The other woman is Auriol Worth, the headmistress, dressed like a headmistress in a good-looking navy suit and white shirt. Her face is precise and professionally observant. She is about fifty. She looks so like a headmistress that it is hard to make anything of her. She says to Alexander, of the poet, as they wait on the pavement, "If I had that one in my class I'd keep a special eye on him."

The Star Primary School is called the Star because of its revolutionary architecture. The committee has come to see it because it is new and exciting. It is wholly glass-walled, and is built in the shape of a star. It is wholly open-plan: the children gather in little, impromptu-looking groups, in one or another arm of the star, bringing with them their brightly coloured bean bags, their plastic stools, their little tables. They are grouped not by age, nor by subject, but by some sort of self-directed choice of activity. A group is making coiled clay pots. Older children are helping younger ones. A group is pouring and measuring water to and from a series of plastic containers, solemnly measuring and recording the heights of the contents. Little ones are pouring. Older ones are measuring. Still older ones are making a graph of the measurements. In another arm of the star children are watching snails climb the walls of a glass tank and are drawing the horns, the mouth, the foot. Small people dart busily and loudly from open space to open space, calling out, "We *urgently* need a wooden spoon," or "Mandy's gone and done it *again.*" Someone is playing the recorder in one star-tip, and someone near her is banging a drum. Because there are no classroom or corridor walls the children's work is on display on easels and noticeboards in the centre. There is a display of portraits of "My Family," and a table with the children's weekly newspapers displayed. There is a book corner in one aisle with a round bookcase, a lot of cushions, and a casual heap of books beside them. There is a lot of noise. It is, on the whole, purposive noise, shrill, variegated, busy, but loud. Alexander—like many of the older members of the committee—is moved by the contrast with his own schooldays. These little children, brightly clothed, free-moving, are different beings from the cowed, subservient, watchful little boy he remembers as himself. One inevitable effect on all the committee members who are not professional teachers, and even on those, like Alexander, who were and are not, is fear, the old cold terror of the school building, of power, of authority, of judgement. In places like this, that is gone. A little girl appears with a piece of bobbin knitting; she says, "Excuse me, I think I've dropped a stitch, it's all gone funny, like moth-holes, I wonder if you could put it right." He takes her darning needle, he prods at the wool. She expects his help as her right. He notes the analogy "like moth-holes."

All the same, he has the beginnings of a headache, from the noise. Where are the corners where a child such as he was might hide, might crouch and read? There are no hiding places. It is all open, all group life.

Auriol Worth is talking to the headmaster, an enthusiastic young man, young for a headmaster, who is able to talk to her quite coherently about the degree to which the children select their activities and the degree to which he suggests and complicates them, whilst keeping up a running conversation with passing children and teachers, like a juggler with a stream of green and orange balls, never confusing them. "I think you're bored with clay, Cilla, I think you should go and join in Miss Morrissey's group, which is talking and writing about amphibians. Everyone always thinks they want to do clay, but actually you need to do a *lot* of things in a day.

"Never mind, Heather. I expect Mr. Dinsdale thought you were upsetting the others. If you come to me at break I'll explain how to measure squares and then you won't feel left out.

"We try to let them dictate the pace and the interest, Miss Worth, but of course we must have things difficult enough to attract and occupy the ablest."

"And what about peer-pressure *not* to attempt the difficult?"

"Ah, there we have to be cunning. We have to disguise the difficulty."

"So you don't encourage ambition, as such."

"We disapprove of competitiveness. We like co-operation. Everyone has his or her talent, which we try to foster."

"And you are not flat on your face with exhaustion at the end of the day?"

"Often." He laughs. "But it's worth it."

Roger Magog is studying the project on "My Family." He says to Roussel, who is passing, "How significant that all these mothers appear to be angry. 'My Mum screming.' 'My Mummy shouted at me.' All these little children draw their mothers with a big, open mouth and a stick body. Only her screaming mouth matters."

"Little children have a very simple scheme of human beings in their drawings," says Roussel. "They learn bodies and hands and faces later. The older children have parents with bodies."

"My dad has a big stik," says Magog. "My dad has a Big ball. He threw the big ball hard at me. It hurt."

"It probably did," says Roussel.

"Sticks and balls and dads," says Magog. "How direct, how innocent, how clear. And the mums screaming. The modern family. Sad."

"Not necessarily."

"Oppressive. 'Go to bed, says Mum. I wont I say I wont. You will says my mum is ther no pease. I hate bed. I want to stay up all nite.' "

"Interesting," says Wijnnobel behind him, "that *e* on nite. The child knows how to elongate the vowel, even in a misspelling."

Alexander is trying to find a group of children who will be doing what Simon Poole might at this moment be doing. He finds a writing group with a young teacher. They have their "newsbooks" and their personal dictionaries, which they carry about in little cotton bags, since there are no desks. They write and talk and take their work to the teacher, who gives them long words for their dictionaries. Alexander asks the teacher what they read, and is shown bright cards with large pictures and a line or two of text. "I read them poems," she says. "I read them Spike Milligan and of course I read them Mickey Impey's *Naughty Poems for Bad Boys and Girls,* they love that. It's great he's actually here."

"Do they learn the poems?"

"Oh no. That would take the pleasure out of them. Learning by rote is very destructive, we know that now, they must *discover* things. Some learn things almost by accident, but we'd never *make* them. They don't learn tables, either, we draw number-squares and they *discover* the relations. That way, it stays in the mind."

"But they learn the alphabet," says Alexander, looking at the dictionaries.

"Oh no. Not as such. Not *by rote.* They sort of assimilate it."

"So how do they find their way round their dictionaries?"

"I show them. Until they know it."

"I used to love chanting the alphabet. Backwards and forwards both. And tables. And French verbs. A sort of pleasure. Like dancing."

The young woman shudders expressively.

Mickey Impey is asked to say one of his poems. The children come out of the arms of the star. He sends two to fetch some big boxes, so he can stand up above them, so they can see. He is a natural showman. He says:

"Children are always being told, come here, go there, do this, do that. They can't help it, they have to. What they get told makes no sense to them, they know what they really want, but the Tellers don't know and don't care, do they, they just go on fixing the world to make it comfortable for themselves, to keep children quiet and nice and sweet and *good.* So I wrote some poems for *bad* children. The one I'm going to read is about some children who go off to a secret country where there are no pushers-around and find all sorts of strange creatures who want to help them take charge of their own lives. Here it is."

The poem was long. The peroration went:

And the Blue Blebs
And the Yellow Yetis
And the Purple Prongs
And the Green Groaners
And the Redundant Reds
And the Great Grey Grunters
And the Picky Pink Pixies
And the Orange Owls
With the horrible Yorubas
And the loathsome Lapps
Come when he whistles
When Mickey the Mad Imp whistles
And they strangle the Grandmas
They annihilate the Aunties
They top-and-tail the Teachers

And truss them in twenties
And trepann them and toast them
And toss them to tigers
Who howl with delight
And dance all the night
In the burning bright light
Of the fire they have made
Of school-uniforms and books and pens and inks, and desks and chairs and blackboards and footballs and hockey sticks and chalk and dusters and chemistry kits and globes and bunsen burners
And they dance and they prance
They writhe and romance
And feed till they choke
On choc-ices and Coke.

"He is out of date in his equipment," murmurs Auriol Worth.

The children roar with applause. Mickey Impey organises them into a long dancing crocodile, and they prance serpentining round the school, chanting loudly after their Piper, whose energies show no signs of flagging, though one or two little ones begin to stumble and cry. Finally Agatha pulls at his arm, and tells him the group must move on: they have other schools to visit. He does not stop immediately: she has to trot alongside, explaining. His lovely face is sulky. He calls to the children, "Do you want to stop?"

"No," cry most. "Yes," cry a few.

"They want to go on," says Mickey Impey.

"Well, they can't," says Agatha, tartly. The rest of the committee group behind her.

"You see," says Mickey Impey, turning to the children as he leaves, "they don't care what you want, they don't *really* let you do as you please, it's all a trick, when they tell you you're free to choose."

A wavering scream, from some of the children, as though he were a pop star, answers this.

The Aneurin Bevan Comprehensive School in Calverley is not a shiny-bright new place like the Star Primary School. It was once the Archbishop Temple Grammar School and the Leeds Road Secondary Modern, and is now one institution on two sites. The old Grammar School is panelled and dark and echoing. The old Secondary Modern is square and shapeless, with pre-fabricated classrooms in its playground, a smell of inadequate sanitation, and exotic salty-looking fungus or chemical rash sprouting on its heating conduits. In this school there is a vigorous discussion of the problems and blessings of mixed-ability teaching. The committee are taken to a fourth-form improvised play, which centres on a family conflict between the women who make Sunday lunch and the men who want to go out to the pub and to football. Parts have been given to the less articulate to make them more articulate, with some success—one girl cries suddenly into the hall:

"And must I spend all my days like this, the same thing time after time, shopping and cooking and waiting till what I have cooked is cold and greasy, week after week after week, and then washing it up and saying it doesn't matter when you come home smelly and sick, smelly and sick, is this what it is to be a human being?"

This eloquence causes her subsequently to blush bright scarlet, and deeply embarrasses her male co-actors, who can only say, "Oh come on," and "It's not so bad as that," and "Women do go on." Magog is delighted with this moment, and congratulates the teacher on bringing out the girl's inner conflicts. The teacher replies that that girl's father is a vicar, and teetotal, and some imagination has gone into her performance. Alexander is bored. He remembers that school is 90 percent boredom. For the good and the bad student alike. Youth is boring, but this is not to be admitted.

The headmaster of the Aneurin Bevan School too is a tryer and an innovator. He has a school council and runs regular school debates in the hall of the old Grammar School. He has staged a debate in honour of the committee.

"This house believes that no good is done by the teaching of English grammar."

There is a hidden agenda to this: the headmaster himself, a geographer by profession, remembers his English language lessons as a boy, the parsing of sentences, the location of dependent clauses, as a form of intense torture, an exercise baffling and pointless. The school week is short, this man reasons, the school year is short, school days in toto are short, and clause analysis is a cruel waste of time. It is probable that most of his colleagues share both his feeling and his opinions. It is probable that most of the children do. Learning English grammar, even to passionate readers, is peculiarly repugnant and somehow *unnatural.*

The headmaster introduces the committee to the school.

"We have the honour to have amongst us a very distinguished group of people who are studying the very question we are debating today. We have Professor Wijnnobel, a distinguished grammarian, we have Alexander Wedderburn, a playwright whose rich language has entranced many of you, we have a young and popular poet, Mickey Impey. We have a scientist, a psychologist and an educational writer, all of whom will bring their own wisdom to the debate. I want them to see that the boys and girls in this school have thought carefully about this subject and I also want them to see that we are in the habit of debating issues that concern us, putting clearly points of view we may or may not agree with, and *listening to what is said by others.*"

The debate is lively. The proposer, a pink-cheeked, darkly handsome sixth-form boy, argues that we all learn to speak grammatically without being taught, that we can understand poems, newspapers, political speeches and each other without always working out what is a noun or a verb, let alone a subordinate noun clause or a subjunctive. When we learn other languages we might need a small grasp of such terminology, but that is the place to learn it.

The opposer, an intense plump girl, argues essentially that grammar is like the names of chemicals or parts of the body. We need to know about the circulation of the blood and the valves of the heart. Language is part of us: it is natural to want to understand it.

The seconder of the proposal destroys this argument. You might die if no one understood your blood or your heart. You would go right on talking if no one told you what a noun or a verb was.

The seconder of the opposer is a nervous boy with downcast eyes and argues that no one will get a job, or pass an exam, if they don't speak and write properly. Rules are there to make life better. People may not like rules but they wouldn't like life without them. Knowing the rules gives everyone an equal chance.

The debate is good. A surprising number of children take part. They are well prepared, with points written out on little cards, which they read. It is quite clear where the passions of these children lie: the anecdotal comments are all one way, the meaninglessness, the injustice, the silliness of particular grammatical problems, the *waste of time.* Such supporters of grammar as there are are rather decorous and dutiful, perhaps even selected by teachers and briefed to support it. "It helps us to write in a more interesting way." "It helps us to see what we really mean."

There is an overwhelming vote against grammar. Wijnnobel congratulates the headmaster on the articulacy of his students. Mickey Impey, who has been wriggling in his seat throughout the debate and occasionally putting his feet up on the back of the chair in front of him (Hans Richter's), suddenly plucks at the headmaster's sleeve.

"Can I say something to these kids? I've listened to them, now I'd like to talk to them. Do you object?"

"I told you," says Auriol Worth to Alexander. "If I had him in my class, I'd watch him."

"Ought we to stop him?"

"Probably. But fortunately it isn't our place."

"Go ahead," says the headmaster to Mickey Impey.

"Listen, you kids. My name is Mickey Impey, I'm a poet. I've listened to what you've been saying and some of it was good, real good stuff, but really you're all herded along by all this way of talking you think is so clever, Mr. Chairman, Ladies and Gentlemen, and all that junk. Listen to me, don't let them brainwash you. Listen to me, think freedom, think *creativity,* think vision. They make you sit there and study all this stuff about Einstein and relativity and so on. You don't need any of that. There was one great man who understood it all—*William Blake.* He saw that if you look at the world properly your imagination inhabits infinity. He understood infinity. Listen to this, it blows your mind.

> *How do you know but ev'ry bird that cuts the airy way,*
> *Is an immense world of delight, clos'd by your senses five?*

Or

> *One thought fills immensity.*

Or

> Energy is the only life, and is from the Body; and Reason is the bound or outward circumference of Energy. Energy is Eternal Delight.
>
> Those who restrain desire, do so, because theirs is weak enough to be restrained, and the restrainer, or reason, usurps its place and governs the unwilling.

"You should be thinking about *this,* about how to use your own energy, about how to see Infinity, not all the stuff they teach you. When

I was at school, no one told me anything like this, so I am telling you."

Some smile. Some titter. Some applaud. Some shuffle, embarrassed. The audience is not one. Those who have spoken are anxious to have their speaking praised. There is always the perennial fear of looking silly which runs in groups of the young. In other places, at other times, Mickey Impey can overcome that fear, can harness and use it, but here his speech goes off at half-cock. Both Mickey Impey and the headmaster are aware of this. The headmaster thanks Impey smoothly "for the message you have decided to share with us," and Impey sits down, frowning.

Alexander says to Wijnnobel, "*Why* do they so hate grammar?"

"It is something we must try to understand. It is a phenomenon we must analyse. Of course, the grammar of which they are complaining is hopelessly out of date, it is Latinate, it has nothing to do with modern thinking. But I do not think that is at the root of the problem. Perhaps a reluctance of the brain to contemplate its own operations."

This last sentence appears at first to Alexander to have nothing at all to do with the teaching of clause analysis. Nevertheless, it is interesting.

Mickey Impey is absent that night at dinner in the Dean Court Hotel. So is Wijnnobel, who has gone back to his university. It is Magog who asks Agatha Mond whether anything can be done about the behaviour of Mickey Impey. A professional *enfant terrible* himself, he does not like terrible behaviour in other, especially younger, men. Agatha replies diplomatically that she is sure that the chairman or the secretary will have a word with Impey about correct behaviour in committee members. In her experience, such problems are usually solved by the unruly member either conforming to the group customs or leaving. She is looking pretty, even beautiful, in a dark red dress which brushes her knees. Her legs are long and thin. She is one of the perhaps 10 percent of women who truly look good in such short skirts. Alexander goes up the stairs behind her and reflects that all the same, it is odd when Civil Servants wear dresses that reveal the movements of their bottoms and the backs of their knees, like schoolgirls, or female commanders of cartoon spaceships. He says, "Do you *really* think our Young Turk will conform or quit?"

"He may well quit. He may get bored. My view is that he will quit. I don't at all want to upset our political masters by complaining about him. He adds a bit of variety. He'll get bored, don't worry." She adds,

"Moreover, he is an excellent group irritant, like the grit in a pearl. He will make the rest of the group cohere, and work together."

He resists the impulse to put a fatherly arm round her shoulder.

The next day is their visit to Freyasgarth. Alexander takes time out in the morning to walk up the road to see Bill Potter, who is expecting him. He is surprised to see Bill's bruised and broken face and asks if he has had a fall.

"No. I haven't. I'm not an old man falling over my own feet yet. I had my head smashed between the door and the wall by a cross young man. My son-in-law. He wanted Frederica. Wouldn't believe she wasn't here. Wouldn't believe I didn't know where she was. Apparently she's done a bolt, taking the boy. I await developments. Never a dull day. I'd be glad if I did know where she was. She needs protection."

"I know where she is," says Alexander, after some thought. "She's being looked after. Sensibly."

"If you see her," says Bill, "tell her we'd be glad to hear from her. Tell her I haven't got so long left on this earth. A daughter's a daughter. She'll come to understand that. Tell her. Oh, I don't know what. You'd better not tell me where she is. In case that lout comes back and tortures the information out of me. He's capable. He'd cry over his handiwork after—he was very spry with damp cloths—but he's got a temper."

"I'll tell her. She's lying low."

"Most sensible thing she's done so far. Though if she'd had *any* sense at all, she wouldn't be in this mess. She should have married a kind man, like Daniel."

"You wouldn't let Daniel in your house."

"No. Well. I've come round. It was his Christianity I objected to, not him, and I've come to the conclusion he's no more a Christian than I am."

"You're a thorough old Puritan preacher, and always were."

Bill smiles at Alexander.

"One of the very few benefits of growing old," he says, "is finding out who's gone along with you, who it is you really share your memories with. We know each other pretty well."

"We do," says Alexander.

Bill has twice said he is old, since Alexander came. He looks older. The battered skin is healing slowly, and is thin as onion skin. The bruises are huge. The blood in them is black. His smile is unintentionally gruesome. Alexander smiles back with love.

Alexander rejoins the committee in Freyasgarth School. They are listening to Miss Godden, the headmistress, telling a fairy tale, *The Great Green Worm,* to the middle class, the seven- to eight-year-olds. The school is made of the local grey stone and is large and simple, a space divided by two movable partitions, dating from the 1930s. The children sit in rows behind long desks, the younger ones at the front, the older ones at the back. The committee sit at the very back. They are not comfortable. Those with small enough bottoms—Agatha Mond, the poet, Roussel, even Hans Richter in his suit—are on infant chairs. Wijnnobel is enthroned high on Miss Godden's shabby desk-chair. Miss Worth and Mr. Magog share a small gym bench, on which they make room for Alexander.

"The Green Worm gave a long hiss (that is a serpentine way of sighing) and without reply, plunged beneath the waves. What a loathsome monster, said the princess to herself; he has greenish wings, and his body is all sorts of changing colours—he has ivory claws and his head is covered with a mane of ugly fronds. I really would rather die than owe my life to that creature."

Miss Godden's voice is quiet. She lingers on the more enticing words: serpentine, hiss, fronds. The children are still. They listen. They do not shuffle. She expects them not to and they do not. She writes up on the blackboard a series of synonyms: *snake, serpent, dragon, worm,* and gets the children to add other words they know: *viper, adder, python, grass-snake, slow-worm* ("A legless lizard, you know, children, not a real snake, a creature that evolved legs and then decided to do without them"), *boa constrictor, cobra, Nag* (one child has read Rikki-Tikki-Tavi), *puff-adder, black mamba, rattlesnake.* This leads to a brief discussion of the difference between synonyms and scientific names designed to differentiate clearly between species and varieties. They talk about the "feel" of words, what is different in *worm* (a "fat, thick, *slow* word," says one red-haired girl) and *snake* ("a kind of quick-sliding but *cutting* word," says the same girl) and *serpent* ("a kind of fairy-thing, or demon out of the Bible," says the girl). They talk about why people don't like snakes and why in stories people are often changed into them. Alexander looks at the girl. She has soft red-gold hair and large dark eyes, and freckles, a soft scattering and speckling of pale coffee on cream. Her brow is wide, her mouth is wide and soft. He knows her, he can read her genes in her face, in her skin, in her lips, even in the movements of attention of her head. She is Stephanie's child, and also Daniel's child, Mary; she carries Bill's flyaway redness and Winifred's old-gold slowness, an alertness that is Frederica (but also dead Stephanie), a slow stare of thought that is her father. She was born within a week of Simon Vincent Poole. Alexander thinks of the boy. He is himself, he has his life ahead of him. Does it matter if he carries Thomas Poole's genes or mine? To Alexander, it does. He wants to *know* Simon. He looks at Mary. He thinks of Agatha Mond's Saskia, who "has no father."

"At the end of these lessons," says Miss Godden, "we always read the page of the dictionary with our word on it—*worm* today, or *snake,* you may choose, Mary Orton, since you have been thinking so hard, which. We look to see all the words there are that none of us know, even me. We think about how many words there are, and what a lot we can do with them."

Wijnnobel nods his head. The poet does not attempt to address this class, partly perhaps because he recognises another charismatic presence in this stout, story-telling middle-aged teacher, partly because he appears to be genuinely interested in the story and the word-game.

He gathers his forces, however, at school dinner. This is eaten at long tables constructed of the bench-desks, and served from large aluminium cans by overalled dinner ladies. The committee sit at the teachers' table, and are served with a sort of lamb stew, some very watery reconstituted peas, some mashed potatoes grey in colour and containing pebbles of solid starch.

Mickey Impey says very loudly, "This stuff is *muck.* Nobody ought to be asked to eat *muck* like this muck. Kids ought not and we ought not, and I *won't eat this muck.*" Alexander can see him thinking: it crosses his mind to incite all the children to throw around, or symbolically refuse, their food. Some are eating busily: some are making listless gestures with their forks. It is not nice food, and it is not completely inedible. He would rather not eat his own, but is embarrassed by the poet into making an effort. The poet stands up and scrapes the whole of his plate into the can of hot water in which the dirty cutlery is soaking. He says, "There must be a pub in this village. Anyone for a sandwich?" Nobody answers. He stalks out. Agatha is right. The rest of the committee becomes markedly more cordial towards each other.

. . .

The committee meets to discuss these and other visits. They sit round a long table in a drab room in the Ministry of Education, which is to be transformed into the Department of Education and Science. They sit on the whole in little professional groups: academics with academics, teachers with teachers, writers and journalists uneasily with each other, no one next to the sweet-faced poet, who sits drawing cartoons on his notepad. Later, these groups will splinter and reconstruct themselves. Alexander sits opposite the chairman, Philip Steerforth, the secretariat, and the other academics, Wijnnobel, Naomi Lurie, Arthur Beaver. He sits there not to catch the chairman's eye but in order to be able to look at Agatha Mond. He does not see himself as part of this group, but as an individual, an observer, present almost by mistake. Other people, as they have done throughout his life, see him as understanding and gentle: a force for cohesion. Auriol Worth and Roger Magog are sitting one on each side of him.

Agatha has written clear reports on the visits they have made. Arthur Beaver, who was not present on the visits, remarks that the Star Primary School and Freyasgarth represent opposing ideas of primary education. He is interested to know if the visiting party has formed any views about their relative merits.

Hans Richter says that it is autumn. He says he says this because in summer the Star School, which appears to be so airy and light, will become intolerably hot, and both teachers and children will be simmering with discomfort. He says architects often ignore people.

Alexander says that that school contains no private places.

Magog says most schools do not contain private places. He asks Hans Richter if his observation is a metaphor.

Richter says no, it is a physical observation. But that mental states flow from physical states, and that when the children are too hot, they will learn less well.

Steerforth recalls his committee from architecture to the teaching of language.

Auriol Worth says that both primary schools were good schools; that the children in them were learning and were happy. She says that unfortunately, perhaps, the good teaching depended in both cases on individual teachers. The headmaster of the Star School had eyes in the back of his head and an unusually good organisational brain. Another head in his place might well, with the same principles, preside over aimlessness and chaos. Equally, Miss Godden was a teacher capable of holding the attention of several age and ability groups at once, and exercising their minds. But a teacher less gifted and inventive could simply lose their attention.

Arthur Beaver says that the committee's report must contain a chapter on the activity of the teacher; the language teaching depends on the ability, and indeed the philosophy, of the teacher.

Magog says that what strikes him is the hatred of grammar demonstrated by the debate at the comprehensive school. It appears that no amount of good teaching can make grammar other than repulsive to the vast majority of kids and probably teachers. When he was a boy—

(All the committee members, all through the committee's deliberations, refer in a certain tone to when they were a boy, or a girl. They trail clouds of past life, glorious or cramped, through the dusty official room. Alexander watches them. He imagines the boy Magog was: fat, thick-kneed, curly, sulky, aggressive, never the *best* boy at anything in the class, always near the best.)

—when he was a boy, grammar was experienced as a trap set to catch you out, as a series of gates in a maze for rats, as an instrument of absolute power and punishment by teachers, as a series of nasty interruptions to any creative flow your writing might get up, as oppression, in short.

He says it doesn't seem to have got much better. He says he is sympathetic to the abolitionists. What that boy said in the debate is true. We speak grammatically without learning grammar.

Naomi Lurie says that without grammar no child can unravel the sentences of Milton, or Donne.

Walter Bishop says most kids will never read Milton or Donne. There is no reason why they should suffer parsing and clause analysis for the sake of the few privileged ones who will. They need to be able to write a job application. To read a government form.

Guy Croom says that human beings, like it or not, need rules. No community can operate without a few simple rules according to which it conducts its business. He is not in favour of new educational methods which attempt to promote discovery at the expense of learning a few facts. He thinks children are being cheated by being made to *discover* all sorts of things they could actually simply learn about and then go on to discover more interesting things. Rules facilitate. Rules create order, and without order is no creativity. The poor little children who didn't know the alphabet are wasting *hours* looking through their dictionaries at random. There is a pleasure in learning ordered rules which seems now to be despised. He thinks no one can cope with the world who hasn't internalised a few simple rules of mathematics. He thinks that football and tennis and games of cards would be intensely boring without rules. Anyone who has a child, he says, who has tried to make up a new card game as it went along, and has been subjected to the *total boredom* of the *ad hoc* and the random, will know that the need for rules is a deep human need.

The poet says, "That's what the Fascists said." He says, "If you *make* people learn old poems they hate them. You should let them just find them. You should perhaps prohibit them, outlaw them. Then they'd be hungry for poems."

The chairman asks Wijnnobel what he feels about rules.

Wijnnobel says that he does not think it is helpful to draw an analogy between the rules devised for political or social control of group behaviour and the forms of the structure of language which can be observed and described in all societies. He says, rather carefully, that he believes in the teaching of the forms of language, because if we have no words to describe the structure of our thoughts, we are unable to analyse their nature and their limitations. Nietzsche, he says, claimed that all Western philosophy studies variations on the same problems in recurring circles because all ideas are "unconsciously dominated and directed by simple grammatical functions" which are in the end, Nietzsche also says, *physiological*. This is not the same as saying that philosophical problems are "only language": it is a claim that *what we can think* is a function of our linguistic competence. He himself—unlike some others in the room—is of the opinion that the grammatical forms and structures we use are innate, are part of the structure of our brains informed by our genes, and that the extraordinary subtlety and reach of human intelligence—*and* its limitations, its recurrent worrying at insoluble "problems"—are a function of this innate order. He also believes that studying this order is hard, and contemplating it is repugnant to many. But if we do not teach words to describe the structure of language, we have no means to consider the structure of thought. This is not a defence, he adds, of the ornate Latinate grammatical exercises now taught, which should be scrapped.

Magog says he agrees with this, and that the rules of grammar desired by Mr. Croom do indeed often turn into petty rules of social oppression and alienation. He believes that the relations between teachers and children are what is wrong. When he was teaching, he got the confidence of his children, he persuaded them to write more and more truthfully, more and more passionately, about the conflicts in their family life—their hopes and desires—as he has recorded in his book *True Life Stories* (an ironic reference to the Agony Aunt magazines, as he is sure he has no need to tell this distinguished gathering)—"and the vocabulary and complexity *and punch,* Mr. Chairman, *and punch* increased with the truthfulness—"

"And after," says Auriol Worth. "After you had stopped teaching these children, whom you had encouraged to speak in this way—to reveal things—I have read your book—afterwards, what happened to them? How long did you stay with them, after you had inspired them to write about abuse and hatred and tension?"

"I was there for a full *two terms.* Before I—before I sold my book. They were strengthened by facing their conflicts."

"A teacher is not a psychoanalyst."

"I have had a lot of flak from people like you, who do nothing much for those *in their care*—"

"I teach them, Mr. Magog. I teach them to read, to write, to think. I teach them *to look outside themselves.* I respect my position. And theirs."

"You are simply an authoritarian—"

"All authority," says Miss Worth sadly, "nowadays, seems to be wrong."

Arthur Beaver says that the present lively exchange of views exemplifies some of the problems he wants to put to the committee about the philosophy of teaching. Martin Buber, he says, claims that the teacher in past times had an accepted authority derived from his culture. He was, in a fine phrase, "the ambassador of history, to this intruder, the child." And the sickness of this system, which intensified as the cultural authority crumbled and was called in question, was a "will to power" which could become domineering and cruel as it became more uncertainly individual. The contrary fault Buber called "Eros," the degeneration of authority into an idealised reciprocity and affection, of a professional relationship into a personal one. Which is not sustainable between all teachers and all children, for it depends on honesty and durability, and all teachers *do not feel* genuine affection for all children, nor do their pseudo-parental relations endure beyond the inevitable parting at the year-end. It is a kind of buddy-buddy relation, which some people believe to be part of child-centred education.

"I see what you are saying," says Magog. "But I can assure you I felt *real love* for every child in my class. *Real love.*"

He glares about the table. Alexander believes him. He also knows that there are charismatic teachers who do occasionally inspire by love.

"For two terms," says Auriol Worth, acid, headmistressy. "You felt real love for two terms. You translated the love into your written words, and you made their private pains public."

"With *every care*—"

"I am sure. Every care the reading public and the law could expect."

A line of division, a set of terms, are set up. The committee will divide, will see its own divisions, in terms of Eros and *Wille zur Macht,* the buddy and the boss. Alexander is fascinated.

After the meeting there is sherry. Alexander moves to the side of Agatha Mond and helps her to hand round glasses. The scientist, Hans Richter, taps Professor Wijnnobel on the shoulder.

"I liked what you said. About order. About describing thought. If *that* is what we are doing, this whole undertaking looks quite different. I thought I was just here to see if science teachers could be got to explain themselves a bit better, in better English, and so on. But what you said changes everything. You said something very fine about the limitations of our thought.

"I am convinced," he continues calmly, as though he were discussing the structure of salts, "that there are intelligences in the universe of which our own are only a very small sub-set."

Gerard Wijnnobel is startled. He has a momentary vision of huge angelic heads, spanning the visible heavens, of an order of serried wings, at once feathered and glassy, at once living forms and geometrically intricate patterns.

He inclines his great head and strokes his thick moustache.

"As to that," he says, "I do not know how we could have any evidence of that. As a two-dimensional paper man could not see or address a three-dimensional clay or flesh man."

"But he could intuit his presence. As we intuit the possibility of solutions to problems before we solve them."

"Or fail to solve them," says Wijnnobel.

"We intuit probable failures, also."

"It is certain that we cannot imagine the languages of such intelligences."

"I shall apply my own intelligence to the language we have. It is more interesting than I supposed."

"Indeed," says Wijnnobel.

VI

Gerard Wijnnobel sits in his official car and thinks about language. He thinks about order and disorder, about form and chaos. He has thought about these things all his life, always with a sensation of an impossible endeavour. His thought is a raft of parallel planks on a darkly swelling sea, it is a most beautiful cone of light around which is the formless, or maybe only invisible and unmapped, dark. He is Hans Richter's paper man, floating on his two-dimensional kite on currents of air, of force, he cannot describe or explore.

He grew up in Leiden, the son of a Protestant theologian, a Calvinist who puzzled, who agonized, daily over the exact relations between virtue, predestination and the words of the one Book. He is not wholly and purely of Dutch Calvinist descent: his mother's father was half-Jewish, a child of a Talmudic scholar and a Dutch Catholic lady who had come to believe that the Church was guilty of terrible cruelty to the Jews, which had come from a misreading and misuse of the Scriptures. Gerard Wijnnobel's grandfather, in his turn, had become obsessed with the language of the Book. He had set out on a doomed attempt, part mystical, part historical, part exegetical, to find the traces of the Ur-language, the original speech of God, spoken by Adam in Eden, and indeed by God, the Word Himself, when He called the universe into being out of chaos, simply by naming it. In the days before Babel, before God punished the human race for its presumption in raising its winding structure towards Heaven by dividing its tongues, by setting confusion amongst its speech—in the days before Babel, the occult tradition went, words had been things and things had been words, they had been *one,* as a man and his shadow perhaps are one, or a man's mind and his brain. Afterwards, after the fall of the tower, language and the world had not coincided, and the languages of men had become opaque, secret, enfolded in an incomprehensible and unpierceable skin of idiosyncrasies. After the fall of the aspiring tower (almost all mythologies held), the original, divine, single speech had been shattered like a smashed crystal, into seventy-two pieces, or into a number which was a multiple of seventy-two. Various words and letters could be read as splinters of this original sphere—each Hebrew letter, each word, each grammatical form. Kabbalists, Hermetics, Hasidic students of the Torah and the Talmud tried to reconstitute the Old Speech, the *Ursprache,* from these lost fragments. Gerard Wijnnobel's grandfather spent his days on the search for this ancient order, occasionally disputing with his grave Calvinist son-in-law over whether or not the Tongues of Flame which descended on the apostles in the upper room at Pentecost had caused them to be able to speak, amongst the unknown tongues in which they babbled, a version, a fragmentary part, of the original Tongue. The fact that Kees Wijnnobel believed that Joachim Steen was doomed to burn in eternal flames after Judgement did not prevent him from finding his linguistic speculations interesting. Kees Wijnnobel was not convinced that the original Tongue had been Hebrew. He thought it was something more natural, more intrinsically part of the nature of things, a tongue in which there were words for *lion, lamb, apple, snake, tree, good, evil* which wholly contained and corresponded to *all* their power and meaning. Elephant spoke elephant, earwig spoke earwig.

The young Gerard Wijnnobel listened and watched. He listened, watched, was revolted, and revolted. The lesson he drew, quite clearly from his father's Bible commentaries, and more reluctantly—for aesthetic reasons—from the speculations of his grandfather, was that it is possible for human beings *to spend the whole of their lives on nonsense.* And not only that, but that perhaps also there was a trap, a quirk, a temptation *in the nature of language itself* that led people, that induced them, to spend the whole of their lives on nonsense. He discovered Nietzsche, who preached against Christianity and its forms with all the delicious fervour and energy of a Christian hell-fire preacher converted, and Nietzsche said, "I fear we are not getting rid of God because we still believe in grammar." Theo-logy, the language of God, grammar, the forms of theology.

Gerard Wijnnobel became a mathematician. He became a mathematician in order to contemplate order and to renounce the mess of language. He worked on the Fibonacci numbers, which describe, among other things, the spiral of the cochlea in the inner ear and the principle that curls the ramshorn, the ammonites, certain snails, certain arrangements of branches around tree trunks. He withdrew into pure form, as though he saw only the relations of quadrilaterals, lengths, and primary colours of Mondrian, when once he had seen the forms of light made and recorded by Vermeer with an image of a rectangular coloured window and the enlightened solid body of a reading, or thinking, or pouring woman.

Perhaps because he came to England in the war and thus had to speak and teach and ultimately think in another language, which, however well mastered, was not his own, the Wijnnobel of the 1940s and 1950s turned his attention back from the forms of mathematics to the forms of language, to grammar. He became interested in Roman Jakobson's theories of "distinctive features" of all languages, in Saussure, who saw language as analogous to a chess game in which words were arbitrary signs to which certain formal functions were assigned, and most recently in Noam Chomsky's claim to have demonstrated that there was a deep universal structure of language, a universal grammar, innate in all human brains, not learned, any more than the beat of the heart or the focus of the eye is learned, not modified by society or experience, but part of human biological identity, capable of constructing the hum and buzz and thought patterns of innumerable tongues. As beavers are born knowing how to make dams, and as spiders are born with the ability to make webs, so human beings are born with the ability to speak and think in grammatical forms. Chomsky's generative grammar, Chomsky's transformational descriptions, still in 1964 new and uncompromising, are mathematical in their exactness and depend on the use of algorithms and mathematical structures for their understanding. Gerard Wijnnobel is convinced intellectually that Chomsky is right: that the human brain is born with a capacity to generate and transform language—that this is innate, not absorbed into some empty bucket or inscribed on some tabula rasa, but there in the folds of the cortex, the dendrites and synapses and axons of the neurones in the brain. The theories, both of learning and of language, that preceded this one are more interested in the way the mind is formed and shaped by society, or by learning, or by random events. To believe that linguistic competence is both innate and unalterable, in the present world, smacks of determinism, smacks of predestinarianism, and of more unpleasant things, a suggestion that heredity, not environment, differentiates between men. Many of the men Wijnnobel meets find that suggestion morally repugnant, exactly as he found his father's ideas repugnant. There is much talk, in his world, of language as either a crystalline, immutable structure, or as order-from-chaos, a flame-like structure that holds its changing shape in the winds of its environment. Aesthetically, Gerard Wijnnobel would like to believe in the flame, in the shifting, variable, changing form. Intellectually, he believes in the crystal. Intuitively, also, he believes in the crystal. Chomsky's descriptions of the human capacity to construct language fit his own sense of his own uses of it.

He believes too, that in some distant future the neuroscientists, the geneticists, the students of the matter of the mind, may find out the forms of language in the forest of the dendrites, in the links of the synapses. The genes are aperiodic crystals, dictating, to the matter they control, the structures, the forms, the substances that matter shall become. Somewhere in the future the understanding of their invariable form may lead to the understanding of the web of grammar and its invariable deep structure. Or so Wijnnobel believes. None of this is exactly helpful with the problem of what to teach to small and not-so-small children, with which the committee is engaged.

VII

Thomas Poole sends Frederica to see his doctor, a cheerful fat man in Bloomsbury Square. The ménage in the flat, after two months, has taken on some aspects of a marriage. There is equable discussion of shopping lists, of the feelings and friendships of Lizzie, Simon and Leo, also of books, of the novels on Frederica's new course, which takes place in a school called Our Lady of the Sorrows, and of ways to dovetail this teaching with the teaching at the Art School. Leo is quiet. He asks sometimes if they will go "back"—he does not say "home"; children can use language with great care. He says, "They will miss me," and specifies, "Sooty will miss me." He watches Frederica for signs of intention, and Frederica attempts to convey settled calm, temporary certainty, trust.

Frederica's wound is healing badly. It festers, it re-opens, it is the wrong sort of shiny pink, there is pus.

Thomas Poole puts a hand on Frederica's shoulder as she leaves.

"Courage," he says. "These things take time."

Frederica turns her face to him. He will kiss her; it seems natural. Leo appears in a doorway, and Frederica shrinks into herself, briefly putting up a hand to ward off a non-existent blow.

"I'm sorry," says Thomas Poole, easily.

"No need," says Frederica.

The fat doctor, whose name is Limass, probes and palpates and dresses the wound. He says, with his cheerful manner, "This is a nasty one, this is a mess, the way it hit you was bad luck."

Frederica says, "There is something else."

"Tell me."

"Something is wrong with my—with my vagina, with all that area. It is very painful. There are what I think you would call pustules. And a sort of crust."

She is precise. She is shamed. She is in pain.

The doctor ceases to smile, does a cursory examination, writes out a chit, and tells her she must attend the Middlesex Hospital clinic for sexually transmitted diseases. Frederica, feeling automatically guilty, because she has gambled sexually in her time and has survived, drops her head.

"When did you last have intercourse?" asks the doctor.

"With my husband. Only with him, since I got married." As this fact establishes itself, guilt is transformed to rage. A vision of the contents of the case in the wardrobe flashes across Frederica's inner eye. She moves her uncomfortable thighs together and feels pain, irritation, discomfort, separate feelings, that accompany all her movements as she walks.

"I see," says the doctor. "You do not seem to have married very wisely."

And Frederica feels a perverse desire to defend Nigel against this easy judgement, even though her own rage does not abate. Or perhaps it is only to defend herself, for having chosen unwisely. She says, "Things turn out different from what you expect."

"They do. Now you trot along to the Middlesex and get analysed before you get any worse. And keep off sex."

"I can't imagine ever wanting—any such thing—again."

"You'll be surprised," says the doctor, with cheery resignation.

"Hullo," says the plangent voice, affable and unpleasant. "Daniel the parson-person, Daniel the Vicarious, Daniel the Representative of a dead preaching-man. Are you well?"

"Little you care. Yes, I'm well. And yourself?"

"I am battered and bruised, my friend, bleeding in invisible places. Last night I went to preach my message, as I make it my duty to do—a man needs to make himself a pretty fantasy of a duty to inhabit human society every now and then, and I thought a modicum of human society was in order, a taste of the honey of human intercourse, sweet Daniel, invisible Daniel—I *yearned* weakly, dear Vicarious, to improve at least one person's understanding. So off I went to my local to preach my little preachment. I told them:

"Woe to all lovers who cannot surmount pity!

"Thus spoke the Devil to me once: 'Even God has his Hell: it is his love for man.'

"And lately heard him say these words: 'God is dead; God has died of his pity for man.'

"So be warned against pity: *thence* shall yet come a heavy cloud for man!

"But mark too this saying: All great love is above pity: for it wants to create—to create what is loved!

" 'I offer myself to my love, and *my neighbour as myself*'—that is the language of all creators.

"All creators however are hard.

"Thus spoke Zarathustra."

"It's better in German, but I don't suppose your education included the language of the ex-enemy, O parson-person, you don't sound like a man of great European culture.

"So I cast these pearls before the locals in my local and they took me by the hair and by the seat of my trousers and inflicted much local damage on my person with their boots, sweet Daniel, their boots and a bicycle chain and a broken pint glass, you would e'en have wept to see it, were you human, which I do often doubt, for you are so unsweet to me, so heel-dragging in the matter of soothing my sores as your dead Master bids you to, for I am the afflicted, O parson, O person, I am your work whether you like me or not, if I understand you rightly.

"Are you asleep, O Yorkshireman? Could you not watch with me one little hour?"

"I am *not* asleep. I am watching with you. You ought to talk to Canon Holly. He reads Nietzsche. He does Death-of-God theology. It sounds to me as though you and Canon Holly could have a fine debate. I am sorry you got bashed, but you do seem, if I may say so, to have asked for it. Indeed, I quite often feel like bashing you myself, if I ever set eyes on you."

"Ah, my sweet friend, my dear Judge come to judgement, at last a moment's true understanding, a moment of *rapport,* worked for incessantly since I began to infiltrate my voice into the passages of your reluctant and unready earhole. I do most deeply, my temporary love, desire to be bashed, as you put it, to be bashed to smithereens and shards and molecules and *pulp* and *broth,* and if you are ready to oblige me I will manifest myself. In the alleys of Smithfield I sought you and I found you not, among hatchets and saws I perceived you not, I turned aside the red robes of justice and saw fearful implements of torture and belabouring but my sweet Daniel, my chastiser in surplice and soutane, I found *not,* although my fessae ached for him, also my lower gut and my labile tongue . . ."

"Listen, you. I do not want to chastise you. Or anyone. I don't wear a surplice or a soutane if you happen to like those things, I wear *boring cords* and a *jumper,* so come off it. Shall I get Canon Holly to talk to you about Nietzsche and the Death of God?"

"There is so much more pleasure in talking about those things to someone who can't bear to contemplate them—so much more skill and difficulty to overcome for the proselytising Prophet. Talking to your Canon sounds like preaching to the converted, a doddle, with no kick to it."

There is a noise in the stairwell of the crypt. Heavy feet descend the spiral stair, quick, sure, hurrying. Behind Daniel, Ginnie Greenhill rises to her feet, holding her knitting needles defensively before her.

A voice, sharp, deep, well-bred. "Is Daniel Orton here? I was told to look for him down here."

"He's working. On the whole we don't see clients down here; there is a sitting-room *upstairs,* where you can have tea."

"I'm not a client, you silly woman. I've got to see him urgently. It's private."

"I don't know—"

"I can hear shouting," says Steelwire's tremolo. "You are distracted. I shall lie down and lick my poor wounds. Think of me licking them, my reluctant friend. Think of a tongue-tip touching blood."

"There is nothing worse," says Daniel, "than people trying to stir your imagination with what doesn't stir it."

"Ah, you are *touché,* I can hear it. How can you be a Christian person and not be stirred by the flow of blood, the *taste of blood,* my dear reluctant friend?"

"Is *that* Daniel Orton?"

"You can see he's talking."

"A moment of your time, Mr. Orton."

"How exciting," says Steelwire as Daniel replaces the receiver. Daniel turns to consider his visitor. A dark, heavily built man, his own height, with well-cut hair, a suit, a silk tie, a blueing chin. Heavy brows, a heavy frown.

Daniel puts out his hand. "Can I help?"

"I think you are hiding my wife from me. I've been looking for her, and I think it might be you who's hiding her. I want her back."

"We don't betray professional confidences—"

"You don't know me. We're related, not really, but in a way. I'm Nigel Reiver. My wife's Frederica. I've not met you but I know about you. You married my wife's sister, who died. I know about you. I think she might have come to you. It's been two months now, and I've been looking, but I've had trouble finding you, too. I've thought it out, she would have come to you, of course. You wrote to her, I saw the letter. I don't want to hurt you, or her, I just want her back. And my son. He ought to be with me. His life is with me. So please, tell me where she is. Tell me where she is. I don't want to hurt her, *I want her back.*"

"I don't know where she is. I didn't know she'd gone."

"I don't believe you. You *must know where she is.*"

"I don't." Daniel adds, unfortunately, "Which looks like a good thing."

Nigel Reiver steps back and punches Daniel in the face. Daniel staggers, and puts up an arm to protect his head. Ginnie Greenhill presses a panic button which starts up a loud angry bell, at earth level above them. They are frequently attacked by clients and have discovered that this bell is enough to deter most of them from further violence. There is also an understanding with the local police that if they hear it sound, they will "look in" to make sure all is well. In this case, the loud noise seems to have a maddening effect. Nigel takes another lunge at Daniel and lands a sideways blow on his ear. There is a sound of ripping inside Nigel's expensively built suit. Daniel thinks briefly of Steelwire, who would be sorry to miss the crunch of bone on skin, the red wet flow of blood. He tries to be a sort of pacifist, but it is not good for people to get away with hurting other people. He advances on his brother-in-law and takes a grip on the knot of his tie.

"Listen, you. I don't tell lies. If I say I don't know where she is, then I don't know where she is. You'd better try to understand that, it'll save time."

He wants to hurt Nigel. His blood drips from his swelling nose on to Nigel's nice shirt. Nigel thinks. Nigel brings up his right hand and slaps Daniel very hard across the untouched ear. Daniel understands that this is all he can do. He *must* strike out. He is overwrought. The bell jangles and howls. A policeman appears at the head of the staircase. Daniel, a little breathless, says it is all all right, thank you, there has been a misunderstanding.

"If you're sure, Mr. Orton," says the policeman.

"A complete misunderstanding," says Daniel.

The two men glare at each other. Nigel makes a conciliatory effort. "I know about your wife. I know how hard you took that. My wife has gone off with my son. I *want them.*"

Daniel sees the dead face, unprepared, unexpecting. His mind reddens. He plunges forward and hits Nigel in the mouth. More blood splashes and drips.

"Christ!" says Nigel thickly. "I'm sorry. I said that wrong. What a godawful mess. Can we sit down?"

"If you insist."

"I told you, I'm sorry, I know I said that wrong, I was trying to—trying to—you know what—and I made it worse. Look, I was the one who comforted Frederica. I held her while she cried. Don't hit me again, I'm just saying—you and I—we know each other and we don't. I know it's private. She cried and cried in my arms, Frederica. I want her back."

He is saying, says Daniel's red mind, that he married Frederica because of *that,* because of Stephanie. He looks at the floor. He scowls. They both scowl. Ginnie Greenhill notes a fleeting resemblance: dark men like dark bulls.

"I'm stepping in deeper, trying to make it better," says Nigel. "Have a hanky, I carry several. They're clean."

Daniel mops blood.

"OK. I accept you don't know where she is. Where can I go? I ought to go after those sodding friends of hers with the Land Rover but I can't remember their sodding names. I *just wanted them out* of my house and out they went. Now I want them, I don't know where to start. I want my boy. He's my boy, he's my blood, *I love him.* A father can love a boy, a father should be with a boy—and a boy with his father. That's true isn't it?"

Daniel drops his head. His son is in Yorkshire. Nigel's son is with Frederica, about whose maternal instincts Daniel, even Daniel, does not feel automatically hopeful. He has never wholly liked Frederica. Part of him does not even want to think of her crying for Stephanie. Who was his. Who was his.

"Every day," says Nigel, "I think, today she'll get in touch. And she doesn't."

"I'll look around. I don't say I'll find her, I don't say I've any idea where to start either. I'll try and give her the message. To get in touch. Then it's up to her."

"I went up to Yorkshire. I smashed the old man's head in a door. I didn't mean to. I've got a temper. I don't mean anything by it."

Daniel laughs.

"What's funny?"

"That's what he always said himself. He didn't mean anything by it. I do advise trying to get her back by peaceful means."

"I love her," says Nigel.

"Love," says Daniel. His work has given him a professional horror of the word. He says to Nigel, guiding him up the stairs, "You've ruined my professional life. You've bashed in both my ears. All I can hear is humming and interference and random noise. Horrible. My work is listening."

"It's funny work. I expect it gets you down. Other people's agonies, nothing you can *do*?"

"It does, a bit. It does."

"How the other half live," says Nigel, emerging. He gives Daniel a card. "In case you hear anything."

"I told you, my ears are out of action."

They part.

"Our great Projector," said Colonel Grim to his almost-crony Turdus Cantor, "is to turn his attention to those tender young sucklings in our midst, to the children whose pretty babble enlivens our dark corridors and sweetly disturbs our contemplations."

"He has none himself," said Turdus Cantor. "None that he acknowledges, none that are known of."

"That has never prevented an enthusiast from pronouncing on the subject. And you must consider, Turdus, my friend, that we were all children once, we are all experts on that state."

"And what we propose for others we derive from our own fears and hopes in that distant time. And so the race goes on."

"But Culvert, save his soul, means to make a new race of children and a new race of men to follow."

"He may do good. Men—and women—love him. They will listen for hours together to his speaking. They would not listen so to you or to me. They would not do as we asked."

"In the old days, which are departed, they did as I ordered."

"But, my dear Grim, the bad old days are departed, indeed."

"And if a man promises happiness, and it is not forthcoming, the people may hate him."

"Or if he has taught them wisdom, they may understand, nevertheless."

"Have you ever known that?"

"No. But hope is a pleasant human failing. Let us go and hear our Projector's blueprint for the liberation of the babes at the breast."

The Theatre of Tongues was crowded to hear Culvert speak on the education of their children. The children themselves, of whom there were perhaps fifty or sixty in the Tower, were not present at this oration, for various ladies had voluntarily taken upon themselves to teach the little creatures the skills of the old civilisation, to wit, reading, writing, figuring, languages, dead and alive, sewing, plain and ornamental, drawing and painting, singing, dancing, playing on flutes, fiddles, tambourines and glockenspiel, making paper carnations, cooking little cakes, observing such humble creatures as spiders, lizards, flies, cockroaches, earthworms and mice; also the growth of beans and mustard seeds. All this activity was admittedly unplanned and haphazard but it kept the little people quiet, and satisfied their driving and exhausting curiosity and activity in what were felt to be reasonable, innocuous ways. But it was known that Culvert had proposals more rational, more profound and more searching for the employment of their long days. ("Who does not remember how long, long are the days of childhood, how the minutes creep, creep, and the hours and the days sink and sough like heavy velvet, and the months are unimaginably far, like other planets, like stars in the black, with dark dust between now and the now to come, perhaps to come?")

I will not give Culvert's speech *in toto*, for although I can assure you that it was most charismatically delivered, that his audience swayed to his periods and parentheses like pink-eyed rats before a cobra, like the faithful at the feet of an inspired preacher, the truth is that on paper it is quite possible that the magnetic quality would be lacking from this oration, as is so often the case with spoken enchantments reduced to flickerings of black ink. And then, he had done so much work, had burned so much midnight oil, with Damian and Roseace bringing him sirops and stimulants, sweets and salts, that his thinking and speaking ran into diverticulated pockets of matter, like those pockets that develop in an overstimulated gut, and retain festering irritants. For he had thoughts on play, and thoughts on the learning of speech and reading, thoughts, most recondite, on the order and organisation of the secret sensual life of infants, which in his view should be uncovered and made public, thoughts on punishment (ah, such finely graded, such delicately apposite, such generously imagined thoughts on punishment), thoughts on group life, thoughts on solitude, thoughts on corruption and so on and so on, thoughts on stubbornness and thoughts on readiness to please, that to recount them all would take more time than any sane reader in this fallen and trivial world would accord me. So I will somewhat brutally summarise his sayings, in order to speed my narration. It is true that the purity and beauty of his ideas were not wholly incarnate in their subsequent application, but I believe they may nevertheless shine through. He meant *well*, he meant *well*, Culvert, and maybe few of us can have a better encomium.

Because the children were not present, many of the women of the Tower were not present, because they were "caring" for the children, as they believed.

But Mavis, wife of Fabian, mother of Florian, Florizel, and the little Felicitas, was present, because she clung greatly to her little children, and feared that Culvert meant to sever their ties.

And Roseace and Damian were there too, and could not keep their hands from each other's body. Culvert had been astonished by the success of his theatrical device where Roseace out of good feeling enacted before the community, in the Theatre of Masks, a passion for Damian's body, which Damian desired her to have and which in daily life she could not feel. And so, as I told you, wearing a sweet-smiling mask and a dishevelled wig, she had submitted in public to the passionate advances of Damian, who had chosen a warrior mask, a stern heroic mask, and achieved his desires to cries of encouragement and pleasure from the audience. But since that time Roseace's flesh ached and yearned for Damian—and he, only a little less, for her—and so they coupled in Culvert's bedroom as he wrote, separated to bring him sustenance, and then coupled again.

This, Culvert believed, was a good result of his intentions.

He had concluded, for himself, that Roseace's breasts were crumpled in texture and that Damian's buttocks were overweening and absurd.

He had proved that a formal enactment of a feeling may lead to that feeling.

He had never noticed that Roseace simpered.

I am about to deflect myself from the summary of Culvert's speech with a vicarious plunge into the pleasurable communion of Damian and Roseace. But I will reserve that for the sweetmeat to follow the meat of his discourse.

A Child, said Culvert, was born to a Woman, and some Man was usually known to have been implicated in the seeding of that Child, though there was less certainty about which Man than many desired to have.

In the corrupt world from which we have fled, he said, this Child was then reared in a Family, made up of a Man, a Woman, and such brothers, half-brothers and female children as were gathered into that group. The social structures of the Society they had fled, to wit, monarchies, the Christian religion, places of education and so on, were all made in imitation of that Family. They were structures of authority, of persecution, of narrow loyalties, of hierarchy, of exclusive and narrow affections and privileges, all of which led to oppression, irrationality and the sense of private property and personal greed.

In their new world, in the Tower, all men would be equal and would care equally for all men. There would be no marriage, no family, and the children of the community would all be the children of every member. Thus envy and favouritism would be abolished. All suckling mothers would give milk indifferently to all suckling children; all would feed equally well or ill, and thus no one would hurt any other.

In order to achieve this, all the children in the Tower would be removed to the new Dormitories which he had had constructed in the last few weeks (even using outside hired labour so as the more rapidly to begin the new order and to abolish the Family). The new Dormitories were constructed in one wing to his own design. In them were cots and cushions, great beds and narrow beds, curtains and coverlets of all kinds of rich and bright colours, for he had observed that children required the stimulation of various colours and textures. Lights, too, he had made, that would shine all night, for he had observed that children were afraid of the dark. And in places these cast shadows, for he had observed that children liked to be frightened by grotesque shadows, and in others they did not, for some children were harmed by fear. And he had observed that some children desired to sleep in heaps like young puppies, and some were of a more solitary nature, and desired to sleep alone, and he had made ample provision for both.

"And if one child desires to heap itself with another who desires solitude, what then?" asked Turdus Cantor.

The children will learn to regulate their own society, explained Culvert. They will learn to respect each other's desires and to offer kindnesses reciprocally. As our society becomes more harmonious, so this will become more natural to them. Grasping and bullying are products of the Family and the Establishment. These will be replaced by reasonable groups, founded on well-established desires.

He went on to education. Children, he said, would learn at their own speed, what they pleased, as they pleased. We should not impose on them early restrictive vices to deform and twist their minds, such as blind, uncomprehending repetition of verses or numbers, such as the laws of perspective or moral saws and sayings. All should be true discovery, all questions should be answered at the time when it was urgent to a child's mind to have an answer, and not otherwise. Books they should have in plenty—their nature to be agreed by the whole community—and adults should always hold themselves in readiness to teach, both how to read and how to understand the contents. For a child, said Culvert, may want to read for fifteen hours together and then not again for a week or two, and it is my belief that those fifteen hours are worth months of forced attention.

Also, he said (remember, I summarise), it is my deep belief that we, who call ourselves adults, grown-ups, reasonable beings, have much to learn from very small children. For we perceive, if we watch attentively, that very small children are full of delighted activity and exploration which we, narrow and shunted, repress in them with smacking and pursing our lips, and threatening with vile things, with castration, with blindness, with dwarfism, with the Fires of Hell. Small children are natural beings, they explode from their mother's wombs full of natural energies and powers which we pervert and suppress. Consider the natural propensity of little girls to raise their skirts and display their round bellies and little bottoms to men and women. Should we not stroke and admire and cherish what they so innocently offer? Consider the natural propensity of both sexes to seek the pleasures dormant in their little organs, in their soft small tails and their hidden sweet beads of flesh. Should we, as now, terrify and hurt them by howling and thundering, or should we not rather smile and play with them? If left to play in innocence, what might they not become, what might they not learn, and in turn teach us, of refinements of pleasure, of ecstasies of perception, of courtesies and reciprocities undreamed?

At this point Culvert's discourse became visionary in its intensity, and hard for some of his more pedestrian or earth-bound companions to follow. For he appeared to be advocating a new kind of school, or theatre (theatre and school, and also church, were part of each other in the forms of his thought), or ritual, even, in which the men and women would set themselves to learn by imitation from babes and sucklings, in which all would be innocently naked on the stage together, and innocently explore all flesh, mature and nubile and milky-new, all apertures, all lips, all teeth, all recesses, all flowings of milk and blood, of seed and sweat, of saliva and tears, of sibilants and labiles, for was not the babbling and lalling of our infant selves and our infant teachers a beginning of language more sweet, more full of promise, than the austere croakings and scratchings and hummings and hawings we had in our fallen state made of it. Oh, cried Culvert, to a great ecstatic sigh of most of his listeners, if we might again approximate our sensibilities to the moment of our birth and learn all afresh, as we shall forge new, freed sensual apparatus and new, unimagined powers of sympathy and pleasure, so shall we forge a new true language, a language of love and playfulness and truth without innuendo or inadequacy or lameness, a language like a sword, a language as immediate as the triumphal song of the seed from the cock, a language before shame and beyond shuffling embarrassment—a new universal speech.

He said also that he had observed that children did not evince the same disgust at the excrement of the human race as was shown by the more squeamish adults, a disgust which had led to the diminishing usefulness of the latrines in the Tower. This disgust might be a distortion of the sensibility induced by our cramped education, but it might also be natural, a natural development. He felt that the childish pleasure in dirt and mess should be set to use, and proposed to found juvenile Troops of cleaners, who should gallop in and out of the Tower with their own little handcarts and ponycarts containing tubs of the offending matter, to the sound of bugles and pipes. He had devised a uniform for these Troops—a subtle olive hessian with scarlet braid at every conceivable juncture—which he now displayed to the assembled company, who applauded courteously.

His ideas on punishment, which are germane to much of what I am to tell, although they were first propounded here, were in a state of some incoherence, and I will save discussion of them for a later point. He would like, he said, to proclaim that there should be no more punishment or chastisement anywhere in their reasonable passional world. But things were not so perfect, not yet, it was hard to see . . . On the whole, he said, it was better for adults never to punish children, whose little peccadilloes should be corrected by their peers, in an atmosphere of tolerance and laughter.

At this point the Lady Mavis asked if she might speak. Culvert had marked this lady as his opposer. She was tall and brown and spoke slowly: she and Fabian, her partner, for husbands there were now *not*, spoke often together and agreed on almost all things, as though they thought each other's thoughts, and communicated sans language. And this state of doubleness, as though they were two trees that had grown together, was highly regarded in the old state, before the Revolution, but was now regarded with suspicion by the people of the Tower, as though she set herself up to have other ideals from them. And although many had availed themselves of the new freedoms, so that sweet orgies of four, or twelve, or twenty took place every night in the little side-chapels and minor dungeons, although more and more were putting themselves forward to act out their desires in the Theatre of Pain and the Theatre of Tongues, no other member had so far approached Fabian or Mavis. And these two had in the early days of escape been all smiles and friendliness; the Lady Mavis had created many gay *fêtes champêtres* for children and adults, with delicious breads and cakes made by her hands, with sweet lemonades, with barley water and fruit fools decorated with cherries and angelica. But now that the pleasures of most were more frenetic and fiercer, these simple feasts were almost shunned, or attracted only the very old and the very young. And on the Lady Mavis's wide brow the shadow of a frown had replaced the wrinkling smile of welcome. One night she and Fabian had discussed, in their stony chamber, the advisability of entertaining other lovers. "It might amuse you," the Lady Mavis had said to Fabian, who had replied, "If I closed my eyes, my dear, and imagined that pink Pastorella or creamy Chloris was in fact your own lithe brown self, with the little scars and the laughing-lines and the secret folds I know so well, I might be able to go through with it, but in truth I doubt it. And it would be a blow *against* freedom of desire to indulge in variety for fear of social disapproval. For such conventional prescription of behaviour is what we fled. And if we desire only each other, whom we know and trust, that too should be possible to accommodate in freedom."

"He may make us act on his stage," said the Lady Mavis.

"I think not," said Fabian. "This is not a monarchy and he is not a king. *All of us* are to do as we please. Let those act who discover themselves by acting."

"He will say, we do not know ourselves," said Mavis.

"And we will demonstrate that we do," said Fabian.

He will hate us, thought the lady, but had not the courage to speak it aloud. Fabian however, heard her thought. And his face too, bore a slight frown.

Culvert had spent time analysing the predominant passions of his people, and writing them down in a table of affinities and oppositions, linked by many little arrows and symbols of swords and crosses, cocks and bulls and open mouths. A truly harmonious world, he concluded provisionally, would need about five times as many citizens to make sure that every possible desire was present and reciprocated. Since the Tower would not accommodate these extra persons and passions, those present in fact must be made to double up, so to speak, to "try out" passions which did not come to them naturally. If a man had a desire to pick off the scabs of another, and no passionate scabbed skin could be found, someone must simulate this passion in the Theatre of Pain and perhaps even learn to feel delight in it.

He had the Lady Mavis picked out as a simple type, the female whose sole purpose was her need to give suck. She was a woman, Culvert's diagnostic pronounced, whose whole sensuous being was concentrated in her big brown nipples and their dark aureoles, whose only delight in life was the drag of infant suction, the love-bites of toothless gums, the steady suck of tiny lips and the kneading of little fingers in her fat round flesh. Since their coming to La Tour Bruyarde she had assumed the freedom of unlacing her clothes and presenting the bursting globes of her breast at every opportunity to her infant's mouth, without shame, which was of course desirable, for shame was abolished. A percipient reader might suppose that the Projector would designate such a person as wet nurse to the whole dormitory of infants, and consider her well placed and useful. But the truth must be told: something in Culvert was disgusted by the sight of these breasts, and of the milk dribbling from the infant lips as it gushed too plentifully forth. He felt a desire, as he saw her placidly feeding her child, to run at her with his hands, or even with a weapon, to pierce or bruise those assertive rounds, to mix hot blood with the pallid milk, to slice, to sever . . . He did not, as a good analyst of desires should have done, consider the whence, the wherefore and the possible satisfaction of his desire to hurt the Lady Mavis. He had not reached that stage in his development which was the deep contemplation of the natural human urge to hurt, to harm, to pierce, to open, to bruise, to stab, to strangle. No, the unregenerate Culvert turned his attention away from his loathing of the Lady Mavis's mammary display, and tried to be rational, to think in the interests of the community. She was not much use, this lady, in terms of reciprocated new delights, for no one appeared to desire her, perhaps because all were repelled by her insistent maternity. He thought she must learn to partake in the polymorphous and manifold pleasures of the flesh, for the good of the greater number. In his secret soul he began to devise a scenario for the transfiguration and *opening* of this austere lady. In the interim he replied, a little testily, that of course she might speak. And he felt a touch of nausea for he knew in advance what she would say, and how it should be countered.

So the Lady Mavis stood up, holding against her breast her little son, Florizel, and said in her milky voice that it was possible to dispute the wisdom of separating small infants from their mothers who had given birth to them. For a child's body grows for a time inside a woman's body, and after it is severed from the umbilical cord, it is still part of her, in that it cannot stand or walk alone for a year or more, and in that its natural economy, its bodily well-being, is dependent on the milk she provides and the care she takes to teach it skills and keep it from harm.

"I do not argue," said the Lady Mavis, "that there is any God who designed or created us so, but I do argue for Nature, for everywhere in the natural world we see such particular bonds and such particular care. Even the female Alligator, who was once thought to be an unnatural and even cannibalistic Parent, has been observed to shelter her tiny offspring in the horrid cavern of her jaw, so that they run in for safety between her terrible teeth. And she does not indiscriminately shelter all such soft helpless amphibians, but only her own, the issue of her own eggs, which she knows and recognises."

"And if this is so," repeated Culvert with patient contempt, "do we not see what evils spring from this partiality, this hotbed of egotism and privilege, this nest of demanding love which holds back the adventurous child from exploring the outer world? It is not only in brute fact, but over and over in analogy, that Mothers have smothered their sleeping infants by rolling over their heavy bulks on their defenceless sleeping faces. No, let us, with a system of checks, balances, reinforcements, subtle affections, extend from each of us to all the others those thrustings and heats of 'maternal' affection, so that all may feel love for all, and the world expand in harmony, for none will compete for what is proffered to all, no orphan child will cry for the breast, no overindulged sprig struggle to evade the strangling maternal clasp—we shall all be one, and one will be all. All will feel *enough* of this mothering-passion, *all*, men, women, castrates and children, and none will emit or endure *too much*."

And they all cried out, Culvert was in the right, nothing would be taken from Mavis's children if they were removed from her exclusive company, but much would be given *as well as* what they had.

And while the company were exploring the new Dormitories, which were opened by the Lady Paeony, who cut a pink ribbon with a pair of scissors, Colonel Grim and Turdus Cantor made their way to the battlements and looked out over the plain. And the company exclaimed over the ingenious sleeping accommodation, the huge circular cushioned beds, decorated with embroideries of lambs in the fields playing sweetly with lion cubs and spotted leopards. And Colonel Grim said to Turdus Cantor, "I see a troop of horsemen approaching. Where is our watch?" And Turdus Cantor said, "Your eyes are better than mine, I see nothing. I am not sure we have a watch, for there is not always a Companion who desires to stand at the post since no one ever comes."

And the company exclaimed over the pretty cupboards for playthings and chamberpots and clothing, all decorated with painted butterflies and smiling lizards.

And Colonel Grim said, "I see a banner with a bleeding tree. The Krebs are riding across the valley in full daylight. They do not usually travel by day. I think you should hurry down and alert Culvert and the others, for it may be they mean to attack us. For there is no way out of the valley to the north now the bridge is cut."

The company had no armed guard and no organised defence for the Tower, which would in fact be difficult, even for a large force, to break into, once the great gates were closed and the bridge down. But everyone bustled to and fro, like insects disturbed in a nest, and found out what swords, pistols, pitchforks, muskets, spits, carving knives and so forth could be brought to bear, as the company of the Krebs approached closer—for Colonel Grim's clear eyes had seen well, they were indeed the Krebs, riding fast and furiously, about a hundred strong, and chanting as they came, in a language no one could interpret.

Their horses were low and ugly, with rough black hair and starting manes; they galloped close to the ground, in a cloud of dust, surprisingly fast. The faces of the riders could not be seen, for they all wore flat leather helmets, with a kind of leather prow projecting over their noses. They wore also black leather jerkins, supple and polished, matt here, glistening there, and leather breeches, also black, so the whole troupe was a moving, singing black shadow, above which sparkled a cloud of silver spear-points on black spears, like monstrous metal midges. Their shoulders were very broad, and their arms very long, but their torsos were squat and their waists narrow, and their bow legs, wrapped round the bellies of their horses, short.

The people of the Tower stood behind their battlements, brandishing their ramshackle collection of weapons, men, women, and a few children. The Lady Paeony declared it was a pity they had not had time to prepare boiling oil, and the Lady Coelia said they had precious little oil to spare, and would be hard put to it if the Krebs took it into their heads to encamp below the Tower and lay siege to it. And when the Krebs came nearer they began to blow great horns, great ramshorns, and circle around before the closed gates.

Then Culvert called down from the battlements, "Do you come here in peace?"

And a high, grinding voice, unaccustomed to the tongue of the Tower, answered thickly, "Neither in peace nor in war. We bring you a thing."

"It is a trick," said Narcisse. "They wish to make us open the door."

"We wish to exchange this thing for things you have. For wine and flour and sugar to make a feast. It is our feast day."

"Show us your thing," cried Culvert.

"You must come down and see," said the Krebs.

"It is a trap," said Narcisse.

"I think not," said Colonel Grim. "It is true that periodically they have great feasts, and like to season their sour beer and their rootcakes with our more refined provisions. Let us go down, Culvert, and see their thing. Fabian will stand over the bridge with a musket, and Narcisse with another, to cover our sally, and we will see this thing."

"We have enough flour and wine for ourselves, and none to spare," said the Lady Paeony.

"And how much shall we have if the Krebs take a dislike to us and camp there to starve us out?"

So Culvert and Colonel Grim went to the mouth of the bridge, and told the Krebs to show their thing to be exchanged.

And they brought a great leather sack, tied with leather ropes.

"Open it up," said Colonel Grim. "So we may barter."

And the Krebs opened the mouth of the sack, and kicked the sack several times, two of them, with their small, sharp, booted feet.

And out crawled a man. He came out with difficulty, his long grey hair matted with blood, his face a mask of blood, his arms bound, and his ankles, so that he could only slide like a snake out of the mouth of the bag. He was gagged too, with a leather strap between his teeth.

"He is a friend of yours," said the Krebs. "Or so he said when we took him."

When they turned their faces up to speak they could be seen to be covered with dark hair, fat faces with mouths lost in the hair, and small glittering black eyes.

"We cannot see him for blood," said Culvert. "Let us see him."

"He is a friend of yours, he says," repeated the Krebs. "If you will not acknowledge him, we will kill him for spying. As you please. Also we will take his ransom as your food parties arrive, for we know where they are and when they will come. But our feast is now, and we would like wine now."

"Stand him up, and untie him," said Culvert.

So the Krebs undid the leathery knots, and helped the man roughly to his feet, jostling him, and leaving his hands tied.

He was a tall man, in a long black cloak. His eyes shone dark in his bloody face.

"Can you see me, Culvert?" he said. "Through all this muck and mire? I am not a gift you would have chosen, but I would be grateful if you would accept me, for the alternatives are not pleasant."

His voice, though racked by pain, was dry and precise.

And Culvert laughed.

"You are right," he said. "You are a gift I would never have chosen, for you and I shall never agree to the world's end. But I can do no other but accept you, old enemy, for I will not have your death on my head."

And no one had any knowledge of the stranger, save Culvert. But they found out food enough, and drink enough, to satisfy the Krebs, and the stranger walked painfully but proudly across the bridge into the Tower. And Culvert said to the assembled people:

"Let me make known to you my old childhood playmate and student companion, Samson Origen. Let me say also, in front of him, as he stands there covered in blood and dust, that he comes as the serpent into our Paradise, for he is the world's great nay-sayer, and there is nothing in the world on which he and I agree. There is no human being worse fitted for our project, or more opposed to our aims, and so we must welcome him with tender loving care and overwhelm him with sweet reason, and seduce him with reasonable pleasures, or he will have us all shivering and chastising ourselves in monastic cells, not because that is our secret delight, but because we must have no delight under the moon. Is it not so, old enemy? Do I misrepresent you?"

"I will keep quiet," said Samson Origen, "for the present, I promise you."

And then he fainted away on the cobbles where he stood, and further philosophical dispute had to be postponed.

Frederica stands on a small platform at one end of a large studio, lit from above. She is dressed in a short black woollen dress and a knitted jacket in black, as long as the dress. Her hair is loose and long: her sharp face looks out from between its curtains. The students sit in chairs with swinging notepad arms, the men in dark jeans, the women in shirts and smocks mostly in dark, fruity colours, slightly acid. They have pale lips and eyes made up like sinister dolls, with long lashes and a bruised look. They are professional waifs. Some are taking notes and some are doodling. Frederica is speaking passionately about paper lanterns on a dark lake, primroses and ruddy sea with crabs, white storks and turquoise sky, and the great sinister cuttlefish "that stared straight from the heart of the light." Everything for

Lawrence, she says, is loaded with *meaning.* She describes the shattered circle of the reflected moon. She talks of the white flowers of evil, the *fleurs du mal,* floating on the sea of death. She is teaching a ten-week course on "The Modern Novel." Art students read with difficulty; choose some *short books,* said Richmond Bly. She has chosen *Death in Venice, La Nausée, The Castle,* all of which are still to come. She has begun with Lawrence and Forster because that was where, in Cambridge, she ended. "The novel is the one bright book of life," said Lawrence, and Lawrence was the point of perfection towards which the novel had been heading, it appeared then. Men asked her if she was "a Lawrentian woman." The sixties are slowly gathering speed, and the sixties do not find Lawrence daring: he has been admitted to the Establishment with the Lady Chatterley trial in 1961. Daring is *Naked Lunch,* is Allen Ginsberg, is Artaud. Frederica by a pure trick of time feels *involved* in *Women in Love,* which is a book about which she feels a fierce ambivalence (it is powerful, it is ridiculous, it is profound, it is wilfully fantastic). Its existence is part of the way she sees the world. It matters to her that these students should see it.

She does not yet know them very well. Later, she will distinguish; potters notice different things from textile designers, painters use language more flamboyantly and more loosely than graphic designers, sculptors are either silent or voluble, industrial designers dislike the culture of the book, jewellers are fey, theatre designers read as though books were blueprints for structures of images. At this early stage, she is a little afraid of them. She is there presenting herself as a *literary critic,* and these students are *artists.* Instinctively, she does not offer them critical categories or moral judgements. She tries to seduce them into seeing that books are complicated formal structures. For they do not like books for the most part. For them, brightness and meaning are elsewhere, are in the studio, in the pub, in bed.

A novel, *Women in Love,* for instance, she says, is made of a long thread of language, like knitting, thicker and thinner in patches. It is made in the head and has to be remade in the head by whoever reads it, who will always remake it differently. It is made of people whose fates are more interesting to its maker than those of his friends or lovers—but who are also an attempt to understand his friends and lovers probably. The people are made of language, but this is not all they are. A novel is also made of *ideas* that connect all the people like another layer of interwoven knitting—*Women in Love* is a novel about decadence, about love of death, about thanatos as opposed to eros. The ideas are made out of language but that is not all they are. This novel is made of visual images—the lanterns, the moon, the white flowers—which you might think were like painted images, but they are not, for they have to be *unseen visible images* to be powerful. They are made out of language but that is not all they are. We must all imagine the broken moon, and she takes her power from *all our imaginings* and their sameness and their difference. She is trying to make the painters and sculptors see how a novel is a work of art and is not a painting. She is trying to understand something herself. A young woman smiles at her: a young man in glasses writes furiously. They are listening. *The group is listening.* She has them: the knitting is a fishnet.

At the other end of the studio, on another platform, another group of students is arranged, less formally, lying on the ground, squatting on the floor, round the model, Jude Mason, who has been reading to them from what appears to be a blood-red ledger. He is partly dressed: below his spare haunches he is naked: he sits on the edge of the platform, his knees drawn up amongst his long grey veil of hair, his balls poised on the dust between his dirty feet. He wears a dirty velvet jacket in a faded speedwell blue, a skirted jacket, from the turn of the seventeenth and eighteenth centuries in style, with filthy lace cuffs and a kind of jabot or cravat. Under this jacket, and beneath the cravat, he is unclothed, his body lean like dark metal. He calls out now, in a sawing voice, "You should teach them Nietzsche. Man in a little skiff on the raging sea of Maya, of illusion, supported by the *principium individuationis.*"

Frederica is angry. The thread of the class attention is broken. Anything she can say will sound school-mistressy or piqued. So will silence. She says, "I am talking about Lawrence."

"I know. I can hear. Bits of it are not uninteresting. The knitting idea is not at all bad, writing does resemble that despised art. Continue. We may yet join your circle."

Frederica stares angrily at him. All imagined retorts sound petulant. He smiles, a self-satisfied, *smart* smile on his drawn, sinewy face.

"Because it is knitting, I should be glad if you wouldn't break the thread of my argument."

"*Argument,* is it? Happy those who earn their daily bread by arguing, as opposed to displaying their flesh and blood for study. I will hear your argument."

This too is a nice provocation: it requires Frederica either to invite him into her class, or to speak up to be heard and interrupted, or to speak low, conspiratorial, so that he cannot hear. The best would be to invite him. But she does not want him. She does not like him. She does not like his look, his smell, or his sawing voice. He is disruption in person. She decides to continue. She opposes herself to him. She wills the attention of her group, the fringes of which turn their heads to see what Jude will do.

"At the centre of *Women in Love,*" says Frederica, "is a mystery, an emptiness. The two women are wonderful both as real women making decisions about love, about sex, about the future, and as myths, as mythic beings willing life or death. But what are we to make of Birkin, who in many ways is Lawrence, in many ways is the central consciousness of the whole tale? We are told, and mostly forget, that he is *an Inspector of Schools.* Indeed, at one moment, we actually see him inspecting a school, when he discusses with Ursula the sexuality of the hazel catkins. But mostly we do not believe in him as an Inspector of Schools. He has the entrée both to the upper-class society of Nottinghamshire and to the Bohemian artistic world in London. There is no reason why this should be so. It feels wrong."

"Matthew Arnold," says the sawing voice, "was an Inspector of Schools."

"Also the author of innumerable books and poems," says Frederica, this time managing to contain and include Jude's contribution. "And part of a cultural dynasty. I was going to go on to say, we experience Birkin, if not as Lawrence's *alter ego* (though he is best when most absurdly insisting on his maleness, for which Lawrence intelligently and complicitly *mocks* him)—if Birkin is not Lawrence's *alter ego,* he is the presence of the *author of the book.* And *Women in Love* is not, is trying very hard not to be, *A Portrait of the Artist.* Lawrence may have said, "The novel is the highest form of human expression yet attained"—which you are in a better position to question than most people are—but I think he felt a kind of sickliness in writing novels about writing novels about writing novels."

"*Tout existe pour aboutir à un livre,*" speaks the Chorus. Frederica gives him a theatrical nod of complicity, covering rage, and goes on again.

"He was in the tradition of realism in which George Eliot wrote of the travails of Lydgate and the moral defeat of Dorothea. He wasn't an aesthete, he didn't want to be. But he was pushed towards it. Because *Women in Love* is a novel about experiencing the world as art—

good art or bad art. It came at the time of the First World War and the trenches, but it does not look directly at those, it is about the forms of vision and the forms of thought."

"And sex."

"And sex. Seen as part of art. But Birkin is not an artist, because Lawrence felt a distaste for writing with his nose in his navel. He wanted to write about death and Europe. And there is an emptiness, a lack of solidity, *because Birkin is not writing a book* when in fact we experience him as though he is. As there would have been an emptiness—a disappointment—if *all he was doing was writing a book*—when Lawrence wants to talk about everything, all life, *not books.*"

She stares at the students fiercely. They stare back. They are all listening. She does not know if she has put it properly this time. It is a question that obsesses her: the unreality of Birkin, Inspector of Schools, who sees the world as a book he isn't writing.

Jude says, "You know what Nietzsche said. He said, 'Only as an aesthetic product can the world be justified to all eternity.' He says *we are all art works* of 'the veritable creator,' 'although our consciousness of our own significance does scarcely exceed the consciousness a painted soldier might have of the battle in which he takes part.' "

"That's a red herring. I don't believe in your 'veritable creator.' "

"No. But maybe your David Herbert does or did, maybe his Birkin does or did or will. I'm afraid you're snarled up in your own narrow little utilitarian roots."

Frederica is about to reply angrily when there is a disturbance at the other end of the studio, and two people come in. The first is Desmond Bull, who says, "Here she is. The class must be finished or almost finished. All these kids must move on."

Behind Desmond Bull is Daniel Orton. His face is an interesting mess, his eyes lost in black bruised pits, his lips split, his nose crimson and florid.

"I've come to tell you," says Daniel, "that your husband is looking for you."

Frederica scrambles off the platform, and embraces him. The students begin to pack up.

"He found me," says Daniel, mildly enjoying the drama of his own appearance. "I hope he can't find you."

Desmond Bull fetches a chair. Daniel and Frederica sit down. Things rush through their minds. Stephanie, William, Mary, Leo.

"He went to see your father, too."

Frederica laughs. "I hope he didn't turn *him* black and blue."

Daniel says, "Don't laugh. He did. He slammed a door on his head. Your father took it calmer than I would. He let him go off with your dress."

"My *dress*?"

"Your dancing dress, your dad said."

Frederica does not like the idea of Bill hurt. Of Bill vulnerable.

"Help me, Daniel," she says, putting out a hand to touch his sleeve. Behind her she senses a whiff of rancid grease, of sour sweat, of fish.

"A Daniel come to judgement," says Jude. "I do believe I have found you at last, my own, my sweet, my only friend, and in the flesh, in the splendidly substantial and generously *abundant* flesh which I hadn't envisaged in all its perfection. Will you acknowledge this thing of darkness, my invisible Master?"

"Oh sod," says Daniel, alarmed out of his manners. "Steelwire." He repeats, "Oh sod."

"Steelwire?" says Jude. "An expletive I do not know."

"What we write in the book at work when we hear your nasty voice," says Daniel. "Descriptive, sort of."

"Is it flattering? Am I flattered? On the whole, yes. It is not bad. A little fame, a pseudonym. Steelwire. It isn't good, either. My name is Jude Mason. It was not, and now is. I am my own progenitor. In my own way. Will everything else be an anti-climax?"

"Probably," says Daniel. "You should start ringing someone else. I've got to talk to Frederica, now. Seriously."

"We shall meet again. I am glad to have seen you. You have an unexpected beauty, parson-person, you do not glitter or gleam but you have a sort of *light* in you. I hope my own appearance was not too disappointing."

Daniel stares gloomily from his chair. His eyes meet Jude's encrusted navel and travel down, across his limp grey member, towards his thin knees.

"You smell like an alley-cat," he says.

"I know several. Resourceful beasts, my friends. Do you know, I was present in the aether when meat was made of our friend's cheeks and ears?" he says to Frederica.

"Go away," says Frederica. "Please. I've got to think. You can talk to Daniel after."

"No he can't. I'm going. You and I can go somewhere and talk and then I'm going."

. . .

Frederica and Daniel talk in a coffee bar. It is a good coffee bar for talking in; it has booths, around Formica tables. Muzak plays. Frederica, who has been avoiding Daniel, who has not attempted to see him or answer his letter, is almost overwhelmed by her happiness in seeing him, by his reality and solidity. Tears rise in her eyes and run over: she puts out a hand amongst the coffee stains and Daniel grips it.

"It's not that your letter wasn't right. It was that I couldn't cope. I have been *such a fool* and now I'm scared. I wouldn't be *so* scared if it wasn't for Leo. I can't do right, for him."

"Tell me."

She tells him. The whole sorry story, the attraction of strangeness, the trap of the country house, the horror of being "a married woman" ("I thought I would still be *myself,* Daniel, and wasn't"), the mistake and the wonder of Leo, the guilt, the guilt, the Conservative canvassers, the friends, the anger, the blood, the axe. She does not tell him about the Bluebeard cupboard or about her visits to the Middlesex Clinic for sexually transmitted diseases.

Daniel listens well. It is his job, and he knows Frederica. She tells him hysterically that *he is real,* tears dripping down her sharp nose.

He says, "He told me he comforted you when she was killed."

"He did. That is true."

They stare at each other.

"It's not really *unusual,*" says Daniel, referring to the pain of grief and memory. "It's all over the place, everybody's got something. It doesn't make it any easier."

Frederica is grateful he is prepared to share any part of his pain with her. She grips his hand on the table.

"What will you do?" he asks her. "Get a divorce?"

"I must. There's Leo. It won't be easy."

"You need a good lawyer. I know one or two—it goes with the job. I'll give you a name and a number. You'd best get on wi' it, get some peace at the end. Where are you living?"

"With Thomas Poole. It works beautifully. He has an *au pair* and we all share the baby-sitting. Leo is not a baby. You must come and see him."

"I should like that. I work long hours, but I should like that. And I wonder—should we all go back to Yorkshire for Christmas? They'd be glad to see you—you know the reasons, beyond that you're their child and in trouble. And I'd like Leo to meet Will and Mary. It's not quite right that they don't know each other. Blood's thicker."

"Not so much these days. I'll think. I'm scared. I want to lick my wounds, I don't want to *discuss* things, the idiotic things I've done."

"You won't need to. Come with me."

They discuss Jude, briefly. Daniel describes his gadfly phone calls. Frederica expresses distaste. So does Daniel.

"He wants us to dislike him," says Daniel.

"Then we will," says Frederica. "We will dislike him *intensely,* if that's what he wants."

Frederica's extra-mural class is not in the Crabb Robinson Institute, but in an old elementary school, in Islington, a Catholic school, red, ugly, with a basement canteen serving ham and cheese buns, doughnuts and potato crisps, watery coffee and tannin-tanned tea, a school which has the beautiful and mysterious name Our Lady of the Sorrows. Frederica's course at Our Lady of the Sorrows has the workmanlike title "Post-War British Fiction." There is one full-length book on that subject, by an American, which states that post-war British fiction is about rebellious working-class lads from the provinces asserting themselves and finding a voice where once they were mute. It says that this subject is entirely new. Frederica questions this view: has the author of this work never read Lawrence, never read Arnold Bennett? She reads this book and takes a certain aesthetic pleasure in the critical attempt to make interesting what is (compared with Lawrence and Bennett) intrinsically *not very interesting,* except that everything is interesting *if you take a run at it,* she tells herself, I will get myself interested in Amis and Wain and Braine and all those others. I will also teach *Lord of the Flies* and Iris Murdoch. I am myself a provincial person become self-conscious but I cannot like the world of these novels. Lawrence was greedy for knowledge, for learning, he was interested in natural history and cultural history, he felt people should get out of mining villages. These people mostly sneer at such things. They have chips on their shoulders. I will say why this depresses me.

Her first extra-mural class resembles an Ionesco play. "If there are fewer than seven students," said Thomas Poole, "the class may have to close. It is pure luck whether people come or not, especially in your area. It is pure luck whether they stay, to some extent. If they don't, the class will be closed."

The class is on the top of the school, up four flights of steep red stone stairs, with an uncompromising metal railing. When Frederica goes into the room, clutching an introductory talk—"Some Trends in Modern British Writing"—she is greeted by the sight of about fifteen people squatting in an uncomfortable circle on small chairs, made for gnomes, for people Leo's size. There are two youngish men in dark suits, a middle-aged couple, a very pretty girl and a stretched-skinned woman who was once beautiful, a small man in a very clean forget-me-not-blue jumper over a tightly knotted green tie, a severe-looking woman, a large comfortable woman, an elderly man in a tweed jacket, and a nun. Frederica stares at this uncomfortable ring of unrelated faces.

"They can't expect you to sit like that," she says.

The nun says, "It has been known. Sometimes the only available chairs are infant chairs. I knew a woman who got down and her bones set into that position, and she had to be carried home bent up like a ladder, most unfortunate."

"My astronomy class," says the elderly man, "has more or less acceptable chairs."

"I think," says the blue jersey, "we should do a raid on other classrooms, Miss Potter, and quickly, and decisively."

The faces, variegated adult faces, with none of the homogeneity of the art student groups, look up at Frederica in a circle, assessing her, assessing the situation. One of the women has amazing blue-and-silver eyelids. One of the men has pince-nez:

"Do you know *where* to raid?" Frederica asks the blue jumper.

"Two floors down, double classroom, nothing in it *pro tem*."

"We shall get into trouble," says the large lady.

"We are all grown-ups," says Frederica.

They organise themselves. They find an empty classroom full of junior chairs, small but tolerable. One of the suits hands them to the other, who hands them to a chain of helpers on the stairs. In ten minutes the group is resettled, the discarded infant chairs stacked neatly at the back of the room. Frederica gives her talk. She is nervous; she has no idea who these people are, or why they are there, strangers who have walked in from the London streets, from a day's work, or perhaps a day's housekeeping, strangers who perhaps want to know about Post-War British Fiction because they want to write it, or perhaps because they are in need of dinner-party conversation, or perhaps because they desperately need to meet someone, anyone, and find

Post-War British Fiction a convenient background noise to accompany these meetings, or perhaps because they have to get out of a house they are shut in, or want to change themselves in some definable or undefinable way.

At that first meeting the group is not a group, and it is only ignorance of their names and natures that prevents Frederica from coming to the conclusion that they are too heterogeneous to form a group. She takes the register:

Rosemary Bell (a dark, thin, pretty woman who is a hospital almoner)

Dorothy Brittain (the large woman, an editorial assistant on *A Woman's Place* magazine)

Amanda Harvill (a beautiful woman, tanned, lined, well over forty, without profession)

Humphrey Maggs (the speedwell-blue jersey, who turns out to work as a clerk in Social Security)

Godfrey and Audrey Mortimer (a retired married couple)

Ronald Moxon (a taxi-driver)

George Murphy (a stockbroker)

Ibrahim Mustafa (a research student)

Lina Nussbaum (an unemployed receptionist)

John Ottokar (a computer programmer)

Sister Perpetua (nun and teacher)

Alice Somerville (retired Civil Servant)

Ghislaine Todd (a young psychoanalyst)

Una Winterson (housewife, mother of four children)

She is new at teaching; she has always said she would never teach; and teaching is in her blood. As she talks, she scans the rows. The two men in city suits sit together at the back (later they will separate). One is dark and one is blond. The dark one meets her eye with a slightly aggressive smile. The blond one stares down at his knees. The married pair smile encouragement. The large lady listens best; she manages to convey an awareness of the rhythms of the structure of Frederica's argument. Amanda Harvill's painted eyelids go up and down, up and down: it is not clear that her listening look *is* listening. Ronald Moxon and Lina Nussbaum fidget and shift. Lina Nussbaum, under a huge frizz of hennaed curls, fidgets worst, and makes a popping sound with her mouth. Sister Perpetua and Humphrey Maggs, accomplished listeners, sit side by side, respectful and thoughtful, and do not move a muscle. Frederica scans them all for signs of interest and rejection. She weaves a web of attention—a mention of Kafka caused a quick movement of interest in Ghislaine Todd; when his name comes back, Frederica meets the other woman's eye. Bit by bit, apart from Lina Nussbaum's popping, and possibly the downward stare of the blond John Ottokar, all the attention is somehow woven together. The questions are at first slow: a kindly one from Audrey Mortimer, a professional one from Humphrey Maggs, who has clearly already read all the proposed Post-War British Novels, a challenging one from Dorothy Brittain, designed to make the atmosphere more electric, a somewhat mischievous one from George Murphy, who has noticed an inconsistency in Frederica's brief account of the Welfare State. They are all talking to Frederica, not to each other. Frederica refers a tentative remark of Rosemary Bell back to the truculent Mr. Murphy, and for a moment the two exchange embryonic views on the effects of the Welfare State on the British people and on Post-War British Fiction. Threads are being knotted. The group walks down to the canteen and eats and drinks, measuring each other, asking "What do you do?" and "What do you think of C. P. Snow?" and "Did you see the *Marat-Sade*?" No one speaks to the nun, who appears unconcerned by her solitude, sipping tea. Frederica looks at them all with an incredulous excitement. She thinks of Olive and Rosalind and Pippy Mammott, of the orchard and the moat. At her elbow, Una Winterson, a quiet, fair woman, inquires socially if Frederica is married, if she has children. Frederica does not want to have that conversation; she turns round in irritation and sees a soft face stretched with anxiety. "I have four: they take up so much time; this is the first time I've come out on my own for thirteen years. I started a degree in classics once, but I got married in the middle and Mike (my husband) thought it wasn't worth going on. I do hope I haven't lost the ability to think. I do sometimes wonder if I have. I don't think I should ever have the courage to talk aloud in class, you know, that's why this coffee-break is such a good idea. If the coffee was only nicer."

Later, like all groups, this class will develop its closeness and splits, its inner circles and its scapegoats, its ritual lines of alliance and alignment, of opposition and passionate disagreement. Frederica is new to it; she has already sensed that the group must come together, and that this has something to do with her own position, standing up in front of them and speaking for an hour and then, after food and drink, listening, making sure.

The adult students are unlike the professional students. They desire knowledge and they come from what they think of as the real world, of work, above all, but also of things lived through, marriage, birth, death, success, failure, which are all phantasms to young students trying to find their shapes in the pages of books. The adults are inclined to measure the books against life and find them wanting. "It made me laugh like a drain," says the taxi-driver of the burning of the blankets in *Lucky Jim,* "but I'm buggered if I can see why I should spend time *talking* about it." George Murphy, the stockbroker, asks with a mocking belligerence why novels are about so little of the world: "the kitchen, forgive me, the *media, academe,* the novel. Just think a minute," he says, "what is going on out there, multi-national companies, people getting killed in very new ways in Vietnam, the discovery of the DNA, men in space, and the novel doesn't seem to have any idea about any of them. Why should I bother?"

"Why do you? Why do you come?"

He smiles. "I joined a class to find out how to mend my Lambretta. And for another ten shillings I could have another class. So here I am."

"Why do you stay?"

"Oh, I like to think a bit about life and death and sex. I expect we'll get on to those things."

Frederica gives a lecture about halfway through the term on "Nostalgia for Tolstoi." She takes her texts from Iris Murdoch and Doris Lessing, both of whom express a sharp dissatisfaction with fragmentary modern forms, and consequent moral simplicities and simplifications. The adults, who tend to talk about characters in books as though they were people whose fates were real, important and interesting, seize on this lecture and attack Frederica. Why, they say, can they not read Tolstoi? Why not read, says Dorothy Brittain, Tolstoi and Dostoevski, George Eliot and Thomas Mann, *Madame Bovary* and Proust? It is agreed that next term this will happen. Frederica does not know, yet, what this decision will do to her.

Frederica sits in the common-room at the Samuel Palmer School with her good friend Alan Melville. She tells him about the extra-mural class and Nostalgia for Tolstoi. She says, "It is funny how the tensions in all groups are sexual, whatever else they are." Alan looks her up and down, and says in his quietly amused Scottish voice, "You seem to be thriving on it. You are beginning to look like the Frederica I remember. Are they all in love with you?"

"There is one very beautiful one, but he never speaks."

"I didn't ask if you were in love with them. That way does no good. You must realise, they will all be in love with you, because of the nature of groups, and you mustn't take it personally."

"We go out in a group now, to the pub, after. At first only a few went, a kind of *inner group,* and then they asked me, and I try to include *all the others,* not just the kind of lively and intense ones."

"A good instinct. You are a born teacher."

"I am not. This is temporary. I am getting back my ambition but I've no idea what to *do* with it. But *I will do such things*—"

They laugh. Frederica thinks what a pure pleasure it is to have a friend who is a man. She looks at his clear-cut fair face and feels full of love for him: he is very attractive, sex is in him, and she has the good sense not to be attracted, for she knows, without knowing how she knows it, that to be Alan's friend is a durable delight, and to be his lover would be a disaster. And how does she know that, and in what unspoken reservations, in what reticence, in what brief sad silences, does she diagnose disaster? She says, "I do love you, Alan."

"I need to be loved. Come to my lecture on Vermeer, after coffee. I have written a wonderful lecture on Vermeer, and I would be glad of your presence."

The painter, Desmond Bull, comes up behind them. He too is a Scot, a craggy-looking Scot with gingery eyebrows like furry caterpillars, a heavy, bristling jaw, sharp blue eyes and diminishing fine red-gold hair in a *faute-de-mieux* tonsure. His chest hair, inside his very open shirt, is abundant and curly and fiery. He wears a matted and unravelling cardigan whose original colour is almost impossible to distinguish: it may have been some sort of blue.

"I shall come, Alan, I shall come and see your slides of Vermeer. You can count me in."

"I'm thinking of applying for a full-time job at Sotheby's," says Alan, apparently irrelevantly.

"You'd be richer. And you wouldn't find *Rituals* in your classrooms."

"Rituals?" says Frederica.

"Happenings. *Old-fashioned* Happenings, organised by Bly. The Calling-Down of Powers. Sub-Golden-Dawn. Most amusing. Here is the man himself."

Richmond Bly approaches smilingly, bearing an exquisite Japanese ceramic cup of some sort of herbal tea. The common-room is a kind of heterogeneous repository of works by students—a zebra-striped sofa, a scarlet plastic bench, a few very comfortable Bauhaus leather-and-steel chairs. The walls are hung with paintings, chosen very fairly from amongst the current student trends: two brilliant hard-edged abstract acrylic paintings; a large soft grey abstract whirl; a painting of stick-like figures in a sombre green park, owing something to Lowry, something to Seurat, something to Nolde; a mystical image of floating figures in conical hats. There is also a reproduction of Linnell's portrait of the mildly agricultural Samuel Palmer, and two of Palmer's prints of sheep, clouds, trees, dark, light, linear insistence and the mystery of space and vanishing behind the lines. The coffee-pots are variable: a silver one, hand-beaten in the jewellery department, with an extravagant rose agate knob, and an austere and functional steel one from Industrial Design, which does not pour very well. All the cups are different, heavy stoneware, thinnest porcelain, comic monkey-heads, lop-sided cabbage-forms, perfect globes of rosy glaze.

"I hear good reports of your classes," says Bly to Frederica. "The students like them."

"I'm glad."

"I am told you are working for a publisher."

"I read for one, in the evenings, yes. Mostly rubbish."

"I am looking for a publisher. I have written a book. A rather *unusual* book, I flatter myself, and such things are, sad to say, hard to place. I wonder if you would care to read it—"

Frederica says she would be honoured. She adds that she does not know *much* about publishing—almost nothing—her opinion is not of much worth—

"You must by now have some inkling of what goes on in the commercial mind. You know the story of J.R.R. Tolkien. His publisher wanted to reject *The Lord of the Rings* and it was published as a profit-sharing venture—to please the Professor—who is now *very rich.* The commercial mind fails to understand the public hunger for the stories of romance and mystery."

"I'm sure that's true," says Frederica, staring at the glass table in front of her, under which Bly's feet are twisting round and round each other in an energy of enthusiasm.

"My lecture is in ten minutes," says Alan. "I must see to my slides."

"You must *take the register,*" says Bly. "These students *cannot have their degrees* without attending art-historical courses. It is a rule."

"I know," says Alan.

In the lecture theatre, he sets up his slides. Desmond Bull and Frederica sit together under the projector. The time for the beginning of the lecture comes, and goes, and ten more minutes go past, and no one comes. At the end of this time, the door opens, and admits Jude Mason, fully clothed in his dirty blue velvet frock coat and a pair of extremely tight midnight-blue velvet trousers. He does not look at them or speak to them, but sits in the front row, as far as possible from Alan, Desmond Bull and Frederica, meticulously swinging out and arranging the flaps of his coat, folding his hands and bowing his head, as though in church.

"As I expected," says Alan.

"We are here," says Bull. "You can show us Vermeer."

"I never went to lectures at eleven in Cambridge," says Frederica practically. "They destroyed the whole morning's work."

"Nor did I," says Alan, who is writing an extremely neat column of *O*s in his class register.

"There's a movement amongst them," says Bull. "They really believe the past is dangerous, is a kind of death. They think it destroys their originality. They think academic talk is anti-art. But mostly they believe in making a rupture, making a revolt, making a new world."

"Vermeer is not my idea of an oppressor," says Frederica.

"Perhaps I am," says Alan. "I tell them I think he solved problems quietly in the corners of his paintings that they take whole pretentious blown-up canvases to explore, and went on, and solved more, and then more—"

"The size is part of the point," says Bull.

"I do know that. I do understand that. It doesn't interest me *much*—"

The sawing voice says from the front row, "Why are we waiting?"

The paintings, or not the paintings, but light shadows of them, thin skins of colour transfused and transfixed by the stream of light, appear on the screen. A woman pouring eternal creamy-white milk from a jug, in a plane of light, a woman weighing gold dust, intent faces closed on their own meditation, knowing somehow, Frederica thinks, that this moment of concentration is to stretch out into eternity, or at least, into an unhuman stretch of time. The geometry of maps, of carpets, of the panes of glass in half-open windows, mediating light, mediated by light. The *View of Delft,* with the yellow patch of roof and the perfect spherical bubbles of light on the wet sides of the ships. A meditation intense, quiet, concentrated and apparently without any touch of anger, or hurt, or aggression. Alan shows how certain lights are made in the *camera obscura.* He does what his own new light-beam, his own lenses, can do, and shows Frederica and Desmond Bull what Vermeer could never have seen, a painted blush, a poised mouth, hairs, the light on a wet eyeball so close that they are resolved into flickering movements of a lost brush in paint now fixed. And then he draws back, and there is a woman, in a room, playing a spinet, weighing gold dust, pouring milk.

When Alan has finished, the sawing voice says, "You could weep, couldn't you?"

It is not clear how this is meant to be taken. Therefore it is not answered. Bull says, "Painters complain, art historians complain, that everyone these days only sees transparencies, which are the colours of light, not the colours of pigment. And so they get the wrong ideas, they see *wrong,* these people say. I say, this is new, it exists, we see all this light—we can learn from it—we could even learn to paint things *to be transparent—*"

Alan says, "They talk about slashing Rembrandts and Vermeers because young painters don't get enough attention. Such *anger—*"

"Just Oedipal," says Frederica. "Possibly."

"Oedipus felt guilty, my dear. These people feel they are waging a holy war. The young against the old and the dead."

"They will grow old themselves," says Frederica, who throughout the increasing youthfulness of the sixties fails to understand how the professionally young fail to understand that they will grow old.

"They may not," says the sawing voice. "They are working up magics to stop time. They are making timeless moments, they are reversing its direction."

The woman pours the milk from her jug. The jug will never empty, her careful wrist will never lift.

"And do you think," says Jude Mason, "that in another thousand years, or two hundred, not to be overweening, my own stringy limbs and my not-very-clean face will shine off screens in theatres in times to come?"

"I should think," says Bull, "that all your images are made in materials with built-in obsolescence, if you want to know."

"Writing is safer," says Jude Mason, "if you want to perpetuate yourself. I am writing a book."

"*Everyone* is writing a book," says Frederica, thinking rather hysterically of Richmond Bly.

Frederica is aware that Desmond Bull finds her attractive. This is not particularly flattering since it is clear that he also finds a good half of the women students attractive, and possibly some of the teachers. But it does stir a flicker of new-old life in her, a kind of readiness. He wanders into her little office, where she is sitting screened off from the Foundation studio, where the students are still experimenting with Jude's grey flesh in an alembic of light.

"Would you like to come and look at the work, one lunchtime? I've got a studio in Clerkenwell, we could go in my van."

"I ought to go home and see my son. I do try to get home for lunch."

"It wouldn't take long. You'd like it. Your son's got all your life."

"I ought not."

"But you will."

She goes with him. He buys a French loaf and a packet of salami and a bottle of Valpolicella and they get into the van. Frederica knows that this is something he does often and often. Only the woman changes. She does not mind this. She likes Bull: she likes the way he knits his brow when thinking. Shut in the van with him, with a faint odour of garlic struggling with a strong smell of exhaust and an even stronger smell of turpentine and white spirit emanating from Desmond Bull, she thinks drily that painters must be at a disadvantage as far as pheromones go. Bull's smile, his strong body, his quick hands are attractive, but the smells are certainly not. She sits upright beside him and discusses Jude Mason.

"Nobody knows where he lives," says Bull. "He picks up his letters from a poste restante in Soho. You might say he was pathetic, tho' he's got a perfect right to his own style, dirt and all—but he isn't, quite, he's got a sort of integrity. Richmond Bly thinks he's mad."

"*I* think Richmond Bly's mad."

Frederica bites back the story of *The Silver Ship.*

"Madder than Blake. Silly-mad. I agree."

The studio is two large rooms built over a warehouse, and is entered up an iron ladder. The smell of paint thinner intensifies, killing the last of Frederica's hunger. The rooms are very large, but the living space is very small, since both rooms are walled in with large canvases on stretchers, several deep. In the centre of each room is a double mattress, with rumpled pillows and a bright Scandinavian blanket. On the floor of one of the studios is a Baby Belling and an electric kettle. In the other is a very small fridge.

"Sit down, make yourself comfortable. It's very basic. You can have a party, or an intimate cuddle, in here. I call these two rooms the Divided Self of Desmond Bull. On your left, modern art post-Rauschenberg. On your right, the Scottish European, the guilty painterly painter. Where would you like to be?"

"How can I tell, if all I can see is the backs?"

"You want me to turn them?"

"That's what I came for, isn't it?"

Desmond Bull pulls the cork and gives Frederica a plastic cup of red wine. It is not very nice red wine. It is sour. He puts an arm round her shoulder.

"Oh, I dunno," he says. "Come and look at my etchings and all that. Why don't we sit down and have a bit of a chat, and so on, and a drink, and then think about the work?"

He puts a hand on her breast. Frederica puts a friendly hand on his hand. Somewhere inside her, her body tries to respond. This arouses a series of protesting tugs of pain and misery in her inflamed interior. Desmond Bull gives her a warm and turpentiney kiss. Frederica says, "I'm a bit off all this at the moment. Just at the moment, it won't go. And I want to see the work. I did come to see the work."

Bull is momentarily disconcerted. Frederica thinks with amusement that he would be much less worried to show her his naked body than these hidden images. And that the idea of sex, of possible sex, has turned her into *a girl, the girl* (at the moment) in his eyes, whereas when they talk, she is someone. He says, "Well, where shall we start?" and then, "It's a bit private, you see, all this. I do it to sell it, but I do it all by myself here, it's a kind of frenzy, I do it *by myself,* and then it has to be looked at, it has to go out and be public." He says, "I'm a bit of a schizophrenic." It is a very fashionable word. But when he turns the canvases round, Frederica sees what he means.

In the left-hand studio, the work is made by someone in the grip of the idea that art is everything and that everything can be seen as art. There is a sense in which it is a junk shop. One work is made of hundreds and hundreds of electric wires, stripped, coiled, layers thick like thick impasto, and all colours, woven red and black fat wires, heavy-duty blue plastic wires, orange, brown, green, acid yellow, like nests, like tangles, like barbed-wire fences, like cartoon roses. Another is rows of pebbles. "One from every garden of every house in my mother's street. Each pebble represents *a* suburban garden. This one is fat and green. That one is rather thin and sort of russet. They are in rows like the houses they come from." He pauses. "The woman who goes with that stodgy grey one wears curlers and has cancer. The one with that quartzy one is a dishy blonde who comes out on her doorstep in a dressing gown."

"How am I supposed to see all that?"

"You can't. But once I tell you, you know it, don't you, you can't unknow it. You can look at the subtle colours of the pebbles, see, the *variety of the colours*—I love this blood-coloured one with blue flecks, the lady who goes with that wears desperate, sad, broken high-heeled yellow shoes and keeps swaggering and staggering. Each of the pebbles has a number, that's the number of the house."

"Which is your mother?"

"That's the right question, you see, do I or don't I distinguish her in that row of pebbles? Which is my mother?"

"Forty-two is dried melon seeds. All the rest are stones. Ergo, forty-two is your mother."

"She's got cancer, too. Of the ovaries. She's shrivelling. I told you, these things are sort of private."

"It's a row of *stones*—" Frederica struggles. "Can it mean anything to me without your talking?"

Desmond Bull is turning things round, bringing colours and forms and objects into the studio, further reducing its open space. He exhibits a gaudy and strangely pleasing collage of flowered shirts, pressed very flat, blue with yellow daisies, pink with red poppies, orange with purple hibiscus.

"You can go out of your mind with looking at these colour combinations," he says. "Shop windows scream at you. You know?"

He turns more. Black canvases, white canvases, some shiny and uniform, some with the black and white smeared over colour, which stares faintly through, a hairstreak of crimson here, a veiled patch of delicious apple green there, yellow ochre under a black stain, indigo under smoke.

"Rauschenberg erased de Koonings, he just painted over them. On the principle that there was art lying around all over the world, and that there was talent all over, you just make what you need, what you see now. These are all erasures of my own work. There are old paintings of mine struggling around under the black and white. I can remember what some of them are—that one was a rather good Cubist self-portrait, that one I think was a Bonnard-ish sort of a window into a garden that wouldn't give up being derivative—yes, look, there's a bit of apple blossom under the black—"

"Did you erase them because you liked them or because you didn't?"

"Both. Both. Paintings I was too fond of and ones that I rather loathed."

"It's all very *theoretical.*"

"It is. It's passionate too, that's what gets me, that's why I do it. It comes out of a sort of idea about art—being *everything*—and *everything being art*—and this is a bit like taking LSD—all the world begins to explode and implode with glittery *meaning.* I'm sorry you won't come to bed with me. It breaks the tension."

"That's a good reason for sex."

Frederica is still baffled by her own relation to the mysterious/ordinary pebbles.

"The thing about the pebbles is, they are no good to me without me being inside your head. All I can do with them, is get *my own* row of pebbles. Or whatever. Shirts, or a collage of chocolate papers, you know?"

"You won't forget my pebbles."

"I won't," says Frederica, almost irritated by this fact. "Of course I won't." And she never does.

"If people *give* you pebbles," says Bull, "it's no good. And for pebbles read anything. I had a girlfriend who always turned up with bags full of shirts she thought I might like. I made a collage once of her offerings—one for each fuck—but it was a half-hearted affair."

When the bottle of wine is drunk, and another, found in the bedclothes, has been opened, Desmond Bull moves into the second studio. This time he does not speak; he moves from wall to wall, humping the canvases and grunting, and offering no more comment than "a painting of masks," "another painting of masks," "another painting of masks," "a painting of masks on fire."

Frederica too does not speak. She does not know enough about paintings to comment on the paint, or even to think accurately about it. She has been in the Art School long enough not to try to convert it into narrative, although the masked figures half-invite this. They are very unsettling; they are articulated skeletons, or studio-articulated lay figures wearing masks that are full of extremely articulated expressions of horror, delight, the rictus of sexual bliss, the smirk of flirtation, the disintegrating template of age, and are at the same time purely flat, purely patterns of well-laid patches of paint, related planes, or a band of dark floating seed-shapes that read suddenly, in another light, as dark hollow eyes in the light, on the paint, in the painted light. Some of the colours are sombre and brilliant, reds, flames, golds, Veronese blues. And some are pale, bluish pinks on thick chalky white, candle-wax colours with touches of transparent blood-pink, and here and there a yellow hand, and here and there a sky-blue foot.

"It's about the impossibility of figurative painting," says Bull.

"About what it feels like to *be* a human body in an abstract world," says Frederica, cleverly, catching his thought.

"I hadn't put it quite that way. I like that. Have some more wine."

"I like the pinks."

"That's Ensor. His pinks are staggering. I'm still learning. You might say the masks are Ensor—but the masks are mine too, they aren't his, his kind of grisly carnival isn't what I'm doing, mine's about Greek tragedy too, about *coming from behind a front.*"

"As though the erased paintings were trying to talk," says Frederica, inspired. He looks at her very sharply.

"Something like that. You're a clever girl. One of these days, when you're not off it, you must come back and we'll have a good long *friendly* fuck, if you understand that."

Can one fuck erased paintings? Frederica thinks giddily. And is a naked prancing man a mask for a brain and a pair of eyes watching and watching and trying to make sense?

"I ought to get back to my son," she says. "I'm glad I saw the work."

Back in the Bloomsbury flat Leo is sitting companionably with Thomas Poole and Simon. He does not run to greet her, but this is a form of punishment; his averted eyes are full of trouble and punishing anger. Thomas Poole, too, looks at Frederica as though she were a desirable woman. He says, "Mr. Parrott rang. And Hugh Pink. You are in demand. And Tony Watson, who thinks he has talked the *New Statesman* into letting you review some books."

"Good. I'm tired."

"I'll bring you a cup of coffee. Sit down and I'll bring you a coffee."

He stands up. She feels guilty. She should have been home hours ago. Thomas Poole touches her hair on his way out to the kitchen. Leo says, "Sometimes you can hate people quite a lot."

"Who? Who do you hate?"

He does not answer. After a bit, he says, "I hate not knowing where people are. I like it when people are where I know where they are. At Bran House, I knew where everyone was."

"I don't go for long. I always come back. I'm earning our living."

"We once *had* a living."

Frederica cannot speak. He creeps to her side, and puts his arms round her waist.

"Never mind," he says, as she might have said.

She bends her head to his. She smells his hair. She has no choices. She imagines suddenly a film in which a sagacious dog travelled hundreds of miles, back along the scent, or the magnetic field, which pulled from what it knew and loved. This hair she could distinguish in a room piled high with other heads. This note she would hear through all others. This person is the centre. It is not what she would have chosen but it is a fact, it is a truth stronger than other truths. It is a love so violent that it is almost its opposite.

"We hate people when we love them," she says. "Sometimes."

VIII

Frederica, Leo and Daniel travel north for Christmas, sitting together on the crowded train like the nuclear family they are not. Thomas Poole is hurt that Frederica and Leo have not stayed to make a family Christmas in the Bloomsbury flat: Christmas is a time when somebody is always hurt. Both Frederica and Daniel are afraid of going back into the family from which Stephanie is absent. Frederica is also aware of having behaved badly to her parents, who do not know Leo. They are fetched to Freyasgarth from Calverley station by Marcus, who says little but seems calm, which was not always the case. As they drive out along the moorland roads Frederica's heart lifts: it is grey, it is dark, it is windswept, it is the north from which she comes.

She is taken aback by the beauty of the new house. It is Winifred, not Bill, who meets her on the doorstep, a Winifred smiling with unquestioning delight and weeping a little—"*Frederica,* Leo," touching both with a warmth that in the earlier days would have been reserve and holding back. Frederica finds that she too is weeping. Leo clings to her leg and watches. Behind Winifred is Mary, who runs at Daniel, and is lifted in his arms. Behind Mary is Bill, smaller than Frederica remembers him, paler and less fiery, waiting to see what his daughter will do. Frederica rushes forward and kisses him too. Marcus carries suitcases to pretty bedrooms looking out on moorland. They are all vaguely aware that Frederica's return from her long sulk or evasion is and is not the restoration of the lost daughter. Stephanie will not return. Winifred embraces Daniel. Bill shakes his hand. Exclaiming with pleasure, sniffing with emotion, the family moves into the living room, which is in the dark of a winter afternoon, except for a tall Christmas tree, shining with multicoloured lights, red, blue, green, gold, white, and decorated, by Winifred and Mary, with the magical golden wire hexagons and polyhedrons made eleven years ago by Marcus for Stephanie's Christmas tree.

Next to the Christmas tree stands Daniel's son, Will, who is ten, with Daniel's dark hair and watchful dark eyes. He stares at his father with angry intensity, and flinches when Daniel approaches to hug or kiss him. Daniel retreats. Frederica says, "You remember me, Will?"

"More or less," says Will, sounding absurdly like Daniel.

Winifred fetches tea on a trolley. There is tea in her wedding-present silver teapot, there are sandwiches of potted meat and egg and cress, there are hot mince pies and a huge Christmas cake. "We made it together," Mary tells Daniel. "Grandma and Will and I made it, we stirred and stirred, we made it *months* ago and left it to *mature*; it's full of brandy and lovely spices. And yesterday we iced it and decorated it for you all to come. We piped everyone's initial round the edge—Marcus helped us put the proportions right—*B* and *W* and *F* and *M* and *D* and *W* again and *M* and *L* for Leo—with silver balls round the letters, and roses decorating them, and then in the middle we made the moors in snow—we put the Fylingdales Early Warning System in the middle because Will wanted it, though it's a funny thing—and snowy trees, and here is a frozen lake—and there is a beck and some crags—Jacqueline says we oughtn't to have the Fylingdales balls but Marcus says it's all right, they're there—they look lovely in icing sugar and we can *eat them up*—"

Daniel says the cake is beautiful, which it is. Winifred says, unnecessarily, that it's a *secular* cake, and Mary says quickly that they are all going to the Carol Service in the church in the village tomorrow on Christmas Eve. "It isn't midnight, it's for the *family,* the teachers at my school go, we sing, I'm good at singing, everyone's going. Except Grandpa, of course."

At teatime Jacqueline Winwar comes with presents for the family to be put under the tree. She is accompanied by the geneticist with whom she works on her snail populations, Dr. Luk Lysgaard-Peacock, half-Danish, half-Yorkshire, with a square-cut jutting gold-red beard, gold-red hair and dark blue eyes under deep eyebrows. Frederica has never paid much attention to Marcus's young friend Jacqueline, whom she always thinks of as one of two, Ruth and Jacqueline, the blonde and the brown, Marcus's religious friends, Gideon Farrar's Young People. She remembers Jacqueline as a nice brown leggy girl with long bunches of hair and owlish glasses. What she now sees is a wiry young woman, about twenty-six years old, who moves quickly and neatly, and has a poised and watchful oval face under a cap of shining brown hair, variable browns, all blending and changing in the light. She has clear dark brown eyes behind black-framed glasses. Will goes and stands next to her. Mary kisses her and so does Winifred. Marcus says "Jacquie," with real pleasure, and is also pleased to see Luk Lysgaard-Peacock. Daniel asks about the snails and Luk says they are hibernating. Frederica watches as they all sit and chat easily. She sees Jacqueline look at Marcus, and then sees Luk Lysgaard-Peacock look at Jacqueline, both with that look that betrays a particular interest, not proprietorial but simply more alive, more alert. She watches Winifred hurry to give Jacqueline tea, mince pies, cake, information about carols. She thinks: My mother would like her for a daughter. She thinks: But it was the *other* one Marcus liked, a much more fey and boring person. The nurse, he liked the nurse, she remembers. She looks at her brother. He is talking to Luk Lysgaard-Peacock. She hears the word "engram," she hears the words "molecular memory," she hears the names Scrope, Lyon Bowman, Calder-Fluss. Jacqueline says, "There has to be something wrong with the planaria experiments, I cannot believe memory is carried that way."

"We could try and repeat the experiment," says Lysgaard-Peacock.

"I'd like to get up something with snails," says Jacqueline. "They have large neurones. You could do something interesting on the chemistry of memory."

Frederica watches Marcus. No, he is not sexually interested in this nut-brown intelligent person. Or does not appear to be—who has ever been able to say what Marcus wanted? Whereas from time to time Jacqueline gives a quick look in his direction. And Luk Lysgaard-Peacock gives a sharp look in hers. Frederica thinks about sex and is quite unaware that she is hearing the first discussion of what will be a scientific advance, an important piece of research.

She thinks: Families pull together and fly apart. Now, I am pleased and excited to see all these faces which resemble mine and each other. But by the end of the holiday we may all feel trapped and impinged on and diminished.

There is a sound of wheels stopping with a whine and a scream. The door bell sounds. Winifred opens the door and stands, puzzled. On the doorstep, in a navy overcoat, shoulders squared, is Nigel Reiver.

"I am hoping," he says, "to find my wife and child. I have brought their presents and thought—since it is Christmas—they might speak to me at least. I have come a long way."

"Come in," says Winifred, uncertainly. It is indeed Christmas; he is the husband and father; hospitality requires that he should be let in; Winifred knows nothing of him or of what has happened.

"Wait—" he says, and fetches from the car two large cardboard boxes, wrapped in Christmas paper, striped in midnight blue and silver, with shiny rosettes of blue and silver paper ribbons.

Frederica stands up in the room with the Christmas tree and moves to stand in the doorway, so that he cannot cross the threshold into the lighted group inside. He puts down his two large boxes, and stands easily there, meeting her eye, ready to move quickly. There is his real face, the dark, dark look, the intentness that always stirs her.

"I did think," he says, "it might be sensible to talk, just to talk. I do think you might at least let me know what you think is happening. I do think I have a right to say Happy Christmas to my son. Don't you?"

The real wrong, Frederica thinks, was hers, was done by her in marrying him when she did not wholly want to, when she could not go through with it. This knowledge makes her tentative, uncertain.

"I don't know," she says, barring the door. "It's no good. It's no good."

"I don't want to impose myself on you if you don't want me," says Nigel. "I won't stay long, though I've come a long way. I want two things: to see my son and give him a Christmas present, and to have a *sensible* discussion with you about where we go from here, even if it's only to arrange a time and place to have a discussion. That's all. I think I have a right to that, I do think so."

Leo appears at Frederica's side. He is white, and staring. He looks from one to the other. Nigel holds out his arms. Leo looks at Frederica, who nods—what? Permission? Understanding? He walks past her, and is lifted in his father's arms. Nigel buries his nose in the bright hair whose scent is the centre of Frederica's existence. There are tears in Nigel's eyes.

"I've missed you," he says to Leo. Leo twists his hand in his father's collar. He looks back at Frederica with Nigel's black eyes in her own sharp white face. She is ready to die, to lose consciousness.

"*Take your coat off,*" says Leo.

"Come in," says Frederica, moving with stone legs, out of the doorway. "Come and meet the family. It is Christmas."

She introduces him. "My father you know. My mother, my brother, Marcus, my brother-in-law, Daniel, Will, Mary, this is a friend, Jacqueline, and a friend, Dr. Lysgaard-Peacock."

"I'll go now," says Luk Lysgaard-Peacock.

"No—" says Frederica. "There is no need for anyone to go. Nigel has just come with presents, he isn't staying, no one must move."

Her voice is sharp. It makes people want to move, and begs them not to. They do not move. Lysgaard-Peacock and Jacqueline do not move. Winifred takes Nigel's coat, and brings him tea and cake. Leo sits on his knee, with an arm round his neck. Bill and Nigel nod at each other with a curious respect: Nigel then nods at Daniel, who smiles and frowns together. No one speaks, so Nigel says, "I brought presents for Frederica and Leo. Perhaps they should open them, since I won't be staying. Perhaps," he says, looking at Will, "you could fetch the two boxes in the corridor."

Will does as he is asked. Nigel tells his son to open his box. Still in the same fiercely cosy voice he tells Will to help Leo. Will helps. The box is opened. A Hornby electric train is revealed, a beautiful thing, a Flying Scotsman engine, carriages, trucks, rails, turntable, station, signals, points.

"He's too little," says Will. He stares almost angrily at Nigel.

"I'm not," says Leo. He clasps the engine to his chest. "I'm not too little. This is *mine*."

"I think you could help him set it up and understand it," says Nigel to Will. "He's not too little if someone works it with him, shows him the ropes, sets it up." He smiles his warm secret smile at Will. "I'll be glad if you'll set it up for him. I'd like to do it myself—all fathers like to play trains at Christmas—but I shan't be here. But you will."

He has somehow acquired a little more territory. He turns to Frederica.

"Won't you open yours?"

"I'll put it under the tree with the others and open it later, on Christmas Day."

"Now," says Nigel. "I may have to take it back, I need to know now if it is what you want."

Nothing, she wants to cry, I want nothing. Leo says, "Open it. I want to see. Open."

Will carries the parcel across. Frederica pulls listlessly at the blue rosette, at the wrapping paper. Leo climbs down from Nigel's knee and comes to help. The shiny paper rustles. There is a large, solid, cardboard box. There is silver-and-pink tissue. There is a dress. It is dark charcoal grey with a high neck and long tight cuffs, woven with red silk braid and embroidery, very rich, very plain. It is a long tunic that goes over a short, slightly flaring skirt. It looks like, it is, Courrèges. Frederica, like most women with red hair, does not wear red, but there is one red, a clear dark vermilion, that brings out the fire in her hair and the gold in her dusting of freckles. This is that red. No one knows what to say. Winifred is wearing a heavy green polo neck and a tweed skirt; Jacqueline is wearing a dark brown double-knit jumper over fawn cord trousers: Frederica herself is in jeans and a checked flannel shirt. Leo says, "Put it on."

"I can change it, or get it altered," says Nigel.

"Put it on! Put it on!" says Leo. "Now. I say, now!"

And Frederica, who has been holding the lid of the box, ready to replace it, suddenly puts it down, picks up the dress, and walks out of the room to put it on.

"I thought," says Nigel to Winifred, "there must be a pub near here, where I could stay—"

"Our bedrooms are full," says Winifred foolishly.

"Completely full," says Bill. "No room at the inn, I'm afraid. None."

Frederica comes back wearing the dress. In its honour she has put on black tights and carefully dressed her hair in a chignon. She is beautiful. Frederica is never beautiful, though often alive with attractive energy, but just for the moment, in the Courrèges dress, she is wholly beautiful, it is the word. The dress fits almost too perfectly: her small high breasts sit neat and elegant inside its beautiful seams; her thin wrists, her narrow waist, her long thin hips, are beautiful where the silk-lined cloth skims past them, making them look like necessary forms in relation to each other. It is a strange style, formal, tailored, severe, ending so far above the knee that the brevity of the skirt should be childish, a gym-slip, a dolly-dress, but is not. Frederica's long thin legs are set off by it; another inch on her thighs would spoil its up-and-down simple complexity. She stands there. Luk Lysgaard-Peacock says, "Beautiful," and Nigel looks sharply at him.

"I can't take it," says Frederica. Every precise inch of it is a betrayal of carnal knowledge, of Nigel's certainty of the nature of her body, of how it works, how it moves, how it is.

"And everyone always says men can't shop for women," says Nigel, as though she had not spoken. "They can if they put their mind to it, of course they can. When I saw that red, I thought, That's the one, it's a risk, but it'll work. And it does. You have to admit it *does something for you,* Frederica. You've got to keep it—no strings—whatever you—whatever we—decide. I want you to have it. It's *yours.* No one else could wear it like that. Leo likes it, don't you?"

"I like it," says Leo.

Winifred makes a new pot of tea for her son-in-law whom she does not know. Leo sits on his knee. Frederica stands there, incongruous and beautiful. The dress isolates her from the company, as though she were in cellophane wrapping. She looks at Nigel with reluctant admiration: there are things he knows how to do. He discusses with Winifred the possibility of local pubs. Luk Lysgaard-Peacock thinks of recommending the Giant Man at Barrowby and then looks at Frederica and does not speak. Leo says, "You might possibly sleep here with us, possibly you might."

"I don't think so," says Nigel, with the same reasonable ease. "Not just now, I don't think that could be managed."

A clock strikes in the village. Mary says, "We shall miss the carol service, we *must go.*"

"Count me out," says Bill.

"We already did," says Mary. "But Daddy will come, and Grandma, and Will, and Jacqueline and Dr. Lysgaard-Peacock, will you come?"

"Why not?" looking at Jacqueline.

"And Marcus will come with *them,* and what about you?" says Mary, looking doubtfully first at Frederica and then at Leo and Nigel.

"Last year we went to carols," says Leo.

"So we did," says Nigel. "In Spessendborough. It was lovely, wasn't it? I love carols. They connect you to your ancestors. Mine are all buried in Spessendborough."

"We don't run to *ancestors,*" says Bill.

"Everyone has ancestors," says Luk Lysgaard-Peacock, looking at the faces with a geneticist's eye.

"Come to the carols," says Leo to Nigel. He turns to his mother in her dress. "You come."

"I'll change this dress."

"*No.* Come in the dress."

Frederica changes her dress.

. . .

They put on their coats, all except Bill, and walk through Freyasgarth to St. Cuthbert's Church, where in the candlelight they sing the old songs: "O Come, All Ye Faithful," "Unto Us a Boy Is Born," "Lullay My Liking," "We Three Kings," "It Came upon the Midnight Clear," "The Holly and the Ivy." Leo stands between his parents, holding both hands from time to time, separating them and connecting them. Daniel stands between Will and Mary. The singing is not much, but there are one or two sweet high voices in the stone, and Luk Lysgaard-Peacock has a clear, unafraid, pleasant tenor. Mary, alone of the Potter stock, can sing, and does, clear and small. Frederica thinks of years of being *trapped* in school singing. And now she is a grown woman, autonomous, and *trapped* by her own nature—her own acts and choices.

Winifred weeps for her daughter Stephanie.

Will cannot weep for his mother.

Nigel's bass is occasionally off-key, but a useful augmentary din.

Daniel thinks of the child in the straw. He thinks of his son, who has a brief life in front of him, and of Mary's son, who was most cruelly killed, long ago. He thinks of the face he does not think of and manages to avert his attention from it in time, by concentrating on song. "The holly bears a berry, As red as any blood, And Mary bore sweet Jesus Christ, To do poor sinners good."

Back in the house, there is a move to leave Nigel and Frederica alone to talk. Frederica does not want this, but everyone nevertheless disappears: Luk and Jacqueline to their own families, Bill to his study, Marcus and Winifred to wrap presents, Daniel and his family to wash up. Nigel and Frederica and Leo sit together in the sitting-room in the evening dark. There is a wood fire.

"We never lived in a beautiful house," says Frederica, wondering.

"Listen," says Nigel. "Come back to our house—not for Christmas, I can see you're here—but come back *for a visit,* say Boxing Day, say the day after—there's the Meet—we could talk a bit and think things out. Sooty is dying to see Leo, and so are Pippy and Auntie Olive and Auntie Rosalind—they are *very sad* at spending Christmas without him, when families ought to be together—"

"This is mine—"

"And I found you, because I knew you'd be here, because *families are important*. So I know you know they are, so I know you know Leo ought to see his."

"I want to see Sooty," says Leo. He says, "I want to see him every day." He says, "Let's go back and just see him, Mummy?"

"I can't," says Frederica.

"Only for a few days. You can bear us for a few days."

"I can't. I mustn't. I can't come."

She cannot, in front of Leo, cry out that she is sorry, she made a hideous mistake, she should never have married, and now they must all suffer for it.

Nigel says, "Well, let Leo come. Let me take him back to see Pippy and Sooty and the aunts. We love him, he's ours, it will be his house, I have a right to see my son."

Frederica bows her head. She thinks she knows that if Leo goes back to Bran House she will never see him again, unless, of course, she too goes back. And she is afraid of going back, physically as well as emotionally. She cannot go there again. It is quite reasonable for Nigel to want to see, to entertain, his son—she believes a child needs two parents, she believes, in principle, in civilised sharing. She also fears, with a sick, exhausted part of her, that Leo may be happier in the end at Bran House, where his life will have a form to which he has been brought up, a form that is his inheritance, on one side. And then she thinks of him being sent away, a little boy, to boarding school, as Nigel was. And then she remembers the clinging body of the boy on the run through the woods.

"I don't know if that would work," she says weakly. She may be being hysterical. Leo could go for a fortnight and come back. He *might* come back.

She is sure in her bones that he would not.

"What do you think, Leo?" says Nigel. "Do you want to come with me?"

"It isn't fair," says Frederica. "How can you make him choose?"

"*You* made him choose," says Nigel with sudden violence. "*You* took him off against his will, against my will, without a word, with your shoddy *friends* in a vulgar way—"

"He *came*—"

"Ah. So *he* came. So in that case you were prepared to leave him then. So you can let him come back now. Bran House is *where he belongs.* So are you coming, Leo?"

"Not without Mummy."

"Just for a week or two, with or without Mummy. If you can persuade her to come, so much the better—if not—"

"You *can't do this to Leo.* Let him go to his grandmother now, let's talk this out without him."

"Leo. Are you coming? Come with me. Come home."

"Listen, Nigel. I *can't ever come back,* I should never have come in the first place, and so far it's *all my fault* because of that. *All.* I think we should get a quiet divorce and think things out *quietly.* As for Leo, he *chose to come with me* and he is with me. Later, when we have a—an official arrangement—"

"There won't be one. If you think I'm going to give you the pleasure of divorcing, you can think again. You are my wife and my son's mother as far as I'm concerned. I don't go back on my word."

"I'm not ever coming back. You know that, really."

"Leo! You come. Now. Get your train, and come."

"Leo—go and find Grandma. I'll try and explain to—to your father—"

"Bitch!" says Nigel. He walks up to Frederica and grabs her shoulders. Frederica flinches and struggles. "Bitch!" says Nigel. "Manipulative bitch." He flicks her about the face with his palm. "Don't you *dare*—" he says, thick with sudden rage. Leo begins to scream. He screams and screams. Everyone appears. Daniel goes up to Frederica, and Nigel lets go. Leo runs to Winifred.

Bill says, "It looks as though you'd better get going."

"It's nothing," says Nigel.

"It isn't nothing," says Frederica.

"Come on," says Daniel, and takes Frederica and Leo away, holding both their hands. Bill continues to glare at his second son-in-law.

"I don't say who's right and who's wrong," says Bill, "for I don't know, and no one's perfect. I do say, you'd better get going, until Frederica says she wants to see you. We are her flesh and blood."

"Leo is *my* flesh and blood."

"We know that. But now isn't the moment. Please go. Christmas statistically breaks up thousands more marriages than it sustains, they say. Try again later. *Please go.*"

Nigel is about to say something belligerent, notices Bill's scars from his last visit, desists, and goes, slamming the door.

Perhaps because Nigel has united them, the family take pleasure in one another's company on Christmas Day. Winifred and Mary have made the house pretty, as the house in Masters' Row was never made pretty. Christmas dinner is traditional and tastes good; the turkey is well cooked, the bread sauce bland and spicy together, the stuffing full of herbs and interest. Frederica and Bill talk animatedly about her next term's novel course. She talks to her father about talking to adults, and about teaching *Women in Love.* They discuss the problem of Birkin, who is a teacher, not a writer.

Bill says, "You can go away from Lawrence and get in a frightful rage with him—a *silly* man, even at times a *bad* man—and pompous—and then you come back and open the book and there's the language, and the vision, *shining* at you, with authority, whatever that is."

"I didn't understand about teaching. I thought it was *dry.* But it isn't. It makes things more real—another world, that is also this world—more real in *this* world—you can't say things like that."

"*That* is what is missing from old Birkin, Frederica. He doesn't have a way of doing that."

"And next term," says Frederica. "*Madame Bovary, The Idiot, Middlemarch, The Castle, Anna Karenina,* I think *Mansfield Park,* perhaps *La Nausée*—"

Life, she wants to say, though it is books she is talking about, and her life, her angry husband, who has a Bluebeard's cupboard full of rubbery pink flesh and has been taught silent slaughter, her life is simmering away elsewhere. She smiles at her father, and imagines his life differently, a class in Scarborough reading *Bleak House,* a class in Calverley coming to grips with *Paradise Lost.* She imagines him imagining dinosaurs striding through the foggy London streets and angels shining in the distance through the trees of the Garden.

In the afternoon she helps Will and Leo to put the train together. The three of them make a good team: Frederica helps Leo unobtrusively, so that he knows the train is his, and can fit the pieces without Will becoming impatient or snatching. At the same time she asks Will's advice, which he gives. Daniel watches them. He offers help, once, but Will snatches the piece of rail from his hands and fits it somewhere quite different. Daniel thinks that there is nothing motherly, even so, about Frederica. She is thin, she is quick, she is nervous: the two boys treat her neither as an adult nor as an equal but as something in between. Leo treats her almost as a prisoner, putting out a small imperious hand to pull her back if she strays too far away. He remembers Stephanie saying that no one *played* in their childhood, and sees that it is a process to which Frederica is applying her intelligence, that does not come naturally to her.

His son, he thinks, will never forgive him. His son, like him, is single-minded. He himself loved one person, and now she is gone, he survives best without feelings of his own. Will intuits this, feels abandoned, and does not forgive. Daniel can foresee a time when they will both regret being so set in themselves, when it might be too late, but he can do nothing. He cannot get through to Will, because they both are as they are. Mary, on the other hand, requires love of him, expects it, creates it where it seemed impossible. He goes off to look for her.

"You ought to talk to your father," says Frederica to Will.

"I don't really want to," says Will.

"Probably you do and don't," says Frederica. "Most people are like that, with fathers."

"I more don't. He went away, just like that. I'm all right without him."

"He was broken up—" says Frederica, as she might to an adult. "He was just broken up, he couldn't go on, they were too close, he and she, he took it worse than other people might. You must *try to understand*. You are very like him. Something in you must understand."

"It almost doesn't matter what I *understand,*" says Will. "I can't be different. I was broken up too. You know."

"I know."

Leo clambers up Frederica, and puts his arms like a vice round her neck. Will watches. Frederica almost pushes Leo away, and then holds him tight. Will says, "I get on as best I can."

"I see," says Frederica, across her son's hair. Will puts in the last piece of rail, completing the circuit.

"Now the power source," he says. "And the engine. Will it go? Will the points work?"

"Let Leo push the switch."

"Come on, Leo."

The train receives its power and begins its rush round the miniature landscape, into a tunnel, through a station, past a platform. Leo switches it on, off, on, off.

"Don't blow it up," says Will. "Gently. Try the turntable."

The two heads bend over the rail. Daniel comes back.

"My father drove an engine," he says to Will. "Your grandfather."

Frederica sees Will think about getting up and going away. He moves the points, instead, rushing the train behind a sofa.

"Will has made an amazing track," says Frederica.

The little train rushes powerfully round, and round, and round.

The good temper persists into Boxing Day. Some of the party are invited to drinks that evening in Matthew Crowe's wing of his Elizabethan house at Long Royston, the rest of which now belongs to the University of North Yorkshire. Alexander Wedderburn has spent Christmas with Crowe, and will be there. It is a long drive from Freyasgarth, but Frederica, Bill and Marcus set out in Bill's car, with Marcus driving. Daniel stays with his children, with Winifred, and Leo.

Crowe serves champagne in his panelled study, under his painting of the flayed Marsyas. He is older: his rubicund face is more hectic, his hair sparser, he has shrunk. Frederica has put on the Courrèges dress, telling herself that she has brought nothing else suitable, telling herself also that by an effort of will she can make it hers, and shear it of its associations with Nigel. Today, too, she looks beautiful.

The room is full of people. Some of them Frederica recognises: there is Alexander, talking to the Vice-Chancellor, Gerard Wijnnobel. There is Edmund Wilkie, dark and rapid, fatter than he was, talking to the philosopher Vincent Hodgkiss, and a slight dark man who turns, and is Raphael Faber. Frederica feels the slight shock human beings feel on seeing a lover, a beloved, unexpectedly. He looks quickly at her, and away. He must be staying with Hodgkiss, his old friend. Crowe takes Bill away to talk to Wijnnobel and Alexander, who are talking about the Steerforth Committee and the teaching of English. Frederica follows: she is unready for Raphael. Alexander puts an arm round her shoulder and asks if she is well. The discussion resumes. The committee, it appears, has become divided into two camps, not so much about the English language as about teaching methods. Alexander describes these camps, following Arthur Beaver's distinction, as those of Eros and the *Wille zur Macht.* Those who believe in love and freedom, and those who believe in rules and authority. Grammar, Wijnnobel says, has somehow become involved in this because of the confusion between rules prescribed by those in power, and rules or laws discovered in what might be called nature. It is an old argument, with a new twist. He is at ease, as far as he is ever at ease. Bill says the secret of good teaching is to know those taught and to care more about what is being taught. Frederica has a sudden memory of Jude Mason interrupting her Lawrence lecture with Nietzsche. "Only as an aesthetic product can the world be justified to all eternity." She begins an anecdote.

"I am trying to teach D. H. Lawrence to a group of art students who don't believe they need to know about the past, don't believe they *ought* to know about the past, and I am constantly interrupted by a kind of naked grey-skinned androgynous model with a sawing voice and long grey hair who recites bits of Nietzsche—"

They laugh. They talk about teaching.

Marcus finds some of his colleagues. Professor Sir Abraham Calder-Fluss is there, a small man with rough white hair and a neat white moustache. He is a biochemist who has worked on protein synthesis in pigeon brain-cells and has a cautious interest in the new disciplines of neuroscience. With him are Jacob Scrope, whose field is artificial intelligence, and Lyon Bowman, who does delicate physiological work on the structure of the cells of the brain, the dendrites, the synapses, the axons, the glia. Scrope is handsome in a carved way, like a mediaeval monk, with a long lined face and cropped hair: Bowman is shorter, and fleshy, with a red mouth and dark curls. Marcus's research, tentatively entitled "The Computer as a Model for the Activity of the Brain," is being conducted under the supervision of Scrope, who is constructing primitive computers with different algorithms to mimic the processes of perception and learning. Marcus does not wholly like Scrope, but he does like Bowman and is both moved and repelled by the Golgi-stained slices of brain tissue with which Bowman works, the complicated branching forest of nerve cells, the spaces. He likes the mathematical work and is good at it, but he is not wholly sure whether what he is doing is what he wants to do. Wilkie is interested in Scrope's computer models, which can be related to his own work on perceptual scanning and the recognition of forms. How much information, he has been finding out, does the eye need before it can say: This is a tree, this is a face. He has been studying illusions: the brain seems to fill in spaces in its own blind spot, left blank in a pattern, like a tablecloth, with more of the same, with *imaginary, hypothetical* tablecloth.

The scientists discuss memory, the chemistry of thought, the mechanics of vision.

The teachers discuss the political connotations of requiring, or permitting, children to learn poems, mathematical tables, the alphabet.

Matthew Crowe detaches Frederica from the teaching group, and takes her over to talk to the Dean of Languages, Professor Jurgen Müller, and the English Professor, Colin Rennie, who is a Scot, and whose subject of study is the novels of Walter Scott. This group is attached to the group containing Hodgkiss and Raphael Faber. Crowe says to Frederica, "I involve myself as best I may in the University which is growing up round me. I try to follow Gerard Wijnnobel's Renaissance ideals and mix the arts and the sciences in some idea of Learning or Thought, but you see how they divide, how they discuss amongst themselves. And then over there is a sociology teacher, Brenda Pincher, and all the wives, they make their own group and talk about whatever women talk about, no doubt. It can't be clothes, their clothes are uniformly horrible, don't you think, whereas you are resplendent. If it isn't an impertinence, which it is, how did you come to be able to afford *that* dress, my dear? I heard you were married, you must have made a very splendid marriage to have that dress."

"I made a disastrous marriage, it has all gone wrong, I am in despair, the dress was a propitiatory present which I shouldn't have put on, because I won't be propitiated, but it was all I had—or perhaps I couldn't resist it. Are you satisfied?"

"No. I want to know *everything.* But later. Look out of my window. See the towers encroaching on my Elizabethan paradise. The Language Tower. The Evolution Tower. The Mathematics Tower. The Social Studies or Social Sciences Tower—they are quarrelling about the name—which isn't finished. They haven't built all the layers of connecting walkways yet. I believe it will look like a beehive."

Müller and Rennie do not want to talk to Frederica. They are having an amicable argument about Lukács's view that Scott is the major European novelist among the British. Müller has written on Nietzsche, Freud, Mann and the end of European cultural continuity. Rennie has written on Scott, Goethe, Balzac and George Eliot. They are heavyweights. They suppose a young woman in a Courrèges dress is a bore. They move closer together and turn their shoulders. Raphael greets Frederica, and asks if she remembers Vincent Hodgkiss. Hodgkiss is not physically memorable; he always appears different, when met again. Frederica smiles at him. Raphael says, "And how is marriage suiting you, Frederica? You appear to be blooming."

"Blooming" is not a word she would have expected from this precise, secret person. It carries a note of hostility, she feels, which is undeserved and irrelevant.

"Marriage is not suiting me. I turn out to be bad at it."

"I see," says Raphael.

There is a silence whilst Frederica thinks about Raphael, whose lectures she attended, at whose feet she sat, whom she loved, in terms of Eros and *Wille zur Macht.* He, like Crowe, for different reasons, seems smaller, as though a light has gone out. It is fearful, the realisation that we no longer love what we desperately loved and desired. It is a kind of death, and also, Frederica sees, a lightness, a beginning of freedom. This face, this intent face, is just a face.

"We were discussing our host's painting of Marsyas," says Vincent Hodgkiss. "Raphael does not see how he could live with it. Raphael thinks he should burn it. Ceremoniously."

Frederica feels a perverse desire to defend the picture, which has always given her a frisson of terror, disgust, and then pleasure of some kind. She looks at it, the faun bound to the tree, his pelt at his feet, his lips drawn back from his pointed teeth, his whole body glistening dark red with the gouts of blood that are about to burst forth into fountains. His anatomy is lovingly accurate; his bloody muscles fold over his shoulder-blades and belly.

"It is about art. And pain—"

"I know *that,*" says Raphael, as though her simplicity is contemptible. "But it is wrong. It is bad."

"Very fashionable," says Hodgkiss. "Have you seen the *Marat-Sade*? Through the howls of the mad and the victims and the executioners, the new world, the new truth."

"Don't be silly," says Raphael, putting down his friend with the same impatient contempt he showed Frederica. "All that is simply disgusting, *Schadenfreude,* something in ourselves we should recognise and look away from. I do not say we do not need to know it. I say we should not indulge bad imaginings."

"It's powerful," Frederica persists.

Raphael smiles sweetly at her.

"It's something that shouldn't be seen. Simply. I shall go and look out of the window at the nice abstract humanitarian towers."

He goes. Hodgkiss lingers a moment, and then wanders over to join Wijnnobel, who has approached the scientists, thus linking the scientific and the language-teaching groups. They are discussing the search for the elusive engram, the trace of a vision, a touch, a voice, a thought, left, where? In a body, to be recalled. The idea of the "molecules of memory" is currently exciting both biochemists and artificial-intelligence workers. Abraham Calder-Fluss explains for Hodgkiss's benefit. "The idea is that it is possible that learned information, as well as genetic coded information, might be retained in and transmitted by very large molecules, such as the DNA and the RNA. And this idea received reinforcement from the immunological study of proteins, since antibodies recognise intruders into organisms, remember them, encode the information in some way, and prepare themselves to resist subsequent invaders. So we wonder, in turn, if the roots of our own memories, the structure of our own consciousness, are to be found in these amazing macromolecules."

Wijnnobel asks what kind of research can be done. Lyon Bowman describes the work of James McConnell, editor of the *Worm-Runners' Digest,* who has trained planaria, flatworms, simple organisms, to avoid bright light, which they associate with electric shock.

"And then he chops up the trained beasties and feeds them to a group of naïve beasties, who absorb their molecules and, he claims, their learning with them—because the cannibals also avoid light, and the control naïve worms rush gaily towards it. I find it hard to credit, myself. What fear of the butcher, what desire for grass pastures, should I not have absorbed from my steak and kidney?"

Hodgkiss says, "The question is, whether the word 'information' means the same in all cases, that of immunology, that of the DNA, that of the mind of the scientist building a computer, or whether you are all thinking by analogy, which is dangerous. I am not enough of a scientist to answer my own question."

Marcus looks quickly at him: he has put his finger on something Marcus has felt to be wrong in all this without having the linguistic interest to sort it out.

Bowman says, "There are physiological changes—very rapid ones—in growing brains—which later cease to happen. I should look *there.*"

Marcus has a momentary sense of the shape of what he wants to know, wants to find out. He feels it as a shape in his own brain, an embryonic form of an idea which cannot be formed in words, or even in a diagram, though it is tantalisingly close to one, it is a sort of a *form* of a thought-not-thought. How does he know it is there at all? Also it is to do with Bowman's work, not Scrope's, but he knows that, before he knows what "it" is that he is looking for. And yet, when he finds it, it will feel like recognition, he thinks, not cognition, not a line scratched on a pale, blank, even *tabula rasa.* He thinks of his brain. He thinks of it as long, powerful feathers curled in a skull shape, layer in layer. He thinks of this wordless thinking as preening, smoothing, until all the little hooks and eyes connect and the surface is glossy and brilliant. He does not know if this analogy is useful or misleading or both at once. He has begun to know enough about science to know that scientific thought moves along in such metaphors and analogies, which it must both use and suspect. He thinks it would be interesting to talk to Hodgkiss. He continues to stand quiet and silent, looking attentive. Calder-Fluss talks about Schrödinger's intuition in the 1940s that genes were crystals—"and there are the aperiodic crystals of the DNA in the double helix. And this raised, in Schrödinger's mind, the idea that life, organic life, feeds on both order—the aperiodic crystals—and also disorder—random atomic vibrations and collisions. And then we begin to see that the *whole universe* might be an information system—of messages flowing through crystals amongst parasitic noise—and human thought then becomes a way of transmitting order between parts of the universe—of *informing* it—"

Their thoughts are interrupted by a crashing noise and a disorderly scuffle at the other end of the room, where the women, the wives, are gathered, quietly discussing, according to Crowe's hypothesis, washing machines and clothes. Frederica is now part of this group, which consists also of Mrs. Bowman, dark and solid in a printed silk dress, Mrs. Scrope, a faded blonde in a little black dress, Mrs. Rennie, a large woman, Mrs. Müller, an awkward woman, Lady Calder-Fluss, a small, sharp, watchful woman, and a tall, square figure, in a burgundy shot-silk cocktail dress with a square-cut low neck, who is Lady Wijnnobel. She has square-cut dark hair with a fringe, large mixed-coloured eyes, a gold bracelet, a cigarette, and a glass of orange juice. Frederica is the only woman in the group who is not surprised to see her. Everyone else has known that the Vice-Chancellor is married, and that his wife never appears in public. She is vaguely rumoured to be "ill," and it is understood that she is never asked after. There is a rumour that she is a Bertha Rochester, mad and shut away. But here she is, in the flesh, contributing nothing to the discussion, staring at the carpet or occasionally at the Marsyas, rocking slightly as though her feet are uncomfortable in the medium-high heels she wears.

The women are discussing, not clothes, not washing machines, but depression. They describe the fear of waking up and the difficulty of getting up, the long days that rush by and the long days that drag, listening to the clock, to the radio, and the washing. They discuss the Calverley doctor, and whether or not he will prescribe pills, and whether or not pills will help, and whether or not one ought to *take* pills, and how bad it is to be bad-tempered with children, and a common feeling that children are like fat jugs into which their life is being poured, like rushing electrical vehicles for which they, the women, provide energy which is not entirely re-generated, like young healthy carnivores (says Fleur Bowman with a smile) who consume the maternal flesh with the Weetabix and Alphabet Pasta in a smiling and automatic way. They say they blamed their mothers for being depressed and that they are now depressed. Brenda Pincher asks, can they not *work,* and they begin a long choral account of the ways in which they have tried this—a bit of typing one did get, one evening class Mrs. Rennie taught, but the baby-sitter never came; Lady Calder-Fluss surprisingly confesses that she wanted to go back to scientific research, to do a Ph.D., but her husband thought it better not.

The sociologist, Brenda Pincher, does not contribute to this discussion, or conversation, or sharing. She listens intently: she is underdressed in brown wool, and has longish pale hair. She does speak, however, to ask Frederica who she is, and what she does. Frederica says she is separated from her husband, and trying to make a living by teaching and writing reports for publishers, and, she hopes, other things. She says it is difficult to look after her son and work. Lady Wijnnobel says, "Your husband should provide for you so that you need not work."

"I don't want to take money from him, not for myself anyway. And I like to work, I need to work, I need to think."

"Did you have the same ideas about work before the birth of your son?" asks the sociologist.

"You should not have had a child," says Lady Wijnnobel, "if you are not prepared to care for him."

She sounds extremely angry: her voice is thick, her face a dark red.

"I can't care for him if I'm *not myself,*" says Frederica.

"You were not created to care for *yourself,*" retorts Lady Wijnnobel, swaying on her heels and looking at the ground. "He who loses his soul shall save it."

Frederica in turn becomes angry.

"I don't think you know enough about me to know what I should do with my life."

"I can see you are not a good woman," says Lady Wijnnobel very loudly.

Frederica finds that her hand is working away in her pocket, to push off her wedding ring. She looks round at the women, who look at the ground with unhappy fixed smiles, all except Brenda Pincher, who asks, in an impersonal sort of voice, "How do you know she is not good, Lady Wijnnobel?"

"I can see round her head a flame of wickedness. She desires to destroy her man and her son," says Lady Wijnnobel, with thick decisiveness. "These things can be seen, if you have an eye to see them."

"I'm sorry," says Frederica. "I'll go away."

"You will stay where you are told to stay," says Lady Wijnnobel, "and listen to what I have to say to you."

Camilla Scrope runs and pulls at the Vice-Chancellor's sleeve, as his wife advances angrily on Frederica, her hand raised, to scratch, to grip, to hold back; it is not clear.

"Eva!" says Gerard Wijnnobel.

"I must speak my mind."

"No, my dear, you must not. You must say you are sorry, and come home now. Now, Eva. Say you are sorry."

He puts his arm round his wife and leads her away.

Mrs. Rennie says, "I knew we ought not to be talking about depression. I knew I'd been told she'd been inside Cedar Mount. I knew I ought to *stop* talking about depression and so the only remarks I could think of were about that."

"I think she'd been drinking," says Mrs. Müller.

"Heavily," says Lady Calder-Fluss. "I noticed. It is a great pity."

Nobody speaks directly to Frederica, who feels that she is somehow branded as "not a good woman" even though something is clearly very wrong with Eva Wijnnobel.

She manages to push off her wedding ring, at last, and thinks of Frodo Baggins, the Hobbit, pushing off his ring of invisibility.

Brenda Pincher says to her, drawing her aside, "And how did you react to all that?"

"Oh, with automatic guilt. I am not a good woman. She saw it. How would *you* react?"

"Much the same, I expect."

She wanders away. Frederica considers her: she is one of the university teachers, an insider, not an outsider, but there she is, relegated to the other halves, the spouses, the merely social appendages. She wonders idly what she is working on, and, as Alexander comes to look for her, forgets Brenda Pincher.

Brenda Pincher retires to Matthew Crowe's panelled lavatory, where she opens her shoulder-bag and takes out a tape-recorder, of which she changes the tape. She has embarked on an interesting research project on the lives and conversational preoccupations of university wives, which she will extend to a larger one, she thinks, on the motherhood and married lives of educated women, in due course. She collects their speech habits, their sentences, their regrets, their hopes, their circular discussions, their pregnant silences, as Lyon Bowman collects patterns of dendrites and glia. She will write a book, in the early 1970s, called *Hen-parties,* which will be a huge bestseller and change many lives, including her own. Now, she wonders whether it would be ethical to erase Lady Wijnnobel's outburst, and knows it would, and cannot do it, out of aesthetic attachment to the disproportionate rage, the moral fury from nowhere. Though she herself does not find the rich redhead in the expensive dress likeable, by any means. Arrogance is recognisable on first sight. She thinks she is *someone,* thinks Brenda Pincher with unfocused distaste, slotting in another tape.

IX

The winter, closing in on the mountains around La Tour Bruyarde, brought on a certain lassitude and disaffection among the inhabitants. Icy draughts whistled and flapped along the twisting corridors and through the great halls, under the doors of stone-walled chambers and down the vertiginous stairs in the turrets and cellars. They huddled in wool and fur and the new pleasures of the flesh seemed less rosy and enticing. The Lady Roseace's face developed a porcelain pallor and her red lips were tinged with blue, cyclamens rather than clove-sweet pinks. The folk still gathered daily to hear the inspiring confessions of the storytellers of the day, to devise playful chastisings and subtle recompenses for pains inflicted and endured, but these occasions too were infected by cold and damp, and many desired not to strive but to sleep, or to go south to the sun and the bright ocean.

Culvert took to walking from room to room in the Tower, always finding a door he had never before opened, a cupboard whose contents were unknown, a glory-hole that breathed decay or a new loft full of hanging bats and thick-twisted cobwebs.

He went also from chapel to chapel, making an inventory of the images of human life therein, the dim limbs and bursting eyes on walls and reredos, the carved, twisted bodies, the empty stares of angels. When he had first come, in the full flush of his zeal for human reason and human passional energies, he had caused many such votive objects to be taken down and carried away, with the object of repainting the walls with lovelier fancies, tributes to beauty of form and freedom of desire, to the joys of copulation and the delights of orgiastic eating, truths, he had said to the other inhabitants, to replace repressive lies and dark imaginings. But now, in the winter, and in the first itching of his first moment of doubt or boredom, he came to ask himself how these images came to be there, what need had created them, to what sick string in the human heart they vibrated.

"Our Projector has discovered Religion," said Turdus Cantor to Colonel Grim, as they stood in furred gowns on a balcony, watching the solitary promenade of their companion deep below them.

"He inveighed most mightily against it," said Colonel Grim, "in his fiery youth. Priests, he said, were poisoners, poisoners of minds and persecutors of young and tender instincts."

"One extreme of passion may become its opposite," said Samson Origen, who was standing at a little distance, unseen in a dark hood. "Hatred may become love. Only a studied indifference can maintain its nature steadily."

"We shall see changes, then?" said Turdus Cantor.

"Our Projector is curious to dissect and galvanise human nature," said Colonel Grim. "Religion is an intrinsic part of human nature."

"I have travelled much," said Samson Origen, "and have met with no society without a religion."

"And you yourself," asked Colonel Grim, "do you hold by any faith, or follow any rite, or pray to any God?"

"I do not. It is natural to human creatures to seek illusion, to tell tales, to make up powers. I make an unnatural effort: I stare into the dark, and abstain from imagination. It is a destructive way, and the rewards are meagre. But I am compelled to it by my nature."

Meanwhile Culvert went from the Mary Chapel to the empty shrine of the Bleeding Heart, and deciphered, candle in hand, the Stations of the Cross in many styles by many artists, from the workmanlike and earthy to the thrilling and rococo. He was, he believed, a reasonable being, a student of happiness and a not-inconsiderable analyst of human nature. It had been his deep belief that the stories of religion were mere lies foisted on a credulous public by fat power-loving priests, bishops and cardinals, and he believed he understood the roots of the desire for power, the desire to control human desires and human hearts. He had been drawn in his rebellious youth to the gay and anarchic tales of Grecian deities, lustful, cruel and capricious, and had been wont to say that their captiousness could never exceed that of a baleful Deity who could complacently equate the slow torture of one man, and that his own son, indeed, his own self in some arcane sense, with the remission of payment for all the centuries of all the evil done by all the torturers of all human tribes and families. But now in the dark days Culvert was revising his understanding, which he now deemed to have been too facile, too youthfully energetic. He wandered from flagellation to flagellation, from bleeding, handcuffed, naked figure to bleeding, handcuffed, naked figure and asked himself to what deep lust in universal human nature these sights corresponded. He did not believe it was so easy as barter of guilt for white-washed innocence, blood spilt for a new infantile freedom of action. No, no, he thought, we desire to see the infliction of pain in order to contemplate its mystery and to stiffen our courage and dread for our day of need, when we shall know it in truth. And then he thought, This too is a superficial understanding. For we take pleasure, if we are truthful, in the observance of the infliction of pain, in the thrill of the knife slitting the nostril, the nates, the veins in the wrists, the anal rose, in the heavy descent of the axe-blade through hair and skin, through gristle and muscle and sinews, through red flesh and spurting blood and pearly bone and soft red-brown bone marrow. And then he thought, This too, is not all, for we are pleased to imagine, to anticipate, the start of our own blood in fresh wounds, the heat of the sheet of it running along thigh and breastbone, the sting, the smart, the lively writhing of the nerve-ends, this we desire, if truth were told. We envy the meek figure with his bruised shanks and his bloody face, we envy him a knowledge we have not.

And so he pursued his quest, from particular to particular constructing the universal. There on ancient cracked boards were Germanic sufferers with snarling agonised lips, with black gouts of blood in hair matted with thorns and oozings, with lacerated rib-cages dripping darkly, with grim, foundering buttocks and knees and calves spattered with thick dark strokes of pain. There by contrast were sweet Italian innocents all prettily crimsoned on ivory and snow and linen, skins laced with trickles and seepings like bright ribbons, down sweetly complacent faces; there were ecstatic Baroque brothers of these initiates, rolling hot eyes to the complicit Sky, panting with red tongues, spreading the cockles of armpit and groin to the gaze and lash of the torturers, who were grave-faced and detached, or greedy and corpulent, or troll-like and toothless, or snarling and canine, or dull and beastly, but always satisfied, always taking satisfaction from the bliss of blood or a job well done. As the artist took pleasure, Culvert told himself, pulling his fur robe tighter with a thrill of horrified pleasure in response, pleasure in the infinity of ways of representing the red lips of a wound or the tender bruised mound of a whip-welt. Is this, the analyst of human nature asked himself, the worship of Death or the worship of Beauty and Pleasure? And he answered himself, to his own satisfaction, The one is the other, and a kind of dark delight invaded his whole frame with a shivering heat, freezing and burning.

So he went on his way, musing on the cruelties of religion, or the religion of cruelty, and came to a winding stair which went down and down, smelling of mouldering growths and old wet stones, down, along, round, down, and his candle flame swayed and bowed and stank in the shadows. And at the foot of the stair was a round door in the stone, which opened with a great key, opened easily, for the wards of the lock were well-oiled, although it appeared forgotten. And inside the door was a Lady Chapel, which, although it appeared to be in the bowels of the earth, was lit fitfully through a stained-glass window, depicting a throned woman in rich blue robes, wearing a golden crown and a sweet smile, with a wheel of seven great swords stuck in her heart and a great apron of blood welling from her wounds to her breast and her lap, and running in tongues of crimson down her blue gown to the flowered mead she sat on. And on the left wall was a great painting of a woman white as stone, and staring, bearing on her knee the bruised and broken body of her son, a foul thing with gaping mouth and dislocated shoulders, with swollen ribs and trailing, piteous pierced hands and feet. And this image was framed in flowers, red roses, white lilies, blue irises, the only colour, where all else was stony and shadowed and veined with grey. And on the right was a painting, tenderly done, of a young girl bending her head over a new-born babe cradled against her naked breast, and the babe was swaddled tight in bandages, and had tight-closed bruised eyes and a mottled, purpled skin, a clammy skin it seemed, as the new-born and the newly-dead have, both.

And before all these women, all these three women, these Mothers of Pain, were row upon row of little lights bravely burning, which, when Culvert considered them closely, could be seen to be helical snail shells full of oil with burning wicks in the oil.

And the pews in the chapel were piled high with old bedding straw, for it was now a storage chamber, and the walls were lined with bales of hay, and in the centre of the chapel, before the altar, was an old woman on a three-legged stool, spinning thread by the light of three fat wax candles, standing in ornate church-silver candlesticks. She had a face like a nutcracker, the old biddy, and a watery, crazed eye and an empty socket of stitched skin next to it, and a mumbling mouth, fallen in, and knobbed, gnarled fingers like twigs, with sore red tips like bright buds. And Culvert had given orders (or suggestions, for the inhabitants were in theory free to reject his instructions) that the members of the community should wear bright, clear colours to signify the new order, but here was this old crone in a black scarf and a black stuff gown, just as the peasants of his childhood had been, and those of his father's childhood, and his grandfather's. And she was spinning a thread that combined scarlet and white, in a fancy twist.

She greeted him familiarly, "Good day, young master."

"Good day," said he, puzzled.

"You don't know me," said she, "and I could take offence at that, for I was your nursemaid once, your little mouth guzzled and sucked at these dry breasts, and before that I was there at your coming into the world, I was the *sage femme* who presided, the midwife who saved you, drawing you all bloody and reluctant out of your sweet mother's bleeding cunt, and slapping life into your backside with one hand, whilst you dangled from your little ankles from my other hand and mewed and howled.

"My name is Griva," said she, somewhat huffily since he showed still no sign of knowing her.

And it seemed to him that he remembered a sweet smell of her laundered undergarments on a sunny day, but he could not swear to it. He felt in his pockets for something to give her and came upon only a wizened little apple, which he looked at, perplexed, until she took it from him, saying, "Thank you," and bit into it fiercely, so that the juice spurted on her chin.

"And what are you doing in the bowels of the Tower?" she asked him, chewing with her toothless gums.

He sat down on the end of a pew, amongst the dusty hay.

"I am thinking," he said, "about religion, and what it means, and about the human tendency to need its practices. I am not thinking very well."

"Thinking," said she, "will not get you far, in that context, my sweeting. What do you think, my nurseling, where do your musings lead you?"

"To ceremonial," said he. "To rites performed. To the question Why? and the deep question Why *in truth*? For it is my observation that all peoples observe certain festivals, to wit, the turn of the year, the feast of the dead, the return to life and such matters. I remember the blessing of the fields, a pretty ceremony, and the candles for the dead souls, all flickering and gleaming."

"I could tell you much," said she, "of the Carnival as it was held in the halls of this house in the days of your forefathers, of the dancing there was, and feasting, and mumming, and ceremonies there were performed."

"Tell me," said he, "for this is what I was in search of. And chance led me to you and your memories."

"Chance," said she, "or something by another name, strong too, chance's sister."

So they sat together in the half-dark, the winter-dark, candlelit and waxy-smelling, and she told him of the old Feast of Misrule at the turn of the year in the Old Hall of the Tower. Of how a Lord of Misrule, the Babu, was chosen from amongst the grooms or footmen—"Sometimes he was a bit lacking, as they say, bats in his belfry, and sometimes he was chosen because he was above himself, an uppity being, a pompous nob, a puffed-up capon, and in the first case, your fool would give out silly orders, as it might be, to wash all the ladies' faces in winelees, or to make pies of live blackbirds, or to dress the hall with bulls' pizzles and pigs' bladders, and no matter what it was, it had to be done, for he was the Lord, but only for a day, only for a poor day. But the uppity lordlings whose come-uppance was near, they was more savage, my young nurseling, for they knew what was coming to *them* and they made sure their pains were paid and their election got its quittance in advance so to speak, so there were roastings and whippings of other young lordlings in plenty, ordered by the Lord of the Day, there was trousers pulled off and spankings performed—and more ingenious punishments, and hangings and danglings and spittings and pokings that would take me a month to retail to you—"

"I should be delighted to hear them—"

"And so you shall, my lovely, and so you shall. But in all cases, whether the Lord of the Day, the Babu, was fool or knave, at the end of it certain things happened as sure as night follows day or death follows life. And these things were: the birth of the new Sun out of the fat body of the Babu—who ate beans and other flatulent things to bloat his belly. And the topsy-turvying of all folk, so that the menfolk danced in skirts and bodices and the ladies had the freedom of trousers and hunting-jackets, and at the end all danced and chased in masks all around the stairs and halls of the Tower, beginning at nightfall of the Shortest Day and ending at the first light which finished the Longest Night and brought the New Year, who was a bloodied babe in the skirts of the Babu.

"And the Yule Log came in—which had been smouldering away for a whole year under the hearth, and the boar's head came in with it, with spiced apples in its snout, dripping with fat, and the Great Pie came in, which was made of snails and pigs' tails in a great spiralling savoury tower, topped with a pastry bird to finish. And they lit the fire in the hearth from the old log, and put in the new, and danced in the light of the flames, and they roasted more snails on its crest in great iron pails, dropping the hot oil into the shells so you could hear the creatures wince and sigh and screech as best they could. The peasants, you know, my nurseling, roast a tower of live cats over the great fire at the year's end, but this was not done in the Tower, for the ladies were squeamish. Indeed in the later days of the Tower they made the little snails from chestnut flour and marzipan but those were soft, sweet parodies of what should be, for there is spirit-life in snails, my dearie, and marzipan is a stolid substitute for succulent flesh."

"Why snails, old woman?" asked Culvert, not because he believed the old creature knew the answer, for it was his opinion that the peasants of modern times did many things of which the original sense was lost in the antiquity of inherited practices. But he thought also that these stunted folk with their repetitive lives might have preserved some wisdom of the earth, some harmonious chord between them and the original Nature in which men and beasts and plants all participated, which might be apparent to a keen intelligence. And the idea was coming to him that their practices, reintroduced, might make in his community a new life of the blood, more subtle and profound as a source of energy than cool-headed local reasonings.

"What spirit-life is in snails?" he asked old Griva, leaning towards her in the half-dark, in the scent of her unclean black garments and the apple-juice of her eating.

"Men say they go between us and those who sleep under the earth," said the old woman. "They weep continuously for the dead, their trails are bright with their tears, they go on their bellies like Him who was punished in the garden, but they are not evil beings, but wanderers, between this world and the next. For the fattest ones are always found in the graveyards—and those we do not pick, or only the naughty boys, in secret—and they hang on fennel, the plant of the dead, and taste of it too, when they are stewed or roasted. They are creatures of the night, making moony trails by starlight, but they are creatures of the Sun too, for when he goes to bed early, they go to their long sleep, and pull a horny window over their shelly, spirally houses. And when he returns, they return from their deathly sleep, their flesh stirs and out they come, cold creatures seeking the warm. They go between, you see, my dear boy, they go between earth and sky, they go between fire and water, they can play the king and the queen too, and their children are like glass and pearls. And when we have sucked them from their hiding place we make little lamps of their dead shells, for that they live in the dark and yet come into the light—they make silvery light with their weeping pathways in life, and hot fiery light in death. They are neither fish nor flesh nor fowl, and so magical, as things undecided are magical, because they are not fixed."

"This year," said Culvert, "we shall hold Carnival again in the Tower. We shall make beautiful costumes, and fantastic masks, and there shall be a rite of the new Sun, we shall welcome the new Sun in our blood, we shall have a Babu and a Woman Clothed with the Sun, and be beasts and men. And I shall send people out to collect snails, old woman, and you shall instruct our cooks in the making of the Great Pie."

"I am already spinning scarlet and white wool for your robes," said the old woman.

"And how did you know that I myself would be the Woman Clothed with the Sun?"

"I knew," said the old woman, shaking her head, whether with grief, or palsy, or grim humour, Culvert could by no means see. "As I know you will prick your finger if you play with my distaff as you are doing."

"Nonsense," said he, wielding the distaff and tangling the thread. "I have an insatiable desire to know how things function in this world."

And he pricked his finger, as she had foretold.

And she took his bloodied finger and put it in her own mouth, and her old, brown, wrinkled lips closed softly on his flesh, and her tongue licked his rough skin and sucked sweetly on his blood. And as his blood ran into the wet saliva and apple-juice on her tongue he remembered everything, his nose up against the warm bag of her breast, the scent of her milk, his little fists kneading her like sweet pastry, the hot swaddling bands between his legs. And tears ran down his cheeks, for the onward flow of time, for the crumpling and drying of flesh and blood, for the singularity of a man shut in his skin as time sucked the marrow from his bones.

"It is odd," said Colonel Grim, "that there should be such a preponderance of scarlet in the costumes or robes for the coming Carnival. Our honoured leader's *name* is evergreen, but his taste runs to flames and blood."

"You should not be surprised at that," said Samson Origen. "For soldiers have always loved to be brilliantly clothed when they parade about, and you yourself have worn a scarlet coat and a scarlet cloak with gilded buttons."

"I have heard it said," said Grim, "that the coats were red so that the blood of wounds should be hidden. But I give that small credence, for our small-clothes were white as driven snow, and there are also green soldiers, like holly trees, and black soldiers, to hide in the night. No, we were red to strike fear of our bloody-mindedness into the enemy, and brassy to glint like the hot sun as we advanced. How we loved our uniforms, and how tender we were to what lay under them."

"Judges are scarlet," observed Turdus Cantor, "and cardinals too have arrogated to themselves that rich colour."

"Also the Whore of Babylon," said Samson Origen. "The original Scarlet Woman on her scarlet beast, swallowing the stars."

"Though our sins be as scarlet," observed Turdus Cantor, "they shall be washed white in the blood of the Lamb. Who is himself woolly-white, with bleaching blood, a paradoxical beast."

"A man in a uniform," said Samson Origen, "or a man in a robe, for they are the same things, is not a man, but a cipher, but a function, but a walking idea; his clothes walk and speak for him. And undercover, who knows who he is, or what he does."

Culvert, all alive with enthusiasm, joined their group and begged that they all take parts in the coming Rite or Play for the New Year on the

Shortest Day. Colonel Grim, he said, was to be the *sage femme,* or Wisewoman, or Midwife to the New Year, and was to wear a specially designed gilded mask and a great coif. And Turdus Cantor was wanted as godparent to the New Year, and he would be clad as an old beldame with a black mask and white woolly hair. And the Lady Roseace would be godfather to his godmother and their names were to be Logos and Ananke, and they were to sing sweetly together at the birth.

"Sweet singing is beyond me," said Turdus Cantor. "My old voice is cracked."

"Then you shall have pan-pipes," said Culvert. "And there will be gongs, and cymbals, and clanging bells, and zithers and flutes."

"And what do you hope to bring about with all this?" asked Samson Origen.

And Culvert told him how he hoped to make the rhythm of the people's blood hum to the rhythm of the turning earth and light the fire of the new Sun in all their hearts. And Culvert told Samson Origen that he desired him to be a Pythoness in the Rite and wear a double mask facing backwards and forwards. And Samson Origen said he would not play, he would not take part, he would neither dance, speak, sing nor mum. "I will watch," said Samson Origen, adding "as long as one man watches and only watches, what you have is art, and intelligent, as opposed to religion, and terrible."

"I do not want you to watch," said Culvert.

Their eyes locked.

"But you do not want to make me act against my will," said Samson Origen. "And my will is to watch, my pleasure is in watching and only in watching. I believe in detachment, Culvert, in the solitary strong mind, as you know. I have seen the Krebs dance for the new Sun, and it is not pretty and not instructive."

"Tell me how they dance," said Culvert, and his eyes glittered.

So Samson Origen, in an even tone, in quietly polished sentences, sipping his hot wine with cinnamon, told his three companions of the great seasonal feasts of the Krebs, of the building of fires and the binding of prisoners, of the brewing of fermented milk with sour barley and pigs' blood, of the drumming of the women, of their wailing voices and averted faces, of the great horns belling and coughing and sounding, of the gongs and the cymbals, the castanets and the tambourines, the bladders and the rattles, and of the long, snaking lines of dancers, all moving as one, stamping with flat feet, rolling their oiled buttocks, faster and faster, of the frightened beasts who were driven into the circle round the fire and torn apart slowly by fingernails and teeth, living haunch from haunch, rib from rib, gut from bloody gut, until the Krebs were clothed in bloody hides and crowned with bleeding horns, or with the heads of wolf or wild-cat, bear-cub or hind, wild ass or mongoose. And the fire would burn brighter and brighter and sputter with fat from the roasting creatures, and then the prisoners would be brought in, and meet the same fate as the beasts, ripped apart and roasted, licked and tasted. And Samson Origen told of the election of the King of the Day who must lord it over all, and was carried on their black shoulders on a wooden throne in the firelight, and crowned with jewels and fed on wine and honey, whose hands and feet were kissed and slavered over, whose rich robes were embroidered in scarlet and golden silks. And he told how, when the sun came over the dark hills at the edge of the plain, this King was whipped, and roasted and torn to fragments and devoured. Samson Origen told this tale coldly, marshalling his facts, but he saw Culvert's eyes bright and wet, and saw the hot rheum in Turdus Cantor's old eyes. Those of Colonel Grim were dry as his own, he saw, and the pulses in his neck and brow were steady as ever.

"And do the Krebs have a God," asked Culvert, "in whose name they roast and consume this unfortunate being?"

"They do," said Samson Origen. "But they may not speak his name, under pain of death, and I do not know it. But the names of his masks are legion: there is a black horse, and a flaming fire, a great worm and a white kid, all of which at different times they dance for and dress themselves to simulate."

"Have you seen this thing?" asked Culvert.

"I have," said Samson Origen. "I watched, endeavouring to feel neither fear nor excitement."

"And did you observe the face of the King of the Day? Did he show fear?"

"He showed smiling vacancy, whether from extreme fear or because he was drugged and unaware, I do not know."

"Or happy, perhaps, in the mystery."

"I think not. You may entertain that idea, but I think not."

. . . So the feasting and dancing, the japes and the singing, went faster and hotter and more lusty. Up and down the staircases and along the corridors they danced, in great human eels, yet not human, for there were bears and boars, horned goats and silly sheep, cunning cats and sly foxes, ravening wolves and hooded crows prancing there, with sweaty human legs and tails, often enough, and little or nothing else, save that the women wore gourds and codpieces and the men wore apple-stuffed breasts, and swishing skirts. And all over the Tower were the brave little snail-lights. And there was no Babo, but at the head of the table was Culvert in the scarlet robes of a priestess, with long, blond curls on his head, and a red mouth and painted fingers. And beside him was the Pope, or Priest, or Bishop, mitred and with a gilded mask, and Colonel Grim, clothed as a beldame, and Roseace and Turdus Cantor as Logos and Ananke, she in a black, studious suit with a silver hawk-mask, and he in many-coloured female robes, with the face of a snake in gold and green. And when the Longest Night was drawing to its thickest, the Yule Log was ignited with great ceremony, and huge trays of snails were put to roast on it, and boiling oil was dripped into their cavities, so that hundreds of tiny boneless bodies writhed and winced and boiled together. And when dawn approached, the ceremony began on the high dais. It was a long and tedious ceremony, for Culvert had not yet got the knack of ceremonies, and did not understand that a mass of men must move, and exult, and engage and if necessary suffer and scream together and as one, if a ceremony is to weld a people. He wished, their Projector, to be all things to all men, Scapegoat and Whore, Mother and Father, Life and Death, Punished and Punisher, and, as will be subsequently clear in this narrative, his folk were not whole-heartedly implicated in his symbolic strutting and groaning, nor were they exempt from that modern saturnalian emotion which is most destructive of religio-aesthetic passion, embarrassed laughter.

He had devised a ceremony in which his eyes were bound, his robes were parted and his posterior fiercely whipped by the officiating Pope, or Priest, or Bishop, to whom he gave a stack of white willow wands and urged her to ruddy them truly and not in jest, for real and not faked blood was required to flow in their new world. Now the Pope under the flammiform cornute mitre was none other than the Lady Mavis, who was quite as reluctant as Samson Origen to perform any role in the Carnival rites, but had not that gentleman's cold blood, or his certainty of rectitude. And Culvert had overridden her demurrings and diffidences with accusations that she was not prepared to sacrifice her private desires for the general life. And when she retorted that it had not been part of the project to enforce people to submit their individual beings to the general will, but to harmonise both equally, he accused her of equivocation and bad faith. It was clear, he said, that she hankered for old orders, for bourgeois fustiness and the servile respect of servants, for hypocrisies and respectabilities and niceties that had been swept away by openness and truth. It was true also, said he, that she inclined still towards the vices induced by that stultifying and crippling institution, the Family. Truly, said Culvert to the Lady Mavis, it appeared to him that perhaps she should consider returning to the world outside. And she thought of the burned and salted fields of her home, of the gibbets and the death cells, of the roving bands of hungry soldiers, and wept bitterly. She thought also of her vision of *fêtes champêtres* and beribboned hats under sheltering trees, and wept more strongly. And she was afraid, for her history had taught her that fear was reasonable and appropriate, and she said she would play a small part. And her child too, the little Felicitas, Culvert insisted, should play a part, she should be the New Year, the Birth of the Sun, a candle to light the whole community to brighter days. Her terror pleased him, for she had always in the past looked at him with a kindly, indulgent, critical look, as though he might grow into a good man in some distant future when he should have discarded certain follies. It pleased him to make her the instrument of his ritual chastisement, for she would hate in principle to see any man whipped for any reason, and yet she would desire, in part, to whip himself for his treatment of her, and yet, too, she would hate that in herself.

And so it proved, for the hand that was raised to whip the white (if pimpled) posterior of the Whore trembled greatly, and fell lightly. Lay on, said Culvert between his teeth, or it will go ill with you. Lay on, said Colonel Grim, in his character of *sage femme*, lay on lustily or you will never be free, and you may reasonably do, dear lady, what both of you desire you to do. Lay on, said the Lady Roseace, laughing behind her hawk-mask, let him see what a Fury a woman can be, when aroused to righteous wrath.

So the Pope laid on, softly, hesitatingly, and then, as Culvert's blood began to blossom, more and more furiously, cutting his backside into a trellis of weals, and continuing even when Culvert's frenzy of pleasure and pain had reached its sighing, sinking climax, so that Reason and Ananke had to pull her back from her task. And then she sat down on the stage, her head nodding under her mitre, and howled like a beaten child. And Reason and Ananke brought great tubs of red winelees, and poured them over Culvert's scarlet posterior, so that the stage was a sea of blood and wine. And out into this red liquid, between the straddled legs, crept a naked child, with a candle, the little Felicitas, who had been cowering under the throne in the stink and turbulence and juices, and now did as she was told, a blood-red naked child, holding aloft a lighted candle, and quite unable to control her bitter weeping. And the people murmured, because both Pope and New Year were so miserable and howling. And Culvert rose in his robes, suddenly deflated, and his eyes darted daggers. And one pair of hands, Samson Origen's, clapped twice, softly. And outside, over the woods, the watchmen saw the first red slip of the new sun, for Culvert's timing had been impeccable.

Tales have been told earlier in this narrative of the delicate and indelicate doings in the Dormitories devised by Culvert. That wise man's conception of childhood was, it is to be feared, somewhat idealistic in its paradisal vision, for he saw the small human creatures in those vaulted sleeping places as rays of pure energy, as beings made of pure, warm, uncorrupted flesh and instincts full of creative kindness, of high inventiveness, of playful spontaneity when not thwarted, perverted and deformed by sick adult inhibitions—prohibitions sprouted from a sick society with stunted desires. It is true that the playfulness, spontaneity and inventiveness of the Lattermen, as the heads of the latrine corps were called, had flourished exceedingly amongst the beds and couches in the juvenile Harem. "To the free judgement of their peers," Culvert had said, "the community would trust the correction of the little peccadilloes, the omissions and hesitancies, of the youthful aspirants to freedom, for they would best know what was appropriate, and how to weigh the offence against the atonement, which might be a small thing, a brief abstention from chocolate, or perhaps a small service, the cleaning of another child's shoes."

What punishments the Lattermen devised in the dark hours has been told, as far as I dare tell. Jojo, Adolphus, Capo and the Grinner have been duly celebrated for the sweet humiliations, the atmosphere of apprehension, the wonderful arbitrariness they devised, so that boys and girls could be induced to punish themselves with sickly fears, and obsessive dreads, not knowing when the jolly mockery might begin, or the process of accusation be set in motion, day or night. For these bright boys were as adept at invading the essence of the closed grey soft matter in the young skull, or the bloody rhythm of the little heart, as they were at invading the beds, and mouths, and bottoms, of the little sleeping figures. And on the day after the Rite of the Solstice they pronounced themselves most dissatisfied with the behaviour of the child Felicitas, and that on two counts; first, that she had *shown herself off* in taking a central rôle in the Rite, she had *sucked up* and abased herself in order to procure this putting of herself on view, all naked with her silly candle. And secondly, that having displayed her meagre little body in this ostentatious way, she had *wept like a baby* and spoiled the whole jolly occasion; she had mightily *let everyone down*.

So they stood the little thing in the middle of the Dormitory, and pulled off her nightgown, and laughed at her nakedness. They wore the pretty masks they had all pranced in during the Carnival, Owls and Pussycats, Tadpoles and Newts, toothy Rabbits and snouty Bears, and pushy little Lambs, and they danced round her, pointing and poking and criticising her little belly and thighs and her trembling little knees. And then Jojo pronounced that she would not be punished *now* for her misdemeanours, but would be given time to think, and reflect, and that the judges would come when they were ready, and do to her what they would do, though they would not say now what it would be.

So they all turned away from her, and giggled together, and the little thing took up her nightdress and crept away to a cot in a corner where she often lay curled like a desperate snail in its shell. And Jojo came after her and snatched at the garment, saying she had wanted to be naked, and naked she should be. So she crawled in under her blanket, and her teeth clattered together like knitting needles, and this noise annoyed Adolphus, who took hold of her jaw and clattered it up and down in good earnest, whilst the others laughed.

And during the night, Felicitas could be heard sobbing and wailing, although these sounds were partly stifled by her pillow and blanket. But Jojo and Adolphus and Capo could not, they declared, sleep in this racket, so they rose up, and took the child from the cot, and put her on her head in the broom cupboard and turned the key. See if you can howl arsy-versy, they told her through the door, but she did not answer, for she could not.

And in the morning the door was opened by her brother Florian when everyone had gone to breakfast, chattering and laughing together. And the child fell out of the cupboard, rigid as a board, and cold as a stone to touch. She was not dead, Florian found, putting his cheek to her grey lips, which breathed a little warmth on his own warm skin. So he wrapped her in a blanket, and nursed her, and lulled her, and after a time she began to shiver, and the blood began to flow through her limbs, and she got to her feet. And she said, "B-b-b-b-b," and "C-c-c-c," but no other word. Nor did she ever again speak word, but crept silently about the Tower, always hugging the wall, for she would not stand freely, and would meet no one's eye, and drooled from the corner of her mouth.

And Florian asked himself whether he should speak to any member of the community about what had happened to his little sister. He saw it would be best to say nothing, for his own sake, and did indeed keep silence for some little time. But one day, finding his mother weeping over her silent child, he could not help himself, and told how it had come about, all of it, only he would give no names. And the Lady Mavis wept bitterly when she heard him, and could not think what was best to do. It might be thought, she should have spoken of the matter openly in the Council of the community, and sought justice for her child. But she judged it best to make peace, for the children were children she had risked her life to save from the soldiers of the Revolution, and she believed they were only children, and had done more harm than they knew. So she asked Jojo and Adolphus and Capo to come to her room, and there she said that no good was done by accusations or retribution; it was part of her creed that no eye should be plucked or tooth extracted in rage or cold vindictiveness. We must love each other, however hard it is, said the Lady Mavis to the meekly downcast boys. Who replied that she was quite right, and also quite wrong to suppose they had harmed her child, who had over-reacted to her rôle as the New Year. Someone, they said, had tittle-tattled, and told lies, but, as she herself had said, forgiveness was of the essence of community living and loving, and they would forgive, naturally.

And the next day, at breakfast, Florian was not to be found. A search was instituted, after twelve hours or so, when it was deemed by the community to be urgent, but the Tower was vast, and the pits and wells and glory-holes and oubliettes so many, and the moat so deep and the ramparts so high that no sign was ever seen again of the foolhardy boy, neither hair, nor bone, nor drop of blood, nor sweet smile.

After the disappearance of Florian, and the unavailing search of the Tower, the Lady Mavis became silent and withdrawn, although she still continued to perform tasks in the community, to peel potatoes, to mend torn clothing, to cook the little cakes, the spiced pastries or mirlitons, which she made better than anyone. She asked to be excused from her duties in the nurseries, and this withdrawal was felt to be graceful and natural, despite the general desire to do away with the feelings of partial maternity which gave rise to it.

But after some little time, the members of the community all received pretty little notes bidding them to a feast in the paved courtyard at the summit of the White Tower, or the Pierced Tower (it went by both names, which referred to the colour of its stone, and the ornamental aspect of its architecture, with many ogive and lanceolate windows). The pretty little notes referred to a *fête champêtre,* which was not so inapposite as it may sound, for the summit of the Tower, surrounded by crumbling battlements, had long been overgrown with tufted carpets of self-sown wild grasses, tenacious barren fig trees and gaudy ragwort, snapdragons and dandelions. And although there was a general opinion that my Lady Mavis's *fêtes champêtres* were now a little tame, a little *passée,* there was also pity for her in the community, and most of them mounted the cracked stairs at the appointed time, jostling each other on the turns, laughing and greedy for the good fare they confidently expected.

It could be seen that the Lady Mavis had prepared her little feast with some care, building a small canopy of red and black silk against the decaying battlements, and setting out on a long damask-covered table beneath it tasty dishes, flagons of pink bubbling wine and garlands of holly, with leaves like needles and berries red as blood. And she herself wore a snow-white robe under a scarlet overdress, with a garland of the holly shining in her hair.

Now the people quickly perceived that with great ingenuity the feast had been laid out on the table in the form of a Man or possibly of a Woman, for the Lady Mavis, in her old-fashioned modesty, had wreathed the joining of the legs in further holly, beneath which sugared figs could be seen nestling, and the breasts were, as we shall see, ambiguous. Now this human feast seemed on first sight like a giant gingerbread man, such as the Witch offered to Hansel and Gretel to entice them into her cottage, a great form composed of smaller forms, custards and tartlets, marzipan sweetmeats and blancmanges, jellies and syllabubs, mincemeats and flummeries, fools and darioles, mirlitons and millefeuilles. Its head was crowned with a circlet of tarts, of cockscombs, and the flesh of its body was all veined and contoured and dimpling, made of peaches and cream here, and slices of quince there, blueberry veinings and blackcurrant flushes. The face was whipped cream and meringue with rosepetal pies for cheeks and huge lips plump and red with apple cheeks and cranberry froth opening on an oval tart of baked larks' tongues, surrounded by sugared almond teeth. The eyes had sloeberry tartlets for pupils, and greengage jelly for the iris, flecked with vanilla, and white syllabub slicked round that, fringed with lashes of burned spun sugar. The Sweet Human had long red shining nails, on its fingers and toes, made of pointed tartlets glazed with scarlet redcurrant jelly, from which dripped pendant tarts like gouts of blood, also glazed scarlet. The breasts of this confected Being were low circling mounds of pink marzipan sweetmeats, with a castle of chocolate truffles for nipples: they were the breasts of a young girl or nubile boy, sweet to touch, sweet to taste. The navel was a deep custard tart amongst the peaches and cream, with a spiral swirl of *crème pâtissière* inside it. The sweetmeat body was, so to speak, naked except for a necklace of round red tarts of currants in scarlet jelly, and a line of these ran also, like Pantaloon's buttons, from chin to belly to crotch, and a further line also dissected this line at the waist, bonds or quarterings of glistening vermilion. "Like flies drowned in blood," said Jojo to Adolphus, of these round tarts, licking his lips.

Between the breasts of the Human Cake was a large shield-shaped exterior heart, composed of a phalanx of tiny, blood-red, heart-shaped tarts. Into the triangle which pierced darkly down between the plump red shoulders of the plump red heart was pushed a dark, triangular slice of cake, like a blade, covered with what appeared to be soot.

The Lady Mavis watched and smiled as the happy horde dismembered and savoured the Baked Human. She remarked smilingly to Culvert that in the early days of their planning of their escape, the dark days of hiding, and mutual trust, and danger, they had imagined a society where sweet things were freely prepared for all comers, where everyone could eat cake, and spiced tartlets, who desired them. Culvert, who had a sweet tooth, bit into a mirliton and reminisced about how he planned to replace wars in the New Order with great contests of gastrosophy, with tournaments of pastry-cookery, with intense trials of skill in the construction of raised pies, or "melting moments" or "bouchées à la Reine" or frangipani, or succotash, or meringues glacées.

And when the limbs of the Cake-Man were scattered and despoiled, when the sweetness had been sucked from its navel and the chocolate nipples had melted succulently in various mouths, when its face and its heart were tattered and disfigured with gaping holes, the Lady Mavis climbed on to the battlement steps, and stood dark against the sky, with the winter wind ruffling the silk canopy at her side, and lifting her somewhat dishevelled hair.

"I have a few words to say," said this Lady, "if you will grant me a few precious moments, before you resume your nibblings and savourings and sippings, which I hope are satisfying as I meant them to be. And my few words consist of a question, and after that, if I have no answer, of a statement."

"She is like the schoolmistress confronting the naughty boys," said Jojo to Adolphus. "But we have no such silly authority here; here are no teachers and no pupils, but freedom."

"My question," said the Lady Mavis, "to which I fear I may have no answer, is Where is my son Florian? For I do not believe that no one knows what became of him. I believe there are those among you who could say, if they chose. And if he is alive, I wish to succour him, to release him, to embrace him, and if he is dead, to weep for him and to bury him decently. This is not much to ask."

The Lady Roseace, flushed with pain, said, "You know well that we have searched everywhere, and for days. We could not have been more diligent if he were our own child—which indeed he was—for we are all part of each other. We have left no stone unturned; we have dragged the moat; we have combed the woods."

"And opened every cupboard," said Jojo, with an air of grave concern. "He was not shut in any cupboard in the castle: we made it our business to investigate every cupboard, every coal-hole, every store-room."

"He was a self-willed little boy," said Adolphus. "He could have wandered into the pig-pen, or the abattoir, or fallen into a well, or been carried off by wolves. He did not listen to advice. I do not think you will see him again."

"We must not lose hope," said Culvert, without conviction.

"In the old days," said Colonel Grim, "I would have known how to find out what had happened. But my old methods are not part of our new world."

"And must never be again," said the Lady Paeony, with scorn. "How many innocents have not confessed to unreal evils on your rack?"

"Just so," said Colonel Grim. "We shall never, I believe, see the bottom of this matter."

"That is the conclusion I too have come to," said the Lady Mavis. "And now, I have a few other things to say."

And she went to the table, and took up the triangular sooty segment of the sugar heart of the Human-Sweetmeat, which had been left untouched on the table. She bit into this, and climbed back to her station beside the battlements, tasting its black taste on her tongue, ingesting its shadowy substance.

"We are told by antiquaries," said she, "that in ancient Babylon, in the chamber at the top of the ziggurat which was reserved for the activities of the God Baal, he came sometimes to sleep with the priestess, and sometimes to share a feast at a giant stone table, and sometimes, in difficult times, to demand a sacrifice. And there are many tales of what this sacrifice was—a red human heart, tastefully roasted, a whole human infant, the first-born, trussed and tossed into the flames of his altar fire. It is told that on his feast days a great cake was baked, and cut into small portions, one of which was blacked with the soot of the eternal Fire of his altar. The people took their cakes blindfold, and he who chose the black square was the Chosen One, devoted to the God. And for a time this Devoted One was fed and fattened, granted his desires of the flesh, sweet cakes and wine, sweet bedfellows and smoky opiates. And when his time came, he was led smiling to the fire, and the God was pleased, and did not wilfully torture or persecute the people for the following year, but let their corn and vines grow rich and their children spring up plump and healthy. We are told that the Krebs still build a Bale Fire and make their offerings, somewhere in the forest, a prisoner, a fool, a goat, a beloved son—the tales vary. And in the religion we have renounced, too, the god-man made himself bread and wine, drank the bitter cup and offered his body to dismemberment, to save the people from pain. He sacrificed himself to himself, as we were all taught.

"We are not gods, we are rational beings in pursuit of happiness. We have no gods, to judge or to comfort, to afflict us or to take away pain. All we are is ourselves, and we have discovered in ourselves in these latter days deep-rooted desires to hurt and to be hurt, ancient instincts of immolation and oblation. I have thought much, over these last weeks, about the desire to hurt. In the farmyard, the sight of blood on a wounded bird, a broken wing, a lame foot, arouses the fat fit hens, the young cockerels and the growing chicks to a frenzy of plucking and pecking. They will peck to death a beast which is injured; they will strip its breast bare of plumage, and expose pimpled purple skin, and then blood, and then bone. This is usual, this is not unnatural in these witless feathered things.

"I do not think there is any god to whom I may sacrifice in order to demand the restoration of my son. I do not believe in vengeance—it is part of the old ways, which we have abjured. Whatever may have happened to my sweet son's eyes and his growing teeth, I ask for no other mother's son's eye or tooth in recompense. All we can punish is ourselves, and the stripped, ridiculous hen, if she could, would hasten her end, if she were rational. If I harbour the idea that my death might propitiate the spirit of cruelty that is abroad amongst you, I know that idea for the sentimentality it is. I should like to think that I can take with me," said she, climbing higher on the battlements, with the wind stronger in her hair and garments—"I should like to think that I can take with me the yeast of blood-lust and malice that is at work, that I could concentrate its energy in my body and extinguish it with my life. Because I go voluntarily, *no one else is guilty* of my death, I kill myself, and restore a kind of preliminary innocence. I mean the pain to stop with me, and the old innocence of flowers and sweetmeats to be restored for a time."

And she ascended another step to the battlements, and stood looking at them. And a strange, strangled sound was heard amongst the skirts of the ladies, and the little Felicitas struggled out and ran across the courtyard, and clambered up the steps, holding to her mother's skirts, and making the raw sounds of the voiceless. The Lady Mavis bent down and picked up her daughter, with tears streaming down her cheeks, and cradled her in her arms, kissing her.

"The child has saved the mother," said the Lady Roseace.

But the Lady Mavis turned again, and climbed, and stood for a moment high and free on the wall itself, crooning to the child in her arms, and then stepped out into the air, crooning and murmuring.

They all ran to the battlements. Culvert alone did not: he ran down. He had an idea of catching his old friend in his strong arms.

Jojo said to Adolphus, "She has decided finally to be a *vol-au-vent*. She is light."

She was light, and the Tower was high, and her skirts were voluminous. The air pressed under her skirts, and lifted her and played with her, like a sycamore seed, like a kite, eddying and spiralling. They could not hear if she was still singing to the child, but they could now hear the child screaming, a rough, shrill sound, as she took account of her slow descent to death.

Culvert was again defeated by his own Tower, whose corridors deceived and delayed. He hurtled and fell: he stood again and found he had run in a circle and was rising where he had been descending. He put his shoulder to a door and found it rusted in its hinges and locks; he ran on, opened another, almost stepped out himself into air.

So the Lady Mavis came down like a great bird, swaying in her skirts amongst the child's raucous cries and her own singing. But when she saw the tree-tops, where she might alight like a bird, or break her fall, she made various ungainly movements with her body, twisting and turning, and managed to project herself downwards head-first, her skirts tumbling around her face, her stately legs scissoring the air in their lace-edged drawers. And her head hit a sharp rock, like a snail dropped by a thrush, and burst apart as Culvert managed to rush across the moat from a side gate with a railed bridge. He was in time to pull the child Felicitas, unharmed, from her mother's twitching grip, and to wipe the blood and brains from her little face.

"She is wrong," said Turdus Cantor, "if she thinks she will terrify those who hurt her son out of their course."

"She will give them a taste for blood," said Colonel Grim. "And for spectacle. As we saw in the old world."

"Hers was an old illusion," said Samson Origen, "that self-punishment will shame the wicked. So many women hurt themselves, thinking their pain will hurt their persecutors, who take pleasure in it."

"And what do you make of her talk of sacrifice?" asked Turdus Cantor. "Her thinking on that matter was deeply confused and deluded, it seemed to me."

"All thinking on that matter is confused and deluded," said Colonel Grim. "But a little blood shed has always been wonderfully fortifying to the energies of judges and soldiers, kings and priests. All such like to seal their pacts with blood."

"Necessity is ineluctable," said Samson Origen. "A self-perpetuating mechanism. Our blood oils its cogs, whether we offer it up or not. Our intention matters not a jot. On the other hand, the absence of this lady is the removal both of an irritant and of a goad to persecution in our little world. It could calm our flushed blood. Or it could arouse further animosity against less vulnerable targets. Blood finds its own level, like water."

Frederica thinks of antechambers, and wonders why, since she is not in an antechamber, but in Arnold Begbie's office, sitting opposite Arnold Begbie, both in tan hide chairs with chrome frames. Begbie is a partner in Begbie, Merle and Schloss. They are on the ground floor of a Georgian house in Sunderland Square, which is, just, Bloomsbury. The room is mostly full of Begbie's large oak desk. Sunlight floods through the window, which is covered with an intricate steel mesh. Beyond are the spearheads of the iron fence of the residents' locked garden. Faint from the garden come voices of children, running and calling.

Frederica looks like a pantomime Maid Marian, in a short green suede dress, mesh tights, high crumpled suede boots. Arnold Begbie's suit is dark, his tie spattered regularly with blood-red dots. He has springing black hair in just-controlled surges. His eyes are black and his skin sultry, his bones—nose, chin, cheeks—jutting and pronounced. His voice is subdued and Scottish. He murmurs, writing, looking down.

"You are quite decided upon divorce."

The meshes make patterns on his blotter.

"I wouldn't have come if I wasn't."

"You know your own mind."

"I didn't mean to sound rude."

"You didn't. So many people come to me, to discuss divorce, when divorce is the last thing they want. Tell me about yourself, Mrs. Reiver, and about your husband."

Frederica gives what she thinks is a precise, dispassionate résumé of her marriage. She has thought out what to say and what not to say. She explains that she was left alone for very long periods, and that her husband opposed her return to any kind of work. She says that she saw no one, but that when her friends visited, her husband was unreasonably angry. She says unemphatically that he became violent. He attacked her, she says. He hurt her. She tried to run away, she says, and he threw an axe after her, wounding her. She is proud of the level, quiet, informative voice in which she says all this. Arnold Begbie writes. He says, "Is that all?"

"We are incompatible." A silly word. An undescriptive word. "It is all my fault. I should never have married him. I know I should not."

This she thinks every day. Mr. Begbie taps his pen on his strong teeth. Incompatibility and mistake, he tells her with practised gentleness, are not grounds for divorce. Grounds for divorce are desertion, cruelty, adultery, insanity and certain arcane and unacceptable practices he is sure they need not go into. It is possible that Frederica is in a position to petition for divorce on grounds of cruelty. Neglect, refusal to listen, can amount, in some cases, to cruelty. Physical violence is certainly cruelty, though the courts take into account the character and circumstances of the partners in deciding what the effects of one particular act of violence might be deemed to be. He imagines she is not used to being struck, or to having things thrown at her. No? Good. And she saw a doctor, perhaps, after the axe wound?

"Of course," says Frederica. "We told him I tripped and fell on some barbed wire."

"A pity. Would he have believed you?"

"I don't know. He stitched it. My London doctor dressed it. I told him how it happened."

"That, unfortunately, would be too late after the event to be very helpful. He might however be able to say that such a wound could not have been caused by barbed wire. The courts do not always look favourably on unsupported assertions of cruelty by the complainant. Did anyone else see the wound?"

"Several people. None of them were people it was any good *telling*—"

Arnold Begbie allows this matter to drop, and asks whether Frederica supposes her husband will contest a divorce, if she asks for one. Frederica says she believes he will: when last seen, she says, he was pressing her to return, and to return her son. He does not like to be thwarted or contradicted, she says. She adds that she knows that if she allowed her son to visit she would never see him again. The solicitor says that the courts may have views on the father's rights of access. Frederica says that she herself believes her child should see his father; that she would encourage this; that she knows in her bones that she would not see him again, if he went there, now. She may need to find evidence, says Arnold Begbie, to support the feeling in her bones in a court of law. Frederica's bones become briefly knobby and obtrusive in the seamless dry run of the language of the discussion: she has a sudden vision of them, quivering and bloody, inside her composed flesh and her green suede. Her bones are not evidence.

Arnold Begbie brings up the subject of adultery. Mrs. Reiver has not herself mentioned any suspicion of adultery. She has said that her husband was often absent for long periods. Has she ever imagined that he might be seeing other women, during those periods?

Frederica says she doesn't know, and hasn't thought about it. She says she believes her husband loves her and adds, flushing slightly, that as far as sex goes, they are happy, they are compatible. That silly word, again. She says her husband is a man who likes women. She hesitates. Arnold Begbie watches her hesitate. He prompts her. "You have remembered something."

"Not exactly," says Frederica. "But I have—I have a venereal infection." She is proud of the precise, unpleasant word. Because she is Frederica, having brought herself to say it, she thinks of irrelevant connotations, Shakespeare's hot Venus, panting for Adonis, Spenser's veiled Venus, medieval Venus, a regal being charioted by doves and accompanied by her winged son and his burning arrows. She shifts in her seat. She says, "There is no other way I could have caught it."

"No other person."

"That is what I said."

"A communicable venereal disease is evidence of adultery. You can produce evidence of that?"

"Yes."

The conversation continues. Frederica dredges her memory. It is agreed that Arnold Begbie will write to Nigel Reiver, saying that his wife intends to petition for divorce on grounds of cruelty, and see what response he gets. In the interim, Frederica must go home and write out an account of her marriage, as fully as possible, listing every example of anything that might be construed as cruelty, and anything she may recall which might be evidence of adultery. Arnold Begbie would like to know what Mrs. Reiver would say to an amicable meeting—in the presence of her solicitor—to discuss the questions of divorce, maintenance, custody, care and control of her child.

"I don't want him to know where I am living."

"That may be difficult. Where are you living?"

Frederica tells him. He says, "And Mr. Poole, in whose flat you are living. Do you hope to marry him, if you obtain a divorce?"

"No—" says Frederica. She says, "It is purely an arrangement—it isn't what you think—it is to share the looking after children—it isn't—"

She cannot tell if he believes her. He says, "If you petition for divorce, you are required to enter a statement asking the court's discretion with regard to your own adultery, if there has been any adultery. Your solicitor is required to bring this matter to your attention."

"There *hasn't,*" says Frederica, with a strong sense of injury. "For one thing, as I told you, I've got this infection . . ." She stops in some confusion.

"And if you had not, you would be tempted."

"I'm not saying that. I don't think—"

"You don't think it is my business. But it is, Mrs. Reiver, it is. I cannot advise you to go on living with an unattached man—even in the presence of an *au pair* girl and several children—if your husband is likely to contest the divorce."

"I can't earn my living if I can't share the child care."

"You could ask your husband for maintenance for yourself, and your son."

"I won't *do* that. I want to earn my own living."

"I would not be emphatic about that if you hope to persuade the courts to allow you custody of your son."

"But my present arrangement—"

"Does not look good, frankly. I advise you to move. Unless you really wish to marry Mr. Poole. Do you think he wishes to marry you?"

Frederica, who has her complex anxieties on that point, is silent.

"Reflect on it, Mrs. Reiver," says Arnold Begbie. He smiles. "We shall find a way. Don't look so downhearted."

"I feel suddenly trapped."

"We shall find a way to free you, don't worry."

This is Frederica's first legal narrative. It is an official tale, told to a partial, official listener. Frederica selected its narrative elements; Arnold Begbie sorted, assessed, rearranged and added to them. It is only the beginning. There will be more. And more, and more.

Coming out of the offices, into the winter sun in the square, Frederica stops to peer through the railings at two blond children, a bigger girl, a smaller boy, riding tricycles on the gravel path round the grass. Two women are sitting with their backs to her on a bench. She can hear their conversation.

"They're all the same. I say, 'You say, "Don't nag." I wouldn't nag if you'd only ever *listen* to what I'm saying and remember it.' But he thinks it's beneath him, he thinks anything I say is bound to be trivial and somehow demeaning, he goes on thinking his *important* thoughts. I tell him, 'I don't want my brain cluttered with questions you can't be bothered to listen to or answer, I could think important thoughts if I didn't have to remember every trivial thing *for you.*' He doesn't care about cluttering my brain, his own's a plane of white frost, an infinite *tabula rasa,* on the personal plane, so to speak."

"I think they feel threatened," says the second woman. "He treats me as though I was a fussing hen, or his mother, who's stopping him doing what he wants, telling him grown-up things are *naughty,* slapping his fingers. I don't want to be his mother, I don't want to be *anybody's* mother as far as slapping people and stopping people goes. But you don't have much choice, if people are to eat and be kept clean. He laughs at me in an indulgent sort of way, but *like a little boy,* if I try to talk about any household thing, and off he goes to the pub. But he gets pretty mad if I do anything he doesn't like while he isn't looking."

"He says, 'Is there any?' or 'Where is the?' all the time. He comes in at any hour, and says 'Is there any food?' He stands there: 'Is there any bread?' He doesn't *look* for it. 'Where is the butter? Where are the matches?' Often he can see them. But I have to run up and down, fetching things. He needs that."

"You don't *have* to."

"It's quicker. More peace, in the end."

"What would happen if you didn't, if we didn't?"

"He might hit me. He might leave."

"Do you really think so?"

"Yes."

A sharp laugh. "So do I."

They are the chorus. All Frederica can see of them are two huge knitted hats, one black, one white, and two fake-fur coats, one orange, one shocking pink. Their voices are pleasant BBC voices, with humour in them. Their husbands are one indistinguishable He, and in the context of those husbands, these women are also one indivisible voice. This is the narrative of women talking, women watching children, talking. Owing to accidents of fate, or quirks of personality, Frederica has never really been part of groups of women talking. She was hated at school; her Cambridge friends are men; she cannot make common cause with Olive and Rosalind and Pippy. But she can recognise an archetypal, anonymous female narrative, and wonders suddenly how this talk affects the relations between the women and the men they return to. Does the speaking of mocking criticism turn Cyril and Fred and Louis and Sebastian into He He He He when they are seen again, does it strengthen opposition to Him or dissolve Him in laughter? She thinks this because she knows already, in a pale and partial way, that the legal narrative she has just constructed has changed several people: Nigel into the Husband, herself into the Plaintiff, Thomas Poole into something he is and is not.

She finds this rather exciting, as an idea about the dynamics of human behaviour.

She finds it frightening as a human experience of her own. She has always thought her life was her own, and she was in charge of it. Even when the axe hit her, she was filled with the rage of the hurt of *her,* with the fury of her own intention to get out, to regain her freedom.

But this narrative is like a fishnet, a trap. It redefines her and so changes her.

She thinks further, as she goes back to Thomas Poole's flat, about antechambers. There are times in life, she thinks, when I am most conscious of being myself, and these are all times of waiting: before journeys, between the first and the worst birth pains, before exams, before going on stage. Times when I was complete because something was about to happen, but was not happening. I have a life which is a string of these moments of completeness, which I remember so clearly, although they are not important, they are nothing. I stand outside a door, and cannot imagine action that will happen.

She cannot remember how it was before she married Nigel. She cannot remember how she came to do so.

She is afraid of divorce, which will free her, as she was not enough afraid of marriage, which trapped her.

I was not thinking, she concludes, thinking now, harshly, of her then self. I was a fool. I gave him something that didn't exist, because I wasn't thinking, a wife, like the simulacrum of Helen who went to Troy whilst the real one did nothing in Egypt.

Why did I?

It was something I thought I had to do.

Why?

It is what people do do.

Why?

She sees in her mind's eye the heavy figure of Daniel, who married her sister. She sees her sister, her head on the café table, crying and laughing and saying she is happy.

I married Nigel because Stephanie married Daniel and died.

Nonsense.

Then, why?

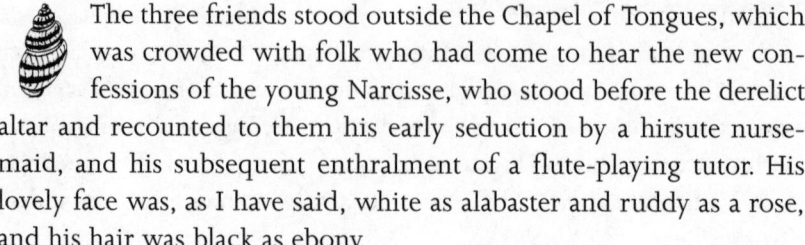

The three friends stood outside the Chapel of Tongues, which was crowded with folk who had come to hear the new confessions of the young Narcisse, who stood before the derelict altar and recounted to them his early seduction by a hirsute nursemaid, and his subsequent enthralment of a flute-playing tutor. His lovely face was, as I have said, white as alabaster and ruddy as a rose, and his hair was black as ebony.

"These tyrants of our childhood," said he, "direct our young inclinations when we have neither force nor knowledge to resist. They teach us titillation, secrecy and control, and in turn become our victims when we learn their lessons too well, when we obtain in our turn power over their desires and their weaknesses. They teach us shame, and treachery, when all should be innocence and freedom. I have confessed before you how I betrayed my friend Hyacinth to the police because his love wearied me: I have confessed how I drove Amaryllis to despair with indifference and neglect. I have reflected much, and see that the creature I was was licked into shape—oh, most *literally*—by that great brutal nursemaid with her hairy lips and her shaggy breasts, in whose loathsome, suffocating, hot embrace I was so frequently and with such taunting endearments *crushed*. She made me desire what revolted me, and as she made me, so I am."

"He goes back and back," said Turdus Cantor. "He began with a man's guilt over the selling of Hyacinth, and called another meeting to say he had found its source in a schoolboy's betrayal of his friend's secret acts to save himself a whipping. Now he says the schoolboy is the son, so to speak, of the too-much tickled nurseling. He will go back and find treachery in the womb, mark me, and they will listen."

"He does not mention the pieces of silver he was paid for Hyacinth," said Colonel Grim. "It is all the body's desire and the perversion of desire. He might speak of the desire for silver amongst his elaborations on tweakings and pokings, lickings and twistings. Cool silver roundels that buy sweetmeats and men's lives, that represent indifferently *any* object of desire."

"And desire shall fail," said Samson Origen. "Our great Projector bids us clarify and examine our desires, acknowledge each dark wriggling thought and appetite, bring them into air and light, and make them clean, and healthy, and innocently wise. But I say that which is crooked cannot be made straight: and that which is wanting cannot be numbered."

"You are a man of few desires," said Turdus Cantor. "What is hard for many is easy for you."

"I have one deep desire," said Samson Origen. "I desire to be at that point when desire shall fail. I desire not to be. Fat Silenus, with grease and winelees oozing from every pore, told the King who caught him that the most desirable state was never to have been born, and the next best was to die soon, for that peace is true peace, which our young friend will not find, whatever he unearths in his memory or his imagination to confess, whatever burdens he unloads into the minds of others, whatever hurts he shares about and about. True wisdom is to stand silent, and neither to give nor to take, but to be still."

"You have not been so silent since you came amongst us," said Turdus Cantor. "You eat and drink. We profit from your conversation. We take pleasure in your company."

"Truly, the gabbing and optimistic atmosphere of this place has had its effect on me," answered Samson Origen. "And your two dry minds, my two friends, have almost made a dent in my resolve to have no attachments. But it cannot last long, as we three all see. The day of blood will come, desire shall be slaked, Culvert will see where he is going, and I shall look on."

Frederica and Alan Melville stand outside the Life Studio, under the glassy lights of the Samuel Palmer School. A group of students are gathered, sitting in a rough semi-circle on the floor, listening to these words, to which Frederica and Alan also listen, at some distance. The reader is Jude Mason, who holds a great heap of untidy typescript on his naked knees. He is wearing nothing but a shiny red dressing-gown which hangs open, revealing his iron-grey body. His face is buried in his long, long iron-grey hair, which is greasy and gleaming. His filthy feet grip the step of the dais on which he is sitting, almost prehensile.

"Here endeth the second lesson," he says, tossing back the curtains of hair. "All is vanity." He beckons to Frederica and Alan, who approach cautiously, entering the perimeter of his pungent smell.

"You no doubt think it is great vanity to read my opus to this captive audience," he says to Frederica, in his clear, sawing voice. "You are a literary person, and I have written a work of literature. But I dare not expect you to take an interest in it."

"I don't see why," says Frederica. "It surprised me. It excited me. I'd like to read it."

The gaunt face peers out between the hair, the deep eyes glittering. "It's not a *nice* book, my dear. It's not a book for nice young women."

"Don't be pretentious. I don't care if it isn't nice. I said, it excited me."

"Books can hurt you."

"I know. If you don't want me to read it, that's OK. I'll go and get on with *Madame Bovary*."

"*That's* not a nice book. That's a mischievous work of despair. My nasty book has more hope in it than that cartload of clay."

He is over-excited by her interest, and unattractive in his over-excitement. Frederica finds herself staring at the defining limits of his taut belly, in order not to meet his eye.

"You didn't think I could write, confess it, you thought I was rubbish, talking rubbish."

"And if I did, you meant me to."

"You can read it. In *manus tuas.* Here." He prances towards her, on a wave of his odour, and thrusts the heap of paper into her hands. "I appoint you my *reader.* Greater love hath no man than this. Though it will require a modicum of love on your part, to go through all that *bumf,* oh, what a word, what a good word, bumf, bumf—I am overcome with over-excitement."

"Is this your only copy?"

"Are you hesitating? Do you regret your commitment? Shall I take it back?"

"Please, stop all that. I daren't be responsible for your only copy."

"You aren't. I sell my body, I purchase carbon paper. I write it all out by hand also, and primarily, I exude, I excrete, little black threads of meaning and bodily *anguish* along feinted lines on scholastic paper. I would not bring my only copy here in this plastic bag, do not think it. It is the child of my body, it is my only delight, I keep copies at my humble *home,* clones, versions. This is my *mundane* copy, fit for crushing with me if I go under a car. At home I have an immortal copy in many-coloured inks. Do not say many-coloured inks are derivative, I forestall you, I tell you freely it is a tribute to him, to Father Rolfe, to the great Baron Corvo, who taught me the bliss of scarlet and emerald inks."

Thomas Poole tells Frederica that an inspector is coming to her evening class. It is February and dark in the evenings. The class has held together, despite Christmas, and the dark days of the solstice. Thomas has told Frederica that it is important to make her students present papers to the class. They are reluctant, Frederica says, they are there voluntarily, why should she make them? If, indeed, she can make them. They like to hear *her,* her cleverness, her passion. She is afraid that they may bore each other. Thomas Poole says that the classes function as therapeutic groups, and that speaking out is part of the therapy. Frederica retorts that she is not a therapist, and that her students are not sick. They are intelligent people, who need to think hard and deep, and don't get the opportunity. She holds it against Poole, later, that he has used this word, "therapy." He persists. She will find that they are grateful to be made to speak, he says. Students, even adults, require you to be the authority that requires effort out of their lassitude and self-mistrust. If he is wrong, in Frederica's judgement, about therapy, he is right about authority. Frederica has learned to make the students speak, and she, and they, are excited by what they say. Nevertheless, the inspector has chosen a difficult day. The evening's presentation is on Kafka's *Castle.* Who would speak on *The Castle,* she asked the class, a month ago. She expected an enthusiastic offer from Ghislaine Todd, the psychoanalyst, who often refers to Kafka, but in fact the one who raises his hand is the quiet blond man in a suit, who never misses a class, and never speaks, except occasionally over coffee to the other suited man, the owner of the Lambretta, whose attendance has become spasmodic.

"Oh, good," said Frederica then. "Are you specially interested in Kafka?"

"Yes," said the blond man. Frederica waited. "Yes, I am," said the blond man.

And now he is about to speak. Thomas Poole and the inspector are in the back row of the circle, which is two rows deep. The lights are dismal. Someone is crunching a Polo mint. John Ottokar stands up, holding a neat white sheaf of papers. His face is classical, broad-browed, blue-eyed, quiet-mouthed, amiable. His hair is massed and thick.

"I think I remember at school being told you must never say 'I think,'" he begins. "But all I can do is say what I think, since there is no other reason for standing here. I am fortunate if you listen. No one in this book listened to K the Land Surveyor, except the official whose bed he invaded by accident, when he had the chance to speak, and he only fell asleep.

"I didn't really read before I came to this class. So I can't make the connections some of you make between this book and other books. This is the book of all the books we have read that has told me most about what it is to be a human being, although what it says is that to be a human being is almost nothing.

"What you notice at first is two things: the Land Surveyor who can't get himself accepted or recognised, and the Castle.

"He can see the Castle in the distance, but there is no way of getting there, or speaking to it.

"In the village, where he seems to have to stay, everything is full of human bodies and human emotions—sex, and competition, silly quarrels and status problems like hens in a barnyard.

"You might suppose the Castle would be fine, or imposing, or a fortress. But is isn't. It resembles the village, or a rock. Or an optical illusion. Kafka tells you several things about it, and the things give contradictory impressions, contradictory feelings. It is in the 'glittering air' in the white snow, it 'soars light and free.' It also resembles his home village he came from. 'It was only a wretched-looking town, a huddle of village houses, whose sole merit, if any, lay in being built of stone, but the plaster had long since flaked off and the stone seemed to be crumbling away.' Also there is a tower, 'graciously mantled with ivy, pierced by small windows that glittered in the sun, a somewhat maniacal glitter.' It is a *mad* tower. Kafka says it seems 'designed by the trembling or careless hand of a child . . . as if a melancholy-mad tenant . . . had burst through the roof.' What is this Castle? It's where he wants to go and can't go, it's the place *where he isn't now,* it's gracious and glittering and mad. Kafka's words don't hang together. Nor does the Castle.

"Life in the village is a muddle and a mess. Like the worst ideas any of us have of life in groups, groups like families or also people who work together, full of sudden hostilities and equally sudden warmth between people which isn't real, hasn't a reason. Everyone talks all the time. They gab and gabble, they explain and excuse themselves, they are shifty and evasive. It is all really power struggles at some level. You don't know if the Castle is different or the same, since you can't go there.

"Everything is like a dream, where you can grasp on to thinking processes or *complicated* human emotions, but only to be denied by the obtuseness of your own sleeping body. Or you are denied by unresponsiveness or *animosity* in the other creatures in the dream world.

"Kafka was a clerk who got pushed about by bureaucracies. He couldn't bring himself to get married. He writes about love and power in a world of struggling maggots and puppies and dreamy muddle. He could be writing about the survival of the fittest. But although the Castle officials are well fed, they're sleepy, too, they can't sit up and take notice, they *don't know what's going on.*

"That's the key to it, really, they don't know what's going on. They have language, but they can't think with it, they fuss about. They talk about love and influence but they mess those words up, they don't *mean* anything. And freedom, what is it? If you're sleepy to death you can't be free. The words of this book are all dilapidated like the Castle itself. When K tries to phone the Castle at the beginning, before he knows better, he hears a funny buzz in the telephone. 'It was like the hum of countless children's voices—but yet not a hum, the echo rather of voices singing at an infinite distance—blended by sheer impossibility into one high but resonant sound which vibrated on the ear as if it were trying to penetrate beyond mere hearing.'

"Children singing is like heaven, but the idea of them humming and buzzing is like the playground, where you can get hurt, where there's no order.

"All the people in this book are in a way no more than cross children. I'd like to discuss this idea more.

"Language gets you nowhere, society seems to be just a mad structure that has only one function—to keep *itself* going in an unthinking sort of a way—not for any reason.

"I read another story by Kafka, 'The Penal Colony,' in which there is a terrible instrument of torture, which has a bed, on which the condemned man lies, gagged, and a Harrow, which writes his sentence on his body with needles, in his own blood, and kills him with writing. It is worked by an official who loves it. He keeps telling the other man, the explorer, that the condemned man *can't read* his sentence but *he can feel it in his body.* There isn't any order except this mad mechanical precision—and the torture machine, like the Castle—isn't so good close up, its cogs make a nasty noise, its felt gag is worn out with earlier tortures. K is a Land Surveyor but he can't get far enough out of the mess to survey. K thinks Barnabas the messenger is an Angel stepping in the blizzard, but he is 'really' only a boy in a dirty jerkin. The messages aren't messages. But Kafka can write in this *non*-language, like an angel, about there not being any angels, and nothing to survey. This is an inhuman book about being human. Or a human book about being inhuman. Or am I just playing with words?"

The discussion is heated. Ghislaine Todd, the psychoanalyst, and Rosemary Bell, the hospital almoner, have developed a running argument about the reasons for male fear of women in the early twentieth century. Todd sees K's impotence as a result of his demonisation of mother-figures, whilst Rosemary Bell sees it as a result of social oppression. Sister Perpetua observes that both these interpretations may relate to the disappearance of God, who was or is both Father and Authority, and whose Presence would make sense of the senseless Castle and the frantic earthly desires and struggles. Humphrey Maggs says Sister Perpetua may be right, but you can't make God exist just because it would make sense of things. Ibrahim Mustafa says that God does exist, and that Kafka knows it, whether he thinks he does or not. An argument develops about K's "assistants"—are they hostile siblings, or anarchic employees in a society without purpose, or perhaps the testicles beside the phallus. Or schizophrenic emanations from K's own damaged psyche, says John Ottokar, or the Id running away from the controls of the Ego and the Superego. He has never said so much before: Ghislaine Todd smiles at him warmly. The inspector is delighted. He makes notes.

Afterwards, they all go to the pub. The pub is called the Goat and Compasses and has a rather clever swinging sign with a Satanic albino goat wielding a compass rather in the manner of Blake's Urizen. It is a dark brown-leather-and-open-fireplace pub, with electric imitation coals; there are a lot of mock-vellum lampshades on mock-candles. They have their own very dark brown table in a deep dark corner, with high settle-like benches along two sides and several mock-mediaeval stools. A good half of the class always go there, and intense relationships are formed. The whole group offers advice on Una Winterson's marital problems, or listens to Humphrey Maggs's views on Harold Wilson, on capital punishment, on homosexuality, the concerns of the day. They do these things in the light of Madame Bovary, of Dostoevski's Idiot, of Proust. Frederica finds she does not want to sit near Thomas Poole, who has come with them and is deep in conversation with the battling Freudian and Marxist. She takes the opposite corner of the table, and finds herself sipping red wine next to John Ottokar. She tells him his paper was splendid. She says, "You never talked, before."

"I don't talk. I thought it was time."

"I don't really know what you do."

"I write computer programmes. For a shipping firm. I am a mathematician."

"George Murphy came to the class because of his Lambretta."

"I came to learn language. I've never used language. I grew up without it."

"I have a mathematical brother who's suspicious of language."

"My situation is complicated. I am an identical twin, and we were both mathematicians. We grew up speaking a kind of private language—almost a silent language—of signs and gestures. We closed everyone out. No one could reach us. We were like a child and a mirror that spoke to itself. I think it frightened us, but when we were frightened, it intensified—our need of each other. We didn't relate outwards. And at the same time, we were each other's prison."

"Did you have the same friends?"

"No friends, until we went to university. We tried to go to different universities, but that didn't work—we started in different places and ended up in the same one. We fought. We both wanted to work in artificial intelligence, and by then we both wanted the other to do something else. It was like being torn in two—being *half* and half. If we saw each other by accident, it was like seeing ourselves when we had thought we were invisible. I can't explain. Anyway. I had a hard time talking to people. Except in computer languages. Algo. Fortran. Cobol. But I saw it wasn't enough. I sat through meal after meal saying nothing. I met girls, and said nothing. Then I got my job."

"And your brother?"

"He went another way. I may tell you, some day, not now. We had problems. He found—a way of talking I don't like. I needed badly to learn language in a—detached?—way. Not *personal* language. You don't follow. I'm sorry."

"You use language with great assurance. Look at your Kafka paper. As you must know."

"I'm interested in whether you think if you don't speak. I felt like—like an ape learning, or Adam in the Bible, writing that paper, making myself think thoughts. I thought, Did I think all those things before I had to write them?"

"Did you?"

"Oh yes. But not in words. In shapes. In feelings. Those words, the word 'shape,' the word 'feeling' don't quite describe what I mean, what I thought."

He has an eloquence, Frederica thinks, which is aware of itself but innocent; he uses words well and with glee because they all appear to him new-minted. She says, "I'm glad you came here to learn language."

"Not only that," he says in a low voice. "I come for another reason."

Frederica looks at him.

"One that does and doesn't need words," he says. "*I want you,*" he says, quickly and quietly.

She is aware of the whole of him, blond smile, fierce intent eyes, his hands on the table, his legs and feet beneath it, near her own but not touching. She responds for a moment, in silence, with a fast flood of blood to her heart and her pale face. He smiles. She does not. He watches her trouble. He stands and walks away to fetch more drinks. He is a grown man, not a student; he is older than she is. The three words have changed everything: and nothing, for she has known, before, how things were. But now they are spoken.

On the way home, Thomas Poole congratulates her on her class. She is a born teacher, he tells her. The group has a life of its own. She remembers that he had used the word "therapy," and is angry. Books are not therapy, she thinks, they are understanding, they are thinking. She is still out of breath because of the fierce certainty of John Ottokar. She says, "My solicitor says I've got to move out, but I don't know where to go. He says I can't go on living with you and hope to get a divorce."

Thomas Poole says, "I had hoped you would stay permanently." His voice does not expect her to say she will.

"I can't," says Frederica, striding along in the dark. "I've got to find somewhere innocent and unexceptionable. I don't see how."

She asks Daniel if he knows where she can live. He does not. She asks Tony, Alan, Hugh Pink, who are also unable to help. It is Alexander, who found her her first refuge, who comes up with her second. He sends her to see Agatha Mond.

X

Two people walk into Hamelin Square on a cold February day. Hamelin Square is not a square: it is a spoon-shaped cul-de-sac, in Kennington, in a part of London south of the river, where there are acres of buildings and no public green spaces that are not small, flat, and surrounded by wire fences. There are many wide, straight, dusty main roads, some of them lined with elegant Georgian rows of houses. There are many small tunnels and mazes of housing of every age, Georgian, Victorian, Edwardian, wartime prefabs in faded pinks and blues, and abutting these tiny homes are tall towers in monumental rectangular concrete, balcony above balcony, grey against the sky. Hamelin Square consists of early-nineteenth-century houses, with elegant long windows, decreasing in size for three floors, and basement areas reached by steps. These houses are quite pretty, in a slightly pinched way; diminished models of the grander Georgian houses on the roads. They are in an extraordinarily mixed state of repair. Some are gentrified, with bright white paint, window-boxes, brass door-knockers and pretty curtains. Some are crumbling, with dirty net curtains on sagging wires, and blistered paint. One or two are gay and incongruous in West Indian mixes of bright dark blues, plum pinks and acid greens. In the centre of the spoon-bowl is a patch of mud that is not a green, on which are two old car-seats, a rotting mattress, a new and bloodstained bright pink baby-doll nightdress.

The two people progress slowly. Frederica's natural aggressive stride is impeded by the slow progress of her companion. She is wearing a long black cloak-like coat over a knitted grey tunic, over green tights and high black boots. She is carrying a dull gold breast-plate and bossed shield, and looks a little like Britannia on the pennies, or the ghost of Britomart. Her companion is wearing corduroy trousers, a blue hooded jacket with silver fur, and a large gold helmet, whose plastic visor descends, imprisoning his head, every few steps, and has to be pushed up again. He is alternately brandishing and trailing a large gold plastic sword with a jewelled hilt, which is too large for him and impedes his progress further. If Frederica offers to carry the sword, he stands still, stubborn with fury, and strikes his head so that the visor falls yet again.

Frederica is a woman who goes everywhere in a rush, in a trajectory. This creeping progress is alien to her. So is the knot of love that winds her round the small figure of her son, so that she feels his steps in her feet, his small angry bones in her gut. She has not been able to work out how far she should consult him on the proposed house-moving. She remembers, she thinks, that at four her own head was whirling with adult thoughts and understanding, all wholly uncommunicated. She supposes Leo must be the same, but does not know. He is happy at Thomas Poole's. He likes Waltraut Röhde, he likes Simon. He has to move or Frederica cannot escape his father. Frederica does not know how anyone can go on bearing so much guilt, so much emotion to be organised and endured. She says, "We could stick the visor up temporarily with plasticine; then you could see."

"I might want it down, if an *enemy* approached."

"We could stick it up in the street, so you could walk faster."

"A street is where an *enemy* might be, I should think." He brandishes the sword, and stands, yet again, stock-still.

If this woman, in this house, doesn't love him, I shall hate her, thinks Frederica.

She has never really had a woman friend. Girls at school disliked her for being clever and she accepted this, as her due, both as a compliment and as a punishment. Cambridge meant men, to love and talk to.

They arrive at Number 42, at the point of the spoon. It is decorously done up: the door is new black paint, the windows are white, the bricks are repaired, there are no window-boxes. Frederica holds up the visor when they mount the steps. It falls again, when they ring the door bell. Agatha Mond sees them, as she opens the door, against the winter light, black-cloaked, gold-gleaming, helmeted and booted. "Come in," she says. "I've made tea."

. . .

Agatha lives on the top two floors of the house. The arrangement they are discussing is that Frederica and Leo should rent the basement and ground floor, for a low rent and some reciprocal baby-sitting. Agatha's part of the house is spotlessly clean. The curtains and sofa are rich, dark and bright with William Morris's Golden Lily; the walls are white and studded with prints and paintings, some abstract, some nineteenth-century, some Doré Dante illustrations, some of John Martin's images of Paradise, Chaos and Pandemonium with swarms of small bright angels like light-emitting bees. In the kitchen Matisse's Jazz prints sit also on a white wall, amongst earthenware jugs and bowls, Sabatier knives, a mixture of old blue-and-white plates on a dresser. In one corner is a playhouse, solidly built of wood and beautifully painted with crimson and white climbing roses and blue columbine. It does not occur to Frederica to think that this order is the result of a frantic morning's cleaning in her honour. She diagnoses the brown jar of graded wooden spoons, large and small, deep and flat; the clean tea-towels on scarlet hooks; the well-used but scrubbed chopping board; the glass jars full of coffee beans, cereals, tea, brown sugar, white sugar. Here is natural order, in which someone takes pleasure. There are two kitchen windows, and two blinds, emerald green and sky blue, which are happy together.

Agatha Mond gives Frederica tea in an old Spode cup and squeezes orange juice for Leo, to whom she also gives a large moon-like biscuit with a smiling face iced on it. For this, he consents to take off his helmet. As he does so, Saskia Mond, dark and wiry in a corduroy pinafore dress and a skinny blue jumper over scarlet tights, appears from her room. She and Leo stare unsmiling at each other and retreat to the sides of their respective mothers. The two women sit facing each other, neither on the sofa, both alone in hard armchairs, as far away from each other as possible.

I can't live here, Frederica thinks. I can't keep this up. I might just as well go now.

"When I bought the house," says Agatha Mond, "which I did very cheaply, because in those days none of these houses were done up, I always intended to share it. So I made two separate entities. There are two kitchens, two bathrooms, although it's so small. And then I've never quite felt I *could*—or that I had to—but I go away so much at the moment, with the committee—and Alexander said he thought you and I might get on . . ."

Her face is composed and severe. She addresses Frederica as though Frederica were a meeting. All her features are perfectly proportioned; her eyes are large and dark but not melting.

"Logically, I thought," says Agatha Mond, "that two women with the same interests—and with children the same age—could make a really sensible arrangement—as long as we thought it out—and built in safeguards for if we didn't like each other—and a reasonable set of rules so we don't start by annoying each other inadvertently. I never have shared—but I'm sure most sharing founders on silly little misunderstandings that could have been foreseen."

Frederica says she is sure that that is quite right.

"It would get harder and harder to discuss difficulties, once the arrangement was established," Agatha Mond persists.

Frederica thinks: She is actually very nervous. She is naturally managing. She is also afraid, for herself, for her daughter. I should perhaps just go. She looks up from her knees and catches Agatha's look directly, and sees her own thoughts being read.

"Of course I am nervous," says Agatha. "It is our children who are involved as well as ourselves. But I am right, we would need rules. If you wanted to come."

"I must go *somewhere,*" says Frederica. "I'm all right where I am, in a way, but it might prejudice my—attempt to get divorced. I think I should say—I don't have much income, but I don't want to earn it by baby-sitting. I will do my share, of course, but I must *work* or I'll die."

"Of course. That is understood. That is why we need to think it out."

There is a silence. Agatha offers to show Frederica the vacant half of the house. This consists of a ground floor—two rooms and a kitchen, and a basement, containing a bedroom and a kitchen. Everything is white, the new bath, the walls, the worksurfaces in the tiny kitchen, the table surrounded by pale wooden chairs. It is surgically anonymous; the floors are sanded and varnished wooden boards.

"I didn't want to impose my taste," says Agatha Mond. "One can hate other people's colours; life can be unbearable with other people's idea of cheerfulness or quietness, don't you think?

"I thought the two households would live separately altogether—apart perhaps from one meal a week, or a fortnight, to be decided; the two women would need to make the acquaintance of each other's children, to know them well. I have a visiting surrogate granny, for difficult evenings, who also irons and polishes; her services could be shared, by arrangement. There should be no feeling that either should ever invite the other to any dinner party or anything—and they would have to be extraordinarily careful about *borrowing* things—though I think arrangements could and should perhaps be made about the Hoover, perhaps only the Hoover . . ."

Her voice is full of doubt. Frederica stares around at the bare white walls, the sparkling white tiles. She has no home-making talents: she has never needed any.

Leo needs a home.

Agatha Mond's voice is full of efficient clarity, fear, and doubt. She is a Civil Servant, vulnerable through her child.

"Do you have parties?"

"Oh no. But that's because I don't like large parties. I'm quite sure, by arrangement . . ."

Frederica says, "I don't think it would work. I don't think I should come here. I don't think my way of life—"

She has no idea what her way of life is. Agatha Mond says, "I quite understand, I do understand—"

Both their voices are drowned by screaming from above. Both women, simultaneously, imagine both children torturing and being tortured. They turn and run, fast. They are young and agile.

Saskia, weeping violently and gesturing with pointy fingers, is dancing round the playhouse. Inside there is a blunted crashing and the fabric is swaying as though it is about to burst. Agatha says to Saskia, "Are you shut out?" and Frederica calls to Leo, "Are you shut in?" Saskia stops crying enough to gasp, "He's *stuck* in. I can't get him out." She then resumes her shrill wailing. Agatha kneels down. Leo is hopelessly entangled, his sword at an angle blocking the doorway, his visor jammed down, his head beating like a giant beetle against the window. Agatha persuades him to keep still. She moves the sword, patiently, inch by inch, manoeuvres the angry small body round it and extricates it. She shows Leo how to take off his helmet in the confined space and wriggle free. She extricates the helmet. The two children sit on their mothers and sob with damp red cheeks.

"I made a cake," says Agatha Mond, smiling now the danger of house-sharing has been averted. "We may as well eat it."

It is a very good cake. It is a golden cake, containing translucent vermilion glacé cherries, shaped into a Hansel and Gretel gingerbread house, thatched with chocolate icing, with blue-curtained windows in yellow brick walls, up which grow climbing flowers on spiralling green stems, surrounding an arched green door. It has barley-sugar twisted chimney-pots, quite Elizabethan, and two doves sitting on the roof. Leo and Saskia carry their slices into the playhouse, into which they both fit, leaving the armour outside the door. Frederica crosses the room to look at the pictures on each side of the chimney-breast. They are facsimiles of the contrary "Nurse's Song" and "Nurses Song" from Blake's *Songs of Innocence* and *Songs of Experience.* Innocence is on the left, the poem contained in the arms of a weeping willow, in a pink-and-gold sunset glow. The nurse sits at the base of the tree, perhaps sewing, perhaps writing. Beside her, two rose-coloured slender girls hold hands in an arch, under which, into the warm light, the rest of the circle are dancing.

When the voices of children are heard on the green
And laughing is heard on the hill,
My heart is at rest within my breast
And everything else is still.

"Then come home, my children, the sun is gone down
"And the dews of night arise
"Come, come, leave off play, and let us away
"Till the morning appears in the skies."

"No no let us play, for it is yet day
"And we cannot go to sleep;
"Besides, in the sky, the little birds fly
"And the hills are all cover'd with sheep."

"Well, well, go & play till the light fades away
"And then go home to bed."
The little ones leaped & shouted & laugh'd
And all the hills ecchoed.

On the right, Experience shows three figures in a doorway, a purple woman bending solicitously over a green-clad youth with long blond hair and a hand laid across his waist to emphasise, rather than conceal, his sex, which is faintly outlined in gold on his green breeches. Behind him a female figure of indeterminate age sits in the angle of the doorstep, head bowed. Vines heavy with grapes climb richly upwards, purple, gold and green, reaching out spiralling tendrils towards both woman and youth.

When the voices of children are heard on the green
And whisp'rings are in the dale,
The days of my youth rise fresh in my mind,
My face turns green and pale.

Then come home, my children, the sun is gone down,
And the dews of night arise;
Your spring & your day, are wasted, in play,
And your winter and night in disguise.

"I wish *I* had these pictures," says Frederica with abstract politeness.

"I wish I had them all. I love their doubleness. One thinks differently about the innocence of children once one has them. And about oneself, one's own childhood."

Frederica looks out of the window, at the mud and rubbish in the centre of Hamelin Square. Some children are chasing and dodging each other between the car-seats, three black, three white children, screaming. It is not possible to tell if they are playing or trying to hurt each other. She says, "At the Art School where I teach, my Head of Department is mad about Blake. He gives lectures on recovering the energies of childish innocence, polymorphous perversity and unrestrained desire."

"That crops up in our committee, too. We have members who talk about learning from the children, letting the children set the agenda, freeing the curriculum. Personally, I find it hard to sympathise with.

"When I was a child I was terrified of other children. They seemed to me like ravening tigers or stupid trolls who wanted to tie you down and poke you. I wanted to be a *real person,* which meant grown-up."

"So did I," says Frederica. "You understand slowly that you understand things that you can't *say* or *use* until you're—'a human being,' I used to say to myself—I felt I was a *person* inside a kind of silly mask and disguise, to whom people spoke in voices suitable for my silly face and silly clothes—*even other children*—"

"And then you wonder—is everyone else in a silly mask, or is it only me—"

"And you don't even know the answer, but you suspect it's only you—"

"And you wait to be a grown-up, or a real person, or a human being—you wait savagely in solitude, guarding your secrets and nursing your—hopes—possibilities—"

"And you find that everyone else, now you're a real person, is saying how much more authentic it is—how much more *free*—to be a polymorphously perverse child—"

"And you wonder if your own child thinks as you thought—"

"Because your child *is* innocent, there is a sense in which you know they *don't* know all the things you are so confident you knew all the time but didn't say—they can so easily be hurt."

"So easily. It's no good saying that childhood is like paradise. It's at least as much like hell. Whatever you do."

"Yet when we get the idea of Paradise"—says Frederica, looking away from Blake to the black Martin engraving of the angel Raphael, made of white light, advancing under black Romantic paradisal trees across a glade towards the softly luminous naked figures of our first Parents—"when we get that idea, it is a memory of a *first state*—we did *once*—when was it?—experience everything more brightly than now—"

They stop, almost out of breath. They smile at each other. Agatha Mond's face is brightened and lifted by her smile; it is less beautiful than it is in repose, more pointed.

"I've never had this conversation," says Frederica.

"Nor have I. More cake?"

A turmoil in the playhouse ends their talk.

Frederica has made a friend.

Three weeks later, Frederica and Leo move into the lower flat in 42 Hamelin Square.

Frederica goes to St. Simeon's to see Daniel. She is restless and lonely, and since Christmas the two have become more friendly than in the past. She stops in the vestry of the half-church, and considers the notices. There is a poster for Gideon Farrar's Children of Joy, "The Christian Embrace. It's Child's Play—the Mums and Dads Are Learning Fast," with a large photograph of a barefooted circle of people of all ages hugging each other and smiling ecstatically. There is a very small card in a corner, with a decorated border in green, red, and blue inks vaguely Gothic, richly elegant, which on inspection contains bleeding red-breasted pelicans and robins, and pointed-toothed bats and monkeys amongst its foliage. It contains a text in beautifully penned Gothic script.

There is a great ladder of religious cruelty with many rungs; but three of them are most important.

At one time one sacrificed human beings to one's god, perhaps precisely those humans one loved best, as in the sacrifice of the first-born.

Then in mankind's moral epoch, one sacrificed to one's god one's strongest instincts, one's "nature." The joy of *this* festival glitters in the cruel glance of the ascetic.

Finally, what was left? Did one not have to sacrifice everything comforting, holy, healing, all hope, all faith in a concealed harmony, in future bliss and justice? Did one not have to sacrifice God himself, and out of cruelty self-cruelty to oneself worship stone, stupidity, gravity, fate, nothingness?

To sacrifice God for nothingness—this paradoxical mystery of the final act of cruelty was reserved for the generation which even now arises: we all know something of this already.

Frederica stands and considers this text, which she cannot place, although it is vaguely familiar. Then she goes down the spiral staircase into the crypt.

Ginnie Greenhill is in her cubicle, listening to the squawk and splutter of the telephone. Her round shoulders, in an apple-green sweater, are tense: from time to time she nods attentively, staring at her egg-box walls.

Daniel is sitting in his own cubicle, reading. His large face is brooding.

From Canon Holly's little sanctum come animated voices. Coming into the crypt, Frederica is surprised to see Rupert Parrott, smoking a briar pipe, woolly-pated and rosy-faced, wearing a greenish tweed jacket and a mustard-coloured waistcoat. He is sitting on the Canon's swivelling chair, turning this way and that, gesticulating. The Canon, also smoking a pipe, and wearing a cassock, is buried in a decrepit leather armchair.

Daniel is pleased to see Frederica. He offers her tea, and goes to fill the kettle. Rupert Parrott swivels energetically and catches sight of her as he comes into view.

"Frederica! I am thinking of publishing a collection of your Reader's Reports. I laugh aloud. I didn't know you came here."

"I come to see Daniel." She sees Parrott coming to the conclusion that she is in Daniel's pastoral care. "He's my brother-in-law."

"You surprise me. I thought you were in training as a Listener."

"I've thought of it. I don't think I'd be any good. I'm not patient, and I'm not self-effacing."

"I'd like to be—" says Parrott, his pink cheeks pinker. "Of course I'm partly here as Adelbert's publisher. But I am interested in the work. The work is important. I'm thinking of publishing a book called *The Helpers,* which I'd like Adelbert to write. About individuals in the caring professions—a psychoanalyst, a psychiatrist, a probation officer, a Listener—and some of the newer leaders of encounter groups and things that are springing up—"

"Tea," says Daniel.

"Please," say Holly and Parrott. It has become a tea party. They chat. Ginnie Greenhill continues her passionate listening to the telephone's babble, in another world.

"Frederica does wonderful work for me, for a pittance," says Rupert Parrott. "I almost never publish anything she reports on, but I *do* appreciate her reporting."

"You did accept Phyllis Pratt's *Daily Bread,*" says Frederica. "I was glad about that, she could write. That would interest Daniel and Canon Holly, it's about a clergyman who loses his faith."

"She came to see me last week," says Parrott.

"What is she like?" says Frederica. "Tell."

"She is *very* large," says Parrott. "In a black broadcloth suit, with a priestlike hat, flat and black with a dull red ribbon. She came into my office and said, 'I have come to withdraw my book.' I said it was already in production, I said the cover was chosen—it has a wonderful cottage loaf on it and a great knife, a shiny knife—a bread-knife—I said we all loved the book. She said in a toneless sort of voice that it was an unpublishable book, not worthy, and she wanted it back. So I said it *was* worthy, and that I should be hurt—one always makes the mistake of supposing *large* people are kindly and concerned—and she repeated that she'd come to withdraw it, it wasn't worthy. She was being the immovable object and for some reason I felt I had to be the irresistible force. So I said she owed me an explanation, she'd wasted a lot of my time and money and emotion, and all that didn't matter, but I thought she was *really good*—I'd at last discovered a *really good* novelist—and as I said it, I saw I really thought it, and I became quite distressed, quite distressed on my own behalf. So she sat there, and repeated her two sentences, about withdrawing the book, and not being worthy. And something made me say, 'If you can honestly *assure* me that this is your own wish—that I should disrupt publication—that you are under no pressure—' And suddenly she was all water, her face dissolved, she said her husband had read the blurb we sent and felt it was all about him."

"Is it?" asks Frederica.

"Probably. How do I know? But I felt somehow furiously determined. So I lectured her on what she owed me—and how good it was—and she got hotter and hotter—steaming hot—and went off to think, she said. I don't know what she'll do. She didn't go into detail. I haven't stopped production. That book *matters to her,* I can sense. I couldn't work out what she was like."

"She can write."

"Oh yes."

"And the other book?" says Frederica. "All that typescript I gave you. *Babbletower.* Have you read it?"

"Oh yes," says Rupert Parrott. "Two or three times." He lowers his voice conspiratorially. "It's a dreadful risk. It could get any publisher into trouble. Even in these marginally more enlightened days. It's not a nice book."

"It sticks in the mind," says Frederica, testing.

"It does. It does stick in the mind."

"Has anyone else seen it?"

"No. I've been thinking about it."

There is a sound above them, and then a sound of feet coming down the stairs.

Black, shiny, cracked patent shoes. Very dirty speedwell-blue socks. Filthy skin between socks and trousers. Tight pin-striped trousers, silver stripe on matt black, calf-clinging, rising to a high waist and old dress-braces. A cloak of iron-grey hair. A velvet jacket, stained midnight blue, partly threadbare, an old white silk evening muffler, a long grey face under the grey hair, an aura, an odour of active staleness and decay.

"I had believed," says the plangent voice, "that you lived here immured and listened to the voices of which the air is so full, the wailing to which I have made my small contributions. I felt a certain inhibition about imposing my corporeal presence on this ghostly converse and so I came secretly and saw that others felt no such compunction, that there is a steady stream of distinctly solid fleshly visitors, of which I thought I might make one. I left a calling card, which was found acceptable, or not immediately torn up or cast into the flames. I wondered if I might be permitted to continue my theological debate with the judicious Daniel in judgement. And I see Frederica, taking tea. This resembles the under-earth hideout of the Lost Boys. Do I interrupt, should I leave, may I stay?"

Canon Holly says, "We welcome all comers. I recognise your voice. We are happy to see you. May I know your name? I am Adelbert Holly, over there is Virginia Greenhill—you have spoken to both of us—and this young man is a visitor, Rupert Parrott."

"I know that name," says Jude. "The arm of coincidence is long."

Frederica's mind has been racing. She does not know whether Rupert Parrott has made up his mind for or against *Babbletower,* but she is fairly sure that the sight and smell of Jude is not likely to influence him favourably. Jude's last remark, however, is decisive. She says, "This is Jude Mason. The author of *Babbletower,* which we were discussing."

"Ah," says Rupert Parrott. He looks at his feet, and twirls in his chair. Jude advances to the centre of the crypt. Rupert Parrott says, "Some of the tortures the little boys undergo in the Dormitories, in your book—"

"Far-fetched, you think? Improbably ingenious?"

"Not at all. Wholly convincing. Traditional, even. I wonder if you were at Swineburn School, perhaps?"

Jude stares; his face closes.

"I even seem to recognise some of the more unpleasant cupboards and places of water-torture. And a few very local slang terms. 'Fessy,' for instance. 'Bullapot.' 'Gullanging.' Were you there in the days of Claude Hautboys?"

Jude stands in his grimy finery and drops his head, so that his face is covered by a curtain of greasy hair. Then he lifts his head, parts the curtain, pushes it back over his shoulders, and says, "No mean French scholar, an excellent guide along the more recondite pathways of French decadence. Heavy-handed, though, and heavy in other ways, very heavy."

This adjective causes a rictus of mirthless laughter in Rupert Parrott's brownie-like face.

"Heavy," he concurs, nodding.

"I matriculated," says Jude, staring intently at Parrott, "and then put an end to it. I scarpered, I quit, I fled, I discharged myself, I disembogued, I ran away betwixt the dark and dawn and was no more seen in that place. Over the hills of Cumberland and far away I wandered, piping wild, feeding on swine-nuts, and so to Paris, a wandering scholar, where I found *protection* and a library."

"A good library," says Parrott.

"The best," says Jude. There is a silence. "May I hope that you found my offering acceptable?"

"A book for our times," says Rupert Parrott. "Strong meat."

"I am a vegetarian," says Jude. "A butcher only in the imagination." It is as though they are speaking in code.

"You realise that this book runs the risk of prosecution? Even after *Lady Chatterley.*"

"I had not considered the matter. I wrote what I had to write. *Lady Chatterley* is a vulgar and improbable book."

"And *Babbletower*—"

"Is all around us," says Jude, casting an arrogant stare around the egg-boxes, telephones and battered chairs amongst the fanning pillars of the crypt.

"It is a challenge," says Parrott. "A challenge I must say I feel I have to accept."

He is worked up. He is sweating slightly around his crinkled hairline.

Daniel recognises the tension in his voice. Daniel spent a long night talking Rupert Parrott out of cutting his wrists, some time ago. He remembers, though he tries not to, a Parrott obsessed by self-disgust and moral despair, a Parrott who finally arrived, tear-smeared and shaking, in St. Simeon's in the small hours, to be consoled by Daniel and subsequently invigorated by Canon Holly's calm acceptance of his secret self, his hidden desires, his ambiguities and equivocations. Daniel told him human beings were infinitely diverse, but Holly commanded him to love his own difference, to admit his dark side into the circle of his fuller Self. And so *Our Passions Christ's Passion* found a publisher and Rupert Parrott became a visiting helper of the Listeners. He is wary of Daniel, whom he does not love but does trust. Daniel can see both why Parrott feels he must publish Jude's book, and why this will not be easy for him, if the book does get into trouble. Daniel knows nothing about book-trouble. But he knows, he thinks, a real suicide risk from a counterfeit or mimic.

"We should drink to this venture," says Canon Holly, producing a bottle of Hungarian Bull's Blood, fashionable at that time. Slugs of Bull's Blood are poured into various unbreakable tumblers, and they drink, including Ginny Greenhill, whose caller has abruptly rung off in mid-sentence, interrupted by despair, a visitor, embarrassment, collapse, she cannot say. Frederica proposes the toast:

"To *Babbletower*!"

They drink.

Frederica sits in the basement in Hamelin Square. She tries to write, and cannot. The paper is blank in front of her. It is early evening. The flat still smells faintly of new paint. She is looking at the area wall through the slats of a buttercup-yellow Venetian blind, which casts a ghostly gold and violet-grey shadowed lattice, or grid, on the white expanse of the paper. She has a new writing table in pale pine-wood and a deep blue plastic chair on chrome legs.

She is surrounded by writing and cannot write. Tony Watson has shown some of her reports for Bowers and Eden to the new literary editor of *Spyglass,* a cultural weekly founded by a minor member of Bloomsbury, surviving with a precarious circulation and a disproportionate reputation for wit and influence. Frederica is now part of a rotating team of four novel columnists, and is therefore surrounded with cardboard boxes of hardback novels. She can review four or even five of these at once, giving the most important perhaps two hundred fifty words and the least a thirty-word sentence. She has learned, the hard way, what you can and can't say in two hundred fifty words. You cannot summarise a plot in that space: you can only hint, at an atmosphere, at an analogy (Amis-territory, Murdochian moral intricacy, Sparkian wit and *bizarrerie,* Storey-north, Snow-corridors). However often they may tell you you should not use adjectives, here you have no choice; adjectives must substitute for discrimination and for narrative: *shocking, flat, murky, torpid, energetic, ferocious, intricate, gripping.* Clichés have become clichés because they are concise, useful and evocative (more adjectives) but Frederica has her standards. She eschews both *vivid* and *vibrant,* both *brilliant, hilarious, maxi* and *mini.* From feeling like an ugly sister clamping a bleeding foot into a glass slipper, she has come to enjoy picking her way precisely through the possibilities. She plays fair. Any really waspish sentence must be balanced by one purely descriptive. Every week two or three novelists write in with at least a thousand indignant words pointing out what she has *not* said. The column makes a substantial addition to her income, more through the sale of suitcases of rejected books than for the words themselves. For every book she reviews, she reads and sells perhaps twenty. She knows a great deal about how not to write a novel.

On the other side of her desk is a heap of books for the novel class. She is constructing a lecture on love and marriage in *Howards End* and *Women in Love.* She has written:

"Margaret Schlegel's credo is 'only connect' but she has to admit failure. Rupert Birkin spends most of *Women in Love* vilifying 'connection' and expressing intemperate suspicion of and antagonism to the word 'love.' But he ends in a mystical vision of oneness and connectedness, beyond language.

"Both writers, both novels, assert an antagonism between 'the machine age' and human passion. Both, in this sense, are pastoral, implying that love was fuller, or easier, or more natural in some primitive, Edenic past, before 'society' became complex, or work mechanised.

"Why?"

She thinks she might abandon her empty page for the lecture, but knows she ought not. This thing must be written. "Just write down everything you think relevant, every example of behaviour you object to, find unacceptable," said Arnold Begbie. "And then I'll formalise it. I'll write it up."

She feels nauseous. She has made three or four attempts. She has written:

> He hit me.
>
> My husband hit me.
>
> Nigel hit me.

This last heavily crossed out.

> He struck me with the side of his hand, intending to hurt.
>
> He is trained to hurt.
>
> He pointed this out.

She has changed the word "struck" to the word "hit." She has a vague idea that this piece of writing should be bare, unemotive, scrupulously neutral, whatever that might mean. "Struck" carries a stronger emotional charge.

> When I locked myself in the lavatory, he turned off the house electricity, to leave me in the dark.

Does this act, which was indeed frightening and humiliating, class as cruelty, or as petty comedy?

> I was frightened. Afraid. Alarmed.

All crossed out.

> When I tried to run away, he threw an axe after me.
> He has had military training. He meant to hit me.

Is Frederica's opinion on this evidence or not evidence? Is it even her opinion? She remembers the smell of the soil in the night, the wriggling horizon, a sound of rushing wings, which was probably only in her head. She does not remember the impact of the blow. She remembers the later seeping and oozing of the wound, the changing colours of the bruising.

> Nigel's horrified face.
> He is not a monster.

The wound hurts her memory less than the refusal, both angry and bland—and how can one man be both at once?—to allow her to *work*. Than the assumption that it was a question of allowing. Though it was. She does not think either Mr. Begbie or the Divorce Court will be interested in these reflections. She writes:

> He steadfastly refused to allow me to discuss my undertaking any work of any kind, though I married on the assumption that I would do so. He claimed to admire my intelligence and independence.

Claimed to? Did he? What do those words *mean*?

> He shut my father's head in a door.
> He attacked my brother-in-law, who is a clergyman.

The document is nauseating because it is the skeleton of a document that could truly plead, that could make its reader weep for pity and laugh grimly at human folly.

The document is nauseating because it is a lie. It recounts true facts, for a valid purpose—to get Frederica out of a marriage that has become a trap—but it recounts these things one-sidedly, in inappropriate (inappropriate? lying? inadequate?) language.

It was really my fault, because he whole-heartedly wanted to marry me, he was *sure,* however foolish this turned out to be, and I did not, I always held back, I always knew I should not have done it.

I married because I was a woman, to get it over with, to stop thinking about whether to marry or not, or what, to know where I was. And then I didn't like where I was, which I should have known if I had had any sense, so it is *all my fault.* I can't write that, for every reason.

We might have worked something out, all the same, if . . .

He was never at home.

What sort of whingeing complaint is that?

I was locked up with his womenfolk, like Mariana in the Moated Grange, but worse.

I can't write this *stuff.* Every ink-blob destroys a bit more of the truthful balanced memory I am trying to hang on to, of a sort of unspoken justice, of a kind of saving not-looking-but-knowing about the whole knotty mess of the experience.

She writes: "Shit." "Fuck." She crosses them out.

I could write it if it was a parody of this sort of document, a work of art or fiction *pretending to be* one of these.

I married him because I was beglamoured by Margaret Schlegel, because I was a reader, dear Reader.

I married him because my sister was dead and he comforted me.

This piece of paper is not about why I married him. It is about what he did, those actions of his, that offer me a way out of the decision I took.

I write things so that someone can sit in judgement on him, and I sit in judgement on myself, the one entails the other; they are both, I was going to say intolerable, but what I mean is, very nasty.

She turns to her lecture. She will work a little on that, and then take another run at the dreadful catalogue.

Howards End, Ch. 22

Margaret greeted her lord with peculiar tenderness on the morrow. Mature as he was, she might yet be able to help him to the building of the rainbow bridge that should connect the prose in us with the passion. Without it we are meaningless fragments, half monks, half beasts, unconnected arches that have never joined into a man. With it love is born, and alights on the highest curve, glowing against the grey, sober against the fire. Happy the man who sees from either aspect the glory of these outspread wings. The roads of his soul lie clear, and he and his friends shall find easy going.

It was hard going in the roads of Mr. Wilcox's soul. From boyhood he had neglected them. "I am not a fellow who bothers about my own inside." Outwardly he was cheerful, reliable and brave; but within, all had reverted to chaos, ruled, as far as it was ruled at all, by an incomplete asceticism. Whether as boy, husband or widower, he had always the sneaking belief that bodily passion is bad, a belief that is desirable only when held passionately. Religion had confirmed him. The words that were read aloud on Sunday to him and to other respectable men were the words that had once kindled the souls of St. Catherine and St. Francis into a white-hot hatred of the carnal. He could not be as the saints and love the Infinite with a seraphic ardour, but he could be a little ashamed of loving a wife. "Amabat; amare timebat." And it was here that Margaret hoped to help him.

It did not seem so difficult. She need trouble him with no gift of her own. She would only point out the salvation that was latent in his own soul, and in the soul of every man. Only connect! That was the whole of her sermon. Only connect the prose and the passion and both will be exalted, and human love will be seen to be at its height. Live in fragments no longer. Only connect, and the beast and the monk, robbed of the isolation that is life to either, will die. . . .

But she failed. For there was one quality in Henry for which she was never prepared, however much she reminded herself of it: his obtuseness. He simply did not notice things, and there was no more to be said.

Women in Love, Ch. 13

"What I want is a strange conjunction with you—" he said quietly; "—not meeting and mingling;—you are quite right:—but an equilibrium, a pure balance of two single beings:—as the stars balance each other."

She looked at him. He was very earnest, and earnestness was always rather ridiculous, commonplace, to her. It made her feel unfree and uncomfortable. But why drag in the stars.

Ch. 27

This marriage with her was his resurrection and his life.

All this she could not know. She wanted to be made much of, to be adored. There were infinite distances of silence between them. How could he tell her of the immanence of her beauty, that was not form, or weight, or colour, but something like a strange golden light! How could he know himself what her beauty lay in, for him. He said "Your nose is beautiful, your chin is adorable." But it sounded like lies, and she was disappointed, hurt. Even when he said, whispering with truth, "I love you, I love you," it was not the real truth. It was something beyond love, such a gladness of having surpassed oneself, of having transcended the old existence. How could he say "I" when he was something new and unknown, not himself at all? This I, this old formula of the age, was a dead letter.

In the new, superfine bliss, a peace superseding knowledge, there was no I and you, there was only the third, unrealised wonder, the wonder of existing not as oneself, but in a consummation of my being and her being in a new one, a new paradisal unit regained from the duality. Nor can I say "I love you" when I have ceased to be, and you have ceased to be: we are both caught up and transcended into a new oneness where everything is silent, because there is nothing to answer, all is perfect and at one. Speech travels between the separate parts. But in the perfect One there is perfect silence of bliss.

They were married by law on the next day, and she did as he bade her, she wrote to her mother and father.

Frederica thinks hard about these passages. There are complicated connections between literature and life. She may have chosen to lecture on love and marriage in Forster and Lawrence because she is snarled in the death of marriage and the end of love: but the marriage was partly a product of the power of these books. Part of Nigel's attraction was Forster's incantation "Only connect." He had Mr. Wilcox's attraction of otherness, but was not, is not, obtuse.

Both characters, both novelists, so passionately desire *connection*. They want to experience an undifferentiated All, a Oneness, body and mind, self and world, male and female. Frederica has tried to want this. Exhortations to want it have permeated her reading. When she was very little she tried to believe in God. She looked at the stars and tried to *think* Someone intelligent, loving, caring, out there, and could not. Forcing herself hurt her head behind her eyes: she remembers the sensation precisely, and it is repeated as she remembers it, and as she tries to desire connection and Oneness. Thinking of her own infantile efforts to believe causes her to think again about something she has noticed in both pieces of writing. They are sustained by what were surely archaisms in their own time, phrases harking back, yearning, for earlier modes of expression.

"Her lord" . . . "the morrow" . . . "Happy the man who sees the glory of those outspread wings." . . . "Only connect the prose and the passion and both will be exalted."

"This marriage was his resurrection and his life." . . . "In the perfect One there is perfect silence of bliss."

And "she did as he bade her," Lawrence's wife echoing the ironic "her lord" of Forster's Margaret, archaic both.

Forster was uneasily mocking, whereas Lawrence was in deadly earnest, thinks Frederica, but both are *imbued* with religious language. Ursula's beauty is "immanent" like a strange golden light. Forster makes love incarnate "the salvation that was latent in his own soul," connecting beast and monk. Sexual love for Lawrence confuses and abolishes grammatical categories, no I and you, no subject and object, but "my" and "her" in a paradisal One "where everything is silent," where language is unnecessary and defeated, thinks Frederica.

She writes:

It is not so simple as supposing that sexual love replaced for the Moderns the mystical experience of the Christian religion. It is more that the narrative of the Novel, in its high days, was built on, out of, and in opposition to the narrative of the one Book, the source of all Books, the Bible. Both Forster and Lawrence use for the joining of lovers the old biblical symbol of God's covenant between Heaven and Earth, the rainbow, even though Forster's rainbow is also a simulacrum of the rainbow bridge built by Wagner's all-too-human deities between earth and Walhalla.

Why bring in the stars? Ursula asks. D. H. Lawrence said the novel is the one bright book of Life. In the one bright book you have to have it all, the Word made flesh, the rainbow, the stars, the One.

Why, thinks Frederica, does it seem so impossible, so far away, so *finished,* this Oneness, Love, the Novel?

Those archaisms were a way of containing and continuing—*just*—the past of the monks, the mystics, the preachers. Now, it can't be done.

Or perhaps, it's only me who can't do it.

. . .

Frederica looks at her markings on her dreadful catalogue of Nigel's sins, or offences, her partial, her lying, summing up of her own story, and asks herself what she thinks about love.

Does the word mean anything?

Did I love Nigel?

He taught me desire.

That destroyed something in me: a separateness that was a strength.

But I did want to *know.*

To know, yes, but not to be *fused* with someone else. The idea is, and was, a little sickening. I am a separate being.

Before Nigel, the men I loved were Alexander and Raphael. They were like unfinished rainbows, they were like Birkin's stars in the sky, they were beautiful and untouchable, and I *liked them that way,* I could put energy into trying to change them, to make them desiring and desirable, but they weren't *for that.* They were what I loved, as paintings are shining. They were the same as each other.

Stephanie and Daniel were part of each other, I think. She knew. He knew. I have had my moments, lately, of desiring Daniel, of imagining his touch, because he knows what it is about.

I don't. I betrayed Nigel because I can't do it.

I recognise John Ottokar. He is *charged,* the way Nigel was, and unknown, in an interesting way.

We could hurt each other. I know that. I am older now.

She thinks: If I don't want Oneness, what is it I want?

She remembers a day, long ago, on the Goathland moors, when a word hit her as a description of a possible way of survival. Laminations. She had been young, and greedy, and acting Princess Elizabeth, the Virgin in Alexander's play, who had had the wit to stay separate, to declare, "I will not bleed," to hang on to her autonomy. And she, Frederica, had had a vision of being able to be all the things she was: language, sex, friendship, thought, just as long as these were kept scrupulously separate, *laminated,* like geological strata, not seeping and flowing into each other like organic cells boiling to join and divide and join in a seething Oneness. Things were best cool, and clear, and fragmented, if fragmented was what they were.

"Only connect," the "new paradisal unit" of "Oneness," these were myths of desire, the desire and pursuit of the Whole.

And if one accepts fragments, layers, tesserae of mosaic, particles.

There is an art form in that, too. Things juxtaposed but divided, not yearning for fusion.

What is really fused is the sperm and the ovum in the zygote, Frederica thought with a certain intellectual rigour. Not man and woman, but cells. Language fails man and woman trying to transcend it and themselves. But the genes go coiling, spiralling, joining, building sentences and phrases of life with their primeval alphabet. Two halves become One.

She remembers her son, who has been suspiciously silent during all this thinking and writing and failing to write. And all the thinking is undone. For it is clear what love is. This flesh which is and is not her own, which was and is not part of her, which completes the circle of the arms.

"Leo. *Where the hell are you?* Leo! Leo! *Where are you?*"

Frederica never invades Agatha Mond's space, but Leo does. Less often, Saskia Mond comes down to play with Leo, to eat supper when her mother is out. So now Frederica goes upstairs, in search of her son. There is no sound of movement, no shrill voices. She turns a corner, and hears Agatha's voice, quiet and dramatic.

" 'It's a house on fire.'

" 'There aren't any houses in this wilderness.'

" 'It's a camp-fire. Soldiers perhaps. Looking for us, perhaps.'

" 'We should hide.'

" 'No, it's a bush, on fire. It's a great thorn bush, burning all by itself on the moor.'

" 'Let's look,' said Mark, who was always impetuous. 'Who could have set a bush on fire?'

" 'Lightning, maybe,' said Dol Throstle.

" 'We should go and see,' said Artegall.

"So the four of them walked over to the burning bush, which could be heard crackling and smelled singeing from a great distance. When they came near it the air was visibly shivering in the heat, and full of flying black specks of burned matter. There was no sign of any human presence, no footprints, no broken stems.

" 'Just a bush, burning,' said Claus.

" 'All the nests,' said Dol Throstle. 'All the young birds will be burned.'

" 'They may well be flown,' said Artegall. 'It is late in the year for them to be still in the nest.'

"He remembered his huge leather books, with page after page of drawings of eggs, speckled and mottled, of nestlings and fledglings, of plumage and claws.

" 'There's something moving in there,' said Dol Throstle.

"The four travellers peered into the smoke. Deep in the heart of the burning bush something stirred and writhed in the heat.

" 'It's a bird burned naked,' said Claus. 'A very big bird.'

" 'It's not a bird,' said Dol Throstle. 'I can see its beaky mouth. It's got teeth.'

" 'It's a snake, a nasty snake,' said Mark.

" 'We must rescue it,' said Artegall.

" 'It's just a nasty snake,' said Mark. 'And badly burned I should think. Better leave it. Rescued snakes always bite you. I read stories too.'

"The two boys, prince and page, glared at each other with brief anger. Then Artegall drew his sword and moved towards the bush. The heat flared in his face: he could smell his own hair burning. He cut away a few branches, in order to get nearer. He was afraid of trying to hook the snake: a sword was not the best implement for that purpose, and if he pushed wrongly the snake might fall from the branch it was on, into the roaring bonfire beneath it. Wrapping his cloak about his face, Artegall pushed nearer to the bush, and pushed his sword under the whole body of the snake, which, to his surprise, seemed to have strength and intelligence enough to coil and cling to the blade.

" 'You've skewered it,' said Mark.

" 'Hold on!' said Artegall to the snake.

"He withdrew the sword and its burden, steel and sinuous flesh, carefully through the flames and smoke. His own hand was scorched, and his sleeve black.

" 'It's *roasted*,' said Mark.

"The snake was very large, and mostly blackish in colour, with a weaving pattern of gold spirals and coins visible under the smoke. Its belly was pale golden, and it had horned eyebrows above a diamond-shaped head. It lay limp for a little time, like a piece of rope, and then a ripple of life ran along its body and it coiled itself, painfully it appeared, raised its head, and opened two great eyes like carbuncles, fiery and burning with inner light."

. . .

"What's a carbuncle?" says Leo.

"A big red jewel," says Agatha. "A big fiery-red jewel. Sometimes also a painful bump on your skin, which can also be red and shiny."

"I don't like snakes," says Saskia.

"You don't know any," says Agatha. "But most people don't." She is sitting on the sofa, with Leo on one side and Saskia on the other. Frederica sits down on the floor.

"Go on," she says.

"And then the snake spoke. It spoke with a kind of hissing, sibilant voice, a voice like leaves rustling, and silk being pulled swiftly through a ring or a buckle, a voice dry and yet sharp and swift. It said, 'I am the Horned Viper, the King of the snakes in this country, and I was thrown into that bush by an angry soldier who set it on fire. I have it in my power to make you able to hear the speech of the creatures that have speech: the birds, and the running and creeping things with legs, and the flying things, and the things that tunnel and burrow. But only you can hear, because only you held out your hand through the flames.'

" 'I didn't believe the creatures talked,' said Artegall. 'I have read it, of course—'

" 'It wasn't exactly talk, in the beginning. Once, we were all one thing, and could hear each other's nature well enough if we *listened,* with no need for speech. And then men made words, and used words for mastery, and we also spoke out what once we had heard and known in our heads, and understood. There have always been a few Men who can hear, or remember in their blood, the old speech—'

" 'And will everything speak to me?' said Artegall.

" 'Why are you talking to it?' said Mark. 'It can't answer.'

" 'No, of course not,' said the snake. 'Most things won't want to go anywhere near you, and most will pretend to be dumb, even if you challenge them. We do not love you. But you may *overhear* things that are useful, even in the gossip of woodlice or the chatter of starlings.'

" 'I should go mad,' whispered Artegall to the King Snake, 'if I could hear everything's voice all the time.'

" 'Well you won't hear it, unless you *listen,*' said the snake. 'And then only if you are patient and persistent. Now I shall go.' And suddenly, like the crack of a whip, he was away, across the heather, and pouring himself into a crack between two great granite boulders.

" 'Did it speak to you?' said Dol Throstle.

" 'I thought so,' said Artegall.

" 'I've heard of that,' said Dol Throstle. 'I couldn't hear it.'

" 'I don't believe it said *anything,*' said Mark."

"Mark is very silly," says Leo.

"No, he's not," says Agatha. "You'll see. He's just a bit cross, at the moment, because he was only a page and a whipping-boy before they escaped, and after the escape he thought that Artegall would be helpless and useless because he'd never come out of his tower. . . . But he'll change. People change."

"Good," says Saskia. "I don't like people who are always cross."

"What are you telling them?" says Frederica to Agatha.

"It's my story," says Saskia.

"I can hear it too," says Leo. "It's all right, Agatha says I can hear."

"You're very welcome," says Agatha.

During the next weeks, Frederica joins the others at the story-telling sessions. She gets a *frisson* of ancient pleasure from watching Leo and Saskia lost in another world; from time to time she is lost herself, for the story is intricate, and Agatha tells it with conviction, inhabits it herself. It is the tale of a prince, Artegall, who wakes one morning in the sunlit tower overlooking a harbour, and finds that everyone has gone. He has spent his whole life in this tower, because his country is at war with neighbouring powers; the town is empty because an enemy fleet has landed. Artegall is rescued by a cook's maid, Dol Throstle, a palace guard, Claus, and his page and whipping-boy, Mark, with whom he has practised soldierly arts, fencing, wrestling, archery. The four escape in a wagon, in disguise, and undertake a journey north, in search of Artegall's dangerous uncle, Ragna, who is neither friend nor enemy. They are pursued by various forces. Artegall is believed by everyone to be useless and simply a parcel, but turns out, despite his incarceration, to be a skilled tracker of game and finder of paths, simply because a princely education has included endless large leather books on venery, woodcraft, geography, navigation and so on. Mark, the page, assumes that he will now assert the superiority denied him by Artegall's position, but Artegall proves "I am *someone,* not just a prince." As they go north, Agatha tells Frederica, the landscape becomes alive: creatures are met that are magical, or from other worlds, and speak other languages.

She says, "I wrote it for bookish children. Like myself, like you. For children despised because they read. To say, you can *learn to live* from books. Not didactically. But the obvious thing would have been to make Mark, the ordinary boy, triumphant. Whereas I think princes and princesses are what we all are in our minds—to be a prince *is* to be ordinary in a fairytale—"

"Isn't it too old for Leo and Saskia?"

"Would it have been too old for you?"

"No. I'd have loved it. I'd have devoured it."

"Well, then. They listen. They ask about the words. I don't know what some of the teachers on our committee would say."

Frederica tells Agatha about her difficulties with the dreadful catalogue. She has been writing a quite different kind of fantasy tale, she tells Agatha, grimacing. Agatha looks darkly composed, and says it must be most disagreeable. She listens, she is sympathetic, but she offers no confidences in return. Frederica wonders from time to time who is Saskia's father. Agatha has visitors: married couples, single friends from Oxford days, male and female, members of the committee, Civil Servants. She cooks elegant little dinners, to which Frederica is sometimes invited. These are the great days of the marathon home-cooked meal, the five-course delicious gourmandising, *pâtés* and prawns in cream, delicate soups and imaginative *hors d'oeuvres,* followed by *estouffades* and *boeuf en croûte,* by *gigot* and ducklings in cider, by stuffed carp and *paupiettes* of sole, followed by delicious salads of endive and oranges, watercress and cucumber, followed by home-made tarts and soufflés, followed by a rich cheese board and possibly devils on horseback. Agatha serves, always, an avocado salad, a roast chicken with garlic, a tart from a French pâtisserie. Three courses, one cooked. The conversation is civilised and quiet. Agatha appears to have no attachments. Frederica notices at one of these dinners that Alexander is interested in Agatha. She notices the warmth with which he looks forward to a Bristol school visit on which he will go with Agatha, whilst Frederica takes care of Saskia and Leo. She thinks: They could do well together. She wonders what she means by this, and decides that she supposes they both have no need of violence. She thinks of Alexander sharing a house with Agatha, quiet and civilised, never quarrelling, never, she supposes, trembling with passion of any kind. She thinks, she does not know Agatha well enough to make any such supposition about her, however well she knows Alexander, by now. Agatha does not want to be known, and some people, Frederica can see, find this quality rebarbative, call her, in their own minds, cold. She is composed, Frederica thinks. She does everything carefully, just so.

She *likes* to live in that story.

But she's not retreating into her childhood, she's grown up. She seems to me much more grown up than I imagine I seem to her.

Frederica feels safe, telling things to Agatha. She trusts her completely, not to gossip, and also not to distort or *seethe* what she's told, in her mind. Because Agatha never reciprocates with confidences, Frederica only tells her things in a slightly ironic, impersonal tone, even if they are very personal and hurtful things, such as how to describe having an axe thrown at her, even, what to say about discovering you have a sexually transmitted disease. Agatha listens, and makes one or two precise remarks about the etymology of "venereal." You can confuse Venus the hot and hurtful with the vernal airs of spring, she says. They seem to go together because of Botticelli's Venus landing in Paphos covered with flowers. But really it isn't that. You must just find some exact words.

"I could leave it out," says Frederica.

"You could," says Agatha. "But it might be very important, as proof of something. What matters is what's evidence. That is."

"It's just the life of some bacteria, really. I feel it's a sort of violation, but really it isn't, really I *don't care* what he did when I wasn't there."

"You might, if you cared more altogether."

"I don't think I care about anything," says Frederica. "Except Leo."

"I expect you will," says Agatha.

Frederica looks at Agatha's neatly drawn face, its clear, elegant proportions. She wants to ask What do you care about? And dare not.

XI

Arnold Begbie has converted Frederica's pitiful narrative into a Petition for Divorce.

In the High Court of Justice
Probate, Divorce and Admiralty Division
(Divorce)
To the High Court of Justice
Dated the 1st of April 1965

The petition of Frederica Reiver showeth:—

(1) That on October 19th 1959 the petitioner, Frederica Reiver, then Frederica Potter, was lawfully married to Nigel Reiver (hereinafter called "the respondent") at the Parish Church, Spessendborough, in the County of Herefordshire.

(2) That after the said marriage the petitioner and the respondent lived and cohabited at divers addresses and finally at Bran House, Longbarrow, in the County of Herefordshire.

(3) That there is one child of the petitioner and the respondent now living, namely Leo Alexander, born on the 14th of July 1960.

(4) That the petitioner proposes the following arrangements for support, care and upbringing of the said Leo Alexander. He will live with the petitioner at 42 Hamelin Square, London SE11, a house shared with Miss Agatha Mond and her daughter, Saskia Felicity Mond. He will start school in September at the William Blake Primary School, Lebanon Grove, London SE11, in company with the said Saskia Felicity Mond; the petitioner intends to apply for maintenance as hereinafter set out.

(5) That since the celebration of the said marriage the respondent has treated the petitioner with cruelty.

(6) That the respondent, who is a man of violent temper, has frequently nagged, sworn at, shouted at and struck the petitioner.

(7) That on September 28th 1964 the respondent attacked the petitioner with several blows to the head, ribs and back; that when she sought refuge in the bathroom, he turned off the mains-electricity to the house, in order to frighten her, and kept her imprisoned therein for several hours.

(8) That on Sunday 4th October 1964 the respondent again attacked the petitioner in her bedroom, so that she ran out of the house in fear and hid in the stables. That when she came out of hiding, the respondent was waiting with an axe, with which he threatened her; that when she ran out into the fields he pursued her, abusing her verbally, and threw the axe, wounding her in the hip.

(9) That before the specific acts of cruelty set out above the respondent treated the petitioner with neglect, spending most of his time away from home, in the company of business friends, beyond the reasonable requirements of the pursuit of his business. That he insisted that the petitioner and child remain at all times in Bran House. That he treated visiting friends of the petitioner with rudeness, and unreasonably refused ever to entertain them or to allow his wife to see them.

(10) That there is reason to believe that the respondent has committed adultery, since the petitioner was diagnosed in November 1964 as having contracted a venereal disease. The petitioner has sworn an affidavit that the disease could have been communicated by no one but the respondent.

(11) That the petitioner discovered a large collection of lewd and filthy publications in the respondent's wardrobe.

(12) That the petitioner has not in any way been accessory to or connived at or condoned the adultery hereinbefore alleged and that she has not condoned the cruelty hereinbefore alleged.

(13) That this petition is not presented or prosecuted in collusion with the respondent.

Frederica considers this document: another narrative of her marriage. She says, "He won't like this."

Begbie smiles. "He cannot be expected to like it."

Frederica tries to cast an analytic look over it.

"You haven't written that he stopped me from *working.*"

"I didn't think it was wise."

"In fact that was the most cruel thing." Frederica's tone is small and dry. "It stopped me from being *myself.*"

"Marriage is expected to have that effect," says Begbie.

"And you have written that I am asking for maintenance. I don't want it. I can work. I want to keep myself."

"You are asking for custody of your son. And for care and control of him. The Court is not necessarily going to look favourably on you as a parent if you put too much stress on your desire to work, if you display too much personal ambition."

"If I were a man—"

"You have a good chance of custody because you are a woman. Women are presumed to wish to stay at home and care for children. Your sex is your principal advantage, if I may put it so. Your husband, as you have described him, has all the other advantages, in the Court's eyes—a beautiful home, several other devoted women who know the boy intimately, the capacity to pay fees at a good boarding school. You will not appear in a good light if you put your own pride before your son's comfort. And if your husband has treated you as cruelly as you claim he has, you must surely wish him to pay you the support to which you are entitled."

"It isn't like that. *I don't* want his money. I don't want a quarrel and a battle. I want Leo, and to be myself, and to work."

"In the adversarial system, both of the British law, and of the marriage relation, I fear a battle is what you must be resigned to. May I ask if your husband has ever been violent towards his son?"

"No. Not really. It counts as violence to Leo to hurt me, I think. It hurts Leo. But no."

"Only towards yourself?"

"Everyone else worships him. Yes, only towards me."

"A pity. A pity." He sits back in his chair, contemplating the disadvantages of Nigel Reiver's lack of cruelty towards his son.

He explains to Frederica that the petition will be served by post; that it will be filed in the Divorce Registry, and that the respondent must enter an appearance in the Divorce Registry if he intends either to contest the divorce, or to cross-petition. If he does not intend to defend the divorce, he must return an acknowledgement to the petitioner's solicitor. He asks Frederica what she thinks her husband will do.

Frederica tries to think. She imagines Nigel's dark face, looking down on the foolscap pages. The blows, the axe, the lewd and filthy pictures. She imagines rage. Nigel's face becomes that of a blue-black demon. She crosses her own arms defensively across her breasts.

"He won't let it pass. He'll fight, and he'll want Leo."

"Then we will fight. We will fight resourcefully. We shall need witnesses to the acts of cruelty—a Court does not always accept the unsupported evidence of an aggrieved spouse. Doctors, family, friends who saw the injuries? It would be a great advantage to be able to prove adultery, which we should be able to do if your account of your—infection—is accurate (and again supported by medical evidence). Are you sure you have no idea where your husband went on his journeys, whom he saw, what he did?"

"I didn't ask. I didn't mind, much. What I wanted was a life of my own. He went around with Pijnakker and Shah, doing business with his shipping, I think. They belonged to a lot of clubs in London, where I certainly wouldn't want to go. There was one called the Honeypot, I remember. And one called Tips and Tassels. I saw a brochure for that once. Oriental waitresses in belly-dancing silk trousers and bras. With tassels. I think Shah had a financial interest in that, I think I heard them saying."

"I know those places," says Begbie, with a note of satisfaction. Frederica watches him sharply. "I know who goes to those places," says Begbie, looking at Frederica. Frederica says nothing. "High-class call girls and tarts," says Begbie. Frederica thinks that she knows this, and has not thought about it, because it was nothing to do with her. She wonders what she meant by "nothing to do with her." She means that she has no proprietary interest in Nigel's body, she thinks to herself in legal words in the lawyer's office. She wants *her own life.* She would not, in theory, mind if he had his, if hers were not house and confinement. Is this so? She remembers her shamed disgust over the filthy pictures. She did not find them amusing. It is very possible that she would not find the Honeypot, or Tips and Tassels, amusing if she were there. Arnold Begbie appears to be hearing her thoughts.

"Evidence of filthy literature in the respondent's possession is admissible as evidence for adultery to be inferred," he says. "If a woman visits a brothel, that is taken as conclusive proof of her adultery. In the case of a man, such a visit provides strong evidence of adultery against him, but is not conclusive."

"Interesting," says Frederica, drily.

She has the impression that Begbie is taking some sort of pleasure in her general discomfiture, which for him is somehow to do with the imagination of the actions of human bodies, and for her is to do with the discrepancy between what caused her pain and what must be adduced as evidence in order legally to end it. If I had cared more about the Honeypot and so on, she thinks, I might not now be here, because I might have cared more *altogether,* and then things would have come out differently.

"If the divorce is defended," says Begbie, "we need to consider the bars to dissolution of marriage. You must consider: denial of the charge, connivance, condonation and collusion. Your attitude to your husband's extra-marital activities could well be taken as condonation, if you are not careful. Then there are the discretionary bars. The ones you must consider here are the petitioner's own adultery or cruelty. Any adultery of your own—I am required by law to put to you—should be recorded in a sealed discretion statement, which will go before the Court."

"I haven't," says Frederica. "I haven't—committed—"

"Both the other side and the Court are likely to wonder whether your relationship with Mr. Thomas Poole was entirely . . ."

"Well, it was. It was for convenience. He had children, and a flat, and a job. We shared baby-sitting. He was a friend and colleague of—*of my father's,*" says Frederica, avoiding Alexander, genuinely indignant.

"Good, good. And now you live with another woman. Good. Are you sure there is no one else? If the other side decide to contest the divorce they will seek to know . . ."

"No."

"And your friends, to whom your husband objected. Were they men, or women friends?"

"Men."

"But he had no cause to be jealous or suspicious?"

"None. They were *my friends.*"

"And always were?"

"Not always, not all. I—slept with some men, at Cambridge."

"Of course. Pre-nuptial incontinence does not come into the domain of public morals. But it may lead to a presumption that you had no objections to sleeping with more than one man: it might lead to questioning about your subsequent conduct."

"I haven't slept with anyone else," says Frederica. It is curious that although this is true, she feels that she is lying and will be found out. This is possibly because Begbie, who is *her* solicitor, is disinclined to believe her. Again, he reads her thoughts.

"Lawyers are temperamentally inclined to question people's statements," he says. "Of course I accept that you have been faithful to your husband."

"It isn't a question of 'being faithful,' " says Frederica. "I'm not sure I know what 'faithful' means. But I haven't slept with anyone else."

"Very good."

Frederica still has the feeling that her solicitor dislikes her. There is something she is not doing or saying that she should be doing or saying. Weeping, perhaps? Lately, any emotion has driven her to dryness. When she was younger, she could scream and weep. But now, she needs to hold herself together. She needs to be competent. And yet she feels that Arnold Begbie does not entirely approve of her dryness and competence.

Out in the square, she sees the same women and children playing on the grass inside the iron railings with their locked gates. They have shocking-pink knitted hats, warm coats, and near-naked legs and thighs. They pursue a shiny pink-and-blue plastic ball into the bushes. The children laugh and hurtle: the women, in their childish garments, admonish them to "be careful." Frederica sees herself as a caged or netted beast. She sees something limp and snarling in a barred cage on wheels, in a hunter's net suspended from a bough. The net is not made by Nigel, who ran after her, panting, in hot blood; and hurled an axe at her, letting her own blood out of her haunch. The net is made by words which do not describe what she feels is happening: *adultery, connivance, pre-nuptial incontinence, petitioner, respondent.* She tries to think out these words. *Adultery* has connotations of impurity (adulterated butter, adulterated white flour) or perhaps of theft? *Incontinence* somehow equates sexual pleasure with lack of muscular control of bowels or bladder: The proper use of the sphincter is to contain, thinks Frederica. These legal words carry with them the whole history of a society in which a woman was a man's property, and also a part of his flesh, not to be contaminated. And behind *continence* and *incontinence* is the alien, ancient, and powerful history of Christian morals. In Cambridge sex was freedom, was individuality, was a gleeful assertion of self-determination, of energy, of choice, however accompanied by an undercurrent of biological terror. We were all cheerfully in revolt, in those days, thinks Frederica, against convention, against bourgeois prudery and caution, against *our parents* essentially, whom for that purpose, the purpose of necessary revolt, we identified with prudery, coldness, respectability. This language is something quite different from prudery and respectability. It is the harsh language of "the domain of public morals." It judges me as a member of society, even whilst offering me a way out of the mess I have got myself into by *joining* society, by getting casually married, because it solved the problem of whether to get married.

This is the day of the extra-mural class at Our Lady of the Sorrows. Frederica goes back to Hamelin Square, where Leo is having tea with Saskia and the surrogate grandmother, Mrs. Alma Birdseye. Agatha too comes in during this meal. The evening darkens; a gang of children scrabble briefly at the basement window and run away; Agatha and Frederica draw the curtains and let down the blinds, making a softly lit warm space inside. Agatha reads from her story. The travellers have been led into a deep thicket by a muddy imp called Yallery Brown, and it is beginning to snow, great slushy flakes which put out their fire, leaving them in the dark, the *real dark,* with a thick blanket of wet cloud between them and the moon and the stars. Artegall hears the speech of shrews and rats in the undergrowth, and of owls staring and listening from thorny branches. He hears the voice of slow worms, beneath the wet leaves, beneath the humus, beneath the earth. The shrews and rats listen for the worms, the owls listen for the shrews and rats, the children in the warm room listen and shiver and imagine the fear of the dark. The creatures speak of hunger, and imagine food. The owls do not like the smell of the humans. Suddenly Dol Throstle sees the glimmer of a cold light, far away in a tangle of brambles and bent thorn-branches . . .

"Go *on,*" says Leo.

"I can't," says Agatha. "There isn't any more, I haven't written any more."

"But you know it," says Leo.

"Not exactly," says Agatha. "Anything could happen."

"Why is the dark?" says Saskia.

"Because we are on the earth, which rolls round and round and at the same time makes great circles round the sun, so that when it is dark we are on the side facing away from the hot sun, which is a great fiery ball—"

"Why?" says Saskia.

"I don't know," says Agatha.

"I'm not afraid of the dark," says Leo, resting his red head on Frederica's knee.

Frederica is afraid. She is afraid of the thicket she is in, of what might happen, of losing Leo, of hurting Leo. These things are in the domain of public morals, now. Someone, somewhere, will judge her. She holds on to Leo.

She arrives at Our Lady of the Sorrows clutching her lecture on Love and Marriage in Forster and Lawrence. She is consoled by the journey on the Underground. There are so many people, so many faces, so many possible lives going on. People who are real, despite the prevalent fashion for looking like round-eyed pale-faced dolls with shining mouths. People with bald crowns and beehive hair, with flowing locks and bristling fans of curls, with Beatle caps and plastic rainhats, semi-circles of transparent plastic, spotted and dotted with crimson and emerald, purple and orange discs, tied with ribbons over grey curls under folding chins. She is safe and anonymous here, and everyone is *interesting.* This is the glory of London, her present London, which is several small worlds, Daniel's church, Hugh Pink's flat, Rupert Parrott's dusty office, the house in Hamelin Square, the staff room, the great studios of the Samuel Palmer School, Arnold Begbie's office and the extra-mural class.

There is a new whiff, amongst the old cabbage and chalk, on the turning of the stair, a rich, rotten whiff which she recognises without naming it. When she arrives in her classroom, she sees what it was: Jude Mason is sitting isolated in the front row, wearing his filthy blue velvet skirted coat and what appears to be a policeman's cape. His iron-grey locks spread over the shoulders of this garment, oiled and gleaming. The other members of the group are talking to each other, and not looking at him.

"I am a vagrant," he tells Frederica. "Come in literally out of the cold. It is cold in my living place, as I have no cash for the meter. It is cold in the streets. Would it inconvenience you if I took refuge here? The British Library also is closed."

"You are not to interrupt everyone," says Frederica.

"Or disrupt, or corrupt. I will say nothing at all, if you let me sit quietly in this corner and listen to you."

Frederica says to the class, "This is Jude Mason. He works at the Art School. He has written a book which is coming out in a few months."

They nod, peacefully. Frederica takes out her notes, and begins to speak of Lawrence and Forster. She speaks of what they have in common: a desire for some kind of whole life, unified experience, complete presence in or on the earth. A dislike for mechanised life, for cities, for fragmentation and dissolution. She speaks of the lost Paradises that haunt Forster's Sussex and Lawrence's Nottinghamshire, that send the one in search of wych elms with pig's teeth, and the other in search of communities of like souls in hot, sunny, "untouched" places. She tries to connect this with the passionate desires of their intelligent women, Margaret and Helen Schlegel, Ursula and Gudrun Brangwen, for liberty and subjection, for thought and instinct.

She scans the class. One of the art students, in a skinny black jumper, a skinny black mini-skirt, thick black tights and laced granny shoes, said to her last week, "We have to be different, we are art students, we have to dress differently." Her friends, all in black on black on black, all with burgundy lips and pale faces, indicated agreement. They are uniformly different. The extra-mural class is heterogeneous. Rosemary Bell has a scarlet woollen shirt and a grey jacket and trousers. Dorothy Brittain has a billowing smock in Liberty wool, patterned with little red and black eyes on fawn. Humphrey Maggs has a collar and tie (white and navy) neatly inside his blue jumper. Amanda Harvill has a long-sleeved, high-necked cream woollen Courrèges-style tunic, stopping well above the knees. She has several gold bracelets on her thin, tanned wrists. Her eyelids today are shining bluebell-blue spangled with gold dust. Ronald Moxon, the taxi-driver, has a donkey jacket over an Aran sweater; Ibrahim Mustafa wears a Beatle-like collarless jacket, navy piped with green, over not quite harmonious grey flannels; Lina Nussbaum has a turquoise long-haired sweater with a cowl neck, Sister Perpetua is black and veiled, Ghislaine Todd has a bottle-green polo-neck under an embroidered waistcoat, Alice Somerville and Audrey Mortimer wear tweed suits over blouses, Una Winterson wears a rust-coloured corduroy shirt-waist dress, and Godfrey Mortimer and George Murphy wear dark suits. Frederica is interested in how much more interesting she finds the suits than the art students' customary solemn black, and looks for the third suit, which is usually John Ottokar.

He is not wearing a suit. He is wearing a rainbow-coloured sweater, made of knitted triangles of every bright colour: violet, purple, crimson, orange, yellow, grass green, bottle green, sky blue, dark blue. It is a beautiful, expansive, expensive sweater, with navy ribbing holding it together at collar and cuffs and welt. In his suit he always appeared contained, discreet, smooth, a little paradoxical under the weight of his beautiful bright sculpted golden hair. Now, to go with the sweater, the hair appears to be looser and livelier, very slightly dishevelled at the edges. His body is at ease in this brilliant jerkin: his large face smiles amiably at the room; his blue eyes, under his broad brow, meet Frederica's fiercely when her look crosses his. He is in a corner, a bright patch, a surprise.

She remembers he said: I want you.

He smiles at her.

She looks at his field of triangles and at Jude's blue velvet, and thinks of dominos, masks, bright disguises. The art students are dressed as art students. The people here are "ordinary people," that is to say, separate and heterogeneous people, all already in some sense acting a part, the part of a child or a student, on a junior chair behind a desk, listening to Frederica talking about Lawrence and Forster and sex and death and the earth. Who is John Ottokar? A computer programmer, a man in a suit, a man who doesn't speak language, a bright patch of triangles? Who is Jude, under his ostentatious disguise? Who is Ghislaine Todd, so neat, so limitedly flamboyant in her flowered waistcoat—a psychoanalyst who hears people's lives in their total disconnected dullness and their total dreamed coherence; is this person, thinking about Lawrence and Forster and marriage, the same, or another? What is her face like, sitting invisible behind her patient? The same? Which is her "real" face? What is the difference between Humphrey Maggs's speedwell blue and John Ottokar's harlequin triangles? Both are brightly *not* their working uniforms. But the speedwell blue breathes allotments and public libraries, whilst the harlequin is dangerous . . . But it is not "dressed up" as Jude is dressed up. Or, for that matter, as Sister Perpetua is dressed up, with a starched white band across her forehead and folds of black veiling around her face and shoulders.

The discussion is wide-ranging. Frederica thinks that an extramural class is carried on in the lingua franca, the Common Tongue, it is truly extra-mural, outside the enclosures of academies, disciplines, sects, factions. What the class speaks is gossip at one extreme and precise philosophical discrimination at the other, and the thread of the language they have to construct to speak to each other connects both extremes with a web of knots and separations. These grown-up human beings speak wisely and foolishly of other human beings:

Margaret and Ursula, Forster and Lawrence, Birkin and Mr. Wilcox, as though they were (as they are) people they know (and don't know). They know perfectly well, if reminded, that four of these six beings are actually made of words, are capering word-puppets, not flesh and blood. Godfrey Mortimer, when Frederica makes this point, makes the point that as far as the class is concerned, Lawrence and Forster are also made only of words: they cannot be touched or tasted, the evidence for their thoughts is considerably more suspect and partial than the evidence for those of Margaret and Ursula. They can talk, they do talk, of what Margaret and Ursula "really wanted" or "should have done" or "might have become," which Frederica knows to be critically illegitimate and guesses also to be what Lawrence and Forster "might have wanted" their readers to discuss. So we learn to understand. So, to quote Forster and Margaret, we "connect" the prose and the passion, in linguistic and imagining eddies of speculation and comment, understanding and bafflement. The class bring themselves to the text. Amanda Harvill, with a moue and a shudder, opines that the Schlegels are "not real women." Sister Perpetua says that on the contrary, they *are* real women, women driven by beliefs about sex and relationships that form and distort their responses. They are not *sexually intelligent* women, says Sister Perpetua, unlike Ursula Brangwen, who understands the language of the body and how it connects to the language of the mind. It doesn't always, says Jude Mason, in a three-word intervention unusual, for him, in its brevity. Sister Perpetua says she *knows* it doesn't always. (Later, she tells Frederica she told Jude to take a bath, as she thought no one else would. "What did he say?" said Frederica. "He said, 'I like my pungency, it's a form of fastidiousness, I keep the People distant,' " says Sister Perpetua. "So affected, you can do nothing with those people, there are many at the back door of our convent.")

The conversation circles round. George Murphy brings up again the question of the novel and the job. During the earlier discussions of "post-war British fiction" Murphy has sardonically pointed out the limitations of most novelists' knowledge of most people's work. Novels, he says, are obsessed with sex and love and God and food, which is fine by him, most people are obsessed by sex and love and God and food. But most people are also obsessed, says George Murphy, by work, by commodities and machines and property, which they do not regard with the contempt and loathing most novelists lavish on these things, but with fascination, obsession, intelligence. Most people, says George Murphy, have relations with groups of people with whom they work, which are not necessarily obsessed with sex and love, though these things come into it. He is interested in Forster's Mr. Wilcox, who is meant to represent the world of work and money—"along with Leonard Bast," says Sister Perpetua—and is a crude and villainous fool, however Forster tries to make him interesting or mysterious. And look at Birkin and Ursula, says Murphy. What do they do, the moment they fall in love? They give up their jobs and look for a pre-lapsarian pastoral existence. As though, says George Murphy, the human ingenuity behind machines and institutions was all evil and destructive. No novelist can know me, says George Murphy. They don't know what I think about all the time.

"They know what you think about in bed," says Amanda Harvill, who clearly finds Murphy attractive. "No, they don't," says Murphy. "I can have the most luscious bird in my arms and be completely *fired up* and part of my mind will be worrying away about share prices and coffee crops and board politics. And the novelist will get the bird right, perhaps, and not have a clue about all the other pockets."

The discussion moves to the Goat and Compasses. Jude Mason continues to accompany the class. They find a long table against a wall, and occupy all of it. George Murphy sits between Amanda Harvill and Rosemary Bell, the hospital almoner, who is a Marxist, and tends to involve herself in ideological conflict with Ghislaine Todd, the psychoanalyst. On this occasion, Rosemary and Ghislaine are almost in alliance against George and his views on life and work. Both are sympathetic, for quite different reasons, to the desire for wholeness and self-identity Frederica has diagnosed in Birkin, Ursula, Helen and Margaret; both are much more ready to accept Mr. Wilcox's complacent stupidity and Lawrence's beetle-miners' animal degradation as truths. George smiles with irritating superiority and says they are utopian pastoralists, the pair of them. His dark suit is well cut but crumpled a little at the waist and inside the elbows. Amanda Harvill stares at him with faded blue eyes under bright blue starry eyelids. Frederica can see her thin hand, caged in its gold circles, resting on Murphy's knees. Jude's smell rises richly from his trousers and his coat-skirts and the lank locks of his grey hair. He is next to Frederica. Opposite them, leaning back into a dark corner, is John Ottokar in his bright domino.

Frederica says to Jude, "Sister Perpetua had a point."

"My *mana?*" says Jude. "I use the flesh against the flesh. I am undesirable and without desire, a good state."

Frederica shifts in her seat.

"Shall I go further away?"

His smell has elements of bacon and elements of rancid butter, elements of sweat and elements of stale beer, though she has never seen him drink, and he is now sipping a grapefruit juice.

"No. I can put up with you. So I might as well."

He considers Frederica. "*You* are not without desire."

"That's my business."

"Not here. You stand up before us, and we watch you, we scan, we surmise."

"I am without desire, because I have to be," says Frederica. "I am required by law to be without desire until I can get divorced." Her eyes lift and meet those of John Ottokar in his bright plumage. It is like being blinded by a torchbeam. She drops her eyes. Jude shifts in his garments, wafting his air around her. She says to John Ottokar, "I like your jumper. A new departure."

"I couldn't resist the principle of its construction."

"Does it have one?"

"Haven't you worked it out? It's the perfect combination of order and chaos. Every *other* triangle—reaching round and round or up and down—is in the strict order of the spectrum, from violet to dark red. And between the building-blocks of order, everything is random, yellow and orange and pink and green in any order, as they come. I like that. When I worked it out, I liked it. I couldn't afford it, but I bought it."

He does not take his eyes off Frederica.

"Frederica is required by law to be without desire," Jude tells John Ottokar.

"Difficult," says John Ottokar, smiling.

"Likely to provoke the opposite reaction, all things considered," says Jude. "Like most things prescribed and required. We want the opposite."

John Ottokar smiles. Frederica stares into her wineglass, slightly flushed, and remembers *Babbletower.* Jude knows about desire and its quirks. She looks at John Ottokar's triangles and tries to imagine him under them. He must not be desired, and Frederica has always wanted what she cannot have. His skin is taut and his shaved moustache glints gold. His eyes are kind, she thinks, but is not sure. She says, "Do you think about your work all the time, like George?"

"It haunts my dreams. I am writing a programme for oil tankers. I plot their courses round the world and work out the optimal deployment of the fleet. My machine speaks to me. Off the coast of Nigeria, I put in a ship and my machine prints out WHAT SHIP. THERE IS NO SHIP. I dream about other things, too," says John Ottokar, looking at Frederica.

"My work is gone from me," says Jude. "Rupert Parrott has my work and I am bereft. I sit in the British Museum, reading about the perfectibility of mankind. It is chastening, chastening."

At closing time, they all go into the street. Frederica sets off for the Northern Line on the Underground. John Ottokar, his radiance concealed under a black PVC raincoat, accompanies her. So does Jude.

"Shall I see you home?" says John Ottokar. Frederica stands on the pavement next to him and finds she is very slightly trembling. "I will see you home, too," says Jude. "I live your way. I live in Stockwell. We will go home together."

"I never knew where you lived," says Frederica to Jude, looking at John Ottokar.

"No one does," says Jude. He says, "I'm not much protection for a lady on the Underground. They attack me, the louts, when they've drunk a little, they take exception to my nature. You, on the other hand, you two, would be protection for me, as far as you go."

John Ottokar says, "Do you look like that because you *want* to be attacked?"

"I look like this because I must. It is my nature to look like this, this is my self-identity and true nature, this is my Birkin-in-Mexico, my costume for crossing the Rainbow Bridge, connecting the prose and the passion, and if I am despised and rejected of men, I must e'en bear it. I cannot *wear a mask,*" says Jude, leering at John Ottokar in his shiny surcoat and his many-coloured jumper.

"And you are asking me to come home with you as protection?"

"No, no, as protection for Frederica. You may leave me to my fate in the Oval. I go down to the end of the black line on my own. But you could significantly reduce the odds in favour of my being stripped and whipped, wounded and set upon."

. . .

They travel together in silence. John Ottokar gets out, with Frederica, at the Oval, abandoning Jude to his possible fate: they see his grey face impassive at the window as the lighted carriages whisk into the dark. Being forced up against Jude's scent in a crowded carriage has an anaphrodisiac effect on the other two: they walk, apart, through the dark streets, into Hamelin Square, and turn, still apart, on the doorstep. Frederica does not invite John Ottokar in. The street lamps make rivulets of golden and silver light on the planes and creases of the PVC.

"I'll give you a ring," says John Ottokar. "If that's OK." His voice is casual.

"That's OK," says Frederica. She goes in, out of the dark. A step has been taken.

But he does not phone, and the next week he is not in the class.

Arnold Begbie receives a reply from Nigel Reiver's solicitor. This states that his client intends to defend the divorce, denies the matrimonial offences with which he is charged, and requests immediate discussions in the matter of access to his son, Leo Alexander. Frederica says she does not want to see Nigel; she is afraid of him, and she does not want to upset Leo. Begbie says she will strengthen her case if she appears to be reasonable, unless she expects Nigel to treat either her or her child with violence. Not Leo, says Frederica. He loves Leo. Images of Nigel and Leo float before her mind's eye; Nigel blown up like a demon, roaring and fire-eyed, blue-black and electric. Leo with her hair and Nigel's eyes, her mouth and Nigel's stocky shoulder-set, with his own white, intent, frightened face. Some small, rigid sense of justice in her points out that a child has only one father, whom it is almost always better to know than to imagine. She agrees to see Nigel, in Arnold Begbie's office.

She expects him to glower with rage and hatred. He sits there in Begbie's chair, with the lattice shadows across his dark face, the set of his body hidden inside his dark suit, and gives her an intent, business-like look. He is a whole, living, complicated human being, not a demon. She does not know him. She remembers the fierce and delightful movements of his naked body. He says, "Of course, I still hope that you will come back to me."

"Why? We weren't happy. I drove you mad. You expected me to be something I wasn't."

"We have Leo," says Nigel, using an unfair verb. "We could try."

"I can't," says Frederica.

They stare at each other.

"Let me see Leo. Anyway. Let him come home for a holiday."

"Home."

"Back to where he was born, then, where he grew up, if you want to be pedantic. Let him run in the country. Let me see him. He's my son. I love him. You can't deny that, you're too straight to deny that."

"I know you love him. He loves you."

"There is no need to hide him from me. I promise not to upset him."

"Mrs. Reiver," says Begbie, "is afraid you will not return the boy at the agreed time."

"I shall not want to return him, of course. But I am not fool enough to suppose I shan't do myself a lot of harm by hanging on to him. And I am not monster enough—whatever Frederica thinks—to hang on to a boy who wants to be somewhere else."

Frederica is not sure that the last remark is true. But it sounds very reasonable.

"Give me Leo for a month in the summer."

"It's too long. He'll worry."

"Three weeks. If I promise never to discuss—what will ultimately happen—and not to try and persuade him to stay for ever. Let him ride Sooty and run in the fields. He'll be happy. He'll think things are better. He must miss Bran House a bit. It will be his, one day."

"OK," says Frederica. "Three weeks." She knows so little about children, so little even about Leo. She has made some sort of instinctive judgement about how long Leo will be happy to revisit his old places before he becomes either afraid of losing her, or afraid of losing his old life again—which, which? *What is best for Leo?*

"If he doesn't want to come at all, you must accept that. I promise to try and make it seem easy for him to come."

"I trust you," says Nigel. Then with a flash of anger. "I don't know why I should, I don't know why I should ever trust you with anything again." And then he bites back the anger and is a mildly smiling man in a suit.

Frederica speaks to Leo. She asks him, would he like to go back to Bran House for three weeks in the summer? With you, he says immediately, as she knew he would. No, she says, with Daddy. Who wants to see you. Very much. She continues doggedly. All over England she imagines people grinding out these sad sentences. We can't get on together any more but we both love you, we both want to see you. Leo pinches his lips together and considers. He closes his face and excludes her from his considerations. She thinks of her nephew, Will, who will not forgive his father. How can Leo forgive her? How long is three weeks? asks Leo, unanswerably, since she cannot return to the imagination of stretches of time in a small child's mind. I shall miss you, in three weeks, she says, drily, casually, desperately. It is in answer to this remark that Leo informs her, equally drily and casually, that he thinks it might be quite nice to go.

He goes in July. He will spend his fifth birthday at Bran House. By then the extra-mural classes are closed for the summer, and the art students are undergoing their final assessments. There are few books, if any, for review, and Frederica's income is reduced to the small sums she is paid by Rupert Parrott for reading his slush heap. Agatha is preoccupied: she is writing the first draft of the Report of the Steerforth Committee. Frederica goes upstairs as usual to prepare Saskia's tea, on the next day when it is her turn to prepare Saskia's tea. Agatha comes home to find her friend and lodger reading Tolkien to Saskia on the sofa where the readings take place. Saskia scrambles down from the sofa and runs to her mother, who gathers her up in her arms. Frederica begins to weep. Her face spreads with salt water. Agatha sits next to her and strokes her hair, puts an arm round her thin shoulders. Saskia touches her wet cheeks. Frederica weeps. She wants to tell Agatha: I have ruined Leo's life. But cannot, in front of Saskia. Agatha gives her coffee, and biscuits with chocolate icing, and suggests that Frederica take a holiday. "Saskia and I are going away, too," says Agatha, not saying where they are going. "So you are free. Eat some more biscuits. You need blood sugar. No one is perfect. Human beings survive. Leo loves you and you love Leo."

"It isn't enough."

"It has to be."

Later, Frederica wonders again about Saskia's father. Are they going to a secret rendezvous with this unknown person? Agatha appears to have solved the problem of the second parent by annihilating him.

XII

When Agatha and Saskia have gone, Frederica is alone in the house. It seems to expand and float, it is full of scattering bright air. London summers are dry and dusty, but inside the white-painted basement Frederica experiences a giddiness, a sense that she is blowing away like an untethered balloon. She cannot sleep. She is racked by desire—for Leo, for whom she weeps, for work (what has happened to her huge ambitions?), for love (there has always been *someone,* Alexander, Raphael Faber, to whom the threads of love could be hooked and pulled taut). She tries to think of work—what does she want to do, to make? She thinks, Perhaps I shall go back to Cambridge and talk to Raphael about doing my Ph.D. after all. Perhaps I will go back into the British Museum and start reading about Milton and metaphor. The moment she has this thought, *Paradise Lost* invades her mind in bright apparitions: Adam and Eve entertaining the angel made of translucent air in the bowery, blossoming, fruitful garden, Satan and Beelzebub floating dull and fiery on the dark infernal lake, the glistening glossy snake wreathing and coiling its sinister way across the enamelled paradisal lawns. This is what it is to be human, thinks Frederica, more than a little mad—to entertain such guests, such mythic beings made of language and light.

All the same, somehow, the idea of Raphael and Cambridge is not entirely delightful. There is something "bygone" about the Cambridge lawns and the Cambridge cloisters, the teacups and the tobacco.

What do I really want? Frederica asks herself, with her blood beating in her empty head in her empty room. And cannot answer. Solitary Frederica is an unreal being, because Leo exists.

. . .

She decides to telephone Leo. It is the second day of his absence. She is afraid to hear Bran House on the end of the line, afraid of all the people there, except Leo, afraid too of what Leo may have become, may think of her.

"Bran House," says the telephone, in a female voice, comfortable, that she cannot place. It is Pippy Mammott.

Frederica says, "Could I speak to Leo, please?"

A silence. Frederica can hear the polished hall, the muted heavy doors.

"I should like to speak to Leo," says Frederica, rather relieved that she does not have to name herself.

"I shouldn't think so," says the voice, answering her first remark.

"I just want to say hullo to him. To keep in touch."

"So did others."

"I know." She does not want to expatiate, or to plead with Pippy. Who also loves Leo. "Is he there?"

"I shouldn't think so."

"Could you look?"

Another silence.

"No, he isn't there. He's out."

"Will you tell him I called? Could he call back?"

"I shouldn't think so."

"He might want to," says Frederica, unable to say "*Please*" to Pippy Mammott.

"He might not," says Pippy. "Best not to disturb, if you want my opinion, as I'm sure you don't."

Frederica, hearing hatred, puts the phone down, carefully. She is shaking. Tears brim.

She decides to call round her friends. She speaks to Hugh, to Alan, to Tony, to Alexander, to Daniel, to Edmund Wilkie. She decides to have a party. She speaks to Desmond Bull and to Rupert Parrott. Rupert has a wife Frederica has never met, Melissa. He asks if she may come to the party. Tony too has now a girlfriend, Penny Komuves. He will bring Penny. Wilkie is back with his old girlfriend, Caroline, of the *Astraea* days. They have both been involved with others, and have now returned. They will all bring bottles, as Frederica has no money. Tony Watson says he has rediscovered Owen Griffiths, who used to love Frederica in Cambridge and is now working in the Labour Party's research department. Frederica decides against inviting Thomas Poole, perhaps out of fear of "the public domain," perhaps out of fear of complications. She does not think of inviting Jude Mason, but is unsurprised when he appears with Daniel, to whom he has attached himself.

It is a good party. The voices mix, mingle and oppose.

"Did you get to the poetry festival at the Albert Hall?"

"No, but some friends did. They said it was wild."

"The audience howled and hooted. And bayed. It was pandemonium."

"It was Nüremberg at times. I was there."

"Jeff Nuttall and John Latham were painted blue. They were dressed as books, which they destroyed. Everyone danced."

"They were all high, they were all spaced out. Adrian Mitchell read a poem about Vietnam."

"It was full of enthusiasm and incredibly tedious."

"The Americans have dropped paratroops in Vietnam. They are on the offensive. It's their war now."

"Wilson should speak against them."

"How can he? Our welfare state is funded by American handouts and subventions."

"They want him to send troops. They urge him to send troops."

"He's cunning. He won't. He won't give them more than words."

"He had no majority in the Commons on the corporation tax. He can't hang on. There'll have to be an election."

"We shall have Reggie Maudling as Prime Minister. He'll succeed Alec Douglas-Home."

"We shan't win the next election. We'll have the Tories back."

"I wouldn't write Wilson off. He's cunning."

"Is it true he's ruled by someone called Marcia Williams?"

"Not ruled. He trusts her."

"Kitchen cabinet . . ."

"Ah, Daniel. Just the man. My theological novelist is trying to take her book back again. First she wanted it back because her husband wouldn't like it. Now she wants it back because he does. He says it's a wonderful picture of the Death of God in our society. He sees the stabbed selfish husband as the sacrificial lamb, I think. He wrote me a letter, saying that when the clergyman loses his faith he *is* the Death of God, and when his wife stabs him, his death opens the way for the Presence of God to be restored, since his Death is incarnate in his doubt."

"It sounds very contemporary."

"Phyllis Pratt says God will be more thoroughly annihilated if she withdraws the book. She's writing another, though. It's got a title. 'Grind His Bones.' It's another theological thriller, she says, about a sexton who composts the vicar and his curate. I can never tell when she's joking. I won't withdraw the book. It's got a cover with a Magritte-like loaf, bleeding gouts of blood."

"Dreadful."

"Saleable, in the present climate. You wouldn't talk to Mrs. Pratt about her theological doubts?"

"I'd rather not."

"*I'll* talk to her."

"Did you hear Patrick Heron at the ICA? He was attacking the Americans. He accused them of cultural imperialism. He thinks it's a kind of chauvinist modishness, all the critics who go round saying everything good comes out of America."

"What he is doing himself," says Hugh Pink, "is incredibly beautiful. All these floating discs and brilliant fields of saturated colour. It's like seeing the elements of creation, it's like seeing angels, except you shouldn't use analogies for it, it simply *is.* It makes me feel ill."

"Ill, Hugh? Why?"

"Because it makes me want to write, as though that was the only sensible thing to do. But I hate poems about paintings, I hate the second-hand. I want to do *something like that* with words, and there isn't anything, or if there is, I don't have access to it."

"How are you, Jude?"

"Ill. Impatient. Lost."

"The printers are trying to bowdlerise your book. They have queried many of your words in red ink."

"I will not have my words touched or changed."

"We'll run it past a lawyer, of course."

"I will not be bowdlerised."

"Don't worry. Your book will either offend, or not, as a whole. There isn't any point in chopping off a few warts."

"You console me."

"I don't mean to, necessarily. Are you writing another?"

"I am too nervous. It is appalling, not to be writing. I have no life. I am no one. So I go to gatherings to which I am not invited."

"I would have invited you if I knew where you lived."

"I can find my way *by other means,* as you see. I like your underground home. You would not like mine."

"What are you doing, Frederica?"

"Nothing much. My son is away. I teach, but the teaching's seasonal. I am trying to get unmarried."

"I can't think why you ever got married. I could find you some work researching at the TV centre. Would you like that? What are you going to do in the long run?"

"I don't know. This morning I thought, I might go back to a Ph.D. I've discovered I can teach."

"Difficult to imagine."

"I *can.*"

"OK. You can. Those that can't, teach. What is it you can't do?"

"Write a novel? Don't be nasty, Wilkie. I *like* teaching. It matters. Ask Alexander."

"What does he know?"

"He's on a royal commission on teaching. He goes in and out of schools."

"Hmm. That might make a good programme. How they learn? What they learn. There are people up in North Yorkshire looking at what the brain does when we learn. Are we a computer, or a jellyfish, or a computing jellyfish? I'm a jellyfish man myself, I think we're made of flesh and blood and neurones *in jelly,* but it's not fashionable. It's all algorithms. Algorithms. Everything analysed into binary dichotomies. Either/or. Whereas you and I know it's both-and, and a few more things as well. Now *there's* something useful to do, study the memory."

"Marcus is doing that."

"So he is. He's turned out well. Surprising."

Tony Watson's new girlfriend, Penny Komuves, is a lecturer at the LSE, daughter of a Hungarian-Jewish economist whose ideas are current in Harold Wilson's Treasury thinking. She and the cheerful Owen Griffiths chatter away about Wilson's kitchen cabinet, to which both have an ancillary access; they gossip about Mrs. Wilson's discomfort in Number 10 and the influence of Marcia Williams. Penny Komuves is short and dark and solid, with a Vidal Sassoon haircut, which suits her. Owen tells stories of George Brown's drinking. Desmond Bull and Hugh Pink discuss Patrick Heron's anti-American aesthetic manifesto as though it was at least as important as Ian Smith's threatened declaration of Rhodesian independence from Britain. Rupert Parrott is different in the company of his wife, who is a rather County girl with a fine-boned face amongst a curtain of silver-blond hair, and angles—rather pretty angles—where less well-bred women have curves. She says almost nothing all evening, turning her head with polite interest from face to face as people speak. The other person who doesn't speak is Daniel, who had hoped to see Agatha, whom he likes; he mentions this to Alexander, who says he had also hoped to see Agatha. "I think she went to Yorkshire," says Daniel. "She said she might see me there, if I go up to see Will and Mary."

"She didn't tell me she was going," says Alexander, with pleasurable sadness. "She sent me a draft of two chapters of our report. She writes very clearly."

Frederica chops up dark bread and French bread and celery and chunks of cheese. Jude Mason looms up behind her.

"You do not appear to be happy. Will you trust me to hand that round?"

"I am not happy; I think that's the first personal remark you've ever made to me."

"I am in your house."

"So you feel you should take an interest in me?"

"No. I feel able to diagnose. You have too many ties. You could have lived as I do, without desire, and then you could have been—"

"What, Jude?" Frederica is slightly drunk. Jude's steely face goes in and out of focus.

"Single-minded. You dissipate yourself. On affections and concerns. Daniel is single-minded. *Tollit peccata mundi,* to speak blasphemously. I prophesy. You will not be what you have the possibility of being."

"That's cruel."

"I am not concerned with kindness. Draw in your tentacles, young woman, all this is trivial, all this chatter. Our deity—I call it Time, Time rules sublunary beings—our deity does not forgive an addiction to the trivial."

"You are pompous. And I am not addicted to it. I am stuck in it. And it isn't trivial altogether. It's like cells breeding, it is *what is.*"

She sees the faces and chatter in her room as a warm brew of potential life and form, infinitely interesting, if only she could find her own proper, her own *real* relation to it. What is "real"?

"I am repelled by cells breeding."

"Your bad luck."

Jude sways. "I have seen things you can't imagine. Horrors that are nothing."

He sits down heavily in Frederica's desk chair, breaking a glass of red wine on the desk, dropping the breadboard on the carpet. Wine drips. Daniel fetches a floorcloth. Jude closes his eyes. "Stoned," says Desmond Bull. Jude falls forward on the desk amongst his grey hair.

"He can't stay here," says Frederica.

"I'll take him away," says Daniel. "I'll stow him in the church."

"I'll help," says Rupert Parrott. "I feel responsible for him, now." Melissa Parrott stands up.

"Get on with it, then. I'll go out and look for a taxi. If we are responsible, do let's get on with it."

"I can manage," says Daniel.

"Rupert says he's responsible. So let's *get on with it.*"

"Masochist," says Jude, through loose damp lips, opening one reptilian eye and closing it again.

The friends go home. Frederica stands on the doorstep and watches them go. The yellow light spills on to the step. Her friends make off towards the Tube, except for Rupert, Melissa, Daniel and the inert Jude, who depart in a black cab. As Frederica turns to close the door, a figure steps out of the shadows of the next doorway, a figure that makes a faint crackling sound. Frederica takes in a gasp of breath and steps up into her own doorway. She cannot see a face: the man wears a soft, wide-brimmed hat, pulled down. She has seen this figure in this hat and the glistening, crackling PVC across the mud-circle a few nights ago, and again, standing motionless on a corner of the square, perhaps a week before.

"Don't be afraid. I wanted to see you."

The blond face turns up into the yellow light.

"I was having a party. You should have come."

"I didn't want to. Intrude. Be at a party. I wanted to see you."

"You'd better come in."

She is afraid, even now she knows it is John Ottokar. He comes up the steps behind her. A car engine in the street coughs into life, and then dies again. Frederica closes them in.

"Come down, have a coffee."

"I don't know."

"Why have you come?"

"You know why."

He takes his hat off; his arms crackle on the way up, and on the way down. There is the thick, yellow hair, lying glossy and bright.

Frederica cannot answer him: she knows, and does not know, and will not say she knows.

"I've been watching your house," he says. His voice is lowered and conspiratorial, although the house is empty. He is a lover, not a thief, yet Frederica is reluctant to tell him the house is empty. He says, "If I can't have—what I want—I shall lose what I have."

Frederica could say, "No, you won't." Or she could ask, "What do you want." She knows what he wants. She asks, "What do you want?"

"You," he says intently. "You are what I want. It's terrible to want anything so much."

"Come in," says Frederica. "You can't stand here—we can't stand here—in the entrance."

They go down the stairs into the basement. His feet are heavy. His face is heavy. In the class, in the pub, it has always been alert, mildly curious and pleased, responsive. Now it is set into an effort of mindless will. Frederica wants to laugh, and cannot. The tension in his body crosses the air between them. They sit down, on the edges of armchairs, staring across the room.

"You didn't come, for weeks. I thought you'd given us up."

"My brother was ill. I had to see to some things. I saw to them. It was a bad time. I could only think about you." He hesitates. "When things went wrong, it became clear to me that I had to—come to you—I'm not making sense." He hesitates again. "I told you, I'm no good at language. I—I have a picture in my mind of you *understanding* it all—"

"All?"

He bows his head.

"My—history. Two people in a room. Bodies and histories."

Frederica has been thinking about his body, though not about his history, which she cannot imagine. She thinks of all the bodies that have just stumbled and strolled and hurried out of this room: Hugh Pink, white and gingery; Alexander, long and bending; Owen Griffiths, bustling; Tony, brisk, and Alan, elegant; Daniel, solid as a rock and jutting with energy; Rupert Parrott, pinkly gleaming; Edmund Wilkie, fin-de-siècle pale, with heavy dark-rimmed glasses; Desmond Bull, muscular and chemical-tinged; the repugnant Jude, grey and scaley. She likes John Ottokar's shoulders. She likes his wide mouth. He is a shape she likes. His skin and hair have for her a kind of delineating glitter of interest and electricity, a field, almost, of force, an almost visible aura of movement in the air.

She says, "I don't know your history."

"No."

He stares at the ground. He does not tell her his history. He lifts his head and stares silently at her. Frederica stares back. The looks are like touching each other; they shock. She says, "I must clear up all this mess." She does not move.

"Later," he says. "Not now."

He stands up. He crosses the carpet, which seems suddenly to be an immense desert space. He puts a hand on the nape of her neck. She thinks, Do I want this? and raises her face to his. He stares down at her and brings down his mouth like a gold bird striking. But gentle. At the moment of touch, gentle.

Frederica thinks: Do I want this, do I want this? John Ottokar touches her face, her hair, her long haunches, her small breasts. He touches lightly, lightly, so that her skin begins to desire, half-irritated, half-compelled, to be touched more violently. She puts her own hands on his shoulders. He kisses her face, again, and his fingers question her clothes, a button, a zip, a strap, so that inside these the naked woman is defined and comes to life. And her mind does not cease: Do I want this, do I want this? She stares out of the basement window at the cone of light falling from the street lamp, frowning slightly, lips nevertheless parted with mindless pleasure, and thinks: Do I want this? She remembers her own young greed, and her need to know—about her body, about sex, about male bodies—her indiscriminate clutchings and searchings and muddles and laughter and disgust. She is afraid now, as she was not, then. Her body is used, not furiously ready. She remembers her childish attempts to attract Alexander's attention and make him want her. She thinks of them as childish now, she thinks of herself as old, on the edge of being undesirable. She thinks that she wanted Alexander because he was remote, the teacher, her father's friend, tabu. And now, she thinks, there is the same thrill: I am the teacher, I am wanted because I am separate and looked at, there is a boundary of the forbidden to cross. She thinks all this whilst she stands there on her carpet in the lamplight, and her clothes fall slowly around her as John Ottokar's fingers find their fastenings and make her into a woman, a woman he wants, and has imagined, and has not seen, and now sees. I am thin, thinks Frederica. I have no breasts to speak of, despite Leo. John Ottokar reaches the warm triangle of her pants, slips a large hand inside them, and takes them gently down to her knees, and then, kneeling, below. Frederica puts a hand over the red-gold triangle of hair, and John Ottokar kisses the hand, and the hair, softly.

He is still wearing all his clothes, including the PVC raincoat. When he moves to kiss her, kneeling before her, his outer casing crackles and whispers loudly, whilst his hair against her hand is sleek and thick and soft and yellow. Frederica is still *thinking*: she makes an effort not to think of Leo and Nigel, who become immediately present in the room. Her nostrils remember the smell of Leo's hair: the closest, the most powerful, the most loved smell of all. She kneels down next to John Ottokar and buries her face in his gold; its smell is good, and alien, and wholesome like bread. She begins to tremble. John Ottokar is shrugging off the PVC skin: inside is a flowered shirt, a shirt like a garden of green chrysanthemums and blue roses, a busy Paradise but well cut, a shirt to go inside a suit, a respectable-shaped shirt but burgeoning with brilliance. Frederica puts timid fingers to its mother-of-pearl buttons. Do I want this? Do I want this? Neither of them speaks. They are separate, and yet intent on connection. The struggle with his shoes is ungainly: Frederica looks modestly away. His trousers are quick, a snakeskin sloughed. His prick is grand and blond and sure of itself. Frederica laughs when it is revealed. They fall together, warm flesh on warm flesh. Do I want this? I want this. I think I want this. I.

They roll laughing on the carpet, near Jude Mason's still damp winestain: they clutch, they touch; it takes its way: it is good. No one speaks, but Frederica hears his voice in a drowse, a series of soft meaningless syllables, full of *z*s and *s*s, a rush of stuttering *t*s, a dreamy hum, and then a final strange whistling, like the sharp thin cry of a bird. She swallows her own cry; she will not let go so far; she keeps her pleasure, which is intense, partly secret.

. . .

In the morning, the two wake naked in Frederica's narrow bed. When, finally, they get up, still almost without speaking, John begins to clear away Frederica's party, still naked, padding in and out of the kitchen with dirty glasses and empty bottles. Frederica sees the bottles and ashtrays and Leo's toys, a tank, a mechanical dinosaur, an articulated wooden snake.

"I can't stay here," she says. "By myself. I can't stay here."

"We could go somewhere else."

"I was thinking of going up to Yorkshire. To see my family."

"We could go to Yorkshire. I don't know Yorkshire. I'm on holiday."

"We can't both go to see my family."

"You could see them—after—when I have to be back. We could have a few days, by ourselves. We could."

"We could just get dressed and lock the house, and go north."

"I've got a car. I could drive you."

"Why not?"

"It is all right, isn't it?"

"It is all right."

Her body hums with happiness. Her mind surveys the place where she lives: books, toys, typewriter, Rupert Parrott's typescripts.

"Let's go *quickly,*" she says.

XIII

There is a moment on the road north when red-brick houses give way to grey stone, and grey stone walls make their appearance. The colour of the sky and the grass changes in relation to these stones: the sky is a bluer blue, the grass a bluer green, and the whole world, to the eyes of a northerner returning, both more solid and more potentially liquid, more serious, less friendly, more real. Frederica sits beside John Ottokar as his dark blue car eats the miles of road, and is surprised by the violence of her sense of homecoming. Most of the houses they see are not particularly beautiful; they are dour enough, though sometimes softened by creepers or climbing roses; the nineteenth-century ones have an air, she thinks, of civic and non-conformist confidence. She remarks on this to John Ottokar, who replies that he grew up in Milton Alfrivers, a twentieth-century Garden City planned by Quaker philanthropists in Essex. "Toy houses in toy closes," he says, "we said they were, in the 1950s. Solid though, with pretty gardens. We wanted to get out."

Frederica, who wanted to leave the north for London, and who likes London, who likes her various displaced London lives, cannot quite describe her sense of belonging to this grey and blue and green, so lapses into silence. They drive into the Dales, and the grey-green hillsides slope up and away from the road to the sky, crazily divided into uneven patchworks by the industrious and energetic dry-stone walls, long snakes of skilfully layered dark flat stones, occasionally staked with bare wooden poles. These craftsmen are my people, thinks Frederica, and then reprimands herself for sentimentality. But the walls are beautiful. "Such skill, such precision," says John Ottokar, looking at the orderly human rearrangement of rocks and stones. "That's what my father always used to say," says Frederica. "I used to wait for him to say it, as he always did. Now I look at the walls, and that's what I think. Such skill."

They are not going to Freyasgarth. They have booked in at the inn at Goathland, where they arrive in the thick blue evening, where the light on the moors is like water or suspended powder. They sign themselves in: Mr. and Mrs. John Ottokar. It is a fantasy, a fiction: Frederica feels freed by it. She is *not* Mrs. Ottokar; nobody here knows who she is. They go up a creaking black wooden stair to a low-ceilinged bedroom with a sprigged wallpaper and a sprigged bedspread. They embrace: John Ottokar's large body is interestingly strange still, and yet warm, and yet connected to hers. They go out of the door and watch the last light flicker and fade over the bowl of hills: they watch the early stars in patches, and the fast rags of cloud blown in darker patches between the starclusters. They hold hands. His fingers are warm; she has the idea that his fingertips make little shocks against her own.

Inside, there is a warren of dark bars, a smell of rich beer, a smell of wine, a smell of paraffin. They eat in a restaurant with peach-painted rough-plastered walls, and have a candle between them in a cobalt-blue pot. They eat roast beef and Yorkshire pudding and are formal with each other, suddenly. They share their histories, or parts of their histories. Frederica describes Bill and Winifred (non-conformism, teaching, common sense), Stephanie (good, clever, dead), Marcus (mathematical, brilliant, difficult), Blesford Ride and Blesford Girls' Grammar (a) liberal and b) stifling and boring). John Ottokar tells of a childhood amongst pacifist Quakers; his father, now retired, was production manager in a chocolate factory, imprisoned during the war for conscientious objection. He describes his mother, but Frederica fails to imagine her, although it is clear that she too is a Quaker and a pacifist. "We went to the local Grammar School in Milton Alfrivers," says John Ottokar. "It was OK. We went to Bristol and did maths. They thought we ought to be separated, so one of us started in Bristol and one in Liverpool, but it didn't work out, so we both went to Bristol."

"Which were you?"

"I was the Bristol one."

"Did *you* think you ought to be separated?"

Frederica is making conversation.

"Yes and no," says John Ottokar, evenly. "I could see why they thought what they did, but it didn't work out."

Frederica thinks of asking, "Why didn't it work out?" and finds she cannot: she is somehow forbidden. There is a silence. He is working out what to say.

"At first we weren't doing the same course at Bristol, but by the end we were, we were doing the same pure maths course." He stops again, and starts again. "Living in the same digs. Solving the same problems the same way."

"Happy?" asks Frederica, who now realises that all this is somehow dangerous ground. There is a long silence. John Ottokar eats and frowns. She remembers him saying that he came to the extra-mural class to learn language.

"Very happy in one way," he says, finally. "I mean, that is, we *knew* each other, you know. That was all we did know. And because—because we were together—we—didn't get to know anything else. We didn't have—friends of our own—that is to say, we did have some friends, we had friends of both of us, and we liked those friends because we were like each other, but we needed—I needed—I needed, I thought, a life of my own, so to speak." He gives a snort of painful laughter. "A girl of my own, for instance. Opinions of my own, I sometimes thought, though an opinion is an opinion, if you happen to share one *genuinely* you can't pretend you don't, that's silly. We were very involved in the CND marches—the whole Aldermaston thing. We marched with our parents and all the Quaker Meeting from Milton Alfrivers. We played in a band. We were part of something much larger than ourselves. That was good." He thinks again. "If you can say terror is good."

"Terror?"

"You march and march, you sing, you link arms, human *solidarity,* but you're doing it out of terror at what some fool can do to the world—of what can't be imagined, but *must.* Every now and then you *do* imagine it. You know? Marching is what you can do, but every now and then you know—that marching might achieve nothing."

Frederica has thought about the Bomb. But, either from self-preservative insensitivity, or from a possibly ill-founded faith in human reasonableness in the last resort, or from individualistic foolish courage, she has always turned away from being obsessed by it. She has a distaste for mass emotion, which she does not admire in herself, but does acknowledge and respect. She has absolutely no desire to spend time demonstrating, and thus is sceptical about the value of demonstrations. She is not sure she wants to involve herself with "all that," though well enough disposed towards it. She takes an internal step back from John Ottokar, and looks sharply at his outer self, across the table. His head is bent over his apple crumble: he is frowning. When he feels her look, he lifts his head, and smiles at her. The smile is full of light and of bright warmth. Frederica is dazzled and touched. She smiles back, a wide smile.

She wants to ask him if, and how, and when, he found a girl of his own, and dare not.

The love-making is more inventive, more collusive, less startled, than the night before. He learns quickly what Frederica does and doesn't like; he stirs her body, he keeps it singing, he is pleased with himself, she is humming with pleasure, with pleasure, with pleasure. They sleep, and wake, and turn to each other and touch hands and faces. Frederica is drowsily alive; she breathes in the air he breathes out and the intimacy is acceptable, is delightful. He speaks in her ear, *tesh, teran, azma,* unknown syllables. And again, softly past her ears, that strange, low whistling note of triumph and ending. He falls asleep quickly and heavily and she raises herself to look at his sleeping face in the moonlight, intimate and strange, a still, sculpted, empty face, fair and beautiful, closed to her. Do I want this? says the insistent serpentine voice. She extends her thin body the length of his, skin to skin, in the fading warmth of their pleasure and each other.

In the morning they eat breakfast in the pink restaurant, now looking out at the moor. There are other guests: a family, a married couple, a solitary spectacled man reading *Lady Chatterley's Lover.* They ask the inn for sandwiches, and set out to walk on the moors. They stride out: their steps go together. The rhythm of the striding, the warmth of her lively skin, bring poems into Frederica's mind, poems she learned when her body ached to be touched, and was not.

> *"Love, do I love? I walk*
> *Within the brilliance of another's thought*
> *As in a glory. I was dark before*
> *As Venus' chapel in the black of night:*

But there was something holy in the darkness
Softer and not so thick as otherwhere
And as rich moonlight may be to the blind
Unconsciously consoling. Then love came
Like the out-bursting of a trodden star . . ."

She thinks of saying this to John Ottokar, and dare not. As a girl she said it to her mirror, conjuring a non-existent face: and now his face, more or less, shines in that space, but the poem is still her secret, is private. I was looking for you, she wants to say to him, and says instead, "Did you find her, the girl of your own?"

"The girl?"

"Never mind."

"Oh, the girl of my own. Oh yes. I found her. She was a French girl. It was—difficult." He pauses. "It was dreadful."

A long silence. Frederica says she is sorry. They walk on. John Ottokar says, "I don't want to—spoil this—by bringing in all that. It's past. It's a—a bad story. Funny and bad.

"When I saw her, Marie-Madeleine, I thought she was beautiful. She was staying in the house we were lodging in: she was a *lectrice* at a school. She wasn't happy. She was out of place. I didn't tell anyone—not anyone—what I felt. I thought about her. I wondered how I could—speak to her. Finally, I went up to her as she was coming back from work—near the school, not near our house—and I said, I wanted to get to know her, to talk a bit. She said, 'Which one are you?' That was the first thing she said. She couldn't tell us apart, then. So I said I was John, and asked her to the cinema. I thought it was dark and secret. We went to see Cocteau's *La Belle et la Bête,* I think. We sat down in the dark. After a bit I had a funny feeling—I knew before I saw—I saw my brother had come in, and was sitting on the other side of her. So when the lights went up, she saw both of us. She had very good manners, she discussed the film with both of us. We went out to coffee, and talked. About CND, about jazz, about the film. She smiled at both of us.

"So then we went out several times, the three of us. I knew what he was thinking, he didn't have to say. He knew what I felt, I wanted Marie-Madeleine, *I wanted her.*

"I don't think he *wanted her,* exactly. He wanted *what I wanted.*

"I told him, I must be alone with her. I told him, we had to separate a little, we had to have individual lives, we had to be two.

"I told her I wanted her. She let me kiss her. And then other things. I could speak to her that way, she knew what I felt.

"But he wouldn't let it be."

"What did he do?"

"He haunted us, at first. He always knew where we were going and turned up, by accident on purpose. One day, Marie-Madeleine told him we wanted to be alone together. She said, nicely, that he should find a girl of his own. He punished her."

"How?"

"He pretended to be me. She couldn't tell us apart. He took my clothes, and took her out, and made love to her, and then mocked her, because she couldn't tell us apart. She went home, she said the situation was too much for her. She was humiliated. And frightened. I shouldn't tell you all this."

"I want to know."

Frederica is greedy to know. She is intrigued. The story is dramatic. They stride companionably along sheep tracks. She says, "You said, when you came, that you brought your history."

"So much of it is *our* history."

"What did you do, when she left, when Marie-Madeleine left?"

She has a very clear mind-picture of Marie-Madeleine, a thin dark French girl with tendrils of ragged curls, downcast eyes and a secretive pointed mouth. Nothing, probably, to do with the real Marie-Madeleine.

"I was furious. I told him *we had to separate.* I said I was going to get an ordinary job and live an ordinary life, on my own, like any other single person, any individual, I was going to make my own life. He couldn't bear it. He—he *pleaded.* He apologised. I packed up in the night, and he crept into my room when I was packing. I said no doubt he knew which train I was leaving on, but I didn't want him on it, he wasn't to come. He said he would make her come back. I said that wasn't the point. I left the house to get in the cab to the station, the next morning, and he came out, he was going to get in, he took hold of me. I stood in the street and shouted. I—I hit him, once, he sat down on the pavement. I went."

The words come awkwardly and painfully. The clouds race in the blue sky: there is a lot of wind, blowing the words into the heather. Frederica imagines the scene. She sees John Ottokar, stiff with grief and rage, closing the cab door. She sees the figure sitting on the pavement, with the breath knocked out of him. She sees this figure from the back, a figure in a space, "he."

"And then?"

"The next I heard, was a phone call from Marie-Madeleine, in Caen. She was desperate. He'd gone there, he was sitting on her doorstep, begging her to come back to me, acting the fool, serenading her with a guitar and a trumpet—he's the musical one—in the small hours.

"I went and brought him back. He had—a sort of breakdown. She said she couldn't take it, she never wanted to see either of us ever again. He's in therapy, now. I—tried that, but I didn't like it, I quit. He—depends on his therapist. He lives in a sort of commune, I think. He was in hospital for a bit. I got my job and my flat.

"If—you and I—go on—you need to know these things."

"It's all *interesting.*"

"That isn't the word I'd use," says John Ottokar.

Frederica is a clever woman, but she is not a woman with an unusually quick imagination. It is not until the two are in bed that night that her imagination really begins to work on the other, the absent brother. She wonders, as she smells the particular smell of his hair, of his chest shining with sweat, of his sex, what it could really be like to make love to another man, indistinguishable from this one, "identical." She measures the length of his arm-bones with the span of her hand, she studies the whorl and spiral of his ears, she touches and tastes their interior with her tongue. Could there be another, the same, who punished Marie-Madeleine through *trompe-l'oeil* and humiliation? The essence of love is that the beloved appears to be unique—*more unique,* thinks Frederica, in whom was instilled (by her father) the knowledge that "unique" is an adjective that cannot be qualified. She tries to imagine another Frederica and her mind shies away in panic.

They set out to walk across the moors to the Falling Foss; they leave the car at Sleights, and walk through Ugglebarnby, Iburndale, Little Beck. The names on the map are ancient and full of life: Hemp Syke, Soulsgrave, Foul Syke, Old Mary Beck, High Bride Stones. At the edge of some woodland they see splashes of scarlet and blue and gold: two people are moving slowly along the hedgerow, pausing and bending; the colour is their thermos flasks, plastic boxes and canvas knapsacks. As Frederica and John Ottokar pass they straighten up and recognise her. They are Jacqueline Winwar and Luk Lysgaard-Peacock. Frederica, held in a kind of glass globe of touch and tension with John, does not want to stop and speak. She wants to greet these two marginal persons and pass on. Luk Lysgaard-Peacock appears to expect this: he inclines his head and returns to his contemplation of the damp grass and the roots of bushes. But Jacqueline greets her warmly and asks if she is on her way to Freyasgarth. She offers coffee from the scarlet flask and John Ottokar accepts. They sit down on large scattered stones, each holding a different brightly coloured plastic beaker. From where they are they can see the new Early Warning System on Fylingdales Moor, three pure white spheres, huge and perfectly round against the sky with its bright blue and slow-moving shifting fluffy clouds, like sheep slowly metamorphosing into cotton-wool, or octopods, or feather beds, or chariots.

Jacqueline asks Frederica if she is on her way to Freyasgarth. Frederica says she does not know: she is taking a few days off on impulse. Jacqueline's bright brown eyes consider John Ottokar. She tells Frederica that Marcus would be pleased to see her. There is something intimate and very slightly proprietorial in her tone: Frederica wonders, as she has wondered on other occasions, exactly what is the relation between those two. Daniel will be pleased to see Frederica, too, says Jacqueline, if she comes. Frederica says she did not know Daniel was there. No reason why she should, she adds. And Agatha will be very surprised, says Jacqueline. She is bringing Saskia to meet Will and Mary. We are all looking forward to her visit. Oh, says Frederica, put out. Jacqueline smiles. We are looking forward to meeting Agatha, she says.

John Ottokar is staring at the three great spheres. It is almost as though they were in another dimension, he says, another reality. Their size is incommensurate with the moorland, their scale is in another world. They are beautiful and sinister. They are so beautiful and simple it is not easy to see them as man-made, and thus they do not seem to spoil the wild landscape as they might be expected to. They are huge yet unobtrusive.

They are monuments to human power, though, says Luk Lysgaard-Peacock. They are listening for the sound of Armageddon. We have built engines that can destroy the world, and we have built these huge, inhuman domes, that watch and listen for the approaching doom. He laughs drily. "I do not suppose they are a very adequate defence," he says, "despite their scale, despite their grace."

No one present can remember how many minutes' warning the radomes give of the approaching cataclysm: four minutes, six? twelve? Prepare to meet thy doom, says Frederica. We shall melt in a flash. Not necessarily, says Luk Lysgaard-Peacock. Death can fall through the air and melt silently and invisibly into grass, into milk, into our teeth and our bones. Though it need not come flying in over the North Sea from Siberia. A local accident is just as sure. There was an accident in Cumberland not long ago; it was hushed up; but the strontium is in the bones of children who were under the blowing cloud. I measure it, in the shells of snails, he says. He shows John and Frederica a box of striped snail shells. In certain snail populations, he says, a band of strontium can be detected in the shells. He has a friend who studied much larger snails—*Partula suturalis,* on the Mooréa atoll, near where the French explode their test bombs. He was using bands of strontium to measure the growth of the shells, and was expelled by the French when this came to their attention. "I've found concentrations of it in Lancashire populations," he says. "You take the shell, and embed it in a transparent gel, and cut it vertically with a fine diamond saw, so that you have a beautiful spiral—a Fibonacci spiral—and you can date events on the spiral, by measuring minerals . . ."

John Ottokar asks about Lysgaard-Peacock's work. He is studying population genetics, he tells them: several populations of the striped snails, *Helix hortensis* (or later *Cepaea hortensis*) and *Helix* or *Cepaea nemoralis* were studied in the 1920s and 1930s to record the predominance or rarity of certain patterns—variations in stripes, their number and thickness, their absence, their colour. "If we look at them now, we hope to see Darwinian selection in action," he says. "We have populations in various habitats—hedgerows and roadsides, various woods, beech, oak, and mixed—and we look for changes in snails with changes in environment. Some are pink, some are yellow, and there is evidence that unbanded snails are more numerous in beechwoods, and striped snails in hedgerows, where they may be disguised from thrushes. We came here because there is a thrush's anvil here where we collect the broken shells—as you see—and count the numbers, and their changes in pattern."

There is indeed a large stone in the roadside verge surrounded by smashed fragments of shell, some open and showing the spiral column, gleaming in the centre, some like crushed eggs.

"But the thrushes are diminishing," says Jacqueline. "Several of the anvils are abandoned: the thrushes have been killed by the pesticides in the food chain, we think; they eat fat shiny worms full of parathion or dieldrin, or heptachlor, and if they are not poisoned they can become infertile, or produce monstrosities, the poisons damage the DNA, change their genes as surely as radiation does—the thrushes we study here are still here and still singing and still breaking snails on the anvil—but in many places they are gone. And then we expect to find changes in the snail populations."

Frederica shivers: there is something uncanny in this conversation about man-made death falling silently through air and water and matter, through leaves and fur and flesh and bones and bony shells, here in the moorland air, face to face with the silent vision of the watching, listening, towering white spheres. John Ottokar and Jacqueline Winwar talk to each other with the indignant fear of their generation, with the wrath against their elders that they are still young enough to feel.

Frederica turns over the shells collected by Luk Lysgaard-Peacock. She looks at the lovely coils and spirals, the helical houses of the vanished creeping creatures, horned, slimy, glistening, seven-thousand-toothed. Lysgaard-Peacock shows them to her—pink and yellow, single-banded and multi-striped. *Helix hortensis,* he tells her, has a white lip—"a lovely, ivory-white, gleaming lip," he says poetically, whilst *Helix nemoralis* can be distinguished by a jet-black lip, "a glossy black." From his chosen language she can see that he loves the creatures he studies.

"They carry their history on their outsides," he says, "on their backs you can read their genetic make-up."

"And you can read that Darwin was right, that natural selection changes the genes of the population?"

"Not exactly," says Luk. "There are puzzling things. If strict Darwinian theory was true, populations under the same selective pressures should become more and more genetically homogeneous—but this isn't so. They show a surprising genetic polymorphism. All sorts of forms persist when strict theory might suggest that they should have vanished. There are fossil populations of *Cepaea nemoralis* tens of thousands of years old with just as much variety of shell colour and banding patterns as we find today."

"Perhaps there are different selective pressures—"

"I like to quote Bacon," says Luk Lysgaard-Peacock. "On diversity, I like to quote Bacon. I try to read the language of the DNA on the backs of my snails, and I think of what he said. 'It is the common wonder of all men, how among so many millions of faces, there should be none alike: now, contrary, I wonder as much, how there should be any. He that shall consider how many thousand several words have been carelessly and without study composed out of 24 letters; withal how many hundred lines there are to be drawn in the Fabrick of one man, shall find this variety is necessary.' The alphabet of the DNA has only four letters, but they can produce an apparently infinite variety. Even in snails."

Frederica considers Lysgaard-Peacock's own face. His beard is very strong and stiff and russet, cut neatly and full of vigour. His mouth amongst the red spikes and spines is soft and secret. His eyes are deep-set. His ears are pointed. He is foxy. He is not unlike herself, in that, and his colouring is roughly related to her own—people might suppose, wrongly, seeing the four human beings together, that these two were related, she thinks. She smiles at him, and he smiles back, not wholly present in his smile, thinking about snails and the DNA. Frederica's glance slides on to John Ottokar, with his wide brow, his shining head, his spine, known and touched vertebra by vertebra. She says to Luk, "Some faces are alike. John has an identical twin. I don't know him."

Lysgaard-Peacock hands her two shells, both yellowish-green and unmarked.

"Geneticists love twins," he says. "Most particularly twins with different histories."

"You must ask him," says Frederica.

"I may," says Luk. He hands her another shell, this one boldly divided by spiral dark stripes on a pale ground. "A present," he says.

John and Frederica come back to Goathland in the evening. They walk in the dusk through the village, where the black-faced sheep stare with yellow, inhuman eyes. Something tugs at Frederica's memory. She came here once, in a bus, on a trip, and had what she has now docketed as an interesting and instructive experience with a traveller in dolls. The sight of a sheep and a thorn bush brings back this person, Ed, in his interesting and repelling fleshiness, but it also brings back a thought. It was a thought about her own separateness, and the power that was possibly inherent in keeping things *separate*—sex and language, she thinks, ambition and marriage, *what* was I thinking? She remembers she was thinking about Racine, and the rhythmic movement of her feet, comfortably in time with the rhythmic movement of the feet of John Ottokar, brings back the couplet in the landscape to which it was wholly irrelevant then, and for *that* reason interesting, for *that* reason compelling:

Ce n'est pas une ardeur dans mes veines cachée
C'est Vénus toute entière à sa proie attachée

She remembers, and with it her delight in the balance of the lines, the way they pivot on the caesura and are both separated and joined by the rhyme. She says the verse out loud, and John Ottokar puts his hand over her buttocks, lovingly, and laughs, and says, "Precisely." Frederica stops in her tracks, dizzy with sex, and puts her arms tightly round him: watched by sheep, and by the man who was reading *Lady Chatterley* in the rosy restaurant, they embrace, they kiss, they walk on. They lean together. Frederica's mind, a dark snake burrowing in darkness, looks for a word which then seemed the key to power and safety. She remembers her distress that Stephanie had apparently found happiness with Daniel. She thinks of Forster and Lawrence, only connect, the mystic Oneness, and her word comes back to her again, more insistently: *laminations.* Laminations. Keeping things separate. Not linked by metaphor or sex or desire, but separate objects of knowledge, systems of work, or discovery. In her pocket her fingers touch Luk Lysgaard-Peacock's snail shells, two greenish and one striped. Are the stripes laminations, or organic growths? The layer of strontium, exposed by the diamond saw in the spiral form, is a *layer*—an accident in Cumberland, a time of fall-out in the air—what is she saying? Partly that even fear of death in the air is not all-consuming or all-pervading. She has the first vague premonition of an art-form of fragments, juxtaposed, not interwoven, not "organically" spiralling up like a tree or a shell, but constructed brick by brick, layer by layer, like the Post Office Tower. The radomes are on the moor and are seen amongst the heather and the neolithic stones and barrows, but their beauty is in the difference as well as in the simultaneity of the vision.

She is feeling for something, and doesn't know what it is, cannot push the thought further. Laminations. Separation. I was thinking about the Virgin Queen, and the power of her solitude and her separation, the fact that her power and her intelligence were dependent upon her solitude and her separation.

"What are you thinking?" says John Ottokar, and takes her shoulders, and turns her face to his. "You've gone away from me. Where? What are you thinking?"

Desire moves round the column of Frederica's spine like the spiral of a helter-skelter, round which she spins screaming with fear and delight.

"I had an idea for a book called *Laminations.*"

"Why *Laminations*?" he says later, in the bedroom. At the time, he simply smiled and nodded.

"I haven't thought it out. It's to do with what was in the lectures, the Romantic desire for everything to be *One*—lovers, body and mind, life and work. I thought it might be interesting to be interested in keeping things separate."

"I know about that," he says, sitting naked on the edge of the bed. The lights are out, but the room is full of pale moonlight. "I know what it is like to be afraid of being two separate creatures confined in one skin."

They are naked and cool in the night, sitting companionably on the edge of the bed. On an impulse she touches his sex, the two balls moving loose and separate inside the cool bag of skin. The penis shrinks like a soft curled snail, and then swings out blindly, a lumbering and supple serpent becoming a rod or a branch. Two in one, thinks Frederica, as his arms go round her. You might think, she thinks, as their bodies join, that here are two beings striving to lose themselves in each other, to become one. The growing heat, the wetness, the rhythmic movements, the hot breath, the slippery skins, inside and out, are one, are part of one thing. But we both need to be separate, she thinks. I *lend myself* to this, the language in her head goes on, with its own rhythm, I *lose myself,* it remarks with gleeful breathlessness, I *am not,* I come, I come to the point of crossing over, of not being, and then I fall away, I am myself again, only more so, more so. His face, *post coitum,* is calm like an Apollonian statue. There is no clue to what is inside his brain-box. I love that, says Frederica's chatty linguistic self, I love not knowing, I love it that I don't know him.

Daniel sits companionably with his father-in-law on the Freyasgarth lawn, making a daisy-chain for his daughter. The fat pink-tipped flowers are scattered across his black thighs, where she has strewn them. The two men sit in deckchairs on the grass and watch the young girl, barefoot in a sky-blue dress, strut and pirouette and swoop in front of them. Her reddish-gold hair falls in a silky curtain about her calm, round face. There are two ways of making daisy-chains. One is to pierce the end of each stalk, and thread the next flower through the green until its head catches. The other is to select a tough daisy with a powerful stalk and thread it through the heads of several others, piercing each at the nape and pushing up through the golden pollen circle, making a thicker, more luscious petalled rod, all pink and white and feathery. Daniel made a bracelet by this method, but Mary exclaimed at the cruelty and extravagance, and he is now making a long green garland, studded intermittently with florets. It goes slowly: split stems curl back and are discarded. Mary runs up and down, bringing handfuls of flowers. Bill says she is denuding his lawn and making it look conventional and respectable.

"There'll be new ones tomorrow," says Mary. "There always are. The more you pick, the more they come."

The blue dress is no more than a floating triangle of cotton, held on by shoe-string straps. Her skin is freckled and new and lovely. She bends down, and straightens. Bill says to Daniel, "She reminds me. She is very like, very like."

"The movements of the neck. The wrists."

The dead woman is dreadfully present. The two men measure each other's apprehension of her absence. Mary jumps high, fluttering her flying feet. They applaud Mary. Bill says, "When you do dance, I wish you / A wave o'th' sea, that you might ever do / Nothing but that, move still, still so—"

"What is that?" says Daniel.

"Nothing," says Bill. "A play I used not to like. I begin to see the point of it."

Mary's dance brings her past in a rush, feet thudding on the grass. She says, "There's a car coming."

Daniel thinks it will be Agatha Mond and Saskia. But it is not. Winifred brings the visitors out: it is Frederica, completely unexpected, and a blond man, completely unknown. Frederica considers Mary, who is slightly out of breath, and looks at Daniel, seeing the same ghost. Their faces twist, and then are stoical.

Daniel sees that Frederica is shining with sex like a sunbather rubbed with butter. Her sharp face has its old edge, a keenness, a glitter, which makes him see that he preferred the recent, more battered, subdued Frederica. He sees a kind of black space walking in the garden, which is his absent wife. Frederica says, "Jacqueline Winwar tells me you are entertaining Agatha here."

"She is visiting Professor Wijnnobel about her committee. She suggested coming over, so Saskia could meet Mary."

Frederica prickles. "It's odd she didn't say anything. To me."

"Is it?"

"It's *my* family. I feel it's odd. I suppose it doesn't matter."

"You are here, now, anyway," says Daniel, equably.

He is being disingenuous. He has noticed, now and then, a speculative gentleness in the way Agatha Mond looks at him. He has thought he noticed (and then dismissed the idea) a particular carefulness of intention when she handed him a plate, or a glass of wine. Nothing much. He likes Agatha Mond. He was, he realises, looking forward to a quiet talk with her in the sunshine, in the north, a step or two forward in discovery. She is a secret woman. He was looking forward to finding out a few things. This—apart from his feelings about Mary and Will (who has gone off on a hike with the local scouts)—is the first *personal* feeling he has had, the first mild *wish* he has formulated, since . . . And now Frederica is here in a great cloud of sex and self-importance like a swarm of bees and a too-sweet smell of honey. Winifred is offering tea to John Ottokar, who is praising the landscape, shyly. He does not look entirely happy. He is standing apart from the family group.

Agatha and Saskia arrive in a hired Mini, a yellow Mini with black trimmings. Agatha is surprised to see Frederica but apparently delighted. She is wearing a woven straw hat and a shift with big, innocent white daisies on a navy ground. Her skin has gone browner in the few days she has been away from London. Her arms are smooth and bare: Daniel wonders what it would be like to run his lips over them, and says, "I'm glad you could make it. Would Saskia like juice? Mary has been dancing."

"I dance," says Saskia.

"It's such a pity Leo isn't here," says Winifred. "On his birthday, too."

Frederica has said nothing about Leo's birthday. She has been trying not to think of it, of him, of what he will be doing. Everyone looks at her, and looks away. John Ottokar wanders off and looks at a rosebush, very intently, as though none of this is to do with him.

Agatha turns to Bill and says that she is in the north because she is drafting the Report of the Steerforth Committee, and has been discussing the technical chapter, the controversial chapter, on grammar, with Professor Wijnnobel. She says she has read the evidence Bill submitted to the committee, with great interest. She would like to talk to him about the relations between reading literature and the new stress on the children's own writing, " 'creative' writing, only I do shy away from that word, I do dislike it."

"Usage will sanctify it," says Bill, "if your Professor Wijnnobel is to be believed. Why do you balk at it?"

"Daniel might agree. It feels blasphemous, it has a faint tainted air of blasphemy hanging around it. I notice you use a religious metaphor, 'sanctify.' "

"On purpose," says Bill, delighted.

"Of course. What do you think, Daniel?"

"Creative? It doesn't seem blasphemous to me. Ugly, though. It makes me think of white elephants at jumble sales, raffia lampshades and pottery rabbits and paper flowers."

They laugh.

Marcus arrives, with Jacqueline. They fetch chairs and make a tea party on the lawn. Birds can be heard, and the hum of bees. John Ottokar is ill at ease. Jacqueline brings Marcus to him, introduces them, says that they have artificial intelligence in common, since Marcus is mapping algorithms in the brain and John is mapping them in shipping traffic. The two men begin to speak of computer languages and their relative strengths and weaknesses. John Ottokar relaxes; he becomes a professional man at a family tea party. Frederica is regretting having come. She had formed some demonic image of Agatha Mond invading her own world, the world of her origins, and this is hard to square with the calm figure discussing teaching methods with Bill Potter, discussing the interesting split in the committee between supporters of Will to Power, and supporters of Eros. "All they are united in," says Agatha Mond, "is opposition to Mickey Impey, who wants to 'liven up the Report' by writing little gnomic epigrams for every chapter." She gives an example:

"A tender love of spit and spot
And mopping up of shit and snot
Is what most teachers have not got."

"True enough, as far as it goes," says Bill.

"But not verse to be *prima donnaish* about," says Agatha Mond.

"He is threatening to lampoon us in the Sunday papers and on the television if we don't print his contribution. He could, too. He could make us look ridiculous in exactly the places we can't afford to look ridiculous in."

It is all very civilised. Daniel notices that Agatha does not address any remarks particularly to himself until Frederica goes away into the kitchen with Jacqueline. She does then turn to him, her face shadowed under her hat, against the red and white stripes of her deckchair.

"I am glad . . . ," she says. "I wanted . . . I was looking forward to seeing you."

"So was I," says Daniel. The two little girls are doing something together at the edge of the garden: Mary, four years older, is showing Saskia something growing, or nesting, between the stones. "They get on," he says, thinking immediately that this remark is fatuous, since there is no real evidence either way. They are not apparently fighting.

"That's good," says Agatha. "I'd like it if . . ."

Frederica returns. Daniel sees her against the sky, so that her hair is brighter and lighter in the sunlight. She looks across at the two little girls, and says to Agatha, "Mary is quite incredibly like her mother."

"Like her father, too," says Agatha. "I think."

"Oh, do you?" says Frederica. "I've never seen that."

"The set of the mouth," says Agatha. "A determined chin. Can a chin be determined? The way it is held, anyway."

"Stephanie's mouth was like that. Mary's mouth is exactly like Stephanie's mouth."

"Married couples resemble each other," says Jacqueline. "Statistically, genetically."

Daniel is deeply annoyed to find that Frederica's voice has come to resemble her sister's. Featureless against the sun, she too is a walking *memento mori,* at least from certain angles; blurred in the light, her edges softened.

"Excuse me," he says, and rises, and walks away into the house.

Frederica and John say good-bye to everyone and drive off. No explanation of John has been offered or asked for. Bill says to his daughter, vaguely, "Be careful," and neither Bill nor Winifred suggests that John Ottokar might come again. They are pessimistic, Daniel thinks, about Frederica's chances of conducting herself sensibly. With reason, he thinks, cross with Frederica almost in the old way. Agatha Mond and Saskia too depart, returning to the Vice-Chancellor's lodgings in Long Royston. Agatha puts out her hand to Daniel: he takes it: there is no *frisson.* Something has not happened. It might not have happened even without Frederica. But Daniel is irritated and feels low.

He is approached by Jacqueline, who asks about his work, and tells him about Ruth, who is becoming more and more involved in Gideon Farrar's Children of Joy. The Children of Joy are a rapidly growing movement in the Church of England. Gideon conducts weekend retreats in seaside barns and country houses, where the Children dance, sing, shout and encounter each other's bodies in loving exploration, acting out infant joys and terrors, anger and tenderness, birth and death. They eat paschal meals, feeding each other around a communal altar table with home-baked breads and home-brewed wines. There are posters of Gideon's benign gold-bearded face above a drawing of robed arms enfolding a flock of naked and aspirant adolescent bodies, a pastoral *couvade.* Daniel does not like either Gideon or the Children of Joy, but is suspicious of his own reasons for this dislike: his is far too inhibited a being, he recognises, ever to be able to sing and shout in communal joy. He asks Jacqueline if Ruth is happy.

"Ecstatically," says Jacqueline.

"I used to think Marcus was in love with her."

"He was. Is, perhaps. I don't understand it. There was a time when they used to make love. Marcus never told me that: she did. She felt she ought to, because he wanted it so much. She said. Then she felt she ought not to, because it was giving off bad messages in the meetings of the Children. They believe they mustn't hide anything. They had a kind of what I call 'emotional stripping session' and someone claimed they could smell bad odours on her body or in her breath or something—I know the phrase 'bad odours' was used. So she gave it up. She thinks she ought to be able to make him go to the Children and she feels she's failed because he doesn't. They still see each other."

Daniel stares over the wall of the garden at the wild land. Jacqueline says, "I know you don't like Marcus."

"That isn't true. I think that isn't true. We've known bad things together and no good ones." He considers Jacqueline. "You like him. That's good."

Jacqueline stands a little more upright.

"I love him. I don't know why. I just one day noticed that I did, that he was *it, the one,* I was even almost annoyed, because you can't say he's a sensible sort of person to fall in love with. Now, Luk Lysgaard-Peacock—he wants to marry me, I think, and he knows what he wants in life—he's ambitious—and kind, and has a first-rate mind, and respects mine. And Marcus is vague and not-quite-there a lot of the time, and doesn't know what he wants, except he wants Ruth, in a funny way, but I think that's because she doesn't *talk,* she's a kind of non-person. I've always just supposed if I waited, he would see I was there, one of these days, and change. You know? In a flash of light, *see* me?"

"It does happen."

"And we were only kids, and he was much more of a kid than I was, and—and I see that *I am* ambitious, too, and I quite like waiting and waiting to be seen, because I can get on with my work while I'm waiting—I've had an idea about neurons and memory—about the nature of learning—a *real idea*—I always talk too much to you, don't I?"

"It's my job."

"I hope not only that. But it does mean I go on at you as I would at no one else—I've *never talked to anyone* about Marcus, I just had it all fitted out in my mind—"

"If I say what I think, you'll be annoyed."

"Say it, all the same."

"I think you should look at Luk Lysgaard-Peacock. In a different way."

"You don't really think that. You know better."

"I have to go on believing in sense, in the possibility of good sense prevailing."

"Not much evidence of *that,* in the world we live in."

"Not much evidence. I agree."

"Whereas love is all over."

Daniel laughs. "All over." He says, "If you are going to work on learning—"

"It's all biochemistry. Love, learning, the lot. Whatever else it is. And don't say knowing that—seeing it that way—doesn't change anything—because actually, it does. It does."

Frederica goes to Paddington. She stands under the Departures and Arrivals. Her mouth is dry, her heart bangs audibly, her blood fizzes.

She is alone. Her brown shoulder-bag hangs below the hem of her bright green cotton shift, which hugs her buttocks. Her long, thin legs tremble visibly. Her eyes are made up like does' eyes. She has had her hair cut, finally: it is a shining bronze cap, or helmet, with pointed tongues licking her cheekbones. At night, in the basement flat, waiting for John Ottokar, she is alive with apprehension, but not like this. This is so extreme, it is abject.

The train comes in. She makes her legs move towards the barrier. It is a very long train, and has come a long way. She jostles for position, she stares. The crowd hurries from the train. From far back she sees the red head bobbing and darting; she hears the running feet scurry and thud; she sees the stout figure weaving its slower way after him. He is wearing a new jacket she does not know, and new, polished shoes. He reaches her; his head butts her crotch; his grasping hands go out and clutch her backside; she bends down; they clutch, they cling, they grip, the small body tries to batter its way back into the thin one it came from. He kicks her legs, he pulls at her neckline, he dislodges her handbag. She kneels on the dirty concrete to contain and support him. He is crying out: she understands the words.

"I hate it. You've cut your hair, I hate it. You *didn't tell me,* I hate you. It's horrible, I think it's horrible, I hate it."

The two small hands scrabble in the smooth cap, dishevelling it, bushing it, tugging, twisting. It is so well cut it falls, raggedly, more or less back into place.

Pippy Mammott arrives, out of breath, with Leo's satchel and suitcase, which she dumps in front of Frederica. She stands and puffs, solid in a red-white-and-blue-checked shirtwaist dress and Clark's sandals. She doesn't speak to Frederica. She says, "Well, good-bye, Leo. Come back soon. We'll miss you."

Leo turns round, still clenching a handful of Frederica's hair, and holds up his face to be kissed. Pippy Mammott bends to kiss him. Her face is very close to Frederica's. She purses her mouth, and Frederica thinks for one dreadful moment that she is going to spit on her. Pippy Mammott's eyes are full of tears. As she kisses Leo, these begin to run out violently, and splash on his small, freckled cheeks.

"We had a good time," says Pippy Mammott to Leo Reiver.

"A *very* good time," says Leo. "Tell Sooty I'm coming back."

He twists his hand, still full of Frederica's hair, to wipe his cheek. He hurts her.

"Thank you," says Frederica to Pippy.

"Don't. Don't thank me," says Pippy. "If I had my way." She does not finish this sentence.

"Come on, Leo," says Frederica. "Let's go home."

Her own tears have come from nowhere and are now falling heavily, dripping from her chin on to Leo's shoulder. She could not find a word for why she is weeping. She cannot control it. Her hands remember Leo's chest, his waist, his weight.

The two women weep, angrily and helplessly. The little boy looks from one to the other, and transfers his attention to a pigeon, swooping in the station canopy, with the light on its wings.

XIV

In September, Leo and Saskia go to school. Both Agatha and Frederica accompany the two, who walk stolidly, hand in hand, through the grey, dusty Kennington streets. The William Blake School has been chosen by Agatha after careful consultation with the school inspectors with whom she works. Lebanon Grove is a treeless crescent of little shops, in the centre of which is the school, a high, gloomy red-brick cube with dusty, barred windows, inside which can vaguely be seen dangling paper parrots and chickens, poppies and clouds. There is a large asphalt playground behind a high, spiked, barred railing, and three entrances—churchy openings with Gothic stone arches and heavy-hasped doors, over which, carved in the stone, are the legends BOYS, GIRLS and MIXED INFANTS. Despite its grim Victorian look, the school has a reputation, Agatha assures Frederica, for progressiveness and innovation. The two women are seized with terror. The two children clasp each other: yesterday Leo said, "The good thing about Hansel and Gretel was that there were *two* of them, I think. They were all right because they were two." Larger children rush in past the smaller ones; pushing, shoving, calling. The children are mixed: black, brown, white, and mixtures of these. The Reception teacher meets the two on the doorstep of MIXED INFANTS and takes their hands. She is a slip of a girl in a strawberry-coloured mini-skirt and high black patent boots. Her hair is dandelion-coloured, her lips painted a ghostly pale cream, her eyes black-rimmed, with false lashes. She resembles a large doll. Frederica had expected a motherly body and sees a child amongst children. Miss Nightingale's voice is kind and sensible. She leads them into the cloakroom, where each child has a hook with an animal and his or her name. Leo's hook has a lion, and the legend: *Leo. Lion.* Miss Nightingale tells him his name means lion, and he says, "I know," and Miss Nightingale says she is pleased. Saskia's hook has a fluffy kitten and says: *Saskia. Cat.* Saskia says she does not want a cat, she does not like cats. Miss Nightingale looks around and offers her a camel or a sheep. Saskia chooses the camel. "They *spit,*" Saskia tells Miss Nightingale, who says, "I know. I've seen them. They are very contrary."

Agatha and Frederica say good-bye. They walk out into the street, bumping against hurtling children. Agatha says it is a good school: the buildings may be grotty, but the children's work is displayed along every corridor; there is a frieze of *The Hobbit,* made by a whole class, with the travelling dwarves with their coloured hoods, Bilbo the Hobbit with his pipe and his furry feet, Gandalf the wizard with his flowing white beard and flaming staff, a mountainous background with peering orcs in cave-mouths and wolves on the skyline, a wood full of fat black spiders and carefully constructed webs, and at the very end, Smaug the dragon in his cave, made out of shining milk-bottle tops for scales, and lying on a treasure made of coloured sweet wrappings and tiny plastic beads. The collage is excellent: Agatha tells Frederica to observe that the children have had to consider how trees grow and spider-webs are woven, to think about perspective and be inventive with materials. On the corridor above this, illustrations to William Blake's poems "The Lamb," "The Tiger," "The Little Boy Lost," "The Clod and the Pebble" celebrate the school's name. There was nothing like this in the schools of Frederica's youth. She finds it exciting and invigorating. But she does not know how Leo will survive group life. In the tiled corridors the shrill voices echo and bay. Frederica was a child pushed aside by, hunted by, other children. A solitary, angry child. Does this hand on? She says to Agatha, "I was no good at group life. I hated school."

"Me too. It seemed eternal. It dragged so. I say to myself, Where are they now, the ones who were so successful, so popular as children?"

At home Frederica has another long, legal envelope. This contains a letter from Arnold Begbie, and encloses, he says, the Respondent's Answer to Frederica's petition. As you will see, says Begbie, the respondent denies all the material facts alleged in our petition. His solicitor has written a letter, of which I enclose a copy, urging you to meet him with a view to reconciliation and restitution of conjugal rights. He also claims custody of your child.

Frederica reads the Answer, on its heavy foolscap paper.

The respondent, Nigel Reiver, by Messrs. Tiger and Pelt, his solicitors, in answer to the petition filed in this suit, says:

(1) That he is not guilty of cruelty as alleged in the said petition.

(2) That he is not guilty of adultery, as alleged in the said petition.

(3) That he claims custody of the child, Leo Alexander, mentioned in the said petition, and proposes the following arrangements for his care and upbringing:—

That he should live with the respondent in the family home, Bran House, Longbarrow, where he will be cared for by the housekeeper, Miss Philippa Mammott, who has cared for him from birth, and by his two aunts, Miss Rosalind and Miss Olive Reiver.

That he should go to Brock's Preparatory School, for which he is entered, and to which his father went, and subsequently to Swineburn School in Cumberland, for which he is also entered.

That he should visit his mother regularly in the holidays and that she should visit him when she wishes to do so, at the family home, Bran House.

Frederica goes to see her solicitor. She sits in the barred light, and hears her own voice, a pleading voice, a panicky voice.

"He can't take him, can he?"

"It would be very unusual for the court to award custody of so small a child away from the mother. Very unusual. Very bad luck. We must ensure it doesn't happen. We must fight. Since your husband clearly intends to fight, we must fight back. I had imagined he might at least have admitted the adultery—if we would drop the cruelty—that would have been civilised, though we would always have to be careful about appearing to collude, or connive at such adultery. For our legal system is oppositional, Mrs. Reiver—the law requires that there be a guilty party and an innocent party, and is hostile to any appearance of *agreement* to divorce, seeks zealously for evidence of manufactured evidence, or lax moral attitudes suddenly conveniently tightened. Not that that appears to be the case here. Your husband is loving and forbearing—"

"Furious and pig-headed."

"As you please. He will say he is loving and forbearing. He condones desertion. He wants you back. You must *prove* that he treated you badly enough for divorce to be a reasonable requirement. I shall instruct Griffith Goatley. He fights like a bull terrier. We need witnesses to the cruelty, and witnesses to his behaviour when away from you. You would not consider instructing an enquiry agent?"

"No. That's a horrible idea. And besides, I can't afford it, I can't afford *anything.*"

"I will ask about those clubs. The Honeypot. Tips and Tassels. There may be a doorman. A barman. An ex-doorman, an ex-barman. They are reluctant to be witnesses. It is not good for their employment. They may know a young woman who may be prepared to say something. It is worth a try. We must have a case."

"He threw an axe at me."

Begbie looks mournful. "We need to *prove* it."

"I have a huge scar. Pink. It throbs in rainy weather."

"We need to be able to *show* what caused it."

"I don't want Leo in a dormitory in a prep school. It's horrible, it's unnatural, I can't bear to think of it—he's *little*—"

"Lots of little boys survive quite adequately." A pause. "I did." Another pause. "The judge probably did."

His face is lugubrious, frowning with what might be anxiety and might be a kind of professional *Schadenfreude.*

"He'd *hate* it."

"We must hope it doesn't come to that. It shouldn't. I'll get Goatley. Meanwhile, think of *anyone* who can describe your husband's unreasonable, cruel, or aggressive behaviour. Maids? We must get on to the doctors. Your friends?"

"They didn't *see* him hurt me. They saw me shortly after."

"Hearsay evidence is not admissible."

"He *can't have* Leo."

Daniel keeps watch in the dark in St. Simeon's Church. Orange street light glares through the jumbled stained glass of the windows, producing a muted glare of acid colours on stone, which occasionally flare differently as headlights pass in the street. He sits in the shadow, behind a Victorian pillar, looking at the faded reproductions of Rubens's *Deposition* and Holbein's *Dead Christ* which Canon Holly has hung over the altar. It is October 28th and Daniel wishes to give thanks for, to contemplate, the ending of an evil. On this day the House of Commons, in a free vote, has passed the Murder (Abolition of the Death Penalty) Bill. Daniel sits in the presence of whatever haunts the dark stone and meditates on the panoply, the grisly ceremony, the ghoulish cruelty, of what has just been done away with. What he has felt, all his life since he first became aware of the pain of death, is not, mostly, a sympathetic identification with the sufferer, though that is part of it. He has seen and he has imagined the man or woman in the dock seeing the judge's black cap, hearing the sentence pronounced, having to do things that belong to the still living, walk back to the cell, eat, speak, defecate, breathe, as a human being certainly dead, a human being whose existence is the knowledge that in ten days, nine, eight, seven, six, five, four, three, two, one day, ten hours, nine, eight, seven, six, five, four, three, two, one, ten minutes, nine, eight, seven, six, five, four, three, two, one, they will come with the hood and ropes, and the dead legs must walk to the gallows and the trap. A death is a death, and this death is a peculiarly horrible death, because of its certainty, because of its public enactment, because it is unnatural, as many other murders are not unnatural. But a death is a death, Daniel knows. Many wait in pain. All human beings come there. What horrifies him about the infliction of capital punishment is the horror it spreads into the whole society which enacts it, connives at it, decrees it. The breath of evil in the court officials, the policemen and -women, the counsel at the bar, the judge, who together must enact the sick drama that leads to the killing. The evil that can be smelled in the cells and in the warders and in the other prisoners who witness the agony, with furtive glee or sick horror. The pleasure in pain that thrills in the press and in the sickened, the profoundly infected, imagination of the people as they imagine what can't be imagined, whether with a murderous delight, or a bloody righteous wrath, or with the unwilling, terrified, *damaged* identification with the sufferer's terror, which was his own response as a child. In Calverley he had met a blabbering man, a shaking man, who was a priest who had attended executions in Calverley Gaol, and had lost his mind in a mixture of guilt, terror and revulsion. A society that can make these mechanisms, Daniel believes, is a sick society, and if it cannot be called an inhuman society, it is only because cruelty is human, cruelty is part of our nature, as it is part of the nature of no other creature. (The warmongering chimpanzee is a discovery of the future.)

Daniel sits in the church and destroys in his mind, one by one, the elements of the narrative and the drama. He thinks of them all soberly, gagging as he always gags as he pronounces in his head "to be hanged by the neck until you are dead. And may God have mercy on your soul." He imagines the black cap and the posy on the judge's desk, the condemned cell and the last walk as Saint Ignatius Loyola taught his followers to picture and meditate on the Stations of the Cross, bringing the agony of the God-Man vividly to life, step by step in the darkroom of the brain, blood, sweat, broken bones, the stink, the roar, the failing muscles, the spitting crowd, the piercing thorns, the failing thighs and knees, the crunching shock of the nails. These things are obscene, and the obscenity is not in the murderous impulse, but in the ingenuity that devised and devises the long-drawn-out agony, the spectacle, the complicity of participants and passers-by. He cannot really see, in the dark, either the heavy, pearly, meat-stiff fall of Rubens's painted flesh, or the grim, stretched, leathery cadaver of the Holbein. Those two knew what flesh was, its beauty and intricacy, its mixtures of rose and wax, blue and grey, shadow and fatty sheen. They painted it at the moment of its dissolution, with aesthetic pleasure in their own power, love of the flesh as it was and would not be, alive in their steady contemplation of death. This is Christ, the divine man, a man tortured and executed, and perhaps, Daniel thinks, it is right after all to find God here, where human ingenuity in evil is most crassly lively and most disingenuously self-righteous. And it is good to thank whatever is for the end of evil, at least in this time and in this place. In later years, when the freedom of the 1960s is spoken of, Daniel will always think of this quiet dark night, when he cleared his imagination's charnel-house and torture-chamber of their gibbering ghosts, and ended sitting in a dark blue silent dome of night darkness, soft and cool and still.

A week before, exactly a week before the Murder (Abolition of the Death Penalty) Bill, in Hyde, in Cheshire, Ian Brady, twenty-six, a stock clerk, and Myra Hindley, twenty-three, a shorthand-typist, were charged with murdering Lesley Ann Downey, aged ten, whose body had been found buried in peat in the Pennine moors six days earlier. Brady was also charged with the murder of Edward Evans, aged seventeen. If the chronology had been a little different, Daniel will think, often, would he have had his quiet night?

Agatha Mond comes down to Frederica's basement to collect Leo for school. It is her day. She has Frederica's post in her hand. There are two fat foolscap envelopes, a small brown one, and one covered with small "Victorian scraps"—angels' heads and bullfinches, a lily and a rose. Leo is struggling with the zip of his anorak, with which he refuses to accept any help. He frowns. Frederica mimes distress and fury over his head to her friend, opens the foolscap letters rapidly, not because she is eager to know their contents, but because she dreads them, and formless dread is always worse than the known and delimited. A letter from Nigel's solicitor, Guy Tiger, is enclosed in a letter from her own solicitor, Arnold Begbie. The letter is about Leo. It is not the first. Nigel has taken to dispatching a steady stream of these legal documents. He does not write letters himself: language is not his medium. He has never written letters to Frederica. She has no box of dead love-letters to consider with incredulity or regret. Begbie's covering note says that the present letter requires careful thought. Frederica, unable to speak because of Leo, snatches up the dressmaking shears with which she has been making chains of paper men for her son, holds up the letter to Agatha, and mimes its destruction.

"Comes the blind Fury with th'abhorred shears," says Agatha. They grin. The quotation makes them both feel better. They do not question why this should be so: they are women who share a certain culture.

"Blind Fury is about right," says Frederica savagely.

"*Courage,*" says Agatha.

Leo zizzes his zip to a triumphant snap. He and Saskia and Agatha depart.

Frederica reads the letter again.

Dear Mrs. Reiver,

I am instructed by my client, Mr. Nigel Reiver, to put to you, through your solicitors, Messrs. Begbie, Merle and Schloss, some considered proposals for the welfare of your son, Leo Alexander Reiver.

My client wishes me to state clearly that the present separation between you is not of his seeking, and that his urgent wish is that you should return, with your son, to the matrimonial home and seek a reconciliation. He rejects entirely the imputations of cruelty and adultery set out in your Petition for Divorce, and seeks earnestly to prove to you that he is prepared to forgive your own desertion, which was entirely without cause, and without any previous warning, discussion or attempt to settle your supposed differences reasonably and amicably.

My client particularly and with great sorrow regrets your unprovoked and unconsidered decision to take with you his and your son, the said Leo Alexander Reiver. He believes that this action was not in the best interests of his son, who was a happy child, living in a cheerful and stable household, in which there were several relatives and a very loving housekeeper prepared to care for him and bring him up in the world into which he was born and where he will, in due course, take his rightful place as owner of Bran House.

My client is informed that you have taken the child to live in a deprived and socially unstable area of London. He is informed that you inhabit a basement flat in what could be described as a near-slum; that you arrange constantly changing and intermittent care for the boy whilst you absent yourself to earn money by part-time employments of various seasonal kinds. My client does not feel that this way of life is in the interests of his son. He has proposed, very generously, paying you a reasonable sum of money as maintenance for his son and yourself, so that whilst the said Leo Alexander is in your care you would be able to devote your full attention to him. My client believes that, if your abrupt departure from the matrimonial home was, as you have stated, to seek employment, your own priorities make you less fit to have the care and control of so small a child than those women who could give him their complete attention, in the comfortable home and healthy country surroundings where he grew up. My client believes that the boy's interests would best be served by his immediate return to the home he has known since birth. He would, of course, if you persist in your present way of life, grant you generous access to the boy, and would always make you welcome at Bran House, as its mistress, or as a visitor, as you may choose.

My client is also extremely concerned and distressed by the provisions you have made, without consulting him, for his son's education. On social and educational grounds, and with the welfare of the child uppermost in his mind, he begs you to reconsider your decision to send the boy to the William Blake School in Kennington, which he does not consider a suitable environment for a boy born into his family, or with Leo's expectations. The sons of the Reiver family have for the past three generations attended Brock's Preparatory School in Herefordshire and Swineburn School in Cumberland. It is my client's heartfelt hope and expectation that he will be able to give his son the excellent education he himself had, and that Leo may be educated amongst his peers, including several of his second and third cousins already at the schools.

In the present circumstances, my client proposes that his son be sent forthwith to Brock's School, where we have ascertained that a place will be held for him. As you are aware, my client will sue for custody of his son if and when your Petition for Divorce reaches the courts. He still earnestly hopes to avoid this eventuality by persuading you to return to the matrimonial home. In the interim, he suggests that it will be the fairest, most appropriate, and most beneficial arrangement if Leo is moved immediately to Brock's Preparatory School, where both his parents will be free to visit him on equal terms. His request is both reasonable and generous, and he hopes that you will give it your immediate and sympathetic attention . . .

She reads the second legal letter, which tells her that the fixing of a date for the hearing of her divorce has been deferred, since the Respondent has asked for time to prepare his case. She opens the brown letter, which contains a very small cheque from the Crabb Robinson Institute, and the one with stickers, which is an invitation to "A Studio Debauchery" from Desmond Bull. Bull has become interested in *collage,* of which the cherubs and lilies are an outpost. He is making a large picture of layers of faces, from past and present, newspapers and paintings, with Robespierre's eyes in Marilyn Monroe's face above Bronzino's Fraud's scaly tail, or with Roosevelt's seated figure cut into Titian's seated Pope. This work is at a chaotic stage, and varies from the banal to the suddenly witty and shocking. Desmond Bull is cheerfully certain that any day now Frederica will join him on his studio mattress. She likes his paintings: she likes him: what follows is obvious. Frederica, because of John Ottokar, cannot claim that she is prejudicing her legal freedom by this move, and is even tempted to make love to Bull to reassure herself that she is not tied to John Ottokar. Because of John Ottokar, she has started to take the Pill, which is making her heavy and bad-tempered, unless it is life that is making her heavy and bad-tempered. She has eaten two packets of pills now, day by day, one in September and one in October, and John Ottokar has vanished for almost exactly that period of time. Desmond Bull's blatant campaign has its attractions for that reason too: it gives the Pills some *point*.

She has not told Arnold Begbie about John Ottokar. There are various reasons for this, involved and at cross-purposes. Begbie will think she was lying when she said she had not committed adultery or incontinence or whatever the law calls it. This matters because she feels judged by Begbie, which ought to be nonsense, but is not. And then, to tell Begbie about John Ottokar is to make the relations with John Ottokar more solid, more real, than either she or John Ottokar wants to think they are. They are not adultery, which is serious: they are just sex. "Just sex" does not stand the glare of legal light upon it. It is as partial a description as "incontinence" or "adultery": it is provisional and does not bear looking at. There *are no words* with which Frederica feels able to explain her relations with John Ottokar to Arnold Begbie.

. . .

Frederica feels wild and oppressed. She takes the sharp shears and slices Guy Tiger's letter in two, vertically, and then again horizontally, and then again, until she has a handful of rectangular segments. This will not get rid of it, she reflects gloomily. More copies can endlessly be quartered, like the heads of the hydra. She picks up the pieces and lays them out on the desk. "A happy child living in Brock's School." The art students are excited by William Burroughs and his cut-ups. Frederica rearranges Tiger's letter into a kind of consequential structure. So.

A happy child living in Brock's School where there were several relations held for him prepared to care for him and will sue for custody of his son which he was born and when Petition for Divorce reaches the rightful place as owner of Bran hopes to avoid this eventuality my client is informed return to the matrimonial home, a deprived and socially unstable environment, suggests that it will be best that you inhabit a basement, the most beneficial arrangement a near-slum; that you arrange immediately to Brock's preparatory intermediate care for the boy, parents will be free to earn money part-time. His request is both kinds. My client does not care for the boy and he hopes that you in the interests of his son immediate and sympathetic paying you a reasonable would best be served by persist in your present way devote your full attention that if your abrupt access to the boy and would always find the matrimonial home as House or as its mistress or as a employment less fit to have the small child who was extremely concerned and distressed by their complete attention without consulting him, for his stable household, in sending the boy to the William Blake relatives and a very loving housekeeper into his family or bring him into the world into the Reiver family he will in due course have taken the child to live in Cumberland it is my client's area of London. he is informed he himself had what could be described as his peers including several constantly changing and sins already at the schools whilst you absent yourself his son be sent forthwith employments of various seasonal proposals for the welfare of Messrs Begbie, Merle and Schloss we have ascertained that the present separation is between his urgent wish for imputations of cruelty in the matrimonial home in the Interim to forgive your own desertion to settle your supposed differences and decision to take with you Alexander Reiver with great sorrow regrets persuading you to return to Swineburn School and to women who could give care and control of so heartfelt hope and expectation may be educated among money as maintenance in the comfortable home environment for a boy born your own priorities make departure from the welfare of the child.

. . .

Lawyers are concerned to make unambiguous statements with unquestionable conclusions; Frederica's cut-up has therefore less beauty than a cut-up of some richer text might have, but it does approximate to a satisfactory representation of her confusion, of her distress, of her sense that the apparent irrefutable clarity of Nigel's solicitor's arguments is a nonsense in her world. She considers it. She finds the Burroughs a student has pressed upon her—"*This* is the voice of now, *this* is where it was going, fragments shored against my ruin and all that, just try this, this is the voice of now, this is *release,* this is the ultimate."

"Cut-ups are for everyone. Anybody can make cut-ups. It is experimental in the sense of being *something to do.* Right here write now. Not something to talk and argue about."

"All writing is in fact cut-ups. A collage of words read overheard. What else? Use of scissors renders the process explicit and subject to extension and variation. Clear classical prose can be composed entirely of re-arranged cut-ups. Cutting and re-arranging a page of written words introduces a new dimension into writing enabling the writer to turn images in cinematic variation. Images shift sense under the scissors smell images to sound sight to sound sound to kinesthetic. This is where Rimbaud was going with his colour of vowels. And his 'systematic derangement of the sense.' The place of mescaline hallucination: seeing colours tasting sounds smelling forms."

Frederica considers this. It is both attractive and repellent as a way of seeing, as a way of acting. Frederica is an intellectual, driven by curiosity, by a pleasure in coherence, by making connections. Frederica is an intellectual at large in a world where most intellectuals are proclaiming the death of coherence, the illusory nature of orders, which are perceived to be man-made, provisional and unstable. Frederica is a woman whose life appears to be flying apart into unrelated fragments: an attempt to tear free from the life of country houses and families; a person who for two months has been a female body chemically protected from the haunting fear of conception; an angular female body symbiotically tied to a rushing, small, male red-headed energy, whose absence itself is sensed as a presence and as a claim; a mind coming to grips with the fact that English literature is a structure half connected to and half cut off from a European literature which was transfigured by Nietzsche and Freud; a person in a basement with not enough money; a memory containing most of Shakespeare, much of seventeenth-century poetry, much, too, of Forster, Lawrence, T. S. Eliot and the Romantics, a chancy baggage which once seemed a universal, reasonable necessity; a Petitioner in a Divorce Court; a wanderer in studios; a judge of the works of such as Phyllis Pratt and Richmond Bly. Frederica is a woman who sits at her desk and re-arranges unrelated scraps of languages, from apparently wholly discrete vocabularies: legal letters, letters about the Initial Teaching Alphabet from Leo's school; Leo's first written words, which are BUS and MAN; the literary texts and the quite other texts that dissect these texts; her reviews, her readers' reports, which do not use the critical vocabulary she has acquired, for this is useless in three-hundred-word segments. She is a being capable of turning her attention from a recipe for an *omelette aux fines herbes* to the *Tractatus,* from Dr. Spock to the Bible to *Justine.* Language rustles around her with many voices, none of them hers, all of them hers.

Like many human beings who feel that they are exploding with grief, confusion, or anger, Frederica has thought of controlling or venting (both contradictory verbs are appropriate) her pains by writing. She has even bought an exercise book in which to record what she feels, in which, she told herself in the stationer's shop, to reduce the lawyers' language to plain expressive English. The exercise book is golden in colour, with a laminated plastic cover, on which is a purple design of geometric flowers, like those we learn to make in school, with overlapping swoops of the compass, shifting the centre and the circumference to make petal in petal, half-moon meeting half-moon. Inside, it Frederica has written a first sentence.

"Much of the problem appears to be one of vocabulary." Which led to no sequel. As far as it goes, this sentence is acceptable, but there is no vocabulary to provide the next sentence. A week later, like a terrier shaking a rat, Frederica wrote:

"There is no vocabulary to provide the next sentence."

A month later, she wrote:

"Try simplicity. Try describing a day."

I woke up too slowly. My tongue was furry. There was a taste of—what? Metal, decay, old wine. I want to write "death" but that's exaggerating. I got up. I went to the bathroom. I did the things you do in the bathroom, piss, shit, replace the death-taste with an alien taste of nasty (?artificial) mint. I hate mint. I have always hated mint but I go on putting it in my mouth. I know I ought in this style to write about the pleasure and relief of pissing and shitting but I don't want to. It is ordinary and satisfactory and writing about it would be shocking, would look as if it were meant to be shocking, which would be the opposite of what I am trying to do. Do I know what I am trying to do? I am not enjoying writing in this style. When I had come out of the bathroom I went to wake Leo. His face was buried in the pillow: it was pink and sweaty where it touched it: it was dry and warm on top. I kissed it. Leo's smell—all his smells—are the best thing I know. I find I don't want to go into what they are like or why they are the best thing. This style won't do that, although it leads you in that direction, it makes you think, aha, yes, now I describe Leo's smell. Keep going. We had breakfast. We had boiled eggs and toast. The bread was a bit old. It always is. I like fresh bread but not enough to go out and get it. If I wrote about the pleasures of fresh bread in this style for long enough I might entice myself to go out and get some, but probably not. We had the usual fight about who ties Leo's shoes because we are late. The usual fight. Describe it. Come on. I can't. This style fills me with a dreadful nausea. People write whole books like this. It looks so clever and it's a cop-out. I wanted to try and think about what had gone wrong and *what I am for* and it is nothing to do with furry mouths or one-verb sentences or noticing things you notice all the time *gracefully,* but as though they hadn't been noticed before, as though they were shocking or surprising. At this rate I could write hundreds of thousands of words and get further and further away from thinking anything out.

Tonight I am teaching *Madame Bovary.* The thing about Madame Bovary was, she didn't teach *Madame Bovary.*

That's banal too. Writing things down makes everything *slightly worse.* Slightly worse, what a fate. Writing is compulsive. And useless. Stop writing.

Frederica considers these abortive beginnings. The desire to write something is still there, accompanied by the nausea. Once, after John Ottokar had made love to her and slept, she had tried to write what she felt about him, about lying with the blond head breathing on her breasts, about wondering whether he would come again, or stay, or settle, or vanish, about whether she herself could bear to hold herself open to him, or would close, would turn her face away, would retreat in a flurry of ink like a cuttlefish (her habitual metaphor for this manoeuvre). Do I love him, she had made herself write, a real question, but the sight of it, and the sight of the rows of sentences beginning with the first person singular had filled her with such distaste that quickly, quickly she had torn the pages out of the book, ripped them into scraps and flakes, and ground them down amongst tea-leaves and sprout-peelings in the bucket under the sink.

"I hate I," she had written in the notebook. This was the most interesting sentence she had written yet. She added the intellectual's question. "Why?" And an answer.

I hate "I" because when I write, "I love him," or "I am afraid of being confined by him," the "I" is a character I am inventing who/which in some sense drains life from me ME into artifice and enclosedness. The "I" or "I love him" written down is nauseating. The *real* "I" is the first I of "I hate I"—the *watcher*—though only until I write that, once I have noticed that, that I who hates "I" is a real I, it becomes in its turn an artificial I, and the one who notices that that "I" was artificial too becomes "real" (what is real) and so *ad infinitum,* like great fleas with lesser fleas upon their backs to bite 'em. Is the lesson, don't write? It is certainly, don't write "I."

This page had not been torn out. Frederica finds it faintly nauseating, but interesting.

She thinks, perhaps cut-ups. She has a vision of controlling the miseries of the divorce and its dragging negotiations by cutting it all up into a kind of nonsense-diary, which produces occasional gems of scrying, like "my client does not care for the boy," though Frederica's innate fairness cannot find much satisfaction in that. The problem is that Mr. Tiger's client *does* care for the boy. That is the problem. And beyond that how anyone as clever as she, Frederica Potter, once was could have got herself into the present mess. She gives a little laugh, rummages through her cyclostyled lecture-notes, and comes up with the quotations about wholeness from Forster and Lawrence. She cuts them away from her text, and slices them up in approved Burroughs-mode. A vertical snip, a horizontal snip, re-arrange. This method produces something interesting and loosely rhapsodic from the Lawrence:

She wanted to be made much of the age, was a dead distance of silence between the immanence of her peace superseding knowledge, height or colour, but something was only the third, unrealized could he know himself what not as oneself, but said "Your nose is beautiful being in a new one, a new, sounded like lies, and she was the duality. How can I say "I," he said, whispering with truth to be, and you have ceased to the real truth. It was transcended into a new oneness of having surpassed one because there is nothing to answer, old existence. How could travels between the separate new and unknown, not him, there is perfect silence of self at all. This I, this old letter.

In the new, superfine bliss she could not know there was no I and you, there to be adored. There were wonder, the wonder of existing between them. How could he tell summation of my being and of beauty, that was not form, or paradisal unit regained from the strange golden light. How love you, when I have ceased, her beauty lay in, for him. We are both caught up and your chin is adorable. But where everything is silent, disappointed, hurt. Even when all is perfect and at one. Speech "I love you, I love you," it was parts. But in the perfect Oneself, of having transcended the bliss.

Which says more or less what it was originally saying, with more or less the same rhythm, as though all the breathings of all the words were interchangeable. The Forster, more tightly constructed, will not deconstruct until cut into considerably smaller segments, when a certain effective contrast of high and low, abstract and solid words begins to work.

Outwardly he was cheerful, could only point out the salvation, all had reverted to chaos and in the soul of every man. By an incomplete ascetic whole of her sermon, only connect husband or widower, he had always, and both will be exalted, passion is bad a belief that is at its highest. Live in fragments passionately. Religion had connect, and the beast and the monk were read aloud on Sunday, life to either, will die. No gift of her own she would only connect! That was the form of a "good talking." The prose and the passion would be built and span their human love which she was never prepared to give. Only connect his obtuseness robbed of the isolation that there was no more to give. It need not take the souls quiet indications the bridge a white-hot hatred lives with beauty. One quality in Henry saints and love the Infinite, however much she reminded could be a little ashamed simply did not notice things she said. He never noticed bothers about my own inside, the sneaking belief that bodily desirable only when held respectable.

She pastes the three cut-ups, the solicitor's letter, the adjuration to connect, the ode to Oneness, next to each other in the notebook.

She thinks: I am being unjust. I am not thinking clearly. I am accusing Forster and Lawrence of making me marry Nigel, out of some desire for Union of Opposites, of Only Connecting the Prose and the Passion. Whereas in fact, at least in part, I married him for exactly the opposite reason, because I wanted to keep things separate. I thought the sex was good, was satisfactory, which is better than good, and I think I thought that because he was rich, I wouldn't have to be a housewife like my mother. I thought all the other parts of myself could go on being what they were, and marrying Nigel would deal with negotiating sex, and with not being a housewife. I deserved what I got, whatever that was: it includes Leo, who is not a question of what I deserve, but of *his own life.*

But the desire to Only Connect, the romantic bit, that was there *too,* we are a mixture of impulses. Here I go again, connecting to John Ottokar, disconnected from him.

She writes a word, underlining it, as a title. *Laminations.* She senses the shape of a possible form, a space where a form will be, that is not yet there to be apprehended. *Laminations.* Cut-ups are part of it. It is a form that is made partly by cutting up, breaking up, rearranging things that already exist. "All writing is in fact cut-ups. A collage of words read overheard." These sentences of Burroughs's sent a spiky thrill of recognition through her brain. *The point of words is that they have to have already been used, they have not to be new, they have to be only re-arrangements, in order to have meaning.* If you write "ragdon" or "persent" those are nothing, but write "dragon" and "serpent" and the thoughts and stories and fears and inventions and colours and stinks and softnesses and violence of human beings everywhere drag and float at the end of them like giant kites sailing from thin strings or monsters of the deep caught on fishermen's lines. Where the cut-ups go wrong is in an over-valuation of the purely random, a too great reliance on the human capacity to insist on finding meaning in the trivial, the flotsam and jetsam of the brain's tick and tock, messages on scraps of paper with one word on. Anything is a message if you are looking for a message. But the glare of an eye looking for a message anywhere and everywhere can be a mad glare, a pointless glare.

She writes down, slowly, under *Laminations*:

> I found my own growing inclination, which I discovered was not mine alone, to look upon all life as a cultural product taking the form of mythic clichés, and to prefer quotations to independent invention. (Thomas Mann, *Die Entstehung des Dr. Faustus*)

Quotation is another form of cut-up; it gives a kind of papery vitality and independence to, precisely, cultural clichés cut free from the web of language that gives them precise meaning. The Mann quotation looks solemn and academic compared to the cut-ups, but it has more life in it. Or a different life. "Only connect" is a cliché, and so is Lawrence's Oneness; also they are ambiguous words of power. You could quote other things, Frederica thinks, as the beginning of the form of what will be *Laminations* goes in and out of focus in her mind's eye. You could quote newspapers. Dostoevski made his novels from the clichés and the reported facts that are newspapers. In this context even the *faux-naïf* style of "I did the things you do in the bathroom" would be one cliché amongst the rustling others, and therefore admissible, contained, laminated. She thinks: I need a card index, not a notebook, I need to shuffle. You could quote your own life. Lawyer's letters amongst lectures on Mann and Kafka. Raw material, worked motifs.

That week, she adds:

> James told of how, when walking on a summer evening in the park alone, watching the couples make love, he suddenly began to feel a tremendous oneness with the whole world, with the skies and trees and flowers and grass—with the lovers too. He ran home in panic and immersed himself in his books. He told himself he had no right to this experience, but more than that, he was terrified at the threatened loss of identity involved in this merging and fusion of his self with the whole world. He knew of no half-way stage between radical isolation in self-absorption or complete absorption into all there was. He was afraid of being absorbed into Nature, engulfed by her, with irrevocable loss of his self; yet what he most dreaded, that also he most longed for. Mortal beauty, so Gerard Manley Hopkins said, is dangerous. If such individuals could take his advice to meet it, then let it alone, things would be easier. But it is just this which they cannot do. (R. D. Laing, *Divided Self,* p. 91)

To this she adds:

> The god ascends the stage in the likeness of a striving and suffering individual. That he can *appear* at all with this clarity and precision is due to dream interpreter Apollo, who projects before the chorus its Dionysiac condition in this analogical figure. Yet in truth that hero is the suffering Dionysos of the mysteries. He of whom the wonderful myth relates that as a child he was dismembered by Titans now experiences in his own person the pains of individuation, and in this condition is worshipped as Zagreus. We have here

an indication that dismemberment—the truly Dionysiac suffering—was like a separation into air, water, earth and fire, and that individuation should be regarded as the source of all suffering, and rejected. (Nietzsche, *Birth of Tragedy*, p. 66)

And:

World declaration hot peace shower! Earth's grass is
free! Cosmic poetry Visitation accidentally happening
carnally! Spontaneous planet-chant Carnival! Mental
Cosmonaut poet-epiphany, immaculate supranational
Poesy insemination!
Skullbody love-congress Annunciation,
duende concordium, effendi tovarisch illumination,
Now! Sigmatic New Departures Residu of Better
Books & Moving Times in obscenely New Directions!
Soul revolution City Lights Olympian lamb-blast!
Castalia centrum new consciousness hungry
generation Movement roundhouse 42 beat
apocalypse energy-triumph!
You are not alone!
Miraculous assumption! O Sacred Heart invisible
insurrection! Albion! awake! awake! awake! O
shameless bandwagon! Self-evident for real naked
come the Words! Global synthesis habitual for this
Eternity! Nobody's Crazy Immortals Forever!

Esam, Fainlight, Ferlinghetti, Fernandez, Ginsberg, Paolo Lionni, Daniel Richter, Trocchi, Simon Vinkendog, Horovitz. Invocation to First International Poetry Incarnation at Albert Hall.

And:

Vladimir:	Rather they whisper.
Estragon:	They rustle.
V.	They murmur.
E.	They rustle.
	Silence
V.	What do they say?

E. They talk about their lives.
V. To have lived is not enough for them.
E. They have to talk about it.
V. To be dead is not enough for them.
E. It is not sufficient.
Silence
V. They make a noise like feathers.
E. Like leaves.
V. Like ashes.
E. Like leaves.

(*Waiting for Godot,* p. 63)

And:

The head Sublime, the heart Pathos, the genitals Beauty, the hands & feet Proportion.

As the air to a bird or the sea to a fish, so is contempt to the contemptible.

The crow wish'd every thing was black, the owl that every thing was white.

Exuberance is Beauty.

If the lion was advised by the fox, he would be cunning.

Improvement makes straight roads; but the crooked roads without Improvement are the roads of Genius.

Sooner murder an infant in its cradle than nurse unacted desires.

Where man is not, nature is barren.

Truth can never be told so as to be understood, and not be believ'd.

Enough! or Too much.

(Blake, *Marriage of Heaven and Hell,* Plate 10)

It is like any student's commonplace book. It rustles with uneasy energies. One night, on an impulse, Frederica adds an anecdote.

After the extra-mural class, in the pub, Humphrey Maggs told us the story of a friend of his whose mother died and left her nothing but debts and a bacon-slicer. She had had a shop which had gone bust, and all that was left was a bacon-slicer. She took it into the cold store of the butcher's shop, which was empty and about to be sold, and tried to slice her wrists with it. It was hard to get her wrists near the blade, and it was too cold in there for her to go on trying: she collapsed in there, in a mess of blood, "a welter of gore, you could say," he said. The cold stopped the blood running and "they" found her and took her to hospital. They tied her up and stitched her up. She liked it there. She became a hospital orderly and after a bit trained as a nurse. She works in an operating theatre. She likes that. She feels needed. No, I don't know what became of the bacon-slicer, he said when I asked him. I expect she sold it. I expect it's slicing bacon somewhere, doing what it was designed for.

This story is interesting because of the words bacon-slicer, and for that matter the thing to which they refer, a whirring blade with a precise function which is not self-slaughter. It is a tale of congruities and incongruities, perhaps spoiled by this excrescent commentary which I may learn to omit.

Two days later, she adds another.

A woman is sitting in Vidal Sassoon's salon, the Bond Street one. She is having her long hair, which she has always had, shorn into one of those smooth, swinging cuts, like blades in their precise edges and points. Two young men are working together on the nape of her neck. Her feet are surrounded by shanks and coils and wisps and tendrils of what until recently was her body. It sifts, it is soft, it pricks between her collar and her skin. One man leans over her and holds the two points of her new hair down, dragged down, to her jaw. He hurts her. If she tries to look up, he gives her a little push down again, which hurts her. The other works above the vertebrae of her naked nape with his pointed shears. She can hear the sound of hair on blade: a silky rasping. He nicks her skin with his points. He hurts her. She is almost sure that the small hurts are deliberately inflicted. Over her neck the two talk. "Look at that one then, look at her strut, she thinks she's the *bee's knees,* the *cat's whiskers* and she's a walking *disaster,* look at that clump he's done at the back, like a great *bubo* all bulging and she can't see it, she can't see it jiggle and wiggle as she walks, she thinks she looks *delicious,* he told her so, he held the mirror at the right angle, so she couldn't see what a godawful *mess* he had made, cutting higher and higher trying to make it better and now there's nothing left to cut, only a gob on the back of

> her *lumpy head.*" They laugh. The woman under their hands tries to look up and is jerked down. She thinks, I will always remember this, but doesn't know why; there are many humiliations, many disasters, why will she always remember this one? They let her head up. She sees her face through tears. The line is like a knife along her jaw. They tell her she looks lovely. All the women in the room have the same cut and all look lovely in the same way, except those who don't. When she moves her head, the curtain of her hair swings and re-forms into its perfect edge. Her neck is naked. She gives the two a tip, though she would like not to. Her hair looks good. Does she?

This is a distinct improvement on "I went to the bathroom": it has no "I" although it is a true story, and a story about Frederica. It gives her a quite disproportionate aesthetic pleasure, both because the words do not immediately nauseate her, and because she has somehow *got it right,* has pinned something down. (As the young men had her pinned down, she thinks, wondering if this is part of the pleasure.) The incident had rankled in her memory but is now pleasing and shapely. It gains something from being next to, but not part of, the cut-ups, the bacon-slicer, Nietzsche, Blake, and *The Divided Self.*

XV

October 1965

The extra-mural class is in full swing. Frederica is teaching Dostoevski and Thomas Mann, Kafka and Sartre. John Ottokar has not signed up for the current session, nor has he said anything to Frederica about this. Most of the rest of the class are there, at ease with each other now, knowing where to look for a response. Couples have formed, jealousies have deepened. Jude Mason has not returned, though his hippopotamus-grey skin can be seen shining under the red lights of the life-class studio at the Samuel Palmer School, and postcards with Nietzschean quotations appear in Frederica's pigeonhole there. Leo has made a friend at school who also lives in the square: a tall black boy with a broad gentle face, whose name is Clement Agyepong; he has a brother called Athanasius, a mother who is a nurse on night duty, and an occasional father, who "sells things." The Agyepongs are second-generation English, whose parents came from Ghana. Frederica likes Clement. Clement belongs to a gang of small boys who race around the square and are suspected of ringing door bells and running away, of twisting off windscreen wipers, nicking milk bottles and vandalising the window-boxes which are beginning to appear on the more gentrified houses, which have new white paint and new brass knockers, which are occasionally unscrewed. Frederica feels an emotion about Clement that she dare not describe to anyone. She is pleased that he and Leo *really like each other,* two boys playing and talking together. She is pleased that she herself likes Clement so much, laughs at his jokes, listens to his stories. She is pleased that her son has a black friend who is *a friend*. She is also pleased because before Clement was

Leo's friend, Leo had been knocked over by-accident-on-purpose once or twice, playing in the square. Dinky cars had gone out and had not come back. His tricycle disappeared and mysteriously re-appeared, without its bell, without the rubber treads on its pedals. These things worry Frederica. She fought her own battles at school, was bashed, bitten, tripped and torn. This is normal. But she always felt safe walking to school in the village as a small child, or riding into Blesford on the bus as a larger one. She wants to see Hamelin Square as an urban village, but it is not. It is less safe. She has not begun to imagine how much less safe she is—along with her contemporaries—going to feel it is. Urban fear in 1965 is a sprout, no more. She is more afraid of Nigel's solicitors finding out about the bicycle and the Dinky toys. Her bruised and tearful son, she thinks, wiping eyes and knees, could be cantering in the paddock on Sooty. Or being tortured by horrid sprogs in shorts in some prep school locker-room, she thinks, more darkly, offering home-made scones and jam to Clement, and reading *The Tale of Mr. Tod* to both boys.

Clement is collecting wood for the bonfire. It is traditional to have a Guy Fawkes bonfire on the earthy tip in the middle of Hamelin Square. The boys rush around to local shops, cadging vegetable crates and broken chairs. Too much cardboard is bad, Clement tells Agatha and Frederica, it flares up and flakes all over, you need wood that will burn steady. Nothing like car-seats that will stink, either, he says, good wood. The fathers, middle-class and working-class, bring contributions. One night the whole collection is stolen in the small hours, and never recovered, though expeditionary forces are sent out to inspect rival bonfires on local bombed sites and football fields. The collecting starts again and guards are mounted, little boys in the daytime, the odd lounging man in the dark. Leo is excited. He does not know what the bonfire will be but it fills his imagination with light on the night sky. He is desolated to find that the great day occurs in fact in the middle of one of his now regular weekend visits to Bran House. He tells Frederica he won't go. This is the first time he has made any demur about his movements between his parents. He comes back from Bran House white-faced and solemn, and says nothing of what he has done or said there. Frederica never asks him, and hopes that those in Bran House maintain the same discretion. She does not like to imagine Pippy Mammott or Olive and Rosalind asking probing questions about the William Blake School, or Clement, or John Ottokar, who has not been introduced to Leo, but has been seen by him, once or twice, sitting with Frederica—only sitting—after Leo has been safely tucked up in bed. Frederica *does not want to know* what Leo is being asked, and this deep desire for ignorance keeps her quiet. But she imagines, and is afraid. Out of what Leo might inadvertently say could be made the evidence on which he will be taken from her.

Leo says: I won't go there when it's the bonfire. *I won't.* Frederica says: You must. Leo says: I won't. I will see this bonfire, I *will be there.* Frederica says she expects there will be a bonfire at Bran House he can see. Leo works himself up into a breathless rage, wheezing and squealing, reminding Frederica of her father and herself. She says, "I *can't* ask your father." Leo says, "You can. You just won't." "Daren't," says Frederica. "You hate me, you don't love me, you don't want me," shrieks her son in his wrath. Frederica telephones Arnold Begbie, who replies, after an exchange of letters, that he is told there will be an excellent bonfire, a positive beacon, in Herefordshire. Leo has another tantrum and ceases to speak. He does not speak for twenty-four hours. The next evening, Frederica comes in with his supper to hear him speaking on the telephone.

"You told me. *You* told me how to make the number. In case I ever wanted you, you said, and I do want you. I want to go the bonfire *here* in vis square. We're building it."

He listens.

"No, Mummy doesn't *want* me to stay here, she says I can't, she says she doesn't want me."

He listens.

"I know. It would be nice there, too. But I've *set my heart* on vis bonfire."

Frederica admires his phrase. I've set my heart.

"I told you, she doesn't want me to stay. Otherwise, I wouldn't need to telephone, would I? She isn't *reasonable,* you know she isn't. She doesn't understand how much I *really need to* see vis bonfire with my friends. She thinks you won't understand I only want to see vis bonfire, but I know you will understand. You do, don't you?"

He listens.

"So I can stay? *Thank you.* I knew you'd understand. I'll find her. You'll talk to her, you'll *tell* her. Just *tell* her. Here she is."

"Frederica?"

"Yes."

"What is all this? What have you been doing to him? Why can't he see this bonfire he's set his heart on?"

"I thought you would want to hold to your weekend."

"And have him think I'm a tyrant. Weekends can be changed, can't they? If he wants something so much, he ought to be able to ask for it, without you riding roughshod over him. *Can't* you have him, or something? What are you doing?"

"Of course I can have him. I can always have him. I just—"

"I expect you had something else on. As far as I'm concerned, he's welcome to stay for the bonfire. I'll have him the weekend before, that suits me quite well, I've got things in Holland . . . Never mind that. Same arrangement, weekend earlier. Put him back on."

"Thank you," says Leo. "I knew you'd make it all right."

The phone makes a gratified quacking.

Frederica goes crossly into the kitchen.

Leo comes back from his next visit to Bran House with his red hair shorn and shaved, so that his pale crown shows through. Frederica is horrified. She catches him up in her arms—he clings, as he always does, tight, choking tight. She says, "Oh, what have they done to you?"

"Pippy said I looked like a little girl. Like a fairy, she said, or one of those hippies. She said she'd make a little man of me."

"Do you like it?"

"Not much. I feel a bit cold. I fink I look a bit silly. Clement's hair's short, though. His is curly. Mine was all floppy. I ought to have gone to the hairdresser, Pippy said."

"You don't like the hairdresser."

"No. I don't like those clipper things on my neck. Pippy did it with scissors and a razor. She said, 'Admire my handiwork.' Everyone did admire it. But it is a bit cold and I look a bit sort of skull-like. But it'll grow, won't it?"

"It will."

Clement and Athanasius, known as Thano, have also made a Guy, which they push around the local streets in a broken pushchair. "Penny for the Guy," they say at the mouth of the local Tube, at the entry to Hamelin Square. The body of the Guy is made from an old stained, tea-leaf-coloured pillow, clothed in a green-and-orange shirt covered with parrots and palm trees. It has a limp pair of pink rubber gloves pinned to its "shoulders," and a pair of diminutive infant's plimsolls, cracked and holed, propped at the base of its lolling trunk. It has a paper mask-face, done on bright orange shiny paper with black felt-tips, round eyes with long, spiky cartoon lashes, a bravado curly moustache. This is tied to a punctured football, on top of which sits an old baseball cap, with the legend SUNRISE RISE AND SHINE! on its brow. Agatha, confronted by this vision at the mouth of the Tube, studies it critically.

"OK, I'll give you a sixpence, because you have done some work. Someone tried to get money out of me for a Daz box with a smiley-face drawn on it. But I can't bear your Guy's horrible armlessness and leglessness. Bring him round this evening and we'll see what we can do." Clement and Thano duly appear with their creaking conveyance, and Agatha helps them to stuff and stitch old tights with waste paper—the Guy's new legs have a certain androgynous curvaceousness, and his arms are plump and solid. Agatha tells Frederica that she was filled with pity and terror at the sight of the dangling gloves, "like parody thalidomide sufferers." She hates the whole business of Guys, she says, the whole idea of celebrating the burning of a minor conspirator, all those centuries ago. I know, says Frederica, but I remember what fun it all was, after the war, when I was little, when we had fireworks again. I don't want them *not* to have what we had. And then you think, how dreadful, a man's fingers and innards all bursting and sizzling, the *pain,* how can we? I know, says Agatha.

The characters of *Flight North* have reached what appears to be an impassable wall of icy rock, sheer, glassy, frozen, louring. They are based in the Last Village, a tiny community which lives in ice huts around a very small geyser in a very small lake in the midst of a frozen waste. In the depths of the lake, in the warm waters, swim shoals of coral-coloured shrimp and steel-blue darting fish, which the people eat sparingly, on certain feast days only. They are globular people, with lovely bracelets of shining fat round their wrists and elbows and knees; they have rose-red faces with round apple cheeks, framed in furry hoods made from the skins of bears and foxes and martens; they look cheerful, but are not. The company of travellers or fugitives has been augmented considerably: they have acquired an ancient, draggled Thrush, who speaks when he chooses, which is not often; a Crow, whose speech is understood only by Artegall, who does not entirely trust it; a strange hound, grey and frequently invisible, which Saskia believes will turn out to be a Wolf; and a strange creature found by Mark in a cave on a moor, which sometimes appears to be a squat toad-like minor dragon, and sometimes is clearly only a lump of flinty stone with glinting silica in the ledges under what appear to be its "brows." It is about the size of a large tom-cat, and in its stony form heavy. Mark, who mostly has to carry it, is often ready to abandon it, but the Thrush says its moment will come, and it has various useful gifts, like the power to start fires in wet wood. The most recent recruit is called Fraxinius, and moves in and out of resembling a human being as Dracosilex moves from stone to reptile. Fraxinius is one and a half times as tall as the men of the party, and skeletally thin and gangling. Everything about him is pale buffs and browns and straw colours—his eyes, his caramel-coloured teeth, his ivory lips, his bushy hay-coloured brows, his barley-sugar smoking eyes, his shoulder-length, knotted, mud-coloured hair "like a hillside which has lain under snow." He can appear to resemble a broom, or a besom, or a clothes pole, and moves, when he can be seen to move, slow and creaking, but when he is not watched, or seen out of the corner of an eye, he appears to bundle along weightlessly, like tangled straw on the wind. The Last Village suits neither Fraxinius nor Dracosilex. Fraxinius spends his time slumped like a broken ladder in a corner of a hut, growing paler and drier in the smoke from the perpetual central hearth. Dracosilex squats like a boring stone. The Thrush has its head under its wing. The Crow reports that the inhabitants of the Last Village are building a great fire on the mountain ledge near the black ice-wall of the escarpment.

Clement and Thano have taken to listening to the story. Saskia originally objected to this but has come round—they share not her private night-time narration but a kind of bumper recapitulation and—almost always—dramatic Shock—which is narrated on Sunday afternoons. Agatha says that the requirement of the Sunday Shock is formally very satisfying, no doubt like constructing episodes of novels like *The Idiot* or *Dombey and Son*. The story does not usually have anything to do with the daily lives of its narrator or listeners, but in this case the Bale Fire has been growing *pari passu* with the bonfire in the mud in the centre of Hamelin Square.

Agatha sits on the sofa, in a black velvet top like a mediaeval page's surcoat, and a pair of silvery knitted trousers. Her dark hair is loose and falls about her face. Saskia is curled up against her. Clement and

Thano sit side by side on the floor by the fire. Frederica and Leo are in an armchair.

"Mark and Artegall offered to help with the collection of wood, but the villagers refused sullenly, saying their fire was their own handiwork. They travelled long distances in search of the wood, which had to be dead and dry; they dragged it back on rough sledges they made from poles tied together with hide. There were not many trees on the Grüner Waste; what there were were stunted thorn bushes, tenacious of life, leaning along the wind which always blew through their fingers, full of ice crystals, which settled there like an encrustation of diamonds.

"Dol Throstle made friends with an old village woman called Throgga, who lay muffled and wheezing in a heap of skins by the fire, toasting fragments of goat-cheese in its embers, or drowsing. None of the villagers talked to Throgga; they brought her beakers of water, and sometimes the leg of a roasted rat or rabbit, but they treated her otherwise as if she was not there. For this reason, perhaps, she was glad to talk to Dol Throstle, and told her tales about the Bale Fire.

" 'It is always set alight an hour before midnight on the Longest Night,' said the old woman. 'In good years, we cook a feast of roots and baked scones and roast ptarmigan in its embers at dawn. If it burns very bright, it is a sign that there will be Spring. We do not have Spring every year here, you must understand. Some of the young things cannot remember Spring. But in *good years* Spring comes and the sun is hot and golden for a day, or a few days, or even a few weeks, and all sorts of herbs and flowers and bushes spring out of the ice, which runs away in little rushing rivers full of cresses—and the sky is the colour of a thrush's egg, not the iron colour it is now.'

" 'It will be hard for the fire to burn at all this year,' says Dol Throstle. 'Out there there is nothing but sleet, icy rain, cold and running and freezing when it gets darker.'

" 'They cover the Wood with skins,' says Throgga. 'But the damp gets in, and a wet wind can prevent the fire from taking hold.' "

There are steps on the stairs. A head comes round the door, blond, smiling a little. It is John Ottokar.

"I knocked," he says. "No one answered."

"We are listening to this story," says Leo, reproving.

John Ottokar takes off his duffel coat. He is wearing his brilliant patchwork sweater. He takes a step into the circle.

"Can I stay and listen?" he says. "Don't mind me. I'll just sit here. Is that all right?"

He is courteous, he looks tentatively at Agatha, he sits down on the carpet beside Frederica's armchair. Her dangling hand brushes the thick pale hair. Agatha is mildly put out. She flushes. I don't know, she says. *Go on,* say Saskia, Leo and Clement. Agatha shrugs and goes on. Throgga tells how the young men must leap the burning fire. The higher it is when they leap it, the brighter the coming year will be. The weather deteriorates.

"Never had the travellers seen such rain, a rain of ice, of hailstones, of sheets of frozen slush, which turned the walls of the snow-huts to dripping glaciers in the brief daytime and to casques of ice at night, which burned any unwary finger that came near their surfaces. The villagers began to look unpleasantly at the Company: they began to say they had brought ill luck and that the Fire would never light whilst they were there. Throgga told Dol Throstle there was secret talk of driving them away, back into the Grüner Waste. Or worse, Throgga said, but would not say what 'worse' was."

John Ottokar sighs, an exhausted sigh, and leans his head back against the arm of Frederica's chair. The story moves on: the villagers mutter, and when the day for the Bale Fire comes, their tinder is wet and the brands they try to take from the huts to the high ledge with the fire on it, sputter and die in the wet wind. The Crow tells Artegall that Dracosilex can light the Bale Fire, and Artegall replies testily that no doubt he could, if he were in his reptile form, but he is a stone and nothing but a stone, and there is no art to revive him.

" 'There is a way,' said the Crow. 'You must take him to the geyser and bathe him in its warm waters, and wash him, and turn him, and he will become flesh again. For he is a salamander and salamanders are at home in the hot depths of geysers: they become lively, there.'

"So the two boys carried the heavy stone down to the geyser lake and plunged their arms into its warm, bubbling depths, holding the stone being very carefully, and lapping the water round him. And their fingers felt the cold stone quicken, and become rough skin, and twitch, and they felt a heartbeat, and the thrum of blood, and the stone toad put out thrusting little legs, and a stubby tail, which had never previously manifested itself, and it twisted out of their clutching hands and pushed off purposefully into the depths.

"There was a long silence, broken only by the bubbling of the geyser in the pool.

" 'He likes it down there,' Mark said. 'It makes him lively. I expect he'll stay for ever and eat shrimps.'

"Artegall hung over the pool, staring down through steam and troubled water and saw two bright golden eyes staring up at him.

" 'Dracosilex, Dracosilex, come up and help us light the fire.'

"And slowly the beast returned to them, lithe now and shining, fiery-crested and gleaming olive-gold. Artegall received him in his arms and wrapped him in his own coat, and hurried across the icy scrub and up the mountain, steaming from exertion and because of the heat of the wet creature in his wet coat in his arms.

"The villagers were gathered in the driving sleet, staring at the great beacon of wood, which was well built, but soaked through in its upper layers. One of the men said that never, even in the worst year in human memory, had the fire refused to light at all. One said that there should be seven different kinds of wood in the fire, and only six were certainly there, with a doubtful twig or two that might or might not be the seventh, horn-wood, a wood of a forest tree rarely found and susceptible to frosts. Artegall came forward and said that if it was permitted for him to intervene, he had a way to light the Bale Fire. One old man said it could only ever be lit by a brand from the ashes of the fire which had been lit last year from the ashes of last year's Bale Fire. One old woman asked Artegall, what was his way, and he opened his jacket, which smelled slightly scorched, and there was the lively creature, glowing red and gold like coals under his craggy grey-green skin. And the old woman said the dragon was a Sending, a magic gift that should be accepted, and the old man said it was dangerous magic which would threaten their traditional ways. But the people were cold and despondent in the rain and snow, and perhaps for that reason the old woman's enthusiasm prevailed over the natural sluggishness of the villagers. So Artegall was permitted to put Dracosilex on the stone ledge near the fire, and he set him down, and asked him to do what he could, to help if he might, and stepped back. And Dracosilex squatted there, glowing on the iron earth, and swayed a little, and opened his mouth, and sighed a great sigh. And out of his mouth, like the tongue of a chameleon, came a sinuous noose of what seemed to be liquid flame, which wrapped itself round the Bale Fire, and again, and again, three times, in a coil. And Dracosilex closed his mouth again, but the liquid thread of flame hung there on the wet wood, and there was a spitting and hissing and a steaming and a sizzling, and the wood began to sprout buds and shoots of flames, which crackled and caught. And soon the whole fire was roaring and blazing so that no force on earth could have stopped it.

"Never was seen such a fire! The villagers roasted meats and made lardy cakes of fat and flour in its outreaches, and from its summit great blades of flame, red and yellow shot with emerald and bright blue, painted the dark sky and flickered bravely in the diminishing sleet, and wrinkled and waved in the wind. All night they danced, and when it was still quite high, towards dawn, the young men began to leap the flames, dropping pebbles, some black, some white, into the embers as they leaped. And some of the women and girls leaped, too—they all wore trousers, in that country, for the cold made nonsense of skirts—and the watching crowd began a growling, rolling kind of song, to a small drum and a bone pipe, as the leaping grew faster and more furious, and a kind of stamping dance took up the new rhythm. And one hot girl took Mark's hand, and made him jump with her; he was afraid, high above the heat, with the tongues of flame reaching up for him from the cauldron of coals, and he came through with singed eyebrows, and smoky lashes, and tears in his eyes. And Artegall took a little run, and leaped, just high enough, and landed in ash, spraying himself with sparking cinders. And two great men lifted Dol Throstle high in the air as though she was an inflated skin bottle, and she closed her eyes, and felt the heat, and opened them, and saw the cold black night glistening against the firelight. And then two of the young men appeared, when everyone had jumped, half-leading, half-dragging, half-carrying the fragile fawn body of Fraxinius. Dol Throstle stepped forward then, and said that it wasn't right to make the creature jump; he wasn't well, as could be seen, and was dry as tinder, and not part of the community. But they said he must jump, he was the last, he must go over. He stood there, drowsed or dazed it seemed, with his knotty locks hanging on his shoulders, and his thin arms dangling at his side. And then he said, in his strange whistling voice, 'I am agreeable.'

" 'We'll drag you out, if you fall,' said the village lads, not too pleasantly, for everyone had in their mind a vision of the conflagration that would follow if this desiccated being were to tumble on hot coals. And Dol Throstle said again, 'He's so dry, he'll *attract* the fire, the flames'll go for him.'

"And the old woman said, 'The flames only go for whom they choose. They will let him pass, unless they choose him.'

" 'I am agreeable,' said the thin creature again, and he shook off the hands of those who held him, and set off in an ungainly shamble towards the Bale Fire.

"And when he came to it, he took a leap, and rose high, high, like a dry leaf in the current of an updraught, and seemed to float and sail against the night sky, which was now paler, deep blue, not black. He hung above the burning logs like a great bat or owl, and they all cried out, at his lightness, at his ease, at his weightlessness. And then he came eddying down, not on the other side, but on to the coals, into the very heart of the fire. And the fire took hold of him greedily, and took energy from him. He blazed—hair, hands, arms—and a wild smoke enveloped his blazing form. Dol Throstle began to weep, and Mark set forward to rescue him, calling for help. But Fraxinius stood there and blazed, and as he blazed, he changed beneath their eyes, drawing energy and form from the flames, which drew energy and form from him. In the red light he became green; his muddy hair became a curtain of new tendrils and new leaves; his outstretched twiggy arms put out shoots of green and his legs became thick, green, living trunks, upholding a body pliable and liquid, emerald and mossy, above which was a smiling green-gold mask from the eyes and mouth of which sprouted young green shoots, and above which twined a crown of shining leaves. And when he was fully grown, he strode out of the fire, with long, sure steps, a tall shimmering green figure with a mane of emerald hair, who wore a cloak of flames which enveloped him and floated after him in the air. And he strode away from the company and away from the folk of the Last Village, and came to the impassable rock face, and put his hand against it. And where he put his hand there was a rushing of green flaming water and melted ice, and thaw of molten rock, which ran away like lava. And the rock face dissolved, or split, into a high, narrow passage, inside which granite steps led into a tunnel apparently walled with thick pillars and, as it were, twisted hanks or root masses all made of green, green ice that gave off light in sparkings as he came near it, and reflected the movement of his flaming leaves as he passed. And he went into the roots of the mountain, and they saw his bright conflagration wink and diminish as he went on into the depths, shining and striding.

"And when he had gone, the fire was dimmed, and the sky was fiery with the dawn, and the crack in the mountain was dark and dangerous, but it was not closed."

Agatha invites everyone to Sunday brunch. John Ottokar says he would love to stay; he and Agatha smile at each other. Frederica is partly pleased—she would like John Ottokar to know Leo in a quiet and uncomplicated and uncompromised way. She is grateful to Agatha. She sees that John Ottokar sees that Agatha is beautiful. She gets up to help Agatha to make the impromptu meal. She herself could not provide one: she has eggs, a little cheese, fruit, two pieces of chicken. Agatha makes a large salad, with fish, and beans, and eggs, and green things and tomatoes. Clement and Thano say they have to go home. They have to go to church, they say vaguely. They are

Catholics, but not Catholics who abjure Guy Fawkes Day. Agatha says she will make pancakes to follow the salad. Frederica beats the batter. Agatha says: "He seems to be a nice young man."

"He comes and goes."

"That's OK, isn't it?"

"I don't know when he will come or go."

"Do you want to?"

"I don't *want to* want to. I don't want him to matter that much, too much. I can't afford . . ." She doesn't finish that sentence. She starts another. "But it isn't very *convenient,* not knowing from one day to the next, whether someone will come or not."

"Can't you ask?"

"I don't think so." She thinks. "I don't know that any answer I'd get would mean anything."

"Things you don't know," says Agatha, "take up energy, they rankle in the mind. Best not to let them. A counsel of perfection, I do know."

"He's nice, though."

"He's certainly beautiful. And seems nice enough, yes."

Frederica thinks that Agatha never has any men visiting, young or old. You would think, she thinks, that Saskia had been produced by parthenogenesis. But that can't be. There is, or was, someone, somewhere. Will she ever be told? Frederica is beginning to doubt it.

In Agatha's sitting-room, John Ottokar is teaching Leo and Saskia a game. Scissors, paper, stone. "You put out your hands together," he says. "*Simultaneously,*" Leo says. "Simultaneously," John Ottokar agrees. His smooth gold hair falls forwards over his brow. He shows them. A flat hand, paper. Forked fingers, scissors. A clenched fist, stone. Scissors cut paper, stone blunts scissors, paper wraps stone. The children are entranced. They play quite differently. Leo changes his shape at each game: he is stone scissors stone paper scissors paper stone paper. Saskia holds on to one form patiently: paper paper paper paper, then suddenly scissors, then stone stone stone stone stone, scissors. John Ottokar laughs and keeps the score. "I played this when I was your age," he tells them. "With my brother."

"Who won?" says Leo.

"No one," says John Ottokar. "We always put out the same thing. Identical. Two scissors, two stones, two papers."

"Boring," says Leo.

"Not exactly. Frustrating, though. Not exactly *playing.*"

"Like when Leo and me make the same noise on the recorder 'cause we only know C and B," says Saskia.

"A bit like that," says John Ottokar. "We used to play the recorder, too."

He stays and plays, quietly, all afternoon. He cuts out newspaper trees with scissors, he glues cut-out dinosaurs in a book, he talks easily to Agatha and Frederica. He stays to supper and helps put Leo to bed, sitting in the corner of Leo's bedroom, out of the light, and listening whilst Frederica reads about Moldy Warp and Fuzzypeg and the old Roman coin. When Leo is tucked in bed, he follows Frederica into her own room, draws the blind, and touches her on the shoulder. Frederica, preoccupied, turns to face him. He puts a hand on her neck, sure, and a hand on her buttocks, sure, and his mouth on hers, gathering her body into his. His skin warms hers and sets it alight. Shafts of lightning run up her spine. She leans back releasing her mouth, to say thickly, "It isn't *fair.*"

"What is? What isn't, what's worrying you, nothing must, nothing must."

He is doing what he can to make their clothed bodies one.

"We *can't.* Leo. Leo. I can't. You can't just."

"OK. Just sit down and keep still with me then. Keep still."

They subside on to the couch. Unsatisfied desire has its own *frisson,* its own bliss. They enjoy it. They do not undress, they do not make love. So that when Leo wanders vaguely in, saying he cannot sleep, there is nothing untoward, no whiff of salt, no exposed organs he should not see, but a large man smiling in a jester's sweater, and a thin red-headed woman in a chocolate-brown shirt over lilac velvet pants.

They do not talk, much. They sit, next to each other. At midnight, John Ottokar leaves. At the foot of the area steps Frederica says, "Leo will be away next weekend. You could come here . . ."

"I can't." At first it seems that he is going to leave it at that. Then he says, "I've got to go on a kind of religious retreat. There's a group. Some of them Quakers, some of them from Ceylon, and some doctors. Some doctors. It's a new thing. I—I go sometimes. I'm expected. Next weekend, I'm expected."

"Where?" says Frederica, who dares not say "Why?"

"Does it matter? There's a kind of Retreat House called Tanglewood, in a Quaker village in Bucks, called Four Pence. I know it sounds dreadfully twee. Names don't matter, words don't matter, if they do, you can change them. I'd tell you about it, but I rather suspect you won't like it, you won't want to know. Religion isn't your thing."

"I'm not *hostile* to religion."

"Aren't you? Think about it, and tell me next time, what you think about religion. I'm hostile to it myself, half the time. But it's there, you can't deny it's there."

"I don't try to."

He looks at her as though she is the world's greatest nay-sayer. He says, "I know I ought not to tell you. I'm under instructions not to—"

"John!"

"You see. You don't like it."

"How do I know what I—? When you don't?"

"We shouldn't have started this conversation. My fault. Come here. Hold on to me. Don't talk. That's better. Now, *this* is real, whatever *that* is. *This* is real."

Her alarmed body does not tingle as it did. He strokes her spine and the flame lies low, flickers sullenly. He puts his warm, mute hand suddenly, swiftly, between her legs, holds her gently, waits for the shift in her pulse, the very slight relaxation of her tense muscles, and says, "This is real. Remember. Now I'm going."

He goes.

Frederica is on the whole pleased that John Ottokar has met Leo in this public, uncompromised way. This is more because she does not enjoy the fact that her relations with John Ottokar have a clandestine and furtive aspect than because she wants to establish any *particular* rapport between son and lover. She does not want to include John Ottokar in any tentative trio, man, woman, child. Nobody wants that. She wants things to be easy and friendly. So she is pleased when John returns once or twice more when Leo and Saskia and Agatha are there. They go once, even, to the Natural History Museum, two women, John Ottokar, the boy, the dark little girl. She feels something discreet and stable and mature is being set up. One evening, over supper, she says to Leo, "Shall we ask John Ottokar to the bonfire?"

Leo says, "No. I don't like John Ottokar."

"Oh, Leo. Why? He taught you scissors, paper, stone—"

"He makes horrible scary faces at me when no one's looking."

"He doesn't—"

"Through the window. Bits of him go white. Sneery faces."

"Why should he do that?"

"And I don't like his smell. He has a bad smell."

"Leo!"

"You asked me. You did ask me. If you want him at ve bonfire, you ask him. I expect the smell won't be too bad out there, not with all the smoke and stuff."

"I won't ask him, if you feel like that."

"I don't feel like anything. I just told you. I just told you, *he stinks.*"

Frederica wonders about discussing with Agatha the possibility that Leo is reacting to herself, John Ottokar, and the smell of sex, even though they have been so careful. Or maybe he simply said the worst thing he could think of—which has certainly been effective, if he did, for Frederica now never thinks of John Ottokar without wondering about the smell, real or fantasised, and of *what*?

Bonfire Night arrives. Agatha and Frederica have been visited by Giles and Victoria Ampleforth, the owners of the pretty white-painted corner-house in Hamelin Square with its vandalised window-boxes, its renovated Georgian shutters, its polished brass knocker. Giles and Victoria want to join in the fun, want to contribute, do not want to be rejected by the other inhabitants of the square, for they know they represent gentrification, which the local Labour Party vociferously opposes, though its councillors, or some of them, and even some Labour MPs are "doing up" the pretty terraced houses in the sallow and sullen squares of south-east London. Giles is an architect, lean and apologetic; his dusty thatched head and horn-rimmed stare do in fact cover a resolute intention to restore, beautify, *save* all the houses in Hamelin Square. Victoria is the proprietor of a children's boutique, Rags, Tags and Velvet Gowns, which sits oddly in the local row of shops between a ferocious Cockney greengrocer and a Pakistani chemist's shop. She sells fancy dresses and sweaters, and a stock of fat and grinning stuffed lions and tigers and polar bears, home-made and full of bounce. Giles wants to be friends with the Agyepongs and the Utters, a huge matriarchal society of the unemployed, who live behind grimy brocade curtains in Number 17, apparently with no furniture and no carpets, though occasional chairs are hurled through windows, some of which now form part of the base of the bonfire. Victoria has made bowls full of hot cider with bobbing frothy apples in it, and trays of dark, burned, sticky toffee. She is afraid it will be rejected, does not want to bring it out. Agatha says, Nothing venture, nothing win, and, Everybody *always* likes toffee. But the middle-class households lurk behind their shutters until the festivities have started, which they do when Kieran Utter sets light to the petrol-soaked brown paper at the centre of the pyre, and a roar of flame leaps upwards. Rockets go up from various areas, and patches of red sizzling light, green fountains of sparks, silver geysers, hiss and flare and vanish into black velvet. Frederica and Leo bring out Leo's box of Roman candles and Vesuvius fountains and peacocks. Leo and Saskia hold sparklers, and wave them solemnly. Someone screams; something hisses. The fire catches and begins to crack and gleam. People come out and stand and stare into it; children run squealing, hide behind cars; Victoria Ampleforth picks up courage and goes round the square with a tray of toffee which everyone accepts happily. She picks up more courage and brings out a stout folding table, behind which she sets up her stall with her hot cider and a collection of Polish enamelled mugs, scarlet and green and blue. The sky is full of puce rain, it is full of silver arrows falling, it is full of humming blue flies. The Guy—Clement and Thano's Guy—has been built into the pyre in a rotting wicker chair, to which he is tied with string and old knitting wool. "Like a Druid sacrifice," Agatha says; he lolls and smiles, the flames not yet near him. "It's a good thing there's no wind," says Giles Ampleforth. "This thing is far too big for this square. We ought to have water buckets around."

"Mrs. Kennet has got her hose attached in her kitchen," says Carole Utter. "As per usual." She takes a swig from a beer bottle. "Two kids got their hair burned last year, and a car got its paint blasted."

"I don't know whose that little Austin is," says Victoria. "It's always parked here, but it doesn't belong to any of the residents."

Frederica brings out a basket of oven-roasted chestnuts, which are also acceptable to everyone. Leo says he wants a banger, and Frederica tells him he doesn't.

The sky is a gold meadow full of crimson serpents; it is a huge fan of silver fronds; it is indigo lit with orange and sepia and hot yellow and scarlet.

They drink hot cider, plastic cups of red wine from a box with a spigot, bottles of ale, Tizer by mistake, Coke and rum, sweet sherry, advocaat. Clement and Thano have got strings of Chinese firecrackers; Brian Utter attaches one to the branch of a tree near the little Austin, where it bangs and splutters and crackles and twists, causing Leo to burst into tears, and a small bald-headed man with a moustache to cry out, "Mind my car!"

The fire is now producing clouds of smoke. It is difficult to see across the square. People are linking arms and singing—"Oh my darling Clementine," the only song the English can ever get very far with. Across the square, through the smoke, Frederica sees John Ottokar, in his many-coloured patchwork jumper; he is bending to set light to something; he straightens up, and waves at her through the grey billows. She makes her way round to him, with smarting eyes. Whatever he has lit does not rush into the air or explode into shimmers of light. It burns sullenly, a tallish thing, producing a blue flame like a cowl around it.

"Skoob," says John Ottokar. It is a new art-form. Book-burning. "Books" backwards. Frederica does not like it. The books are lurid paperbacks. The top one has a pair of breasts bursting out of black lace and a vanishing face above them. The next one down, however, is Tillich's *The Ground of Our Being* and below that, Bishop Robinson's *Honest to God*.

"I don't like book-burning," says Frederica.

"That's why Skoob," says John Ottokar. "No point burning things nobody cares about."

He raises a glass of ink-dark wine to the Guy.

"Here's to him. He had the right idea. Explode it all. From underneath. Then there's a chance of living a real life. Up in flames. Theophany."

"You're drunk."

"Oh no. You may be. Let's dance."

He links arms with a swaying line of residents, and pushes his other arm through Frederica's. She smells his armpits, acrid, sour, and another smell, thick incense, musky, sweet, sweet. She tries to pull away, and he pulls her tightly to him, his head back, his lovely face ruddy in the reflected flames.

"Let's dance."

Through the smoke, on the other side of the bonfire, she sees John Ottokar in his multi-coloured sweater.

She has failed a test she was waiting for.

. . .

Little black boys, little white boys with sooty faces, rush like imps, widdershins, as John Ottokar comes round and links arms with Frederica on his left, and the population of Hamelin Square sway, amiably drunken, and sing. "We'll take a cup of kindness yet/For the sake of Auld Lang Syne."

XVI

Towards midday on the second day, the Lady Roseace and the young Narcisse paused in their headlong flight to allow their horses to breathe, and to give some relief to their own bodies. It was a late spring day, full of hope; they had come through the neck of the mountain pass, and were on a fair plain, where delicious little bosky groves mixed with springing cornfields and hay meadows. In every tree the birds sang as though their tiny throats would burst with the passage of the trills and whistles and gobblings and gurglings of their invariant musical phrases. Butterflies fluttered from flower to flower, or floated along the meadow borders. Crickets rubbed their dry legs monotonously against their thoraxes. The travellers found a stone basin, into which a fountain ran between mossy stones, and a wild cherry tree, full of fruit, with which Narcisse filled his hat, whilst the Lady Roseace brought out the wine and water flasks, their stock of biscuits and sausages and dried cheese. They were out of the environs of La Tour Bruyarde. They were free, and expected their free food to taste delectable, and so it did. They were free, and so they looked at each other with a new curiosity, dusty and travel-stained as they necessarily were. In the old days, the young Narcisse's face had been almost too extravagantly lovely, a gold-skinned shield-shape surrounded by luxuriant blue-black curls like clustering grapes. His huge dark eyes, too, had been like grapes, with those long, glistening lashes and perfectly curved wine-dark brows which many women would give much, in cash or kind, to have naturally, and which are almost always the prerogative of the male sex. His cheeks were lovely planes and his chin a perfect, gravely pretty triangle, above which, in the old days, his mouth had had a suspicion of a sulky swelling, a youthful push of a pout. But hard experience had ironed out the roundnesses and plumpnesses and soft dimple-pits of that boyish beauty and replaced it with a melancholy gentleness, a droop of the upper lip, a tension in the lower, that the Lady Roseace found more interesting and more attractive than his primitive self-conscious loveliness. His teeth, as he bit into his biscuit, were as white and even as they had ever been. His neck was strong now; there were muscles under the skin, like a young stag rather than the soft fawn or silken porcelet he had then resembled.

As for the lady herself, she had worn less well, and kept her face in the shadow of her hood, and her back to the sun as she ate. Her flesh, too, had tightened and pulled, in the curious and wonderful and terrible days of La Tour Bruyarde, and she had visible tendons and moving muscles where no woman was expected to have them who had been properly nurtured in milk and silk; she had lines on the surface that were more *indecent*, that is to say, *improper*, than the exposure of pretty nipples or a round white belly would have been, for youth is and was a woman's best ornament, and this should never be forgotten, particularly by women no longer young. And those pretty nipples, to tell the truth, those rosy buttons of bliss, were not now what they had been, but had slipped, so to speak, down the slopes of the blue-veined alabaster mounds of her breasts, which had themselves slipped, slipped, so that there were fissures and tiny ravines, declines and cuts and crackings in the heaving surface, which was now more like chamois leather (a pretty substance) than heaped snow, or ripe peaches, or whatever other delicate simile excites my reader. But under her travelling gown, her corset gave a youthful apple-shape to these hidden blown roses, and her waist was wonderfully trim, and her thighs, too lean perhaps for the taste of that time, promised for that reason a performative agility, a delectable grip and spring. So thought Narcisse, considering what he could see, and imagining amiably (and generously) what he could not.

"We shall come to look back on these past days as a bad dream," said the Lady Roseace, nibbling a sausage, toying with a cherry.

"We must not forget them, ever," said the young Narcisse. "For there is a lesson to be learned—about excess, about the metamorphosis of freedom into humiliation and slavery. We must go into the world and preach moderation in all things."

"As for me," said the Lady Roseace, "I mean to become a Quietist, a Retired Person in a rosy cottage far from the rut and muck of human conflict. You may preach if you will, but I shall abstain, from everything, *everything*, including preaching."

"You are too lovely to abstain from *everything*," said the young Narcisse, congratulating himself on abstaining from the treacherous phrase "*still* too lovely."

The Lady Roseace met his eye sadly and sweetly.

"Truly *everything*," she said with her lips, and who knows, with her will too, but the young Narcisse read a different message in the disposition of her limbs on the grassy bank where she sat. And he rose up, and went off into the wood, to relieve his bladder and prepare his instrument for singleness of purpose.

And the Lady Roseace lay back peacefully in the grassy hammock and thought she heard laughter in the air. She thought she heard a kind of yelping laughter, and the babble of many excited voices, and a kind of interwoven music of song and cry and howl. And the clear note, liquid and clamant, of a horn. And she thought, lying there, It is the lord of these fields, out hunting for his pleasure. And she knew it was not. And she hoped, as the excited babble grew nearer, that it would pass by the grove where she was partly hidden. And she knew it would not.

When Culvert rode into the clearing the Lady Roseace's dress was covered with the bloody slaver of the hounds' jowls, and her sleeve was torn and bloody where she had fought them off, and her dress too was torn, between her bubs, to her crotch. And she tried to hold it together, and he said, "I have seen you, more than enough, there is no need for modesty. Let it flap."

"Not modesty. Decency," said the Lady Roseace.

"You have no right to be decent, and no need, where you are going, which is where you have come from, where the idea of *decency* was long ago done away with."

And the Lady Roseace said, "My dear friend Culvert, whom once I loved as I love my own skin, to save whom I would once gladly have died and thought my life well given, why do you seek to prevent me from leaving La Tour Bruyarde? I am not going to your enemies, for your enemies are my enemies, and if they find me, they will do to me what they would do to you, for we were once one, as you well know. I am going merely because I feel myself old and tired, my sweet friend, and unable any longer to play my part in your grand design of free life within the walls of La Tour Bruyarde. My idealism is quenched, dear heart, but not my sympathy—I desire only to live alone in a country cottage and think of our great hopes, and our great days—and your great achievements in the world you have created. Others can play the part you projected for me, others with stronger hearts and stronger limbs and steadier visions. I am a spent force, Culvert, and not worthy to be in your company. But I remember how in the old days you said—when we planned our freedom in hiding from the Revolutionary Armies—you said that the true principle of our new society should be perfect liberty, to fulfil in harmony every least desire, of body or soul. And now, my dear lord, every least desire of my body and my soul is renunciation. I desire solitude, poverty, inertia, quotidian boredom, things we mocked and despised in our high days, but things which now I believe have a certain value for such as myself, wrung out like old cloths, cracked like dry posts. O Culvert, O magnanimous, subtle Culvert, liberty must include the *freedom to leave the group*, harmony of desires must include the desire to abstain from desiring? Let me go now, and the people will praise your wisdom and gentleness for generations."

"This is simply flattery," said Culvert then, staring down from his shifting horse, which danced uneasily, and which he controlled completely with the iron resolve in his grim knees. "You should hear yourself, your weak, lying, flattering voice, saying what you do not believe, to save your skin, which is no longer worth saving, which disgusts me. You do not think me magnanimous or wise. You do not think what I have made in La Tour Bruyarde is just or beautiful. You have murmured against me and despised our work; you have sneered and doubted and made our path difficult from the very outset of our Project. We cannot afford to let you go loose and tell lies about us to the weak, unstable outside world. We cannot afford to let you weaken our resolve by opening chinks in our defence, to let you water the strong wine of our purpose with the spittle of fear and indecision and vacillation. Where one weak link parts, the whole chain springs loose and the other links rattle to the ground. No, you must return, foolish woman, and meet the punishment I have designed for you.

"Where is that young fool, Narcisse?"

"He is gone. We quarrelled and parted. He is far away."

So spoke the Lady Roseace, in her despair, to give the young man a chance.

Now Narcisse in the deep thicket was frozen in mid-piss, his organ in his hand, scarce daring to breathe or move, lest he discover himself. And when he heard her thus attempt to save him, he debated with himself whether he should sally out of the thicket to defend her (which was not very possible, with the hound pack and the huntsmen still gathering) or whether he should stay where he was and accept her gift of hiding. But he might have saved his moral niceties, for the hounds picked up his scent and followed him into the brush, where they leaped up at his unbuttoned garments and tore viciously at those parts over which he held his lovely hands, and at the hands too, so that both were mangled to shreds of dangling flesh. And then Culvert came and took him, and bound him upright in his saddle, all bleeding as he was now, and bound the Lady Roseace also, with her torn clothes, and so they rode back to La Tour Bruyarde.

"We might try to save her," said Turdus Cantor to Colonel Grim.

"We must do what is possible," said Colonel Grim, "which might barely include saving ourselves."

"She will be better out of this," said Samson Origen. "Provided it is quick."

It was not quick . . .

"And now," said Culvert to his captive lady, "I shall show you the machine I have prepared for you. I shall explain its intricacies and its sinuosities and its delectable and devilish resorts and triggers, one by one."

And he clapped his hands, and a trolley was wheeled on to the stage, on which stood a small, shining, pointed tower or turret, a conical affair, perfectly plain on the surface. And from its base, like the elastic of a dunce's cap, dangled a leather string, with stirrups.

"Now," said Culvert, "when the leather tongues at the base of this ingenious turret are pulled tight in their eyelets round your ankles and securely spiked on their steel prongs; when the tip of the turret has been inserted into that soft place it is designed for, then this smooth cone will open a myriad tiny mouths, from which will issue a myriad tiny tongues, that will lap and lick and titillate, but which are also made of fine steel and tempered blades, and will shave and slice and carve and work, bit by bit, inch by inch." And Culvert explained to Roseace that this instrument was designed to enter her, and to expand inside her, and blossom at its summit and along its sides with an ingenious series, a veritable forest, of little brushes and soft, probing glove-fingers, which would give intense pleasure, and then of little penknives, and forks, and tweezers, and scissors, and revolving cheese-wires, and whisks, and pincers and probes, which would be triggered by motions, and fluids, and belches, and each other . . .

"We shall take notes," he said, "on the variables, the optimal applications of pleasure and pain, the alternations of each, whether pleasure is involuntary in the presence of fear, as some have argued, whether in death, the female orgasm is as violent as that of a hanged man . . ."

The Lady Roseace had heard and read of the great courage of heroes and heroines in the face of unbearable pain. She believed, rightly, that such courage cannot be maintained if its opponents are truly determined it shall not. She believed, rightly, that she had perhaps one more chance to speak before, in some sense, she ceased to be, although *something*—which she devoutly hoped would not much resemble Roseace—would in some sense live through the attentions and ministrations of the instrument. She said, "This is a most ingenious device."

"I think so. I have given it much thought."

"It must have taken ingenuity and practice."

"Even so. I have laboured."

"You must have planned the Instrument, from the earliest days of our coming here, or even from before . . ."

"It has always been in my mind, yes."

"Tell me, Culvert, was it designed in the abstract? Or always for me—"

"Always for you. Its proportions are constructed to fit the proportions of your interior cavities, as I have often and often measured them."

"So when we came, you knew it would end here?"

"It has not ended," said Culvert. "But you will end here, yes. Unless my machine is defective. Which I am very sure it is not."

"Irony is a useless weapon against Projectors," said Colonel Grim.

"Irony is a useless weapon when they are inserting a biting and scratching and sawing metal device into your cunt," said Turdus Cantor.

"Irony is the last satisfaction," said Samson Origen. "Before death. Death will be very satisfactory to that poor lady. But her death will not, I think, be as satisfying to our Projector as he supposed it would when he projected it. And I do not know if he is clever enough to see that the satisfaction will not be greatly—if at all—increased by constant repetition of the experiment. It is time to prepare our own evasion. Would you not say? With a little more cunning and a little more aggression than those two innocents?"

"I thought," said Colonel Grim, "that you believed it was best not to have been born, and next best to die quickly. I can't see why you would want to stir from this Tower, where your second-best fate impends even more insistently."

"I abstain from sexual bliss myself," said Samson Origen. "And I would rather not die as part of another man's desperate search for its vanishing lineaments in my pain or anyone else's. I think we will find a way of gratifying our Projector and pleasing ourselves."

"You will act against your principles."

"But not against yours, *mon Colonel*. So you must be active in this."

Babbletower has a cover with a black tower on the midnight-blue sky, with a white moon riding on one of the rather Disneyish turrets, and white arched windows winking in its gloom. A trail of scantily clad people, mostly women with flowing hair and exposed breasts in Empire-line clinging dresses, winds its spiral way round the lower levels of the mass, and vanishes through a heavy doorway. The people bear some resemblance—partly owing to the way their diaphanous clothing clings to their limbs—to Samuel Palmer's churchgoers winding their way to Evensong in a Kentish vale. Only three colours have been used in the printing: cobalt blue, black, and pink. The lettering is black and Gothick. BABBLETOWER, by Jude Mason. Inside, the title page says "*Babbletower: A Tale for the Children of Our Time.* By Jude Mason." The book appears in March 1966. Frederica receives two copies, one from Rupert Parrott ("Thank you for bringing this book to my attention. I am sure it is worth publishing it. We must hope it will do well.") and one from Jude, inscribed "For Frederica, who thought I couldn't, and then decided that I could. In one of the most improbable interpretations of that phrase the Onlie Begetter. I babble. I salute you. Jude."

Frederica finds the cover passable, no more. It is striking. But simple. And has a misleading Tolkienish-science-fictionish look.

She notices a few reviews. The *Daily Telegraph* (brought home from the Ministry by Agatha) has a headline A FURTHER SYMPTOM OF OUR DECADENCE, and says that the book, occasionally quite powerful, reflects the sensationalism, desire for perverse stimulation of jaded palates, determination to shock at all costs a cynical public increasingly difficult to shock or to rouse except by extreme crude measures. "We are a sick society, in which apparently anything goes, in books, in behaviour, in style of dress, in pointless posturing. In a more robust society, this book would not have been published, for the publisher would have had convictions, and the courage of those convictions. In the present climate of slimy liberalism, anything is allowed to creep out from under a stone and preen itself in the common sun."

The *Guardian* headline is THE WOUNDED SURGEON PLIES THE STEEL and its critic concludes that we live in a sick society and the only way to confront our sickness is to explore, to inhabit, to hunt out every last hiding place of our shames and our subterfuge, our divided and blunted consciousness, working our way bravely through disgust to a new understanding. We are in a state of breakdown, and only by breaking down all inhibitions will we come to see our sick selves as we really are, and embark on the difficult and dangerous project of reintegration. "*We must accept that we are loathsome,*" says this critic, "and Jude Mason has taken a fearless step forward on all our behalfs."

In *Encounter* there is a long article by Marie-France Smith, who is described in the Contributors' Notes as "Carlyle Professor of Comparative Literature at Prince Albert College in London University." Professor Smith is learned, and treats *Babbletower* as a learned treatise, exploring the explorations of liberty and license of those post-revolutionary French thinkers Charles Fourier and the Marquis de Sade, "who urged on the crowd that besieged the Bastille where he was imprisoned, through a speaking trumpet made out of the fall-pipe of his latrine." "There is considerable interest amongst current French thinkers, the heirs of surrealism and anarchism, both in Fourier's gentle belief that indulgence of every natural (i.e., every possible) human desire could be harmoniously ordered into a new paradise, a new Jerusalem, and in the darker belief, of Sade, who also believed all existing natural passions should be admitted and permitted by the state, but had a further belief in the *unnatural act* which could be an instrument of power over Nature and a deep insight into her ways. Sade's philosophical interest in transgression may be related to that of Nietzsche, who remarks that the wisdom of Oedipus and the understanding of Hamlet are bought by *unnatural acts* . . ."

. . .

Frederica encounters Jude himself outside the male lavatories in the Samuel Palmer School. He is wearing his blue velvet Caroline coat, which looks as though clouds of greasy dust would rise from it if he were tapped with a carpet beater. His hair swings and swings, iron-grey and knotted and gleaming with its own ancient oils, ending at the hem of his coat-skirts. It has pale flecks like a small flock of clothes moths on it, minute shredded scraps of pink lavatory tissue, improbably electrified. He is preceded by his own rancid smell, and succeeded by the wafted air of the latrine. Frederica thanks him for the book, congratulates him on it, and asks if he is happy with the reviews.

Jude's long grey face folds lugubriously. He pulls a sheaf of reviews from his pocket and begins to read.

"How can I be pleased," he says, "when I am treated as a *symptom* of other people's swinish *malaise*? I am *myself,* I hope, and my book is mine, and a work of art, I do believe and maintain, contrary to their insulting insinuations."

"At least they're talking about it. If they think it's a symptom, they'll talk about it a lot. Come away from the loo, Jude, and tell me what you think about Marie-France Smith."

"A cold philosopher who would unravel the rainbow. Nowhere in her whole disquisition on Sade and Fourier and *les philosophes* does she use an active verb of my people, my personae. *Nowhere* does Culvert *do* or Samson Origen *think* or Turdus Cantor *speak.* It is as though we *were not.* All of us, who peopled my poor skull and rode across its plains and savaged each other so incessantly and ingeniously, *we are nothing,* Frederica, but a few concepts. We are Liberty and the Id, we are the fraying backcloth of the Theatre of Cruelty."

"For God's sake, Jude Mason, are you trying to say the critics should have discussed your characters *as though they were real people?*"

"As though they were *real characters,* my sweet. A lot more real than Mr. Philip Toynbee or Mr. Cyril Connolly or Professor Marie-France Smith."

"You are an ungrateful sod. They've done you proud."

"Not a sod. A total abstainer. In mourning for a world."

Frederica understands. She says, "You miss them. You've lost them. Are you writing anything else?"

She is dragging him by the elbow up the stairs out of the basement, away from the lavatories.

"Hush. Tell no one. I'm thinking of a story of Artists. And a lot of poisonously fatal Young Things. But artists disgust me, rather. They're too simple. Soldiers, now. I might write a tale set in a barracks. A fortified barracks under siege, no ingress nor egress."

"Like *Babbletower.*"

"In no way. On the shore of a salt sea, with a desert behind its back, defending a space where life may not flourish. That's promising. I've thought of that just talking to you, here, now. But in truth, my angel, I am flummoxed and bereft. I am a *one-man* wake and I am lost. I am to be interviewed by the *Evening Standard* tomorrow. I have no opinions to offer their young woman."

"You have lots."

"Just as bad. They want one or two simple ones. A line. I am not a line. I am a tangle."

Frederica asks whether Rupert Parrott is happy with the book's reception. This evokes further plaints.

"I had *supposed* that some festivity would have been forthcoming. A few glasses of champers, which of course I don't *drink* but I do like to look at the bubbles going up, and some *canapés.* You know, when I first read about a party with *canapés* I was in my *indigenous French* phase—so imagined a *Roman orgy* where everyone lay around on *canapés,* couches, all different colours, salmon pink and sky blue and *bronze*—a delectable rolling-around on sofas, an ogling. I do feel I might have had a minor or minimal orgy for my debut, even if the *canapés* were all bite-sized, and made for teeth and gullet rather than fundament."

"We could all go to the pub today and drink to *Babbletower,*" says Frederica. "Alan and Desmond Bull and you and me and a few others. No *canapés* in pubs, but we could raise a glass to you."

"Conciliating your Eeyore with burst balloons in honey-pots," says Jude, revealing an unusual aspect of his reading. "Very well, I will permit you to console me, we will take a *jar* together."

He does not take a jar, when the celebratory group is gathered in the local, which is a rather opulent scarlet-leather-and-gleaming-brass-and-engraved-mirrors-and-fat-frilled-glass-lampshades place called the Griffin. He takes "a Bloody Mary without the Mary, *all blood,* dear, with several shakes of that dark brown fluid which I believe is made like the Roman *liquamen* from rotted fish." He is high on excitement; his smell is hotter and ranker than its usual cold dustbin air.

The party consists of several painters and a few art historians and some students, as well as Frederica, Alan, and Desmond Bull. They all inspect the book and deprecate the cover. Gareth Larkin, who teaches graphics, says he will set Jude's book as a project for his second-year students—"and that way you'll have twenty or thirty alternatives to choose from. I like to give them something to bite into, in the second year, something real."

"Jude could pose for the torture scenes," says one of the female students, who is wearing a purple shirt with a frilled high collar, scattered with sprigs of daisies, above a black hobble skirt and laced granny boots.

"You'd enjoy that," says Jude, automatically. His face is a mask, a skin stretched over something; he is *going on rather,* today, Frederica thinks, wondering what he is "really" thinking or feeling.

Later, when the artists have drunk a large number of pints, and Jude has imbibed several more "simply Bloodies, thank you, dear," there is a potential moment of ugliness when it becomes clear that there is a feeling that Jude should buy a round of drinks. It is not clear to Frederica whether Jude is aware of the muttering and growling. Someone says *sotto voce* that having a sold book in the hand is worth a studio of unsold canvasses when it comes to the liquid. Jude goes to the lavatory and Frederica offers to buy the round; these are the days before the women's movement, when it is still quite difficult, though not impossible, for a woman to buy a round in a pub. Alan helps her to carry and offers to help her to pay. She refuses the offer, and becomes irrationally annoyed with Jude herself, as he re-arranges his coatskirts on the tubby red stool he is occupying. Fourteen pints and a simply Bloody makes quite a hole in her own small resources.

The interview in the *Evening Standard* is conducted by an up-and-coming trendy young journalist (these are the freshly shining, newly hitched days of the word "trendy") called Marianna Toogood.

Jude Mason insisted on being interviewed in a Soho teashop: La Pâtisserie de Nanette, a tiny cubby-hole of a café, behind thick lace curtains, where there are three little round tables with white lace cloths flung over dark red plastic cloths, and rickety little bentwood chairs. It seemed an odd place to meet the author of "a tale for the children of our time," which has been described as disgusting, sadistic, pornographic, intellectual, profound and "a mirror of our present disorders."

I did not know what to expect, and at first took my interviewee for a tramp who had wandered in by mistake, an impression I am sure he meant me to have. He wears his hair very long; it is dark grey and centrally parted; his clothes, a sort of velvet frock-coat which was once pale blue, and velvet britches, could charitably be described as well worn. There are holes in his shoes. His face is long, his bones prominent, his eyes hooded. He could do with a wash, but has a certain fancy-dress *panache.* He is a fairytale figure, a cross between Captain Hook, Gollum, and the Marquis de Sade, from whom he claims to have learned his craft.

He is difficult to interview, since he answers most conventional questions with a simple "no" or a resolute silence. He prefers not to divulge where he was born, where he was educated, where he lives, or whether he has any family or friends. His voice is extremely "cultivated," with a clipped twang which is more BBC than the BBC, a Brideshead bray. He did reveal that he had run away from school—a boarding school, one assumes, since he said "I absconded in the deep darkness"—to sit at the feet of the surrealists and anarchists, and of the playwright Jean Genet, who he says is "the Master" but not a model for his own way of life. "Genet believes that stealing is a good and easy way of encouraging the flow of goods in a community: since I have and want no possessions I neither steal nor am stolen from."

He earns his living, he tells me, as an employee in an art school. When asked what he does there he is surprisingly forthcoming. "I offer myself. I display my puny musculature. I let them trace the lineaments of my absence of desire." He has an affinity for the art students, perhaps? He tells me he read his book *Babbletower* aloud to selected groups of them, during which he was overheard and "discovered" by "someone" who showed his manuscript to his publisher, Rupert Parrott, of Bowers and Eden.

Parrott obviously has an eye for the *risqué* and unlikely success—he published Phyllis Pratt's *Daily Bread,* the best-selling story of stabbings and *crises de foie* amongst the rural clergy.

He has ordered several *pâtisseries,* which he consumes with greedy deliberation, biting into them with long yellow teeth. During the interview he devours a meringue swan, biting off its head with a decisive snap, a kind of choux pastry called a *religieuse* (a nun) which has a chocolate-veiled "head" on a fat, cream-filled body, and two *feuilles de palmier.* He says he does not often get the chance to eat *pâtisseries.* He likes eating, but does little of it—"indigence is a great staver-off of *embonpoint.*" He does not drink, or smoke. I wonder whether this is because, like Timothy Leary, he believes psychedelic drugs to be healthier than the normal psyche-deadeners of our society, alcohol and nicotine. This suggestion makes him indignant. He remarks oddly that he needs "neither mind-expanders nor chest-expanders nor sock-suspenders nor a trouser press." I get the feeling that he considers me to be intellectually so far beneath him that it is not worth giving serious answers to my questions.

Many of the reviews of *Babbletower* have suggested that it is likely to become cult reading among the young and turned on, the disciples of Artaud and Peter Brooke, *Gormenghast* and Burroughs. He is, I suggest, a proto-hippy or Flower Person. He repudiates this, quoting Peter Pan about being a little chicken sprung from the egg. "I am what I am and was, my hair is what it was and is, my book is my book and sprang from my head fully armed, *sui generis.*"

But he likes the art students? I would like him to like *something* besides decapitated sugar swans and nuns.

"They are revolting," he says. He corrects himself. "They are in revolt. They are breaking their chains. They will not submit to be made to crassly imitate or even look at the drawings of Michelangelo or the techniques of Ruskin. They will all be original in their own ways, which are all new and unsullied by contact with the boring and *complicated* past, and which therefore all resemble each other in their freshness and innocence and simplicity." He appears to mean what he says, but it is hard to be sure.

I ask him if he thinks *Babbletower* will attract a large following. Yes, he says, he should think so. I ask him why, what about his book will attract them?

"Oh," he says, "the world is full of people doing horrible things to other people for love, and people love to read about people doing horrible things to other people because they want to learn how to do horrible things themselves to the people they love and they want to learn to write about that, naturally, it is part of it, writing it down. It keeps the world going, like Genet's movement of goods from place to place."

He bites into a great pastry cabbage and smiles at me through spurts of cream.

Rupert Parrott, when he sees this, shouts at Hugh Pink. His shouting always has a breathy quality, as though the shouter himself is trying to suppress it. He shouts that Mason must be prevented from giving any more interviews. He is making them all look ridiculous. Hugh Pink replies pacifically that the chances are that he gave a perfectly reasonable interview, but that the journalist took against him, or against the cake shop, or something. Or against his smell, says Hugh Pink, which she did have the good grace not to mention, though it can't have gone down very well with the meringue. Hugh says he supposes the interview will be good for sales, which it is. *Babbletower* passes three thousand and continues to sell.

. . .

Frederica is stopped by Jude outside her office. He pulls out the growing sheaf of reviews from his inner pocket and peels off the interview. He is outraged. He is particularly outraged by Marianna Toogood's reporting of "*crises de foie*" in the novel of Phyllis Pratt. "They are illiterate, these young *things,*" he says. "*Crise de foi,* sans *e,* crisis of the Faith; crise de foie, *with* an *e, liver attack,* as in foie gras, *fat liver.* Pig-ignorant."

"It could be a joke. A pun."

"Don't be silly. She's not capable of any such refinement. Pure pig-ignorance. Look what she did with my remarks about the revolting students' revolting reluctance to learn the rudiments or study the great who have gone their way. She can't recognise *irony.*"

"Journalists never can. Most people can't. Rule One. As she should have known, since you can't see it's *her* joke about the *crise de foie* or *foi.*"

"She made me look a fool. She didn't report any of the things I actually *did* say about my book, about my people, about my meaning. Only made animadversions on my teeth."

"You do ask for it, you know."

"Ask for what? I ask for nothing."

Frederica catches sight of another, newer review.

"Is that Anthony Burgess? Can I look?"

Burgess's review opens with a disquisition on evil. He quotes Golding's oracular saying "Man produces evil as a bee produces honey." He suggests that the English have always been uneasy with evil—"They don't go beyond right and wrong, they lean naturally towards the comedy of manners, where virtue is inextricably entangled with Class, whereas on the Catholic and Calvinist continent, writers are not afraid to acknowledge the whiff of sulphur from the Pit, the eternal confrontation between Good and Evil." He cites Al Alvarez's rousing introduction to his anthology of modern poetry prepared to measure up to the horrors of our history (the Holocaust, the Bomb): "Beyond the Gentility Principle."

Jude Mason, says Burgess, is far out beyond the Gentility Principle. In the battle between Saint Augustine, the Bishop of Hippo, who believed that fallen man was naturally evil, and Pelagius, the hopeful Hibernian heretic, who believed that man could by free will and reasonable exercise of virtue achieve salvation, who, asked Burgess, is not instinctively on the side of Pelagius? And who, who ponders long and deeply, does not come to fear, to accept, that the grim Bishop was nevertheless in the right of it, that there is some quasi-mechanical system of destructiveness, betrayal, cruelty, in which we are entrapped, however we struggle?

Jude Mason, says Burgess, is that new kind of 1960s artist, the Fabulator. His Fable enacts the battle between Augustine and Pelagius but in a society more like the post-Revolutionary France, where the sardonic Marquis de Sade promulgated his theories of freedom and terror, a renegade Augustinian, whereas the "sweetly dotty" Charles Fourier constructed a Utopian vision of Harmony where the stars would sing together because human passional and sexual freedom and bliss had heated the universe and changed the music of the spheres, had turned the oceans to a kind of agreeable lemonade, sharks to supertankers and supertigers to supertransport. Jude Mason's people, says Burgess, are trapped in their Projector's Fourierist utopian project, which is a mechanical conveyor-belt to Sadeian subways and dungeons.

This book, says Burgess, portentously, mischievously, is in great danger of being prosecuted for obscenity, for a "tendency to deprave and corrupt." Can it be acquitted on that account? True pornography, he says, is *kinetic,* it moves to action, it titillates, it irritates and excites flesh and spirit to seek relief. It does not follow that because a writer's concern is deeply moral, deeply concerned with right and wrong, that what he writes will necessarily lack this *kinetic* quality. "The value of art is always diminished by the presence of elements that move to action: the pornographic and the didactic are, in a purely aesthetic judgement, equally to be condemned." Jude Mason is both didactic and pornographic: it is to be supposed that he believes his own stance to be that of his creation Samson Origen, who professes a Nietzschean eschewal of the libido and all its works. But he has chosen to construct his fable, his *machine,* his clockwork, in parody of the drives and devices it criticises, the sado-masochistic panoply of straps and knives, the pornographic relish of human surfaces and orgiastic contortions. Does his titillation titillate? Do his switches set in motion cogs which turn on switches which set imitation in motion? The greatest works of art are not kinetic but static. *Ulysses, Lady Chatterley's Lover, The Rainbow* "discharge their emotions inside the book itself, producing the catharsis of art." Jude Mason, though he has considerable talent and ingenuity, is working in a more dubious and dangerous mode. Freud and Mephistopheles might smile mockingly at this Projector as he smiles mockingly at his own Culvert.

Babbletower appears in March 1966. In April Harold Wilson wins a General Election with a greatly increased effective majority of ninety-seven. *Babbletower* has now sold six thousand copies and aroused much discussion. Alexander Wedderburn reports to Frederica that Naomi Lurie, the Oxford don on the Steerforth Committee, has told him in confidence that the Director of Public Prosecutions has asked her to read and report on *Babbletower,* to give an opinion on whether a prosecution under the 1959 Obscene Publications Act would be appropriate, and whether expert opinion would be heavily in favour of the book. Dr. Lurie, says Alexander, doesn't like the book but believes it can be argued to have literary merit, and should be in print.

One of the new Labour MPs in the new Parliament is Dr. Hermia Cross, a physician and Methodist Lay Reader whose Liverpool constituency contains both a smart suburb and a racially pullulating series of council estates. Dr. Cross, surprisingly, asks the Attorney-General in the House whether he intends to take any steps about a dangerous and disgusting book which has received misguided praise in some quarters. The Attorney-General, Sir Mervyn Bates, replies that he believes that the peak of the book's sales is past, that it is priced too high to be widely circulated, and that Literary Criticism, on the whole, appeared to believe the work had some merit. Dr. Cross retorts that she believes the book presents acts of cruelty in a seductive light, and that we are living through a time of horror when it is unfortunately clear that literary works *can* influence minds predisposed to evil to commit acts of cruelty and degradation. The trial of Ian Brady and Myra Hindley is being heard as she speaks, though she makes no direct reference to it. She is backed up by Sir Evelyn Maiden, a Tory MP from Suffolk, who says he has seen the book, "and it is filthy, filthy, filthy muck." She is also backed up by other Tory backbenchers. In the Sunday papers that weekend there are articles mocking the protesting MPs, and a cartoon of Dr. Cross dressed as a governess brandishing a whip over a crawling bare-arsed figure who is presumably Rupert Parrott, since it is clearly not Jude Mason. There is also an article entitled "Sticks and Stones May Break Your Bones" by Roger Magog, which argues hotly and passionately that it is always wrong to restrict the written or the spoken word, "because precisely, *words cannot hurt you,* every man has the right and the freedom to make up his own mind how to react to incitements and temptations and actions of whatever kind, and what we should do for the weak and wrong-headed is *educate them to judge better,* not suppress other's freedoms. We must be vigilant, but not repressive . . ." On the following Monday, Dr. Cross announces that if the DPP will not act as it should, she will take out a private prosecution against the publishers and author of *Babbletower* under Section 3 of the 1959 Act. This—and the unfortunate coincidence of the Moors Murders trial—brings about a change of heart in the DPP, which announces that it now intends to bring a prosecution against the book.

Frederica hears this news from Rupert Parrott himself. She goes round to Elderflower Court with a heap of reports, and a basket to carry away further books. Parrott is sitting behind his desk. He says, "Now see what you have brought upon me!" and hands Frederica the official letter. "They have seized my stock," he says. His round cheeks are pink, his eyes glittering. "We shall fight," he says. "We shall fight, no matter what the cost, no matter what the pain. It is a matter of principle, of freedom of conscience, of the right to free speech. If people like this are allowed to win, we shall be back in a society where burning books is a step on the way to burning people."

He looks an unlikely martyr for free speech, with his little curls, his mustard-coloured waistcoat and his tartan tie. Frederica says, "What will you do?"

"Elect for trial by jury when we come before the magistrates. Assemble a team of expert witnesses who will make it once and for all impossible to attack literary works. Demolish Mrs. Whitehouse and Dr. Cross and their pro-censorship movements. Start a Defence Fund with appeals to other publishers for solidarity. Bear witness."

"What does Jude say?"

"To tell you the truth, I could do without Jude. He is our weak link. He will make a dreadful impression on a jury. Apart from the way he looks, he has a tendency to counter-productive frivolity. I count on you, Frederica, to keep him in order, that is, to make him see sense. We must have a good Brief. I thought of Augustine Weighall. We must talk to the solicitors. We must explore *every possibility.* There can be no question of losing. We cannot afford to lose."

He purses his mouth and looks directly at Frederica. "We need all the help we can get."

"I'll do what I can," says Frederica, not sure what that is, what role she can have.

"But screw your courage to the sticking-place," says Rupert Parrott, "and we'll not fail. Who said that?"

"Lady Macbeth, I think."

"Ah," says Rupert Parrott. He laughs, a warm, rueful laugh. "Not a good choice. I must be careful. You can't make mistakes like that, under cross-examination."

"She didn't exactly *fail.*"

"In the long run she did. She got damned spots on her hands and died in a nightmare. I intend to *win this case* and die contented in my bed."

Frederica in the first part of 1966 has her own problems. Her divorce is apparently no nearer being heard, and she is besieged by a long series of letters from Nigel's solicitors about Leo's education. "If the boy is to go to Swineburn, as is to be hoped, or to some other Public School, he should already be studying Latin and French, in order eventually to be prepared to sit the Common Entrance examination. Mr. Tiger's client is reliably informed that no such preparation is or will be available at the William Blake Elementary School. He is perfectly prepared to pay his son's fees at a local Preparatory School to be agreed, and would be glad to be informed as expeditiously as possible of any arrangements that could be made for his satisfaction in this regard." Frederica snips and pastes these messages into her *Laminations*—"French facilities Latin elementary all confusion opportunity languages"—and sends off spirited messages to Mr. Begbie, who translates them into lawyers' *lingua franca.*

"Tell him that as far as I know he himself never passed an exam, doesn't speak any languages and never reads a book, whereas I have distinctions in four languages at A Level and a First Class English degree from Cambridge, and share a house with a Principal in the Ministry of Education, so might be thought to have my son's educational interests at heart. Tell him my father is a distinguished schoolmaster and no one could care more than we do about education and civilisation, neither of which are my husband's *strong points.* Thank you."

She describes this situation with indignation to Alan Melville and Tony Watson, the chameleon and the fake of her Cambridge days. Alan, the chameleon, whose elegant manner covers a ferociously competitive struggle to break out of a Glaswegian working-class world, wonders whether Leo might not be quite happy in a boarding school in the country, "with educational *standards*" and civilised boys. Tony, who is the son of a rich socialist man of letters and was sent to prep school and public school, who pretends to be a working-class chap, with woollen shirts and donkey jackets, is all for leaving Leo where he is. "If they bash him in the playground, you'll see. If he isn't learning anything, you'll notice. Alan doesn't know what he's talking about. Thirty little boys in a locker-room, all of them wanting to cry for their mummies in bed at night, is nevertheless like a crocodile pond, with jaws snapping and the fattest getting fatter. And you just don't know what sort of pervert's putting your son to bed at night. I do."

"You survived," says Alan.

"So did you, all your wasteland gangs and playground battles."

"Some don't," says Alan.

"I know," says Tony, who is reporting the Moors Murders trial, and living in a hotel in Chester. The discussion of where Leo will be least vulnerable has a new edge because of the fates of Lesley Ann Downey and John Kilbride, whose ordinary, gentle, childish, vanished faces appear daily in softened grey newsprint everywhere. Tony has heard the home-made tapes of the little girl crying out to be released, to go home to her mother, saying that she is frightened, being told to shut up and keep still. At the end of these tapes are children's voices singing Christmas music. On the reverse, Tony tells Frederica and Alan, is the crazy humour of the "Goon Show." Don't tell me, says Alan. I don't want to know any more. I don't myself, says Tony. I don't want to go back there, I don't want to be a reporter, I don't want to know. Frederica, her heart thumping, her gorge rising, distressed by the juxtaposition of this and Leo, by fear of losing him, by fear, by fear, finds she is weeping. Alan and Tony put their arms around her as she sobs. A car coughs in the street. Tony puts down the blind.

Frederica has also received several visits from Paul Ottokar. John Ottokar appears less frequently, and never telephones. So that when Frederica sees the blond face with its sweep of gold hair at the basement window, or the figure standing waiting in a black PVC mackintosh when she comes home from her shopping, she learns to assume it will be Paul, who, unlike John, has no regular job to go to. Even so, it is difficult to tell. They hunch their shoulders the same way. They stand with their feet at the same angle. Their grave, tentative, charming smile is the same smile.

"I thought I'd drop in. I hope you don't mind. I'm at a loose end."

"I don't mind, no. But I've got a lot of work to do. Essays to correct. Some writing. Have a cup of coffee."

"Thank you. I will."

He does not keep still. He prowls around her basement room, taking books out of the bookshelves, putting them back differently. He picks up paperweights and balances them, and makes a feint of dropping them, and smiles, and restores them. He says, "Where's your record-player? Where's your music? Let's put on some music."

"I don't have a record-player. I'm tone-deaf. I like silence. I can't think in music."

"You won't get very far in swinging London. You'll need to know about music to know my brother. We've always had music. We played in a group, did he tell you? We played in the Aldermaston marches. He plays the horn and I play the clarinet. We're good. I'm forming a new group. I want him to come and play. Neither of us is *really* good without the other. We anticipate. We hear each other's thoughts. It's got a lovely name, my new group."

"Has it?"

"It's called Zag and the Ziggy-Ziggy Zy-Goats. Clever, don't you think?"

He prowls.

"You should come and hear us. When we play, we're good together. Other times, we aren't. I took it hard, Frederica, that my brother should have signed up for all your book classes without so much as a word to me. I took it hard, but I understood it. Both of us feel both things, you know, the need to be *two,* and the need to be *one.* We don't always feel them simultaneously. I read all your books from your class, when I was in the—when I was in retreat. *Dr. Faustus* and *Death in Venice, The Castle* and *The Idiot, The Birth of Tragedy from the Spirit of Music,* I read all that. I made sure you'd be interested in music."

"No. It's been left out of me."

"I'll play to you, one day. We'll play to you. *Everyone* now, *all the time,* understands the world through music. Books are like little scratches on the window. Inside, your soul spreads out in music. Music is wiser than *pyramids* of books."

"Sit down, you're making me nervous."

"I'm nervous myself. I'm intruding. I'm being rude, I'm doing what John won't like. Forgive me."

"Sit down."

"If there was any music, I could keep still and listen."

"There isn't."

"I'm making you angry. Look into my eyes. I am the one you haven't kissed, the body you don't know. Is it delectable or terrible to look at the *same thing* and know you don't know it, although you do?"

"I think you'd better go. I have things to do."

"Aren't you curious to see if it's the same, or different? Same face, same voice. Same kiss? Shall I kiss you, so you *know* whether it's the same, or different?"

Frederica sits and sips Nescafé out of a black mug with a rose-pink lining, salvaged from Cambridge, retrieved from Freyasgarth. What is disturbing is the sameness, not the difference. John Ottokar can be still and gentle, like a great lazy cat, and this one cannot, his fingers move nervously on his knees, which tremble together; his head tosses imperceptibly to some tune that twangs in his brain. But the smile is John's smile, and the eyes are John's eyes, and the fingers are John's fingers, and the voice, with its clarity and warmth, the voice is John's voice.

She says, "I don't want to know. I think you ought to go. I'll work out what I feel about John *with John,* if that's what he wants."

"He won't mind, if you kiss me. He'll expect it. We come as two sides of one coin, two faces of one herm. He knows that. Dear frowning Frederica, his kiss is not *complete* without my kiss, either for him, or for you, and he knows that. Don't be cross. Kiss me. He knows I am here, now, he *knows I am here,* he expects this. We always know. Take one, take both. He *knows I will be here.* Reject one, reject both. It might be better. We might be too much for you."

"You might," says Frederica. "You well might. But I'll discuss that with John."

"When I'm gone," he says, rising abruptly, "you'll be sorry, you'll desperately want to know what I'm like, you'll *ache.*"

"I'll take my chance."

"You don't take chances. You're cold, you're canny, you'll never hold him with that grismal frown. You'll bore the pants off him."

"I really do think you'd better go."

He goes.

Next time he comes, it is as if this conversation had never taken place. The figure waiting by the steps of Number 42 is sober-suited, in one of those collarless suits made fashionable by the Beatles, but in sober midnight-blue, over a white polo neck. Frederica, at the same instant, experiences a lurch of sexual delight, and makes an intellectual observation that this is almost certainly Paul.

"I'm sorry to bother you," he says. "I'm sorry to intrude, but I should be grateful for some professional advice, if you could spare me a moment or two."

"Come in," says Frederica.

"The thing is," says Paul Ottokar, once they are well in the basement, resuming his prowling, "the thing is, that the little group I belong to—not Zag and the Zy-Goats, which doesn't interest you, because you aren't musical, but the little spiritual splinter-group or spearhead—we are having a Poetry Weekend, and as my brother has no doubt told you, we—he and I—are dreadfully ill-read animals, and I don't know where to start my reading for this weekend. We are going to be called the Spirits' Tigers, I think, and someone called Richmond Bly is going to come and talk to us about 'The Visionary Aspects of English Romanticism.' Now I haven't the *vaguest idea* what all that is—but I do pick things up very quickly, as you may have observed—I got a lot out of *The Birth of Tragedy from the Spirit of Music,* I nicked dear John's copy—*he knows,* of course, I expect he *felt* it rising off his desk and going into my satchel, we're like that, we have kinetic knowledge of each other. So I thought I'd come to you for a reading list of *essential* English Romanticism for this weekend. So I can surprise Elvet Gander—I *love* surprising Elvet—there will be a poet there called Fainlight, I think, and a performance artist called Silo, who plays the drums with Zag and the Zy-Goats. Is it an impossible request? Can you make me a shopping list or batting order of English Romanticism? It will be good for my rather unenlightened soul."

"I could do that," says Frederica.

"I can't make head or tail of the *Visions of the Daughters of Albion,* I thought of *chanting* them. Like mantras. With bells and a drum and a wailing of thin horn music."

. . .

Frederica sits and writes. She writes down "Kubla Khan," *The Ancient Mariner,* "The Immortality Ode," "The Death of Hyperion." Paul Ottokar says, "I hope I wasn't offensive, last time. I was high. If I was offensive, please don't be offended. I should like us to be friends. In a minor key."

"Do you want a list of criticisms, or just of texts?"

"Whatever *you* think. I am in *your* hands."

Frederica writes. She wants to ask: And will John be coming to your Poetry Weekend? She does not ask.

"I'll make you a cup of coffee, whilst you write," says Paul Ottokar. He finds her kettle, her coffee, her cups, her milk, without hesitation. He finds Leo's biscuits iced with smiley faces, cherry-coloured, lemon-coloured, coffee-coloured, chocolate. He puts them out on a plate with Peter Rabbit and Benjamin Bunny. Frederica writes: Thomas de Quincey: *Confessions of an English Opium-Eater,* and accepts her own smiley biscuit, on her own plate, from the gently courteous intruder. She feels like crying.

John Ottokar telephones. He sounds strained. He talks about nothing much for a good five minutes and then says, "Can I come and see you?"

"When?" says Frederica.

"Over the weekend," says John Ottokar.

"Leo is going to his father this weekend."

"Then I'll come," says John Ottokar.

Frederica does not say then: "But there is a Poetry Weekend in Four Pence." She feels wise, and restrained, not to say this. She washes her hair, and makes the bed with clean sheets, and buys supper, supper that won't spoil, smoked trout and salad, a lemon tart. When John Ottokar arrives he is wearing his Liberty shirt with the green chrysanthemums and a collarless jacket in green baize, bottle-green, bound in dark blue. He has, despite these bright garments, a faded look to Frederica's eye. As though the other were brighter, sharper, clearer, more extreme than this one. Frederica searches his face for differences, and he sits there, over the dinner table, a little stony, a little guarded, undergoing her scrutiny as though it was exactly what he expected. He speaks rather doggedly of events in his world of work: Tony Benn's policy on North Sea oil, the balance-of-payments problems that loom. He looks around the basement room and says, "It's good to be here."

"I thought you would be busy with a Poetry Weekend."

"Ah," says John Ottokar. He puts down his knife and fork. He stands up and goes over to the basement window and looks out at the dark well.

"I think, Frederica, it might save us all a lot of pain and trouble if I were to put on my coat now, and go, and never come back. The alternative is pretty dreadful for both of us. It starts here. Either I ask you—what's he been saying, what's he been doing, what did you answer, what did you do?—or I don't, I keep quiet, and *both of us imagine*—you and me, that is—and he becomes a huge—a huge—a *demon* between us. I know now, you aren't looking at me—not *me*—you're looking at both of us, comparing, wondering. Your memories are all mixed up—which one smiled *that* smile, which one liked that poem, perhaps. Probably both did. Tearing ourselves apart is an act of violence, Frederica, an *unnatural* act in a sort of a way. You don't want all that. And I want you to myself, or not at all."

"What does he want?"

"To have what I have."

"At the same time as you, or instead of you?"

"That's a good question. At the same time, but *better.* He'd like both of us to make love to you, and he would be the one to do it *better.*"

"And none of that is up to me?"

"Oh, some of it is, yes. But some of it isn't. I thought I would get away—from him—and I *can't*—there are reasons why I can't—good reasons—but I want my own life."

"Can't he get a girl of his own?"

"He wants mine. Whoever she is. And I—don't want that. That is between us, that *is* a difference."

Frederica says, "You can't just let him win. That isn't good for either of you."

"But you must see—as for *you—I want you*—and what I don't want, is for you to have to fight him—or be fought over—or *have anything to do with all that.* I want you to be you—as I first saw you—all thin and nervy standing there talking about the 'form of consecutive prose' wasn't it, with your eyes lit up, and your mind following a thread with a kind of *single-minded glee*—I thought, if I could get her to look at me, like that, to think about me with that sort of concentration."

"I do. I am. I do."

"You might have done."

"I do."

She stands behind him, and puts her arms round him. He is trembling.

"I won't be beaten," she says, "I'm a fighter, you know that. We can't be beaten. We must think our way *through* all this. I can lock him out."

He trembles more violently. "No," he says, "that won't work."

"*You,*" says Frederica furiously, "*you* have got to know where I stand. *You* have got to stop being gloomy, and fight. You can't just walk out on me, having just walked in, because he's trying to walk in too. Did you let him have everything he was trying to take, when you were little? The cake, the tricycle, the little knife?"

"Oh yes. I always let him. There was always another, somewhere, I could have, until he came and wanted it."

"Well, *there isn't another Frederica Potter.* There is one of me and one only. I am I, and inseparable from myself, and indivisible into equal or unequal halves. And at the moment I want *you,* and you are what I want, unless you go on being gloomy and renunciatory, in which case I shall get depressed—but then *he* won't get me, John Ottokar, *neither of you will.* It's up to you. Only, I warn you, I warn you, I will not be a soft ball you toss between you, I will not be talked about or shared out in my absence, I will live my own life, which, just at the moment, I choose shall include *you.* End of speech."

John Ottokar turns away from the window and takes her in his arms. He sighs.

"Come to bed," says Frederica. She turns to pull down the blind and for a moment thinks she sees a blond figure in a dark PVC raincoat standing patiently outside the window. She puts her face to the glass, and there is nothing. She pulls down the blind, and holds out her arms. Whoever wants to see two merged shadows on the translucent cloth can see them. She begins to unbutton John Ottokar's shirt.

They make love. Most of that night, and most of the next day, with the blind drawn down, they make love. They make love in deepening silence, broken only by the odd squeak and suck of skin, the odd bird-like cry, the odd rustle of hair on cotton sheet, of finger- and toenails braced against flesh and bedclothes. They explore each other's bodies, diligently, companionably, leisurely, with little fits of reciprocal fury, with slow, slow holdings back and rapid provocations. She learns his many tastes, his dryness and damp, his sleekest surfaces and his roughest. She learns him as though he were inside her skin, as though she were inside his. No two can be closer, no two assemblies of living cells can be so confounded, so intertwined: they wind sinuously about each other like snakes, they buck like goats, they swallow like silent fish in the deep, they follow delectable rancid scents like cats in the jungle. They eat, are eaten, fling back free a while and separate on drenched bedclothes. Both the body's hope and the mind's fear of the fusion of cells somewhere in there, in the pulling and gripping dark, are absent: they may do as they please, only to please, because they are protected by the Pill. What Frederica delights in most is the warmth of flat belly against flat belly, the push of pelvis against pelvis. When they pull away in the morning light, she touches his skin and finds it is bloody; she touches her own, and her fingertip is scarlet. "Look at us," she says. They are like painted savages, streaked and smeared with warm and drying blood, spread thin like ruddy paint, in whorls and runnels, palm-prints and traced loin-cloths, which reflect each other, body and body. It is her own blood, the blood of the seeping, "break-through" bleeding produced by the Pill in odd gouts and sprinklings, nothing to do with the old rhythms of fertility. Frederica looks to see if John Ottokar feels distaste for this body-paint, but he is tracing its contours with his own finger, smiling.

"Signed in blood," he says. "You can read me on you and you on me."

"Like savages. A rite of passage."

"Does it hurt?"

"No. It's lovely. It's warm. A glow."

They are whispering. Above their heads, Saskia's footsteps trot and stop: Agatha calls out, the words inaudible.

"I've marked you," he says. "We've marked each other."

"Let's never move," she says, but this is an artificial note, this breaks the spell, for in the end they must move, and they know it.

"Are you happy?" she says, like all lovers, and he answers, "Completely," one lovely hand heavy on the sharp edge of her haunch.

For whatever reason, this visit of John's puts an end to the visits of Paul, at least for a time. Frederica wonders if Paul *knows,* in some way, and the knowledge keeps him away. Knows what? she wonders, a week or two later, when the red glow has been washed off her skin and has cooled and faded a little—only a little—in her memory. For she does not know, she does not exactly want, or need, to know, what she and John Ottokar intend, or desire. Frederica has told no one but Agatha about John Ottokar, and Agatha very little. John Ottokar as a secret, as a hidden pleasure, is nothing to do with her and Leo's future. But she is not free, as once she was, to feel her way in and out of loves and likings. For Leo watches her, calculating, jealous, wondering what she wants, what she plans, and his watching, like Paul's quite different watching, weighs on her. And although in the early summer Frederica does not see Paul, she realises that Leo does, or has.

"I smelt that bad smell of that smiley man again today," says Leo. And, "That man with the smell came by and looked in."

She cannot mention this to John. She does not know what to make of it. She is nervous.

She dreams she is in bed with two men, one red, one white, made of hot stone, with stone erections tipped with drops of blood (the white man) and white drops of semen (the red one). They turn to her, they lay their heavy arms across her chest, crushing her. They mount half of her, a thigh one side, a thigh the other. They are heavy, they crush her, she cannot cry out. She wakes. She is afraid. She is rather pleased with the energy and simplicity of the dream-forms, as though they were a work of art she had deliberately constructed.

XVII

Dear John,

I write this letter only after much deliberation. There is a convention amongst psychoanalysts to put it at its lowest—in certain circumstances it bears a resemblance to a TABOO—there is a convention that it is "not done," may be injurious, to approach the relatives and lovers and associates of any "patient," with or without that "patient's" consent. Conventional psychoanalytic treatment is a relationship between two people, analyst and analysand—other relationships are worked out within that framework.

As you know, and as I know you know, I am "treating" your brother for what have been diagnosed as "manic-depressive episodes." As I believe you also know, I am in considerable sympathy with those new, and I believe promising, I will go so far as to say *exciting* ideas, thought-patterns, hypotheses, which suggest that we should look on unusual manifestations of the psyche not as aberrations from a specified *norm* (What is normal? Who dictates what we shall take as our *norm*?) but as ways of exploring the spirit, of exploring the pain, the Experience of the soul in a damaged and damaging environment. I do not, in other words, see your brother as a "sick man" in need of a "cure." But he is undoubtedly a perturbed spirit, undergoing, passing through, a kind of psychic electrical storm, in which great bolts of lightning "all sweating, tilt about the watery heaven," and he could be empowered or destroyed by these fiery currents.

I was pleased—pleased is a trivial word, I mean to say, and *should* say, *joyful,* to find Paul, or Zag as he prefers to be known, as a participant in the Meetings of the Spirits' Tigers. The good old Quaker word "Meeting" does suggest what these gatherings are meant to be, and one of the purposes of the Meetings is to restore to the spiritual group the energy, the *violence* even, which, as Christopher Levenson said in his poem from which we took our name, has slowly over the centuries leached away from the original Pentecostal waitings on the Inner Light. The Quakers no longer quake: the disciples no longer speak with tongues: the Inner Light is dimmed: "the Spirits' Tigers are grown tame." It is entirely good that we few should come together to reverse this entry, to generate energy, heat and light, to make each other as far as possible *whole* in the spirit, at least to *empower* those of us who are lost, or wandering, or crashed. I believe Zag's choice to make one in these Many is a wise choice and to be supported. I believe the group—the Meeting—has been constituted by a wisdom and a purpose beyond the random needs of its individual members.

Now, what has this to do with me? you will ask. Or you will not ask, you will despise my rhetorical attributed question, for you know very well in part—*but not I think, in its wholeness*—what I am going to say to you, to request of you, to lay on you, in the vulgar tongue of our times.

As I was delighted to see Zag bathed in the light of the silence of the Tigers, so I was, on the two brief occasions when we met, overjoyed to see you. Your presence relaxed and calmed him; you brought a serenity to the Meeting which was good for others besides Zag; I think maybe the depth of the silent contemplation did you some good too, or so it appeared.

But you have not come to the last few meetings, and you have not answered the letters that have been sent to you. Zag says he believes you have "given up on him" and also "given up on the Tigers."

I have been a cabin attendant on Zag's spiritual voyage long enough to know that he believes it is your wish to put a distance between you. This is a sane wish, worthy of respect. There are three things I would nevertheless say to you—after great deliberation, as I say.

1. Your retreat is directly endangering Zag's progress—he feels bereft, he feels angry, he feels many many negative things, which he turns against himself, like a child who cuts his own skin. When he does not see you you become in his mind a fantasy spectre or emanation, powerful, to be fought. When he does see you, he sees that you are a complex, separate human being, with *real* needs and a *real* life with which he can come to terms.

From Zag's point of view, steady contact with you—above all, perhaps, in the sane and controlled emotional "field" of the Spirits' Tigers—is necessary for the preservation of some sense of "reality." And however much I may believe that "reality" is not the same thing as common-sense *convention* or *normality,* I do believe it exists. There is a real world—even if infinite—and there is an unreal world, and Zag is in great danger of being trapped in the latter.

2. Your retreat is, I suspect, endangering you, John. For you are *part of* Zag, and the separation must be a subtle unravelling, not a brutal and bloody teasing. You know that in your heart of hearts. Your "dailiness" you cling to is

an unreality as dangerous as Zag's bad trips to the Aurora Borealis. If I overstep the mark, burn this letter. If I speak to any flicker of recognition in any anxiety anywhere in your head or your heart, consider further, come and talk to me, come back to the Spirits' Tigers and bring the problem into the white light of our joint watchfulness and dreamy unknowing.

3. The world is changing before our eyes. Consciousness is changing. We can move into a state where *we do not hurt each other.* You were drawn to the Spirits' Tigers for reasons beyond even your mysterious positive and negative charge to and from your brother. We can say these things, these days, without sounding mad, or cranky, but soberly and truthfully.

Again, if this says nothing to you, burn this letter, forget you received it.

With best wishes.
Yours very sincerely,
Elvet Gander

John Ottokar shows this letter dumbly to Frederica. He holds it out, over the table in a coffee bar where they are meeting in his lunch-break. He is wearing his suit, and a blue-and-white-striped shirt, and a dark blue tie with small emerald spots on it. Frederica is irritated by his portentous and apprehensive expression. She is more irritated by the content of the letter.

"*His* problem," she pronounces, "is logorrhea. Some of those sentences mean almost nothing."

"It's partly a question of religious language," says John Ottokar. "It tends to be kind of portmanteau and empty at the same time. I do rather hate it. The Quakers avoid it if they can."

"He's meant to be a psychoanalyst."

"It's not exclusive. You can be both."

They are bickering about language, in order to avoid discussing the letter.

"What do you think?" says John Ottokar.

"It's nothing to do with me," says Frederica. "It's *your* letter, and *your* brother, and *your* Quakers and *your* Tigers. And *your* psychoanalyst."

"I see."

He stares gloomily at the tablecloth. He puts together his papers, as though he is about to leave.

"I'm sorry. I sound spiteful. I don't mean to be. It scares me. All these things you seem to be involved in, to *belong to.*"

"I don't say that. The point is, I haven't gone to the Spirits' Tigers, not since . . . not since we . . . I know you don't like it. I want—I want to give—what *we* have—a chance."

"If you think I think I've got any right—am in any position—to stop you being a spiritual Tiger—please reconsider. I don't have any such right—I'm not asking for it."

"I know."

And don't look gloomy and submissive, Frederica wants to cry out; what I liked was your independent *prowling.* John Ottokar says mildly, "Elvet Gander has got a point. He won't say Paul is sick, because he doesn't like the word, but Paul is whatever Paul was when everyone said he was sick. He can't cope with normal life, I do know. And I do know that I could help. He's right there. I know."

"Well then, you must help him."

"But if I help him at the expense of my own life—if I get all *snarled*—"

Frederica feels she ought to say, "We'll deal with this together, we'll see it through, don't worry." Those are the lines that are written into the script, but she doesn't want to say them. She doesn't know where she and John Ottokar would or would not be going *without* Paul/Zag and Elvet Gander and the Spiritual Tigers.

"I don't want to bore you," says John Ottokar, responding accurately to this unspoken communication.

Frederica laughs.

"I don't see how anyone could find all this *boring,*" she says. "Frightening, yes. What will you do?"

"I shan't go to the Tigers. I do want peace and quiet—the normal. I find them *heady* and—and intensely satisfying. But I ought perhaps to write to Gander and try and say what I feel, why I don't think it's a good idea. And I don't want to write, I hate writing, I hate putting things down, it's all lies, it's all *approximate* . . ."

"I'm going to meet Gander myself," says Frederica. "Rupert Parrott's having a meeting 'In Defence of *Babbletower.*' He's asked all his trendy authors—Gander, and Canon Holly and Phyllis Pratt. He's asked me, because he says I can make Jude behave better. He says a recent graduate gave evidence in the *Lady Chatterley* case, just a young girl, to show she was unsullied. I can't see me making a good impression in the witness box as an unsullied young girl who had read *Babbletower* and was still unsullied. He's terribly worked up. In a crusading sort of way. Whereas Jude is terribly worked up in a *personal* sort of way, and doesn't look well."

The June end-of-the-year exhibition at the Samuel Palmer School is still known as the Dip Show, though the students are now taking a degree, not a diploma. This is why they must pass a literature exam, and why Frederica has been working hard, invigilating and marking papers. Frederica and Agatha go to the Dip Show together, on a sunny Sunday afternoon. Leo and Saskia go with them, and Clement and Thano attach themselves to the party. So does John Ottokar, who turns up "for the fairy story," and stays to lunch, as he sometimes does.

Frederica enjoys the atmosphere. The great studios are divided into spaces, and there are abrupt changes of identity from space to space. A series of stormily menacing rural landscapes is juxtaposed with a box containing brilliant demi-lunes and diamonds of purple and yellow spots and stripes. This is next to a series of collages—balloon-breasted bearded men in fishnet tights and stilettos wrestling or embracing giant carrots and stuffed rabbits, which is in turn next to a painterly series of portraits of men and women in the act of peeling soft plastic masks off their faces. Frederica now knows enough about painting to see that what makes these interesting is the virtuosity and variety of the troughs and channels and folds and texture of the different surfaces, the perspectives of the doubled eyes and twisted sockets. She can also see that the student (Susie Blair) has been taught by Desmond Bull. Susie Blair writes decorous little essays for Frederica on "Show the different methods by which Jane Austen invites and discourages the reader's sympathy for Emma Woodhouse and/or Fanny Price"—these essays show no sign of the savage intelligence that imitates flesh and plastic in oil paint. Frederica enjoys the gaps between the painters' writings and their inventions, which she could never have thought up, or begun to imagine, even the weakest. In the next cubicle are a series of dream-worlds somewhere between Claude and Arthur Rackham, entitled *Faery Lands Forlorn*. They ought to be kitsch, and are not, not quite. Saskia says, "Look at the little greeny lights."

The painters are dispensing red and white wine in crinkling plastic beakers; everything is spread with a faint dust of trodden potato-crisps. The party hurry past a room with nothing in it but a red canvas, a white canvas and a blue canvas, with the predictable rubric "United?" They come to the graphics department, where everything is display-conscious. Here they discover that the design teacher has been as good as his word, and has set *Babbletower* as an exercise in jacket design and poster production. Here too they find Jude himself, patrolling the display like an Ancient Mariner ready to pounce and expound. He hurries up to Frederica, John and Agatha.

"Here you have the Artwork for a work of art *temporarily,* we hope, suppressed. What is your opinion of all this? Who carries away the palm for *suggestiveness*?"

"Vis man," says Leo to Saskia, *sotto voce,* "is ve *other* smelly man. My mum knows lots of really *stinking* men."

"This one *pongs,*" agrees Clement, equably.

"Be quiet," says Jude. "Little children should speak when spoken to, you must know that. How fortunate that you are all too short to see my collection of turrets. Go over there, where a well-meaning young woman has done a pretty Perrault and give me your opinion of her Puss-in-Boots and her Little Red Riding Hood. Marks out of ten, please."

Some of the *Babbletower* covers are banal. Others are clever and suggestive. One has Hockneyish drawings of a man in a wig and a woman in hoops, leering at each other half-heartedly. Two or three have Disneyish Germanic castles. One has a long procession of maggot-like infants, carrying rose branches, passing under a portcullis into blackness. One has three Blake-like Elders or Wise Men standing on a battlement amongst flocks of big black birds. One has Brueghel's beautiful painting of the unfinished, crumbling, weed-ridden Tower of Babel, with brilliant little droplets, or tongues of scarlet shiny blood dripping out of its orifices and down its ledges. Jude points this one out with approval. "The lettering is a bit fancy," he says. "If you look closely you can see it's made of needles and pins, I don't like that. But it's better than these dreadful *people* who aren't my people, who stop you *seeing* the people in the book, who *interfere.*"

"This one's clever," says Agatha.

It is semi-abstract and very bright—a tomato-coloured double-apple-cheeked fruit, with a serpentine pointed conical tube in very bright green, coiled round it and penetrating it.

"I hate it," says Jude.

"It's a good joke," says Agatha, in her mild, dark voice. "Cul-vert. Rose-Arse. It's all there, in *purely visual language.*"

"I can see that. I hate it."

Agatha considers.

"I might hate it, if I were you. But since I'm not, I find it very witty. I hope it got a good mark."

"It did," says Jude.

He takes them "to see my glory and my shame." He hurries them down flights of stairs and into the refectory, where there is a display of the Foundation Course Life Studies, which include Jude naked, in chalk, in charcoal, in pastel, in gouache, in pencil, in acrylic, in oil. He is a faceless skinny length of bone in a tent of hair, he is meticulously delineated nipples and prick in bronze and green on grey paper, he is soft, soft lead, uncannily recalling the exact tone of his hippo-grey skin, sitting regally in a gilt chair, lying foetally coiled on plumped and depressed cushions. He is tendons and knobby knees and chilblains and scraggy neck; he is aquiline disdain; he is gloom with downcast eyes. The three little boys go from image to image; they do not say so, but everyone can see they are comparing the depictions of his genitals. Leo points and whispers: Clement nods.

"I am instructive," says Jude.

"Do you *enjoy* seeing these?" says Agatha.

"It convinces me I exist, I suppose. And that we do not see ourselves as others see us, which I know. And that my shins are not proportionate—at some moment, from some angles—with each other or with other parts of my anatomy."

Far away, in the bowels of the building, they hear music. It is a jazz clarinet, wooden and liquid, a clear long, long wail, a run of chords, a desolate repeated complaint. They wander in its direction. One or two canted notices, hung on door-knobs, say in red letters on white card: PERFORMANCE THIS WAY. Performance art is not—not yet—really on the agenda of the Samuel Palmer School. Not many people are following the signs, but the children pull the adults along. In a sculpture storeroom, abutting the garages and car park, a small dais has been set up. It is shrouded in black velvet, hazed with chalk dust. Behind it is a long and welded sculpture, painted in pillar-box red, with a series of blade-like forms suspended from a series of ladder-like forms. To its right is a huddled crowd of chipped and cheesy-surfaced classical plaster casts: a bland Apollo tipped off-balance against a smiling, hoofed Pan, a headless Athena with her Gorgon breastplate, a horsehead, a very small centaur. On the left of the dais is Paul Ottokar, in tailcoat and white tie (he looks classically beautiful), playing the clarinet, with his music propped before him on a very pretty gilt stand. On the right is a kind of cage-like edifice made from multi-coloured playstraws, inside which is a human being dressed like a large bird, with a bright yellow bulging rump, a feathered tail, wrinkled yellow tights, large clawed feet constructed from wire, insulating tape and putty, a tarred and feathered torso, and a head crested with green feathers, masked like an American Indian bird-man, over which is strapped an aluminium contraption with a very long, proboscis-like stabbing beak with a strip of Day-Glo-pink fluorescent paint running its whole length.

With this he monotonously taps a large metal plate, painted with a black-and-white spiral pattern, at his feet. The tapping is not in synch with the clarinet music. At irregular intervals the bird-man raises and lets fall his wings/arms in an impotent way. When he does this, a rattle whirs briefly. Saskia says, "It is the Dong with the luminous nose." Leo says, "It is *ve other* smelly man, ve *other* John." He looks at John, to make sure there are two. Frederica looks at John, to see what they should do. John stands in the shadow of the plaster casts and smiles slightly, listening. The only other person in the room is Desmond Bull, who kisses Frederica and smiles at Jude.

Paul Ottokar pauses in his playing, without acknowledging his audience. His companion does not pause in his manic tapping. Paul Ottokar bows, sits down, and begins to play the Adagio from Mozart's Clarinet Concerto. The man-bird taps, mechanically. The beautiful sounds bubble and flow. The beak stabs and taps. Frederica tries to shut out the tapping and cannot. The bird-man raises his wings and whirs. The music gathers power. The bird-man ceases to tap and for a moment a small trill is alone in the silence. Then the bird-man begins a virtuoso imitation of a hen laying an egg. The children laugh. It is a very good imitation. The music sings away. The bird-man taps again. He stops. He makes a series of sounds which can be interpreted as a hen trying frantically to escape pursuit, failing, and having its neck wrung. He strangles, he gags, he croaks. The lovely music runs on. Frederica thinks: There is *not enough point* to all this, or else I am missing something. It is a thought she is often to have, in those years.

When the music has come to an end, Paul Ottokar closes his music book, folds his music stand, takes out a box of matches and sets fire to the straw cage.

"Watch it!" says Bull.

The base flares, blackens and dies. The structure collapses. Clarinet player and bird take a bow. They step off the dais. "Is vat all?" says Leo.

"That is all," says Paul Ottokar, unsmiling.

"It was *quite* funny," says Clement judiciously.

"It gives a headache," says Saskia, more musical than Frederica and Leo.

The brothers are side by side.

"You burned the cage," says Leo. "How can you start again?"

"We aren't going to," says the bird-man, with a Liverpudlian voice under his mask. "We've done that, now. We're going for a spaghetti. It's the end of the day. Anyone coming?"

"Yes," says John Ottokar. "That would be a good idea. Anyone else?"

Everyone goes to the Spaghetti House around the corner. It seems quite natural, quite ordinary, two brothers have met by accident, a group of friends have decided to have spaghetti after a Dip Show.

The bird-man is introduced as Silo. Under his aluminium dong-beak and his formal mask he is pale, scrawny-necked and bespectacled. Frederica asks John Ottokar, who appears to know him, if Silo is anything to do with Silence. John says no, his name is Sidney Lowe, it's the first syllable of his names. Paul Ottokar says, "You could take it as a sign, though, that the syllables come out like that. It might have a meaning."

"Most syllables can be made to mean *something,*" says John.

"Empiricist, nationalist," says Paul, as though these words were delicate insults.

The meal goes well. The Spaghetti House is made with barn-like booths and red-checked tablecloths; all the booths are full of celebrating art students drinking Chianti. The children become restive, waiting for their dishes of carbonara and bolognese, and John Ottokar organises a kind of round-table serial game of scissors-paper-stone. Leo says, "Is it *true,* what you said, you two always put out ve *same thing,* always?"

Paul smiles at John. "Did you tell him that?"

"It was true, then."

"And now? Try now?"

It is like arm-wrestling, a trial of strength in a pub; it is amiable, but tense. John and Paul are sitting opposite each other. They put out a hand each. Flat, both. Paper, paper. Again. Clenched fists. Stone, stone. Stone, stone. Stone, stone. Scissors, scissors. Paper, paper. Scissors, scissors. Stone, stone. Stone, stone. Frederica watches with alarm. Bull says, "This is nothing to do with the law of averages." Silo says, "Do you read each other's minds?"

"No, no," says Paul. "We just *know.* Quick as a flash, we *know.*"

Scissors, scissors. Paper, paper. Stone, stone.

They look pleased with themselves. Paul says, "Do you remember, we used to sing?" He hums. "Anything *you* can do, I can do *better.* I can do *any*thing, *bet*ter than you." John joins in.

"No you can't." "Yes, I can." "No you can't." "Yes, I can."

"It was true and not true," says Paul.

Frederica has not seen them together since the bonfire night. Leo and Clement and Thano start singing. "Anything *you* can do, *I* can do *better.*" Frederica thinks: I thought the problem was, the two of them, fighting over *me.* She has the sexual self-confidence, over-confidence perhaps, of her curious historical position, brief and anomalous, a Cambridge woman when there were eleven men for every woman. They were princesses, those women, though ordinary enough, in fact. Now she sees that it is not that, not so much that, that is the problem. She is in competition with each brother for the attention of the other, and must lose. They sit at ease, smiling at each other, thrusting out their identical fists, paper, scissors, stone, with no winner, no loser, no difference.

She thinks: They are like the two blades of a pair of scissors. She thinks: If we are two, we are two so, as stiff twin compasses are two. She thinks, with an internal mad laughter, "Those whom God hath joined together let no woman put asunder." She has a brief memory of their joined bloody bodies, John's and hers. She feels Desmond Bull's hand, making a firm secret curl behind her buttocks, strong, steady. She does not push it away.

They sing another song. Everyone joins in.

"I'll sing you one-oh.
Green grow the rushes-oh.
What is your one-oh?

One is one and all alone
And ever more shall be so."

Saskia and Agatha raise clear voices. Thano sings strongly. It is a good, friendly party. "I'll sing you two-oh. Two, two, the lily-white boys, clothed all in green-oh. One is one and all alone, and ever more shall be so. I'll sing you three-oh. Green grow the rushes-oh. What are your three-oh? Three, three, the Rivals."

"You're out of tune, Frederica."

"I expect I am, Paul. I always am. I told you, I'm not musical. I'm tone-deaf."

"We could teach you. You probably aren't *really* tone-deaf. Almost no one really is incurably tone-deaf. You could learn."

"No, I couldn't. I can't. I'll shut up, since my singing offends you. I'll be the audience."

Desmond Bull's fingers wrinkling the cloth on her buttocks. The two faces opposite, both with eyebrows quizzically and ruefully raised, the charming expression identical, *the same.*

"Go *on,*" says Leo, crossly.

"Three, three, the Rivals. Two, two, the lily-white boys, clothed all in green-oh. One is one and all alone and ever more shall be so."

Laminations

Instructions for use. Your Pills are presented in separated bubble-strips, clearly marked with the days of the week. Press each pill out of its bubble and swallow it with water at the same time each day. It is important not to miss a day: if you do, you may not be fully protected. When you have taken three weeks' supply of pills, you must take none for the next week, during which bleeding may occur. This bleeding may be scanty, though occasionally it may be copious, more than your usual menstrual bleedings. This bleeding is break-through bleeding, and cleanses the womb: it is not a "period," and should cause you no discomfort. If heavy bleeding occurs and persists after several cycles of the Pill you should see your doctor, who may prescribe an alternative dosage.

The herald brought the little glass slipper to the house of the three sisters, and there was great excitement there. The eldest stepsister claimed that the slipper was hers, and would fit her; the stepmother measured her foot against the delicate shell and declared that it would never go in. "It is a small price to pay for the hand of a Prince and half a kingdom," said the stepmother then. "Be resolute, and I will take a slice from your heel with this knife, and the foot will slide in." So they did as she suggested, and the eldest sister came before the herald and the young Prince and stretched out her fat leg proudly and turned her foot in the shining shoe. But the herald observed that gouts of dark blood were welling up inside it and brimming over, and he asked the sister to take off the shoe again, and she did so, and her wound was visible to all, and she was shamed and disgraced. Then the second sister, no whit discouraged by her sister's failure, tried to force the pretty shoe over her knobby foot, but it would not go, no matter how she struggled and shoved. So her mother took the little axe with which they killed the hens, and quick as a flash chopped off her big toe, and bandaged it, and then they were able to force the foot in, and the second sister hobbled proudly into the presence of the Prince. But the brown bird in the tree that flowered on Cinderella's mother's grave called out, "There is blood in the shoe, there is blood in the shoe," and when the herald came near he saw that the shoe was full of blood and the second sister was faint with pain. So she too was disgraced, and went away to weep and sulk. And the herald asked, "Are there no more young women in the house?" And the stepmother said, no, but the father said, "There is only Cinderella, in the ashes, in the kitchens." So Cinderella was sent for, and she came, and stretched out her pretty little foot, all grimed as it was with ashes, in its cheap stocking, and the shoe fitted exactly, like a glove. And when the Prince saw that the shoe fitted exactly, he recognised his beautiful dancing partner in the little skivvy, and said, "What was lost is found, and this is the bride my heart is sworn to." And they both rode away together, past the brown bird singing in the weeping tree.

Quaere. Who cleaned the coagulated blood out of the shoe, twice over, before Cinderella inserted her virginal toes?

> *Under a Tree I saw a Virgin sit*
> *The red and white rose quartered in her face.*
>
> *Just at the stroke when my veins start and spread*
> *Set on my neck an everlasting Head.*

"I take no such pleasure in life that I should much wish it, nor conceive such horror in death that I should greatly fear it; and yet I say not, but if the stroke were coming, perchance flesh and blood would be moved with it and seek to shun it." (Elizabeth I)

The Trial: Day 11

"You had a conversation with Gran, did you not?"

"No, she shouted down: 'What is all the noise?' I said: 'It is just the dog barking'—not that the tape-recorder had dropped on my toes as was alleged I had said."

"But this was during the shouting?"

"No, it wasn't."

"It is very odd that she should ask the question after the noise had ceased."

"No; she was probably awakened from her sleep and had got out of bed to come to the bedroom door."

"You were quite determined that the old lady should not interfere?"

"Yes, I shouted up so that she would not come down. If she had come down she might well have dropped dead with shock."

"There were spots of blood on your shoes?"

"Yes. It was probably splashed on. Possibly because the shoes had been left in the living-room. I had been out in my high-heeled shoes."

"The trial is now in its eleventh day. Have we heard this suggestion before, that the shoes were in the room, and that you were not wearing them that night?"

"No."

"Let me see the shoes, please. Is there any trace of blood inside those shoes, as far as you know?"

"No."

"Your feet were inside the shoes and your feet were taking whatever blood fell upon that area?"

"No."

"Are you now wearing the high-heeled shoes you were wearing that night?"

"Yes."

"May I see one of them, please?" (*Shoe handed to the Attorney-General*). "Is that the shoe you were wearing to go on the moors?"

"Yes, I went in the car. I always wear high-heels outside. We were not going to walk on the moors. We were just going to park."

The Story of Stone

Peter Stone, a sculptor, a student at the Samuel Palmer School. A slight, bowed young man, with a pitted, ashy skin, loose lips, and a shock of colourless hair always full of stone-dust. He was working, I was later told and shown, on a kind of minor marble menhir, white with pinkish veinings, which was in the Dip Show, or Degree Show. It was an erect cylindrical form, with a gently rounded top, which had been chipped and worked into a crazed, dimpled, sinewy surface, so that the marble glittered here and there, and did not have the smoothness one easily associates with marble. It was not very big; three feet perhaps. Having learned to look for subversion and opposition in new works of art, I decided that this was an act of defiance against the welded metal or moulded plastic and fibre-glass sculptures: Stone's carving was the only *carved* work in the Show, that year.

I invigilated the final examination he took: final in every sense. He must have been sitting in about the third row back: one of the big studios had been set out with temporary desks. He came in smiling broadly, and sat down staring around, and writing nothing. He was twitching and fidgeting. He began to write. His handwriting was very large and vacant. He kept coming up to the front for more paper. He asked to be excused, left the room briefly, came back and wrote a few more large words, asked for more paper, rushed out to be excused, dust falling from his hair, came back, wrote more words. Because they were all art students, no one paid much attention to this behaviour. Finally he reached a point where he was writing one large, childishly formed word per sheet, rushing back and forwards, writing another. A sheaf of paper rose in front of him. Finally he rushed out and did not return. "Stoned," one of the other students said. We laughed, and finished our work. I gathered up his papers at the end of the exam. He had written only one sentence, over and over, in huge round letters. YOU CAN'T GET BLOOD OUT OF A STONE.

Later we discovered that he had run down the Holborn up escalator, on to the Central Line platform, and had opened his arms and jumped into the path of an approaching train. He was killed, instantly they said, as they always do. Perhaps he thought he could fly. Perhaps he was in despair over his exams. No one knew. There must have been a great deal of blood. The train driver collapsed and has been unable to start work again. This story is almost too neat, as though the language had constructed it, not it the language, blood and stones, but it is a true story, a story of our times, uncanny only because of the too great, glittering precision of the language.

Why a Tongue impressed with honey from every wind?
Why an Ear, a whirlpool fierce to draw creations in?
Why a Nostril wide inhaling terror, trembling and affright?

Why a tender curb on the youthful burning boy?
Why a little curtain of flesh on the bed of our desire?

The Virgin started from her seat, and with a shriek
Fled back unhindered till she came into the vales of Har.

But Shelob was not as dragons are, no softer spot had she save only her eyes. Knobbed and pitted with corruption was her age-old hide, but ever thickened from within with layer on layer of evil growth. The blade scored it with a dreadful gash, but those hideous folds could not be pierced by any strength of man, not though Elf or Dwarf should fuse the steel or the hand of Beren or of Túrin wield it. She yielded to the stroke, and then heaved up the great bag of her belly high above Sam's head. Poison frothed and bubbled from the wound. Now splaying her legs she drove the huge bulk down on him again. Too soon. For Sam still stood upon his feet, and dropping his own sword, with both hands he held the elven-blade point upwards, fending off that ghastly roof; and so Shelob, with the driving force of her own cruel will, with strength greater than any warrior's hand, thrust herself upon a bitter spike. Deep, deep it pricked, as Sam was crushed slowly to the ground.

No such anguish had Shelob ever known, or dreamed of knowing, in all her long world of wickedness. Not the doughtiest soldier of old Gondor, nor the most savage Orc entrapped, had ever thus endured her, or set blade to her beloved flesh.

Observer May 8th, 1966 (Maurice Richardson)

"If those two were sane they'd have gone mad long ago." I was rather impressed by this comment—by a local hall porter—on the psychology of Ian Brady and Myra Hindley. Behaviour so atrocious can only be described in terms of Irish or Hegelian logic, the logic of contradictions. How does one begin to explain it?

It is all very well to say that we were all once polymorph—perverse infants, and that Mr. Everyman's unconscious teems with sado-masochistic impulses. True, of course. But there is nothing impulsive about their dreadful calculated performances and the elaborate decoying that must have preceded them. I find it less difficult to empathise with Jack the Ripper than with these two. Odd how one always calls them Brady and Myra.

The other peculiar feature here is the dual element. *Folie à deux* in which two people go mad together is not unknown. An hysteric who falls in love with a psychotic will share the psychotic's delusions as long as they are together. Separate them, and the hysteric recovers, while the psychotic remains insane. And according to Freud hysterical women may share the perversions of their lovers. . . .

In the dock: Brady is thin, bony, rather gangling. Lean face with straight nose jutting out under his rather flat forehead. His dark brown hair is neat and tidy, yet looks faintly dusty. His clothes—grey suit, pale blue shirt, ultramarine, mildly artistic tie—are dateless, not like those of David Smith, who goes in for the gear. One of the first things you notice about him is his bad colour: pale mud. He really does look terribly sick.

Myra by contrast is blooming. Her hair, naturally brown, has been changing colour from week to week. First silver-lilac, then bright canary blonde. She is a big girl with a striking face: fine straight nose, thinnish curved lips, rather hefty chin, blue eyes. Full face she is almost a beauty. The Victorians would have admired her.

She wears a black-and-white speckled coat and skirt and a pale blue shirt open at the neck: it matches Brady's. I suspect she imitates everything he does, even to always keeping her handkerchief neatly folded. At a glance she looks as smartly turned out as a duchess, but when you look closer you see at once that this is mass-produced supermarket chic: there is an ambience of bubblegum and candyfloss.

Both take copious notes and lean over the front of the dock to prod their solicitor, the eupeptic Mr. Fitzpatrick, with a pencil. Occasionally they offer each other a packet of mints. Once during David Smith's evidence Myra flashes Brady a quick bright smile. When he goes into the witness box she gazes at him. When it is her turn, he draws faces on his scribbling pad.

Tea—yes—with some of the hosts of detectives working on this case. We talked about modern youth, violence, censorship, permissiveness and all that. One of them, who is a bit of a sociologist and has a highly specialised knowledge of swinging Manchester, thought there was a dangerous current of perversion in the air. "Kinky" had become a household word. He'd seen a shop advertising: NEW LINE IN KINKY RAINCOATS. Why, he said, don't they label them raincoats for sexual perverts and be done with it? He said it twice over. This may be an unduly puritan reaction: it is quite a common one. We shall encounter it more often as a result of this case. . . .

I haven't myself dreamed about the case at all, but occasionally in court towards the end of the afternoon I've caught myself lapsing into fantasies. These have taken the form of carrying out vengeance on the accused, which shows how careful you have to be. Once, I said to myself: If I were to put on Batman's gear, swoop down on the dock, which I could easily do from my seat in the gallery, what would the *News of the World* pay for my life story?

I lie awake at 2 a.m. because some race-going son of Belial—there are night clubs now even in Chester—has jammed the horn of his car. I try to find a suitable text in Sartre's *Saint Genet* which a kind local friend has lent me: he thinks that Brady might conceivably turn into his opposite. I'm afraid he has a long way to go, and he lacks Genet's talent. How about this?

"Thus the evil doer is the Other. Evil—fleeting, artful, marginal evil—can be seen only out of the corner of one's eye and in others . . . The Enemy is our twin brother, our image in the mirror . . . For peace-time Society has in its wisdom created what might be called professional evil doers.

"These evil men are as necessary to good men as whores are to decent women. They are fixation abscesses. For a single sadist there is any number of appeased, clarified, relaxed consciousnesses. They are therefore very carefully recruited. They must be bad by birth and without hope of change."

H'm. I think I know what Mr. Justice Fenton Atkinson would say to that. And I rather think I agree with him. We've had rather a surfeit of evil up here.

The summer holidays return. Leo will go to stay at Bran House; it is as though there were a regular pattern of life, and Frederica half-hopes that Leo thinks there is, but it is no such thing, it is all provisional and full of violence and threats of violence. The lawyers' letters fly. She cuts them up and pastes them into *Laminations.* She considers her own summer plans. Perhaps she will go back to Yorkshire.

Whilst she is thinking this out, John Ottokar telephones. He is at work; she has never seen where he works or where he lives, which she believes is somewhere in Earls Court. She imagines his place of work as a large space full of huge, clean, quietly humming machines, with walls of glimmering blue-grey screens showing graphs, and the columns of the strange binary language they print out on interleaved concertinas of pristine paper. She imagines him surrounded by other decorous, suited people, some of them—she is not sure about this—in surgical white coats. She imagines cool, metal venetian blinds, and shining steel furniture. It is probably nothing like this, but this is what she imagines. He says, "Can you come out to dinner with me?"

"I should think so. I can get a baby-sitter. Agatha's working late, I know. I can ask a student."

"Chez Victor," he says. "Eight o'clock."

Frederica likes Chez Victor. It is small, and dark, and simple and sophisticated, and truly French; the food is French French food and reminds her, amongst dark green paint and etched glass, of the heat of Provence, M. et Mme. Grimaud, wine and garlic. She wears a black linen shift, well above her knees, and a silk shawl, black, embroidered with creamy cabbagey roses and golden lilies, with a long, shimmering fringe. She has learned to line her eyes with a black, surprised stare, and to lengthen her lashes; nothing can make her angular quickness look doll-like, but this is as near as she will ever get. She has painted her wide mouth creamy-brown, a pale colour, which does not wholly suit her. John Ottokar is wearing his suit. Frederica loves to see him in his suit. She is afraid of having to live her life amongst the unkempt, the meagrely bearded, the sagging and woolly, the deliberately ill-defined. She likes edge. John Ottokar in his suit, with his long, blond, well-cut hair, has edge. He looks good in Chez Victor: a serious man eating a serious meal. They have *pâté, soupe de poissons,* skate in black butter, an *entrecôte sauce béarnaise, pommes dauphinoises,* an excellent salad, a perfect *tarte au citron.* They discuss the coming summer.

"I am thinking of going back to Freyasgarth."

"It is beautiful, up there."

"We had a good few days in Goathland."

"More than good."

There is a constraint in him.

"Do you want to come for a bit? Do you have any holiday?"

She never invites him: she always waits for him to move. This time, she has exposed herself.

"Of course I want to come. Of course I do."

"But?"

"I have ten days owing to me."

"But?"

"You *know* what the 'but' is, Frederica. The Spirits' Tigers are having a month-long Retreat, at Four Pence. They've got people coming from Timothy Leary's League for Spiritual Discovery. And some

Buddhists. And Elvet Gander. And of course Paul. He wants me to come. Gander's writing again."

He looks at the starched white tablecloth. He does not look at Frederica. He says, "Paul asked me to ask you if you'd come."

"God, no," says Frederica, quick as a flash, with automatic revulsion. She looks at his brooding face, turned down, lit a little by the shine of the clean cloth in the dark green room. "I'm sorry, John. I don't mean to sound nasty. But I'm not religious and I *hate group things,* I hate them, I hate pressure on me to lose myself, I can't bear it, I won't."

"I told him you wouldn't. I told him why. I told him what you've just said."

"And?"

"He said, that's exactly why she *ought* to come, she doesn't know what she doesn't know."

"Probably he's right. But I'll go on not knowing, if you don't mind. I'll put a lot of books in a bag, and go north, and read and write, and be part of my family, which is a group I've got no choice about belonging to."

"I shall lose you."

"Who can tell? We have to decide what's important. I can't imagine *you*—not the you I know—in some sort of ecstatic group love-in, all moaning and humming and confessing, if you want to know. But everybody has all sorts of sides to them. There are things about me *you* can't possibly imagine."

"It isn't like that. It isn't moaning and humming."

"I know. I'm unfair. I think we ought to stop talking about it."

"The Quaker silence," says John Ottokar, and does not finish the sentence.

"The Quaker silence?" says Frederica.

"When I was a boy, the silence made other people bearable for me. And more than that. You could sit there—they were all quite ordinary—and after a time, after a time of silence—everyone was quiet—you lost—not your *self* exactly—but all the mess of—the *fuss* of your life—you were all quiet together. It wasn't that everyone became one, or anything—I couldn't bear that any more than you could. It was just that they were *true*—*truer*—than before—to be truthful, I don't really want them to be Tigers—I just liked the quiet, the truth. Look, Frederica, this really is a thing words can't deal with. I keep saying 'true' and you don't know what I'm talking about, it doesn't *represent* what I'm talking about."

"Perhaps I do."

"It's something I can't really do without, anyway. Not having known it. I don't think there'll be much of it—if any—at Four Pence this summer. But there's the other thing too, I've got to look after Paul, that's how it is."

"I understand all that."

At this moment, she loves him, she would use the word "love," for what she feels about his careful truthfulness.

"I shall lose you," he says.

"I don't know," she says, trying to be as honest as he is. "I shouldn't have sounded so nasty, but it is true, I can't really bear it, all that, Tigers and chemical ecstasy and hugging-encounters, I really feel—"

"Repelled."

"Yes."

"So do I. Really. I shouldn't go. For myself. Only Paul—"

"You wanted to be separate."

"I do. But *really.* Sometimes I think Gander could help us through."

"Do you?"

"Not with much conviction. I don't know *what* I think. The trouble with Paul is, he does. I'm the tough one, in one sense, but he's the one with convictions, and feelings, he *dives*—"

"I can't cope with both of you."

"Fair enough. I shall lose you."

He stares at the tablecloth. Frederica bites lemon tart. Her tongue tastes sweetness and sharpness. She has no need of any chemical: the tart is sweet, is sour, is unforgettable.

"It is up to you," she says.

He lifts his head.

"I shall come with you. I won't lose you. It matters to me. We'll make our own quiet, up there on the moors."

His hand moves to touch hers, on the white cloth. She has a moment of fear—has she promised more than she can give, has she *taken on* the complicated coils of the brotherhood?

"No promises," he says, hearing this thought in the silence. "Just a summer holiday. A good one."

She takes hold of his hand. His skin is dry, and warm, and good. They get the bill, and go on the Underground, back to Kennington.

When they come back to Hamelin Square, there are more people than usual on the pavements. The Agyepongs are out, and also the Utters, and the small man with the little Austin is standing behind it. The door of Number 42 is open—not the area door, but the upper door, and framed in it are Leo, Saskia and their substitute-granny, peering anxiously out. As John Ottokar and Frederica emerge from the pan-handle, so to speak, of the square, into the frying-pan itself, a golden figure leaps up the area steps, three at a time, and crosses to the central mud patch in three long balletic, scissor-like jumps. This figure has flying gold hair and a long, shimmering, shining robe, a kind of sleeved gown in transparent plastic shot with rainbow colours, like oil spilled in a puddle on the road. The plastic makes a hissing and swishing noise. The figure's arms are full of something which he places carefully in the old chair which lolls against the broken bedstead on the mud, where the bonfire's charred traces can still be seen. He bends over the chair, and Hamelin Square is suddenly full of music, not pop music but Brunnhilde's fire music from the end of *The Valkyrie.* It is not clear why no one moves forward, but no one does. He produces a straw-cased Chianti bottle, from which he pours libations into the chair, and then, sweeping in a great circle round the edge of the mud patch, over various towers of books, which can now be seen to ring the whole circle. He is singing, or humming, not Wagner, but some ecstatic blending moan. He dances, extending his arms in the light of the street lamps. It becomes clear that inside his plastic robe he is naked except for a swirling design of gold and burgundy body paint, spiralling round his arms and legs, making targets of his nipples, crossing in arching branches over his belly under his erect cock in its golden bush. As they watch, he produces a cigarette lighter and sets fire to the skoob turrets, of which there are seven, all of them quite high. His face too is painted, a snarling cat mask under the blond flying hair. He skips from burning books to burning books, making obeisances, mopping and mowing. He sings, he dances. "Ite Bacchae. Io Zagreus." It is absurd and frightening. The books flare and then burn sullenly, smelling bad and smoking. He returns, pouring more paraffin from the Chianti bottle. Frederica, at first paralysed like everyone else by the noise and the flickering flames and the strangeness, is suddenly galvanised by a dreadful fear. She pulls her hand away from John's and runs forward, kicking at the nearest skoob tower, to demolish it. The books are somehow fused together, and fall together, a falling tower, spitting sparks. Frederica can read their spines. They are her books, and not only her books, but part of herself, the books she has been teaching to her civilised extramural class. *The Castle, The Trial, The Idiot, Madame Bovary, Anna Karenina, Mansfield Park, La Chute, The Age of Reason, Lord of the Flies, Free Fall, Women in Love, Howards End.*

Rage takes hold of Frederica, rage unreasoning and wild, rage all too reasoning and justified, for all her notes, all her work, are written into the flyleaves of these burning books. She tries to kick the books apart to extinguish the flames, she rushes to the next tower—*Paradise Lost, Euripides, Dr. Faustus*—and the cloaked figure swoops at her from behind the bedstead, *yowling,* as she puts it to herself, finding *le mot juste* even in the conflagration.

"*I'll kill you,*" she howls at Paul-Zag, "let me get at you, *I'll kill you*—"

"I can't be killed," he intones. "I am born from the flames I don't burn I am not consumed."

"Rubbish," says Frederica. *"You will pay for this—"*

She tries to grasp him: his skin is hot and slippery under her hands, which are now smeared with gold and wine-dark grease. She grabs hold of the flying plastic, which is now very hot and limp and feels as though it will melt. He leaps back towards the centre of the square, and sets light to the old chair, in which is the Chianti bottle, which explodes, sending a tower of flame at the dark sky, singeing the blond locks badly and melting one side of the robe, which, as plastic does, shrivels and shrinks in the heat, producing its own stink and its own thick smoke. Frederica is divided between murderous rage and the desire to retrieve, to extinguish, to protect her books. She moves towards the next tower and is forestalled by Paul-Zag, who dances forwards, bends down, and before her horrified eyes clasps the whole structure protectively to his breast. There is now a terrible smell of burned flesh, as well as burned plastic and burned books. Paul falls over backwards in the mud. Frederica kicks her sullenly smouldering books away from his charred breast and belly. John Ottokar—too late, weeping—arrives at Frederica's side. Paul lies on his back and looks up at the haze of streetlight, the black-let-down-with-orange-and-sodium-silver sky, the very distant, diminished stars. He is not yet in pain; that will come. Marie Agyepong appears with a pot of zinc-and-castor-oil ointment. Paul looks at Frederica out of sly and inhuman eyes, their lashes painted and weeping black and red tears on his gilded cheeks. The sky, he announces, is full of great spiders spinning, it is swarming with octopods in every colour, it is thick with crawling worms and maggots who eat flesh and spit blood, they must all hide, but there is nowhere to hide. Brunnhilde shrieks defiance and submission. Frederica thinks she can see her enemy summing up, cannily, the effect of his pronouncements on the assembled company, all now creeping up on the mud patch. "He is high," says Marie Agyepong, "that's most of it, he's on a bad trip."

"I am high," says Paul. "I am in a high place, I shall leap down and my angels will hold me up, you'll see, I am on a bad trip and the spiders are coming after me, I shall fall and great will be the fall thereof and when I fall it will all fall, all that's holding it *up* will drag it *down,* you'll see, whether you want to or not, you'll have to see."

"It *hurts,*" he says suddenly, and begins to moan frantically.

"I sent for an ambulance," says Marie Agyepong. "He's burned quite bad, they'll have to take him to the burns unit in Roehampton."

And indeed, the sirens can be heard, coming round the corner, into the square.

John Ottokar says he will go with his brother, in the ambulance.

Frederica, having comforted Leo, spends the night sorting the burned books from the almost intact, the black paper from the scorched brown and yellow, the ashes from the written words. She weeps quietly, once the kindly neighbours have gone home. John Ottokar does not ring from the hospital. He does not ring the next day, either.

XVIII

After Paul-Zag's demonstration, there is no further word from the Ottokars. Frederica listens for the telephone for a day or two, and then flares into something resembling her old anger. She goes to visit Desmond Bull, in his studio. She admires the masks and the collaged staring eyes; she drinks beakers of Bull's Blood, she falls, queasy with red wine, turpentine and anger, into the arms of Bull on the mattress on the studio floor. Bull is a no-nonsense lover, like a steam-hammer, she thinks, which is what she needs. A bang, a bonk, abandon. She bites his shoulder, she scratches his ribs and buttocks, she urges him on, like a wild woman. She is under the protection of the Pill; they meet, theoretically, as equals. No finesse, no holding back, no exploration, no discovery. But a reasonable amount of pleasure, a not unpleasant throbbing and bruising, a salutary moment or two of oblivion. Followed, in due course, by a meal of pasta asciutta, rigatoni seeping hot tomato and melted creamy cheese, and a heated discussion of Patrick Heron's striped paintings. It is equality, possibly, Frederica thinks, pushing the twins back into her mind's caverns. She wonders if she is behaving like a man. She can feel the marks of her own teeth in her lips; she can feel the swelling where his cheekbone has ground on hers. The lineaments of satisfied desire, she does not say. Desmond Bull asks after Jude Mason and his book. It has gone quiet, Frederica says, it's the fallow season for lawyers.

She goes north, alone. She is fretting; she does not know what to do, with her summer, or with her life. She misses Leo, and yet, guiltily, feels free without him; she will not think about the Ottokars, and has nothing to do with her freedom. It is a warm summer: she sits on the lawn behind the Freyasgarth house, looking onto the moors, and reading novels for review (there are not many, the supply dries up in the summer) and the texts for her next year's teaching. *Death in Venice* and *Daniel Deronda*. It takes her a day or two to realise how much older her father looks; he is becoming a little deaf, his steps are careful, even tentative, his opinions are advanced, also, more tentatively. Daniel arrives, two days after Frederica, to see Will and Mary, to rest for a few days. He too thinks Bill looks older.

A drama is going on which neither of them quite understands, since it is largely kept from them when its actors are present in Freyasgarth, and much of it takes place at Long Royston or in Calverley. It is to do with Marcus and his two friends, Ruth and Jacqueline. Frederica, lying in her deckchair on the lawn, watches these three pass, in twos, in threes, in fours—sometimes including Luk Lysgaard-Peacock—arguing, vehemently or gloomily, staring at the ground or gesturing, frozen into silence by Frederica's look. Once, Frederica comes upon Marcus and Jacqueline, standing by the gate. Jacqueline, brown, determined, severe, is berating Marcus.

"You've *got* to. Only you can do anything to stop this wickedness. You know it's wickedness, and you know *you* can do something. Why are you so *wet*?"

"It isn't any of my business. And I wouldn't change anything. Only make it worse."

"But it's *horrible,* Marcus."

"Possibly. Possibly."

They see Frederica, and freeze into silence. She broods for a moment, and returns to the intricacies of Thomas Mann's vision of liveliness and decay in Venice.

Marcus and Jacqueline come to Sunday lunch at Freyasgarth. It is not clear to Frederica whether or not they come as a couple; she even goes so far as to ask Daniel, who says he has no idea, but rather thinks it alternates, on-off, "to everyone's dissatisfaction." Winifred makes a good lunch, a roast, a salad, a raspberry soufflé. Afterwards, they have coffee in the garden. A figure approaches the group from the house; the door bell has not rung. It is Ruth, the nurse, with her pale plait hanging between her shoulders, wearing a cotton gingham dress, blue-checked with a crisp white collar. She looks very young. She says to Winifred, "Please forgive me for intruding, please forgive me for coming in without knocking. I've come to say good-bye to you. I'm leaving Calverley—I've resigned my job, I'm going away."

"I'm so sorry," says Winifred. "I hope you'll be happy. Where are you going?"

"You said you hadn't decided," says Marcus. "You said you were thinking."

"Well, I've thought. And I've prayed. And it has all become quite clear. Quite clear. And once it was clear, there wasn't a moment to lose. So I've given in my notice, and packed things, and here I am to say good-bye."

She continues to smile brightly at Winifred. She does not look at either Marcus or Jacqueline. Daniel says, "Where are you going, Ruth?"

"I'm going to take vows. Oh, nothing like the old nunneries, nothing enclosed like that. But the Children of Joy are forming a little residential community—the Joyful Companions—and I'm to be one of the first Companions. I'm suitable, I have skills I can bring to the work."

She smiles her little white, composed smile. Daniel offers her his chair, which she accepts, still not looking at Jacqueline or Marcus.

"It is a wonderful opportunity," she says, in her clear, composed little voice. She folds her hands in her lap, and looks down at them.

"Is this to do with Gideon Farrar?" asks Daniel.

"Of course. The community will begin in Gideon's vicarage near Bolton. It is ideally situated, there is plenty of quiet country round, and the parish is a country parish, but we will be able to receive—guests, people in need—from the industrial cities—we will be able to go out and find them . . ."

Marcus says, "You were doing good where you were, in the children's ward."

"Oh yes, but that is a place of death and despair. A terrible place, where I couldn't go out. With the help of the Children I can be much *more* use—we can help each other, and the sick and the unhappy, we can *show* people. We can heal. Gideon can heal. I've seen him. We can work together."

"Vows?" says Daniel.

"Oh, not like vows used to be. New vows. I can't tell you them, but they're simple, fidelity to the community, perpetual watchfulness, complete trust."

Jacqueline says, explosively, "You can't do this, Ruthie. It's dangerous. You *can't.*"

"It isn't dangerous. It's saving. I knew you wouldn't understand."

"Gideon Farrar may have charisma, but *you know,* Ruthie, he's dangerous—*you know* and I know you know."

Ruth rises to her feet again, and smooths the gingham dress carefully.

"I knew you'd be like that. I won't let you upset me. I know you don't understand. I know—I'm afraid—you won't understand. That's why I came—now—to say good-bye—where everyone could see—so you couldn't—make it hard. You don't understand and I know you don't understand."

"Nor do I," says Marcus.

"I know. I thought you might. You so easily could. But you don't. I think I'll go now. There's no point in letting anyone upset me."

She stands. She shakes hands with Bill, who looks gloomy, and Winifred, who smiles mildly. She tries to kiss Jacqueline, who turns away, kisses Daniel, who says, "Look after yourself, Ruthie," and attempts to kiss Marcus, who suddenly takes hold of her wrist.

"Don't go, Ruthie." It is not clear what he means, don't leave now, or don't go to the Children of Joy.

She pulls her hand away. She walks quickly away, into the house. Her head is bowed. It is possible she is crying. Marcus goes after her. She begins to run. They both disappear into the house. Jacqueline stands up, sets off, thinks better of it. Luk Lysgaard-Peacock appears at the back gate, from the moor, dressed for walking. Jacqueline pays no attention. She says to Daniel, "*You* know Gideon Farrar. *You* know what he does. Stop her."

"I can't. What do you know about the Children of Joy?"

"Nothing. The whole thing is entirely distasteful. But I do know Gideon, and where Gideon is, love means sex. He *uses* his—his *presence*—his separateness—all those young girls—*he works them up*—I've been there, I know—"

"Does he hurt them?"

Jacqueline thinks about this. She says, "I think so, yes. I think he makes a kind of horrible fantasy of sacrifice and communion and really it's just lust—"

"Those are all just words."

"Are you trying to excuse him?"

"No. I know him, as you say. I think your words are accurate words."

"Well, then, stop Ruth."

"It's hard. She's grown up. She's made a choice."

Marcus reappears. He walks past his family, past Luk, out on to the moors. He begins to walk away, fast. Jacqueline stands up and runs after him. She catches him up at some distance; they can be seen as they embrace. Marcus bows his head on her shoulder, they walk on, arms entwined.

Luk Lysgaard-Peacock comes into the garden and is offered coffee, which he accepts.

Frederica and Luk Lysgaard-Peacock find themselves alone in the garden. Bill has gone to sleep; Marcus and Jacqueline have vanished; Daniel is taking Will to visit a friend, and Mary has gone along for the ride. Winifred is stacking dishes. Luk Lysgaard-Peacock does not ask about the drama, but Frederica tells him, briefly.

"Ruth came in and announced she is going off to live in a holy community and take vows. They are all upset. Jacqueline went off to cheer up Marcus, or vice-versa."

"In that case, I will save my own news."

"Your own news?"

"I have been invited to be head of a research institute in Copenhagen. It's an honour."

"So you're going?"

"I'm thinking. There are reasons for and against."

He considers the now empty moor beyond. Frederica has seen him look at Jacqueline. She wants to tell him, waiting never works. This would be impertinent. So she says, "Are there *Helix hortensis*—or should I say *Helices hortensis*—over there?"

"I imagine so. Not the particular population I am studying. And not my two slug populations on the moors, which are so strangely different."

Frederica becomes mildly interested in both Lysgaard-Peacock and his snails. She is interested because she suspects him of being another laminated being, a creature capable both of giving his entire attention to small, pearly, convoluted crawling lives, of thinking thoughts about genes and DNA of which she has no conception, and of furious but not incapacitating sexual devotion. She is trying to turn the jottings of her own *Laminations* into a coherently incoherent work. She has had the idea that she is many women in one—a mother, a wife, a lover, a watcher, and that it might be possible to construct a kind of plait of voices, with different rhythms and vocabularies. But it will not work. The story of Stone is one thing. The legal cut-ups are quirky new *objects.* But the moment she tries to write anything tinged with her own *feelings,* she is disgusted, as though she had touched slime, a metaphor she undoubtedly finds because of her temporary contact with *Helix hortensis.* If she writes what she feels truly—Leo's strangling arms, the memory of Nigel's blows, John Ottokar's blood-stained belly, disgust overcomes her at its falsity; it is false because it is *banal,* a cliché. She looks again at Luk Lysgaard-Peacock. He is a watcher, a collector, a thinker, a walker—he is "in love" with a brown girl who is "in love" with her brother, Marcus—inexplicably, to Frederica's mind—and this love makes him, too, more banal, more ordinary. She dare not speak these thoughts to him—he has a great deal of reserved dignity. But she does observe that the sex lives of the snails are no doubt less complicated, less anguished than those of human beings. She says she believes snails are hermaphrodite, and can manage the whole business by themselves. Lysgaard-Peacock replies that there is still some dispute about whether they do, in fact, ever keep themselves to themselves. The general belief is that they require another snail to reproduce—there is, as he puts it, some courteous dispute and jostling about who shall put what where. Snails, he says, are equipped with a curious organ, known as a *gypsobelum,* or love-dart, with which they apparently excite each other. Indeed, the differences between these organs are one of the clear ways of distinguishing *Helix hortensis* from *Helix nemoralis.* He describes the work he has done on two populations of large slugs, *Arion ater,* one on the moorlands and one from the valley lower down. These creatures, he says, are interesting because the moorland population, although identical in appearance to those of the valley, are self-fertilising, and genetically identical, whereas the valley slugs are sexually propagated, and genetically diverse. Odd, he says, that the upland, hermaphrodite, celibate slugs have preserved, over presumably thousands of years of disuse, enormous genitalia. Not in line with Darwin. Frederica asks him whether all this genetic science has changed his attitude to human behaviour. He thinks.

"I was going to say, no. But I think, yes, when I think about it. Love, and all that, is human, like language, which is purely human. I've never liked the idea of teaching apes human language—it diminishes them, in some way, like putting them in knickers and bonnets. But when you begin to understand how we are all constructed by the coded sequences of the DNA—hermaphrodite slugs, sexed slugs,

Cepaea hortensis and ourselves—when you realise all the things that go on busily in your cells all the time with which your language-consciousness appears to have nothing to do—I think it does change you, yes. I think it does diminish your sense of your own importance rather comfortably. Love is love, and all that, but sex is a blind drive, like—oh—antibodies breeding round diseased cells, or viruses hurrying along our blood."

"I thought that might be comforting."

"Oh well. At times. To the head."

"Perhaps one has to make do with that?"

"Ah, but the *luck,* if one didn't, if things went well."

"In my experience," says Frederica, "they *don't* go well. Or not for long."

"Are you trying to tell me something?"

"No. Well, no, not really."

"Nothing I don't know."

Frederica copies part of an article lent by Luk Lysgaard-Peacock into her *Laminations,* partly because she likes the idea of the snails wearing their genetic code for all to read on the spiral of their shells. She also copies out a description of the love-dart of *Helix hortensis* and its difference from that of *Helix nemoralis.*

Laminations

Habits and habitats. Helix hortensis is described as a somewhat indolent yet moderately sensitive animal, carrying its shell obliquely upright when crawling. It is less nocturnal in habit than its congener, though said by Nagel to be deeply skioptic or responsive to shade, and does not conceal itself so deeply and carefully during the day.

Diagnosis. H. hortensis is distinguished from *H. nemoralis* by its smaller size, more globose shape, white aperture and thinner and more glossy shell; moreover there is much less band variation, there is a larger proportion of bandless and 5-banded shells, and the commonness or rarity of the band formulae is quite different in the two species.

Internally, the differences are striking, the chief divergence being the structure of the gypsobelum or "love-dart" which in place of presenting the four simple longitudinal blades with connecting crescentic films, as in *H. nemoralis,* has the four blades deeply cleft and widely reflected along their entire length, forming thus eight sharp, divaricating blades; there are also no crescentic films between the blades, which terminate abruptly at the base, and not gradually, as in *H. nemoralis*; the vaginal mucus glands are also usually more branched than in *nemoralis,* and instead of being simply and uniformly digitate, are swollen or sacculate at the extremities.

Frederica cuts Luk Lysgaard-Peacock's information into her reading of the documents of the counter-culture.

Timothy Leary, *The Molecular Revolution,* lecture delivered at LSD conference sponsored by the University of California. Extracts.

Lecturing to a Turned-On Audience

If any of you have smoked marijuana in the last two hours, you are listening not just to my symbols. Your sense organs have been intensified and enhanced, and you are also aware of the play of light, the tone of voice. You are aware of many sensory cues beyond the tidy sequence of subjects and predicates which I am laying out in the air. And there may even be some of you in the audience who decided that you'd put over your eyes that more powerful microscope and find out, "Well, where is this fellow at, anyway?" Perhaps you have taken LSD tonight, in which case my task is not to wake you up but rather *not to pull you down.* I have often had the experience in lecturing to psychedelic audiences of having my eyes wander around the room and suddenly be fixed by two orbs, two deep, dark, pools, and realise that I am looking into someone's genetic code, that I have to make sense, not to a symbolic human mind, not to a complicated series of sense organs, but I have to make sense to many evolutionary forms of life—an amoeba, a madman, a mediaeval saint.

Iron wheels revolved there endlessly, and hammers thudded. At night plumes of vapour steamed from the vents, lit from beneath with red light, or blue, or venomous green.

There stood a tower of marvellous shape. It was fashioned by the builders of old, and yet it seemed a thing not made by the craft of Men, but riven from the bones of the earth in the ancient torment of the hills. There upon a floor of polished stone, written with strange signs, a man might stand five hundred feet above the plain. This was Orthanc, the citadel of Saruman, the name of which had (by design or chance) a twofold meaning; for in the Elvish speech *orthanc* signifies Mount Fang, but in the language of the Mark of old, the Cunning Mind.

Helix hortensis—Scalariform and sinistral monstrosities
Irregularly grown and anomalous shells.
Helix hortensis monst. scalare Ferussac [picture]
Shell with elevated spine and partially dislocated whorls.
Monst. sinistrorsum Ferussac
Shell reversed or sinistral in coiling.

We must realise that evolution is not through, that man is not a final product, and just as there are many species of primate, there may be just as many species evolving from what we now call man, *Homo sapiens.* It may well be that we'll have two species. One species, which is the machine species, will like to live in metal buildings, and skyscrapers, and will get their kicks by just becoming part of a machine. That species of man will become an unnecessary, easily worn-out part of the whole technological machinery. In that case, man will become anonymous—just like the anthill or the beehive. Sex will become very depersonalized. It will become very promiscuous. You won't care who you make love to because they're all just replaceable parts. You know, she's the new pretty blond girl who runs the electronic typewriter; so that we may well get a new species who will be technological. But I do know that our seed-flown species will continue. And we may hang out in new pockets of disease which the machine people haven't cleaned up with their antiseptics. And we'll be somewhere out in the marshes, or somewhere out in the woods, laughing at the machine and enjoying our senses and having ecstasies and remembering where we came from and teaching our children that, believe it or not, we're not machines, and we weren't designed to make machines, and we weren't designed to run machines. I think you have to be a very holy man to appreciate and understand and run a machine because the machine is a beautiful yoga and a beautiful ecstasy. I've nothing against machines; it's just incredible that the DNA could produce us and then produce those machines.

(Timothy Leary, *Soul Session,* p. 221)

Frederica's thoughts run uneasily on genetic similarities and differences, machine-men and seed-flower species, stones, paper and scissors. She thinks that the DNA which is the fetish of the turned-on has probably very little, though not nothing, to do with the DNA of *Helix hortensis,* in the food-processor, on the slides, under the microscope, of Luk Lysgaard-Peacock. She would rather know what Lysgaard-Peacock knows, but is closer, even when trying to understand the snails, to the language of Leary.

. . .

Long legal envelopes continue to arrive, even in the summer, even in Freyasgarth. Frederica opens one and finds a thick document, with a covering letter from Arnold Begbie, who says, with studied neutrality, that it appears that, upon reflection, "your husband, the respondent" has decided to add to his Answer, already filed, "a prayer for counter-relief" on the grounds of desertion, mental cruelty and frequent adultery. The respondent has applied to the registrar for leave to amend his answer and to enter the cross-petition, and this leave has been granted.

Mr. Begbie says that he wishes to point out to his client that her husband is required to make specific allegations of her own misconduct, but is not required to divulge the evidence upon which he will rely to prove this misconduct. The question of desertion is clear, and the question of mental cruelty is related to this and to the removal of the child, Leo Alexander. The allegations of adultery are numerous and precise. Mrs. Reiver has not elected to include a discretion statement in her own petition, and has assured Mr. Begbie that the question did not arise. He would therefore be grateful to know how she would like him to proceed. She will note that the new prayer for counter-relief does include a prayer for the court's discretion in the matter of the cross-petitioner's own adultery.

Mr. Begbie also wishes to inform Mrs. Reiver that all the persons cited in the cross-petition's allegations of adultery must be named as co-respondents and served personally with notices of the petition; they may then choose whether to enter an appearance, if they wish to defend the proceedings, or take part in any other way. If these persons do not wish to contest the proceedings, they need do nothing.

Mr. Begbie will be grateful to receive Mrs. Reiver's further instruction as soon as possible.

Frederica looks at the counter-petition. It is long, and detailed. It is fact and fiction. It names Thomas Poole, Hugh Pink, John Ottokar, Paul Ottokar and Desmond Bull, and speaks of acts of intimacy, public embraces, and nights spent under the same roof. It claims custody of the child of the marriage, Leo Alexander. It is a snake of black language, tied with red tape in an impeccable bow. Frederica's first, easiest, simplest emotion is that she has made a fool of herself in not *telling* Arnold Begbie about what she calls, to herself, "the end of my celibacy." Her second is rage that Begbie, whom she neither really likes nor really trusts, should need to know where she has lain down, whose skin she has touched, by whom she has been penetrated. It is *private,* she thinks. She then takes in the implications of the serving of the petitions on Thomas Poole (who may simply be ruefully sensible) and on the Ottokars. Can Nigel claim damages against John Ottokar? Can Paul be called to give evidence? They have vanished into the Spirits' Tigers: she cannot see John wanting to maintain their uncertain, delicate, tentative love or liking in a witness box before a judge. He is not ready, and may never be, and she may not want him to be, now, or yet, or ever, how can she tell, but the law and Nigel will make it be solid, be cut and dried—*cut,* and *dried*—gone . . . And some, though not all, of this, is true, and will the court, whose ways are not her ways, suppose she is a woman sensible enough to keep Leo? It is the Swinging Sixties, but the courts are run by old men in eighteenth-century wigs, with nineteenth-century outward morals, and she will be pulped, mashed, humiliated, *destroyed*.

She has taken the horrid envelope to her bedroom, to read in peace. She cannot speak of this to her parents. She begins to weep, blindly, uselessly, furiously. The door opens. It is Daniel.

"What is it, Frederica?"

"Look!"

He looks.

"Half of it's lies. *Lies.*"

"You'll get your divorce, one way or the other."

"Yes, but *Leo.* Who will get Leo?"

Daniel sits on the bed.

"They usually give the child to the mother."

"But I look *horrible* in that document, feckless and frightful. And they've got everything, the pony, the Right School . . ."

"But you want him with you?"

"It isn't a question of want or not want. We *have* to be together. He saw that. I thought I could leave him, but I couldn't, I couldn't have, not ever—"

She thinks of Daniel, a good man, as she is not a good woman, walking away from Will and Mary. She has always wondered how he could have done that, and has not asked, and will not ask. But she looks at him, red-eyed, stricken with guilt.

"Oh, Daniel."

He holds her. She lies on his shoulder and weeps, with more and more abandon. He strokes her hair, his mouth set grimly. They hear Mary pass, singing, singing in tune and clearly, as no Potter ever has.
"Your daughter can sing in tune."
"My dad could. He used to sing th' *Messiah*, in the big choirs."
"She sounds happy."
"Human beings are tough."

The Council of the Wise (1)

Frederica finds herself, almost by accident, at a meeting in the offices of Bowers and Eden in Elderflower Court to discuss the organisation of the defence of *Babbletower.* Rupert Parrott's solicitor is a cautious small man called Martin Fisher; another solicitor has been found to represent Jude, also a small man, called Duncan Raby. Martin Fisher is dapper and silvery; Duncan Raby is sleek and dark and can bend his fingers backwards, which he does, with little cracks, in moments of agitation. Godfrey Hefferson-Brough, QC, is to lead for Parrott's defence; Samuel Oliphant, QC, has been retained to represent Jude. Hefferson-Brough is large and craggy, with tree-trunk bones and red-veined cheeks and sharp eyes under tangled eyebrows. Samuel Oliphant is one of those whippet-like lawyers who look as though they are on the scent of a fine point even in repose; he has colourless, apologetic hair, and fine bones which are transformed by a wig into blades and edges. These four and their clerks are present at this meeting—other lawyers will come and go from time to time during the succeeding months. When Frederica arrives at Bowers and Eden with a heap of annotated manuscripts from the slush heap, she finds Jude in the entrance lobby, surrounded by his miasma, asserting in his sawing voice that decisions are being made without him, behind his back, undercover. Parrott is protesting, pink-faced and tense, that Jude would not be here if things were being hidden from him. The sawing voice rises: "I overheard your *secretary,* Parrott, saying to *someone,* it would be *easier* without the *author present,* he can be very *temperamental,* very *difficult*—"

Frederica says, "Oh, shut up, Jude. You are having your cake and eating it. If ever you do overhear things like that it's your *civilised duty* to ignore them, and anyway, you know in your terms it's a compliment, you *like* to be thought temperamental and difficult. Everyone's doing their best."

"What do *you* know about it?" says Jude, still truculent, but milder.

"I know you," says Frederica. "I know how much Rupert has done for you. I think you should shut up."

"We are having a Council of the Wise," says Parrott. "I think you should join us. I think your advice would be of help. This is just a little preliminary gathering—some experts, mostly Bowers and Eden authors—Professor Marie-France Smith has agreed to come along, and Roger Magog. They wrote well of the book, very well, they will advise us. And I've persuaded Phyllis Pratt to give us her thoughts, yes. You are a part of our deliberations, and you brought both Mrs. Pratt and Jude to our attention. You could come and help on the Eng. lit. front."

They sit round a shiny oval mahogany table in an upper room Frederica had not even known about; it smells musty and unused, but with an overtone of past nuts, and old apples. Rupert Parrott sits at one end, flanked by pairs of lawyers. Frederica and Jude sit at the other. Also present are Canon Holly, representing the Church, Elvet Gander, representing mental health and the sciences of the soul, Marie-France Smith and Roger Magog, and a squat person with red ringlets and a red beard, both mildly matted, with merry blue eyes behind gold-rimmed glasses and an open-necked madras-checked shirt, who is introduced as Avram Snitkin, an ethnomethodologist. Jude lays his long grey hands on the mahogany and asks earnestly, "What is an ethnomethodologist?"

"That is hard to say," Snitkin replies cheerfully, "since no two ethnomethodologists can agree on a definition of ethnomethodology. We have very beautiful conferences, discussing the meaning of the term 'ethnomethodology.' "

"And you can't give me a working definition?" says Jude. "A court will require a working definition."

"We study what people actually think they are doing when they are in the process of doing whatever they do. As opposed to the things sociologists think that people think they do when they perform acts already classified and categorised by sociologists, in certain ways."

"You are sociologists?"

"Many of us, most of us, spring from that discipline. The classic ethnomethodological study was the bugging of a jury room in order to observe, without any interference in the data by *overt* observers, what function jury members believe themselves to be performing *in qua* jurors—what jurors think jurors are. Do I make you any wiser?"

"Oh yes," says Jude.

"And where did you 'bug' this jury room?" asks Samuel Oliphant, articulating the inverted commas.

"In California, don't worry," says Snitkin, smilingly.

"Dr. Snitkin has made a study of the uses that people—men—make of—of *risky* published material," says Rupert Parrott. "That is why I invited him to this gathering. He believes that pornography performs a useful social function. That it, so to speak, *siphons off*—"

"An unfortunate metaphor," says Jude. "Very. I must point out that my book is not pornographic. It is in that context *emetic.* It will be better if we do not use the word 'pornographic' about it."

"Let me call this meeting to order," says Parrott. "The idea of this meeting is to exchange ideas between lawyers and persons who might be thought to be experts, in the new fields of 'expertise' in the literary and social value of works of art which are supposed to 'tend to deprave and corrupt' the general public. When *Lady Chatterley* was triumphantly acquitted, the defence produced an impressive file of the great and the good, poets, professors, bishops and one young girl, to say that the book was full of tenderness and sweetness and light and advocation of married fidelity. The prosecution relied on reading aloud 'bouts' of explicit sexual description, and rhetorically and famously asking 'Is this a book you would allow your wife and daughters, or your servants, to read?' It is my opinion, and the opinion of the legal advisers who are here today, that the prosecution of *Babbletower* will be different from the prosecution of *Lady Chatterley,* because the book is different, but not only for that reason. There is scope for 'experts' who are not simply literary critics or respected public figures. I won't go on, now, but will hand over the conduct of proceedings to those who will guide us."

Frederica looks round the table. Marie-France Smith is a surprise; she is a tall, slender, blond, elegant woman, with a strikingly beautiful face, long hair tied back with a black velvet bow, and an expression of gentleness and wary tension combined. Phyllis Pratt, the novelist, is the shape of the cottage loaf she described in her novel, *Daily Bread;* she has little fat curls, dark and silver, on her ample head, smile-lines moving up into round cheeks from soft mouth and eye-corners; she wears a serviceable jersey trouser suit in bottle green with a flowered Liberty shirt under it, sprinkled with honeysuckle. Canon Holly's ragged silver mane and his smoke-stained, lupine teeth she knows well. Magog is meaty and energetic and restless. Elvet Gander has a bald head and a precise, distinguished, long-nosed, carved-looking face, with a wide, controlled mouth and deep-set dark grey eyes above high, clean-cut cheekbones. His head is the head of a tall man, a grandee, though when he stands, his body is surprisingly short and slightly bowed, with long hanging arms and bowed legs. His skin has a grey cast—not an unhealthy putty-grey, like Jude's, but a polished granite, stony.

The subsequent conversation is conducted by the two solicitors with occasional comments from the two silks. Preliminary discussions are held of lines of argument in defence of *Babbletower*: psychological, political, literary merit, usefulness as emetic, religious depth. One of the lawyers—Raby—says he feels clergymen can "backfire" as witnesses. It might be possible to agree with the other side not to call clergymen. Canon Holly says that would be a pity, since there is great and genuine theological suffering and profundity in the work. "Convince me," says Samuel Oliphant, mildly, enticingly, dangerously. "There was a Bishop in the *Chatterley* case," says Hefferson-Brough. "Got rather mangled. Said the book promulgated marriage. Got reprimanded by the Archbish, I hear. Cantuor. Not a good precedent, on balance." Canon Holly says he knows a better Bishop, a radio Bishop with a large following, who might appear, who has thought much about the experience of pain and desolation. Raby says he is against bishops. Martin Fisher says, if they have a Bishop, we should have a Bishop. Jude says bishops are sods and buggers like everyone else. Phyllis Pratt tells Jude that the assembled company is trying to *help* him; her tone is that of the chairman of the Mothers' Union (this is before chairwomen and before personified Chairs). Jude says, "I simply thought—" Phyllis Pratt says, "Don't. Don't simply think. You have a task to perform, part of which is not to make things difficult for your friends." Jude says, "Who is my friend, when all men are against me?" "And *folie de grandeur,* dear," says Phyllis Pratt, "and premature martyrdom, are both *unhelpful.*"

Hefferson-Brough says, "Naturally, your appearance will have to be regularised."

"Regularised?"

"You will have to be tidied up. Short back and sides. Suit. Tie. A good wash. *Sine qua non.*"

"Oh no," says Jude. "I am a poor bare forked thing, and such as I am, I am, and as such you must e'en take me, for a man and his clothes are *one flesh* and cannot be parted. I have as it were and to my own secret deities *vowed* that neither hair of my head nor nail of my feet and fingers shall I wilfully cut with scissors or injure with files and this state I propose to maintain come hell come high water."

"Short back and sides," says Hefferson-Brough.

"It might be best," says Oliphant, "not to call you into the witness box at all. It might be the most advisable course."

"It would be extremely foolish not to call me," says Jude. "I will speak. I will appear and expound and defend my book."

"I can tell you now," says Hefferson-Brough, "that if you insist on going into the box looking like that, we may as well go home now. That is what I have to say."

Duncan Raby changes the subject. He asks about witnesses to literary merit. It is agreed that Anthony Burgess shall be sounded out, since he wrote well of the book. Also Professor Frank Kermode, Professor Barbara Hardy, Professor Christopher Ricks, William Golding, Angus Wilson, Una Ellis-Fermor, and "that chap at Cambridge," says Hefferson-Brough, "that chap everyone's always talking about." "Dr. Leavis," says Frederica. "Him, yes." "He wouldn't appear for *Lady Chatterley,*" says Martin Fisher. "Although he's a Lawrence man. I can't see him liking *Babbletower.*"

"I was his student," says Magog. "As a postgraduate. He is cranky and paranoid, though undoubtedly a genius. I think I myself will better represent his critical approach. He is not easy to deal with, and I don't think he'd agree."

"We are glad of your support," says Martin Fisher.

"You represent the teaching profession also," says Duncan Raby, bending back his fingers.

"I want to put the case that *nothing* should be suppressed, that censorship is ludicrous and unworkable."

"Here you must argue for the merits of *Babbletower,* as an expert on its merits, literary or social," says Raby.

Magog does not answer this remark. It occurs to Frederica that he has not actually read *Babbletower*: as a teacher, she is now experienced in the eye-movements, the judicious nod, of those who have not read something they claim to have read. Magog says there are writers on the Steerforth Committee of Enquiry who might have the requisite *gravitas.* Alexander Wedderburn, for instance. He himself thinks there is little merit in Wedderburn's *writings* but Wedderburn has a good presence and is taught at O Level and A Level, he will impress. Hefferson-Brough says he is exactly the sort of chap who will go down well with a jury.

Tea is served, by Rupert Parrott's secretary, from a silver teapot into pretty little Crown Derby china teacups. A plate of biscuits is handed round: bourbons, custard creams, squashed flies. Avram Snitkin, sitting next to Frederica, murmurs, "Fascinating."

"What is?"

"Your British rituals of decision-making. Tea and biscuits. I am thinking of writing a study of the compiling of lists. Who compiled the list of the people who are here to compile the list of the people who will be invited to give evidence for *Babbletower*? How far is this list a ritual list of people who must be asked but won't appear? And so on."

"I suppose an ethnomethodologist would be interested in what happens to a person who defines himself for the duration as an expert witness for the defence of a book, of this book?"

"Indeed. Including an ethnomethodologist."

On the way out of the publishing house, Frederica finds herself between Jude and Elvet Gander. Jude is morose and unusually silent. Gander says to Frederica, "We have not officially met, I believe, but I know *of* you."

"What do you know *of* me?" Frederica asks, truculent and rattled. Nothing has been heard of John Ottokar since the service of the counter-petition and prayer for relief. He has vanished from her life as though he had never been. A date has been set for the divorce hearing in November. She is afraid.

"Nothing but good," says Gander, in reply to her question. "You were much in question at a difficult series of sessions in Four Pence this summer. I break no confidences if I say so, I think, and I assume that you too find your situation, shall we say, *difficult*? Forgive me if I speak out of turn."

"Perhaps you do. I don't know that I want to think or talk about—about *them,* about all that."

"One of the two brothers took the same line. The other was voluble. I attempted to mediate—to make the silent speak, and the roarer be still. The results were unfortunate."

Frederica is silent.

"Midnight arson," says Gander. "Midnight arson, minor explosions, damage to property."

"The path of excess leads to the palace of wisdom."

"You mock. I do believe there is much truth in that. I would like to help you, but you are not ready to let me. You think I am a charlatan."

"I don't." He waits. "Perhaps I do."

"You don't know."

"I don't know that I *want* to know."

"You may suddenly, quite suddenly, decide that you need me. I am here, if you do. You interest me."

"Don't listen to the tempter," says Jude. "He'll blow your mind."

This is an un-Jude-like phrase, in an un-Jude-like vocabulary. It sounds different. It evokes small mines, arson again, explosions.

Gander laughs. "Fair is foul and foul is fair. You do right to mistrust the chance-met. We shall meet again, in easier circumstances. As for you, Jude Mason, I would like to say, this process, this legal process, is going to be a severe test of your exiguous survival machinery. If you need help, I am here."

"You will help the whole world," says Jude. "Indiscriminately."

"No, no. We meet those who need us. We gravitate to them. Karma brings us where they are. We three are walking along this road together for a reason. Or, if we were not, we now are. So I tell you what I see in your face and your stars and your body language, in case that may be the reason. If not, no harm done, forget it."

As the divorce hearing approaches, Frederica grows thinner and sharper. She is obsessed by the fear of losing Leo, a person who makes her life difficult at every turn, who appears sometimes to be *eating* her life and drinking her life-blood, a person who fits into no pattern of social behaviour or ordering of thought that she would ever have chosen for herself freely—and yet, the one creature to whose movements of body and emotions all her own nerves, all her own antennae, are fine-tuned, the person whose approach along a pavement, stamping angrily, running eagerly, lifts her heart, the person whose smile fills her with warmth like a solid and gleaming fire, the person whose sleeping face moves her to tears, to catch the imperceptible air of whose sleeping breath she will crouch, breathless herself, for timeless moments in the half-dark.

She thinks, perhaps, she might be able to talk to Agatha about this terror, but Agatha is preoccupied and evasive, is uncharacteristically short with her. Frederica takes note of her own friends, her particular old friends, Daniel and Alexander, going up Agatha's stairs, rather than down to her own basement, and tells herself it is natural, Agatha is beautiful and clever, Alexander has always been easy prey for mysterious silence, Daniel needs to get out of himself. Agatha is "working late" a lot, too, which Frederica, asked to baby-sit, regards with sour suspicion. One evening she is baby-sitting when Agatha is still out and Alexander arrives. He comes down to talk to Frederica—"*faute de mieux,*" Frederica says, jokingly to him, and crossly to herself. Alexander accepts a cup of coffee and tells Frederica what he sees she needs to know and has not bothered to discover, that Agatha is strained to breaking by the practical and political difficulties of the drafting of the Steerforth Report.

Agatha does not discuss her work with Frederica. Frederica does, or did, discuss hers with Agatha—it interests both of them. Alexander leans back on Frederica's sofa and talks about the committee.

"It's very difficult for a *group* to write something. It's quite interesting to see what kinds of manoeuvres we go through to get it done. We've got two people in overall charge of the writing—Agatha and myself—we co-ordinate what will be the chapters. Then we've got little sub-groups, working together on different areas—we've got a group on 'Spoken and Written English,' and one on 'Classroom Conduct—Love and/or Authority,' and one on 'The Class Problem in the Class—the Question of What Is "Correct" and What Should Be *Corrected,*' and one on 'The Principles of Education—Is It Child-Centred or Community-Oriented, and Can It Be Both?' And one on what sort of grammar to teach, and how much, and why. And that one has a sub-heading, language as an *object of study,* like zoology, or mathematics. It's amazing what terrible passions it all arouses—real, important passions, mind you, about real, important things. You get evidence in from schoolteachers saying they want to create 'whole personalities,' 'friendly atmospheres,' 'full and satisfying lives,' 'full development of potentialities,' 'satisfaction of curiosity,' 'confidence,' 'growth,' 'perseverance,' 'alertness,' and that sort of thing—and when you actually start looking at what they do, how they behave, what they *mean* by these phrases, you find that the words are like sand slipping through your fingers, you feel you're staring through a microscope at a lot of life-forms that suddenly look like great thick snakes curling round and *biting* each other. We're writing about teaching language and the language we write about teaching language won't stick to the thing we're writing about. Won't describe it. Steerforth himself said almost nothing for months of our deliberations and then suddenly made a little speech about how profoundly *resistant* the mind was to studying its own operations. He and Hans Richter and Wijnnobel are writing a kind of preface pointing out how 'children' and 'language' have both been profoundly changed in our time by becoming objects of intense study, of focused attention."

"Agatha never talks about all this. It's fascinating. Go on."

Alexander goes on. He describes the drafting groups, and the unexpected alliances, oppositions and alignments. The journalist, Malcolm Friend, who has contributed almost nothing to the debate, turns out to be a brilliant drafter of pellucid paragraphs and is in charge of the "child-centred, community-oriented?" debate. The teachers are divided on the question of classroom authority—some oppose learning anything by rote, and are in favour of the child "discovering naturally when he needs to," using the model of language acquisition by untutored two-year-olds. Some believe equally strongly that children *need* to know things they are reluctant to learn, as a store for when they will be glad of them, or because "society" needs them to know these things. The word "society" is not yet the problem it will become, but it is a problem. A majority of the committee, probably, dislike grammar and teaching grammar: the minority in favour of it are ferociously moved by its order, its beauty, its complexity. Emily Perfitt believes in learning poetry, but in eschewing grammar, which she defines as "mental cruelty," quite simply—an *interesting locution,* according to Wijnnobel, Alexander says. He describes how Agatha keeps the drafting groups in order by threatening to second Magog and Mickey Impey to join them. These two are part of no group and act as ambassadors "from one to another."

Frederica says she met Magog at Bowers and Eden. She recounts the meeting of that committee. She says the lawyers were endlessly qualificatory and endlessly subtle about the nature of expert witnesses. She says life is full of lawyers and committees defining the indefinable, like childhood, tendencies to deprave and corrupt, language, pre-nuptial incontinence, adultery, guilt. She says she feels terribly guilty towards Nigel, because she should not have married him, but that she is not technically guilty of most of the things of which she now stands accused. Some, yes, she says. But it's *nobody else's business.*

Alexander says he knew before he joined the committee that there would be one lucid moment when he *knew* what teaching was, and children were, and language did, and that this knowledge would disappear in a welter of study and definition and complexity. He says it has happened exactly so, and that the complexities are real and substantial. He says that the good teachers they have observed *know,* as he knew then, what teaching and children and language are, and act on their knowledge.

He says he is sorry Frederica feels guilty but he is sure she will soon be able to put it all behind her.

Frederica tries to say: I am afraid of losing Leo. She is so afraid of losing Leo, that she cannot utter the sentence.

So she says, "They were discussing asking you to give evidence for Jude."

"Do I want to?"

"You ought to. He'll *die* if they condemn his book."

"I don't like it."

"No. But you don't want it suppressed."

"I suppose I don't."

They hear Agatha come in. "Well," says Frederica. "Off to your drafting then."

Laminations

My mother groan'd! my father wept.
Into the dangerous world I leapt:
Helpless, naked, piping loud:
Like a fiend hid in a cloud.

Struggling in my father's hands,
Striving against my swadling bands,
Bound and weary I thought best
To sulk upon my mother's breast.

William Blake,
Songs of Experience

Our work has been concerned with two things, or concepts, which have in recent history become both absorbing subjects of study, and *problems,* as perhaps they were not in the past. We refer to "the child" and "language." Before the nineteenth century the child was either an infant or a small adult, wearing the same clothes as his parents, subject to the same legal penalties, including hanging by the neck, and controlled by the same moral codes. Now we take account of the length of time it takes a human creature to become an independent, responsible being, both physically and mentally. We take an intricate interest in the processes—including the learning of language—by which such independence and responsibility are achieved.

Language, too, has become, not merely the glass through which we see "the world outside" but the instrument with which we shape and limit our purposes and our apprehensions. Our philosophy is a philosophy of language: Wittgenstein sees philosophy, indeed, as "language-games" which are "forms of life," whereas the school of "Language, Truth and Logic" sees linguistic forms as productive of both facts and fictions about the nature of things. There is a growing belief in some schools of thought that "language is divorced from the world," that it is perhaps simply a partial system which best describes only its own interrelations and structure. At the same time, there is a proper and increasing interest in language as an instrument of power, of subjection and manipulation, and a concomitant belief that even young children should be familiarised with and alerted to language's manipulative potentialities. There is, in this context, the vexed question of the relation of such political uses of language to the ingrained British habit of defining "correct" speech and writing in terms partly of the speech habits and linguistic structures of a particular group or class, of identifying the "rules" of grammar with the rules, both helpful and restrictive, of prevailing interests and power-structures.

(Draft, subsequently heavily revised, of the Introduction to the Report of the Steerforth Committee of Enquiry on the Teaching of the English Language)

We are likely to withdraw our willingness to listen when we are told that infantile sexuality is polymorphously perverse. And Freud must mean that polymorphous perversity is the pattern of our deepest desires. How can this proposition be taken seriously?

If we divest ourselves of the prejudice surrounding the "perverse," if we try to be objective and analyse what infantile sexuality is in itself, we must return again to the definition. Infantile sexuality is the pursuit of pleasure obtained through the activity of any and all organs of the human body. That this is Freud's notion becomes abundantly clear if we examine the specific nature of the "perverse" components in infantile sexuality. They include the pleasure of touching, of seeing, of muscular activity, and even the passion for pain.

Freud and Blake are asserting that the ultimate essence of our being remains in our unconscious secretly faithful to the principle of pleasure, or, as Blake calls it, delight.

In man the dialectical unity between union and separateness, between interdependence and independence, between species and individual—in short, between life and death—is broken. The break occurs in infancy, and it is the consequence of the institution of the human family. The institution of the family means the prolonged maintenance of human children in a condition of helpless dependence. Parental care makes childhood a period of privileged freedom from the domination of the reality-principle, thus permitting and promoting the early blossoming, in an unreal atmosphere, of infantile sexuality and the pleasure-principle. Thus sheltered from reality by parental care, infantile sexuality—Eros or the life instinct—conceives the dream of narcissistic omnipotence in a world of love and pleasure.

But if the institution of the family gives the human infant a subjective experience of freedom unknown to any other species of animal, it does so by holding the human infant in a condition of objective dependence on parental care to a degree unknown to any other species of animal. Objective dependence on parental care creates in the child a passive, dependent need to be loved, which is just the opposite of his dream of narcissistic omnipotence. Thus the institution of the family shapes human desire in two contradictory directions, and it is the dialectic generated by the contradiction which produces what Freud calls the conflict of ambivalence.

But the contradiction in the human psyche established by the family is the contradiction between the life and death instincts as previously defined.

(Norman O. Brown, "Death and Childhood,"
Life Against Death, p. 113)

When they finally woke, it was already dark night. Gretel began to weep, and said, "How are we now to get out of the Forest?" Hansel, however, comforted her: "Wait a little while, till the moon has risen, and then we will find out our way." And when the full moon was up, Hansel took his little sister by the hand and they followed the flinty pebbles, which glittered like newly minted groats, and showed them the way. They went on all night and at daybreak came to their father's house.

Other echoes
Inhabit the garden. Shall we follow?
Quick, said the bird, find them, find them,
Round the corner. Through the first gate,
Into our first world, shall we follow
The deception of the thrush? Into our first world . . .

Go, said the bird, for the leaves were full of children,
Hidden excitedly, containing laughter.
Go, go, go, said the bird: human kind
Cannot bear very much reality.

T. S. Eliot, *Four Quartets*,
"Burnt Norton"

A Dream

A woman, waiting for a divorce hearing, finds herself on the banks of a quick little stream, very English, overhung by trees, with sun and shadow chasing each other along it, and a breeze, too, stirring the leaves and the water. She is walking in a meadow in long grasses, by this stream, wearing her engagement ring, which is a row of alternating blue and white stones, sapphires and moonstones. The clasps of the setting spring open and the stones of the ring fall and roll in the grass, blue and white stones rolling everywhere, tiny and glittering, more than the ring ever contained. She tries to gather them up: they slip like drops of water through her fingers and bounce, as tears bounce when wept with great force. The dreamer, who is not the woman now, "sees" the woman's face with empty eyeholes like the empty sockets of the ring, and blue and white stony tears pouring down her cheeks.

In the river, hidden under the bank, are "water-babies" wrapped like caddis-grubs in shreds of old leaves and broken snail shells, glued into a housing; they peer out, they hang in the current which rushes and bubbles past them but does not detach them.

The tears and stones trickle into the river and melt like waterdrops on water.

The thought of our past years in me doth breed
Perpetual benediction: not indeed
For that which is most worthy to be blest—
Delight and liberty, the simple creed
Of Childhood, whether busy or at rest,
With new-fledged hope still fluttering in his breast:—
Not for these I raise
The song of thanks and praise;
But for those obstinate questionings
Of sense and outward things,
Fallings from us, vanishings;

Blank misgivings of a Creature
Moving about in worlds not realized,
High instincts before which our mortal Nature
Did tremble like a guilty Thing surprised . . .

William Wordsworth,
"Ode: Intimations of Immortality"

From the moment of birth, when the stone-age baby confronts the twentieth-century mother, the baby is the subject of violence, called love, as its mother and father have been and their parents before them . . . We are effectively destroying ourselves by violence masquerading as love.

(R. D. Laing)

At least 83 people, mostly children, are dead, and 46 were still entombed early today on the hillside at Aberfan, near Merthyr Tydfil, after a rain-soaked coal-tip avalanched on Pantglas Infants' School, a farm and a row of houses yesterday morning. Eighty-eight children are safe and 36 are in hospital.

Mr. S. O. Davies, Labour MP for Merthyr Tydfil, said that debris from a local colliery was still being tipped on the slag heap when the disaster happened . . .

Among those brought out alive and taken to hospital was the headmistress, Miss Ann Jennings, 64. The body of the deputy head-teacher, Mr. D. Beynon, was found, with five little children in his arms, all dead . . .

. . . Because of early morning fog, 50 children from the neighbouring village of Mount Pleasant escaped the tragedy. Their school bus was delayed and they arrived at the school 10 minutes late, and just after the landslide had occurred. The mother of one of them, Mrs. Olwyn Morris, said, "If there had been no fog, my boy, Joel, 14, would have been in the school. He ran home crying and told me what had happened."

The desires of the heart are as crooked as corkscrews,
Not to be born is the best for man:
The second best is a formal order,
The dance's pattern; dance while you can.
Dance, dance, for the figure is easy,
The tune is catching and will not stop;
Dance till the stars come down from the rafters;
Dance, dance, dance till you drop.

W. H. Auden, "Death's Echo," 1936

XIX

"Put your coat on, Leo, hurry up."

"I don't go to school today."

"Oh yes, you do. Agatha and Saskia are waiting."

"But we are being divorced today. I am coming to be divorced."

Frederica has said nothing to Leo about this event.

"You can't come," she says. "Little boys don't go to the divorce courts."

"*I* do."

"No, you don't. You must go to school."

He holds her dressing-gown: she means to change for her court appearance when he is gone. He stamps. He shrieks. "I will, I will, I will."

"You won't," says Frederica, raising her voice to match his. Both are near tears, white with anxiety.

"I am coming with you."

Agatha appears in the doorway.

"We are going to be divorced," says Leo.

"You aren't. You are going to school, with me. Don't upset your mother."

Leo glances from one woman to the other, weighs up the effect of further demonstration, and takes Agatha's hand, refusing to meet Frederica's eye.

"See you later," says Frederica, adding "alligator," on an uncertain, quavering false note.

Leo does not reply. He stomps off with Agatha. It is a bad beginning.

. . .

Frederica puts on a black dress. It is a black wool crepe shift with a pointed shirt-collar and buttoned cuffs at the end of long sleeves. She looks at her face in the mirror and thinks she looks respectable and urban. She thinks about make-up, sees that she would be better without it, fox-faced and clean-cut between the knife-blades of red hair. She applies the make-up nevertheless, to mark the occasion, perhaps, to hide behind it, perhaps, because the natural look of unmade-up skin has not yet come in, perhaps. As she always does on important occasions, she makes a dab with the mascara brush at her red-pale eyebrows, which normally she never touches, and as she always does, botches and blotches it, leaving gouts of black in the ginger, scrubbing them out, raising red welts. She wonders about relieving the black with a necklace or a brooch—she is not given to wearing jewellery—but the only thing she can find is a pretty Indian string of garnet and pearl beads, given to her by Nigel, which seems tactless.

She has refused offers to accompany her to the Court. She has tried not to think about it too much—she is not, she thinks, afraid of appearing in public, even in the witness box, for is she not a good public speaker, a charismatic teacher, an articulate person? She has been afraid of losing Leo, but not of losing him because of anything she may say or do. She has her confidence. She puts on a pair of black, shiny high-heeled shoes, slings her bag on her shoulder, and sets off for the Underground. The time ahead is a kind of blank. But at the end of it, something will be over, will be settled. She will be—not free, the word is beginning to be meaningless—but responsible for herself to herself again. The inside of her mouth is dry.

Inside the Court building she meets Arnold Begbie, who has with him her Counsel, Mr. Griffith Goatley, holding her brief and a whole heap of other briefs. Mr. Goatley is a blond, clean-cut, fastidious-looking person, with a beautiful pale skin and beautifully manicured hands. He tells Frederica not to be nervous, and she says she is not. He tells her to speak out, and to say everything she has to say, clearly—"Even what you may find it distasteful to say, Mrs. Reiver, just speak out." He says that she is the only witness he will be calling, in her own suit. "We have signed affidavits from your doctor, in the matter of the little infection you unfortunately had, and from a barmaid at the Tips and

Tassels Club, and from a waitress and the doorman at the Honeypot, in the matter of your husband's probable adultery. This should be quite enough—would certainly have been quite enough—had the counter-petition not been brought. My colleague Laurence Ounce, who is appearing for the opposition, seems to be calling a considerable number of witnesses in person. Only one of the persons named as co-respondents has entered an appearance—"

"Who?"

"Mr. Thomas Poole."

"There was nothing wrong—that is, there was *nothing*—he will say so—"

"Of course. That is Mr. Ounce, over there, with your ex-husband, I assume—"

Frederica gazes distractedly around the stony corridor she is standing in. There is Nigel, stocky, fierce, in his dark suit and a blood-red tie, with the faint hint of blue on his strong chin, even at this time in the morning. There too are both Olive and Rosalind, in tweed suits, one honey-coloured, one green-and-mauve, both slightly seated, over sensible flanged suede shoes, and there is Pippy Mammott in rust, with her face scrubbed pink and shining and her hair full of iron pins.

There is Mr. Ounce, and Nigel's solicitor, Mr. Tiger. Mr. Ounce is portly and billowing, with vinous cheeks and a mouth with all sorts of fluent and savorous curves in it; he has not got much hair, a struggling dark, thinning thatch, but that will vanish under the wig. He is wearing his gown, which billows about his billows. He laughs, and Nigel laughs with him. The three women ostentatiously do not see Frederica. Nigel genuinely does not.

It is like waiting in an examination hall. A clock ticks, somewhere. Dust motes are suspended in long tubes of pale November light. Frederica thinks: I am too thin to be convincing. It is an odd thought, not real, a product of unreal air, full of old pain, old terror, old triumphs and despair, old dust.

And then suddenly they are all in the Court, and there is the judge, Mr. Justice Hector Plumb, under his wig, a man not plummy but the opposite, chalky, with a yellow note to the chalk, a man with a thin, semi-transparent hooked nose and deep-etched lines running down and down in papery skin to a folded neck under his bands, a man whose hands, lifted to cover his mouth as he coughs, show bones through softly folded, shimmering, ancient skin above thick pale nails. A man with glaucous eyes under extravagant white eyebrows, a man patently not well, saving his strength, watching from inside the bright cocoon of his purple robes.

Griffith Goatley explains, in a melodious and pleasant voice, that the two suits, between Frederica Reiver and Nigel Reiver, and between Nigel Reiver and Frederica Reiver, have been consolidated and are to be heard together. "I appear for the wife, Frederica Reiver, and my learned friend, Laurence Ounce, appears for the husband. The petition of Frederica Reiver, being the leading suit, is to be heard first."

Frederica's petition, with its charges of cruelty, mental cruelty, adultery, is read out. She is called to the witness box, and finds herself standing looking out over the court, where she sees Nigel, Arnold Begbie, a spattering of complete strangers.

Griffith Goatley takes Frederica through her marriage. He addresses her courteously, as though she was a very young woman who had found herself in a world that turned out to be unpredictable and dangerous.

Q. And in the beginning, your marriage, this marriage which you say you made after reflection and after some three years of acquaintance, your marriage was happy?

A. Yes. In many ways, yes. It was not quite what I expected.

Q. What did you expect?

A. I thought he liked me for what I was. But afterwards, he seemed to want me to stay in his house and never to go anywhere, or see any of my old friends. Or work.

Q. You have a first class degree from Cambridge University?

A. Yes.

Q. And you were a popular and successful undergraduate?

A. Yes. I think so. I am an intellectual. I intended to go on and do a Ph.D.

Q. Your husband knew of this ambition?

A. I believe so. He often said he admired me for my independence, for my self-reliance, things like that.

Q. But when you were married, this changed?

A. Yes. When my son was born, of course, it was more reasonable to expect me to stay at home, perhaps.

Q. Did you feel that your husband's attitude to your independence was only because he felt you should look after your son?

A. No. I felt he was jealous. I felt he felt I should stay put, in the house, where I was. I felt he felt that that was what women did.

Frederica hears her voice. It is not her voice, it is the voice of a quiet young woman, acting out the lives, making the plaints, of intelligent women everywhere.

Q. Was there any lack of help in the house?

A. No.

Q. Would it have been possible for you to see your friends, to work on a thesis, perhaps, without harming your son, or your marriage?

A. I think so, yes. My husband is very well off, and there were many people looking after Leo, anyway.

Griffith Goatley's gentle, reasonable questions continue. He takes Frederica through her shock that her letters were being opened, through Nigel's telephone insults to her friends. He takes her also through Nigel's increasingly lengthy absences.

Q. You felt he was neglecting you?

A. You could put it that way, yes. I felt he thought I was shut up there, now, that part of his life, the wooing, was finished. He went back to his world, but I couldn't, I mustn't.

Q. Would you say your marriage was sexually happy?

A. At first, yes. Very. (A pause.) That was the best thing . . . the language that worked . . .

Q. Did that change, in later times?

A. Yes.

Q. Can you tell us why?

A. Partly, I think, because I withdrew. I began to see I ought not to have got married.

Q. And was there anything in your husband's behaviour that led you to reconsider your marriage?

A. He became increasingly violent.

Q. When you say, increasingly violent, do you mean as a lover, or as a jealous and unreasonable husband, Mrs. Reiver?

A. I mean both. He began to hurt me. In bed. And then he began to attack me. Out of bed.

Q. I believe on one occasion, you looked into his boxes in his cupboard, when he was away.

A. Yes. I did.

Q. Can you tell us why you did this?

A. He had stolen one of my letters. From my brother-in-law, who is a clergyman, and had written to cheer me up. I was trying to find it.

Q. And what did you find?

A. A collection of—of pornographic pictures. Dirty magazines.

Q. You were shocked?

A. It was very interesting. I was horribly shocked. I felt—quite ill. I felt—*dirtied*. I was surprised to feel so bad.

Q. Can you say what the pictures were like?

A. They were sado-masochistic. (Frederica senses that this precise technical term was not what was required.) There were women being tortured and made filthy. Chains and leather and knives. And lots of flesh. I felt dirtied. I was surprised.

Q. And did your husband ever attack you? Physically?

A. He began to, yes.

Griffith Goatley takes Frederica blow by blow through the battery, the ridiculous confinement in the lavatory, the chase through the stables, the axe, the wound. The healing.

Q. And did you, at any time, tell anyone else that this wound had been caused in this way?

A. No, I was ashamed.

Q. What had you to be ashamed of?

A. I think people are often ashamed of being hurt. Of having got themselves into a position where . . . anyone should want to hurt them so much.

Q. And what was your husband's attitude?

A. He was very affectionate.

Q. He was remorseful?

A. He was sorry, yes. But he was excited by the—the drama. I knew it would happen again.

Q. So you decided to leave?

A. I thought I would have to. I was very disturbed. I was afraid. It was out of control. I thought I would get away and think things out.

Griffith Goatley takes his witness through her flight in the woods, through her search for somewhere for herself and her son to live, through her decision not to return. He asks her if during her marriage she believed her husband to have been faithful, and she says that, on reflection, she sees she did not, that she had not wanted to understand his prolonged absences, his visits to clubs "with topless waitresses" with "business associates." Griffith Goatley refers to signed affidavits from the barmaid at the Tips and Tassels, from the doorman at the Honeypot, which state that Nigel Reiver has been seen leaving with certain women, whose profession is to "entertain men all night." "The doorman, as you will see," says Griffith Goatley, "deposes that Mr. Reiver is a well-known customer of the club, who enjoys the shows and the ladies. The doorman says," reports Griffith Goatley, "that Mr. Reiver's tastes are well known, slap more than tickle, so to speak, not averse to a few risks."

Q. Do you know what the doorman may mean by that, Mrs. Reiver?

A. No. Not exactly.

Q. Are you surprised by this evidence?

A. No. Well, yes, in a way, I didn't know. But no, on the other hand, I did know there was something and was trying not to. I don't know how much such things matter.

Q. They may matter very much. I will turn, if I may, and I apologise for speaking frankly, to the evidence of your doctor. On two occasions in November 1964 you were treated at the Middlesex Clinic for sexually transmitted diseases.

A. I was.

Griffith Goatley goes through the medical evidence.

Q. And how do you believe you came by this infection?

A. From my husband.

Q. You are sure of this?

A. Quite sure. He was the only person I slept with, between marrying him and leaving him. I was furious.

Q. Furious?

A. Well, I know now, it could have hurt—the baby, it could have—hurt his eyesight. *Or his brain.* I ought to have been told.

Judge. Are you offering this evidence in support of a charge of adultery, or of cruelty?

Griffith Goatley cites several precedents for both.

He concludes his examination of Frederica with a few questions about her present way of life, her home, Leo's school, his friends. He sits down. He has told the story of an intelligent, perhaps over-confident, perhaps over-educated young woman, who has found herself in deep water, socially and sexually, who may have provoked reasonable irritation but has been attacked and abused out of all proportion to her faults.

Laurence Ounce asks if he may put a few questions to this witness at this point, on behalf of his client, in answer to her petition. The judge gives him leave to proceed.

Q. Tell me, Frederica Reiver, why did you marry Nigel Reiver?

A. Why?

Q. Yes, why. You are a clever woman, you had a life-plan of sorts, you had known your husband some time—known in every sense I believe—before you decided to marry him. You were not, I take it, swept away by sudden passion. So why?

A. He wouldn't take no for an answer.

Q. But you are a very strong young woman, strong-willed, clever, we are always being told how clever you are. I am sure you have given no for an answer to several other young men?

A. Yes. I have.

Q. So why were you suddenly ready to marry this one? You were already sleeping together, I believe?

A. Yes. As I said, that worked. That was the thing I was sure about. I thought all the rest would follow.

Q. An odd view, for an "intellectual," as you labelled yourself.

A. Not really. All intellectuals these days read D. H. Lawrence, who says we should listen to—to our passions—to our bodies. To our feelings. I had strong feelings. Good ones.

There was nothing but cool respect in Griffith Goatley's eliciting of information. Laurence Ounce meets Frederica's eye with sexual intelligence; he implies, with a twist of his clever lip, with a cock of his large head, that they understand each other.

Q. Ah, D. H. Lawrence. The immemorial magnificence of mystic, palpable, real otherness. You felt *that.*

A. I don't know why you're asking. But yes, in a way. The prose is dreadful. But why not? Yes, that. It did seem to work.

Q. You married for good sex. Despite the fact that Mr. Reiver in no way shares your intellectual tastes, may never have opened Lawrence?

A. It was the attraction of opposites. I didn't know anything about him. He seemed—you quoted it—*other.* I liked that. I thought he was more—more self-sufficient and grown up than most of the men I knew.

Q. And you knew a great many?

A. I was in a position to.

Q. An odd phrase. You refer, no doubt, to the privileged position of Cambridge women. You were not sexually inexperienced when you married Nigel Reiver?

Griffith Goatley objects. Pre-marital incontinence is inadmissible as evidence in a divorce suit. The judge over-rules him, when Ounce explains that he is seeking to establish how likely or unlikely Mrs. Reiver was to have been surprised by "sexual peccadilloes and so on, on a husband's part."

"You may answer," says the judge.

"You knew quite a lot about men, when you married," says Ounce, wrinkling his eyes at Frederica, waiting to re-establish the fleeting sexual connection between them.

"Yes," says Frederica.

"How many men had you slept with?"

Goatley objects; his objection is sustained; the judge and the Court have seen Frederica hesitate, not knowing the answer.

"Moving on," says Ounce, "moving on to the question of these feelthy pictures. Do you not think—as a sophisticated woman, as you are, that you may have been exaggerating your reaction to them? You have a degree in English literature, a good degree. You must have discussed Shakespeare's bawdy, Chaucer's naughty tales, Rochester's lyrics, with aplomb, in your day, I imagine. Are you really shocked by a few filthy pictures, however deplorable—are they not an unfortunate phenomenon like smoking-room songs, like the lavatory jokes indulged in by all little boys, including your own son, I have no doubt."

"I can only say I was terribly shocked. It does interest me that it was such a blow. I agree, if you'd *told* me I'd react like that, I'd have said I probably wouldn't. But they made me sick."

"A real foray into Bluebeard's cupboard. Perhaps best to leave cupboards shut, you might think. All marriages need private places, private cupboards, you may think. The pictures were not forced on you, were not left about to upset you?"

"Oh no."

"Going back to your evidence. My learned friend asked you why your sexual happiness changed. I believe he expected you to reply, 'Because my husband neglected me and was cruel to me' or some such answer. But I wrote down what you did say. It was 'I think it went wrong because I withdrew. I began to see I ought not to have got married.' Would you care to comment on that observation, Mrs. Reiver?"

Frederica looks down at her hands. She cannot quite speak. He has heard her thoughts. She knows the answer, and knows she should not give it, and cannot speak.

"Come, Mrs. Reiver, you are usually so articulate, so clear. It is a simple question. 'I began to see I ought not to have got married.' "

"I began to see I had promised something I couldn't give," says Frederica, temporarily relieved by having at last said what is in her mind. She pauses again.

"You had married in bad faith?"

"Not exactly."

"Not exactly. But it might look like that. You might be thinking, I have made a mistake, maybe even, a dreadful mistake, and a sensitive man, even if not the most articulate man, might become irascible, sensing this reserve, might have fits of blind irritability, in response to this withdrawal."

"I didn't withdraw."

"Forgive me, Mrs. Reiver. It is the word you used."

"*Withdrawing* doesn't excuse axe-throwing."

"It does not. But we do not admit that an axe was ever thrown. Tell me again, Mrs. Reiver, why you married Nigel Reiver."

"I have told you. Sex. Sexual happiness, that is. And persistence. His persistence."

"The fact that he was very rich had nothing to do with it?"

"Almost nothing. I like—I liked—good restaurants. But it was more the glamour of the opposite, of the unknown, how the other half live. Bad faith, again. I am not asking for maintenance, not for myself. I hope I am allowed to make that clear at this point. I didn't marry for money. A bit for the glamour of the difference."

"You *are* very articulate," says Laurence Ounce, somehow diminishing Frederica.

Q. If we may turn to your precipitate flight from Bran House, for a moment. It was very convenient, was it not, that your friends, a group of male friends, were visiting at the time, were able to hang around with a Land Rover and wait for you?

A. They were not welcome. They might never have come again. I was very frightened. It seemed like then or never. At the time.

Q. And how did you prepare your son for this midnight exodus? Did you tell him you were leaving Bran House, his father, who loved him, his aunts, the housekeeper who had been responsible for his upbringing, his pony, to whom he was so attached? Did he come willingly?

A. (The witness is visibly shocked by this question.) He decided himself.

Q. What do you mean? You put it to him, to a little boy in his bedroom, a *very small* boy—you asked him to decide between his parents?

A. No. I would never do that. No. I didn't tell him. I didn't wake him. I didn't think I could. I didn't think it was fair. I didn't mean to go for long, for ever, then, at that moment. I felt he was better where he was.

Q. You felt he was better where he was.

A. Well, then, in a sense, obviously, yes, he was.

Q. How did he come to go with you, then?

A. He ran after me. He said he was coming. He seemed to know I was going.

Q. He wanted you to stay?

A. No. He said he was coming. I would have gone back in with him, and stayed. But he said he was coming.

Q. He was a desperate, confused little boy, in the middle of the night?

A. Yes. But he was determined. You don't know him. He has a strong will.

Q. You are not going to tell me that a little boy of—four years old—has a will strong enough, in the middle of the night, to impose a decision on a loving mother who has—with some self-renunciation it would appear—decided that *he was better where he was*? Was it not rather, Mrs. Reiver, the case that a little boy, whom you had been content to leave in his bed, sensed inconveniently that you were leaving him, and came out to remonstrate, to plead? And you, fearing that your rendezvous with your young men would be missed, snatched up this little boy, *as an afterthought,* and carried him away as an unplanned piece of luggage?

(The witness is silent.)

Q. Would you not say it was more or less like that?

A. (In a whisper) No. It was not like that. I love my son.

Her voice is small and dry. She cannot utter, she cannot speak. She licks her lips, a nervous gesture which the Court notes.

Griffith Goatley asks his client a few calm questions after this. He then produces signed affidavits from Bill Potter and Daniel Orton, describing violent assaults made upon them by Nigel Reiver on two occasions after his wife's departure.

Laurence Ounce's first witness is Miss Olive Reiver. He establishes that she is the unmarried sister of Nigel Reiver and lives in the family home, Bran House. He takes her through her brother's marriage.

Q. Were you surprised when he married Frederica Potter?

A. Not by then, no. She had often been staying with us. They were obviously very much in love. I was happy to see Nigel so happy.

Q. And Frederica. Was she happy?

A. It was hard to tell. She didn't find it easy to fit in to our way of life. She wasn't from our sort of background.

Q. Do you think she found you intimidating—the close family—the lifestyle of the country, to which she was not used?

A. Oh no. I think perhaps she rather despised us. She thought we were a bit slow and boring, I think. She lived for the moment when Nigel was there. She didn't try too hard with the rest of us.

Q. She perhaps missed her old friends?

A. I wouldn't say that. She had lots of visitors. All the visitors she wanted. Mostly young men from London. We made them welcome, of course; that was good manners.

Q. Was any attempt made to prevent her friends from coming, or to discourage communication with them?

A. Oh no. We keep open house. I think they found us a bit stick in the mud. Tweedy types. (Laughs.)

Q. And when your nephew was born—young Leo—did she seem more settled?

A. Oh no. Perhaps the reverse. She began to seem quite sulky and unhappy. We couldn't cheer her up. She took to sitting in her room.

Q. She was depressed?

A. You could call it that. It was a good thing there were so many of us to give a hand with the baby.

Q. But she loved the baby?

A. Oh, I think so. But I don't think she's the sort to whom looking after a baby comes naturally. She didn't hold him naturally, you know, she was kind of awkward. *Reserved* with him.

The evidence moves on to the alleged acts of cruelty.

Q. Did you ever see your brother express anger towards his wife?

A. They had the odd row. They both gave as good as they got. Shouting matches on the stairs. Kiss and make up, I've seen it several times. Normal, I'd say. She did sulk rather a lot, and that provoked him. But they were happy after their rows, all smiles and hugs.

Q. Did you ever see your brother strike his wife?

A. No. Never.

Q. But he might have done?

A. I don't know what went on in their private quarters. But I wouldn't think it was like him. We'd have seen, if she'd been bruised, and she wasn't.

Q. On a certain occasion, in 1964, the doctor was called to dress an extensive gash in your sister-in-law's thigh?

A. She told us she'd tripped over the barbed wire in the paddock field, going about to look at the moon.

Q. Did that strike you as an odd story?

A. Not really. She was always running around at night and wandering off. She was bored, poor thing.

Q. And the injuries were consistent with the barbed-wire story?

A. The rips in her trousers were. I didn't get a close look at her leg. That wasn't my concern.

Q. The wound didn't happen when she was wearing a nightdress?

A. I know nothing about a nightdress. I never saw a nightdress. I did see trousers with bloodstains and barbed-wire rips.

Q. Did you ever think your brother might have caused the injury?

A. No. I'm surprised to hear it suggested. He loves her—well, anyway, he loved her. He was very tolerant of her ways, in my opinion, and has made great efforts to get her to come back and live in the family home, with the little boy. It's not surprising he got a bit irritable—she made him look a bit of a fool, you might think, just going off like that in the middle of the night, with a pack of arty types from London. But he wouldn't *hurt* her. What good would that do?

Q. And what do you think should happen now, after she has stayed away for three years?

A. I don't approve of divorce. I'm a regular churchgoer, I know the Church's teaching is that marriage is once and permanent. I think a child should live in the family home with both his parents. But if she won't come back and try again, try a bit harder, I think she should let Leo come back to us, to the home he grew up in and will inherit, where he's loved and safe.

Laurence Ounce calls Rosalind Reiver. The witnesses have not been in the courtroom before they give evidence. Rosalind Reiver too reports that Frederica had frequent visitors, made no attempt to settle in Bran House, "sulked" and enjoyed quarrelling with her husband. She also states that the wound in Frederica's thigh was said at the time to be caused by barbed wire, and that she has seen ripped trousers with bloodstains consistent with this story. She too knows nothing of a nightdress.

The two sisters are impressive because of their solid, unimaginative ordinariness. They are reasonable, circumscribed, English country gentry. They frown as they appear to try to be fair to their errant sister-in-law. They make it clear that they are devoted to Leo; their heavy mouths smile, their dark eyes open with love when he is mentioned. Rosalind adds to Olive's evidence a moving image of the two of them teaching the enthusiastic little boy to ride Sooty, of the mother refusing to come out and watch his exploits, "reading a book" all the time, when he has learned to post at the trot. She too thinks Nigel has been very patient.

Laurence Ounce calls Pippy Mammott. Pippy's face is pink and shining with generous indignation. She is a more volatile witness than the stolid sisters, in that she has an air of having worked herself up to make an appearance, state a position, fight for a cause. Pins are working their way out of her head: now and then, during her evidence, she puts up her hands to put them back, looking as though she is trying to hold her head together. Ounce puts to her much the same series of preliminary questions as he put to the sisters, about the early days of the marriage, about Frederica's friends, or lack of friends, about their way of life, about Leo.

Q. She seemed happy to be pregnant?

A. I wouldn't say that, no. Oh no. I would say it came as a blow to her.

Q. It wasn't a planned pregnancy?

A. I overheard her talking to one of her friends on the telephone. She was always talking away on the telephone, all the time. She said, "Guess what, I'm preggers, it's an absolute disaster, it ruins absolutely everything, my life is in ruins."

Q. Are you sure these were her words? Or is that just the drift of what she was saying?

A. I was dreadfully shocked to hear her. It was a terrible thing to say. So naturally I remember it.

Q. But perhaps when the baby was born she felt different? Many women are shocked to find themselves pregnant, but love their child when he comes.

A. I don't think she felt any different. She wasn't natural with him. I tried to show her little things—how to soothe him, how to do his little nappies, how to get him to take his milk, but she was very irritable, very sulky, very sluggish, she didn't want to know. I caught her looking at him as though she wished he weren't there.

Q. That was your interpretation.

A. I know who did everything for that child. I know who put plasters on his knees and who he turned to when his guinea-pig died. I know who knew how he liked his eggs and his toasted soldiers . . .

Q. Perhaps she felt *de trop*?

A. What did you say?

Q. Perhaps she felt you looked after him so well, she was superfluous?

A. I don't think that was so, not at all. She plain *wasn't interested.* She was always *reading a book* when she wasn't walking *by herself* or phoning her friends. I've seen her feeding the little boy with one hand and holding up some book with the other, and her eyes were on the book, I can tell you, not on the baby. I've heard him howl his little heart out, and I've run and run to see what the matter was, and he's been hurt with a penknife, and there she was upstairs, *reading a book,* and didn't seem to hear a squeak. Not a squeak.

Q. But the boy loved his mother?

A. Naturally he did. He was always trying to get her attention. Mostly he failed. But I was there—his Pippy—and his aunts were there, and so he was well looked after.

On the question of Nigel's attacks on his wife, on the question of the trousers, the imaginary nightdress, the nature of the wound, Pippy's witness coincides precisely with that of Olive and Rosalind. It goes further.

Q. Did you see the wound in question?

A. Naturally I did. If there's anything to be dressed, or cleaned, or tended, I'm the one—even when it's her.

Q. How would you describe the wound?

A. Very jagged, very uneven. Typical barbed-wire, like you see in hunting. Dr. Roylance said so immediately. Typical barbed wire, he said. Silly girl tried to scramble over a hedge without seeing there was wire the other side, and fell. She doesn't have country instincts. We all knew the hedge was wired. Nigel was very upset. He sat with her all day, soothing her, and chatting.

Frederica writes a note to Goatley. "She's lying. They're all *lying.*"

"Exaggerating?" he writes back.

"No, *lying.* Flat, magniloquent *lies.*"

"Perhaps she believes herself?"

"She *can't*—none of it was *like that.*"

"The judge might notice she's full of animosity. It does come through. But it's hard to credit her with the imagination to lie on a large scale."

"But she *is*—"

"Ah, yes, but what does the court believe?"

Ounce does not ask Pippy, as he asked Olive and Rosalind, what she thinks should happen now. He does say, "Do you think there is any hope of reconciliation after three years' absence?"

"As to that, I couldn't say. I know Nigel wanted things to be as they were and should have been. Families should be together. But I say, if she won't do as she should, the little boy should come back where he's at home, and happy, and loved. There's an abundance of love, a *sufficiency* of love, I do want to make that clear. She could see him all she wants, she knows she could, but he needs his proper things in the proper place. He can't be happy in a basement in *south London,* he's a country child, born and bred . . ."

The court is adjourned for lunch after Pippy's evidence. Frederica drinks a half-pint of shandy. She cannot eat. She does not like beer, but needs alcohol and is thirsty. She tries to joke; she says to Arnold Begbie, "I feel I'm on trial for reading books."

"You are. Partly."

"I wouldn't be if I were a man."

"Perhaps not. I know a couple—early thirties, can't have children, desperate to adopt. The social worker concerned in vetting them sent in a report saying, 'Plausible couple, well-intentioned. Too many books in the house. Wife reads.' "

The next witness after lunch says his name is Theobald Drossel, known as Theo. He is very small; only his head can be seen above the box; he is almost entirely bald and his skin is unhealthy. His face is long and lugubrious. He wears a brown suit and a checked shirt. Frederica finds him faintly familiar, and then, as he says what his profession is, recognises him in the same instant. He is the little man from Hamelin Square, whose Austin coughs continuously. He says he is the director of the Sharp Inquiry Company.

"I watch people. I find things out. Anything, really. I find out. I do mostly marital work. In the nature of things."

Q. You have been in the employment of Mr. Nigel Reiver?

A. Yes. Since December 1964.

Q. What were you asked to do?

A. Follow that lady. Mr. Reiver's wife, see where she went, what she did. See what the little boy did.

Q. And where was Mrs. Reiver living from October 1964?

A. She was living in Bloomsbury, in a mansion flat owned by a Mr. Thomas Poole. I watched her go in and out of the flats, and I watched her go to work with Mr. Poole and come back with him. In the nature of things, I did not gain access to the flat to see what went on there.

Q. Did you form any impression of the relationship between Mr. Poole and Mrs. Reiver?

A. It was very loving, very affectionate. I saw them kiss and cuddle on various occasions, when they separated in the street, and so on. I saw them go shopping with all the kids, his and hers. They was very like a married couple, you know, easy with each other, very affectionate.

I engaged their *au pair* girl in conversation on two occasions. I pretended to be a neighbour who wanted to borrow a drill. I find a drill is a more plausible thing to try and borrow than sugar. Lots of people don't have drills. The young woman—very prudently—wouldn't let me into the flat, so I couldn't ascertain the sleeping arrangements. I pretended to think that Mrs. Reiver was, so to speak, Mrs. Poole, and the young woman in question, Miss Röhde, (referring to his notebook) enlightened me, as she thought, as to the real situation, but said she supposed they would soon marry, *everything pointed that way,* she said, they would make a lovely family.

Q. Later, Mrs. Reiver moved house?

A. Yes. She went to live in Hamelin Square, Number 42, with a Miss Agatha Mond and her little girl. Miss Mond appears to be unmarried and to have few visitors.

Q. And Mrs. Reiver? Did she have few visitors?

A. No. She had a great many. She had many male visitors, both single ones and in large groups. I kept a record, the days I was there—I wasn't always on this job, you must understand, I had other commissions, there are gaps in my information. I counted about seven or eight very regular male visitors, to whom she was very affectionate, kissing and hugging and stroking.

The witness reads out a list: Tony Watson, Hugh Pink, Edmund Wilkie, Alexander Wedderburn, Daniel Orton, Desmond Bull, Jude Mason. He reads out a rough count of observed visits, singly and in groups. Frederica stares. Her private life is a spectacle for this little man in an Austin. He describes her friendly evenings as "wild parties—the neighbours used to *murmur* about them as they passed my car. She was felt to be a bit outrageous, in the square."

Q. Did you feel that any of these visitors were more than simply intimate friends?

A. I followed the lady on various occasions when she visited Mr. Desmond Bull in Eagle Lane, Clerkenwell. I got friendly with his landlady, who is rather proud of having a Bohemian painter lodging in her house. This landlady—Mrs. Annabel Patten—told me—he reads from his notebook—"he has a mattress in his studio where he screws his models and students and women who come." It was her opinion that Mr. Bull was "an insatiable sex maniac." I do not think she meant by that that he was mad or perverted, merely that he enjoyed sex. She herself took a vicarious pleasure in his activities, and . . .

The judge points out that what the landlady said is inadmissible, since it is hearsay. Ounce asks his witness if he himself observed anything in Mrs. Patten's house.

A. I was able to gain her confidence enough on July 28th, 1966, to be allowed to peep in through a glass panel—one of those frosted things—on Mr. Bull's door. There I observed Mrs. Reiver holding a glass of wine in a state of undress.

Q. Undress?

A. Stark naked. Very much at her ease.

Q. Perhaps she was modelling for Mr. Bull.

A. If she was, that was not all, because I saw Mr. Bull, also stark naked, with his member erect, walk towards her and push her down. On his mattress, you see, the one on his studio floor. I was able to persuade Mrs. Patten to sign a statement as to what we had witnessed—she said she didn't mind, as Mr. Bull "doesn't give a fuck who knows what he does, he's proud of it."

Judge. Mr. Bull has made no answer to the service of the Petition naming him as co-respondent.

Clerk. No, my lord.

Judge. He has not put in an appearance.

Clerk. No, my lord.

Judge. He is content to let this matter go forward and not to contest it.

Q. Are there other men with whom you observed Mrs. Reiver to be on intimate terms?

A. There is Mr. John Ottokar.

Q. When did you first see Mr. Ottokar?

A. That must have been in May or June 1965. He used to come regularly to the square and stare at her lighted windows like a love-sick male dog. At first I thought he might be a burglar—I was sitting quiet in my car, quite unobtrusive—I sit for hours, often, sometimes I read a bit, by torchlight—but I saw his look, the way he looked. And one night she let him in. So I crept across the square and looked down into the basement. She sleeps in the basement. Often she doesn't draw the curtains. Even when she does, since it's a fairly thin blind, you can see quite clearly from the shadows what she is doing, what anyone else in there is doing. I was able to satisfy myself that intercourse had taken place. I saw it take place again on July 5th and July 14th and on at least fourteen subsequent occasions.

Q. And did you observe Mrs. Reiver with Mr. Ottokar anywhere else?

A. I followed them to Yorkshire in the summer of 1965, where they signed into a hotel under the names of Mr. and Mrs. John Ottokar.

Judge. Was that necessary, given how much you said you had seen?

A. Oh, I think so, my lord: I was able to obtain signed affidavits from the hotel staff there, and also my brief was to follow her everywhere she went, not to lose sight of her.

Ounce. Are there more men you have seen with Mrs. Reiver in compromising situations?

A. There is Mr. Paul Ottokar.

Q. Mr. Paul Ottokar.

A. The problem with Mr. Paul Ottokar is that he is Mr. John Ottokar's twin. His identical twin. I did not realise at first that there were two young men of this description—blond young men with long hair—so to speak *haunting* Hamelin Square, because you don't expect it, do you, you don't expect two vagrants hanging around in the small hours to be watching the same window and look alike. But on one occasion I have observed one brother to be watching from the basement area from which I have watched myself on occasion when Mrs. Reiver was so to speak amorously engaged within with the other brother, so I did a bit of thinking and realised there were two. Mr. John Ottokar works for the Eurobore Systems Analysis Centre. Mr. Paul Ottokar is a pop singer called Zag who sings with a group called Zag and the Szyzgy Zy-Goats. S-z-y-z-g-y, my lord. Pronounced "Ziggy."

Judge. Say that again.

Witness. Zag and the Ziggy Zy-Goats.

Judge. Clever. Very clever.

Witness. My lord?

Judge. Continue. So you found two brothers, twin brothers, taking an interest in Mrs. Reiver?

Witness. Yes, my lord. It is more difficult to tell them apart than you might think. For sometimes both of them wear respectable suits, and sometimes both of them wear, kind of *costumes*—harlequin things, and shiny cloaks and stuff, and painted bodies. And when they watch at night, they wear black PVC raincoats, and it's beyond me to know which one is inside and which is out watching.

Judge. What do you mean, painted bodies?

Witness. Well. They go in for very weird behaviour, very ostentatious, self-advertising kind of stuff. There was one night, one of them set fire to a lot of books, with paraffin, on the bit of waste ground in the middle of the square. He was wearing nothing but a long glittery plastic cloak and he was painted all over in all sorts of colours on his naked body. I formed the opinion he was under the influence of some sort of drugs. Mrs. Reiver had a battle with him over the fires. It was her books he was burning, I think, perhaps. They wrestled, and he fell in the fire, and got quite burned. They called an ambulance. She was holding on to his naked body and screaming and crying.

Ounce. Was Mrs. Reiver's son in the company of these painted young men?

A. Often and often, both when she was there and when she wasn't. He plays a lot with a gang of little black kids that run around in the street doing silly things like steal milk and ring people's door bells, and one of the brothers encouraged them to set firecrackers under my little car. It did quite a lot of damage.

Q. Is there anything that leads you to feel certain that Mrs. Reiver did have intercourse with both brothers, and not only with Mr. John Ottokar?

A. Well. Once I could see they were arguing and so I crept up and listened. No one can see you in the area outside the basement window if you keep in the shadow of the steps. And he was shouting at her, he was telling her they both always shared women, that he was the *real* one and his brother was "the shadow" and a lot of stuff like that. I wrote one phrase down. "This is the real flesh you have imagined." He seemed to be trying to say the experience wasn't complete without both of them, so to speak.

Q. And what was her response?

A. I saw them lying on the bed. I saw him undressing her, before I had to run, because I heard Miss Mond coming home.

Part of the Evidence of Thomas Poole, examined by Laurence Ounce.

Q. And why did you invite Mrs. Reiver to share your flat?

A. Because I was sorry for her—she had been very frightened, was at a loss, and needed, she believed, to hide from her violent husband. It seemed a sensible arrangement. We were both single parents, with the care of children, who needed to work for our livings. I was able to help her find work. We were able to share housekeeping and baby-sitting.

Q. And you enjoyed having her?

A. Very much. We knew each other well. I was a colleague of her father, as a schoolmaster, at Blesford Ride School.

Q. So you were *in loco parentis*?

A. To an extent.

Q. Although your children were the same age. Or almost.

A. There are more generations than two.

Q. Indeed there are. You are not old enough to be her father. Did you find her—do you find her—attractive?

A. Yes. She is an attractive woman.

Q. Did it occur to you that things might work out very well if you married, if you worked together, harmoniously, and shared your lives as you were, in fact, already doing?

A. It did occur to me, yes.

Q. Would you have liked to marry Mrs. Reiver, had she been free?

A. The question is purely hypothetical.

Q. Would you?

A. Yes. I would. I admire her greatly and feel love for her.

Q. To the point of making love to her, in earnest of your hopes, when she was in your flat?

A. No. She didn't want it. She had been much hurt. She needed peace, and a time to reflect. I tried to give her that.

Q. Why did she leave, Mr. Poole?

A. Because she decided to ask for a divorce, and felt that our co-habitation might compromise her. She may have been right. I am very sorry it had to be so.

Q. Perhaps she left you for younger men, and a racier life?

A. Perhaps. She was determined to divorce her husband and take charge of her own life. I don't think she would do anything to jeopardise that.

Q. Would it surprise you to learn that she has been reported as giving "wild parties" and entertaining a pop singer called Zag?

A. Nothing would surprise me about Frederica. She has a streak of recklessness. But she is also an adult, and an intelligent woman, who made a mistake she is paying for.

Q. You refer to her marriage as "a mistake."

A. She was much cast down by the sudden death of her sister. I think she married whilst deeply involved in that grief, that terrible pain. I think she should not have made any decision, in that state. But there it is.

Nigel Reiver is the last to give evidence. He stands in the witness box, watchful but relaxed, his face a mask of courteous attention, his body "ready to spring," is the phrase that comes into Frederica's head. he does not look at her, either with defiance or with regret. His hair is smooth and longer than it used to be; he too is entering the Swinging Sixties.

Frederica is suddenly invaded by a total memory of the first time they made love, in his bachelor flat amongst the dust and dirty shirts; she remembers his body above hers, and his intent face, looking darkly down; she remembers her surprise at the vanishing of her own habitual detachment, the surprise of her hot pleasure, her complete presence in his hands, under his weight. From time to time, with other men, inconveniently, she has been visited by the ghost of this completely unghostly moment of life, this excess of delight. Now is a bad moment to remember it; she looks down, and feels the hot blood running up her neck. All these words, all these lies and equivocations and painful approximations and truths are to do with this, which cannot be described.

She listens to him describing their marriage, in his usual blocked, cautious words. He is not indignant, as his sisters were on his behalf. On his own, he might not move an arbiter to think him greatly wronged. Frederica is moved.

Q. Your wife has complained that you were absent for unreasonable periods, that you prevented her from having a life of her own.

A. I expected her to be my wife. Her idea of what that meant and mine weren't the same. With hindsight, I think both of us could have given way a little.

Q. You were surprised when she suddenly left.

A. Very. I didn't think things were that bad. I knew she was a bit upset. I thought she'd come back.

Q. You hadn't hurt her, or frightened her?

A. I lost my temper, once or twice. I was worried. Normally, I pride myself on keeping my temper. So when I do shout and hit, it frightens people, it frightened her perhaps, more than it ought.

Q. You say you shouted. Did you hit her?

A. I pushed her about a bit once in the bedroom. She provoked me.

Q. Provoked you?

A. I got the sense she wasn't *with me* and didn't want to be. Her thoughts were somewhere else. It was like living with a—with a—with a walking corpse. That isn't what I mean. She was there, but there wasn't anyone there. I wanted to shake her, to get her attention back, and once or twice I did, that's all.

Q. Did you ever throw an axe at her?

A. No.

Q. She has claimed you did. Can you remember any episode which she might be referring to?

A. No. (Pause.) She must have just made it up. She's got the imagination.
(He gives the impression that he has not.)

Q. When your wife left, did you hope she would come back?

A. Of course. I thought it was a silly misunderstanding.

Q. Did you make any efforts to get her back?

A. Yes. I looked everywhere I could think of. I went to see people—friends—and family. She hid from me. When I found her, she'd clearly decided to live in a different style.

Q. But you still wanted her back?

A. I believe in marriage. We have a child. A woman's place is with her husband and child. She wouldn't talk, she wouldn't discuss, she wouldn't entertain the idea. I'm not a saint, I'm a reasonable being. I've waited and hoped. Now, I think I give up. I'd like to remake my life: but I do want my son. I love my son, he's happy at home, where he belongs.

Griffith Goatley questions Nigel about the obscene pictures, about the Tips and Tassels, about the Honeypot. Nigel replies that the pictures were given to him by a schoolfriend who thought "they were a good joke." "I put them with my rugger things and forgot them. I expect they're still there." He is open about the Tips and Tassels and the Honeypot.

A. Certain sorts of business entertaining does go on in places like that. With foreigners, you know, people who expect this kind of thing. It doesn't mean much to me, either way, but I go along with it. I admit once or twice I did go off with women from there. It isn't very nice, I see, but it isn't what I think of as "adultery"—

Q. It *is* adultery.

A. Here it is, it's named so. It is, I see that. But it's just horsing around, you know, naughtiness. I never thought of it as anything to do with my marriage. It's not like paying serious attention to another real woman.

Q. Real?

A. Woman out of one's own class, one's own world, who might make claims, distract your *feelings* . . . (He stops, apparently at a loss for words. He says) I don't think all that has anything to do with why she left me. I don't think it was important.

Goatley. She may hold a different view on that.

A. I bet she doesn't. *That* isn't what's at stake. It's her idea of her independence, that's what's the real issue here. I give in on that now, I'm asking for a divorce, being a wife isn't her idea of how to live, I accept that now. If we'd both been a bit wiser in the beginning, it would have saved a lot of tears. But we do have a son, and for his sake I would try to keep it up, I would have tried, because I think he comes first and he will be best in Bran House, in his own place. I wanted her to stay, but she went off with all these men, and a man can only take so much of that.

Laurence Ounce produces a signed affidavit from Nigel's doctor, Dr. Andrew Roylance, who says that he has never at any time treated Mr. Reiver for any venereal infection, and that he remembers the occasion of Mrs. Reiver's flesh wound, which he was told was, and which was in his opinion consistent with, a tear caused by falling on barbed wire scrambling over a wall or hedge with a concealed strip of the wire.

Frederica is recalled to the stand, and examined by Laurence Ounce about the evidence of Theobald Drossel.

He takes her through the evidence about Thomas Poole, and through Thomas Poole's own evidence. Frederica replies confidently enough that she lived chastely at Poole's flat, and adds tartly, "I would have had to in any case, even if I had not wanted to, since I had caught the infection."

Q. If you had not had the infection, you might have slept with Mr. Poole.

A. I do not think I would, no. I am just pointing out, it was out of the question.

Q. But you *thought* about it being out of the question.

A. Mr. Poole has said that he himself thought we might consider—a closer relationship. I didn't. He says I didn't. He is quite clear.

Q. So it matters to you to be thought chaste, to be a woman who does not sleep with all and sundry?

A. I have never done that, and don't intend to.

Q. What are your relations with Mr. John Ottokar?

A. Private, I hoped. I have made love to him. I admit that. On several occasions, more or less as Mr. Drossel says.

Q. Do you love Mr. Ottokar?

A. I don't know what that word means, any more. I don't know how to tell a Court what I feel about him. I think I do feel—have felt—love for him. Yes. It is—it was—a serious relationship.

Q. It is—it was? How do things stand at present?

A. I don't know. I haven't seen him since the summer.

Q. I believe he is your student.

A. Was my student.

Q. You were, as it were, in a position of responsibility towards him?

A. Hardly. He comes to an *adult* class I teach. We are all grown-up people, in that class.

Q. And sleep with each other?

A. No. This is different.

Q. Mr. Ottokar is not here today. He has been served with a petition, and has not entered an appearance.

A. That is so.

Q. Was there, is there, any question of your eventually marrying Mr. Ottokar?

A. None that I know of. None, that is. All this—these proceedings—have probably put an end to it. I mean to the relationship, not to the idea of marriage, which never arose, until you mentioned it.

Q. Never arose. Never arose. It was simply an affair, under your son's nose, but not serious.

A. It was serious. It was not frivolous. I tried to see him without upsetting or involving Leo.

Q. And his brother?

A. I have never slept with his brother.

Q. What is your relationship with his brother?

A. I should like to say, none. His brother—his brother—he invades my flat, without my consent. He invades his brother's relationships. It is hard to explain briefly.

Q. Mr. Drossel describes a scene in which he claims one Mr. Ottokar burned your books whilst under the influence of drugs.

A. I think he was. Yes, he did. It was Paul and I tried to stop him. I don't want him in my house, or near my son. It is all very unfortunate.

Q. It is all very unfortunate. Very unfortunate, I would agree. You feel a little out of control of these brothers and their passions and their way of life?

A. I may never see them again. I haven't seen them, either of them, for months. It's past.

Q. But you feel love for Mr. Paul—I'm sorry—for *Mr. John* Ottokar.

A. I did. I don't know what I feel now. I *don't know.*

Q. And Mr. Desmond Bull. You heard Mr. Drossel's evidence.

A. That was the only time.

Q. The only time?

A. The only time I made love to Desmond Bull.

Q. But you go there often?

A. He is a colleague. I like his pictures.

Q. But the only time you made love to him on his mattress, to which he invites many women, was the time when Mr. Drossel happened to have his eye to the etched window?

A. Yes. That one time.

Q. We may find that hard to believe. Why did you break your rule, if it exists, on that one occasion?

A. I needed comfort. I was in a great rage, after Paul Ottokar's skoob activities.

Q. Skoob?

A. Books, backwards. Towers of burned books. A new art-form.

Q. So one artist burns your books and your natural reaction is to make love to another because you "needed comfort," because you were "in a great rage."

A. Yes.

Q. And that is what you normally do, when you are in need of comfort, make love to some man?

A. No.

Q. You say you have never made love to Mr. Hugh Pink?

A. No.

Q. Nor to Mr. Tony Watson nor to Mr. Alan Melville?

A. No. That is, no, not since I was married.

Q. And Mr. Edmund Wilkie?

A. Not since 1954. A long time ago.

Q. Tell me, Mrs. Reiver, do you think the act of sex is sacred, or just a kind of quick source of comfort or assuagement of rage?

A. "Sacred" is a word that isn't in my vocabulary. I think sex varies with people and times. I think it can be very serious—very important—and now and then not important, just something that happens. One should never hurt or cheat people. This isn't a good answer, I know, when I'm in this court, which calls sex adultery, and sees every man as a potential husband and father. But the truth is, *I was faithful to my husband until I left him*—as he was not, even if it was only tips and tassels and honeypots, so to speak. *Sex isn't*—

Q. Sex isn't?

A. It doesn't matter.

Q. You were going to say?

A. Sex isn't the root of the matter. The root is unkindness and cruelty.

Q. You will have read Sigmund Freud, being so clever. Everything has a sexual element, according to him. Unkindness and cruelty may spring from the sexual insecurity of a man denied and at some deep level rejected, frustrated, trivialised?

A. (Silence.)

Q. You have no response to that?

A. It wasn't a question. It was a statement.

Q. A statement on which you don't wish to comment.

A. No. I think not. No.

The lawyers make their final speeches. Griffith Goatley speaks first. He presents his client as a brilliant and generous young woman—he emphasises the "*young*"—who married in good faith someone not from her own background, someone socially more privileged, from a class with very well-defined ways and expectations, into which she was expected to fit—to fit gratefully, he might suggest, as might be clear from the evidence of her sisters-in-law and housekeeper. There was no suggestion of compromise, says Mr. Goatley. "From the moment of marriage this young woman's husband treated her primarily as a fourth member of his household of adoring women. The reasonable expectations she might have had of any continuance of the friendships or conversations she valued in her own world were disappointed. Her husband's absences were longer and longer, and as he himself has admitted, concerned not only with business, but at least as much with convivial pleasures, and more reprehensible activities—some of which endangered his young wife's health, and, as she has pointed out, might well have endangered the health of their unborn child. She felt herself unwanted and superfluous in this apparently idyllic home—and whatever Your Lordship may make of the factual side of the evidence of the Misses Reiver and Miss Mammott, it seems abundantly clear that there was never either liking or sympathy or understanding shown towards my client."

Griffith Goatley, with clarity and reasonable precision, sums up Frederica's tale of violence—the blow to the spine, the terror in the lavatory, the axe-throwing. "Her husband and his family deny that any of this took place: they have closed ranks: their evidence, you may think, is almost remarkably consistent and homogeneous. My client is, as she has been throughout her married life, isolated and unsupported." Frederica is not, he says, a saint or a heroine—"she is a young wife who got out of her depth—both as to social class, and, you may think, despite some juvenile peccadilloes, as to sexual cruelty, as to the interest in hurting and humiliating women represented by the nature of the pornographic material she discovered, and by the kind of entertainment provided at least by the Honeypot, and by precise services offered by the particular call girl, Myra Thanopoulos, with whom Mr. Reiver does not deny that he has associated."

He asks that Frederica Reiver be granted a divorce on grounds of cruelty, both mental and physical, and on grounds of adultery.

Laurence Ounce describes his client as a serious, dynamic young man—much involved in his business, but this is normal, is not a fault or a sin, who has married a girl met whilst she was a Cambridge undergraduate, happy and flourishing amongst the admiration lavished on her in this world of young men. He was aware of her reputation as a sophisticated and *experienced* young woman—though not, perhaps, of the extent, or, one might say, the indiscriminate nature of this sophistication and experience.

He felt, perhaps, that he had carried away the princess for the ball under the eyes of the suitors. He believed, perhaps, the story of the fairytale—"The most surprising people do believe it, my lord, and act upon it, and learn to adjust their naïve expectations with good and bad humour as the case may be." He believed that they would marry and live happy ever after, that the princess would become lady of the manor and live as her predecessors had lived. But she did not want to, had no intention of being happy ever after. Adjustment was certainly required on both sides—when was it ever not? But Mrs. Reiver would not adjust—she needed her court of young men, her "career," her books, her "independence," just as though her marriage vows had never been made, and even though she has a small son who might be thought to be enough occupation for the next few years of the happy ever after. She has admitted, strikingly, that she "withdrew" and "realised she should never have married." She puts this realisation as *preceding* the cruelty she claims her husband exercised—she is involuntarily honest, even though unstable. She invents a story, of acts of violence committed by her husband. Of acts so suddenly cruel, out of the blue, that she is forced to make a dramatic midnight flight through the woods—"The story is now Bluebeard's Castle, and the grisly exhibits have been duly viewed in the cupboard"—snatching up her son *as an afterthought* "although she thought he would be better where he was." What are we to make of this tale? It is confidently rejected by my client, by the Misses Reiver, by Miss Philippa Mammott. Mrs. Reiver has a first class degree in English. She is an expert in the European novel, on which she has been lecturing with some success, it appears, to Mr. John Ottokar, amongst others enchanted by her rhetoric. She is at home in Dostoevski, Stendhal and Sir Walter Scott. She knows all about axes and women in white robes fleeing through the woods in the dark. My client's sisters, more prosaic, see *trousers* with hedge-tears typical of barbed wire's jagged ripping. Are we to believe that these taciturn, churchgoing ladies—"tweedy and boring" as they put it themselves, got together and concocted a foolproof coherent story? And that they then suborned the excellent Dr. Roylance to commit perjury? This is not feudal England, and he is not a retainer. No, the unstable, creative imagination, the *literary cleverness,* is all Mrs. Reiver's." Mr. Ounce submits that Mr. Reiver has no case to answer as to the alleged cruelty. Look at these two, he says, and decide who it is safe to believe. In all marital problems there is a balance of right and wrong and it is very rarely all on one side. But in this case it is clear where the guilt lies, as it is clear from Mrs. Reiver's subsequent behaviour what sort of lifestyle she would naturally choose, left to herself.

When the judge begins to speak, Frederica thinks again: I am too thin. She *has not enough weight.* She is nothing. The things she knows she cannot say and the things she says are not descriptions of what she thinks was and is what happened or is happening. He has not heard her. He will find against her. He looks down from his height, sourly she thinks, wet buried eyes in a sick skin.

He says:

"We old men have to remember that marriages change, that social customs change, that expectations change. You are here in a Divorce Court, in a Christian country where the established Church, to which one of you belongs, believes marriage is for ever and indissoluble. You both desire divorce, although our law requires that you must neither connive nor collude in seeking it, but show cause why you should be divorced, give evidence of matrimonial offences which are sufficient reason for divorce. Mrs. Frederica Reiver, the wife, first sought relief alleging cruelty and adultery. Mr. Nigel Reiver was for some time long-suffering, sought restoration of his conjugal rights in the matrimonial home, and has now, perhaps for sufficient reasons, decided that his patience will lead nowhere, that his hopes are unrealistic, that his best help is to accept the situation with a good grace.

"I have carefully considered the evidence set before me. Mr. Reiver admits to the adultery of which he is accused, but denies the charges of cruelty. The major charges—the blows and the story of the axe-attack—depend entirely on Mrs. Reiver's own uncorroborated account. She appears to have complained to no one about this alleged attack within the time which is allowed to make this complaint admissible as evidence of the attack. She appears not to have complained specifically of this attack to the shadowy young men who waited for her in the Land Rover after her flight, though we do have the affidavit of Mr. Hugh Pink that he was told—*eleven days* later—that an axe had been thrown. This evidence we must weigh against the very clear evidence of the Misses Reiver and Miss Mammott, and whilst it is not beyond the bounds of credibility that these respectable bodies should have agreed a story to support their brother and employer, it is my belief that the balance of probability is against it. The same balance of uncertainties applies to the sorry tale of the venereal infection. Mrs. Reiver claims that she could have caught it only from her husband. He does not deny that he has consorted with women from whom he *could* have caught such an infection, but he presented medical evidence that he did not. Mrs. Reiver claims to have seen no friends, male or female, since her marriage, until she ran away. This is contradicted by the evidence of the Misses Reiver and Miss Mammott. Her recent behaviour does not suggest that physical chastity is high enough on her scale of values to render it entirely improbable that she could have contracted the infection elsewhere.

"Her own adultery—subsequent to her desertion, which she does not deny—is amply witnessed and supported. She denies several counts and admits others. We need not go into the truth, or lack of truth of the contested allegations, since what is admitted is enough to show the nature of the case.

"I have some sympathy with both parties to this divorce. Both misunderstood the nature of each other's commitment, though this might have been more easily remedied than Mrs. Reiver's petition melodramatically assumes. Mr. Reiver expected to find a wife who behaved like a wife and accepted the constraints upon her freedom inevitably incurred by becoming a wife. Mrs. Reiver assumed that Mr. Reiver admired her as she was, for her intellectual virtues perhaps, and would allow her a latitude he was far from admitting. The higher education of women has in many ways, I have observed, been very hard upon both men and women. It has encouraged skills and raised expectations which society as it is at present constituted is incapable of fulfilling or satisfying—skills and expectations perhaps incompatible with the fulfilled life of wife and mother. Other women, faced with the realisation of this problem, have perhaps been more patient, more tractable, more resourceful. Mrs. Reiver was young and volatile. She chose to run away.

"Much turns on the alleged axe attack, which is the only substantial act of cruelty alleged. I feel that it is unsafe to accept Mrs. Reiver's evidence on this point—the balance of probability, which this court is allowed to consider to be adequate—lies with the husband's account, and the evidence of his household. Mrs. Reiver's desertion is undeniable.

"Mr. Reiver's attempts to persuade her to return are well documented and wholly convincing. Both parties have committed adultery: neither has any prospect, apparently, of a second marriage, which might offer a family to the little boy.

"I find for the husband, whose prayer for counter-relief the Court accepts. He is granted a decree nisi. The wife's petition is rejected.

"In the matter of custody of the son, Leo Alexander. The Court will institute custody proceedings as soon as is reasonably possible. The Court Welfare Officer will visit both parties, and both houses, and will also talk to the boy himself, who is, I understand, articulate and bright. I should like to be able to institute the custody hearing before Christmas, but the Clerk fears that because of pressure of cases this may not be practicable. The Court directs that for the present the child shall stay where he is, with his mother, to disrupt his life as little as possible. Since it is clear that he has been happily travelling between households, the Court also directs that he spend Christmas with his father, arriving on December 24th, returning to his mother on December 27th promptly."

Frederica stands outside the courtroom in her little black dress. Her visible knees beneath its high hem tremble and knock together. She feels she has been watching a film about a woman whom she rather despises, a silly woman who has been judged and found wanting. On top of this, she feels obscurely, the story of her life has been changed by the way it has been told today—both the true bits, and the velleities, and the flat lies, one part of a new fiction, a new story, in which she—who is she, does she exist?—is entangled as in a fine, voluminous net. She thinks she does not care who wins the divorce, as long as the divorce happens. She thinks that the story that was told is the story of a woman unfit to have charge of a small boy, whom she does not love enough. She feels she has stepped into a world where the codes, the rules, are different: reading is wicked, is neglect, a movement of love or comfort to one man is simply defined as depriving another of his *rights.* She stands by herself and her knees knock. Words come into her head. "Who is it that can tell me who I am?" Who said that?

Someone comes up behind her and puts an arm round her shoulders. "That was pretty dreadful. Are you OK?" It is Nigel. She flinches, and then turns to meet his eye: he too is involved in this linguistic net laid over bare limbs in a bed, over the axe, over the little boy sleeping, over what can't be named or defined or understood.

"I'm shaking," she says.

"You know you don't have to worry about costs. I'll pay."

"Thank you."

"We'll talk about Christmas."

"We will."

"All's fair in love and war, heh?"

"No. It isn't. It isn't. Some things aren't. Lies aren't."

"I want my son, Frederica."

"So do I. So do I."

"I don't think you do, not really, not deep down. That's what all this is about. That's what I'm fighting for."

He is telling the truth. She bows her head.

"We'll see," she says, in a small voice.

"We will. If he comes home, you can come whenever you want, you can take him on holidays, we'll make it *good,* we won't exclude you."

"He wants to stay with me."

"We'll see about that."

He pats her shoulder again, and again she has the double movement of flinching and turning to him.

That night, she dreams. She is outside a high gate, with barbed wire wreathing its top. The weather is darkly hot and stormy. She is not tall enough to peer in through the keyhole, which is high above her head and massive. She knows no one will come. She looks around for something to stand on, to see in, and finds a kind of rolling platform on wheels, which she knows, as dreamers know, is what is used to roll condemned men, unable to walk, close enough to the hangman. She pushes it towards the keyhole. Its wheels are wooden, and crank and grumble. She mounts the steps and grips the bar in front of her. She can see in. The keyhole is like a long telescopic tunnel. Dark. Beyond is a garden. It is in many ways the Long Royston garden where she played the young Virgin Queen in Alexander's *Astraea*. It has wide lawns, with croquet hoops and rose trees, and is bordered by a forest of dark boughs, with beautiful ashy black leaves, and golden fruit covered with soot, so that the gold shines dimly, fitfully, through the black dust.

Over the lawns pad great cats. Lions, tigers, black panthers, with gold eyes, with green eyes, with blood on their white fangs, silent and pacing. She knows she has to try and let them out, and that if she lets them out, they will devour her. There is no key. She has the idea that she can pour herself through the keyhole, but this is nonsense. A voice in the head says, "You are thin, you are thin." She sees that she is indeed thin, she is two-dimensional, a paper woman, a cardboard woman. She watches herself insert herself between the great gates, insubstantial inch by inch, and float above the garden like a kite. At the end of the garden is a kind of shrine, a cave with a stone bed in it, on which is a stone lion, a small lion, which emits a kind of pulsing light, a hot, bright glow. She manages to alight on the grass, and walks towards this creature. All the other great beasts pad behind her. She is in a dress made of red and white paper, which shreds and falls in drifts like petals as she goes forward. She is as she was the young Elizabeth, pursued with scissors by her stepmother, Catherine Parr, and her stepmother's jocular, amorous husband, Thomas Seymour, intent on shredding her petticoats for fun, or so it was said in Seymour's trial for treason, for which he lost his head. He lost his head, the voice says in her head, as the grass becomes full of floating red and white fragments between the croquet hoops. Her dress is no longer a dress, it is a paper band round her waist from which hang red and white ribbons, which do not cover the ruddy triangle of her pubic hair. Now, as in the play, she cries out the line of the beggarwoman in the ballad whose red flannel petticoat was cut away—"Lawks a mussy on me, this is none of I." Figures are hurtling after her, large stone women, red women, white women, howling, "Off with her head." If she can reach the stone lion she is safe. The garden grows as she runs. She trips on the hoops, her feet bleed. A red woman pronounces, She thinks she is Una with the lion, but everyone knows that is a lie, a whopper, a terrible tarradiddle, Una was a virgin and virgins don't have lions.

Virgins have stone lions, she says. That isn't right. They don't. The stone lion snarls and begins to grow a stone pelt, bristling. Its eyes are red. It yawns. She must reach it.

She isn't a virgin, say the pursuing three. They are all red now, all three, and she is white with fear, with cold, she shivers in the cool evening in the garden and tries to cover her nakedness with her hands. They have the faces of Easter Island gods, carved in red stone, in bloodstone, in carnelian. They say, She can't do anything, she's made of paper, she's cardboard, she's just cardboard, she's thin, she's a line.

Paper wraps stone, she says, falling towards the glowing creature couched on the stone bed. And everything falls, showers of red and white paper roses, showers of cards, the heavy stone figures. Everything falls, and she is under, and the stone lion is under her.

She wakes.

XX

"Members of the jury," says the Clerk of the Court, "the prisoners at the bar, Bowers and Eden Limited, and Mr. Jude Mason, are charged that on the 13th day of March last, they published an obscene article, to wit, a book entitled *Babbletower: A Tale for the Children of Our Time.* To this indictment they have pleaded not guilty and it is your charge to say, having heard the evidence, whether they be guilty or not."

There is only one prisoner at the bar. He is wearing a charcoal-grey flannel suit, a white shirt, and a neatly knotted dull-crimson tie. His hair is a smooth skullcap of iron grey shot with silver; his face is gaunt, his eyes downcast. He has the look of someone released from confinement, a rehabilitated prisoner, a monk returned from contemplation to the "real" world. His clothes, precisely observed, fit very well; nevertheless, at first glance, they have a look of hanging on him, a suggestion of the clothes hanger, the scarecrow. His neck is thin and grey inside his collar. His bones have a mediaeval look, the cheekbones high and carved, the nose prominent, the eyes half-shut, a little sunk.

Frederica is in Court, with Daniel. She does not at first recognise the prisoner, although she has been part of the meeting which argued for his transformation, and indeed produced the argument that prevailed.

"It's only a *mask,* Jude, for God's sake. A court trial is a fiction, we play parts, it's a game of chess. You have to play the White Knight, you have to *look like* a respectable member of society, as the court will think one ought to look, that's what matters, you have to *look right,* it's part of it."

"It isn't a fiction. It's a truth. I am on trial and I am as I am. My appearance is a true statement of what I am."

"*I don't* know what your appearance states," said Duncan Raby, Jude's solicitor.

"You are not skilled in the semiotics of clothes," said Jude. "My coat is sky blue, the colour of truth, and it is the dress at once of the Enlightenment philosophers and the licentious beaux of the courts. My coat is sullied, as truth is sullied. My hair is nature, untended. As is my skin."

"That's nice to know," said Raby. "But it won't cut any ice with Mr. Justice Gordale Balafray and it's a tactical disaster."

"Come on, Jude," said Frederica. "You must wear the mask appropriate to the rite you find yourself in. You must play their game. You must look respectable. Hair grows and a coat can be put in a cupboard. You expose your naked body happily enough for gain—"

"That is also a form of integrity."

"Do you want to win this case?" cried Rupert Parrott. *"Or not?"*

But Frederica is shocked to see the prisoner at the bar. He does have a look, she thinks, of the virtue having gone out of him. He looks ill.

The jury sits in its box. There was some discussion, before it was empanelled, about whether it should be an all-male jury, as used to be customary in obscenity cases. The judge declared himself possibly in favour of such a jury: both Counsel for the Prosecution and Counsel for the Defence were agreed that there was no necessity for such a ruling in their view, and that the presence of one or more women on the jury would make it more representative of the public opinion, the community at large of right-thinking persons, which is represented. As a result there are three women on the jury, none of them young, one the owner of a beauty salon and a widow, one a retired physical training instructor from the Women's Royal Navy, and one a housewife. The men are all middle-aged except one, a swarthy young man in a leather jacket who owns a gramophone record shop. There are a bank manager, an accountant, a swimming-pool manager, a technical college lecturer (in physics), an electrician, a restaurant owner, a tailor and a teacher from a comprehensive school. Most of them read the oath with no stumbling; the tailor is Jewish, wears a skull cap, and swears by the Old Testament.

Some procedural discussion takes place. It is agreed that, following the precedent of the *Lady Chatterley* trial in 1960, the jury shall hear the speeches both for the Prosecution and for the Defence before they retire to read the book itself: this provision was then made because it was felt to be unjust that they should read it having heard only one side, with the Prosecution's comments sharp in their minds. Mr. Justice Gordale Balafray is a very large man, long-faced, darkly handsome under his white wig, which therefore shines whiter. He has a reputation for fairness both to barristers and to witnesses. He has a reputation for liking the arts, too.

It is also agreed, that since the witnesses both for the Prosecution and for the Defence are "expert witnesses," they have the right to remain in the Court during the trial and not be excluded.

Sir Augustine Weighall, QC, begins his case.

"If Your Lordship pleases. Members of the jury, I appear with my learned friend Mr. Benedict Scaling to prosecute in this case. The defendant company, Bowers and Eden Ltd., is represented by my learned friends Mr. Godfrey Hefferson-Brough and Mr. Peregrine Swift; the defendant Mr. Jude Mason is represented by Mr. Samuel Oliphant and Mr. Merlyn Wren."

Sir Augustine has a pleasant, aquiline face, with a thin mouth shrewdly pursed when he is in repose. He has the gift of keeping still when he is speaking, looking attentively and considerately at the jury, meeting eye after eye, impartially, with concern. He speaks clearly, unemphatically, practically. He tells the jury that they are here to decide whether the book *Babbletower: A Tale for the Children of Our Time* is an obscene book within the meaning of the Obscene Publications Act, 1959. The word "obscene," he tells the jury, is defined by the *Oxford English Dictionary* as "offensive to modesty or decency; expressing or suggesting unchaste or lustful ideas; impure, indecent, lewd." It has other meanings, including "lack of perspicuity in language; uncertainty of meaning; unintelligibleness," and it is the case that the previous law against "obscene libel" did perhaps lack perspicuity, and was uncertain in its meaning. The 1959 Act elucidates the matter in Section 1(A)1, where it defines "obscenity" as follows:

"For the purposes of this Act an article shall be deemed to be obscene if its effect . . . is, taken as a whole, such as to tend to deprave and corrupt persons who are likely, in all circumstances, to read, see, or hear the matter contained or embodied in it."

"This elucidation provides other problems of perspicuity in language, meaning, and intelligibleness. You may think you need guidance on the precise force and meaning to attribute to the words 'deprave' and 'corrupt.' The same dictionary gives as the current sense of 'deprave': 'To make morally bad; to pervert, debase, or corrupt morally.' The definition of 'corrupt' is longer and more complex. The 1959 Act no doubt intends the third meaning of the verb as given: 'To render morally unsound or rotten; to destroy the moral purity or chastity of; to pervert or ruin (a good quality); to debase, defile.' "

In practice, Sir Augustine tells the jury, the phrase "deprave and corrupt" has been taken to mean "to cause to behave badly," to incite to actions which are contrary to the law, to ideas of decency or propriety which are generally current in the community. He gives precedents for this understanding. He goes on to quote Mr. Justice Stable, who exhorted a jury to "remember that the charge is a charge that the tendency of the book is to corrupt and deprave. The charge is not that the tendency of the book is either to shock or to disgust. That is not a criminal offence."

Counsel in past cases have rightly emphasised this, and have said to the jury, as he himself is now saying, that the fact that they find a book unpleasant, or shocking, or disgusting, is not in itself a reason to consider it "obscene." But he believes that the phrasing "*tend to* deprave and corrupt" does give the jury the right, and possibly the duty, to consider the effect of the book on the soul, if that word is permissible, on the state of mind and health of the spirit, of those who may read it, whether or not it may lead directly to action which is depraved, corrupted, or unlawful.

He tells the jury that they are the only judges of whether or not the book is obscene. Evidence will be led from expert witnesses, by both the Defence and the Prosecution, as to the nature of the work in question, and as to whether it has any literary or other merit. But the opinion of these witnesses will be relevant only as to the merits and demerits of the book, not as to the point of obscenity, on which their opinion should not be asked; if they offer opinions on whether the book is obscene, the jury should disregard them. The matter of obscenity, of whether the book tends to deprave and corrupt, is for the twelve men and women in the jury box, representing humane and civilised society and common sense, to decide.

When they have decided that, and only then, the question of the literary or other merits of the book may arise. Section 4(2) of the Obscene Publications Act entitles the defendant to an acquittal if the jury is satisfied that notwithstanding the obscenity of an article, its publication is justified as being for the public good in the interests of "science, literature, art or learning, or of other objects of general concern." The Defence have given notice that they intend to raise the Section 4(2) defence and prove it through the testimony of experts. They will argue that the book has literary merits and other important values—social, psychological—which justify its publication in the public interest. "You will make up your own minds as to that, on hearing their evidence. His Lordship has ruled that, exceptionally, the Defence witnesses should be heard first in this case, so that the Prosecution will know upon what grounds they defend the book before calling witnesses in rebuttal."

Sir Augustine tells the jury that Mr. Justice Byrne, in the case of *R.* v. *Penguin Books,* the *Lady Chatterley* trial, ruled that the prosecuting counsel should not read out passages of the book before the jury themselves had read the whole of the book. Mr. Gerald Gardiner, QC, in his objection on that occasion said, "I am not objecting to my learned friend putting before the jury the nature of the story, or the grounds on which the Prosecution contends it is obscene. . . . I submit the Prosecution are not entitled to try to prejudice the jury's mind as to particular passages before they have read the book as a whole."

Sir Augustine says that he will therefore summarise his case against the book at this point, and examine particular passages later. In the old days when books were tried for "obscene libel" and there was no defence of literary merit, or public interest, it was often sufficient for "purple passages" to be read out and to be found unacceptable, to secure a conviction. Here, it is the whole book which is on trial and must be judged, as to whether it tends to deprave and corrupt. Sir Augustine says he is very happy to accept this ruling, since, although *Babbletower* contains many very explicit descriptions of lewd actions, of explicit sex, of unnatural acts, and most gravely, detailed and superfluous descriptions of cruelty and torture, it is the tendency of the book itself that is in his view finally obscene, corrupt, that is, rotten, and depraved, that is, unnatural and degrading. He believes that the jury will find that such literary merit as it has—and he does not intend to deny that it has some—does not outweigh the unpleasantness, the perversity, of its actions and its conclusion.

"It has been said," says Sir Augustine, "that in the trial of D. H. Lawrence's *Lady Chatterley's Lover* it was Lady Chatterley herself who was on trial, for her adultery, for the fact of her sexuality. In the case of *Babbletower* it is the prisoner in the dock who is on trial, his imagination, the world he created, the tendency of the messages he offers. *Babbletower* is a book without hope. Its slender narrative turns on the decision of a group of people with vaguely French names to go and found a community in 'freedom'—'freedom' in this case meaning complete freedom of sexual expression, no matter how disgusting or perverted that expression may be. This 'freedom' degenerates into licence and into cruelty, madness and destruction. The tortures and humiliation—not only of grown men and women, but of little children—that follow, are described in lurid and superfluous detail. The word 'pornography' is derived from two Greek words, *porno,* a prostitute, and *graphein,* to write. It has been defined as writings about whorehouses and prostitution. It has also been defined as 'the writings of prostitutes.' You may think, when you have read *Babbletower,* that it is simply the product of a depraved and dirty imagination. You will be told, I am sure, by the Defence, that it is a very *moral* book, showing that licence leads to cruelty and repression. You will make up your own minds about this. You may come to the conclusion that the so-called 'moral story' is no more than a thread on which to hang writings that titillate, that exacerbate, the darker and nastier imaginations of men. You may be told the story is tragic and terrible; you may wish to retort that it completely lacks what Aristotle called *catharsis,* the purging of pity and terror. It is a book that begins, and remains, merely nasty and disturbing. In the opinion of the Prosecution, it arouses unpleasant, worse than unpleasant, feelings—it stirs up the worst instincts of men, where the sexual urge meets the urge to be cruel. You will hear psychological evidence from both sides about this matter. I will say no more now.

"*Lady Chatterley's Lover,* ladies and gentlemen, was felt to be an offence to public decency because it described sexual acts explicitly, and because it used four-lettered words which are felt to be part of a vocabulary proscribed by our society as a whole. It was mixed up with feelings about class and the nature of marriage. Many eminent witnesses argued that it was tender—"

Mr. Hefferson-Brough objects. Comparisons as to obscenity between one book and another are not admissible.

The judge says they are admissible if the point in question is one of literary merit, and not simply of comparative obscenity.

Sir Augustine says that in practice this is a very fine tightrope to tread. He says that he wished merely to observe that the kind of problem raised by *Babbletower* was different from the problems of love, marriage and language raised by *Lady Chatterley,* who was acquitted. It was a problem of cruelty and perversion. He will move on to his next point, which is one concerning the possible or probable readers of the text. The Act speaks of "persons who are likely, in all the circumstances to read, see or hear the matter contained or embodied in it."

He reminds the Court that the country has just lived through the trial of the Moors Murderers. He asks the jury, when they listen to the arguments that they will undoubtedly hear about literature, about fiction, not inciting readers in general to bad acts, to remember the library of Ian Brady, to remember Myra Hindley's participation—learned from Brady, who learned it from books, at least in part—in acts derived imaginatively from books, from *The Scourge of the Swastika* and from the Marquis de Sade. Myra Hindley was possibly a normal young woman before this relationship. The works of the Marquis de Sade are certainly in Mr. Jude Mason's library. His *Babbletower,* his isolated "Tour Bruyarde," is plagiarised from the terrible Marquis's Château de Silling in *The 120 Days of Sodom.* "Do not think, ever, ladies and gentlemen, 'Well, it is only a book.' Men and women are greatly moved by books, their lives may be enriched, changed, or ruined by books. Dictators seize and burn books, because books are dangerous. That fact too will be advanced, no doubt, as a reason for not condemning *Babbletower.* But they are right, the dictators. Good books are dangerous to bad men, and by the same token, bad books are dangerous to good men."

Godfrey Hefferson-Brough rises to open the case for the defence of Bowers and Eden. He is a fleshy man, a red man, a hairy man under his false hair. He is not humorous, he is not beguiling, he has a tendency to thunder. He appears throughout the proceedings to be a prosecuting counsel who has strayed into the realm of defence, and is happiest attacking the opposition. Augustine Weighall's style is sweetly reasonable and understated: Hefferson-Brough would like to make rhetorical flights. It is significant that he, like Martin Fisher, the Bowers and Eden solicitor, is an "Erstwhile Hog," which is the arcane term for an Old Swineburnian. Rupert Parrott, too, as we have seen, is an Erstwhile Hog.

He speaks a panegyric about Bowers and Eden. They are an old firm, a respectable firm, dating back to the old days of John Murray, John Blackwell, and George Smith. A specialist firm, whose field has always been religion, theology, social thought, with a lighter section of belles lettres and fiction, fiction appropriate to the *gravitas* of the house, not salacious fiction, not avant-garde fiction, not shockers and penny dreadfuls. A few donnish detective stories, with perhaps an inquisitive vicar, or vicar's lady, as the sleuth, a few novels lately like Mrs. Phyllis Pratt's excellent *Daily Bread* about the daily lives of the clergy. Mr. Rupert Parrott, the recently appointed managing director of this small firm, is young, but old for his years, a churchgoing Christian, a happily married husband and father, the dynamic successor to a perhaps dozy, perhaps out-of-touch board of directors. He has tried to expand his list to include burning concerns of the moment, things nowadays hotly debated, new strains of theology, works on the Holocaust and its causes, works on the Samaritans, on new forms of social help for the despairing, works also on psychoanalysis and psychiatry, on sociology and philosophy, on the pros and cons of new things like psychedelics and pop music, serious analyses of these things, up-to-date and responsible.

Babbletower and its author came to Mr. Parrott's attention through a literary friend who read for him, and whose judgement he trusted. He saw immediately that it was a controversial book, a book that would arouse strong feelings, a book that was strong meat, yes, very strong meat for readers to digest. But he formed the view—"and it is a view I believe you will share, ladies and gentlemen, when you have read the book"—that it was a powerful and original work, a satirical work about the follies of utopian projectors, and about sexual optimists who believe anything goes and all is permitted. He formed the view that it was—despite its frankness, its full-blooded depiction of the consequences of folly and wrong thinking—he formed the view that it was an *intensely moral* work, a work attacking just those aspects of our society which the 1959 Obscene Publications Act is itself designed to attack, the vacuously pornographic, the licentious, the depraved and the corrupt. For the depraved and the corrupt in *Babbletower,* as you will see, ladies and gentlemen, receive short shrift, they meet a terrible reckoning. This is a book designed to bring home to you the disgusting nature of the world of the depraved and the corrupt in our own society—in all societies—and if you are disgusted, the book has worked its work, for it is not designed to give you a warm and comfortable glow of pleasure. No, it is designed to warn, to alarm, to *avert.* There are episodes, there are tendencies in our society which it is needful for wise men to know about, shun, and do away with, and it is the knowledge of these tendencies—and a righteous horror—that *Babbletower* promulgates.

Hefferson-Brough, like Sir Augustine, discourses on the meaning of "tend to deprave and corrupt." The Act, he says, was designed to stop pornography, the filth dirty old men use to masturbate with, the slime oozing from the gutters of brothels, the puerile jokes about torture which we all know, and which the author and publisher of this book abominate as much as you do, ladies and gentlemen. The Act was not designed to stop works of literature—even *daring* works of literature that take a fearless look at a real social problem, the decay of social and sexual controls that leads precisely to a flood of true pornography, trivial, rotten and rotting to the fibres of our community. The Act was designed to make it possible for works of literature to be published in freedom and without fear of prurient attacks. We shall lead evidence to show that there is overwhelming support for the literary, psychological and social importance of *Babbletower.* Bad books do hurt good men, as my learned friend wisely said. But good works hurt nothing but bad books.

"As good almost kill a man as kill a good book; who kills a man kills a reasonable creature, God's image; but he who destroys a good book, kills reason itself, kills the image of God, as it were in the eye."

Frederica wonders if this quotation is not excessive. She looks at the jury to see how many of them react to *Areopagitica*; one man frowns with recognition, one woman gives a beatific smile of assent and nods; most others stare, puzzled and stolid, into space.

Samuel Oliphant, QC, then speaks on behalf of Jude Mason. He says that his client is a young man, an artist, who lives in poverty in order to practise his art. He is not a pornographer, and in his view *Babbletower* is a complex work of art, the subject of which is the relation between erotic freedom and community, between repression and cruelty. His work is, and will be shown to be, in a great European tradition of satirical flouting, of moral outrage working *through* the outrageous. In cases where a work of art is being prosecuted as an obscene publication, it has been held—he cites precedents—that the *intentions* of the author or publisher are irrelevant to the jury's decision as to whether the book is obscene. In other cases—he cites other precedents—it has been held that in the case of literary merit, intention can and must be discussed. "In the *Lady Chatterley* trial, D. H. Lawrence's intentions invariably and inevitably came into the evidence and the debate. It was suggested by many Defence witnesses that Lawrence was a Puritan. He had written a frank book about sex, but his intentions were puritanical. The same, ladies and gentlemen, could be argued of my client. One of his characters—perhaps the only wholly sympathetic character in the whole tale of excess and punishment—is a figure with the strange name of Samson Origen, who preaches abstemiousness, indeed abstention from all activity, a kind of asceticism. Strange though it may appear, in a book so full of plain-speaking sexual descriptions and even orgiastic behaviour, the ruling atmosphere is one of asceticism and abstemiousness. There is a certain humour, a certain irony, in Mr. Mason's work, which is on the side of Samson Origen. It would be possible to miss this humour, this irony, particularly when you are reading with an eye to looking for depravation and corruption: I therefore bring it to your attention as perhaps the saving grace of this sorry tale. Mr. Mason's intentions are to mock folly, and worse than folly, through exposing and depicting it mercilessly. This is an art as old as time, and as honourable as any other."

During these speeches, Frederica is aware of a strange whirring and clicking coming from behind, or under her seat. As the judge says, "The next question, is it not, is to arrange for the reading of the book?" she turns, and sees the gingery hairy face of Avram Snitkin behind her, bright blue eyes peering between sandy lashes.

Mr. Justice Gordale Balafray asks what arrangements can be made for the jury to read *Babbletower.* How long should be set aside? Where should the reading take place?

Frederica whispers, "Are you recording this on your tape-recorder?"

"Of course."

"Is it allowed?"

"I've got permission from the Court. I didn't say it was ethnomethodological research. I said it was for the publisher's records. I'm baffled they don't use it for the official records but they don't—there's their shorthand writer, over there, with a *pen*. But they don't mind me making a recording; they say that's fine."

She hears the snake of tape rustle on its reels, digesting the words.

The barristers and the judge discuss the reading. Samuel Oliphant says that the book could be taken home and read in quiet domestic surroundings, at a reasonable speed. Hefferson-Brough says that for *Lady Chatterley* a special room was found at the Old Bailey, with armchairs. Juries have been known to retire to hotels. The jury foreman reports that the chairs in the jury room are hard. The judge seems decided by this last complaint; he retorts that they are the chairs in the jury room, where the jurors are doing the work they have been called to do. We have all sat on hard chairs, in our time, says he, in schools, in libraries, and been none the worse for it. Indeed, he himself finds himself more alert, sitting on a good solid hard chair, than sunk on cushions. No, the jury-room chairs must suffice, will suffice.

The jury set off to read the book at two-fifteen. The Court waits. Elvet Gander says to Adelbert Holly and Avram Snitkin that perhaps the judge is a person with sadistic inclinations. That could, of course, go either way, for or against *Babbletower.* Frederica thinks of going to speak to Jude, but he has disappeared, apparently into the belly of the Old Bailey. Rupert Parrott repeats several times that the Counsel for the Prosecution is formidable. Parrott's face is pink and shining. He is wearing a peacock-blue waistcoat under a fine blue-grey worsted suit.

At four-fifteen the judge sends to enquire of the jury how much longer they will need to read the book. Three or four claim to have finished it already. The foreman—the swimming-pool manager—says that he has been asked to request a dictionary—a *large* dictionary, my lord, and also, if it's not too much trouble, a *French* dictionary, as well as the English one, that is. Several more jurymen say they will soon be through. Hefferson-Brough asks that the jury be told to read the book carefully and thoroughly, or alternatively be dismissed and replaced. The jury returns to its room and its hard chairs, and its copies of *Babbletower* with the black, pink and cobalt covers. Twelve men and women, twelve readings, or skimmings, or stumblings, or approximate scannings. One woman takes the book home to bed, reaches the death of Roseace, and wakes her husband, gagging. This is later known, because her husband is "in the Print," a member of a print trade union, and tells a journalist on the *News of the World,* who prints this information when the trial is over.

The Court reassembles the next day. The first witness for the Defence is called. He says he is Alexander Wedderburn. His profession, he says, is that of a playwright. He is a member of the Steerforth Committee Enquiry into the teaching of the English language. He has worked in cultural radio—the Third Programme—and educational television. He has been a schoolmaster in a boys' boarding school. His plays are set texts at O Level. He is described in the Press as "a very handsome public figure, wearing a well-cut corduroy suit in a dark green, with a lemon-coloured shirt and a blue tie with green carnations on it. He has a mane of silvering hair, a pleasant tenor voice, and an expression of cautious courtesy and helpfulness which never failed, even under pressure."

His evidence lasts three hours, and is solid and, on the surface, calm. Hefferson-Brough takes him through the text of *Babbletower,* reading out long passages—mostly not sexual, and none of them cruel—asking him if he feels these passages have literary merit as pieces of English prose, if he thinks the characterisation is subtle, if he thinks the content is serious. Alexander says that *Babbletower* is not part of a genre that requires subtle characterisation. Hefferson-Brough asks him to explain "genre" to those members of the jury "who do not know any technical literary terms." He reminds his witness "not to be technical if you can help it." Alexander says that the point about the characters in *Babbletower* is that they are *types,* like the characters in an allegory, or a satire, or a comedy of manners. They don't need depth. Their actions are what is important. He is asked to explain "allegory," "satire," "comedy of manners." He is asked to say that to say that characters are "types" is not to say that they are vulgar or crude. He replies, "Of course not," and hears a ripple of laughter, laughter against either him or Hefferson-Brough, with whom he is meant to be agreeing. They *represent qualities,* says Alexander. Good qualities? Not necessarily. Many qualities. As in life.

The trial is to be characterised by Hefferson-Brough's paucity of vocabulary for discussing literary merit. Alexander thinks at first that this is due to an excessive concern for the jury's sensibilities as common readers, or "ordinary men and women," whatever those are. But his experience of Hefferson-Brough's questions, which is very similar to that of the specifically *literary* experts who follow him, is of struggling through a suffocating cloud of wool, trying to find air, trying to find light, trying to make a precise sentence and being told again and again that his vocabulary—his expert vocabulary—is inadmissible in this place, must be rephrased. Scrupulously Alexander tries to say that one passage is more successful than another, that one scene is almost tragic whereas another is merely blackly comic, Grand Guignol. "And what do you mean by Grand Guignol, Mr. Wedderburn? Tell us in

English, please, tell us what that is, so we may share your thought." And of the scenes that Alexander says are "less good than others," Hefferson-Brough immediately asks, "But would you say that this scene is well-written? Does it have literary merit? Is it good, or is it not?" And Alexander says again and again, because he must, that it is good. *Babbletower* is flattened in his hearers' minds to a series of "good" passages.

In answer to Samuel Oliphant he reiterates that *Babbletower* is a serious work, by a promising young writer, with a moral purpose.

Sir Augustine Weighall then cross-examines.

Q. Mr. Wedderburn. You are a man of very wide reading, a man whose life has been devoted to great writing. Your own verse drama gives me intense pleasure, I may say, on the page as on the stage. I do not flatter: I am glad to take this opportunity of speaking of your "lovely inchanting language." I want to ask you a simple question. Did you *enjoy* reading *Babbletower*?

A. Enjoy? Yes, and no.

Q. Let us discuss both halves of that entirely comprehensible answer. Let us start with the "yes." *What* did you enjoy?

A. Vivid descriptions. The successful depiction of a world part fairytale, part dystopia.

Q. Dystopia?

A. Anti-utopia. Depiction of a not-ideal world. Good writing. The sentences are lively. The atmosphere is brooding.

Q. Did the book—I know you will answer clearly, for you are a thoughtful man and a writer yourself—did the book give you any *sexual* pleasure?

A. (After some thought) Some, occasionally. Not much. All writing is connected with sexual pleasure. Wordsworth said the rhythms of language are the rhythms of the human body, of "the grand principle of pleasure in which we live and move and have our being."

Q. That is very interesting. The rhythms of all writing are in your view connected to sexual pleasure. That is indeed very interesting and illuminating. Did the book give you any more specific sexual pleasure—such as you might feel looking at an erotic painting, for instance?

A. Not much.

Q. Yet you said it was well written, and "vivid," you said, and "lively." A very large proportion of this book is descriptions of sexual acts, of naked bodies. Yet they gave you no pleasure?

A. Not much.

Q. Are you perhaps denying the pleasure, out of a desire to defend the book?

A. I don't think so. I think the author meant me to experience only a limited pleasure. Meant me to imagine pleasure, and then to find he had cut it off, so to speak.

Q. He tried to disgust you?

A. That is the *unpleasant* side. He had good reasons.

Q. He may well have had. So, in so far as you responded sexually to his writing, it was with disgust?

A. It is more complex than that.

Q. More complex. Perhaps the writing was meant to have an *emetic* effect, to disgust you with the world and action of the book?

A. It is more complex than that, too.

Q. It seems to be very complex. The only certain thing is that you are resolute to deny that he meant you to experience any pleasure in the infliction of pain, any reprehensible pleasure in the infliction of pain?

A. I did not say that.

Q. And you do not think that?

A. You have me in a grammatical snarl.

Q. But you know what I am asking?

A. I do not think that the intention of the author was to make me feel reprehensible pleasure in the infliction of pain.

Q. And you did not feel any?

A. No. Or almost none.

Q. You are a man who has to be truthful, I see, Mr. Wedderburn. Not none. *Almost* none.

Tell me, as to the question of literary merit. *How good* do you think *Babbletower* is, in literary terms? We are not allowed to compare books as to relative obscenity, but we are allowed to make comparisons of *literary merit.* D. H. Lawrence, when *Lady Chatterley* was tried, was taught in many university courses, throughout the world, as was abundantly testified. My learned friend Gerald Gardiner, on that occasion, made the point that some of the early works of Chaucer might be thought to be risqué without that great name attached to them. Tell me, Mr. Wedderburn—as a teacher, as a writer—*how good* is Mr. Jude Mason? As good as D. H. Lawrence? As good as William Burroughs? As good as Mickey Spillane?

A. It is his first book. It is a serious literary book. It is not a shocker, like Mickey Spillane, who is unreadable, in my view. It is well written and seriously meant. You can't really come to any conclusions about the final status of living writers at the outset of their careers.

Q. You can't really come to any conclusions about the literary merit of young living writers at the outset of their careers?

A. I said "final status."

Q. But judgements of literary merit are *provisional* in this kind of case, as opposed to that of D. H. Lawrence.

Samuel Oliphant objects. The judge overrules him. Alexander says they are of course provisional, compared to D. H. Lawrence, but that does not mean they cannot be made.

The next witness to be called is Dr. Naomi Lurie, Reader in English Literature in Oxford University, and a Fellow of Somerville College. She says that she is the author of various books, including *Dissociated Sensibility, Myth or History?* (1960). She says she is in charge of the studies of many young women, and would be quite happy for them to read *Babbletower.* She would, she says when pressed, encourage them to do so. No, she would not positively *teach* the book. She is opposed to the teaching of contemporary writing; Oxford University until very recently taught *nothing* written later than 1830.

She is a dark-haired woman in serviceable tweed, in her mid-fifties. Hefferson-Brough says to her, "You are a maiden lady, living in an exclusively female college, and you write on devotional poetry. But you admire this book, you have said, you have said you believe it has literary merit?"

Dr. Lurie says, "I am certainly unmarried, and I certainly teach women. I don't believe women make any different literary judgements from men."

There is a ripple of laughter in the Court. Dr. Lurie smiles primly.

Sir Augustine tempts Dr. Lurie into the statement that Swift's *Modest Proposal* for solving the Irish problem by roasting and stewing the infant Irish is shocking in the same way as *Babbletower.* "Or worse." He asks Dr. Lurie if Swift makes the prospective taste, "the culinary delights," of the broiled babies attractive. No, says Dr. Lurie. And the loathsome practices in *Babbletower,* the sodomy, the torture, the orgies, says Sir Augustine. "They are unattractive in the same way?"

"I think so," says Dr. Lurie. Sir Augustine's fine face takes on an ironic smile, which he turns on the jury.

"You find the descriptions of Narcisse's juvenile peccadilloes, of Damian's love-making with Roseace, as repugnant as Swift's broiled babies?"

"I do not say that. Swift is a pure satirist. He writes with *saeva indignatio.*"

"Savage indignation," Sir Augustine translates kindly for the jury.

"Whereas it is part of Mr. Mason's plan to, so to speak, put the reader through the pleasures of the *Babbletower.*"

"To *put the reader through*. Not to stir, not to titillate, not to seduce? Your verb is austere and pedagogic."

"He does wish to titillate, at the time, of course. But temporarily."

"He turns titillation on and off, like a tap."

"If you like," says Dr. Lurie.

Anthony Burgess is the next witness. His face is craggy; his voice is round and beautifully produced. He praises *Babbletower* in musical terms: *brio, appassionata, fugue.* He says in answer to Hefferson-Brough that he believes that *Babbletower* is a deeply moral, almost too moral, book.

Q. How can a book be too moral, Mr. Burgess?

A. Well, as I have said before from time to time, the value of art is always diminished by the presence of elements that move to action. This book is didactic. The didactic is lesser than the purely aesthetic. It has *designs on you.* Never trust a book that has designs on you.

Q. *Babbletower* has moral designs on you?

A. Yes. It moves by disgusting and frightening you.

Q. But it is a work of literature.

A. I don't know what you mean by "but." It *is* a work of literature. It is a very promising, serious piece of writing. It ought to be praised. It isn't *Ulysses* or *The Rainbow* but it ought to be read, it ought to be discussed.

Sir Augustine rises to cross-examine. He measures the novelist with his eye.

Q. You quoted yourself just now. You said that the book was a lesser art-form than the purely aesthetic because it had designs on you, it moved to action.

A. It is didactic, yes.

Q. In your review—your very perceptive and brilliant review of the book—you do not only say that the book moves to action because it is *didactic.* You associate the didactic and the pornographic as "moving to action." You associate them *in this book.*

A. That is so. You have understood the review.

Q. So the book is pornographic as well as didactic.

A. It is not high art, in which everything is resolved in a balance, a form that can be contemplated with aesthetic pleasure. It is a mixed form, a hybrid form, which makes its effect by moving to action. That does not mean it is not a work of art, or that it should not be published. We can't suppress every book that isn't as good as *Ulysses*. Or *The Rainbow*.

Judge. Indeed not. I must remind the jury that the opinion of literary experts on whether or not the book is obscene should not be taken into account.

Q. Mr. Burgess, I am going to ask you, as I have asked others, whether the book gave you any sexual pleasure? Moved you sexually?

A. Oh yes. It did. It's a good book, it does its work. It stirs you up. Most good books do. Reading and sexual excitement are intimately connected.

Q. Except in *Ulysses*?

A. In *Ulysses* of course, too. That's an unworthy question. But differently.

Q. Differently?

A. It's rawer, here. In *Babbletower*.

Q. Mr. Burgess, you are a writer. A daring writer, you take risks. When you write about sexual excitement, or even more, about cruelty, do you imagine your reader as you write?

A. Yes.

Q. How do you imagine him or her?

A. As like myself. Excited when I am. Detached as I am.

Q. Do you imagine the effects of your writings on the less educated, the more imaginatively restricted persons who may also read your books?

A. That is harder. It would be silly to pretend everyone reads in the same way. It would be silly to pretend one could gauge the effect of a piece of writing on all its potential readers.

Q. Do you feel responsible for the weak, the uninstructed, the excitable readers of your books?

A. You can't be, wholly, responsible for all readers. But up to a point, yes, I do. And, in answer to your unspoken hint or question, I am quite sure that Jude Mason is not trying to *work up* ignorant readers into a state of irresponsible excitement. But you can't predict that that will never happen.

Q. You can't predict that that will never happen.

The next witness is a novelist too, who is also lead reviewer for a serious Sunday newspaper. He is a dapper, pretty man called Douglas Corbie; he is little, with a melodious but insistent voice, and time is beginning to etch nutcracker lines in his cheeks. His hair is the cream colour of metallic blond hair going white. He has written many thick and well-received novels—*A Pernicious Influence, Hengist's Horse, The Voice of the Mock Turtle, Life in a Glass House*—and has sat on the committee of the Society of Authors and the Literature Panel of the Arts Council. He is examined by Samuel Oliphant. Douglas Corbie agrees that he is himself a novelist of some importance, that he is a leading critic, that he has read *Babbletower,* and admires it.

Q. It is a serious work of literature, in your opinion.

A. Without any doubt. The young man is extremely promising. He has much to learn but he is extremely promising. He should be encouraged; young writers should be encouraged, as I know to my cost, having found the going hard.

Q. Can you say why it is a serious work of literature?

A. Oh yes. Because it treats of evil. We don't consider evil, in our society, you know. We are English and *ever so nice* and we are obsessed with problems of right and wrong *manners,* with little details of social correctness, yes, with silly things like fish-forks and *placements,* and whether people have the right *accent,* or whether their shoes are or aren't nasty. And this in the time of Auschwitz and Hiroshima, so shaming in many ways, all our fuss about flowerbeds and whether white flowers ought to be in herbaceous borders, or whether they are vulgar, you know?

Q. But does Jude Mason tackle the problem of evil?

A. Oh, well, yes, he does, *indeed he does,* and with gusto, with such gusto almost *too* enthusiastically, all those Gothic chains and dungeons, a bit bathetic, in a way, but very effective, very effective, no doubt. William Golding has treated evil. *Lord of the Flies,* a book about the evil of schoolboys let loose, very revealing. Mr. Mason's dormitory life in *Babbletower* is the evil of schoolboys let loose too, a Grand Guignol version. *I myself* prefer to embed my depiction of evil in the day-to-day, in drawing-rooms and theatre bars and suburban kitchens and school staffrooms, I prefer to embed it in *felt life,* as James said, yes, to notice the social detail. As Auden said, "A crack in the teacup opens / A lane to the land of the dead." Teacups will suffice, though Mr. Mason appears to think not, he chooses the full panoply, beatings and hangings, a more *dangerous* way, difficult to bring off—he *does* bring it off, very largely, of course—but *I myself* believe the study of evil is more effectively embedded in *felt life.* The people at Auschwitz, you know, the torturers, they went home at night to suburban kitchens and pink lampshades and knuckles of pork, all that stuff, you can do it through lampshades and pork, you don't need . . .

Q. What do you say of Mr. Mason's book? Is it serious? Is it good?

A. Oh yes, as I said, he's good, he's learning, he will be very good, it's important to let him keep trying, very important. Yes.

Sir Augustine says, "No questions, my lord."

The next witness is Professor Marie-France Smith, from Prince Albert College. She wears an elegant suit, in fine black wool piped in white.

Hefferson-Brough is gallant with this witness, who is both lovely and fragile. His gallantry rattles Professor Smith, who is trying to produce a dry, scholarly account of what she believes to be the intellectual background of *Babbletower.* Hefferson-Brough takes her through her *Encounter* review of *Babbletower* step by step.

Q. You say in this article, Professor Smith, that this book which the ladies and gentlemen of the jury have just read is "in the mainstream tradition of European intellectual history and philosophical debate." That is a large claim.

A. I could prove critically, I think, that the author has a very wide acquaintance with French thought, with French controversy, at the time of the Revolution and later, about how far human beings should be free and how far it was necessary for them to be restrained.

Q. You mention the names of certain thinkers in your review. A certain Charles Fourier, for example. Can you tell us about his thought, and about how it is to be found in this book?

A. Fourier was a gentle and eccentric thinker who like many thinkers at the end of the eighteenth and the beginning of the nineteenth centuries believed that a revolution in human feelings and lifestyles could introduce an age of Harmony. He believed "civilisation" (the last few centuries) was evil, repressive and decadent. He believed human harmony could be achieved by indulging all human passions and desires, of which he identified, I think, 810. He believed "civilised," decadent men thought all human beings were roughly the same, but that in fact they differed greatly. He felt that lesbians, sodomites, flagellants, fetishists, nymphomaniacs and so on could and should be accommodated rather than punished. He wrote a *Nouveau Monde Amoureux* which depicts the journey of a group of colonists to Cnidus in Asia Minor, where they found a community, a *phalanx* of erotic freedom. They organise sexual orgies, and also gastronomic orgies—Fourier saw warfare, in Harmony, as a civilised contest between chefs as to the making of little pastries, of which he was very fond. He liked inventing hierarchies—he had a court of love with high priests, pontiffs, matrons, confessors, fakirs, fairies, bacchantes . . .

Q. And all this, you say, was very gentle?

A. Oh, wholly, yes. It was like Watteau's *Embarkation for Cytherea,* a dream world with a serious political imagination behind it. Fourier *really believed* that the Terror in the French Revolution might, pushed a little further, have ushered in one desirable further breaking down of rules and conventions—the abolition of marriage, which made almost everyone, in his view, unhappy. "In Harmony," he wrote, "every mature man and woman must be granted a satisfying minimum of sexual pleasure."

Q. And you see *Babbletower* as in that tradition?

A. The first part, yes. The characters are setting off to found a Nouveau Monde Amoureux, a New World of Love. What happens owes as much to de Sade as to Fourier.

Q. Tell us about de Sade. You take him seriously as a thinker?

A. You must. He is important. He represents the line from the Enlightenment philosophers who extol human reason and free will, in its cynical vein. He asks, If we are free to follow our passions, who can prevent us from following our desire to hurt others, to kill, to rape, to torture? Those are, he says, human passions; they are *natural*. Voltaire, Rousseau, Diderot, the freethinkers, lead, according to one view, to the guillotine and the Sadeian *boudoir.* Mr. Mason has understood this. He has shown it.

The prisoner looks at his hands. He does not look at Professor Smith. Some of the jury notice this.

Q. What is your evidence for this diagnosis?

A. Well, let us start with the title. *La Tour Bruyarde* translates as the noisy, or shouting, or howling tower—the word "bruyard" suggests the noise made by hound dogs. It is an image of the Tower of Babel, which was constructed to displace God from Heaven, and was punished for its presumption by having a spirit of discord sent amongst its members, so that their languages were confused, they could no longer understand each other. It is a communal enterprise, set against the Authority of God. The *Babbletower* community is Fourier's Nouveau Monde Amoureux. It is also Sade's Château de Silling, where the libertines cut the bridge that connects them to the outer world so as to perform their terrible deeds.

Hefferson-Brough thanks Professor Smith for her clear exposition of the *gravitas* of *Babbletower.* He sits down. The prosecutor rises.

Q. Thank you for your charming lecture, Professor Smith. You have painted a very convincing picture of a very French intellectual document, a philosophical dialogue called *La Tour Bruyarde.* These books you speak of, de Sade, Fourier, they are in print in France?

A. Yes.

Q. Freely available?

A. Yes. Not all of Fourier. Much was never edited, the manuscripts are in the Bibliothèque Nationale.

Q. These preoccupations are very *French* preoccupations, are they not? Your country has always given more latitude to sexual freedom?

A. In some ways.

Q. English people have had to go to France and buy books thought unsuitable for English readers, to see the Folies Bergères, and so on. Some people think it is a good thing to have these latitudes. Some believe that our greater care for our own public morals, our greater concern for restraint of the things M. Fourier was so anxious to promulgate, has something to be said for it. Those who drafted the British Act of Parliament according to which this case is being tried might have been of the second party, you may think.

Samuel Oliphant rises to object that this is a statement, not a question.

Q. Tell me, Professor Smith—you have spoken with such cool clarity, such French analytic vigour, both of de Sade and of *Babbletower.* You do not, if I may say so, *seem* like a natural devoted reader of the lucubrations of the satanic Marquis. Do you *enjoy* de Sade?

A. Enjoy? No, I do not. (This is clearly a true statement of revulsion.)

Q. But you read him because you think you should?

A. Yes. As I said, he is important. I prefer Fourier.

Q. The gentle, the dotty, the permissive Fourier. The verbal Watteau of fairies and flagellants. And *Babbletower,* Professor Smith. Did you *enjoy* Babbletower?

A. No. I admired it.

Q. But the author would have liked you to enjoy it?

Both the beautiful professor and the prisoner at the bar cast down their eyes, flushed.

A. We are taught, these days, that authorial intention is something we cannot know, and is irrelevant to our critical judgement.

Q. And—forgive me—you felt no *frisson* of sexual pleasure during your reading?

A. (Very flushed) I may have. I do not remember. It was neither my primary nor my predominant response.

Q. Thank you, Professor Smith.

The next witness is a theatrical director, Fausto Gemelli, who has worked with Peter Brook and Charles Marowitz, who speaks with enthusiasm of Edward Bond's *Saved,* which presents the murder of a baby in a pram as an acting out of Blake's "sooner murder an infant in its cradle than arouse unacted desires." He speaks of Genet's *Maids* and *Balcony,* of Artaud's Theatre of Cruelty, which aims to be, in Artaud's words, "like victims burned at the stake, signalling through the flames." Samuel Oliphant asks him if, in the time of Genet, Bond, Artaud, the *Marat-Sade* and Peter Brook's *Lear,* he finds anything culturally out of bounds in *Babbletower.* He replies that he does not. He is passionately enthusiastic, gesturing, crying from a cloud of long black hair. Sir Augustine says, "No questions," judging perhaps that Mr. Gemelli speaks to his own audience and alienates others in about equal proportions.

The trial is now in its third day. The Defence calls Elvet Gander, who says he is a medical doctor, a psychiatrist, and a psychoanalyst. He agrees that he works with schizophrenics, with disturbed adolescents, and that he writes general books on language and society, on the psychic health and sickness of the community in which he lives. He agrees that he is the author of *Language Our Straitjacket, The Oppressor's Tongue, Am I My Brother's Keeper?,* and that he has a particular interest in the links between language and repression ("and *expression,* of course," he adds).

Elvet Gander in the witness box has a hardness and polished look. His skull shines, his nose shines, his long teeth shine brightly. His eyes are huge, sculpted and hooded; he speaks, as he gives his evidence, in an increasingly incantatory flow, even, towards the end, swaying slightly like a snake-charmer, and tapping gently with his hand on the ledge of the box. He wears a crumpled corduroy jacket—black—over an off-white polo-necked jumper and cord trousers. Frederica sees him, fancifully, as polished ivory, polished creamy marble. Hefferson-Brough asks him a series of questions designed to establish that he believes *Babbletower* to be important as a depiction of *private psychic disintegration* and of a more important malaise in society at large.

Gander speaks at length, plangently, musically, weaving his audience briefly into an assenting union, although afterwards many, most of them, cannot remember all he said, cannot, some of them, remember almost anything. He says human beings are divided creatures, more and more divided, more and more cut off from each other and from any sense of themselves and their identity. He says that *Babbletower* reflects both dividedness and a deep desire for unity of self and of community, as indeed does the original myth of the Tower of Babel. He says that human beings experience themselves as projections of other people's ideas (primarily their families'), or of their own fears and hidden wishes. He says that we live in a world where we are labelled, judged and punished as criminal, madman, pervert, sadist, when other words might apply as well, or better: desperate, affectionate, logical, confused. Language destroys us as language creates us—Lady Chatterley was condemned for honest no-nonsense four-letter *words* describing bodily functions we have erected a whole cage of euphemisms and evasions to avoid naming, so dividing ourselves from ourselves. There are physical ailments—Tourette's disease—where the body, the nerves, involuntarily ejaculate the unspeakable, "fuck," "shit," "piss." He does not apologise to the Court for the use of these words. They are nocturnal emissions of the human corpus, to be wiped away like stains, like the *ejaculations* they are in truth. Yes, we muck about with the language of our bodily selves at our peril, and Jude Mason has shown us the consequences, the leather tongues and steel tools we make when we are forbidden to use tongues and tools.

Godfrey Hefferson-Brough, faint but pursuing, tries both to stem the flow and to concentrate his witness's attention on "the book in hand, so to speak." This coincides with Gander's intent and rapturous comparison of dialogue to coition and masturbation to interior monologue. "There is evidence that the sexual discharge in male onanism is greater than it is in intercourse."

"Is this relevant?" asks Mr. Justice Gordale Balafray. "How does this connect to the matter in hand, to the question of the subject-matter of this book?"

"I am saying it is onanistic babble, consciously and conscientiously *exposed,* my lord. I am saying it is a product of isolation and a sense of unreality."

He rushes on. He talks of the community of *Babbletower,* La Tour Bruyarde, in search of a lost primeval unity. "An *impossible* identity, polymorphously perverse, *one.* I could quote Rilke, my lord, who prays to be made a self-sufficient hermaphrodite."

"Does he indeed?"

> *"Mach Einen herrlich, Herr, mach Einen gross,*
> *bau seinem Leben einen schönen Schoss,*
> *und seine Scham errichte wie ein Tor*
> *in einem blonden Wald von jungen Haaren."*

"I do not know," says the judge, "whether I want to ask you to translate that for the benefit of the jury, Mr. Gander, or whether I want to ask that it be struck from the record as irrelevant. My German is a little rusty. In so far as I can follow your quotation it seems a little—a little—well. Perhaps Mr. Hefferson-Brough can enlighten us on whether we should ask for a translation."

Mr. Hefferson-Brough says that the general argument was, if he has understood Mr. Gander correctly—Mr. Gander's enthusiasm, though infectious, has carried him away perhaps—the point appeared to be that the community was sick and that it desired, and failed to achieve, unity.

Judge. What has this to do with "onanistic babble" and quotations from Rilke?

Gander. May I answer? D. H. Lawrence said he would make his world—his novel's world—healthy, by inviting into it every little black snake that coils and curls at the edges of the marshes of the unconscious. The French surrealist Leiris said, "Masochism, sadism, almost all vices in fact, are only ways of feeling more human." I am saying Culvert, the hero of *Babbletower,* like Fourier, as Professor Smith has pointed out, sets out to *include everything* in his Tower, in his community, so there shall be no lost soul, no sour rejected creature prowling, but *all shall be one.* It doesn't work, of course, in his book, but the desire is noble, is noble, is sane and healthy. I offered Rilke's metaphor because it amused me, as an image of wholeness—of the impossibly yearned-for hermaphroditic polymorphously perverse beautiful self-satisfying *wholeness.*

Judge. I am not sure I ought to; we may be wasting the Court's time, but I am going to ask you to translate it.

Gander. Thank you, my lord. It goes—let me see—it goes

> *Make* One *beautiful one, Lord, make One big one,*
> *build a beautiful womb inside for its Life,*
> *and erect its Shame like a Pillar,*
> *in a blond forest of young hairs.*

Judge. Thank you. Thank you very much. I am sure the jury would rather know that that was what it said than not know.

Gander. It is very strong. Very beautiful.

Judge. It may be. It sounds better in German, it is true. Mr. Hefferson-Brough, I do think we should return to the *gravamen* of this matter.

Hefferson-Brough. Certainly, my lord. Mr. Gander—can you say, in your own words, what you think are the purposes and effects of what have been called the—the sado-masochistic passages that become more frequent as the story becomes, so to speak, *darker.*

Gander. Certainly, I can. They have been well defined as degradation ceremonies. I would refer the jurors to an article by H. Garfinkel in the *American Journal of Sociology* LXI (1956) on "Conditions of Successful Degradation Ceremonies." In modern society these ceremonies are part of our alienation and take place in all our institutions—R. D. Laing in his article in a book called *Ritualisa-*

tion of Behaviour in Animals and Men—a Royal Society publication—defines many modern psychiatric diagnoses as ceremonials of alienation, degradation ceremonies precisely. Some public confessionals are the same thing. I think the institutions of the confessional and the theatre in *Babbletower* function as degradation ceremonies. You could compare them to the rituals enacted in certain brothels where men are compelled to dress up as naughty children or martyrs in chains and *be degraded*. As Genet has shown, people also need to enact the masters of ceremony, degraders, judges and bishops and generals, yes. In brothels as in real life. A movement of violence, of bloody revolt, is often necessary to pierce through to our authenticity.

Judge. I am not quite sure I understand you. You are saying that courts and psychiatric hospitals and perhaps the Church are designed to degrade people? You are saying that Mr. Mason says this?

Gander. No, no. Only that from certain angles such institutions can be *perceived as* degrading, and *Babbletower* deals, profoundly, brilliantly, *fluently,* with the riddles and ambiguities of our degradation of each other. You could say, my lord, that the desire to degrade is an aspect of Original Sin, an aspect of that force of *division of people* which is represented by the Lord God in the Bible smiting the presumption of the original inhabitants of Babel.

Judge. Your own expressions are precise and convoluted, Mr. Gander. Do I understand you to be accusing the Lord God of a kind of sin in dividing people by smiting them?

Gander. The Lord God is a human myth, a human projection, so yes.

Judge. You were sworn in, I must remind you, on the Bible.

Gander. I said, I swear by Almighty God. I did. I do. But that God is a force of unity, a field of light, of beauty, not a harsh judge smiting people.

Judge. You enlighten me.

Gander. I have a quotation, my lord, from Simone de Beauvoir on Sade which makes quite clear what I am saying.

Hefferson-Brough. It may be that we can dispense with this quotation, and return to *Babbletower* and its depiction of cruelty, which, you were saying, I think, is a profound study of human misery, *malaise,* you said, exactly, a French word, meaning sickness or misery.

Gander. But my quotation does just that, it explains Sade and also Jude Mason. Listen. Simone de Beauvoir is very clear. She is a major writer, a respected thinker. She says: "To sympathise with Sade too readily is to betray him. For it is our misery, subjection and death that he desires; and every time we side with a child whose throat has been slit by a sex-maniac, we take a stand against him. Nor does he forbid us to defend ourselves. He allows that a father may revenge or prevent, even by murder, the rape of his child. What he demands is that, in the struggle between irreconcilable existences, each one engages himself concretely in the name of his own existence. He approves of the vendetta, but not of the courts. We may kill, but we may not judge. The pretensions of the judge are more arrogant than those of the tyrant; for the tyrant confines himself to being himself, whereas the judge tries to erect his opinions into universal laws. His effort is based upon a lie. For every person is imprisoned in his own skin, and cannot become the mediator between separate persons from whom he himself is separated."

Hefferson-Brough. You are not saying, Mr. Gander, that Mr. Mason is arguing that "we may kill, but we may not judge."

Gander. Oh no. He *rejects* de Sade, he *rejects* him. But he gives the argument a run for its money. We live in a free society, a serious argument has a right to a run for its money.

Judge. A serious argument. "He believes in the vendetta, but not in the courts."

Gander. It is an argument. You are a wise man, this is a wise Court, you must see—I am sorry, I put that badly—*I know you know* that is a serious argument. You, and Jude Mason, must both reject it. Even I, with all my scepticism about judgements, labelling, projections, emanations, spectres—even I prefer *this Court* to a vendetta, to a simple killing. I reject Sade. But I recognise his profound importance. You cannot *ban* him. Or Jude Mason.

Judge. Very well, Mr. Gander. Very well. Mr. Hefferson-Brough, your witness has taken us into deep water.

Hefferson-Brough. It is clear that we are speaking of a deep novel, my lord. Not a pleasant novel, but not a trivial one. One that goes deep.

Sir Augustine asks Elvet Gander whether there are *any* books he would suppress, if it were up to him. The witness replies that he would suppress the novels of Barbara Cartland, which are lies, and bring untold misery to those who believe them. Sir Augustine says that even these are surely evidence of some human velleities, some mind-set worthy of serious study. Gander smiles and agrees. "I was hasty. I was making a rhetorical point. You are right. There is no good reason for suppressing anything at all."

Q. Anything goes, in the end?

A. Oh yes, I think so. Anything goes.

Q. No further questions, my lord.

Godfrey Hefferson-Brough is beginning to look red and heavy. He consults with his junior and with Rupert Parrott, obviously in doubt about further witnesses. Nevertheless, he calls Avram Snitkin, who entrusts his tape-recorder to Frederica for the duration of his evidence.

Snitkin has been called, essentially, to describe various pieces of sociological research which claim to show that those with a propensity to offend, sexually, are less, rather than more, likely to do so if they have access to "explicit literature." He is a bad witness, because he can hardly bear to make a statement without enclosing it in a cocoon of "on the one hand" and "on the other hand," and "so to speak" and "in some very precisely delineated circumstances." He is also a bad witness because it is easy for the Prosecution to enquire whether the writings used in the experiments referred to were classifiable as "pornography." Snitkin speaks for a long time about this, saying at vast length that the term depends on the definition of the word "pornography," which itself depends on the uses to which the material described is put by the people whose habits in the context of the use of what might be defined as pornography are being studied . . .

The judge cuts him short, perhaps already rendered irritable by the jousting behaviour of Elvet Gander.

Snitkin also argues that there are studies that have shown that obscenity is traditionally a weapon of the alienated and frustrated. He is prevented by the judge, and by Hefferson-Brough, from defining "obscenity," "alienated" and "frustrated" at great length. He describes the beliefs of "the young, the idealistic who hope to remake our society." He says:

"If anarchy is an essential precursor to the creation of an alternative society, so the deflowering of language, rendering it obscene and useless, is part of the process of structuring a new one."

Sir Augustine asks him if he is saying *Babbletower* IS "obscene."

Hefferson-Brough objects—the witness's opinion as to the obscenity of the book is inadmissible.

The objection is sustained.

Sir Augustine asks him if he considers *Babbletower* an example of the "deflowering of language desiderated by the young."

Snitkin says no, not at all, quite the opposite. It's *against* the deflowering of language, it's hyper-articulate. It's *literary.* "I was simply saying," he says, "that we live in a climate of opinion where it's not particularly shocking. That's what I'm saying."

Sir Augustine. Some of us live in such a climate. Some of us try not to.

The next witness is Canon Adelbert Holly, white mane flowing, nicotined fingers gesticulating, dog-collar shining. He is identified as a Canon of St. Paul's, a writer on theology and psychology, a trained "sexual therapist" and the director of a charity which mans telephone lines to provide help to the despairing.

Hefferson-Brough asks him if he finds *Babbletower* to be a well-written book with a moral message. Canon Holly agrees that it is both well written and moral.

Q. You would, in your capacity as a Christian pastor, encourage people to read this book?

A. Oh yes. It is a deeply, a profoundly Christian book.

Q. Can you tell us why you are able to describe it in this way?

A. It is a book about suffering and the infliction of suffering. Suffering and the infliction of suffering are at the centre of the Christian religion. We venerate the dead body of a man who has been whipped, tortured, crowned with thorns, pierced by a sword and hung by his hands, pierced with nails, until he is dead. We claim, moreover, that our God exacted all this suffering from this Man—who was part of Himself, who was Himself—as payment for our sins. Our God is a cruel God and a jealous God. The Bible tells us so persistently. Cruelty and suffering are *at the centre* of our creed and our ritual. The Christian religion is an expression of the perception that what we now call sado-masochism is a central truth of our existence.

Judge. You are telling us that you, a Christian priest, believe that God is essentially cruel, and that this book says so?

A. *Part* of what we used to call God is cruel. The other part is Human, is Christ. I am with William Blake, who wrote, in his *Vision of the Last Judgement,* "Thinking as I do that the Creator of this World is a very Cruel Being, and being a Worshipper of Christ, I cannot help saying: 'The Son, O how unlike the Father!' First God Almighty comes with a Thump on the Head. Then Jesus Christ comes with a balm to heal it." We must worship Christ's Humanity. We must eat his battered body and drink his spilt blood in remembrance of Him, as he adjured us to do.

Hefferson-Brough leads, or attempts to lead, his witness back to a moral analysis of some of the events in *Babbletower,* the hunting of children, the death of Roseace. He attempts to get his witness to say that these episodes are morally shocking, not sexually titillating. He does not quite succeed, as Canon Holly's responses to his questions are rapturous and wild—"Oh, *superbly* horrible, *brilliantly* effective, *beautifully* dreadful." Canon Holly divagates into general reflections on children and death, drawn, according to him, from the profound psychoanalytic insights of Norman O. Brown. *Babbletower,* the Bible, and the works of Norman O. Brown, cries Canon Holly, deal with the generation of love and death in the human community. Neither the germ cell nor the One Spirit of the human community know death, says Canon Holly.

Death comes with individuation, when the infant is separated from the breast that suckles it and becomes a separate sexual being—at the moment when, within the family, the individual *separates* and starts a *new* nuclear *family,* death is born—when the Son becomes the Father, the Father can die, must die. "The human family is created by an intense mode of love and creates an intenser mode of death, that's what Brown says, my lord, that's what Jude Mason demonstrates."

Judge. Is it? You have lost me, Canon, I fear. I can understand your individual sentences, but your general drift I find hard to follow.

Holly. I can clarify.

Judge. No, don't. I trust the jury to have understood as much as they need. I trust the members of the jury to see whether this theological interpretation concurs with their reading of the book in question.

Samuel Oliphant questions the Canon on behalf of the author.

Q. You are acquainted with Jude Mason?

A. I have known him some little time.

Q. How would you describe him? Is he a serious writer?

A. He is a very gifted young man, with very severe difficulties, as the very gifted often have. His relations with society have not always been easy, and his living is hard, but he struggles to communicate his messages, to create his art.

Q. He has persisted with his writing despite severe personal difficulties?

A. He has lived on the edges, at extremes, in poverty. His attitude is a symptom of a sickness—he has been socially persecuted and derided, he is a scapegoat and a victim.

Mr. Oliphant, who has not quite expected this answer, hesitates, and then decides that to go on is better than to go back.

Q. You are saying he lives in difficulties, and knows the pain of modern life?

A. I always think of him as a kind of Holy Fool, like Jean-Paul Sartre's Saint Genet, in his book of that name. Or Dostoevski's Idiot, an innocent at large in a cruel world. Sartre sees Genet as a *shaman,* he is dismembered, chopped to bits, by the spirits in death and is reborn, wise. Jude Mason has the wisdom of the resurrected. His life has been hard, but he has been reborn, renewed, in his work.

Jude Mason does not look grateful for this odd encomium. The Defence barristers look intensely embarrassed. Sir Augustine rises to cross-examine.

Q. I am interested in your observations on Christianity and sadomasochism. Are you saying that the tortures in *Babbletower* are presented as a religious experience of the cruelty of the world, or of its Creator?

A. I am, yes. I am. I do believe it is so.

Q. You think that the motive for describing these explicit sexual cruelties is one of pure religious fervour, a desire to bring the reader to know every depth of degradation of pain, of sexual pain?

A. The divine Man knew every depth—he died in pain—and we need to know.

Q. He was not, I think, subjected to sexual degradation.

A. *All* degradation is sexual. He was a Man; he suffered as a Man.

Q. And you think the reading of this book—with its recondite sexual horrors—is in some—distant, perhaps—some way *related* to the Passion of Jesus Christ?

A. I cannot think we are not meant to know what is *possible* in this world.

Q. Let us be quite clear—you think it a *Christian act* to encourage the reading of this book?

A. I would quote John Milton's *Areopagitica:* "I cannot praise a fugitive and cloistered virtue, unexercised and unbreathed, that never sallies out and sees her adversary, but slinks out of the race, where that immortal garland is to be run for, not without dust and heat."

Q. But did not Our Lord Himself say, and tell us to pray, "Lead us not into temptation"?

A. The translation has altered. We say now—"Do not put us to the test."

Q. Do we indeed? No further questions, my lord.

Frederica misses several further witnesses, as she has to spend time with the Court Welfare Officer, who comes to interview her before the custody hearing. The Court Welfare Officer is a Mrs. Anthea Barlow, a middle-aged lady in a Persian lamb coat, with a fur hat and bright, wide-apart eyes. She has greyish fair hair and a slightly ecstatic expression, which does not inspire confidence in Frederica, who sees her as the same sort of churchy woman as Charity Farrar, the wife of Gideon, who has founded The Children of Joy. Mrs. Barlow asks sensible enough questions in her light, rushing voice. Has Frederica thought that Leo might be happier in Bran House, in the fields, in the paddocks and orchards? Frederica says yes. She says she nearly left him behind, for those reasons. Mrs. Barlow asks why she did not?

"Because *he* wanted to come, and for the first time really I saw he was *mine,* my child, I am the mother he *has,* his genes are *mine,* not Pippy Mammott's, he needs *me* with all my imperfections, we look at each other with the same look."

"And his father?"

"Him too. That's the disaster. But he is a *little boy,* and a clever boy, and a sharp-willed boy, and he does know what he wants."

"Do you love him?"

"More than anything else, including myself, including my books, whether I want to or not. It's just the nature of things. It's a ridiculous question."

"I know. I just like to see what sort of answer I get to it. You'd be surprised what some people say. They make it a function of a battle, or they say, 'I've got to, haven't I?' "

"Well, I have got to, haven't I? It's part of my biology."

"I have no doubt that you love him."

"What will happen?"

"It's not in my hands. I must talk to his father, and his aunts. I must talk to him. May I talk to him alone?"

"If he wants to."

"I'm experienced in talking to children. I won't worry him."

"He's a bit on edge. I want to say—I don't approve of sending little boys away to school, I think it's dangerous and horrible, such *little boys*—but he's like me, he's a loner, he needs to run his own life, *he'd hate it.* Please understand that. *He'd hate it.* I hope I don't sound shrill."

"No. Reasonable. Can you look after him?"

"I've got all these good arrangements. I've got Agatha and Saskia. And a good school."

"It is. I know it."

"What will happen?"

"There is always a predisposition in favour of the mother. Less, maybe, with boys. But judges tend to assume women will care better for little children. Rightly, in my view."

"There are a lot of other women, in his case. But I am his mother."

"You are. And I do see how much you care."

Back in Court, Hefferson-Brough has called Rupert Parrott to the stand. Parrott says he is proud to have published *Babbletower,* that it is an important, if controversial, book, that its message is deeply moral, and is a message for our times. He speaks in a light, pleasant, very slightly pompous voice, with exaggerated courtesy, a little old-fashioned. His blue eyes shine, his round cheeks are flushed and shining, the attention he gives to his questioners is just too intense, too considered. Hefferson-Brough asks him if he thought the book ran any risk of being thought outrageous, unacceptable, obscene, when he took it on.

A. Well, yes, naturally. It's strong meat, it's strong stuff, it doesn't pull its punches. But I was quite confident that the reading public, *and* the authorities, would take it for what it was—a serious and ambitious literary work. I felt its moment had come, and that I was there to bring it into the world. It says things about our society that need saying, need bringing into the light.

Q. What sorts of things are these?

A. Much has been made, by the Prosecution, of the scenes of sadistic treatment of little children in the dormitories. Those are in fact one of the things that made me recognise that the book had to be published. I recognised the dormitories and the tortures from my own schooldays—

Q. You are an Erstwhile Hog? That is to say, an old boy of Swineburn School.

A. Yes, I am. As you are yourself, I believe, and as is Jude Mason, the author of *Babbletower.* There are many fine things in *Babbletower,* but one of the finest is the depiction of what went on routinely in the dormitories of big schools—almost certainly still goes on.

Q. Let me be clear. You are not claiming that murder took place in the dormitories of Swineburn?

A. No, but almost, and nobody said anything. There is a conspiracy of silence. A climate of acceptance. Boys are thought to be nice, and teachers are supposed to be kind and considerate. This book tells the truth. It seems like wild fantasy but quite large chunks of it *that I know about* are sober fact. That is why I was so struck by it, initially. Later, I understood its other great merits. But it has an element of sober realism people lucky enough not to be Erstwhile Hogs may not assess properly.

Q. You believe it is for the public good to know that things happen in real life which are not very far from the fantastic events depicted in *Babbletower*?

A. On balance, yes, I do. I mean, I think public innocence about such things is no longer possible. Anyone who heard Fausto Gemelli's evidence will agree that we live in a moral climate now where things are pretty generally discussed rather than hidden. We are less easily shocked—as a nation—than we were in the days of Christine Keeler and Mandy Rice-Davies. I think there are good and bad aspects to all this—I think Press reports can upset certain people, vulnerable people, almost certainly much more than imaginative works like *Babbletower.* Sir Augustine mentioned the Moors Murders. I think the reporting of them was terrifying and disturbing in a way this literary work isn't. But I think we admit generally *now* that certain things go on that we once used—as a public community—to pretend didn't exist. When Oscar Wilde was sent to prison the judge said, "It is the worst case I have ever tried," and claimed that Wilde's crime was "so bad" that he had to put "stern restraint" on himself to suppress the language he would rather not use, "which must rise to the breast of every man of honour who has heard the details of these two terrible trials." There was one lone voice in the Press then that said the judge must have tried worse crimes, murders and extortions, and that society was guilty of hypocrisy. "Why does not the Crown prosecute every boy at a public or private school, or half the men in the Universities? In the latter places 'coederism' is as common as fornication, and everyone knows it." There is a gap between what many or most people now *know* about human nature and what we are allowed to say. Those of us who suffered at school—as I did, and as I can see Jude Mason did—suffered also from the little boys' normal conspiracy of silence. I think the public conspiracy of silence is as bad as the frightened conspiracy of little boys in dorms. We are grown-up men now. We live in a grown-up time. We have a right to responsible grown-up descriptions of the actions of which we are capable.

(Scattered applause in the Court.) The judge asks for silence and requests that the interruption not be repeated.

Sir Augustine asks Rupert Parrott only a few questions.

Q. Mr. Parrott—you are a generally respected publisher. You have a reputation for being intellectually up-to-date, even *avant-garde.*

A. I would say so, yes.

Q. You publish Elvet Gander, who has enlightened the Court about degradation ceremonies and polymorphous perversity.

A. You need not sneer at him. He is a serious thinker, much respected and admired, and I am proud to publish him. (Scattered local applause.)

Q. I hope I was not sneering. You publish also Canon Adelbert Holly, who has told us that the essence of Christianity is masochism and the suffering and infliction of pain?

A. I do. And am proud to publish him. I do not agree with all his points of emphasis. But he is a daring and a subtle theologian.

Q. No doubt. No doubt. You feel a considerable sense of mission about *Babbletower,* do you not? You feel it represents a blow for sexual freedom, fearless, explicit description of hidden vices and horrors, do you not?

A. I do. You try to make these feelings sound misguided or absurd, but they are not. It is a serious and beautiful and courageous book, confronting the dark fearlessly. I am, as I said, proud to be associated with it.

Q. You feel also a sense of mission, I sense, about the revelation of the squalid school secrets you shared with Jude Mason and perhaps with that other Erstwhile Hog, my learned friend, the Counsel for the Defence.

A. To an extent, yes.

Q. To an extent. You do not think your judgement of *Babbletower* is perhaps twisted, perhaps vitiated, by your recognition of your schooldays in parts of it, in the dorms of La Tour Bruyarde? As Dr. Gander has reminded us, childhood wounds lie deep and fester. Might they not cloud your judgement?

A. I don't think so. I think they reinforce it. I would like to do away with the hypocrisy which made those sufferings possible and prolonged.

The next witness for the Defence is the accused in the dock, Jude Mason himself. He stands in the box, eyes downcast at first, holding his fists close together in front of him; Frederica suddenly intuits that he is wearing imaginary manacles. She looks at his thin face and his eye-hollows and imagines the fall of his hair as it used to be before he was sanitised and tidied. He looks insubstantial, grey-skinned after his publisher's pink, bony and brittle. Frederica wonders what has become of his smell, the frying grease, the rancid sweat, the body fluids. Does he now emit carbolic soap or Old Spice? Her nostrils imagine the sniff of fresh newsprint. She smiles. Samuel Oliphant rises to examine his client.

Q. Tell us your name.

A. Jude Mason.

Q. Is that your real name?

A. Yes. It is not the name my parents gave me.

Q. What was that?

A. Julian Guy Monckton-Pardew. (A ripple of laughter in the Court.)

Q. You changed your name?

A. Many people do. I changed my name, and my life.

Q. What sort of a family do you come from?

A. I have none. They have cast me off. My father made a lot of money selling pork and veal pies to pubs. I am a vegetarian. Not out of virtue or anything. Out of squeamishness. My mother was a photographic model. Her name was Poppy. I called them Poppy and Pappy. We lived in Wiltshire. They had enough money to pay nannies and nurses and send me away to prep school at five and to Swineburn at thirteen so I can't be said to have known them very well before we mutually cast each other off. I don't know if they're alive or dead. They don't know if I am. That suits all of us.

The sawing voice is monotonous but conveys an uneasy urgency: these are things the speaker has rehearsed and wants to say, not things reluctantly drawn from him.

Oliphant. Mr. Parrott has already spoken about your experiences at Swineburn. Were you happy there?

Jude. Oh, from time to time, blissfully and disastrously happy. It was those times that ruined my character and my life. Mostly I was miserable, frequently I was terrified. There was a great deal of refined cruelty in that school, as has already been suggested. A great deal.

Oliphant. Cruelty exercised by whom?

Jude. Oh, routinely by the masters. We were whipped all sorts of ways by all sorts of men, for all sorts of reasons. You survived better if you developed a taste for it, if you learned to cater to those who had a taste for it. Also the boys were cruel, in thumping, bashing ways and in subtle, teasing, nasty ways, as is no doubt normal everywhere. I imagine it was all quite *normal.*

Oliphant. Did you survive?

Jude. No. In short, no. Contrary to appearances, I have no taste for being hurt, just a lot of enforced experience of it. I did think it was inevitable and immutable and eternal, as little children do, and most adults conveniently forget.

Oliphant. Were you a good student?

Jude. I believe so. I was very good at languages. Poppy-mommy, my sweet mother, glimpsed perhaps half a dozen times a year, was, or is, I am told, partly *French.* She modelled rather *naughty* clothes sometimes. My French was good.

Oliphant. And English literature and language?

Jude. Ah. When I was a *little boy* the English master predicted a glorious future for me. Scholarships, university, poetry of the profounder kind. I was a *stellar student* in my early days. I was the star in all the plays, you know, in all the Shakespeare plays.

Oliphant. What parts did you play?

Jude. I was a delicious squeaking Cleopatra. The English master, Dr. Grisman Gould, was good enough to say that he had never seen a better one. I believed him at the time. Later, I took to doing *friends.* Horatio, you know, Kent, steady souls. I'd have liked to do Iago, but you don't get school productions of *Othello.*

Judge. Where is all this questioning leading, Mr. Oliphant?

Oliphant. I am hoping to establish Mr. Mason's literary background. As a help with the question of the literary merits of his book.

Judge. I see.

Oliphant. And my learned friend Mr. Hefferson-Brough has already linked Mr. Mason's experiences at school with the seriousness of his purpose as a writer.

Judge. Your client's *intentions* are not relevant as to the question of obscenity.

Oliphant. I understand that, my lord. But they are relevant as to *literary merit,* and the two are linked here, are very much linked, in the formative years of my client's mind.

Judge. Very well. But I do not think we need to examine closely all his lessons or amateur dramatic performances. He obviously enjoyed his dramatic performances.

Jude. Not always, my lord.

Judge. Indeed? Not always. Continue, if you please, Mr. Oliphant.

Oliphant. You did not go to university, Mr. Mason?

Jude. No.

Oliphant. Although you might have been expected to?

Jude. I was very unhappy. I ran away from the school. I ran away rather classically, or perhaps romantically would be a better word, in the middle of the night. I stole a bicycle and went all the way to Harwich. I got on a boat and went to Amsterdam. I messed around there a bit and then someone took me to Paris.

Oliphant. You were sixteen?

Jude. Yes. I don't think my parents looked for me. I never heard of it if they did. I sent a postcard from Paris with a Poste Restante address and got a postcard back saying they didn't want to know.

Judge. Are we really to believe that is all the contact you had?

Jude. I don't know why you shouldn't believe it. It's true. It's quite easy to stay hidden, my lord, if people have no real desire to find you. I was a disappointment, it has to be admitted. Poppy said continually I was a disappointment. She said it on the postcard. She can't spell. She wrote it with one *p.* I probably sent a disappointing postcard. It had a sphinx on it, by Gustave Moreau. They were afraid I was decadent.

Judge. So you sent the postcard to provoke them?

Jude. It wasn't *much* of a provocation, my lord, from a sixteen-year-old boy who had been living pretty rough for six months.

Judge. That is as may be. I am interested in your veracity, you see.

Jude. I am telling the truth, and nothing but the truth.

Judge. But not the whole truth?

Jude. You can't tell the whole truth in one-line answers, my lord. I don't think you'd like the whole truth if I told it. I really don't. It isn't very nice. But I haven't told you anything untrue. I swore not to.

Judge. Mr. Oliphant, please continue your questioning.

Oliphant. In Paris, did you attempt to continue your studies?

Jude. I decided to get a ticket to the Bibliothèque Nationale. I made various friends—various people looked after me a bit—I talked to people in cafés—I worked a bit in theatres and cinemas, showing people their seats. I got interested in French literature. A man I met told me about Fourier. He seemed odd, you know, and interesting, so I said I was working on him and went to the library and did work on him, and got interested. I am an auto-didact. I believe in auto-didacticism. Auto-didacts tend to study one thing at once, study it to death. I did Fourier, and then I went on to Nietzsche.

Oliphant. And when did you start your own writing?

Jude. There was never a time when I was not writing. I was writing when I was a very little boy, and before that I was telling stories to myself. I used to dress up in front of the mirror and act the stories. Once I acted a whole pantomime for Poppy and Pappy—it was *Cinderella,* I made all the costumes and played all the parts, I didn't have any friends, though I did have a Nanny at that point who acted the Fairy Godmother and the Narrator. They clapped a bit, but they had to go out before I got to the glass slipper. I'm sorry, I see I'm boring you and being irrelevant, but you did ask for the whole truth and that was my first bit of writing. I've never ever told anyone all this before—not ever having been under oath—except one person. And *that* was a mistake.

Oliphant. When did you start writing *seriously*?

Jude. All that was serious. It was deadly serious. It was my real life. Much more real than the horrible school *cells* and *teams.*

Oliphant. When did you start writing *Babbletower*?

Jude. Well, in a way, then, when I was a little boy. Who was it said there are only five or six good plots? Anyway, I was always writing the same story. The story about the *group of friends* who *run away* to a *better place* and make a better life, a more beautiful life, a freer life, where they can do what they want. It's the story of *Cinderella* and the story of *Pilgrim's Progress* and the story of *The Coral Island,* I suppose. Getting out of the dungeon and the cinders and going to the ball or to heaven and sleeping in feather beds and eating off gold plates. Only as I got older and more suspicious I saw that the place you make might turn out to be much like the place you ran away from.

He is now, Frederica thinks, acting the great writer accounting for his great talent, modestly. Oliphant says firmly,

Oliphant. But *Babbletower* is a grown-up book, not a childish fantasy.

Jude. It is a grim grown-up book about childish fantasy. And about grown-up fantasy. It is also a grown-up fantasy itself, I have to admit. That's not wicked. Fantasy is natural to human beings as honey is to bees. People are always saying things are as natural as honey, these days. Now what was . . .

Oliphant. You have heard the very clear evidence of Professor Marie-France Smith. What did you make of her arguments?

Jude. (The sawing note more pronounced.) Professor Smith is an *academic* and her account *smells of the lamp,* as they say, I believe. She makes my book sound all cut and dried, a trussed-up little plump *thesis* waiting to be roasted and consumed. I don't recognise the terrible passions of my book in Professor Smith's arid little "explanation." *I lived that story, Mr. Oliphant, I have lived through all those things—*

It is at this point that the first fleck of white foam, or crust, appears in the corner of Jude's mouth. He pokes at it nervously, with the tip of his tongue.

Oliphant. Well, you may dislike the emphases. But you did read Fourier, you say yourself, and you do maintain that *Babbletower* has a serious moral point, do you not?

Jude. Does art ever have a "serious moral point"? It moves, it appals, it makes you chuckle, it delights, it despairs. All right, you don't like my answers. You are right not to. I am behaving stupidly. I can't help myself. But my book is not a stupid book, it is a good book, and is meant to enlighten and to move, not to harm and disgust. Those who cannot see that can't read properly.

For several more repetitive minutes, Jude and his Counsel joust around the ostensible "purpose" of *Babbletower.* Oliphant is patient with his client's natural tendency to contradict, for rhetorical effect, points that are designed to help him. Jude is got to agree that his vision of human nature is "dark" and "pessimistic," but not "perverted," not "twisted." He complains briefly about meaningless adjectives and is brought again to the point. He says that like Nietzsche he desires a "strong" pessimism, a "gay" despair. He asks if he may quote Nietzsche and is told to go ahead.

Jude. He says: "Whenever anyone speaks, without bitterness, rather innocuously, of man as a belly with two needs and a head with one; whenever anyone sees, seeks and *wants* to see only hunger, sexual desire and vanity, as though these were the actual and sole motives of human actions; in brief, whenever anyone speaks '*badly*' of man—but does not speak ill of him—the lover of knowledge should listen carefully and with diligence, and he should in general lend an ear whenever anyone speaks without indignation. For the indignant man, and whoever is constantly tearing and rending himself with his teeth (or instead of himself, the world, or God, or Society), may indeed morally speaking stand higher than the laughing and self-satisfied satyr, but in every other sense he is the more commonplace, less interesting, less instructive case. And no one *lies* so much as the indignant man."

May I say, my lord, that the "English vice" is not what it is always said to be, but precisely *indignation.* We get furiously upset about everything—the price of stamps, the state of public lavatories, the behaviour of schoolboys and politicians, the weather, books that are written with the heart's blood and fuelled by real passion. It is *indignation* that has put my book on trial, seeing things that are not there, making hypotheses about its effect that are *quite unjustified.* My book thinks badly of man, but so do quite a lot of other writers, including Saint Augustine. *Indignation* is prurient and suspect, my lord, it is unworthy to be heard. Do not hear it.

Judge. You should perhaps have read for the Bar, Mr. Mason, instead of devoting your time to Fourier and Sade.

Godfrey Hefferson-Brough, perhaps wisely, asks the defendant very few questions about *Babbletower.* He returns almost compulsively to the state of affairs at Swineburn School in the late 1940s. Later, the Press is to remark that just as it began to appear that Lady Chatterley herself was on trial for adultery in the trial of Penguin Books, so it seems, from time to time, in the *Babbletower* case, that the real defendants are the masters and boys of Swineburn, the Erstwhile Hogs and the erstwhile Swineherds. One journalist, asking why Hefferson-Brough returned so compulsively to the charge, to the school, when the advantage to his client was, to put it nicely, dubious, will conclude that he was compelled to do so by some unresolved business of his own. "Everything in England," this journalist writes, "comes back to the inextricable links between our educational system, privilege, or lack of it, and sex. De Sade was abused by the Jesuits, but Fourier was sublimely innocent of the snares and puerile disasters of the Public School dorm."

Q. You say, Mr. Mason, that you were taught by Dr. Grisman Gould.

A. That is so.

Q. He was a good teacher?

A. In his way, sublime.

Q. So I believe. He had favourites?

A. Not *obviously.* But yes. He singled out particular boys. He gave them an extra-curricular literary education. He disabused their innocence, you might say.

Q. Were you one of his favourites?

A. For a time. Later, I was not. That was a normal pattern. First he loved you. Then you "disappointed" him. Then he began to find fault. Then he destroyed you.

Q. That's a strong word. "Destroyed."

A. Most of his favourites came to grief. There were scandals. They were said to have cheated. Or were caught in the lats with little boys. Or got drunk. Or killed himself, one. They were going to be wonders and something always happened.

Q. Were you yourself involved in any scandal?

Judge. Where is this line of questioning leading, Mr. Hefferson-Brough?

Hefferson-Brough. It is all to do with the realism of the subject-matter of this apparent fantasy, my lord.

Judge. It is hard to see how.

Jude. I don't mind answering. I am telling everything, today.

Judge. That is for me to decide. Continue, Mr. Hefferson-Brough.

Hefferson-Brough. Does the question stand, my lord?

Judge. I think not. I think Mr. Mason need not answer that question.

Jude. I don't mind.

Judge. You must speak when you are asked to.

Jude. How can I explain, if I may not speak?

Judge. You are not here to explain your life, but to defend your book. Mr. Hefferson-Brough.

Q. Did Dr. Grisman Gould ever interfere with you, Mr. Mason?

A. I wouldn't call it *interfering.* That is quite the wrong verb. He was a person of infinite subtlety and charm. Oh dear, yes.

Q. Are you aware of the Erstwhile Hogs' Round Robin, Mr. Mason?

A. No. Tell me. I should like to know what that was.

Q. Do you know what became of Dr. Grisman Gould?

A. I think he is dead. I am not sorry if he is.

Q. He committed suicide in 1952, Mr. Mason. He was dismissed from the school, dishonourably, after the composition of the Round Robin.

A. How?

Q. How?

A. How did he kill himself?

Q. He slit his wrists in a hot bath.

Judge. I do not think you can pursue this topic further, Mr. Hefferson-Brough. The witness has said he knows nothing of these facts.

Hefferson-Brough. Certainly, my lord. I would like to ask Mr. Mason if he believes that Dr. Grisman Gould was a corrupter of youth, the centre of a circle of corruption and perversion at Swineburn in the 1940s and early '50s.

A. Not a circle. It was never more than one at once I think. That's how he kept going. Each one thought he was the first and only. And his successor thought the predecessor was a *disappointment,* as Dr. Gould said he was. He looked like the Archangel Michael, you know. Austere, pure, golden. I suppose you knew him, too. I don't like to think of him bleeding in a bath. Ugly. Better than a bullet in the brain, but ugly.

Q. Mr. Mason, is it from Dr. Grisman Gould that you first learned of the—the sado-masochistic practices described in *Babbletower*?

A. It may well be. He gave me Rousseau's *Confessions.* Rousseau couldn't reach orgasm without being whipped. The things in my book happen everywhere. Dr. Grisman Gould's speciality was *confession* afterwards. Verbal recapitulation.

Q. Indeed. Are we to recognise the model for your Projector, Culvert, in Dr. Grisman Gould?

A. Not *culvert,* Mr. Hefferson-Brough, as in the English *drainage system.* Cul-vert, as in French, green or verdant cul or—orifice. Hmm. Do you know, I had never thought about whether Culvert was Dr. Grisman Gould. He is so many, Prince Charming, the Scarlet Pimpernel, Rousseau, Charles II, James I, Fourier, myself—I think he may also be Dr. Grisman Gould. Dr. Gould might have acknowledged him as Prospero acknowledged Caliban, to whom he taught language. "This thing of darkness I acknowledge mine." I could have confessed *for hours,* having invented Culvert. You distress me. I did not invent Culvert to propitiate Dr. Grisman Gould.

It can be seen that the defendant is trembling. The crumb of white in the corner of his mouth is extending into a fine white crust that runs along his lips. From this point on in his evidence his words are accompanied by the sound of a fluttering or beating, which is his knees knocking gently and rapidly against the wooden box, which is his hands playing on the bar before him. It is like a wing-beat, or a heart-beat, not quite regular, but persistent. His answers, written down, may seem jaunty, foolhardy, but to those in the Court the plangent voice had also a fixed, raucous note which is disturbing and irritating.

Sir Augustine Weighall rises to cross-examine. He rearranges his gown with care. His face is grave, concerned and almost friendly.

Q. You have told my learned friend that you were christened Julian Guy Monckton-Pardew. Did you give up that name as a rejection of your parents, or as a rejection of the connotations of the name itself?

A. Both.

Q. What do you dislike about the name?

A. Every aspect of it. The pretentious double-barrel. The romanticism in Guy is all crusaders and Old England (or Old Norman Conquest) and Julian is a name no pretty boy should be asked to bear. Also, I have to tell you, my parents made it up. He was Monckton, and she was Pardew; it comes from the French, Pardieu, I suppose. It's a burdensome sort of name. Like a plaster imitation of an effigy in a church.

Q. That is a very articulate rebuttal. And the name you chose has its own romantic poetry, too, in opposition, I take it. Would I be wrong in suggesting that you chose Jude as a tribute to Thomas Hardy's hero Jude the Obscure?

A. You would not be wrong. I meant to be obscure. I am obscure.

Q. Hardy's Jude was an auto-didact, a workman, an intellectual excluded from the inner circle of university life?

A. He was. It seemed appropriate. Romantic, as you say. There's nothing wrong in romanticism.

Q. Indeed there is not. Hardy's Jude was called Jude Fawley, as I recall. But you chose the name Mason. Hardy's Jude was a mason, a stonemason by trade, I believe.

A. He was. He was an honest craftsman, and he saw the poetry in stones. I believe art is craft first. I meant always to be an artist. "Mason" seemed a good place to start.

Q. Your name is indeed precisely crafted. I believe *Jude the Obscure* was received with considerable criticism when it first appeared?

A. With vituperation. It was burned by a bishop. Hardy said the general idea was "We Britons hate ideas, and we are going to live up to that privilege of our native country. Your picture may not show the untrue, or the uncommon, or even be contrary to the canons of art; but it is not the view of life that we who thrive on conventions can permit to be painted."

Q. You have that by heart. It obviously means a great deal to you. How long have you had that by heart?

A. Since my schooldays.

Q. So you chose your name, long before the writing of *Babbletower,* for its associations with an obscure auto-didact and an unconventional, rejected book?

A. That is so. There is nothing wrong with that.

Q. Was it Dr. Grisman Gould who drew your attention to *Jude the Obscure*?

A. Indeed it was not. I found it quite by myself. Quite by myself. He did not like Hardy. He found him heavy-handed and improbable. His tastes ran to poetry.

Q. Can you tell us which poetry?

A. Shakespeare. The sonnets. The early poems. *Venus and Adonis. The Rape of Lucrece.* He was very subtle on lacerated skin. He had his little games with rosy cheeks and threads of blood. We knew all about the dirty Dark Lady and the fair young man. He was good on paintings of martyrs, too. Crawshaw. Oscar Wilde, by extension. *The Ballad of Reading Gaol.* "Each man kills the thing he loves." He knew about that. When you knew him very well, he would read you Bosie's sonnets about Shame.

> *"I am Shame*
> *That walks with Love, I am most wise and turn*
> *Cold lips and limbs to fire . . ."*

"I am the Love that dare not speak its name." Bosie was a dreadful poet. Dreadful. I nearly gave Grisman Gould up when he started on that stuff.

Q. Bosie was Lord Alfred Douglas?

A. Yes.

Q. To whom Oscar Wilde addressed passionate letters?

A. Yes. They were silly letters, badly written.

Q. You admire Wilde?

A. As a writer, in moderation. As a man, no. He was a fool. A snob. He made a fool of himself over worse fools.

Q. Dr. Grisman Gould admired Oscar Wilde?

A. In moderation, too. Why are you going on about Oscar Wilde? Are you trying to draw an analogy?

Q. Do you accept an analogy?

Samuel Oliphant objects and his objection is sustained. Sir Augustine turns to another line of questioning.

Q. How do you make your living, Mr. Mason?

A. With great difficulty. I expose my body in public places. I achieve sempiternity in charcoal, in acrylic paint, in oils. In short, I model in art colleges. It is an honest trade, and humbling.

Frederica can hear this roll off Jude's tongue: it is his practised party piece.

Q. And did you pursue this trade in Paris?

A. No. I did not know how to set about it. I did not think of it.

Q. So how did you live?

A. I made myself useful to various people. I was a *protégé,* from time to time. People took an interest in my career, in my mind, in my future.

Q. Where did you live?

A. In many places. Backstage. Under bars.

Q. With the kindly protectors?

A. No. As a matter of fact, no. If you mean, was I a kept boy, no. *I was not.* Never again. No.

Q. Never again?

A. I sleep by myself. I live by myself. I am a private person. I do not see how this is relevant to your enquiries, or whatever the phrase is, *but I have no sex life.* It is over-valued. Sex is better in the head, *pace* D. H. Lawrence, who knew a lot less than he thought he did about a lot of things.

Q. Are you saying, Mr. Mason, that after your schooldays you have lived chastely and written vivid sexual fantasies, for choice?

A. Not always, and not entirely. But that has been the general idea, the ideal state of affairs, yes. Nietzsche said philosophers were always "irritable and rancorous" towards their senses. He said sex was very damaging to spiritual and artistic preparation. "Those with the greatest powers do not need to learn this from experience, from unfortunate experience." He was right.

Q. Let us turn to your writing, Mr. Mason, now we understand a little better what you believe in. Despite your admiration for Nietzsche, you were a little unhappy with Professor Smith's definition of your book as a philosophical exploration of freedom and restraint?

A. She was *so dry.* So *logical.* A book is a passionate thing, it is made of experience, it is lived as it is written, it is more immediate than reality.

Q. More immediate than reality.

A. I think if most people were honest, they would admit that imaginary experiences are more real than actual ones. It is like the smell of coffee—the thing itself is never so good, it is always a bit musty. I began to write to avoid life as it is lived, and found I had found it more abundantly.

Q. Life. You are quoting the Bible there, Mr. Mason, as you are no doubt well aware. But the life *you* offer your readers is not a very usual life—it is, as has already *abundantly* appeared in evidence, a life of manacles and ingenious tortures, pederasty, orgies, coprophilia, flagellation and slow murder for pleasure. What do you wish to do to your readers, Mr. Mason? Do you wish to make them take pleasure in the images of these horrors? To make them shun them? To incite them to copy them?

Jude is silent. He is silent for some time, licking the crust round his dry lips. He says, finally,

A. I don't know. I don't consider readers, particular readers. I write what I have to, what I see. These are the fantasies people have, some people live by. This is how people are, more people than you think. I don't know *why* people need fantasies, any more than I know *why* they dream. I only know, if you stop a man dreaming, you destroy his mind. If you shut off his fantasies, I think, you make him dangerous.

Q. But Culvert *indulges* his fantasies and becomes a killer.

A. It does him no good.

Q. It does his victims no good. Did you take pleasure in the death of Roseace, Mr. Mason? In the writing of that death?

A. Pleasure?

Q. Do not stall, Mr. Mason. It is a simple question. Did you take pleasure in the slow death by sexual torture of the Lady Roseace?

A. Did Shakespeare take pleasure in Cornwall's pleasure in the putting-out of Gloucester's eyes? Did he mean to incite Elizabethan noblemen to go about putting out people's eyes? They did, and enjoyed it. Now we don't, much. He put us off the idea, I believe.

Q. *King Lear* is a great and terrible tragedy. Are you comparing *Babbletower* to that kind of work?

A. No. Oh no. I am a mere Marsyas. A minor artist, a pipe-player who was flayed by Apollo.

Q. Explain your reference.

A. He was a goat-foot, a satyr, who challenged Apollo to a musical contest. He lost, and Apollo flayed him alive. He pulled him, Dante says, out of the scabbard of his limbs, "*della vagina delle membre sue.*" He had no more song, after that. Oscar Wilde says that modern art is the cry of Marsyas, bitter and plaintive and sad. Not tragic. Tortured but not tragic. Tragedy is past.

Q. So your art is not tragic, it is a satiric piping. You wish to blow a raspberry at convention?

A. Raspberry? I don't understand raspberry.

Q. Come, Mr. Mason. You must have heard the term. A rude noise.

A. Don't say "Come" to me in that tone of voice. I don't see why a rude noise is called a raspberry. For the little rosette of anal veins around a fart, perhaps?

(Some laughter, some irritable restiveness in the courtroom.)

Q. Would you accept, Mr. Mason, that it is difficult in some ways to reconcile the savagery of many of the comments in *Babbletower* with some of your own attitudes and statements during the course of your evidence?

A. I do find it difficult myself. Giving evidence is much less pleasant than writing. You are not in control, giving evidence. You are tempted into saying silly things.

Q. You have, so to speak, "presented" yourself to the Court. You pose as an unsophisticated auto-didact, a victim of the public school system. You are constructed of literary images, references—Hardy, Wilde, Marsyas. It is as though you were self-designed as a player in a drama where you were a victim, unjustly accused of writing a corrupt book—long before this trial ever took place, or this action was brought. You are a bit of a *poseur,* Mr. Mason.

A. Is that a question? (The witness is shaking so much that his answer is croaked.)

Q. I am trying to get to the bottom of the purpose and nature of the book you have written. Mr. Avram Snitkin, a witness called by the Defence, has talked about the modern desire to shock, to break taboos, to use "bad" words to create anarchy—

A. I reject all that. I am not interested in anarchy. I am an artist. A lot of nonsense is talked about those words, those words you don't use—you can't do *anything* with those words, it's like studding your pages with gobs of exudations—*those two words,* "gobs" and "exudations," are better words than "shit" and "snot," they're words you *react to.* If I want to upset you I can write in perfectly legitimate words a description of bliss, or hurt, or evacuation, which will leave a trace on your memory as though a knife had slid across your brain; I can leave a *trace* of these that won't go. Poor old Lawrence tried to accommodate and tame those words, like old copper coins with the faces rubbed off, bum pennies for bun pennies. It won't work because they only exist to shock. And no, I don't write to pose or to shock, Mr. Weighall, *I don't.*

Q. You don't. You write to hurt—to slice our brains and our memories—

A. That is not illegitimate.

Q. Let me finish. You said earlier, and I quote: "I write what I have to, what I see. These are the fantasies people have . . ." You write the kinds of fantasies that are enacted in brothels and written down badly in dirty books in brown wrappers, Mr. Mason, but you write them in better words and make them more powerful. Do you not agree that they might hurt people just as much as these other pornographic works?

A. Hurt? Hurt? I don't think those other things *hurt,* Mr. Weighall. I have been in those places, and I know, I have been amongst the incense and the poppies and the tawdry bits of silk and satin and tulle. I have seen grown men making fools of themselves in nappies with bottles, or loaded with heavy chains. I have seen judges pretending to be housemaids in frilly aprons and black stockings and I've seen postmen pretending to be judges and an eminent surgeon pretending to be a fire that could only be put out in a particularly disgusting way. If I wrote you a scientific treatise on these things, you *couldn't touch me*—but I am an artist—meretrix, meretricious I may have been as a boy, porno-grapher I am not, *I am an artist.*

Q. You protest eloquently. You have not answered my question about your readers, Mr. Mason. You have not answered it. I put it to you that when you were a boy, Dr. Grisman Gould hurt your body and depraved your mind with a mixture of literature and cruelty—and that you are intent on passing on that hurt to the world, to your readers, to the possible victims of those of your readers who resemble your own betrayer.

A. You understand nothing. I loved him. He was not a tawdry Svengali. He was—he was—he is dead, it doesn't matter what he was, he is not on trial, though he appears to be. He is dead, and I loved him, and I have not loved since, and shan't.

Q. You have not answered my question. Hurt was done, you were depraved and corrupted, and you are *passing that hurt on.*

Jude. (to judge) Do I have to answer that? It—isn't—a question. This is all nonsense.

Judge. It is a question of opinion. You need not answer it.

Jude. He need not have asked it.

Judge. The jury will please ignore the question.

Snitkin's tape-recorder whirs. Augustine Weighall says he has no further questions, thus leaving the deleted question, the struck question, the non-question, indelibly engraved on the jurors' minds as the climax of his case against Jude Mason.

Frederica leaves the court during the evidence of the next witness, a schoolmaster who confirms the stories of excesses at Swineburn, and asserts that he would have no objection to his charges reading *Babbletower.* She meets Alexander Wedderburn, wandering along the corridors. Alexander thinks the case is going badly for the Defence. He says that Augustine Weighall is much cleverer than Godfrey Hefferson-Brough. "He must have known something about Jude's history," says Alexander. "More than his own people did."

"Probably met him in some brothel in Piccadilly," says Frederica tartly. "They all dress up and *port about,* as my father used to say. Jude is an idiot. Why must he *show off*?"

"He said. He's an artist."

"So are you. You don't."

"The dreadful thing is, he's potentially a better one. And they might put him in prison. He's got no common sense. That's his tragedy. I have. Abundantly. That's mine."

"Don't you start talking in cheap epigrams. I *hate* Oscar Wilde."

"So does Jude."

"With the hate that dare not tell its name, I guess. Now I'm doing it."

"You're worried."

"I never thought I'd say it, but I've got kind of *attached* to Jude. I never thought I'd agree with Canon Holly, but he is a kind of holy fool, a real *idiot.*"

. . .

The Defence's final witness is the novelist Phyllis Pratt, Bowers and Eden's only bestseller. Mrs. Pratt is wearing a pink suit over a floral shirt, and an amethyst cross on a silver chain. She addresses both the Counsel for the Defence, and later Sir Augustine, in a sensible, complicit, lemon-and-honey voice, tart and warm. She states that she has much enjoyed *Babbletower*—"quite a *satisfactory* experience, like a fairy story, with the punishment of folly and a few thrills to it, but never real enough to *alarm* anyone." She says that as a vicar's wife she has met "many tortured souls who have harmed others, or who would have liked to harm others" and believes that reading *Babbletower* would "on the whole, merely cheer such people up. That somebody knew, and could make fairytales out of it. Fairy stories and detective stories do much less harm than real reports of what went on in concentration camps, I think you'll find. They put a kind of pink glow round it all, that takes it out of the sordid real world."

Would she, Hefferson-Brough asks her, give it to her children to read?

"Any mother knows that some children can take *anything* and some cry and cry over the death of a seal or a Bambi and never quite recover. I think Mr. Mason made a little mistake calling his work a tale for children. It isn't. Children don't like explicit sex. They like dirty noses and dirty bottoms, not genitalia doing what genitalia are made for, or can be contorted to do. No, I'd be careful who I *recommended* it to. But one must be sensible, that goes for every grown-up book."

Sir Augustine asks her, as he has asked all the defence witnesses, whether she was sexually moved by the book.

A. Of course I was. He's a clever writer. I was moved by the bits that appealed to my particular fantasies, as I expect you were, and I laughed at some of the others, and I skipped some of the others, as I expect you would in normal circumstances.

Q. It can't be normal reading for you, Mrs. Pratt. Your own books are grounded in realism, in village life, in domesticity, in the Church.

A. I heard you grilling Mr. Mason about fantasies. The heroine of my first book stabbed her husband in a real *welter of gore* when he pushed her too far. That was a fantasy, Sir Augustine, which would perhaps have become a fact, if it hadn't got out on paper and cheered up a multitude of other vicars' wives and other women indulging similar fantasies. What Mr. Mason said about fantasies and dreams was very wise. They save us, they save us from action.

Q. Even the warning dreams, the premonitory dreams, of murderers?

A. Come, come, Sir Augustine. You are not going to tell me that anything as accomplished and fastidious and in places downright *funny* as *Babbletower* bears any relation to the deranged vision of murderers? Or that poor Mr. Mason wants *to kill someone*? He is a good writer, and he's half-dead with anxiety, and I think it's a pity.

Augustine Weighall has considered other obscenity trials, and believes that previous prosecution witnesses have been ill chosen. He has decided, also, that his witnesses, coming after the long file of defence luminaries, must be succinct and convincing, carry weight. In the event, he calls five: Hermia Cross, who began the public agitation against *Babbletower,* a chief superintendent from Staffordshire, a suffragan bishop from a difficult part of Birmingham, Roger Magog and Professor Efraim Ziz, a historian of Judaism.

Hermia Cross is disturbingly sensible. She is an MP, has been a local councillor, has worked with recidivist adolescents and with the Marriage Guidance Council, is a Methodist lay preacher and a school governor. She is solid and stolid, with dark straight hair and a firm straight mouth, short but full of presence. She says that she agrees that *Babbletower* is better written than most pornography, but doesn't believe it is literature. Literature, she says, is complex and varied. *Babbletower,* like all pornography, is simple and repetitive—"like a good wank, if you'll forgive the expression." It repeats pain and hurt, and is offensive because it puts ideas into the heads of those who like hurting children. "A good wank is one thing, my lord. Hurting children's another. We live in the permissive society, I'm told. We see where that leads. It leads to Brady and Hindley hurting children. Killing children. All the rest is trappings. This book is offensive and dangerous."

Asked whether she agrees with Phyllis Pratt that fantasy might provide a beneficent release, she says she does not. "Not in my experience, it doesn't. I think that's *her* fantasy, if I may say so. Airy-fairy. I think it does more good to watch and pray, if you feel temptations, than to set pen to paper and indulge your imagination. Watch and pray." Asked by Oliphant if she believes that this goes for stabbing people with bread-knives too, she replies that that is not the issue in question. "But yes, quite probably. Watch and pray. Somebody somewhere may wield a bread-knife in earnest, as a result of reading about one." The Court stirs: they are Phyllis Pratt fans. Samuel Oliphant pushes his advantage.

"You are not a great reader, Miss Cross? You do not have a passion for literature?"

"No. I don't. I think a lot of time is wasted by a lot of people, reading rubbish, and talking rubbish about books. But I *do* know the difference, I think, between a book that is just nasty and a book that is positively hurtful."

"How do you know?"

"I know quite a lot—pragmatically—about the sort of people who are vulnerable to that sort of book. It's common sense."

"And do you consider *yourself* depraved and corrupted by *Babbletower.*"

"Sickened. Disgusted."

"That is not what I asked."

"No. But I am not its expected audience. I watch and pray."

Superintendent Wren is a large, ferociously groomed wax-skinned man, with a surprisingly light voice. His evidence is dull and cumulative, a list of cases in which it is his understanding that crimes were incited, or suggested, by reading matter. "Those that are content with reading," he says, "don't stay content, they start thinking, Why *not,* and then they go on to try it out. Like Ian Brady. They try it out." One of his examples is a man who, hearing *The Brothers Karamazov* read on the wireless, was suddenly seized with an impulse, snatched up an axe from his coalshed, and murdered his mother-in-law in her bed.

Augustine Weighall, to pre-empt the Defence, asks him, "You are not suggesting that *The Brothers Karamazov* should be banned."

"No, sir. I am not. I am just explaining, that those vulnerable to suggestion, do act on it. Now this book is not like *The Brothers Karamazov,* a difficult book, that makes you think, a human book, that makes you feel. It is a book in which nothing happens except sex and death, a typical pornographer's book—"

"Objection. The witness's opinion as to whether the book is pornographic is inadmissible."

"Objection sustained."

The suffragan bishop's name is Humphrey Swan. He is thin and sad and bespectacled and insubstantial. He says that *Babbletower* is evil, and far from presenting a Christian view of the world, as Canon Holly has argued, is quite possibly open to prosecution for blasphemy in connection with its dubious presentation of Our Lord's sufferings. He expatiates on this at some length. He says that the book *does* lead the weak into temptation, temptation to great evil.

Asked by Hefferson-Brough if he considers that he himself has been depraved and corrupted by the book, he replies that he has been dragged through dirt and made to see horrors.

Q. I did not ask if you felt disgusted. I asked if you felt you had been depraved and corrupted.

A. If I must answer that question, yes or no, I must answer yes. I am a worse man, a sicker soul, for having read that book. I shall take time, I shall need effort, to recover from the experience. An element of good in my soul has been slaughtered and is festering.

Q. That is strong language, Bishop.

A. So is the disgusting language of that book, sir. Strong and bad. Worse than bad, because it is *truly* tempting in its sensuousness. Evil. Evil.

Rupert Parrott's face is red with fury when he sees the jaunty figure of Roger Magog in the witness box. He says in a stage whisper to his solicitor, "He thought there was more attention in it for him, this way." The judge stares reprovingly. Magog states that he is an educator, a writer on matters social, literary and educational. He states that he is a member of the Steerforth Committee of Enquiry. He is wearing a red bow-tie and a kind of navy blazer. He smiles around the court, including Parrott in his benignity.

Weighall. People may be surprised to see you in this court, Mr. Magog, appearing as a witness for the prosecution. You have,

I believe, a reputation as a liberal thinker, a defender of our liberties?

Magog. Indeed I have. I am proud of it. I have written essays on freedom of speech. I spoke in favour of *Lady Chatterley.* I wrote articles in support of the Sexual Offences Bill, which is, as we speak, before the House of Commons, and will, I trust, reach the Statute Book this summer.

Weighall. You wrote an article in the *Guardian,* I believe, when *Babbletower* was first published.

Magog. I did.

Weighall. Tell the Court about this article.

Magog. It was called "Sticks and Stones May Break Your Bones." It argued that the written word could harm no one—no adult—and that there should not be any prohibition of any written text depicting any lawful act, as it is impossible in practice to distinguish pornography from literature, and it is more important that literature not be repressed than that pornography is *suppressed.*

Weighall. Admirable sentiments, you may think. Yet you are prepared, now, to argue before this Court, that the tendency of *Babbletower* IS to deprave and corrupt those who may read it?

Magog. (very firmly) I am.

Weighall. What brought about this change?

Magog. It was quite simple. I read the book. (Gales of laughter in court.) I knew you would laugh. You may laugh, you may all laugh, you have a right to laugh. I made a fool of myself, but I have learned something. When I wrote the article I genuinely believed *no book* could harm someone like me, someone normal and sensible and well read. It was a matter of principle. Then I read the book. It was a dreadful experience. I know now what it is to feel depraved and corrupted. This book—you may laugh—revealed things to me about myself that horrified me—that if I were a weaker man, if I were some of the unfortunate children I have taught—might have tempted me. In short—I saw the light. I deliberately use the religious language of a conversion experience. It was a sign. It is better *not* to live in a society which indulges and admires depictions of cruelty. I was made deeply uncomfortable by the *Marat-Sade,* I was disgusted and dirtied, but I believed it was for the good of my soul to see those horrors. I am told there is a writer who has made what he believes is art out of *enacting* the horrors of the Moors Murders for audiences. I am told he claims he is taking "crucial anxiety" and "turning it upside-down in creative play." I have heard that they are arguing that they should have access to corpses and disembowel them in Harrods' windows—artists have as much right as anatomists to corpses, they say. I have no doubt Mason would find it easy to justify the horrors of *Babbletower* on the same grounds. But I do not want to live in a society that can find anything—*anything at all*—playful or creative in these horrors. I have come to believe they should be—not swept under the carpet—but incinerated. Burned with flames of fire. I have had enough of the Permissive Society and before long those who advocate more and more of it will come to feel as I do, to weep for their lost cleanliness and innocence. True freedom is not freedom to hurt others.

Samuel Oliphant takes up this phrase in cross-examination.

Q. Mr. Magog. You said, "True freedom is not the freedom to hurt others."

A. I did. It isn't a fashionable thought, these days. I stand by it.

Q. But, Mr. Magog, is not that—according to Professor Smith, according to Dr. Gander, according to Mr. Wedderburn—is not that the central message of *Babbletower* itself?

A. *Babbletower* is a text that twists round and round itself like the snake round the tree. What *is* its true message? We have heard that the Marquis de Sade felt we should be free to murder and rape. The devil can dress his texts with a little morality. The message I get from *Babbletower* is Sade's message, the modish message of the moment. The author kills off his murderous hero to give his readers another sadistic kick. It is clever and disgusting and infectious.

. . .

Sir Augustine's last witness comes into the witness box slowly, and when he is there, is hardly visible above its rim. He is tiny, old and frail; he has a sweet, small face, with a parchment-coloured skin traced like an ancient map with fine lines and the brown islands of age; he wears gold-rimmed spectacles on a beaked nose, and a black silk skull cap above a fringe of baby-fine bright white hair. He wears a loose black jacket, under which his spine is humped and twisted; his hands are twigs, claws, knots of bone and vein, which grip the bar in front of him. He says that he is Professor Efraim Ziz, and teaches in Cambridge. He is an expert on Jewish history and rabbinical writings. He is a survivor of the Treblinka death camp, where he lost his wife, his children and his sisters. He is the author of *Babel and Silence,* and of *The Tongues of Men and of Angels,* studies of Jewish mystical histories of language and silence, of a book on Kafka and the German language, and of *A Private Place.* This last, he explains in a small, clear, precise voice, is an account of that sense of "an inner private, silent place" which made possible the survival of some "fortunate or unfortunate inmates of those places."

He is asked by Sir Augustine if he has read *Babbletower.*

A. I have.

Q. Can you give us your opinion of it.

A. It is written by a writer of talent. It is a clever and tormented book. In the last resort, it is pornography, not literature.

Q. Can you justify that opinion? So that the jury may understand how you arrived at it?

A. Pornography is confined to certain aspects of human nature; it is to do with one person's power over another person's body. It reduces human beings to bodily functions—certain repetitive, emphasised, selected functions which are made public without any remnants of privacy, or secrecy (the places of imagination, gentleness, the unspoken, kindness and delight). Pornography tears away veils from shames which then fester and destroy. It diminishes humanity.

Q. You have written about these matters, I believe.

A. I have. I should like, if I may, to quote a passage from Maurice Girodias's *Olympia Reader,* which I criticised in my book.

"Moral censorship was an inheritance from the past, deriving from centuries of domination by the Christian clergy. Now that it is practically over, we may expect literature to be transformed by the advent of freedom. Not freedom in its negative aspects, but as the means of exploring all the positive aspects of the human mind, which are all more or less related to, or generated by, sex."

This is obviously a foolish statement, an exaggeration. But it is an exaggeration of a position which is taken by respectable people, including those who have eloquently defended *Babbletower.* Nothing should be hidden, nothing should be silent, nothing should be unspoken. And what should be spoken is sex, is the body *as body.* A society with no religious beliefs may reach this position logically. Nietzsche, to whom Mr. Mason is so attached, wrote, "Once Spirit was God, then it became man, now it is becoming mob." Mob is public man as pure animal, as pure body. I have seen the power of totalitarian states; I have seen the power of those who had total freedom—total *permission*—to do as they pleased with the bodies of others. There are limits to this power. There are *not so many things* you can do to bodies. But those who "enjoy" this freedom—in all senses of the word "enjoy"—resemble each other.

It is not only—perhaps not mostly—what Efraim Ziz says that has its effect on the crowded courtroom, perhaps on the jury. It is his physical presence, his frailty, his age, his survival, his gentleness, his sweet seriousness. Samuel Oliphant rises to ask him, as he has asked Magog, whether he cannot accept that *Babbletower* is on his side, is making his own points, is "opposed to total or totalitarian freedom."

Ziz replies:

"Mr. Mason has used the myth of the Tower of Babel, which is a myth about language and God, to make a modern point about the human body and its freedom and its sufferings. There is a long tradition of rabbinical commentary on the fact that the inhabitants of the Tower were not all destroyed, as the inhabitants of Sodom and Gomorrah were, or the whole generation before the Flood. And this was, according to Rabbi Juda ha Nassa, because they loved each other. They worked together. After their presumption they were not destroyed, but were taught eighty languages by the eighty angels around the throne of God. Speech and writing were made *more difficult* for them, but they were saved. Whereas Mr. Mason's people are not saved, because there is nothing but total freedom and the body in his book. They are not dignified. There is no hope."

Q. You sound as though you are describing a pessimistic book, but a work of literary merit?

A. I do not say there is no literary merit. I say there is not enough. Not enough to save the book from doing more harm than good to those who read it.

Q. Your view is that of a religious teacher?

A. Yes. And it is that of an expert in pain, who wishes to see less of it in the world.

The barristers make their final speeches. Sir Augustine is clear and on the whole unemotional. He reiterates the point that *Babbletower* is repetitive and constricted in its subject matter; he quotes one or two of the most distressing passages; he quotes also a passage from Sade.

> Is murder a crime in the eyes of Nature? Doubtless we will humiliate man's pride in reducing him to the ranks of other productions of Nature, but nevertheless he is merely an animal like any other, and in the eyes of Nature his death is no more important than that of a fly or an ox. . . . Destruction is Nature's method of progress, and she prompts the murderer to destruction, so that his action shall be the same as plague or famine. . . . In a word, murder is a horror, but a horror often necessary, never criminal, and essential to tolerate in a republic.

Who, he asks, copied out and studied this passage? Who referred to the innocent victims of his sadistic crimes as animals? Ian Brady, the murderer, who shared his reading matter and the nihilism, the desperate vision derived from it, with his dazzled victim and fellow criminal, Myra Hindley. "Do not believe, members of the jury," says Sir Augustine, "that cruel acts and cruel visions cannot be passed on, from one human being to another. The well-intentioned 'experts' who have amused and bemused us with their academic dissertations on the harmless pleasures of sado-masochism and their determined cheerful *liberal* willingness to say that 'everything goes,' refused, almost to a man and woman, to admit that they were sexually or viscerally stirred by the excesses of *Babbletower.* They refused to admit that their flesh tingled or crawled when they read of the torture of little Felicitas or the ingenious death of the Lady Roseace. They are expert witnesses, they are specialist witnesses. Professor Marie-France Smith is a beautiful woman, a cool Frenchwoman, who, for reasons best known to herself, chooses to spend her time studying the sexual dottiness of M. Fourier and the nasty doctrines of the evil Marquis. Canon Holly, a Christian clergyman, is willing to equate the most grotesque fancies of Jude Mason with the sufferings of his Lord. Dr. Gander is harder to follow, but it is clear that his normal responses to depictions of pain, of sexual excitement, of the desire to hurt, are hopelessly entangled in abstract words to which he can give any meaning he chooses—words like 'liberation,' words like 'freedom,' words like 'oppression'—words which can only have the odd meanings they have for him because in fact he lives in a decent society where he is free to say what he pleases because his rights are protected by the vigilance of courts like this, and juries composed of sensible people such as yourselves.

"You have read the book, members of the jury. I do not know how you responded to it. You may have been disgusted, you may have been sickened, you may have been stirred in ways that disturbed you. Your flesh may have crawled, as mine did. I have appeared in many obscenity cases, ladies and gentlemen, and I can tell you that most pornography is sickening in quite a different way from *Babbletower.* It is sickening because it is boring, it is grotesque, not threatening, it is against life because it appeals from dead imaginations to dull imaginations. I will grant that *Babbletower* is better written than the trash which normally, in horrible bulk, appears before the courts. It is more disturbing for that reason. It is more potent. The expert witnesses have told you at some length that this is because of its literary merit. They have also told you that it is hard to assess the literary merit of contemporary works. They have told you their reasons for wanting this book published, and they have told you—most of them—that it has not stirred them up. I think you know better than that, members of the jury. I think your responses are simpler and more honest, not tied up in abstract languages and doctrinaire beliefs. I think you are better judges of what Ian Brady and Myra Hindley might make of *Babbletower*—and not only them, but smaller sadists, ready to do smaller hurts that are nevertheless hurts.

"I believe that Mr. Parrott is a good man, an honest man, a well-intentioned man, and a slightly foolish man, who has been misled by modish rhetoric and mistaken libertarian idealism to take risks that he would have been better to have turned away from. I believe Mr. Mason is a man whose mind and body were depraved and corrupted in his youth—even in his childhood—and I feel a great deal of sympathy for him. My learned friend Mr. Hefferson-Brough obviously feels personal sympathy for the sufferings of this Erstwhile Hog, and I extend mine to him. I believe that Mr. Mason's early experiences did lead directly to his later way of life, his acquaintance with the seamier aspects of our society, and to the form and content of *Babbletower* itself. I believe you may have read, as I have, that it is an accepted understanding, nowadays, that child-beaters have been beaten children, and that those who exploit innocent children sexually have themselves, often, been so exploited as children themselves. It is known as a circle of deprivation—or perhaps a circle of depravity—and it is our duty, as responsible human beings, to break it. Mr. Mason has been hurt, and he is trying—perhaps even unconsciously—to hurt others.

"You have been told—and I tell you again—that discussion of motive, of intention, is irrelevant in deciding whether a work has a tendency to deprave and corrupt. Mr. Parrott may be a good man, and Mr. Mason may believe he is a serious artist, but the first question for you is whether *Babbletower* has a tendency to deprave and corrupt—to deprave and corrupt not *literary experts,* but ordinary men and women, trying to live their lives, men and women who can be tempted or crushed by despair. If you decide that the book has such a tendency, you must then consider whether it has sufficient literary or other merit—sufficient gravity, grace, seriousness, beauty—to outweigh the detrimental effects of this tendency on ordinary readers. Whose testimony will you trust in this? Those long-winded experts, who see the whole thing through a cloud of their own complex terms and good intentions, or the wise Professor Ziz, who believes the book is a dangerous book, is 'pornography not literature' and is himself 'an expert in pain who wishes to see less of it in the world.' "

Hefferson-Brough's speech is longer, noisier, and more repetitive than Sir Augustine's. He says frequently that "in this day and age" much is acceptable that would once have been thought obscene libel, and does not give the impression that he is sure that this is for the best. He says that it is right to publish serious studies of sadism and masochism, and it is right also to make serious literary representations of them. He speaks passionately, and at too great length, in the general perception, of the harm done by secrecy and silence at places like Swineburn, by people like Dr. Grisman Gould. He uses tired words—"brilliant," "outstanding," "promising," "talented"—of Jude Mason, and speaks warmly of the responsibility of Rupert Parrott, of the unlikelihood of Bowers and Eden being found in the position of publishing anything that tends to deprave and corrupt. He praises the good sense of Alexander Wedderburn and Phyllis Pratt; he demolishes Roger Magog with his only literary reference.

"Mr. Facing-both-ways was a character in *Pilgrim's Progress.* Mr. Magog likes to pronounce upon issues of the day. No doubt you will find him pronouncing in favour of *Babbletower* at some point in the future, as he pronounced in favour of it last week." Of Efraim Ziz's evidence he says, perhaps unfortunately, that concentration camp guards can no more be thought of as typical probable readers than can Ian Brady or Myra Hindley. "Ordinary, responsible English people are not like that, ladies and gentlemen. They are like you and me. They can take these things in their stride. If we are to ban all books that might encourage monsters to be monstrous we should start with the Brothers Grimm and the giant who cries fee-fi-fo-fum, I smell the blood of an Englishman. Because some people in some places have ground up bones and made bread we mustn't forbid fairytales. And the eminently sensible Mrs. Pratt has told us that that is what *Babbletower* is—a fairytale."

Samuel Oliphant reads out various passages of *Babbletower,* none of them sexual or sadistic: the descriptions of the woods, the remarks of Samson Origen, the descriptions of the tower and its daily life. He reads well. He says, "Is this depraving or corrupting? Or is it good writing, by a young man whose career stands in danger of being mined by the enthusiasm of moral zealots, out of touch with the times. A young man whose life has been hard, but who has, in circumstances of pain and difficulty, written a brilliant, daring and moving book, for which he should be being rewarded, rather than castigated and punished? A young man, who, far from being a seducer and a tempter, is a stern moralist and a tragic poet."

The jury look at their hands, at the ceiling, at the prisoner in the dock.

Mr. Justice Gordale Balafray sums up. His summing up is dry, and he thanks the jury for their patience, giving the impression that his own has sometimes been tested. He tells them that they are to decide the question of obscenity—of whether the book, as a whole, has a tendency to deprave and corrupt. If, and only if, they come to the conclusion that it has, they must decide on whether the work has sufficient literary merit—or other quality of value to society—to outweigh the tendency to deprave and corrupt. "The Defence has raised a defence under Section 4, which entails, as we have seen, the calling of expert witnesses. As we are all aware, the world these days is a world of specialised knowledge and is full of experts on everything under the sun. But English criminal law is based upon the view that a jury takes of the facts and not upon the view that experts may have. You, ladies and gentlemen of the jury, are the sole judges of the facts in this case. It is my place to put the law to you, but the facts—both as to the tendency to deprave and corrupt, and as to the literary or other arguments which may outweigh that tendency—are yours and yours alone to decide. You have heard the dictionary definitions of the words 'deprave' and 'corrupt.' I do not know if I can improve on those definitions, or elaborate on the meaning of the word 'tendency.' "

The judge goes on to recapitulate the evidence. On the whole, he is fair and appears to lean to neither side, though he becomes testy when faced with the evidence of Canon Holly and Elvet Gander, and says, "You may think that the Prosecution has a point when it refers to the obfuscating language of some of the so-called experts, their use of words in ways contrary to commonsense interpretations of those words, and so on. You are here to uphold the commonsense virtues, to represent ordinary men and women." He remarks, also, that in Canada only five witnesses may appear for each side, and states that "there is some attraction in this restriction, you may think, in this concentration of witness."

He speaks of the jury's solemn duty to balance the decision as to whether the book is obscene against the difficult assessment—"more difficult, as both sides admit, in the case of a new book, by a living author—of its literary or other merit." He reiterates, "You, the jury, are to be the sole judges of these things. You are to decide, on the basis of what you have read and heard, whether this book is obscene, and, if it is, whether its merits outweigh this obscenity sufficiently for the publication of the book to be in the public interest."

The jury retires. The Bowers and Eden people discuss whether or not the judge's summing up was hostile or friendly: the fact that they cannot decide is felt to be on the whole a good sign. Canon Holly ventures the opinion that they have put up a strong fight, and Rupert Parrott says, "Shut up," and then apologises. The judge sentences some prisoners who are already convicted. Jude Mason has disappeared somewhere. Frederica cannot imagine his feelings. Avram Snitkin tells her that no jury will convict for obscenity "in this day and age." Frederica snaps, "I don't want to hear that phrase again." "Why?" says Snitkin. "It's a pompous cliché." "Its got a precise meaning." "Its connotations are horrid. Anyway you're wrong. I've been looking at their faces. They hated Canon Holly. They thought Jude was putting them down. They didn't like him." "Juries don't work on 'like' and 'not like,' you know. They take their duties very seriously. They aren't coming back."

After three hours, the jury return to enquire whether they have to decide the question of obscenity separately from, and before, the question of literary merit. The judge tells them that this is indeed so. The foreman says that this is difficult, given that they have, so to speak, heard everything at once, both sides of the matter. The judge agrees that it is difficult, and says he wishes he could help them further.

After five hours, they return. Jude Mason returns to the dock. The clerk speaks into the silence.

Members of the jury, are you agreed upon a verdict?

Foreman. We are.

Clerk. Do you find that Bowers and Eden are guilty or not guilty of publishing an obscene article?

Foreman. Guilty.

Clerk. Do you find that Jude Mason is guilty or not guilty of publishing an obscene article?

Foreman. Guilty.

There is a general hesitation in the Court. The judge says, "Let us be quite clear. You find the publishers and the author guilty of publishing an obscene article. A defence has been raised under Section Four of the Obscene Publications Act, arguing that the book has literary and other merits that outweigh the alleged obscenity of the book. Do you find such merits in the book in question?"

Foreman. No, my lord. We do not.

Clerk. And that is the verdict of you all?

Foreman. It is.

Frederica finds she is weeping. Rupert Parrott listens white-faced to the judge, who says that the book has been published in good faith by an honourable firm, imposes a small fine (£500) and orders all copies of the book to be seized. The judge then turns to Jude.

"It is possible for me to impose a sentence of imprisonment upon you, but it seems to me that it would be wrong to do so. Evidence has been given, including your own, that you see your work as a serious work of art, although the jury has found otherwise. I shall impose a fine of fifty pounds, having regard to your clear lack of means to pay any greater fine."

"I knew you were all against me," says Jude.

XXI

Rupert Parrott declares his intention to appeal. The lawyers advise against it, on grounds of expense, of the unlikelihood of success, of waste of time and effort. It will take a long time, they say, and a great deal of money, to acquire the court records, which are in any case only selective. Parrott says that he has a complete record of his own, recorded by the diligent Avram Snitkin, and sets his secretary to the transcribing of this document. He speaks of engaging a new barrister, since Hefferson-Brough is firmly set against going any further. Mention is made of John Mortimer, a young playwright and divorce lawyer who is also having some success in this field. A correspondence of some acrimony begins in *The Times* about jurors, and exactly what, or who, the commonsense common man is whom they are supposed to represent. A fund is started for the Defence of the Arts against legal onslaughts from the Establishment. It is not very well subscribed. Samuel Oliphant is more in favour of an appeal than Godfrey Hefferson-Brough, and spends some time perusing the typescript of Snitkin's tapes as it piles up in Miss Patty Stott's out-tray. There is a snag. His client has disappeared. He went to the lavatory whilst Parrott was making statements to the Press at the end of the trial, and has not been seen since. Letters to his convenience address remain unanswered. His slots before the art students are filled by an ex-boxer, chocolate-coloured and muscular.

Frederica does not really listen to Parrott's troubles about the loss of Jude, because she has troubles of her own. The custody hearing approaches, and Jude's trial has made Frederica even more despondent than she would have been. She feels that both she and Jude are naughty children whose naughtinesses have found them out, have been judged by the inscrutable rules of the inscrutable grown-up world to be not naughtiness but grave crimes. She feels too, as children do feel, that what she thought was the grown-up world, and believed to operate by logic, operates in fact according to the system created out of its own prejudices and emotions, which cannot be second-guessed. She and Jude have been made to recite travesties of their life stories, in language they would never have chosen for themselves. They have been judged and found wanting. In a sense, it does not matter. Who cares, Frederica thinks, what those twelve stolid and baffled people think of *Babbletower,* what His Honour Judge Plumb makes of educated women or sex after the Pill? But these things do matter. Jude's book will not be read, and worse, worse, Leo will be taken from her.

At first she draws comfort from the frequent visits and reassurances of Anthea Barlow, who exclaims brightly that she has established a real *rapport* with little Leo, who is "wise for his years," who is "a constant surprise to me"—"You must be so proud of him, Mrs. Reiver." Later Frederica begins to feel irritation with Mrs. Barlow's over-frequent quotations from Julian of Norwich. "All shall be well, and all shall be well, and all manner of thing shall be well, Mrs. Reiver."

"You don't *know* that."

"I believe it. Dame Julian was talking of the long term, of course. You don't have any religious beliefs, Mrs. Reiver?"

"No," says Frederica, reflecting that even here, where she is simply being intellectually truthful, she is open to judgement, judgement which may take her child from her. "My brother-in-law is a clergyman," says Frederica lamely.

"All shall be well and all shall be well and all manner of thing shall be well. By the purification of the motive in the ground of our beseeching. That's how Dame Julian goes on. By the purification of the motive."

"I'm not quite sure what you mean."

"Oh, I'm just chattering. You must want what's best for Leo, for dear Leo, Mrs. Reiver."

Frederica has a vision of fields and paddocks, of woods and hills, an English vision. She sees Sooty's stolid black figure swishing through meadow grass in a slight drizzle.

"Nothing is altogether best," she says. "It's not black and white. It's a mess. Most of life is. Courts don't seem to know that."

"Oh, of course they do. They don't see life at those rare moments when it isn't a mess, you must remember. Mess is their business. You must have faith."

"They believed all those lies those women told. Olive and Rosalind and Pippy Mammott."

"It may not be the same judge, Mrs. Reiver. Have faith."

But it is the same judge. The custody hearing takes place before His Honour Judge Plumb. This time Leo is taken to the courtroom, and sits with Mrs. Barlow whilst his parents tell the judge what arrangements they have made for his welfare. Nigel's barrister has brought photographs, of Bran House, of the orchard, of Leo's room; he has also brought photographs of the pile of bed-heads and rotting chairs in Hamelin Square, luridly lit by the bonfire, in whose shadows the black children dance. He explains that Leo's place is assured at Brock's and Swineburn. "I need not assure Your Honour that the Swineburn of the 1960s is a very different place from the Swineburn that has been so much in the press since the *Babbletower* case. It is a traditional but forward-looking school, with high standards and a kindly regime." He explains that the three women of Bran House are in the Court and ready to speak, or to give any help they can to describe the loving home that awaits Leo—as it always has—since he was snatched away from it.

Nigel speaks. He is brief, he is sensible. He says his son is his son and he is fortunate enough to be able to provide for his security and loving care. He says he does not doubt that his ex-wife loves the boy in her way, but he does not think she is the type to be interested in kids, not really, and she will find she can do very well by visiting and so forth, which she will be free to do. He says he doesn't like the look of the place where she is living or the kinds of friends she has, and he doesn't want Leo to grow up there. He speaks brusquely, man to man, looking the judge in the eye, confident but anxious *enough*.

Pippy Mammott speaks. She says that the boy's mother has never loved him, that she isn't maternal, that she only wants the boy to spite his family, that she herself is his real mother, has looked after his sicknesses, taught him to tie his little shoes, done *everything* whilst "she" looked on, or "sulked," or "read books."

Frederica speaks. Or tries to speak. She is inaudible. The judge peers down at her, his long white face creased into a frown.

"Speak up."

"I'm sorry. I wanted to say, the square isn't like that, now. It's gentrified. We've got a circular lawn, with a yin-yang pattern in bricks. The dump's gone. We all contributed."

"I see."

"It's important not to make it look worse than it is. Because any arrangements I make can't compete with Bran House. I wouldn't want Leo not to go there. But he wants to be with me, and my arrangements are good, and will work—though it is harder for a woman to work, and look after a child, than a man. But we are two women, two responsible women, Your Honour, two efficient women. I know the Bran House people love Leo—he loves them—but I too have feelings about tradition and family. My family is a bookish family, a *thinking* family—it matters as much to me that Leo should grow up in a house *full of books,* as it does to his father that there should be a pony and woods. And I care about schools and I happen to think it's *wicked* to send away little boys to sleep in dormitories when they could be at home with their mothers. You may not agree, but it is a belief I do hold, and Leo is my son. My father was a schoolmaster in a boarding school, a very liberal one, so I know what I'm talking about.

"I know I've been criticised. You criticised me, when you heard the divorce. Some of the evidence you heard was lies, but that's over, that's done. It isn't ideal to have to try to earn your living and bring up a son—and I won't take maintenance for me, I don't want it—it isn't ideal, but it can be done. If I were the person they say I am, I wouldn't even be *trying* to keep Leo. When you heard the divorce, you asked if I meant to take him when I left. I said I thought of leaving him because it would be better for him, but he insisted on coming. Please understand—*that is what happened.* I thought of leaving him, and he came, and—he's a little boy, but he knows what he's doing. I wouldn't think of it again. Unless he asked."

Judge Plumb says: And if he asked?

Frederica: I'd listen, I suppose. He's his own—

She cannot speak.

Judge Plumb asks to speak to Mrs. Barlow, alone. Mrs. Barlow comes out of the Court and says the judge wants to see Leo, who has been taken away to "play" somewhere else. There is a long wait. Then all the parties file back into the Court. Frederica feels ill. Her life has passed, in this moment, entirely out of her control. She was proud and fierce and independent: she was clever and free and wild. And now she is in a room full of people all of whom exercise control, influence, over her future, because of the existence of an absent small boy whose rights and desires are more important to her than her own. She thinks, briefly, that sex made Leo, and remembers pleasure with Nigel, which seems to have nothing to do with Leo. She feels emptied, and knows that everything will be taken from her. She does not even hear the beginning of the judge's remarks.

". . . there had to be substantial doubt in this case whether the very strong presumption in the favour of the mother, the biological presumption that she would care for the child, that the child needed her physical presence, at least in the early years, would apply. Mrs. Reiver has been described—by those unfriendly to her—as 'not the maternal type,' and it is true that she is not an archetypal mother-figure. But few real women are, yet most bring up children. Miss Mammott is extremely motherly, and whereas Mrs. Reiver showed no signs of resentment towards Miss Mammott for her role in the little boy's upbringing, Miss Mammott displayed a spitefulness towards Mrs. Reiver, a possessiveness about the boy, which I did not find wholly encouraging. It has been eloquently argued, on Mr. Reiver's behalf, that his family is old and has traditions his son may inherit. I was however struck by Mrs. Reiver's argument that her own more modest family also has traditions, which she may reasonably expect her son to adhere to. It takes all sorts to make a world, the sporting and the bookish, the entrepreneurial and the intellectual.

"I am entirely convinced that both parents love Leo very deeply, and are primarily interested in his welfare. In this he is a fortunate little boy, compared to many who appear before me. It is clear that he would be less comfortable living with his mother than with his father, but comfort is not everything. And as an old boy of a particularly spartan prep school and public school I am inclined—which may surprise her—to agree with Mrs. Reiver that little boys, at least, are best at home, with those who love them.

"I have been very impressed with the clarity and perceptiveness of Mrs. Barlow's accounts of her conversations with both the father and the mother, the people at Bran House and the people in Hamelin Square. She herself is very impressed with the intelligence of the little boy, and after speaking to her, I have myself spoken this morning to Leo. I always take off my robes on such occasions, so as not to frighten the children more than can be helped. It is quite clear to me from talking to Leo—and, indeed, from what Mrs. Barlow reports—that he wishes to stay with his mother. He does not wish to lose contact with his father or his old home but he fears the loss of his mother as the worst thing—"the *bad thing*" that could happen to him. Mrs. Barlow has suggested that there may be an element of fear *that his mother would leave him,* in his fear that he will be taken from her. These are deep waters. They need not concern this Court, since it is quite clear what the boy wants, and he is able to state his wishes fearlessly, and in the expectation of being listened to—on which his parents are to be congratulated.

"I therefore award joint custody of the boy to his father and his mother—with an expressed wish that his mother's wishes should prevail on his early schooling at least. I award care and control of the boy to his mother, Frederica Reiver."

Outside the court again, Frederica stands giddy, looking round for Leo. There is a scuffling sound, and a shrill cry, and she feels a violent pain on the right side of her head. Pippy Mammott has rushed up and swung her heavy handbag at Frederica's face. The sharp clasp cuts her eye-corner: her cheek begins to swell into a grazed, bleeding bruise. The Bran House people gather round Pippy, who is crying hysterically, and pull and hustle her away. Nigel stops to study Frederica, but Mrs. Barlow has taken Frederica in charge, has a Persian lamb arm round her shoulder—she smells of Je Reviens—and is drawing her away down a corridor. In some curious way, this moment of violence is a release. Nigel calls, "I'll see you," Frederica nods, her head bowed over a bloodied handkerchief. Heels tap on stone: the opponents hurry apart. In a kind of antechamber Frederica finds Leo. She begins to cry. Anthea Barlow brings a bowl of warm water, with cotton wool, and dabs at Frederica's cheek. Tears run into the water. Leo sits beside her, his body pushed against hers. Frederica smells disinfectant, Je Reviens, and Leo's hair, Leo's warm red hair. He does not discuss his experiences. He does not ask how she hurt herself. He winds his fingers in hers, and says, "When can we go home?"

Spring 1967 runs into summer. The gentrification of Hamelin Square continues: tubs of geraniums and tiny cypresses appear and are stolen, more windows are painted white, a park bench appears on the grass, is stolen, and is replaced with a more stolid one, bolted to the earth, with a bright green waste bin, also bolted to the earth, next to it. Homosexual behaviour (in private) and abortion are made legal. The world explodes in colour: the Beatles produce *Sergeant Pepper's Lonely*

Hearts Club Band, with its Peter Blake cover on which the four moustachioed majordomos in brilliant satin uniforms stand beside their suited waxwork selves of 1963, under the cardboard eyes of Karl Marx, Laurel and Hardy, Alistair Crowley, Cassius Clay, Mona Lisa, W. C. Fields and Tarzan. The songs are full of brilliance, "Lucy in the Sky with Diamonds," tangerine trees and marmelade skies. BBC2 begins to transmit in colour. Frederica has a colour TV because she has acquired a small TV column in a women's magazine which flares briefly under the name of *Boadicea,* with mini-skirted, glacé-booted, gold-macintoshed career women striding through it. She cannot stop watching, and neither can Leo. The colours are rich, are jewelled, are electric and psychedelic after the small grainy grey worlds of *Muffin the Mule, The Virginian* and *Batman.* An orange cut in half is a glistening revelation, an open rose is a visual drama, the Queen's pink and blue and green and yellow outfits seem absurd and inappropriate, as they did not in mere black and white. The *Report of the Steerforth Committee* is published. It is a fat document in two volumes and arouses a storm of protest—*Charter for Permissiveness, The Beginning of the Age of Ignorance, Fetter Our Children with Rote Learning, Why Do They Not Realise That Education Is Oppression, Out of Touch Committee, Committee Unacceptably Child-Centred, Where Are Our Verbs and Conjunctions, Participles Depart* and so on. Roger Magog adds a note of protest saying that the committee has failed to understand the need for partnership and trust between pupils and teachers. Guy Croom adds a dry note predicting that certain skills are about to disappear for ever. No journalist reads the document through, and its conclusions are often stated to be the opposite of what their authors believe they are. Alexander commissions a series of modern-dress Shakespeare scenes for educational television, and thinks of writing a Brechtian play about the French Revolution.

Cassius Clay tears up his draft papers and refuses to join the war against the coloured people of Asia in Vietnam. In June the Israelis win an efficient and passionate Six-Day War against the Egyptians and the Jordanians: they take possession of Jerusalem, and process to the Wailing Wall, despite booby-trap bombs which explode amongst the trumpets.

In July the Round House is given over to a Congress on the Dialectics of Liberation, which is addressed by anti-psychiatrists who believe that the human race is being destroyed by illusion and mystification; by

Stokely Carmichael, who believes the Third World and the American blacks must get the guns from the white man and use them; by Herbert Marcuse, who is happy to see flowers and believes in a Marxian liberation of the instinctual self from technology. Violent attacks are made, verbally, on mass suicide and mass murder, and David Cooper sums up, calling his summing up *Beyond Words,* calling for an end to "the opposition between subject-object, white-black; oppressor-oppressed one; colonizer-colonized; torturer-tortured; murderer-murdered one; psychiatrist-patient; teacher-taught; keeper-kept; the cannibal-the one who is eaten up; the fucker-the fucked; the shitter-the shitted upon." There is an orchestra of piano frame, metal pipes, milk crates, tin cans. There are flowers everywhere, blooming and wilting.

Plans proceed to appeal against the *Babbletower* decision. There is concern over the non-appearance of Jude Mason; there is a theory that he has fled to Paris again and an underlying, suppressed fear that he may be dead. Another person who has not been seen is John Ottokar, who has made no sign of life since he was called a co-respondent. Frederica has given him up; she is proud, she will not telephone his place of work; if he does not want to see her, she has other things to do. She goes back once or twice to Desmond Bull's studio, goes dancing with Hugh Pink, who dances badly, but has sold a volume of poems—*Orpheus Underground*—to Rupert Parrott. It is a strange, hectic time. It will come to seem much longer in memory than it is, as though Flower Power went on and on. To most people the noise, the smells, the brilliance, are peripheral, are words only, go past whilst they cook or push pushchairs or nurse the elderly, or work in shops and banks and laboratories, wandering into clubs or festivals, once, or twice, or more often. In June 1967 the "spontaneous underground" UFO sprouts the Electric Garden in Covent Garden, which opens with a fight between supporters of Yoko Ono and the Exploding Galaxy. Avram Snitkin is now conducting ethnomethodological research into flower people, electric gardens, Technicolor dreams and alchemical weddings. He has taken a fancy to Frederica and invites her to come along with him from time to time, but she does not go until August, when the Electric Garden has folded and re-opened as the Middle-Earth.

In July Leo is seven and Frederica is summoned to see his teacher at a parents' evening. She sits with Agatha in the school hall, under a dangling forest of paper streamers of paper flowers, pinned to cotton threads attached to the paint with blue-tack and drawing-pins. They wait in line, until the teacher—a young woman in a kind of suede tunic, with long hair like Minnehaha's and eyes painted round in black—can give them their ten minutes. Frederica sits, when her moment comes, hunched over the low desk.

"He's doing just fine, Mrs. Reiver. Such a bright little boy."

"He is, isn't he?"

"His relationships with the others are good, no problems there, he has lots of friends."

"I'm so glad."

"He hasn't started reading independently yet, of course, he's a bit late with that. I expect he's a slow developer."

"What?"

"I expect he's a slow developer. As far as reading goes."

"There must be some mistake. He has an enormous vocabulary. He said 'incandescent' the other day. He talks about 'prototype' jets and 'machinations.' "

"I expect he does. He probably doesn't have the motor skills. Don't worry."

"Listen—he can read *all Beatrix Potter.* He reads them *to me.*"

"Reads, or recites, Mrs. Reiver? He's probably too clever for his own good, for his reading, that is."

"He reads them to Saskia."

"Saskia is a fast reader. Don't worry, Mrs. Reiver, all children develop at different speeds. He'll learn."

"But my family is a reading family—"

"I expect you put him off. A bit, you know. Too much emphasis, too many expectations. Go easy on him."

"But if he *can't read*—he can't learn *anything*—"

"Don't worry, Mrs. Reiver."

She looks at her watch.

Frederica talks to Agatha. She says, "He can't read, I didn't *notice,* he talks all the time, I'm dreadful—"

"I did wonder," says Agatha. "I tried him out once or twice. Saskia's quick. He's impatient. He can't be bothered with the little words, and he can't run at the big ones. They teach them with all sorts of methods, look-and-say, ITA, all sorts of experiments, some of which work with some children, some of which don't. Don't worry. There are people I know who can help. It's early days."

Frederica is desolate. She says nothing to Leo. She listens to him "read" *The Tale of Mr. Tod* and feels, when he goes to Bran House for his summer holiday, that she deserves to lose him. It has not occurred to her that Leo could be *her son* and not read.

August comes. The Beatles go to meditate with the Maharishi and Brian Epstein kills himself. The Beatles return. They say the Maharishi has told them not to mourn. Jude Mason is still lost, and Frederica, restless and lonely, goes to the Middle Earth with Avram Snitkin. Avram Snitkin is observing, not dancing. He has brought with him a notebook with an *art nouveau* cover in purple and gold and silver, and a paper bag full of fudge. He takes out the pieces of fudge and arranges them in a row on the edge of the table in front of him. "Have some," he says. "It's hashish fudge, it's a good recipe, it'll do you good." His eyes are moist with happiness, his hair floats gingery towards his shoulders, his beard bunches, his bare crown gleams purple and green, orange and rose, yellow and crimson, in the strobe lighting. He squats like a stolid dwarf in a corner and smokes his own rolled cigarettes, reaching out meditatively from time to time and ingesting the hashish fudge. Frederica wants to take a piece, and does not. She is a northern Puritan, getting back control of her own life. She has a little flowered shift, with cut-away armpits, a little girl's shift, covered with great innocent white daisies and brilliant blue convolvulus, on a black ground. The points of her red helmet of hair lick her white cheeks.

"Do dance," says Avram Snitkin, "if you feel like it." He takes another chunk of fudge. Frederica looks around. The place is like a warehouse, or a hangar. It is concrete, coloured only by the moving lights, which weave and dance and swirl, giddy and violent. It is full of scented smoke; the smoke changes the light, thickening it, filtering it, catching it and twisting it. The noise threads through the light. Somewhere, a long way away, a band is playing, a group is singing. Avram Snitkin likes to be marginal; they are in an alcove, round a corner, they cannot see the players.

Frederica is not musical. She is a not a child of her time in this. She is torn apart by the noise. By the amplification of the throb, by the howl, by the blast. By the thrum, by the beat, by the rhythm, by the reprise, by the clash. It gives her no pleasure. It explodes the blood in her ears, it appears to be jabbing through her kidneys, it is pain, it is pain, it is pain.

They are dancing. They are gyrating, dreamily, in their conical witch-shifts, in their elven robes, in their falling black layers of cheesecloth, in their silver-and-white net, in their *fleurs du mal,* purple and black, in their white roses and moonflowers. They sway like snakes piped to, they twist and turn slowly, they move all together to the rhythm, smiling slightly, intent in their incantations and evocations. They are all dancing together, but there are no couples. Frederica is good at jiving—she can twist and turn at the end of a man's arm, spiral away and stamp and laugh and come back. Jive is sex, jive is a swing, jive leaves you laughing and breathless. These creatures—most of them are girls—are like mushrooms, like twining flowers, they go round and back, all together, all separate, a group, no individuals, no pairs.

"I do empathise with these people," says Avram Snitkin. He pops in another cube of fudge. His smile is beatific. "I do empathise with these people." Frederica looks at his notebook. He has written, "I do empathise with these people," drawn a smiley-face, added a copperplate alphabet and a series of loops followed by another, round which he has drawn a snake.

He repeats, "I do empathise with these people."

Frederica gets up and walks carefully round the dancers, looking for the loo. The noise increases. It is a not-unsubtle noise, turned up to a howl, to a screech, to a scream. She catches a glimpse of the group that is playing. The lead singer has a loose coat of multicoloured satin patches with huge silver cuffs and lapels. His trousers are white satin and he wears a kind of Augustus John hat in white satin. He is waving a white stick wound round with flowers and ribbons. His head is thrown back, his throat throbs with his ululations, his face is John Ottokar's face.

Frederica turns round and starts walking back again. She thinks she must go home. Her teeth are blue, her hands are green, her hair is murky purple. She sifts smoke, she slides between dreaming figures.

She makes her way back to Avram Snitkin, who says or shouts, "I do empathise with these people."

Frederica cannot speak. Two lines of Herbert come into her head.

> *Thus thinne and leane, without a fence or friend*
> *I was blown through, with ev'ry storm and winde.*

She begins to say them to herself like a mantra. Later, whenever anyone says "the sixties," this is what she will think of, Zag and the Szyzgy (Ziggy) Zy-Goats singing in the Middle-Earth, the hum become a howl, the maze of light, the crowd of single dancers. Thus thinne and leane, without a fence or friend, *I do empathise with these people,* I was blown through, by every wand'ring wind. Blown through, blown through, blown through.

"We need Jude to sign the appeal form," says Rupert Parrott. "Frederica, you were always our lead to him. Can't you find him?"

"There's not been a squeak out of him. All the Press fuss, no one has had any idea."

"You don't think he's jumped in the river?"

"I would have thought," says Samuel Oliphant, "that he'd have made sure we saw him jump, or at least found his floating body."

"I thought that at first. I'm not so sure now. Don't we know *anyone* who might know where he is?"

"Daniel," says Frederica. "He used to phone Daniel, in that crypt. Daniel and Canon Holly."

Frederica and Rupert Parrott go round to St. Simeon's. Daniel is sitting in his egg-box cubicle, talking to a schoolboy who has failed his A-levels and taken six codeine pills. He is persuading him to go to a hospital. After a bit the boy puts the phone down, whether because he is bored or because he is sleepy or because he has despaired is not quite clear. Daniel writes up the conversation, ending, "I think he knew six codeines won't kill him but I may be wrong." He says, "What brings you here?"

"Jude. We can't find Jude. We need him to sign the appeal form. And we're worried about him, of course. We'd like to be sure he's all right. Obviously we would."

"He hasn't been here."

"Has he called?" says Frederica.

"That would be confidential, if he had. But he hasn't, no."

"Do you have *any idea* of where he lived?"

"Not really. South London, I had the impression, I don't know why."

"He came 'home' on the Tube with me once."

"South London's very big," says Rupert. "And he might have gone elsewhere. Anywhere else, except he had no money."

"No bank account?"

"No. He took postal orders. Or cash."

Daniel turns over the log of the early days, when Jude Mason was the anonymous and irritating Steelwire. Whilst they are doing this research, Ginnie Greenhill comes in, offers tea, and asks what they are doing.

"I remember something," she says. "I do remember something." She thinks.

"I almost had a conversation with him once, when Daniel was away, in Yorkshire. He talked about living at the top of a tower."

"That was his book."

"No, no. He said, 'No one wants to live where I live because a child fell from here, from the top of the tower.' "

"That was *his book,*" says Rupert Parrott. "A child fell from the top of Babbletower."

"Well, perhaps he put the fall in his book," says Ginnie Greenhill, who has not read the book.

"He says all sorts of things," says Daniel.

"We could try," says Ginnie Greenhill. "We could ask the local newspapers and the social services about children who fell from the tops of towers. In South London."

This search takes time. More children have fallen than they expected, from towers in Rotherhithe, in Brixton, in Peckham, in Stockwell. They ask the councils who lives in the flats from which the children fell, and find no one resembling Jude Mason. The most hopeful is the Wastwater Tower in Stockwell, on an estate called the Wordsworth Estate, where all the towers are mysteriously and perversely named after lakes—Grasmere, Derwent, Ullswater. A small girl did fall from the top of this tower in 1962; she was two years old, the daughter of a seventeen-year-old mother who was accused and acquitted of pushing her. Her name was Diamond Bates. This is all anyone knows. The flat is now occupied by an unemployed man—"a bit simple," called Ben

Leppard. Frederica frowns in thought. She says "Monckton-Pardew. Benedictine Pards. It could be him." "He's lived there since 1962," says the council official they are talking to. "Let's try it," says Daniel.

The Wordsworth Estate has, though it is already unfashionable to say so, a certain presence, a certain style. Its concrete towers are uncompromising and erect; wide open spaces spread between them. There are little balconies and the windows vary in form—some are circular, some are small rectangles, some are large. Their frames were once painted pale blue, but are now smeared and peeling. The idea of the architect was to expose the natural materials, the concrete, the metal, so they would weather as granite weathers. But concrete does not weather as granite weathers, and the smears and stains on the tower-surfaces look like great expanses of splashed and drained dirty dishwater. The space between the towers, which on the maquette was green, with bushes and trees, is cracked asphalt, with the odd spike of a ripped-off sapling, dying in its round hole; there is green between the cracks, where the earth bulges, the green of moss, green of algae. It is a grey day in early autumn when Daniel and Frederica arrive. The wind blows fish-and-chip papers across the asphalt. The entry to Wastwater Tower stinks of urine and is stained with smeared faeces. These are clichés, and like clichés, are depressing most of all because they are commonplace and inescapable. It would be nice if the lift worked, but it does not. Frederica skips up several floors, and then, the hare to the tortoise, waits for the steadily toiling Daniel. They are both completely out of breath when they reach the thirteenth floor. Frederica's lungs are bursting, her heart is hammering. Daniel wipes his face with a handkerchief.

They are in a bare concrete landing outside a blue door with peeling paint. On the landing is a plate with a chicken bone (the rib cage) and a smear of tomato ketchup. They knock. No one answers. They knock.

A voice from the floor below says, "Ben doesn't come out."

A girl is standing there, neatly dressed in a pleated skirt, a jumper, and white school socks. She is perhaps ten years old, round-faced, and has a mixed inheritance, wiry African hair, dark red in colour, dusky cheeks, a large mouth.

"Do you know him?"

"We feed him. Mum does. We put his food, and he fetches it in when we aren't looking. He doesn't like to come out. Mum says he's a bit simple."

"What does he look like?"

"We haven't seen him for yonks. He used to be a weirdo. A long-hair. He used to get beat up. Now he don't go out."

"Can we get to see him?"

"Not if he don't answer."

"Has nobody got a key?"

"It isn't locked. No one wants to go in there. It stinks something dreadful."

Daniel tries the door. The hall is empty, the floorboards bare. There is a smell. A decaying version of Jude's lively odour. They go through a dark passageway into a largish room, which has a whole wall of glass, and is therefore full of grey light, which shows old wall-paper covered with autumn leaves, stained and sprouting salt and fungi. There is almost no furniture. A mattress, with a heap of blankets, in one corner. A table, with a row of coloured ink bottles and a pot of calligraphic pens. A Baby Belling, on the floor, encrusted with layer upon layer of burned food like the crust of an extinct volcano, black, mouldy, verdigris, soot-brown.

In another corner is a very neat heap of books, arranged in several flat towers, by size.

There is someone curled in the blankets, but he does not move.

"Jude," says Frederica.

"Out," says the ghost of the sawing voice.

"It's us. Frederica and Daniel. Your friends, we hope. We want to talk to you."

"Out."

Daniel advances and turns back the blankets. Jude is lying there in the respectable shirt he wore to the trial, which looks as though it has never subsequently been taken off. His hair is growing—it is tousled and filthy, but it is a good nest of grey wires, not a grey skull cap. Daniel sees that Jude is dangerously thin. He says, "We'll have to get you out of here. You'll have to come with us. I could get you into a hospital."

"You—need not strive. Officiously. To keep alive."

Frederica says, "They need your signature. For the appeal."

"There is no need. They will lose."

"Jude—come on—you used to *fight,* in your way—"

"And now I am dying in my way. Go away."

In the end, they carry Jude, more or less, down the twisting stairs of the tower, and into a taxi, whose driver sniffs Jude's smell, thinks of rejecting him, looks at Daniel, and accepts. Jude begins to cry when Daniel suggests a hospital. In the end they take him to Daniel's own bedsitter, which is in Clerkenwell, and is spartan in a more cluttered way than Jude's echoing eyrie, is small, and overfurnished. Jude is bathed, by both Daniel and Frederica, moaning a little. His hair is washed, and becomes oddly floating and electric, giving him the air of a Blakean sage. He closes his eyes throughout the operations, and is dressed in Daniel's pyjamas, and put into Daniel's bed. Daniel will sleep on the sofa. "Not for the first or the last time," says Daniel. Frederica says she would have Jude, but there is Leo, there is Agatha, there is Saskia. "No," says Daniel, "he's my job. For the present."

"He's got to sign the appeal form."

Jude opens his eyes. "If you keep them from me, I will sign it." He closes them. He opens them again. "I wonder, did you find my original garments?"

"No," says Daniel.

"They were in a paper box somewhere there. They are all I have."

"You want me to go and look for them?"

"I have no others. Yours will not do for me, and you would not care to lend them. Thank you."

He closes his eyes again, and settles back into Daniel's pillow. He murmurs, "You are a man of God." There is a note of satisfaction in his voice.

Daniel lets Frederica out. He says, "I wonder how long I've got *him* for."

Frederica says, "You're both as tough as old boots. You'll get him out, when the time's right."

"Aye," says Daniel. "I will."

The Space is mysteriously hung with silken draperies, painted with symbols, cups and swords, suns and moons, sunflowers and compasses, crowns and chains. It is lit by glancing rays of coloured lights, and scented with strange smoky perfumes. Two parties of travellers advance across it and meet. One party are fair tall folk, cloaked in shimmering grey cloaks over flowing green robes belted with silver belts wrought of leaf-shapes and clasped with emeralds. All wear crystal wings that flash in the changing light and silver bands in their flowing hair, from which simple jewels hang to rest on their brows. They are led by a white-robed figure, hooded, with a tall stave in his hand, and they are singing quietly.

A Elbereth Gilthoniel
Silivren penna miriel
O menel aglar elennath!

Their feet are sandalled or shod with fine boots in pale leather.

The second party are white-robed and masked with sun and moon masks in silver and gold. They are crowned with mistletoe, and in their midst are figures partly naked, but with bright metallic sunbursts and crescents covering their sex. They are led by a Bard who introduces them:

These, the Twenty-four in whom the Divine Family
Appear'd; and they were One in Him. A Human Vision!
Human Divine, Jesus the Saviour, blessed for ever and ever.
Selsey true friend, who afterwards submitted to be devour'd
By the waves of Despair, whose Emanation rose above
The flood, and was nam'd Chichester, lovely, mild & gentle! Lo!
Her lambs bleat to the sea-fowls' cry, lamenting still for Albion.
Submitting to be call'd the son of Los, and his Emanations
Submitting to be call'd Enitharmon's daughters and be born
In vegetable mould, created by the Hammer and Loom
In Bowlahoola & Allamanda where the Dead wail night & day.
I call them by their English names: English, the rough basement,
Los built the stubborn structure of the Language, acting against
Albion's melancholy, who must else have been a Dumb despair.

The Bard steps forward. He says:

"Let us celebrate the mythopoeic imagination of Albion. Let us celebrate the Makers, who made systems and were not enslaved by those of other men, but broke through to the Vision of what lies beyond Language, to the eternal symbols and the unchanging Light. Let us celebrate the sevenfold vision of William Blake and the true Jerusalem; let us celebrate also J. R. R. Tolkien, who single-handed forged the Elvish languages and the myths of Middle-Earth and the lands beyond the Western Sea. What you are about to see is a Rite and an Invocation, a Calling and a Dance, and who knows what shadowy forms, or creatures of light, may not come into our ken as we weave together these two powerful nests of language, text and textures, into the warp and woof of a new Cloth of Dreams . . ."

The figures on the stage begin to chant, and to pass long, shining threads from one to the other. The Elves sing of Earendil and Luvah. The Bard describes the work of the Emanations.

The Feminine separates from the Masculine and both from Man
Ceasing to be his Emanations, Life to themselves assuming:
And while they circumscribe his Brain and while they circumscribe
His Heart and while they circumscribe his Loins, a Veil and Net
Of Veins of red Blood grows around them like a scarlet robe.

The threads are now mixed with red threads, and one of the Bards is turning in the weaving like a bobbin.

Covering them from the sight of Man, like the woven veil of Sleep
Such as the Flowers of Beulah weave to be their Funeral Mantles;
But dark, opaque, tender to touch, and painful and agonising
To the embrace of love and the mingling of soft fibres
Of tender affection, that no more the Masculine mingles
With the Feminine, but the Sublime is shut out from the Pathos
In howling torment, to build stone walls of separation, compelling
The Pathos to weave curtains of hiding secrecy from the torment.

The Elves sing of the terrors of Orthanc and Minas Morgul; of the web of Shelob and the Eye in Barad-dur. A soft voice sings of the hope of severing the bonds, breaking the bounds, making a bridge of rainbow light.

Happenings are happening all over London. Frederica has come to this one with Alan Melville. The Bard is Richmond Bly, and Alan and Frederica are present out of morbid curiosity. It is hard to see what is happening as the stage is full of smoke and threads of silk and swirling garments and weaving, and it is hard to hear, as there is an accompaniment of breathy flute music, pan-pipes and tinkling bells. There is also a vague noise of disturbance from outside, from the car park which adjoins the theatre-department building where Richmond Bly's Rite is being performed. It is a noise of motor bikes revving, and drumming, African drumming, Frederica thinks vaguely, and gongs, and tambourines, and cymbals. This noise swells. The mythopoeic celebrants of Albion dance meditatively on. A voice says, "I am the Lady Galadriel, I wear the Ring of Water." The noise from the car park has diminished, and appears to have gone away, but then returns in a much louder burst. It is clear that the noisemakers have left the car park and entered the building through the basement. A kind of rhythmic drumming and stamping begins to mount from the depths. Alan Melville says, "I knew we ought to come, I knew it would be interesting." Frederica says, "Interesting might be the wrong word."

The invaders swarm through the theatre. Many of them are naked, painted with flame-shapes in red lipstick, or corkscrew patterns in what looks like woad. They are carrying posters on sticks, most of which depict the Buddhist monk who immolated himself by fire in Vietnam, a cross-legged seated body clothed in saffron, clothed in flame, clothed in smoke, keeling over on stone. Others are carrying stout staves on which are impaled pigs' heads, sliced in half, showing teeth and vertebrae and brains. They run up to the stage. They are many, they are male and female. The drumming intensifies. They fight with the robed figures. They seize the pipes and little bells, they play their own rhythm. A figure in black, a kind of blond demon, leaps to the front of the stage, swaying to the drumming, and takes the microphone from its place beside the Bard. "Let's have a poem," says the poet. It is Mickey Impey. "Let's have a poem! Zag is coming! Let's have a proper poem." He begins to chant:

The Zy-Goats dance
To the ziggurat
They dance and prance
For the Cat in the Hat
The great gold Cat
In his shiny Hat
In his super-sleek sanguine
Shiny Hat.
By the light of the skoobs
They waggle their boobs
Wiggle their pubes
Snort in their tubes
For the glittering Cat
By the ziggurat.

Goat and compasses
Cat and fiddle

Lush farrago and Tarradiddle.
Amphisbæna
And alley-cat
What's the meaning
Of this and that?
Scallywags
And Pleiades
Orthoptera
Helicoptera
THE BEES THE BEES THE BEES KNEES.

Spirally spirally spirally twirl
Widdershins widdershins widdershins whirl
Coil recoil
Trouble and toil
The cosmic pot on the cosmic boil.
Shimmy your pelvis
Twirl your toes
Rotate the honey pot
Roger the rose.
Come and dance
Dance and prance
To the ziggurat
And the great gold Cat
In his super-sleek sanguine
Shiny Hat.

The audience laugh and chant with him. Paul-Zag in his white satin trousers and jester's jacket comes through the audience, unsmiling and beautiful. He steps up on to the stage. He is followed by his Group, all in white satin, carrying baby-baths, pink plastic baby-baths full of something dark and slopping. Richmond Bly, masked and robed, steps forward to confront the intruder, tripping over the microphone wire attached to Mickey Impey, recovering himself.

"Excuse me," says Richmond Bly, behind his sun mask. "This is a serious Rite."

"I know," says Paul-Zag. "It's a Happening, It's all happening. You're happening, I'm happening, we're happening, it's really happy. Take delight in the unforeseen. Allow me to make you an honorary member of Zag and the Szyzgy (Ziggy) Zy-Goats."

He waves forward his followers. The stage is crowded with grinning half-pigs'-heads on sticks, with burning monks, with singing and dancing.

"You are a jolly good fellow," says Zag to Richmond Bly. "And I am a jolly good fellow. Let us be joined."

A young woman wearing a dead poppy and a few feathers dips her arms into the baby-bath, which is full of pale intestines in dark blood. Zag lifts a string of them above his head and winds them round the neck of Richmond Bly, round his own neck. The red runs down their white clothes, both their white clothes.

"No," says Richmond Bly. "I always—faint at the sight of blood."

"Loss of consciousness is good for you," says Mickey Impey. "Dissolve the one in the many."

"No, really," says Richmond Bly, plucking at his fleshy necklace without being able to bring himself to touch it.

"You are not the Wizard of Oz," says Mickey Impey, snatching off Bly's sun mask. Paul Ottokar stands smiling, grave and lovely, dripping blood.

The followers are stuffing their trousers with offal, with intestines, and drawing them dripping out through their flies.

Richmond Bly's heavy face goes lemon-coloured, goes candlewax. He falls heavily forward, fulfilling his word. His face slides in pigs' blood. Some of the audience laugh. The drummers drum. The drummers drum. The drumming makes it better, increases the laughter.

"Make things *happen,*" cries Mickey Impey. "Happenings don't have *audiences.* We are all *actors.* Move, you tubs of lard, get off your bums, come and dance."

"All the same," says Frederica. It's not *real.*"

"The pigs' heads are real," says Alan. "And the monk was real."

"Oh hell," says Frederica. "I'm going home. I've got to relieve the baby-sitter. No one in the future will think there was anyone who had to leave a Happening to relieve a baby-sitter."

A smell of burning begins to mix with the smells of butchery and incense. A smell of burning paint. There is the soft sound of an explosion. Someone begins to call out, "Clear the theatre. Fire! Fire!" People push and cry. The drums drum. It turns out later that someone has set fire to various small skoob towers in the corners of the studios, and that a can of acrylic paint has exploded. Frederica hurries down the stairs amongst clouds of smoke through a river of foam. She does not wait to see whether the building will burn down—the baby-sitter is waiting. She goes down into the Underground, on the long, plunging escalator down which the sculptor Stone wandered wildly to his death.

The escalators are crowded. Frederica sometimes studies every face, looking for the differences, the similarities, the thoughts, and sometimes glides past, seeing all the white spaces as identical. Tonight she sees nothing, no faces, a white procession. A voice cries, from below, "Frederica!"

She sees his face coming up to her from the dark. Clean-cut, well-groomed, blond over a black suit and a black plastic raincoat, John Ottokar. As they pass, she shouts, truculent, "What have you got to say for yourself?"

"I was scared."

"No excuse."

"But true. Wait for me."

"No, I won't." She is enraged. But when she reaches the bottom she regrets this. She hesitates, turns, runs round, and gets on to the up escalator. She meets John Ottokar, again about half-way, coming down.

He says, "I said Wait!"

"And I said No. And then I changed my mind."

They pass and sail on. They are very long escalators, the longest in the Underground. She thinks she hears him call "Wait" again, and does wait, stands at the head of the escalator, looking down at the faces coming up, all different in the unearthly lights, none of them his. After a long time she makes her way down again. He is not at the foot of the escalator either. And the baby-sitter is waiting. She walks through arches, she gives a coin to a singer who is softly asking, "Where have all the flowers gone?" She waits on the platform, looking under the dark arch, smelling old, old soot, thinking of the dead Stone and the living Ottokar.

There are plenty of seats in the train. She sits by herself, thinking that this is not her time, she did not enjoy the Happening, though it had its interest. She looks at her shadowy face in the dark window. White, staring, with dark eyes, darker than they are, smudged with exhaustion. A transparent paleface, a ghost, more elegant than the real flesh in a shining mirror. She meets her own eyes and catches the look of someone standing, farther along, someone reflected, by an angle of the light, two or three or four times, his face upon his face upon his face, like fine paper masks, but really only one, one face, John Ottokar. She smiles tentatively at him in the dark glass. His mouth lifts in an equally tentative smile. She moves her head, fractionally, the ghost-light in the red hair, and he nods. She hears the rustle of PVC, she smells, amongst the soot and cigarette smoke, faintly, the blond hair, the presence. She does not look round. She says to the glass, "I've learned to do without you."

"I never doubted that. The question is, Can you be doing *with* me?"

"I might."

"That's good."

They touch hands, and smile at each other's shadow in the glass.

After all the trouble, the announcement in the Press in December is curt.

Babbletower wins appeal. Judge misdirected jury. He dropped them in at the deep end and left them to swim with no directions.

"The appeal judges found in favour of the publishers Bowers and Eden, and of Jude Mason, author of *Babbletower: A Story for the Children of Our Time.* The publishers had appealed on eleven grounds. The appeal judges dismissed most of these, but agreed that the trial judge had been unnecessarily disparaging of 'expert' witnesses, and had not given the jury sufficient direction concerning the defence of literary merit, 'dropping them in at the deep end and leaving them to swim as best they could' in the words of one of the appeal judges."

There are photographs of Rupert Parrott, drinking champagne with his legal advisers. There are only old photographs of Jude Mason. Daniel brings these newspapers to Jude, who is still lying in Daniel's bed. He is less skeletal and is wearing new pyjamas, provided by Ginnie Greenhill. Jude sits up and scrutinises the papers expressionlessly.

"So that's all right," says Daniel. "You can get up now, and make a lot of money, and be famous."

"No. I want none of it. They've picked me clean, I want none of it."

"You've been justified."

"Some said one thing. Some more have said another. It is not good to be *talked over,* picked over."

"Well, however that may be, my friend, you've got to get up now, and go elsewhere."

"You should have thought of that before you brought me here."

"I did. I said you could stay until you were better. Now, I think you'd better go."

"I may not be better."

"That's a risk we've got to take. You can get up and buy me a drink."

"I might," says Jude. "I'll think about it."

The three friends looked at the heap of bones, white bones, fresh bones, skulls and ribs and shins and carpals and tarsals chucked together, with a rag of cooked flesh here and there upon them.

"The Krebs have come, and gone," said Samson Origen.

"We must not touch these," said Colonel Grim. "In case they return, and learn we are still alive."

"Let us go away from here," said Turdus Cantor. A beast began to howl somewhere far away in the forest, and a great bird turned and turned above them in a hot blue sky. So the three old men began to walk away across the valley, looking back from time to time at the Tower, and the grim mound at its foot, until it was so far away that its human origin could not be distinguished, and it looked like a chance heap of rocks, sprouting green here and there, with what might be shells or pebbles clustered palely at its foot. And they went on walking, and if the Krebs did not catch up with them, they are walking still.

ACKNOWLEDGEMENTS

A great many people have encouraged my curiosity about a great many things, from snails to obsolete legal forms to ethnomethodology. I am indebted to Steve Jones, Steven Rose, Arnold Feinstein, Fran Ashcroft and Lawrence Razavi for help with matters scientific, to Richard du Cann, Andrew Pugh, Steve Uglow, Arthur Davidson, Razi Mireskandari, Simon Goldberg and Marion Boyars for legal aid, to Laurie Taylor for instruction in ethnomethodology, to Carmen Callil, Martin Asher, Steve Fountain, John Forrester and Lisa Appignanesi for help with the ideas and fashions of the sixties, to John Sutherland for help with the history of trials for obscenity, to Claudine Vassas and Daniel Fabre for information on birdlore and the folklore of the snail, and to Claudine for the myth of the ziz, to Ignes Sôdre, Michael Worton, Jean-Louis and Anne Chevalier, my husband, Peter Duffy, Jenny Uglow and Jonathan Burnham for helpful discussions of ideas. Randolph Quirk and fellow members of the Kingman Committee provided ideas about language. Hazel Bell's indexes to *The Virgin in the Garden* and *Still Life*, though not designed as author's aids, were very helpful for that purpose. I am also deeply indebted to all the members of my extra-mural classes in Kensington and Marylebone. Jonathan Barker made indispensable suggestions for reading. David Royle talked to me about art in the sixties and lent me books in the nineties. Helena Caletta and John Saumarez-Smith are both more research guides than booksellers. Books I have found particularly helpful are Jeff Nuttall's *Bomb Culture*, Robert Hewison's *Too Much*, Richard Neville's *Playpower*, Bernice Martin's *A Sociology of Contemporary Cultural Change* and James Britton's *Language and Learning*. Bryan Clarke's article "The Causes of Biological Diversity" drew my attention to the remarks of Sir Thomas Browne on faces, alphabets and diversity. Writers whose ideas changed me in the sixties and are still important to me are Iris Murdoch, Doris Lessing and George Steiner. I have briefly borrowed a character from one of Iris Murdoch's sixties novels.

I would like to thank Humphrey Stone for designing the text, and drawing the snails.

I am particularly grateful to Elizabeth Allen for legal and archival research on obscenity, the Moors Murders and on divorce, and to Gill Marsden for work on the manuscript and for keeping things in order. I am, as always, not sure what I would do without the London Library.

Any mistakes in this book are all my own.

ABOUT THE AUTHOR

A. S. BYATT is the author of *Possession,* winner of the Booker Prize and a national bestseller. Her two novels that lead up to *Babel Tower,* tracing the fortunes of Frederica and her family through the 1950s, are *The Virgin in the Garden* and *Still Life,* and her other fiction includes *The Shadow of the Sun, The Game, Angels and Insects,* and two collections of shorter works: *Sugar and Other Stories* and *The Matisse Stories.* She has also published three volumes of critical work, of which *Passions of the Mind* is the most recent. She has taught English and American literature at University College, London, and is a distinguished critic and reviewer. She lives in London.

ABOUT THE TYPE

This book was set in Bembo, a typeface based on an old-style Roman face that was used for Cardinal Bembo's tract *De Aetna* in 1495. Bembo was cut by Francisco Griffo in the early sixteenth century. The Lanston Monotype Machine Company of Philadelphia brought the well-proportioned letter forms of Bembo to the United States in the 1930s.